David W. Cescon and Lea A. Harrington dedicate this sixth edition to Ian F. Tannock and Richard P. Hill, who published the first edition of this textbook in 1987.
Their accomplishments as scientists and editors have expanded the frontiers of scientific knowledge, and have inspired countless trainees, clinicians, and scientists around the globe.

The Basic Science of Oncology

SIXTH EDITION

Notice

Medicine is an ever-changing science. As new research and clinical experience broaden our knowledge, changes in treatment and drug therapy are required. The authors and the publisher of this work have checked with sources believed to be reliable in their efforts to provide information that is complete and generally in accord with the standards accepted at the time of publication. However, in view of the possibility of human error or changes in medical sciences, neither the authors nor the publisher nor any other party who has been involved in the preparation or publication of this work warrants that the information contained herein is in every respect accurate or complete, and they disclaim all responsibility for any errors or omissions or for the results obtained from use of the information contained in this work. Readers are encouraged to confirm the information contained herein with other sources. For example and in particular, readers are advised to check the product information sheet included in the package of each drug they plan to administer to be certain that the information contained in this work is accurate and that changes have not been made in the recommended dose or in the contraindications for administration. This recommendation is of particular importance in connection with new or infrequently used drugs.

The Basic Science of Oncology

SIXTH EDITION

Editors

Lea A. Harrington, PhD
*Professor
Department of Medicine
University of Montreal
Institute for Research in Immunology
 and Cancer Pavilion
Montreal, Quebec, Canada*

Richard P. Hill, PhD
*Professor Emeritus
Department of Medical Biophysics
Princess Margaret Cancer Centre
University of Toronto
Toronto, Ontario, Canada*

Ian F. Tannock, MD, PhD, DSc
*Emeritus Professor of Medicine and
 Medical Biophysics
Princess Margaret Cancer Centre &
 University of Toronto
Toronto, Ontario, Canada*

David W. Cescon, MD, PhD
*Medical Oncologist and Clinician Scientist
Princess Margaret Cancer Centre
University of Health Network
Assistant Professor of Medicine
University of Toronto
Toronto, Ontario*

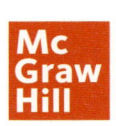

McGraw Hill

New York   Chicago   San Francisco   Lisbon   London   Madrid   Mexico City
New Delhi   San Juan   Seoul   Singapore   Sydney   Toronto

The Basic Science of Oncology, Sixth Edition

Copyright © 2021, 2013, 2005, 1998, 1992, 1987, by McGraw Hill. All rights reserved. Printed in the United States of America. Except as permitted under the United States Copyright Act of 1976, no part of this publication may be reproduced or distributed in any form or by any means, or stored in a data base or retrieval system, without the prior written permission of the publisher.

1 2 3 4 5 6 7 8 9 LWI 26 25 24 23 22 21

ISBN 978-1-259-86207-6
MHID 1-259-86207-0

This book was set in Minion Pro by KnowledgeWorks Global Ltd.
The editors were Karen Edmonson and Christie Naglieri.
The production supervisor was Catherine Saggese.
Project management was provided by Garima Poddar, KnowledgeWorks Global Ltd.

This book is printed on acid-free paper.

Library of Congress Cataloging-in-Publication Data

Names: Harrington, Lea, editor. | Tannock, Ian, editor. | Hill, Richard P.,
   1942- editor. | Cescon, David (David W.), editor.
Title: The basic science of oncology / editors, Lea Harrington, Ian F.
   Tannock, Richard P. Hill, David Cescon.
Description: 6th edition. | New York : McGraw Hill, [2021] | Includes
   bibliographical references and index. | Summary: "Covers cancer
   causation, cancer biology, and the biology underlying cancer treatment,
   for trainees in both clinical and research areas of oncology"-- Provided
   by publisher.
Identifiers: LCCN 2020017240 | ISBN 9781259862076 (paperback ; alk. paper)
   | ISBN 1259862070 (paperback ; alk. paper) | ISBN 9781259862083 (ebook)
Subjects: MESH: Neoplasms
Classification: LCC RC263 | NLM QZ 200 | DDC 616.99/4--dc23
LC record available at https://lccn.loc.gov/2020017240

McGraw Hill books are available at special quantity discounts to use as premiums and sales promotions, or for use in corporate training programs. To contact a representative please visit the Contact Us pages at www.mhprofessional.com.

Contents

Contributors   viii
Preface   xi

1   Introduction to Cancer Biology   1
Lea A. Harrington, David W. Cescon, Richard P. Hill, and Ian F. Tannock

2   Methods of Molecular Analysis   5
Paul C. Boutros, Lea Harrington, and Thomas Kislinger

3   Epigenetics   51
Kyaw Lwin Aung, Stanley Zhou, and Mathieu Lupien

4   Cancer Epidemiology   69
Matthew T. Warkentin, Lidija Latifovic, Geoffrey Liu, and Rayjean J. Hung

5   Carcinogenesis   97
Denis M. Grant

6   Cellular Signaling   113
Lea A. Harrington

7   Oncogenes and Tumor-Suppressor Genes   139
Previn Dutt and Vuk Stambolic

8   Cell Proliferation and Death   163
Kelsie L. Thu, David W. Cescon, and Razqallah Hakem

9   Genomic Stability and DNA Repair   193
Guillaume Laflamme, Yahya Benslimane, and Damien D'Amours

10   Tumor Progression and Metastasis   223
Virginie Defamie and Rama Khokha

11   Angiogenesis   247
Janusz Rak and Urban Emmenegger

12   Tumor Growth, Microenvironment, Metabolism, and Hypoxia   275
Neesha Dhani, Richard P. Hill, and Ian F. Tannock

13   Cancer Heterogeneity   305
Craig Gedye

14   Imaging in Oncology   329
Mattea L. Welch and David A. Jaffray

15   Molecular and Cellular Basis of Radiotherapy   349
Marianne Koritzinsky and Scott V. Bratman

16   Tumor and Normal Tissue Response to Radiotherapy   369
Scott V. Bratman and Marianne Koritzinsky

17   Discovery and Evaluation of Anticancer Drugs   403
Kyaw Lwin Aung, David W. Cescon, and Aaron D. Schimmer

18   Anticancer Chemotherapy, Pharmacology, and Mechanisms of Resistance   429
Eric Chen and Ian F. Tannock

19   Molecular Targeted Therapies   461
Zachary Veitch and Philippe L. Bedard

20   Hormones and Cancer   487
Nathan Lack and Etienne Leygue

21   The Immune System and Immunotherapy   515
Samuel D. Saibil, Ben X. Wang, and Marcus O. Butler

22   Guide to Clinical Studies   547
Eitan Amir

Index   573

Contributors

Eitan Amir, MBChB, PhD
Staff Physician
Princess Margaret Cancer Centre
University Health Network
Associate Professor of Medicine
University of Toronto
Toronto, Ontario

Kyaw Lwin Aung, MBBS, MRCP (UK), PhD
Assistant Professor
Department of Oncology
Livestrong Cancer Institutes and Dell Medical School
University of Texas at Austin
Austin, Texas, USA

Philippe L. Bedard, MD, FRCP(C)
Clinical Director, Cancer Genomics Program
University of Health Network
Staff Medical Oncologist, Princess Margaret Cancer Centre
Associate Professor of Medicine, University of Toronto

Yahya Benslimane, PhD
IRIC – Institut de recherche en immunologie et en cancérologie
Faculté de médecine
Université de Montréal
Montréal, Québec

Scott V. Bratman, MD, PhD
Dr. Mariano Antonio Elia Chair in Head and Neck Cancer Research
Senior Scientist and Staff Radiation Oncologist
Ontario Cancer Institute and Princess Margaret Cancer Centre
University Health Network
Associate Professor of Radiation Oncology and Medical Biophysics
University of Toronto
Toronto, Ontario

Paul C. Boutros, PhD
Professor, Human Genetics and Oncology
Director of Cancer Data Science
Associate Director Cancer Informatics
University of California
California, Los Angeles

Marcus O. Butler, MD
Medical Oncologist
Clinical Head, Immune Monitoring Team
Princess Margaret Cancer Centre
Departments of Medicine and Immunology
University of Toronto
Toronto, Ontario

David W. Cescon, MD, PhD, FRCPC
Medical Oncologist and Clinician Scientist
Princess Margaret Cancer Centre
University of Health Network
Assistant Professor of Medicine
University of Toronto
Toronto, Ontario

Eric X. Chen, MD, PhD
Medical Oncologist
Princess Margaret Cancer Centre
University Health Network
Associate Professor of Medicine
University of Toronto
Toronto, Ontario

Damien D'Amours, PhD
Professor, Department of Cellular & Molecular Medicine
Principal Investigator, Ottawa Institute of Systems Biology
Faculty of Medicine
University of Ottawa
Ottawa, Ontario

Virginie Defamie, PhD
Research Associate
Princess Margaret Cancer Centre
University Health Network
Toronto, Ontario

Neesha Dhani, MD, PhD, FRCPC
Medical Oncologist and Clinician Investigator
Princess Margaret Cancer Centre
University Health Network
Assistant Professor of Medicine
University of Toronto
Toronto, Ontario

Previn Dutt, PhD
Research Associate
The Princess Margaret Cancer Centre
University Health Network
Toronto, Ontario

Urban Emmenegger, MD
Medical Oncologist, Division of Medical Oncology, Odette Cancer Centre
Associate Scientist, Biological Sciences Platform, Sunnybrook Research Institute
Associate Professor, Department of Medicine, University of Toronto
Toronto, Ontario

Craig Gedye, BSc (Hons), MBChB, FRACP, PhD
Senior Staff Specialist, Department of Medical Oncology, Calvary Mater Newcastle
Director, HMRI Clinical Trials
Chair, Renal Cancer Subcommittee, ANZUP Cancer Trials Group
Conjoint Associate Professor, School of Medicine and Public Health, University of Newcastle
Callaghan, Australia

Denis M. Grant, PhD
Professor
Department of Pharmacology & Toxicology
Temerty Faculty of Medicine
University of Toronto
Toronto, Ontario

Razqallah Hakem, PhD
Senior Scientist
Princess Margaret Cancer Centre
University Health Network
Professor of Medical Biophysics and Laboratory Medicine and Pathology
University of Toronto
Toronto, Ontario

Lea A. Harrington, PhD
Professor, Faculty of Medicine
IRIC-Institut de Recherché en Immunologie et en Cancérologie
Université de Montréal
Montréal, Québec

Richard P. Hill, PhD
Senior Scientist Emeritus
Ontario Cancer Institute and Campbell Family Institute for Cancer Research
Princess Margaret Cancer Centre
University Health Network
Professor Emeritus of Medical Biophysics and Radiation Oncology
University of Toronto
Toronto, Ontario

Rayjean J. Hung, PhD, MS
Head, Prosserman Centre for Population Health Research, Lunenfeld-Tanenbaum Research Institute of Sinai Health System
Canada Research Chair in Integrative Molecular Epidemiology
Professor, Division of Epidemiology, Dalla Lana School of Public Health, University of Toronto
Toronto, Ontario

David A. Jaffray, PhD, ABMP
Professor of Radiation Physics and Imaging Physics
Chief Technology and Digital Officer
MD Anderson Cancer Center
Houston, Texas
Professor of Radiation Oncology, Medical Biophysics, and IBBME
University of Toronto
Toronto, Ontario

Rama Khokha, PhD
Senior Scientist
Princess Margaret Cancer Centre
University Health Network
Professor of Medical Biophysics
University of Toronto
Toronto, Ontario

Thomas Kislinger, PhD
Senior Scientist
Princess Margaret Cancer Centre
University Health Network
Professor of Medical Biophysics
University of Toronto
Toronto, Ontario

Marianne Koritzinsky, PhD
Scientist, Princess Margaret Cancer Centre
University Health Network
Associate Professor, Departments of Radiation Oncology and Medical Biophysics
University of Toronto
Toronto, Ontario

Nathan Lack, PhD
Senior Research Scientist
Vancouver Prostate Centre
Assistant Professor of Medicine
University of British Columbia
Vancouver, British Columbia

Guillaume Laflamme, PhD
Postdoctoral Fellow
Department of Laboratory Medicine and Pathobiology
Faculty of Medicine
University of Toronto
Toronto, Ontario

Lidija Latifovic, MSc
PhD Candidate, Epidemiology
Dalla Lana School of Public Health, University of Toronto
Princess Margaret Cancer Centre, University Health Network
Toronto, Ontario

Etienne Leygue, PhD
Professor
Department of Biochemistry and Medical Genetics
Max Rady College of Medicine
Rady Faculty of Health Sciences
University of Manitoba
Winnipeg, Manitoba

Geoffrey Liu, MD, FRCPC, FISPE
Alan B. Brown Chair in Molecular Genomics and Senior Scientist
Princess Margaret Cancer Centre
Professor of Medicine
Medical Biophysics Pharmacology and Toxicology, and Epidemiology
University of Toronto and Dalla Lana School of Public Health
Toronto, Ontario

Mathieu Lupien, PhD
Senior Scientist
Princess Margaret Cancer Centre
University Health Network
Associate Professor of Medical Biophysics
University of Toronto
Toronto, Ontario

Janusz Rak, MD, PhD
Jack Cole Chair in Pediatric Hematology/Oncology
Professor, Department of Pediatrics
McGill University
Montreal Children's Hospital and The Research Institute of the McGill University Health Centre
Montreal, Quebec

Samuel D. Saibil, MD, PhD
Staff Oncologist and Clinician Investigator
Princess Margaret Cancer Centre
Assistant Professor, Department of Medicine
University of Toronto

Aaron D. Schimmer, MD, PhD, FRCPC
Director of Research
Senior Scientist and Staff Physician
Princess Margaret Cancer Centre, University Health Network
Professor of Medicine and Medical Biophysics, University of Toronto
Toronto, Ontario

Vuk Stambolic, PhD
Senior Scientist
Ontario Cancer Institute and Princess Margaret Cancer Centre
Professor of Medical Biophysics
University of Toronto
Toronto, Ontario

Ian F. Tannock, MD, PhD, DSc
Emeritus Professor of Medicine and Medical Biophysics
Princess Margaret Cancer Centre & University of Toronto
Toronto, Ontario

Kelsie L. Thu, PhD
Staff Scientist
Keenan Research Centre for Biomedical Science, St. Michael's Hospital
Assistant Professor, Department of Laboratory Medicine and Pathobiology
University of Toronto
Toronto, Ontario

Zachary Veitch, MSc, MD, FRCPC
Staff Medical Oncologist – Clinician Teacher
St Michaels Hospital – Unity Health
Department of Medical Oncology and Hematology
Li Ka-Shing Knowledge Institute
University of Toronto Department of Medicine
Toronto, Ontario

Ben X. Wang, PhD
Scientific Associate
Tumor Immunotherapy Program
Princess Margaret Cancer Centre
University Health Network
Toronto, Ontario

Matthew T. Warkentin, MSc
Lunenfeld-Tanenbaum Research Institute, Sinai Health System
Division of Epidemiology, Dalla Lana School of Public Health
University of Toronto
Toronto, Ontario

Mattea L. Welch, PhD
Scientific Associate
Princess Margaret Data Science Program
University Health Network
Toronto, Ontario

Stanley Zhou, PhD
Princess Margaret Cancer Centre
University Health Network
Department of Medical Biophysics
University of Toronto
Toronto, Ontario

Preface

Since the publication of the fifth edition of *The Basic Science of Oncology* our knowledge about the molecular basis of cancer has continued to grow, as a result of the continued rapid development of powerful techniques to study the genome and epigenome, as well as the levels of gene expression and the proteins that are produced. Concurrent with understanding of the molecular pathways that drive the development and progression of cancer, and the heterogeneity of the changes in these pathways in individual cancers, new molecular-targeted agents have been developed and are being tested, with variable success, in attempts to treat cancers selectively. The sixth edition of *The Basic Science of Oncology* places these major advances in the context of previous studies that have generated the important background to cancer biology. Many of the chapters have new authors and have been extensively revised and rewritten to reflect our new knowledge. We have added new chapters on Epigenetics (Chapter 3) and Molecular Targeted Therapies (Chapter 19).

As in previous editions we have attempted to bring together the contributions of experts into a book that, we believe, is suitable for fellows, residents, nurses, medical students, graduate students, and senior undergraduates who are interested in the biology of cancer. We have maintained a format that allows the reader to investigate a particular interest selectively and included references that can be used as a guide for those seeking information in greater depth. We believe that the book will be useful as a teaching aid and as a broad introduction for those interested in the study and treatment of cancer.

We are grateful to Dr. Robert Bristow, our former co-editor for the fifth edition of this book, as well as many people for their assistance in producing this sixth edition. To our authors, including former and new contributors; to our publishers and their affiliates, who have encouraged us and accepted with good grace our failure to meet various deadlines and whose artists have redrawn many of the figures; to our colleagues, students, and trainees who have provided us with helpful and constructive criticism, and to our families who have continued to provide support and encouragement during the several phases of writing, rewriting, and reviewing.

L. Harrington
I.F. Tannock
R.P. Hill
D. Cescon

Introduction to Cancer Biology

Lea A. Harrington, David W. Cescon, Richard P. Hill, and Ian F. Tannock

Chapter Outline

1.1 Perspective and History
1.2 Recent Advances in Oncology
1.3 The Future of Oncology and Cancer Treatment
References

1.1 PERSPECTIVE AND HISTORY

It is recognized increasingly that cancer is a genetic disease that occurs because of mutations in critical (driver) genes and that the development of a cancer, especially in adults, is often a long process taking many years. Epidemiologic studies have identified many environmental factors that can cause mutations and are carcinogenic. When Sir Percival Pott carried out his epidemiologic study in 1775, suggesting that the causative agent of scrotal cancer in young chimney sweeps might be chimney soot (now known to be tar), he not only identified the putative carcinogenic agent but also demonstrated that a cancer may develop years after exposure. Another dramatic example is mesothelioma, which is a rare cancer arising from the pleural membranes around the lungs, that develops decades after exposure to asbestos (Lemen, 2016). Epidemiologic studies have also identified tobacco smoke as a major environmental cause of several types of cancer: Doll and Hill (1950) showed that heavy smokers over the age of 50 have a 1 in 2 chance of dying from a smoking-related disease such as lung cancer. On the positive side, individuals who quit smoking at an early age exhibit a gradual return to a near-normal risk of lung cancer (Doll et al, 2004). More recently, obesity (which is increasingly a health concern throughout the world) has been associated with increased risk of certain types of cancer (eg, breast, colorectal), and reducing weight is associated with a lower cancer risk (Iyengar et al, 2015; Hopkins et al, 2016). These and other studies underscore the possibility that, with some types of cancer, a degree of prevention may be achieved via changes in lifestyle.

Other historically important contributions to the understanding of cancer include an appreciation that cancer is, in part, heritable. Studies of geographically or socially isolated populations, such as the Mormons in Utah, and of changes in cancer incidence in migrant families demonstrated that both genetic predisposition and environmental factors are important in cancer causation. Analysis of cancer-prone families have assisted in the identification of genetic abnormalities that can lead directly to malignancy, such as mutation of tumor suppressor genes, including the retinoblastoma gene (*RB*) in children, the *TP53* gene in Li-Fraumeni syndrome, and the *BRCA1* and *BRCA2* genes, which are associated with familial breast and ovarian cancer. Viruses have also been identified as causative in the development of some common human cancers, including hepatitis viruses (B and C) as precursors of hepatocellular carcinoma, and human papilloma viruses (HPVs) as a causative agent for a range of cancers including those of the cervix and the oropharynx. The development of vaccines against HPV (Future II Study Group, 2007) and of vaccination programs against hepatitis B virus (HBV) and hepatitis C virus (HCV) in regions where these viruses are endemic (Luo and Ruan, 2012) holds promise for marked reduction in the incidence of these cancers.

Early advances in understanding of biologic properties of cancer followed the development of the microscope, which allowed Virchow, a nineteenth-century pathologist, to declare: "Every cell is born from another cell." This property is true of both normal and cancer cells. Microscopic examination of tumors and normal tissues established many important properties, including the characteristics of the cell cycle, the hierarchical organization of cells within normal tissues and to a lesser extent in tumors, the requirement for angiogenesis in tumor growth, heterogeneity among tumor cell populations, and relationships between histopathologic characteristics of tumors and their prognosis. Development of methods to culture cells, including colony-forming assays to reflect longer-term survival, allowed quantitative studies of the response of cancer cells to radiation and drugs, and allowed the therapeutic response of tumors to be related to the sensitivity of individual cells within them. The establishment of inbred (syngeneic) mice allowed tumors to be transplanted between them, while subsequent development of immune-deprived mice has allowed study of human cancers in an in vivo environment as xenografts (established either from cell lines, or directly from patient tumors—patient-derived xenografts or PDX models). Methods for the culture of large collections of molecularly characterized cancer cell lines has permitted screening of drugs and facilitated the development of agents targeting specific genetic changes. However, current cancer treatment strategies are still dependent on some of the earlier-developed chemotherapy drugs.

1.2 RECENT ADVANCES IN ONCOLOGY

The underlying biology of cancer can be conceptualized as a process of many small changes, in a manner akin to evolution. Genetic changes that affect growth potential provide an environment permissive for further changes that are selected for (or against) by environmental conditions. Increasing knowledge of cellular signal transduction pathways has revealed that many aspects of cellular function, including proliferation and death, are controlled by a balance of positive and negative signals received from inside and outside the cell. Thus, a decreased or increased ability to respond to a specific signal may allow the cell to proliferate in the face of other signals that would normally prevent such proliferation. Interaction of cancer cells with their surrounding microenvironment (stromal tissue, microvasculature, infiltrating hematopoietic cell populations) that comprises a substantial proportion of the tumor mass is also a key factor in cancer progression and metastasis. For example, the development of vascular networks in tumors (angiogenesis) is necessary for tumor growth, and the behavior of cancer cells is influenced by external signals from circulating molecules (hormones and growth factors) and from neighboring cells and their surrounding cellular and extracellular microenvironment. Changes to the environment in tumor cells (such as poor oxygenation) can cause changes in gene expression that enhance the development of more aggressive tumor phenotypes. Investigation of these processes has led to a better understanding of how and why cancer cells can spread from the primary tumor to grow at other sites in the body as a (*metastasis*)—a property of malignant cancer that is a dominant contributor to morbidity and mortality in affected individuals.

Although cancers are typically clonal, indicating an origin from a single cell, they become heterogeneous in their genetic composition and cellular properties, and cells within different regions (or indeed within the same region) of an established tumor may express different genes (Gerlinger et al, 2012). One aspect of tumor heterogeneity is the development of cellular hierarchy, as in some normal tissues where there is a limited number of cells with a high proliferative potential that replenish mature cells that are lost from the tissue. Tumor cells with high proliferative potential, known as cancer stem cells (CSCs), are those that can regenerate the tumor after treatment. Surface markers have been identified that appear to characterize CSC in some cancers, but the stability of these markers and the exclusivity of the CSC phenotype to only a small population following treatment is uncertain and may differ within and between tumors. The plasticity of cancer cells may allow them to develop or select for a CSC phenotype as well as develop resistance to therapeutic agents. This plasticity remains a major challenge to treating tumors by targeting specific genetic pathways.

The availability of increasing levels of genomic analysis (eg, through The Cancer Genome Atlas) has led to a model in which cancer development and progression are believed to result from successive mutations or other genetic changes that destabilize the genome and permit unregulated cell growth, which in turn elicits further alterations in the surrounding tissue that permit growth and invasion. These genetic alterations may arise directly or indirectly from inherited genetic mutations, chemical- or radiation-induced DNA damage, incorporation of certain viruses into the genome, or random errors during DNA synthesis. Such mutations can be classified as those responsible for cancer growth (driver mutations) and passenger mutations that arise as a result of the unstable state of the genome but are not responsible for its uncontrolled growth. Different types of cancer can carry very different numbers of mutations, and a greater burden of mutation (with the potential to encode new protein antigens) has been associated with increased probability that a tumor will respond to immunotherapy (Chan et al, 2019). The behavior of both normal and cancer cells is also dependent on epigenetic modifications that influence the expression of genes. Such changes may also contribute to transient changes in properties of cancer cells, including those that convey resistance to therapy (Dawson, 2017).

Modern cancer treatment employs a combination of surgery, chemotherapy, and radiotherapy, increasingly in combination with each other and with drugs that target specific biologic networks. Drug therapies are focused increasingly on genetic changes in cancer cells and on targeting driver alterations. Two examples are vemurafenib, which improves survival by inhibiting the BRAF kinase in the ~50% of human melanomas that have a *BRAF* mutation (Chapman et al, 2011), and larotrectinib, which targets fusion proteins expressed in various solid tumors that harbor a C-terminal fusion with one of the 3 tropomyosin kinase receptors TRKA, TRKB, or TRKC (Drilon et al, 2018). These and other examples build on a paradigm first established in the treatment of chronic myelogenous leukemia with an inhibitor (imatinib) of the binding site of the BCR-ABL protein kinase, the protein that is aberrantly expressed as a result of the Philadelphia chromosome translocation (O'Brien et al, 2003). Another successful approach uses monoclonal antibodies to target aberrantly expressed surface receptors. A well-established example is trastuzumab, a monoclonal antibody that recognizes the HER2/NEU receptor overexpressed on some aggressive breast cancers; incorporation of this (and related) agents in treatment regimens has been shown to improve survival rates when used in conjunction with surgery for localized disease, and increases survival and quality of life for patients with advanced disease (Loibl and Gianni, 2017). Recent additions to the therapeutic antibody armamentarium include immunotherapy agents that inhibit immune checkpoints (eg, PD-1/PD-L1); development of these agents was enabled by characterization of the interactions between immune T cells and tumor cells, work that was recognized in 2018 by the Nobel Prize in Physiology or Medicine awarded to James Allison and Tasuku Honjo. These agents, which inhibit the negative signals suppressing antitumor immunity, have shown benefit in many cancer types, including melanoma and lung cancer (Haanen and Robert, 2015; Chowdhury et al, 2018).

Traditional methods of treatment have also undergone substantial refinements. New methods for the delivery of radiotherapy such as image-guided, intensity-modulated, and stereotactic radiotherapy have allowed higher doses to be delivered to the tumor with increased precision and with lower doses to critical normal tissues. These techniques have improved local control of primary tumors, such as those in the prostate, and new combinations of radiation with surgery and chemotherapy are also improving patient survival. Development of these techniques has paralleled that of enhanced methods of imaging tumors in the body with high resolution including computed tomography (CT), magnetic resonance imaging (MRI), and positron emission tomography (PET).

1.3 THE FUTURE OF ONCOLOGY AND CANCER TREATMENT

The ability to sequence the DNA and RNA of cancer and normal tissue genomes has provided insights into the molecular signals that are associated with various types of cancers. Molecular profiling of key oncogenic factors has allowed many types of cancers to be divided into subcategories and is being used to define better treatments for subpopulations of patients. Breast cancer, for example, has for many years been defined not just by "stage" (size of the primary tumor, and whether the tumor has spread to the lymph nodes) and grade (the extent to which it differs from normal breast tissue) but by whether the tumor is estrogen-responsive (ie, estrogen receptor or ER-positive or ER-negative) and whether it overexpresses or exhibits genetic amplification of HER2. These features guide the selection of available agents that interfere with estrogen-mediated growth (tamoxifen or aromatase inhibitors) or target the HER2 receptor (trastuzumab). Gene expression classifiers (eg, OncotypeDX, MammaPrint, and others) have enabled further stratification of ER-positive early-stage cancers to better predict outcome, and identify patients who can benefit from, or should be spared the toxic effects of, chemotherapy (Cardoso et al, 2016; Sparano et al, 2018). More recently, knowledge of germline (eg, BRCA1/BRCA2) or somatic mutations has been used to identify patients who may benefit from particular types of therapy, eg, platinum chemotherapy or poly (adenosine diphosphate [ADP] ribose) polymerase [PARP] inhibitors in HER2-negative breast cancer. Other features of cancer genomes, such as the presence of certain patterns of mutations (microsatellite instability, related to deficiency in DNA mismatch repair) can also be identified diagnostically and used to guide the application of effective therapies, in this case immune checkpoint blockade with pembrolizumab (Lemery et al, 2017). One concern regarding the use of biomarkers based on gene expression or somatic alterations is that tumor heterogeneity may limit the utility of assays performed on single biopsies. An emerging area is the use of circulating tumor DNA (ctDNA)—identifiable in the peripheral blood—as a minimally invasive tool for diagnosis, molecular stratification, and assessment of treatment response (Heitzer et al, 2019).

A positive aspect arising from the sequencing of cancer genomes is the realization that some cancers may have an Achilles' heel. In single-celled organisms such as the budding yeast *Saccharomyces cerevisiae*, the concept of synthetic lethality is well established. This phenomenon is based on the observation that a mutation in a gene pathway "A," though not lethal on its own, becomes incompatible with survival when combined with another nonlethal mutation in a separate gene pathway "B." Because cancer genomes possess many mutations that differentiate them from surrounding normal tissue, it should be possible to exploit this unique complexity of the cancer cell (O'Neil et al, 2017) and enable the development of strategies to target cancers that have lost tumor suppressors. One well-known example is the identification of PARP inhibitors as a synthetic lethal treatment in cancers deficient in homologous recombination repair because of loss of BRCA1 or BRCA2 function (Lord and Ashworth, 2017). Several potent PARP inhibitors have been developed and are approved for use in BRCA-deficient ovarian and breast cancers (Farmer et al, 2005). The advent of powerful high throughput functional genomic and drug screening platforms enables ongoing efforts to identify and develop new synthetic lethal strategies, for example, Aurora kinase inhibitors for cancers deficient in the retinoblastoma (RB1) protein (Gong et al, 2019).

The examples above suggest that there are increasing opportunities to harness the knowledge of specific tumor alterations to direct precision therapeutic approaches, and indeed there is an increasing trend in large cancer centers to employ what is termed personalized medicine, where the goal is to provide treatment of an individual's cancer tailored to the genetic profile of their cancer. It is now relatively inexpensive to sequence an entire genome (or more focused regions of relevance) and identify somatic alterations and patterns of mutagenesis. However, understanding and acting on the results of such tests is a greater challenge, for which knowledge of the relationship between tumor alterations and drug response is incomplete. In addition to lineage-dependent differences in responses that may be exhibited between tumor types when they share the same molecular alteration (eg, *BRAF* mutant melanoma vs colorectal cancer), the tumor microenvironment (eg, hypoxia) may further alter gene expression and tumor biology and both microenvironmental and genetic heterogeneity need to be addressed to provide a "true" state of an individual's cancer. Another problem with matching drugs to tumors is that genetic analyses of cancers have identified many more potential targets than there are drugs available to use for such treatment, with the result that truly personalized medicine remains confined to a small fraction of patients (Tannock and Hickman, 2016).

In the face of this genetic complexity, it has become important to pursue research into the fundamental principles of how cancer gene networks interact with one another and how they affect cell growth, signaling, and response to the environment. The goal of the chapters that follow is to provide a succinct but comprehensive summary of the basic science underlying oncology.

REFERENCES

Cardoso F, van't Veer LJ, Bogaerts J, et al; MINDACT Investigators. 70-gene signature as an aid to treatment decisions in early-stage breast cancer. *N Engl J Med* 2016;375:717-729.

Chan TA, Yarchoan M, Jaffee E, et al. Development of tumor mutation burden as an immunotherapy biomarker: utility for the oncology clinic. *Ann Oncol* 2019;30:44-56.

Chapman PB, Hauschild A, Robert C et al; BRIM-3 Study Group. Improved survival with vemurafenib in melanoma with BRAF V600E mutation. *N Engl J Med* 2011;364:2507-2516.

Chowdhury PS, Chamoto K, Honjo T. Combination therapy strategies for improving PD-1 blockade efficiency; a new era in cancer immunotherapy. *Cancer Treat Rev* 2018;63:40-47.

Dawson MA. The cancer epigenome: Concepts, challenges, and therapeutic opportunities. *Science* 2017;355:1147-1152.

Doll R, Hill AB. Smoking and carcinoma of the lung; preliminary report. *BMJ* 1950;2:739-748.

Doll R, Peto R, Boreham J, Sutherland I. Mortality in relation to smoking: 50 years' observations on male British doctors. *BMJ* 2004;328:1519.

Drilon A, Laetsch TW, Kummar S, et al. Efficacy of larotrectinib in TRK fusion-positive cancers in adults and children. *N Engl J Med* 2018;378:731-739.

Farmer H, McCabe N, Lord CJ, et al. Targeting the DNA repair defect in BRCA mutant cells as a therapeutic strategy. *Nature* 2005;434:917-921.

Future II Study Group. Quadrivalent vaccine against human papillomavirus to prevent high-grade cervical lesions. *N Engl J Med* 2007;356:1915-1927.

Gerlinger M, Rowan AJ, Horswell S, et al. Intratumor heterogeneity and branched evolution revealed by multiregion sequencing. *N Engl J Med* 2012;366:883-892.

Gong X, Du J, Parsons SH, et al. Aurora A kinase inhibition is synthetic lethal with loss of the *RB1* tumor suppressor gene. *Cancer Discov* 2019;9:248-263.

Haanen JB, Robert C. Immune checkpoint inhibitors. *Prog Tumor Res* 2015;42:55-66.

Heitzer E, Haque IS, Roberts CES, Speicher MR. Current and future perspectives of liquid biopsies in genomics-driven oncology. *Nat Rev Genet* 2019;20:71-88.

Hopkins BD, Goncalves MD, Cantley LC. Obesity and cancer mechanisms: cancer metabolism. *J Clin Oncol* 2016;34:4277-4283.

Iyengar NM, Hudis CA, Dannenberg AJ. Obesity and cancer: local and systemic mechanisms. *Annu Rev Med* 2015;66:297-309.

Lemen RA. Mesothelioma from asbestos exposures: epidemiologic patterns and impact in the United States. *J Toxicol Environ Health B Crit Rev* 2016;19:250-265.

Lemery S, Keegan P, Padzur R. First FDA approval agnostic of cancer site—when a biomarker defines the indication. *N Engl J Med* 2017;377:1409-1412.

Loibl S, Gianni L. HER2-positive breast cancer. *Lancet* 2017;389:2415-2429.

Lord CJ, Ashworth A. PARP inhibitors: Synthetic lethality in the clinic. *Science* 2017;355:1152-1158.

Luo Z, Ruan B. Impact of the implementation of a vaccination strategy on hepatitis B virus infections in China over a 20-year period. *Int J Infect Dis* 2012;16:e82-88.

O'Brien SG, Guilhot F, Larson RA, et al; IRIS Investigators. Imatinib compared with interferon and low-dose cytarabine for newly diagnosed chronic-phase chronic myeloid leukemia. *N Engl J Med* 2003;348:994-1004.

O'Neil NJ, Bailey ML, Hieter P. Synthetic lethality and cancer. *Nat Rev Genet* 2017;18:613-623.

Sparano JA, Gray RJ, Makower DF, et al. Adjuvant chemotherapy guided by a 21-gene expression assay in breast cancer. *N Engl J Med* 2018;379:111-121.

Tannock IF, Hickman JA. Limits to personalized cancer medicine. *N Engl J Med* 2016;375:1289-1294.

Methods of Molecular Analysis

Paul C. Boutros, Lea Harrington, and Thomas Kislinger

Chapter Outline

2.1 Introduction
2.2 Principal Techniques for Nucleic Acid Analysis
   2.2.1 Cytogenetics and Karyotyping
   2.2.2 Hybridization and Nucleic Acid Probes
   2.2.3 Restriction Enzymes and Manipulation of Genes
   2.2.4 Blotting Techniques
   2.2.5 The Polymerase Chain Reaction
   2.2.6 Fluorescence in Situ Hybridization
   2.2.7 Comparative Genomic Hybridization
   2.2.8 Spectral Karyotyping/Multifluor–Fluorescence in Situ Hybridization
   2.2.9 Single-Nucleotide Polymorphisms
   2.2.10 Sequencing of DNA
   2.2.11 Variation in Copy Number and Gene Sequence
   2.2.12 Microarrays and RNA Analysis
   2.2.13 Technologies For Studying Epigenetic Changes
2.3 Creating and Manipulating Model Systems
   2.3.1 Cell Culture/Cancer Cell Lines
   2.3.2 Manipulating Genes in Cells
   2.3.3 MicroRNAs and RNA Interference
   2.3.4 Site-Directed Mutagenesis
   2.3.5 Transgenic and Knockout Mice
   2.3.6 Other Methods of Gene Editing
2.4 Proteomics
   2.4.1 Mass Spectrometry
   2.4.2 Top-Down or Bottom-Up Proteomics
   2.4.3 Gel-Based or Gel-Free Approaches
   2.4.4 Quantitative Proteomics
   2.4.5 Challenges for Biomarker Discovery with Proteomics
   2.4.6 X-Ray Crystallography
   2.4.7 Nuclear Magnetic Resonance Spectroscopy
   2.4.8 Cryogenic Electron Microscopy
   2.4.9 Protein Arrays
2.5 Translational Applications with Cells and Tissues
   2.5.1 Laser-Capture Microdissection
   2.5.2 Tissue Microarrays
   2.5.3 Flow Cytometry
2.6 Bioinformatics and Other Techniques of Data Analysis
   2.6.1 Statistical Analysis
   2.6.2 Unsupervised Clustering
   2.6.3 Gene Signatures
   2.6.4 Network Analysis
Summary
References

2.1 INTRODUCTION

Advances in understanding the biology of cancer have transformed the field of oncology. Although genetic analysis was limited previously to gross chromosomal abnormalities in karyotypes, DNA and RNA in cells can now be analyzed at the individual base-pair level, and there is increasing knowledge about the structure and interactions of proteins. This intricate knowledge of the molecular properties of cancer increases the possibility that personalized treatment for individual cancers might be achieved. To appreciate the relevance and nature of these technological advances, as well as their implications for function, an understanding of the modern tools of molecular biology is essential. This chapter reviews the cytogenetic, nucleic, proteomic, and bioinformatics methods used to study the molecular basis of cancer, and highlights methods that are likely to affect its future management.

2.2 PRINCIPAL TECHNIQUES FOR NUCLEIC ACID ANALYSIS

2.2.1 Cytogenetics and Karyotyping

Cancer is thought to arise from a stepwise accumulation of genetic changes that confer a selective growth advantage to the involved cells. These changes may consist of abnormalities in specific genes (such as amplification of oncogenes or deletion of tumor-suppressor genes). Although molecular techniques can identify specific DNA mutations, cytogenetics provides an overall description of chromosome number, structure, and the extent and nature of chromosomal abnormalities.

Several techniques can be used to obtain tumor cells for cytogenetic analysis. Biopsies of leukemias and lymphomas from peripheral blood, bone marrow, or lymph node are easily dispersed into single cells suitable for chromosomal analysis. Cytogenetic analysis of solid tumors is more challenging. The cells are tightly adherent and must be dispersed by mechanical means and/or by digestion with proteolytic enzymes (eg, trypsin, collagenase), which can damage cells. Second, the mitotic index in solid tumors is often low, making it difficult to find enough metaphase cells to obtain good-quality cytogenetic preparations. Finally, lymphoid, myeloid, and other (normal) cells infiltrate solid tumors and may be confused with the malignant cell population.

Chromosomes are usually examined in metaphase, when they become condensed and appear as 2 identical sister chromatids held together at the centromere, as DNA replication has already occurred at that stage of mitosis. Exposure of the tumor cells to agents such as colcemid arrests them in metaphase by disrupting the mitotic spindle fibers that normally separate the chromatids. The cells are then swollen in a hypotonic solution, fixed in methanol-acetic acid, and metaphase "spreads" are prepared by physically dropping the fixed cells onto glass microscope slides.

Chromosomes can be recognized by their size and shape and by the pattern of light and dark "bands" observed after specific staining. The usual way of generating banded chromosomes is proteolytic digestion with trypsin, followed by a Giemsa stain. A typical metaphase spread prepared using conventional methods has approximately 550 bands, whereas cells spread at prophase can have more than 800 bands; these bands can be analyzed using bright-field microscopy and digital photography. The result of cytogenetic analysis is a karyotype, which, in written form, describes the chromosomal abnormalities using the international consensus cytogenetic nomenclature ((Brothman et al, 2009); see Fig. 2–1 and Table 2–1). Table 2–2 lists common chromosomal abnormalities in lymphoid and myeloid malignancies.

The study of solid tumors has been facilitated by new analytic approaches that combine elements of conventional cytogenetics with molecular methodologies. This new hybrid discipline is called *molecular cytogenetics*, and its application to tumor analysis usually involves the use of techniques based on *fluorescence in situ hybridization* (FISH; see Sec. 2.2.6). These techniques can be used to "paint" each chromosome with a false color, thereby facilitating their recognition (see Sec. 2.2.8).

2.2.2 Hybridization and Nucleic Acid Probes

DNA is composed of 2 complementary strands (the sense strand and the nonsense strand) of specific sequences of the 4 nucleotide bases that make up the genetic alphabet. The association (via hydrogen bonds) between 2 bases on opposite complementary DNA or certain types of RNA strands

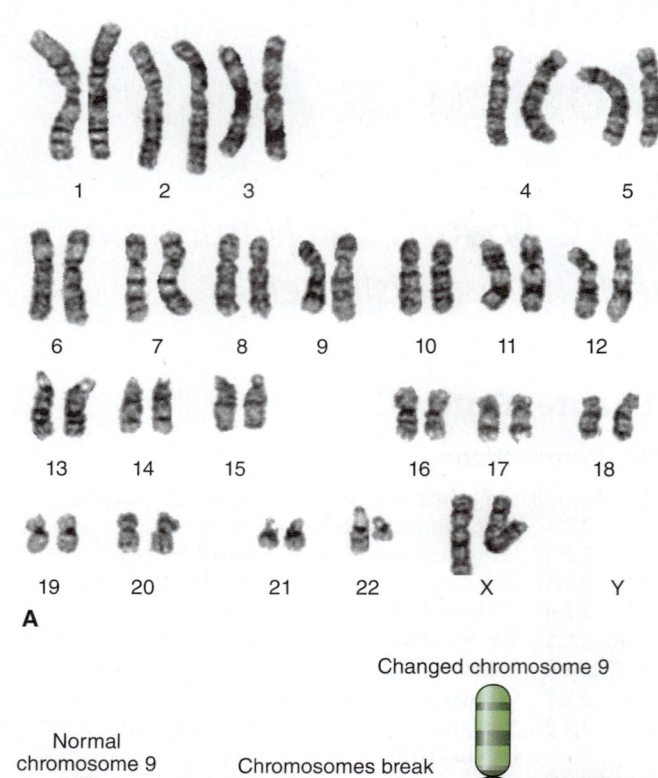

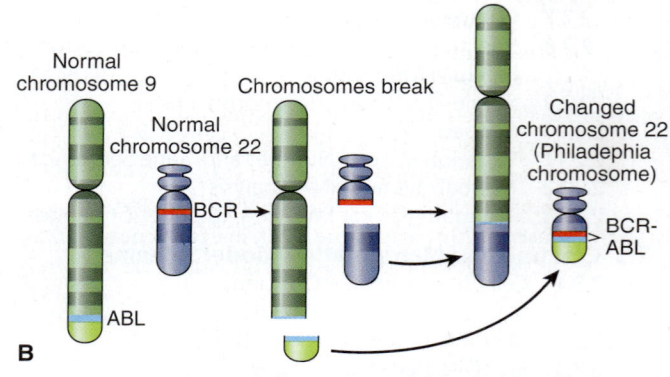

FIGURE 2–1 The photograph on (A) shows a typical karyotype from a patient with chronic myelogenous leukemia. By international agreement, the chromosomes are numbered according to their appearance following G-banding. Note the loss of material from the long arm of one copy of the chromosome 22 pair (*the chromosome on the right*) and its addition to the long arm of one copy of chromosome 9 (*also the chromosome on the right of the pair*). B) A schematic illustration of the accepted band pattern for this rearrangement. The green and red lines indicate the precise position of the breakpoints that are involved. The karyotypic nomenclature for this particular chromosomal abnormality is t(9;22)(q34;q11). This description means that there is a reciprocal translocation between chromosomes 9 and 22 with breakpoints at q34 on chromosome 9 and q11 on chromosome 22. The rearranged chromosome 22 is sometimes called the Philadelphia chromosome (or Ph chromosome), after the city of its discovery.

that are connected via hydrogen bonds is called a *base pair* (often abbreviated as bp). In DNA, adenine (A) forms a base pair with thymine (T) and guanine (G) forms a base pair with cytosine (C). In RNA, thymine is replaced by uracil (U). As DNA replicates during the S phase of the cell cycle, a part of the helical DNA molecule unwinds and the strands separate (see Fig. 2–2). DNA polymerase enzymes add nucleotides to

TABLE 2–1 Nomenclature for chromosomes and their abnormalities.

Description	Meaning
–1	Loss of one chromosome 1
+7	Gain of extra chromosome 7
2q⁻ or del (2q)	Deletion of part of long arm of chromosome 2
4p⁺	Addition of material to short arm of chromosome 4
t(9;22)(q34;q11)	Reciprocal translocation between chromosomes 9 and 22 with breakpoints at q34 on chromosome 9 and q11 on chromosome 22
iso(6p)	Isochromosome with both arms derived from the short arm of chromosome 6
inv(16)(p13q22)	Part of chromosome 16 between p13 and q22 is inverted

the 3′-hydroxyl (3′-OH) end of an RNA/DNA primer that is hybridized to a template, thus leading to synthesis of a complementary new strand of DNA. Transcription of messenger RNA (mRNA) takes place through an analogous process under the action of RNA polymerase, with one of the DNA strands (the non-sense strand) acting as a template; complementary bases (U, G, C, and A) are added to the mRNA through pairing with bases in the DNA strand so that the sequence of bases in the RNA is the same as in the "sense" strand of the DNA (except that U replaces T). During this process, the DNA strand is separated temporarily from its partner through the action of topoisomerase I. Only parts of the DNA in each gene are translated into polypeptides, and these coding regions are known as exons; noncoding regions (introns) are interspersed throughout the genes and are spliced out of the mRNA transcript during the RNA maturation process and before protein synthesis.

Synthesis of polypeptides, the building blocks of proteins, are then directed by the mRNA in association with ribosomes, with each triplet of bases in the exons of the DNA encoding a specific amino acid that is added to the polypeptide chain.

Many techniques used in molecular genetic analysis depend on the specificity of hybridization and the action and fidelity of DNA polymerases. When double-stranded DNA is heated, the complementary strands separate (denature) to form single-stranded DNA. Given suitable conditions, separated complementary regions of specific DNA sequences can join together to re-form a double-stranded molecule. This renaturation is called *hybridization*. This ability of single-stranded nucleic acids to hybridize with their complementary sequence is fundamental to techniques used in molecular genetic analysis. Using an appropriate reaction mixture containing the relevant nucleotides and DNA or RNA polymerase, a specific piece of DNA can be copied or transcribed. If radiolabeled or fluorescently labeled nucleotides are included in the reaction mixture, the complimentary copy of the template can be used as a sensitive hybridization-dependent probe.

2.2.3 Restriction Enzymes and Manipulation of Genes

Restriction enzymes are endonucleases that have the ability to cut DNA only at sites of specific nucleotide sequences and always cut the DNA at the same place within the designated sequence. Figure 2–3 illustrates some commonly used restriction enzymes together with the sequence of nucleotides that they recognize and the position at which they cut the sequence. Restriction enzymes allow DNA to be cut into reproducible segments that can be analyzed precisely. Many restriction enzymes create sticky ends, because the DNA is cut

TABLE 2–2 Common chromosomal abnormalities in lymphoid and myeloid malignancies.

Malignancy	Chromosomal Aberration*	Molecular Lesion
Acute myeloid leukemia (AML)		
M1, M2 subtypes	t(8;21)(q22;q22)	*AML1-MTG8* fusion
M3 subtype	t(15;17)(q22;q11.2)	*PML-RARA* fusion
M4Eo subtype	inv(16)(p13;q22) or t(16;16)(p13;q22)	*MYH11-CBFB* fusion
M2 or M4 subtypes	t(6;9)(p23;q24)	*DEK-CAN* fusion
Therapy-related AML	~5/del(5q), ~7/del(7q)	
Chronic myeloid leukemia (CML)	t(9;22)(q34;q11) (Ph¹ chromosome)	*BCR-ABL* fusion encoding p210 protein
CML blast crisis	t(9;22)(q34;q11), 8, +Ph¹, 19, or i(17q)	*BCR-ABL* fusion encoding p210 protein, *TP53* mutation
Acute lymphocytic leukemia (ALL)	t(9;22)(q34;q11)	*BCR-ABL* fusion encoding p190 protein
Pre-B ALL	t(1;19)(q23;p13.3)	*E2A-PBX1* fusion
Pre-B ALL	t(17;19)(q22;p13.3)	*E2A-HLF* fusion
B-ALL, Burkitt lymphoma	t(8;14)(q24;q32)	Translocations between *myc* and *IgH*, *IgL*κ and *IgL*λ loci
	t(2;8)(p12;q24)	
	t(8;22)(q24;q11)	
B-Chronic lymphocytic leukemia	+12, t(14q32)	Translocations of *IgH* locus

*For an interpretation of the nomenclature of chromosomal rearrangements, see Table 2–1.
Data from Sheer D, Squire J. Clinical applications of genetic rearrangements in cancer. *Semin Cancer Biol* 1996 Feb;7(1):25-32.

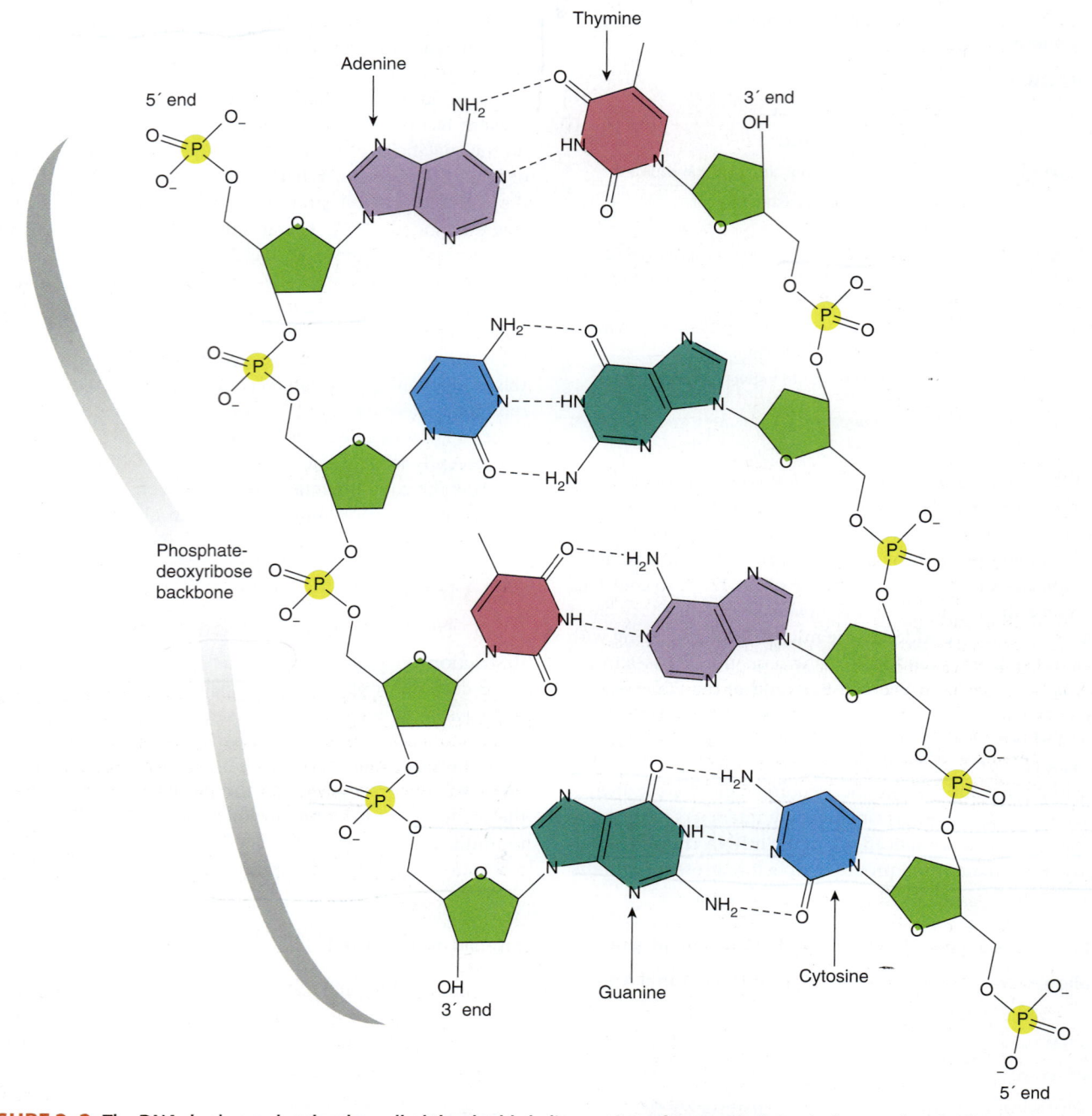

FIGURE 2–2 The DNA duplex molecule, also called the *double helix*, consists of 2 strands that wind around each other. The strands are held together by chemical attraction of the bases that comprise the DNA. A bonds to T and G bonds to C. The bases are linked together to form long strands by a "backbone" chemical structure. The DNA bases and backbone twist around to form a duplex spiral.

in a different place on the 2 strands. When the DNA molecule separates, the cut end has a small single-stranded portion that can hybridize to other fragments having complementary sequences (ie, fragments digested using the same restriction enzyme), thus allowing investigators to cut and paste pieces of DNA together.

Any DNA segment of interest can be inserted into a bacterial virus or plasmid to facilitate its manipulation and propagation using restriction enzymes. A complementary DNA strand (cDNA) is first synthesized using mRNA as the template by a reverse transcriptase enzyme. This cDNA contains only the exons of the gene from which the mRNA was transcribed. Figure 2–4 presents a schematic of how a restriction fragment of DNA containing the coding sequence of a gene can be inserted into a bacterial plasmid that also contains a gene that confers resistance against a drug that would otherwise kill host bacteria (eg, ampicillin). The plasmid or virus is referred to as a *vector* carrying the passenger DNA sequence of the gene of interest. The vector DNA is cut with the same restriction enzyme used to prepare the cloned gene, so that all the fragments will have compatible sticky ends and can be spliced back together. The spliced fragments can be sealed with the

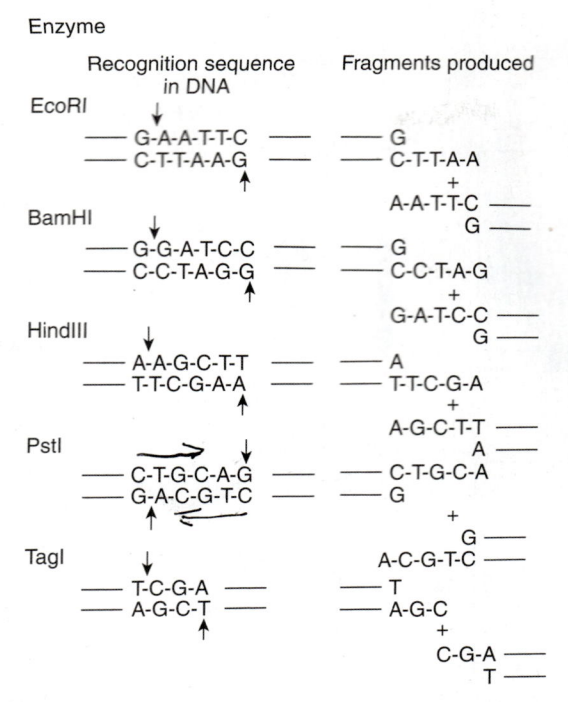

FIGURE 2–3 **The nucleotide sequences recognized by 5 different restriction endonucleases are shown.** On the left side, the sequence recognized by the enzyme is shown; the sites where the enzymes cut the DNA are shown by the arrows. On the right side, the 2 fragments produced following digestion with that restriction enzyme are shown. Note that each recognition sequence is a palindrome; that is, the first 2 or 3 bases are complementary to the last 2 or 3 bases. For example, for EcoR1, GAA is complementary to TTC. Also note that following digestion, each fragment has a single-stranded tail of DNA. This tail is useful in allowing fragments that contain complementary overhangs to anneal with each other.

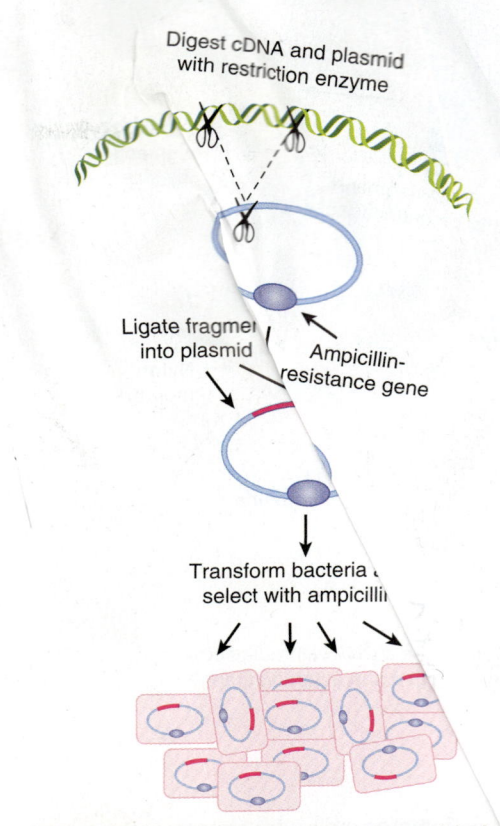

FIGURE 2–4 **Insertion of a gene into a bacterial plasmid.** cDNA of interest (*pink line*) is digested with a restriction endonuclease (depicted by *scissors*) to generate a defined fragment of cDNA with "sticky ends." The circular plasmid DNA is cut with the same restriction endonuclease to generate single-stranded ends that will hybridize and to the cDNA fragment. The recombinant DNA plasmid can be selected for growth using antibiotics because the ampicillin-resistance gene (*blue oval*) is included in the construct. In this way, large amounts of the human cDNA can be obtained for further purposes (e.g. for use as a probe on a Southern blot).

enzyme DNA ligase, and the reconstituted molecule can be introduced into bacterial cells. Because bacteria that take up the plasmid are resistant to a drug (eg, ampicillin), they can be isolated and propagated to large numbers. In this way, large quantities of a gene can be obtained (i.e. cloned) and labeled with either radioactivity or biotin for use as a DNA probe for analysis in Southern or northern blots (see Sec. 2.2.4). Cloned DNA can be used for nucleotide sequencing (see Sec. 2.2.10), or for transfer into other cells. Alternatively, the starting DNA may be a complex mixture of different restriction fragments derived from human cells. When a large number of different DNA fragments have been inserted into a vector population and then introduced into bacteria, the result is a *DNA library*, which can be plated out and screened by hybridization with a specific probe. In this way, an individual *recombinant DNA clone* can be isolated from the library and used for most of the applications described in the following sections.

2.2.4 Blotting Techniques

Southern blotting (Fig. 2–5) is a method for analyzing the structure of DNA (named after the scientist who developed it). The DNA to be analyzed is cut into defined lengths using a restriction enzyme, and the fragments are separated by electrophoresis through an agarose gel. The smallest DNA fragments migrate farthest in the gel and the largest remain near the origin; pieces of DNA of known size are electrophoresed at the same time (in a separately loaded well) and act as molecular size markers. A nylon membrane is then laid on top of the gel and a vacuum is applied to draw the DNA through the gel into the membrane, where it is immobilized. The nylon membrane containing the fragments of DNA is incubated in a solution containing a radioactive or fluorescently labeled probe that is complementary to part of the gene (see Sec. 2.2.2). Under these conditions, the probe will anneal with homologous DNA sequences present on the DNA in the membrane. After gentle washing to remove the single-stranded, unbound probe, the labeled probe remaining on the membrane will be bound to homologous sequences of the gene of interest. The location of the gene on the nylon membrane can then be detected either by the fluorescence or radioactivity associated with the probe.

An almost identical procedure can be used to characterize RNA species separated by electrophoresis and transferred to

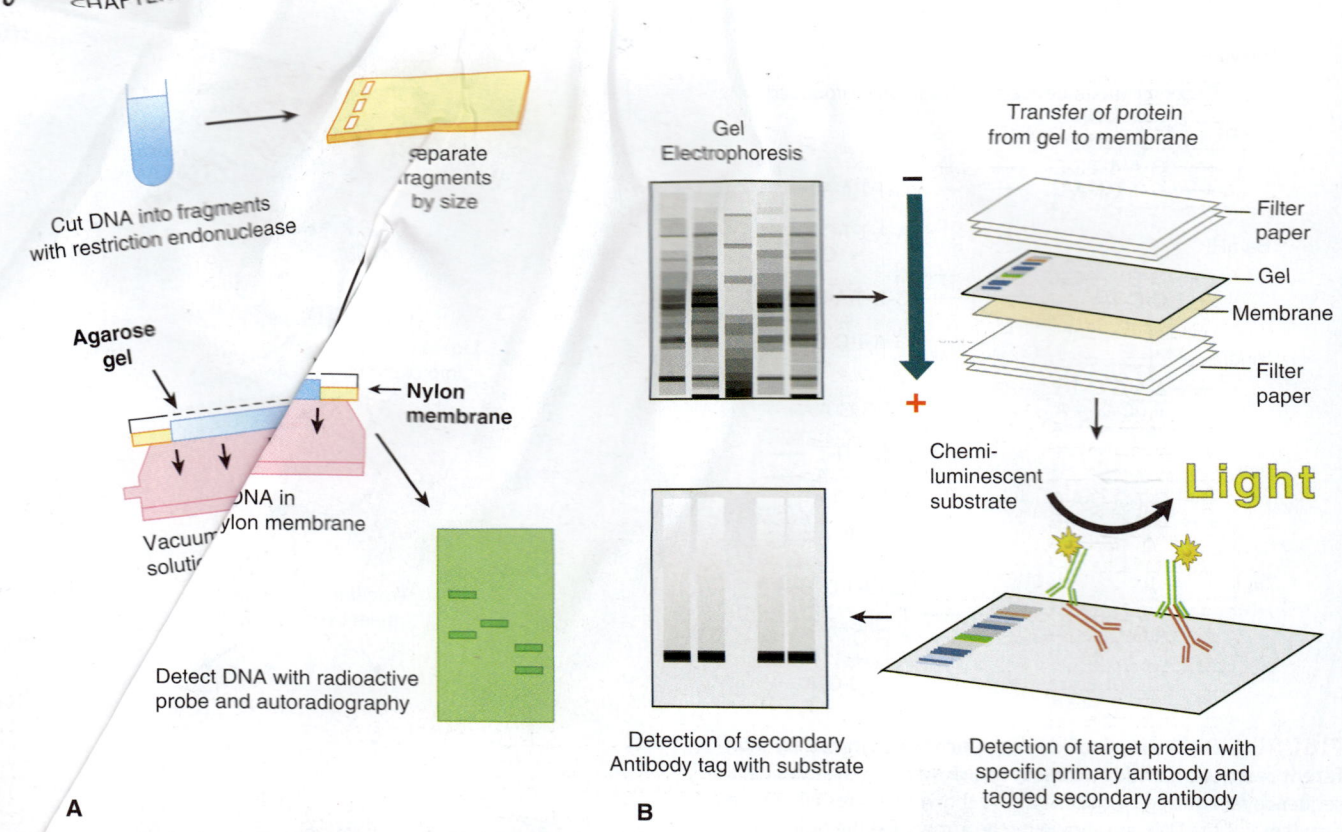

FIGURE 2–5 Common molecular biologic techniques: Southern, and western blotting. A) Southern blotting. Schematic outline of the procedures involved in analyzing DNA fragments by the Southern blotting technique. A less commonly used but similar technique, called northern, is used for the detection of RNA instead of DNA. Only Southern is capitalized (after its discoverer, Ed Southern), whereas western and northern are not capitalized. **B) Western blotting.** This method involves transfer of a protein gel (eg, SDS-PAGE, upper left corner) onto a membrane (upper right), probing the membrane with an antibody specific to the protein of interest followed by a secondary antibody conjugated to a fluorophore (e.g. as in LICOR detection) or an enzyme that will generate a chemiluminescent signal (eg, as in ECL) (lower left). (Reproduced with permission from Ghosh R, Gilda JE, Gomes AV. The necessity of and strategies for improving confidence in the accuracy of western blots. *Expert Rev Proteomics* 2014 Oct;11(5):549-560.)

a nylon membrane. The technique is called northern blotting and is used to evaluate the expression of genes.

An analogous procedure, called western blotting, is used to characterize proteins. Following separation by electrophoresis in the presence of detergent (to ensure their migration is primarily a function of mass rather than charge), the proteins are immobilized by transfer to a charged synthetic membrane. To identify specific proteins, the membrane is incubated in a solution containing a specific primary antibody either labeled directly with a fluorophore or incubated with a secondary antibody that will bind to the primary antibody and is conjugated to either horseradish peroxidase (HRP), biotin, or a fluorophore. The primary antibody will bind only to the region of the membrane containing the protein of interest and can be detected either directly by its fluorescence or by exposure to chemoluminescence detection reagents.

2.2.5 The Polymerase Chain Reaction

The polymerase chain reaction (PCR) allows rapid production of large quantities of specific pieces of DNA (usually about 200-1000 base pairs) using a DNA polymerase enzyme called *Taq* polymerase (which is resistant to denaturation at high temperatures). Specific oligonucleotide primers complementary to the DNA flanking the region of interest are synthesized or obtained commercially and are used as primers for *Taq* polymerase. All components of the reaction (the target DNA, primers, deoxynucleotides, and *Taq* polymerase) are placed in a small tube and the reaction sequence is accomplished by changing the temperature of the reaction mixture in a cyclical manner (Fig. 2–6A). A typical PCR reaction would involve (1) incubation at 94°C to denature (separate) the DNA duplex and create single-stranded DNA; (2) incubation at 53°C to allow hybridization of the primers, which are in vast excess (this temperature may vary depending on the sequence of the primers); and (3) incubation at 72°C to allow *Taq* polymerase to synthesize new DNA from the primers. Repeating this cycle permits another round of amplification (Fig. 2–6B). Each cycle takes only a few minutes. Twenty cycles can theoretically produce a million-fold amplification of the DNA of interest. PCR products can then be sequenced or subjected to other methods of genetic analysis. DNA polymerase enzymes with greater heat stability and copying fidelity can allow for long-range amplification using primers separated by as many as 15 to 30 kilobases of intervening target DNA. The PCR is exquisitely sensitive and its applications include the detection of tumor-specific DNA sequences that

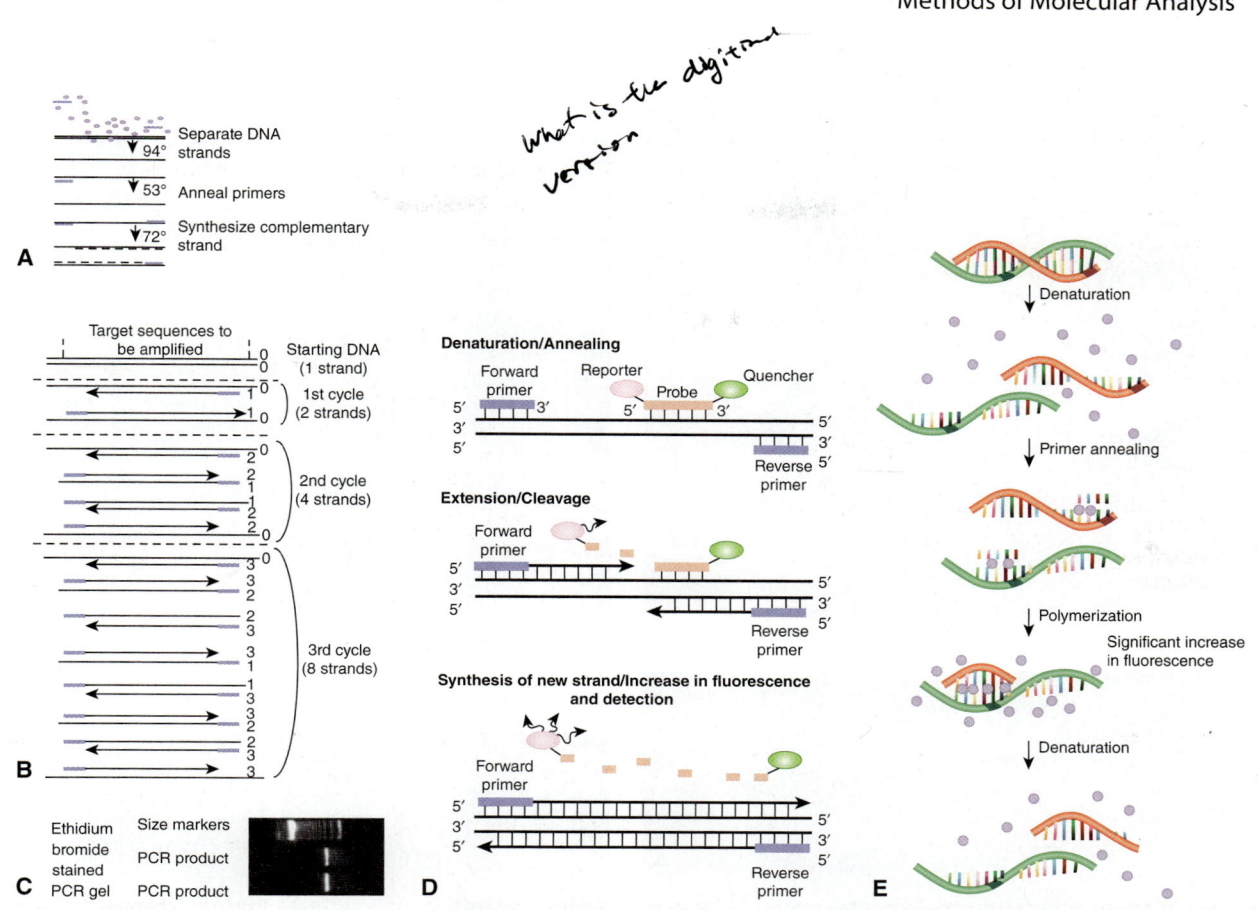

FIGURE 2–6 **A)** Reaction sequence for 1 cycle of PCR. Each line represents 1 strand of DNA; the small rectangles are primers and the circles are nucleotides. **B)** The first 3 cycles of PCR are shown schematically. **C)** Ethidium bromide–stained gel after 20 cycles of PCR. See text for further explanation. **D)** Real-time PCR using SYBR™ Green dye. SYBR™ Green dye binds preferentially to double-stranded DNA; therefore, an increase in the concentration of a double-stranded DNA product leads to an increase in fluorescence. During the polymerization step, several molecules of the dye bind to the newly synthesized DNA, and a significant increase in fluorescence is detected and can be monitored in real time. **E)** Real-time PCR using fluorescent dyes and molecular beacons. During denaturation, both probe and primers are in solution and remain unbound from the DNA strand. During annealing, the probe specifically hybridizes to the target DNA between the primers (*top panel*) and the 5'-to-3' exonuclease activity of the DNA polymerase cleaves the probe, thus dissociating the quencher molecule from the reporter molecule, which results in fluorescence of the reporters.

indicate minimal residual disease in hematopoietic malignancies and of circulating tumor DNA from solid tumors.

PCR is used widely to study gene expression and to screen for genetic alterations. Reverse transcriptase is used to make a single-strand cDNA copy of mRNA, and the cDNA is used as a template for a PCR reaction as described above. This technique allows amplification of cDNA corresponding to both abundant and rare RNA transcripts. The development of quantitative PCR techniques to assess species abundance during PCR, as a function of product accumulation (called *real-time qPCR*), has allowed improved quantitation of the DNA (or cDNA) template and is a sensitive method to detect low levels of mRNA (often obtained from small samples or micro-dissected tissues) and to quantify gene expression. Different reagents are available for real-time detection (Fig. 2–6C, D). There is a very specific 5' nuclease assay, which uses a fluorogenic probe for the detection of reaction products after amplification, and there is a less specific but much less expensive assay, which uses a fluorescent dye (SYBR™ Green I) for the detection of double-stranded DNA products. In both methods, the fluorescence emission from each sample is collected by a charge-coupled device camera, and the data are processed automatically and analyzed by computer software. Quantitative real-time PCR using fluorogenic probes can analyze multiple genes simultaneously within the same reaction. The SYBR™ Green methodology involves individual analysis of each gene of interest but, using multiwell plates, both approaches provide high-throughput sample analysis with no need for post-PCR processing or gels.

2.2.6 Fluorescence In Situ Hybridization

To perform FISH, DNA probes specific for a gene or particular chromosome region are labeled by incorporation of biotin, digoxigenin, (fluorochromes are now more commonly employed), and then hybridized to (denatured) metaphase chromosomes. The DNA probe will reanneal to the denatured DNA at its precise location on the chromosome. After washing away the unbound probe, the hybridized sequences are detected using avidin directly (which binds strongly to biotin) via antibodies to digoxigenin that are coupled to fluorescent secondary antibodies, such as fluorescein isothiocyanate, or directly via the coupled fluorophore. The sites of hybridization are then detected using fluorescent microscopy. An advantage of FISH for gene analyses is that information is

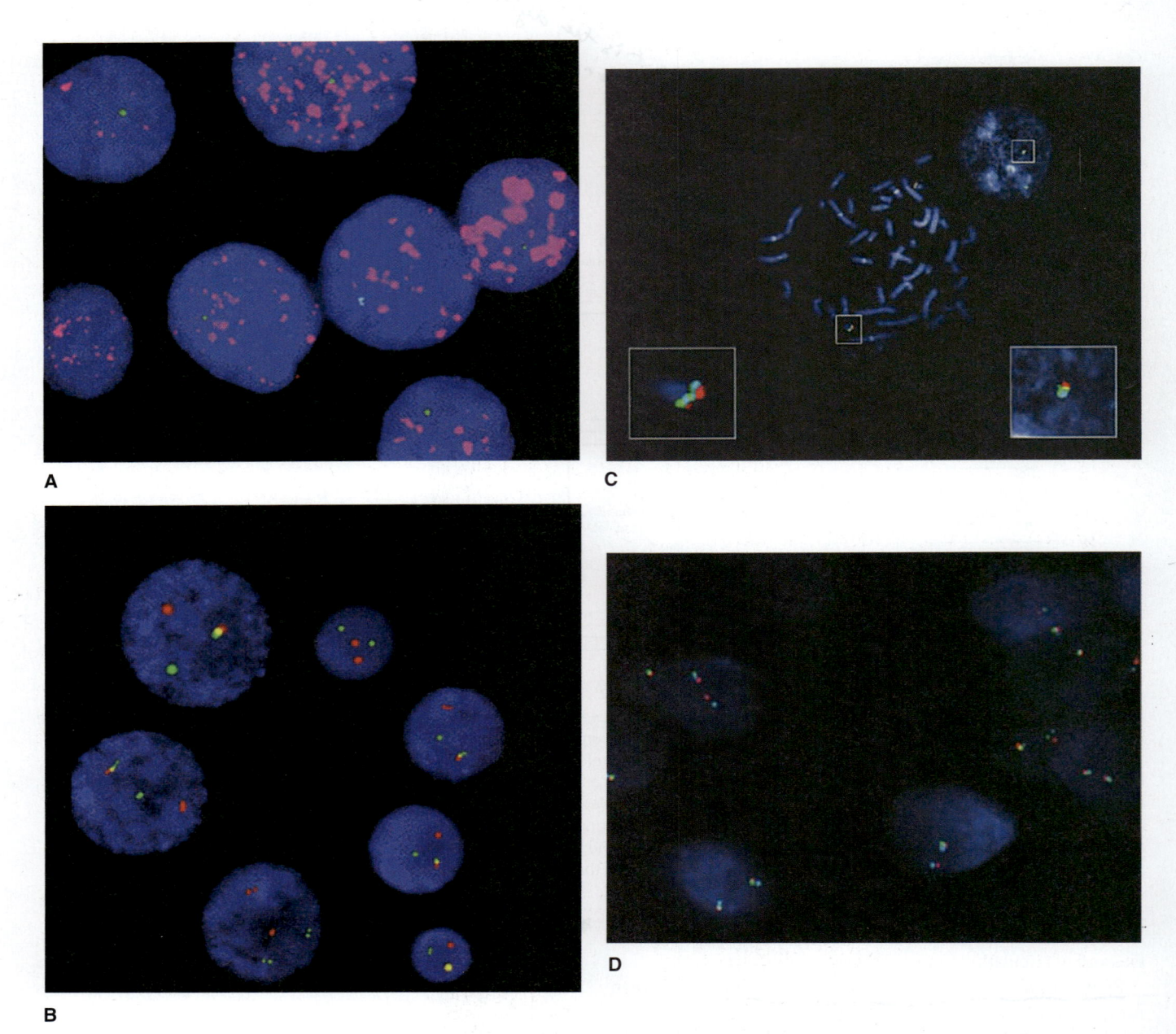

FIGURE 2-7 Fluorescent methods to detect gene amplifications and rearrangements. **A)** MYCN amplification in nuclei from neuroblastoma detected by FISH with an MYCN probe (magenta speckling) and a deletion of the short arm of chromosome 1. The signal (pale blue-green) from the remaining chromosome 1 is seen as a single spot in each nucleus. **B)** Detection of the Philadelphia chromosome in interphase nuclei of leukemia cells. All nuclei contain 1 green signal (BCR gene), 1 pink signal (ABL gene), and an intermediate fusion yellow signal because of the 9:22 chromosome translocation. **C)** FISH analysis showing rearrangement of TMPRS22 and ERG genes in PCa. FISH confirms the colocalization of Oregon Green–labeled 5 V ERG (*green signals*), AlexaFluor 594–labeled 3 V ERG (*red signals*), and Pacific Blue–labeled TMPRSS2 (*light blue signals*) in normal peripheral lymphocyte metaphase cells and in normal interphase cells. **D)** In PCa cells, break-apart FISH results in a split of the colocalized 5 V green/3 V red signals, in addition to a fused signal (comprising green, red and blue signals—which looks white when overlapped) of the unaffected chromosome 21. Using the TRMPSS2/ERG set of probes on PCa frozen sections, TMPRSS2 (blue signal) remains juxtaposed to ERG 3 V (red signal; see white arrows), whereas colocalized 5 V ERG signal (green) is lost, indicating the presence of TRMPSS2/ERG fusion and concomitant deletion of 5 V ERG region. (Reproduced with permission from Yoshimoto M, Joshua AM, Chilton-Macneill S, et al. Three color FISH analysis of TMPRSS2/ERG fusions in prostate cancer indicates that genomic microdeletion of chromosome 21 is associated with rearrangement. *Neoplasia* 2006;8:465–469.)

obtained directly about the positions of the probes in relation to chromosome bands or to other previously or simultaneously mapped reference probes.

FISH can be performed on interphase nuclei from paraffin-embedded tumor biopsies or cultured tumor cells, which allows cytogenetic aberrations such as amplifications, deletions, or other abnormalities of whole chromosomes to be visualized without the need for obtaining good-quality metaphase preparations. For example, FISH is a standard technique to determine the HER2 status of breast cancers and can be used to detect N-*myc* amplification in neuroblastoma (Fig. 2–7A). Whole chromosome abnormalities can also be detected using specific centromere probes that lead to 2 signals from normal nuclei, 1 signal when there is only 1 copy of the chromosome (monosomy), or 3 signals when there is an extra copy (trisomy). Chromosome or gene deletions can also be detected with probes from the relevant regions. For example, if the probes used for FISH are close to specific translocation breakpoints on different chromosomes, they will appear joined as a result of the translocation generating a "color fusion" signal or conversely, alternative probes can be designed to "break apart" in the event of a specific gene deletion or translocation. This technique is particularly useful for the detection of the *bcr-abl* rearrangement in chronic myeloid leukemia (Fig. 2–7B) and the *tmprss2-erg* abnormalities in prostate cancer (Fig. 2–7C, D).

2.2.7 Comparative Genomic Hybridization

If the cytogenetic abnormalities are unknown, it is not possible to select a suitable probe to clarify the abnormalities by FISH. *Comparative genomic hybridization* (CGH) has been developed to produce a detailed map of the differences between chromosomes in different cells by detecting increases (amplifications) or decreases (deletions) of segments of DNA.

For analysis of tumors by CGH, the DNA from malignant and normal cells is labeled with 2 different fluorochromes and then hybridized simultaneously to *normal* chromosome metaphase spreads. For example, tumor DNA is labeled with biotin and detected with fluorescein (green fluorescence) whereas the control DNA is labeled with digoxigenin and detected with rhodamine (red fluorescence). Regions of gain or loss of DNA, such as deletions, duplications, or amplifications, are seen as changes in the ratio of the intensities of the 2 fluorochromes along the target chromosomes. One disadvantage of CGH is that it can detect only large blocks (>5 Mb) of over- or under-represented chromosomal DNA, while balanced rearrangements (such as inversions or translocations) can escape detection. High-density single-nucleotide polymorphism (SNP) arrays can overcome some of these problems (see Sec. 2.2.9).

2.2.8 Spectral Karyotyping/Multifluor–Fluorescence in Situ Hybridization

A deficiency of both array CGH and conventional cDNA microarrays is the lack of information about structural changes within the karyotype. For example, with an expression array, a particular gene may be overexpressed but it would be unclear whether this is secondary to a translocation placing the gene next to a strong promoter or an amplification. Universal chromosome painting techniques make it possible to analyze all chromosomes simultaneously. Two commonly used techniques, spectral karyotyping (SKY) (Veldman et al, 1997) and multifluor–fluorescence in situ hybridization (M-FISH) (Speicher et al, 1996), are based on the differential display of colored fluorescent chromosome-specific paints, which provide a complete analysis of the chromosomal complement in a given cell. Using a combination of 23 different colored paints as a "cocktail probe," subtle differences in fluorochrome labeling of chromosomes after hybridization allow a computer to assign a unique color to each chromosome pair. Abnormal chromosomes can be identified by the pattern of color distribution along them, with chromosomal rearrangements leading to a transition from one color to another at the position of the breakpoint (Fig. 2–8). In contrast to CGH, detection of such karyotype rearrangements using SKY and M-FISH is not dependent on change in copy number. This technology is particularly suited to solid tumors, where the complexity of the karyotypes may mask the presence of chromosomal aberrations.

2.2.9 Single-Nucleotide Polymorphisms

DNA sequences can differ at single-nucleotide positions within the genome. These SNPs can occur as frequently as 1 in

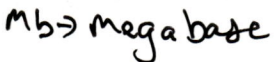

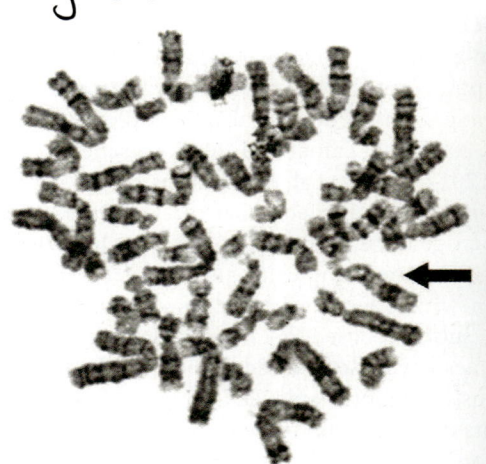

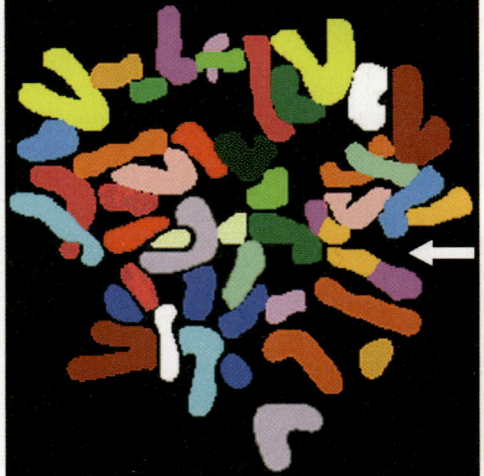

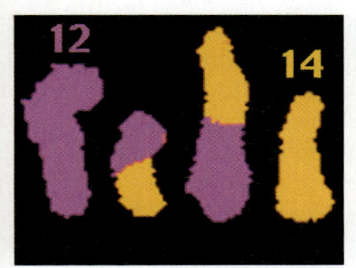

FIGURE 2–8 SKY and downstream analyses of a patient with a translocation. One of the aberrant chromosomes can initially be seen with G banding, the same metaphase spread has been subjected to SKY and then a 12;14 reciprocal translocation is identified.

every 1000 base pairs and can occur in both introns and exons. If these events occur in exons, they can influence protein structure and function. For example, SNPs may be involved in altered drug metabolism because of their modifying effect on the cytochrome P450 metabolizing enzymes. They also contribute to disease (eg, SNPs that result in missense mutations) and disease predisposition. Most early methods to characterize SNPs required PCR amplification of the sample prior to sequence analysis, but modern methods of gene sequencing and array analyses have largely replaced this older technique. Probes to some of the 50 million SNPs in the human genome can be used with DNA microarrays to interrogate genomic architecture. For example, SNP arrays can be used to study loss of heterozygosity (LOH) and amplifications. An advantage of SNP arrays is that they can detect copy-neutral LOH (also known as uniparental disomy or gene conversion) whereby one allele or whole chromosome is missing and the other allele is duplicated.

2.2.10 Sequencing of DNA

To characterize the primary structure of genes, and thus of the proteins that they encode, it is necessary to determine the sequence of their DNA. Sanger sequencing (the classical method) relied on oligonucleotide primer extension and dideoxy-chain termination (dideoxynucleotides [ddNTPs] lack the 3′-OH group required for the phosphodiester bond between 2 nucleosides). DNA sequencing was carried out in 4 separate reactions each containing 1 of the 4 ddNTPs (ie, ddATP, ddCTP, ddGTP, or ddTTP) together with dNTPs. In each reaction, the same primer was used to ensure DNA synthesis began at the same nucleotide. The extended primers terminated at different sites whenever a specific ddNTP was incorporated: the method produced fragments of different sizes terminating at different 3′ nucleotides. The newly synthesized and labeled DNA fragments were heat-denatured, and then separated by size with gel electrophoresis and with each of the 4 reactions in individual adjacent lanes (lanes A, T, G, C); the DNA bands were then visualized by autoradiography or UV light, and the DNA sequence could be directly interpreted from the x-ray film or gel image. Using this method, it was possible to obtain a sequence of 200 to 500 bases in length from a single gel. The next development was automated Sanger sequencing, which involved the development of primers and ddNTP terminators each labeled with a different fluorescent dye. The reactions are performed in a single tube containing all 4 ddNTPs, and a laser then reads the gel to determine the identity of each band according to the wavelengths at which it fluoresces. The results are then depicted in the form of a chromatogram, which is a diagram of colored peaks that correspond to the nucleotide in that location in the sequence. Then sequencing analysis software interprets the results, identifying the bases from the fluorescent intensities (Fig. 2–9).

Next-generation sequencing (NGS) automates the sequencing process by creating micro-PCR reactors and/or by attaching the DNA molecules to be sequenced to solid surfaces or beads, allowing for millions of sequencing events to occur simultaneously. Although the analyzed sequences are generally shorter (~21–400 base pairs) than in previous sequencing technologies, they can be counted and quantified, allowing the identification of mutations in a small subpopulation of cells that is part of a larger population with wild-type sequences. The recent introduction of approaches that allow for sequencing of both ends of a DNA molecule (ie, paired-end massively parallel sequencing or mate-pair sequencing), make it possible to detect balanced and unbalanced somatic rearrangements (eg, fusion genes) in a genome-wide fashion.

There are several methods used for NGS. Each technology involves (1) template preparation, (2) sequencing/imaging, and (3) data analysis. Initially, all methods involve breaking genomic DNA randomly into small sizes from which either fragment templates (randomly sheared DNA usually <1 kbp in size) or mate-pair templates (linear DNA fragments originating from circularized sheared DNA of a particular size) are created. These methods have, until recently, used short sequence reads. There are at least 10 methodologies that employ short-read NGS, including massively parallel signature sequencing (MPSS), Polony sequencing, 454 pyrosequencing, and Illumina (Solexa) sequencing, among others (Fig. 2–10A–C). More recently, these techniques are being supplanted by long-read sequencing methods, which overcomes many of the limitations in completeness and accuracy of genome assembly that was encountered with short-read NGS methods (Alkan et al, 2011; Midha et al, 2019). An example of a long-read NGS method is shown in Figure 2–10, D. As one example, the Oxford NanoPore sequencing platform has been gaining appeal for its rapid sequencing capability, long read length, and portability for near–real time analyses (Ip et al, 2015; Loman et al, 2015; Quick et al, 2016; Faria et al, 2017).

The ability to sequence large amounts of DNA at low cost makes the NGS platforms useful for many applications such as discovery of variant alleles, de novo assembly of bacterial and lower eukaryotic genomes, cataloguing the mRNAs ("transcriptomes") present in cells, tissues, and organisms (RNA sequencing), and gene discovery. These techniques have also been applied to most major tumor types to identify recurrent point mutations, copy number aberrations and genomic rearrangements (Puente et al, 2015; Bailey et al, 2016; Fujimoto et al, 2016; Nik-Zainal et al, 2016; Fraser et al, 2017; Hayward et al, 2017; Scarpa et al, 2017) (https://www.genome.gov/Funded-Programs-Projects/Cancer-Genome-Atlas). In cancers, pan-genome sequencing analysis has yielded major insights into the complexity and diversity of cancer genomes, even within what was traditionally viewed as a single cancer subtype based on histopathologic analysis. These techniques have also allowed an unprecedented view of the previously unappreciated DNA recombination and rearrangements that underpin these genomic abnormalities, including chromothripsis, whereby many clusters of chromosomal rearrangements can be clustered in a single rearrangement event, or kataegis, a more commonly seen pattern

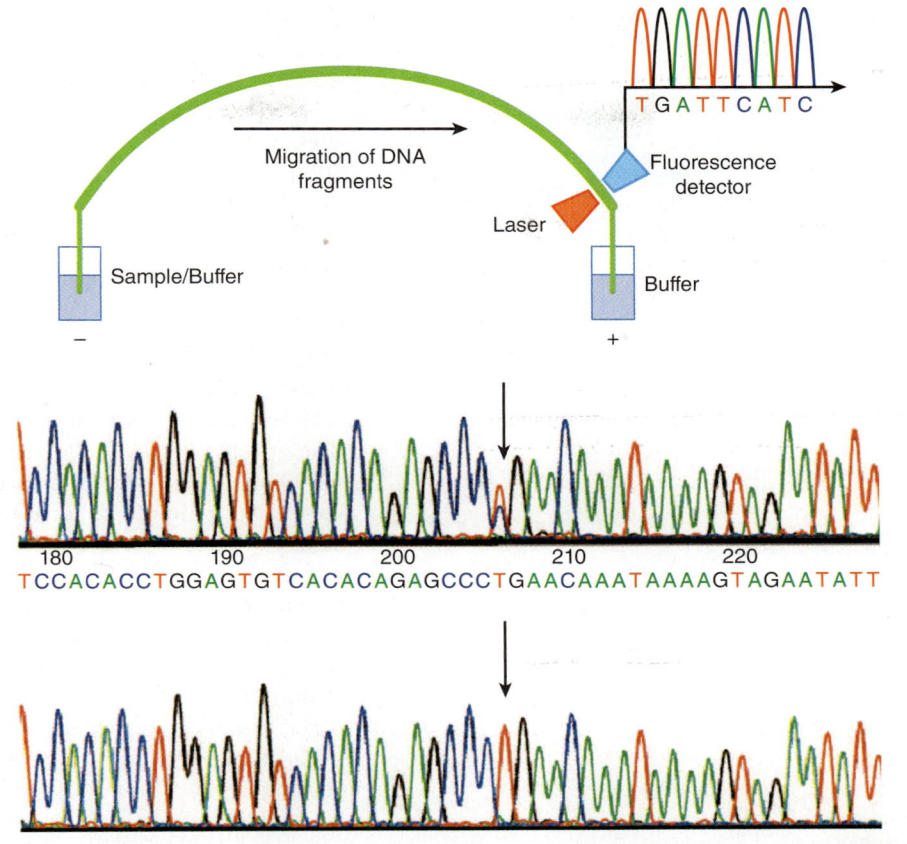

FIGURE 2–9 Outline of automated sequencing and thereafter automated sequencing of *BRCA2*, the hereditary breast cancer predisposition gene. Each colored peak represents a different nucleotide. The lower panel is the sequence of the wild-type DNA sample. The sequence of the mutation carrier in the upper panel contains a double peak (indicated by an *arrow*) in which nucleotide T in intron 17 located 2 bp downstream of the 5′-end of exon 18 is converted to a C. The mutation results in aberrant splicing of exon 18 of the *BRCA2* gene. The presence of the T nucleotide, in addition to the mutant C, implies that only 1 copy of the 2 *BRCA2* genes is mutated in this sample.

of hypermutations that occur within a small genomic region (Cieslik and Chinnaiyan, 2020).

In the analysis of DNA sequencing, the raw data are typically in a file format called a fastq file. Algorithms that align multiple input fastq files usually store these data in a binary format called a bam file. There are several tools used for alignment, and most exploit an algorithm called the Burrows-Wheeler transform, with the algorithm BWA being the most widely used in large-scale consortia (Li and Durbin, 2009). The alignment process identifies the best match within the genome for each read—in some cases, there is no good match and in others, multiple matches to repetitive regions of the genome for a single read. This process allows identification of the full set of reads that cover each base of the genome, and is repeated for both the tumor and a normal tissue reference. Then, different variant-detection algorithms are executed to identify specific mutation types. For identifying somatic mutations, the set of reads covering a base in the tumor and in the normal reference are compared. Changes in this distribution can correspond to either a loss of heterozygosity or a somatic point mutation. Similarly, the number of reads covering an individual base in the genome can be used to identify copy number changes through depth-of-coverage analysis. There are many algorithms available to perform somatic variant detection, and several large-scale benchmarks of them have been developed to identify best practices (Boutros et al, 2014; Ewing et al, 2015; Cai et al, 2016; Bohnert et al, 2017).

2.2.11 Variation in Copy Number and Gene Sequence

Genome-wide analysis applied to human genomes has led to the discovery of extensive structural variation, ranging from kilobase pairs to megabase pairs (Mbp) in size, that are not identifiable by conventional chromosomal banding. These changes are termed copy-number variations (CNVs) and can result from deletions, duplications, triplications, insertions, and translocations; they may account for up to 13% of the human genome and may reflect as much genetic diversity as do single-nucleotide changes (Redon et al, 2006; Sudmant et al, 2015) (Fig. 2–11).

NGS technologies have allowed new insights into the total number, position, size, gene content, and population distribution of CNVs in normal and cancer genomes. There are several

16 CHAPTER 2

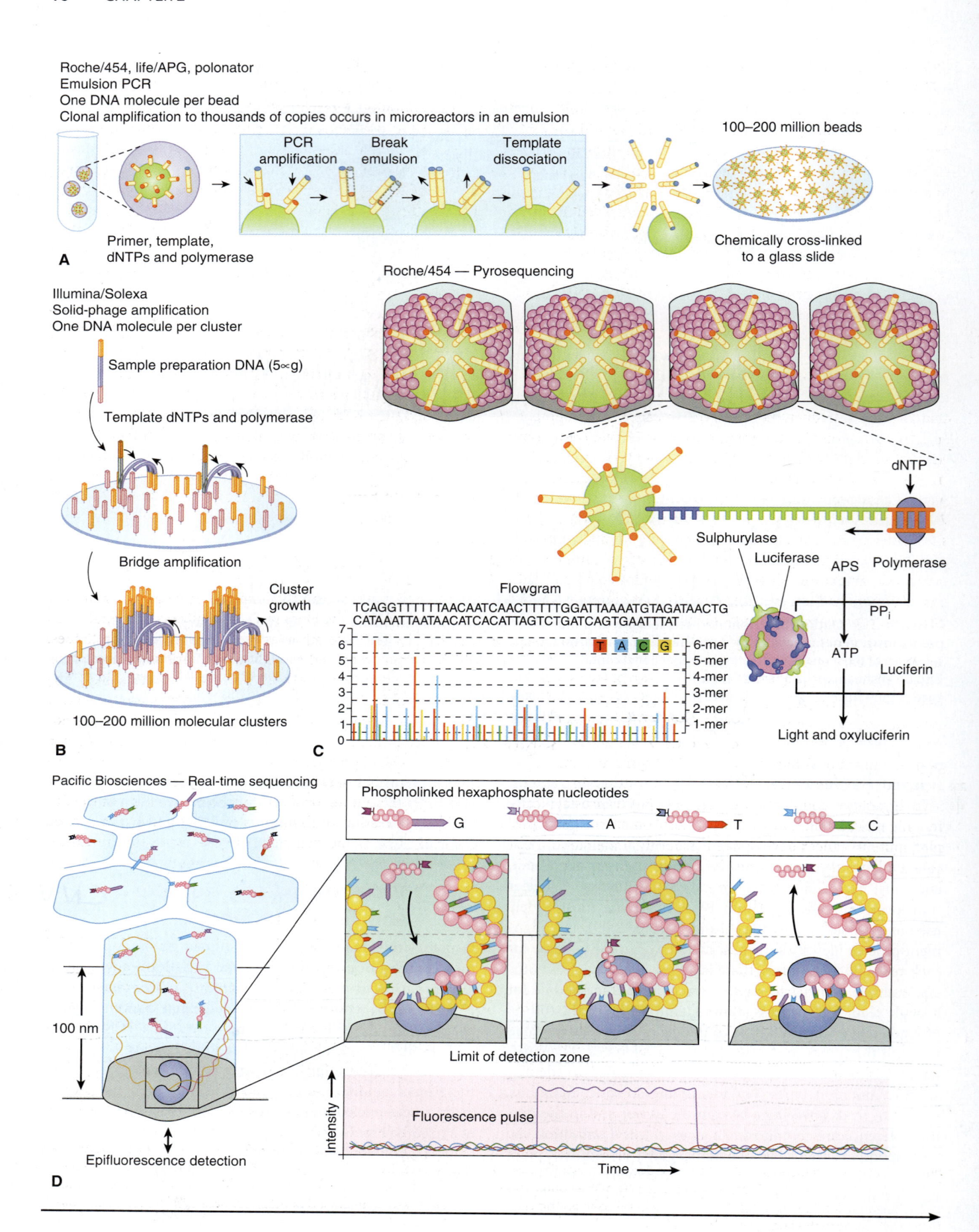

Roche/454, life/APG, polonator
Emulsion PCR
One DNA molecule per bead
Clonal amplification to thousands of copies occurs in microreactors in an emulsion

PCR amplification | Break emulsion | Template dissociation

100–200 million beads

Primer, template, dNTPs and polymerase

Chemically cross-linked to a glass slide

A

Illumina/Solexa
Solid-phage amplification
One DNA molecule per cluster

Sample preparation DNA (5∝g)

Template dNTPs and polymerase

Bridge amplification

Cluster growth

100–200 million molecular clusters

B

Roche/454 — Pyrosequencing

dNTP
Sulphurylase
Luciferase
APS
Polymerase
PP$_i$
ATP
Luciferin
Light and oxyluciferin

Flowgram
TCAGGTTTTTTAACAATCAACTTTTTGGATTAAAATGTAGATAACTG
CATAAATTAATAACATCACATTAGTCTGATCAGTGAATTTAT

T A C G
6-mer
5-mer
4-mer
3-mer
2-mer
1-mer

C

Pacific Biosciences — Real-time sequencing

Phospholinked hexaphosphate nucleotides
G   A   T   C

100 nm

Limit of detection zone

Epifluorescence detection

Intensity
Fluorescence pulse
Time

D

different classes of CNVs. Entire genes or genomic regions can undergo duplication, deletion, and insertion events, whereas multisite variants (MSVs) are more complex genomic rearrangements, including concurrent CNVs and mutation or gene conversions (a process by which DNA sequence information is transferred from one DNA helix, which remains unchanged, to another DNA helix, whose sequence is altered). CNVs can be inherited or sporadic; both types may be involved in causing disease, including cancer. However, the phenotypic effects of CNVs are unclear and depend on whether genes transcribed into proteins or regulatory sequences are influenced by the genomic rearrangement. It is clear, however, that CNVs are a distinguishing feature of all human genomes. One study that genotyped 873 volunteers in Canada showed an average of 81 CNVs per person (71,178 in total), many of which had been previously undescribed (Uddin et al, 2015).

High-resolution SNP arrays in cancer genomes have shown that CNVs are frequent contributors to cancer development. In adenocarcinoma of the lung, a total of 57 recurrent copy number changes were detected in 528 cases (Weir et al, 2007). In 206 cases of glioblastoma, somatic copy number alterations were also frequent, and gene expression analysis showed that 76% of genes affected by copy number alteration had expression patterns that correlated with gene copy number (Cerami et al, 2010). High-resolution analyses of copy number and nucleotide alterations showed that individual colorectal and breast tumors had, on average, 7 and 18 copy number alterations, respectively, with 24 and 9 as the average number of protein-coding genes affected by amplification or homozygous deletions (Leary et al, 2008).

Heritable germline CNVs may also contribute to cancer. For example, a heritable CNV at chromosome 1q21.1 contains the NBPF23 gene, for which copy number is implicated in the development of neuroblastoma (Diskin et al, 2009). Also, a germline deletion at chromosome 2p24.3 is more common in men with prostate cancer, with higher prevalence in patients with aggressive compared with nonaggressive prostate cancer (Liu et al, 2009). How CNVs, either somatic or germline, contribute to cancer development is poorly understood. Possible explanations come from the Knudson's 2-hit hypothesis (Knudson, 1971): tumor-suppressor genes can be lost as a consequence of a homozygous deletion leading directly to cancer susceptibility. Alternatively, heterozygous deletions may harbor genes predisposing to cancer that become unmasked when a functional mutation arises in the other chromosome resulting in tumor development. Rare tumor-suppressor genes can be altered by homozygous deletion (Cheng et al, 2017) and the pan-cancer landscape of somatic gains and losses is being cataloged by large consortia (Zack et al, 2013). Duplications or gains of chromosomal regions may result in increased expression levels of 1 or more oncogenes. Germline CNVs can provide a genetic basis for subsequent somatic chromosomal changes that arise in tumor DNA. For example, a recently developed database that reports on genome-wide CNV in cancer genomes shows that CNVs associated with cancer can have large cis-associated regions of genomic diversity, or these boundaries can be very narrowly defined, for example, surrounding the MYCN locus (Dalgleish et al, 2019). In neuroblastomas, up to 25% of patients have amplified MYCN, and these patients exhibit a poorer prognosis. Our emerging understanding of CNVs within normal and cancer genomes will no doubt have major impacts on our ability to identify, classify, and treat cancer.

2.2.12 Microarrays and RNA Analysis

Microarray analysis evaluates expression of genes, including those identified by the Human Genome Project. Several commercial kits facilitate RNA extraction from cells or tissues, which is then converted to cDNA with reverse transcriptase; this may be combined with an RNA amplification step. The principle of an expression array involves the production of DNA arrays or "chips" on solid supports for large-scale hybridization experiments. It consists of thousands of microscopic spots of DNA oligonucleotides, called *features*, each containing specific DNA sequences, known as *probes* (or *reporters*). This approach allows for the simultaneous analysis of the differential expression of thousands of genes and has enhanced understanding of the dynamics of gene expression in cancer cells (Fig. 2–12).

FIGURE 2–10 Examples of next-generation sequencing (NGS) methods. **A)** In emulsion PCR (emPCR), a reaction mixture is generated compromising an oil-aqueous emulsion to encapsulate bead-DNA complexes into single aqueous droplets. PCR amplification is subsequently carried out in these droplets to create beads containing thousands of copies of the same template sequence. EmPCR beads can then be chemically attached to a glass slide or a reaction plate (From Metzker, 2010). **B)** The 2 basic steps of solid-phase amplification are initial priming and extending of the single-stranded, single-molecule template, and then bridge amplification of the immobilized template with immediately adjacent primers to form clusters (From Metzker, 2010). **C)** Pyrosequencing. After loading of the DNA-amplified beads into individual PicoTiterPlate (PTP) wells, additional beads, coupled with sulfurylase and luciferase, are added. The fiberoptic slide is mounted in a flow chamber, enabling the delivery of sequencing reagents to the bead-packed wells. The underneath of the fiberoptic slide is directly attached to a high-resolution camera, which allows detection of the light generated from each PTP well undergoing the pyrosequencing reaction. The light generated by the enzymatic cascade is recorded and is known as a flow gram. *PP*, inorganic pyrophosphate (From Metzker, 2010). **D)** Pacific Biosciences' 4-color real-time sequencing method. The zero-mode waveguide (ZMW) design reduces the observation volume, therefore reducing the number of stray fluorescently labeled molecules that enter the detection layer for a given period. The residence time of phospholinked nucleotides in the active site is governed by the rate of catalysis and is usually milliseconds. This corresponds to a recorded fluorescence pulse, because only the bound, dye-labeled nucleotide occupies the ZMW detection zone on this time scale. The released, dye-labeled pentaphosphate by-product quickly diffuses away, as does the fluorescence signal.

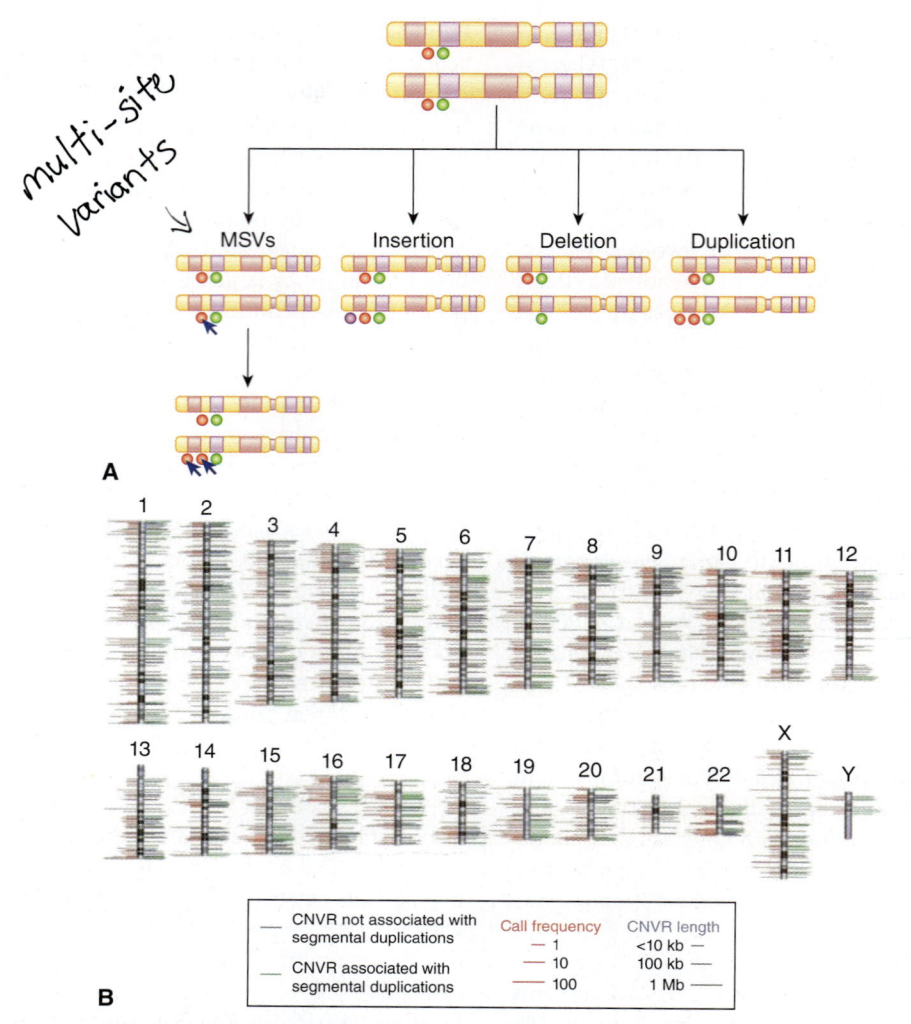

FIGURE 2–11 A) Outline of the classes of CNVs in the human genome. B) The chromosomal locations of 1447 copy number variation regions (a region covered by overlapping CNVs) are indicated by lines to either side of the ideograms. Green lines denote CNVRs associated with segmental duplications; blue lines denote CNVRs not associated with segmental duplications. The length of right-hand side lines represents the size of each CNVR. The length of left-hand side lines indicates the frequency with which a CNVR is detected (minor call frequency among 270 HapMap samples). When both platforms identify a CNVR, the maximum call frequency of the two is shown. For clarity, the dynamic range of length and frequency are log transformed (see scale bars). (Reproduced with permission from Redon R, Ishikawa S, Fitch KR, et al. Global variation in copy number in the human genome. *Nature* 2006 Nov 23;444(7118):444-454.)

Microarray platforms include (1) Spotted arrays where DNA fragments (usually created by PCR) or oligonucleotides are immobilized on glass slides. The size of the fragment can be any length (usually 500 bp to 1 kbp), and the size of the oligonucleotides range from 20 to 100 nucleotides. These arrays can be created in individual laboratories using "affordable" equipment. (2) Affymetrix arrays, where the probes are synthesized using a light mask technology and are typically small (20–25 bp) oligonucleotides. (3) NimbleGen, the maskless array synthesizer technology that uses 786,000 tiny aluminum mirrors to direct light in specific patterns. Photo deposition chemistry allows single-nucleotide extensions with 380,000 or 2.1 million oligonucleotides/array as the light directs base pairing in specific sequences. (4) Agilent, which uses ink-jet printer technology to extend up to 60-mer bases through phosphoramidite chemistry. The capacity is 244,000 oligonucleotides/array. There are now a number of web-based resources that describe in detail how microarray data is analyzed, for example: https://www.biointeractive.org/classroom-resources/how-analyze-dna-microarray-data.

All the sequencing approaches described in Section 2.2.10 can be applied to RNA, in some cases by converting the RNA to cDNA before analysis. This approach, known as RNA-seq or whole transcriptome sequencing, is used increasingly. The technique has advantages when compared to expression microarrays in that it obviates the requirement for preexisting sequence information in order to detect and evaluate transcripts, including intron/exon boundaries and other unusual transcripts; for example, it can be used to characterize fusion transcripts that arise from genomic rearrangements. The technique has been applied to RNA populations other than mRNA, such as total RNA, tRNA, rRNA, microRNAs (miRNAs), and other long noncoding RNAs (lncRNAs) (Wang et al, 2009). This method has also been applied to single cells, called scRNA-seq.

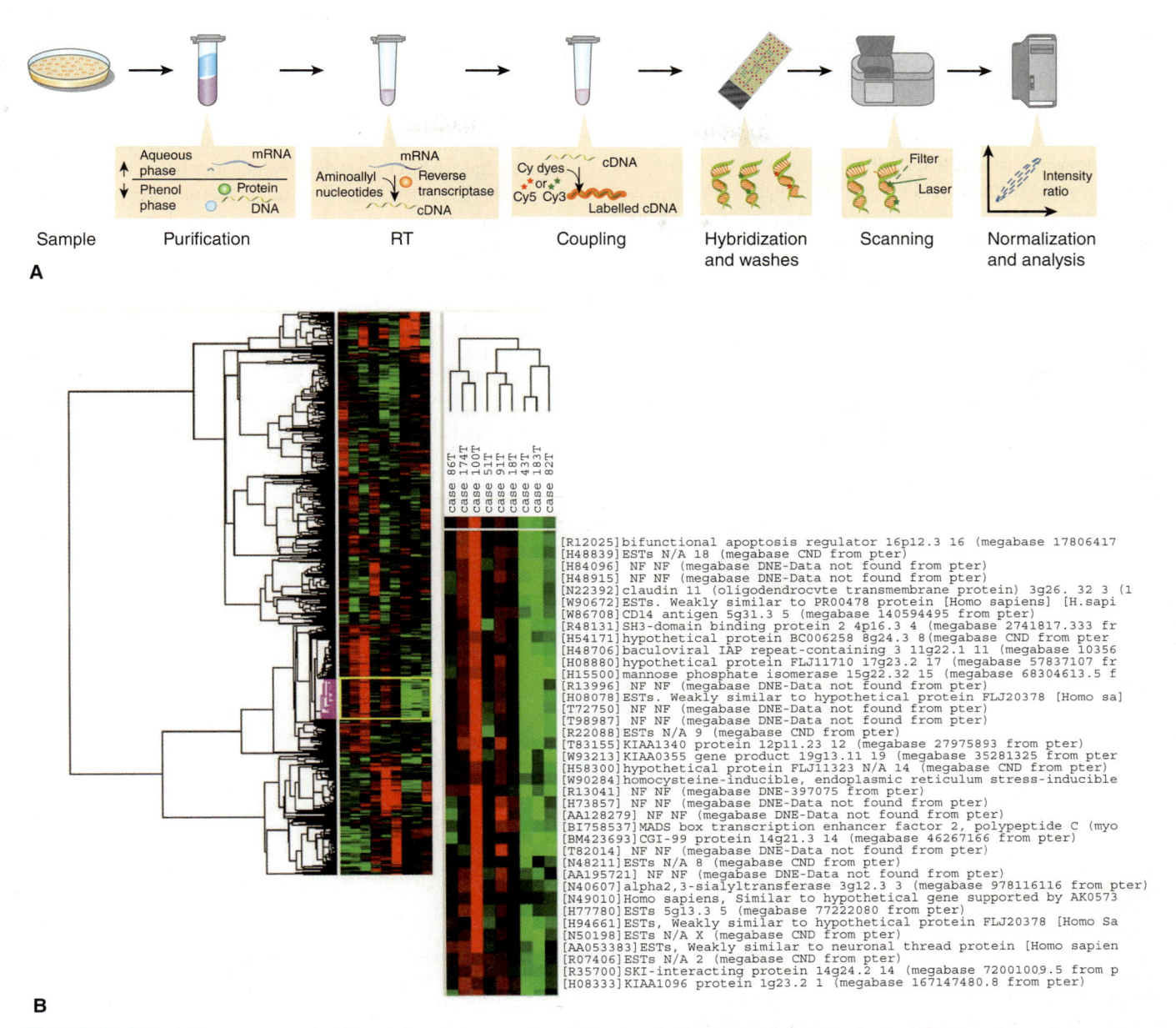

FIGURE 2-12 A) The steps required in a microarray experiment from sample preparation to analyses. *RT*, Reverse transcriptase. For details, see text. Briefly, samples are prepared and cDNA is created through reverse transcriptase. The fluorescent label is added either in the RT step or in an additional step after amplification, if present. The labeled samples are then mixed with a hybridization solution that contains light detergents, blocking agents (such as COT1 DNA, salmon sperm DNA, calf thymus DNA, PolyA or PolyT), along with other stabilizers. The mix is denatured and added to a pinhole in a microarray, which can be a gene chip (holes in the back) or a glass microarray. The holes are sealed and the microarray hybridized, either in a hybridization oven (mixed by rotation) or in a mixer (mixed by alternating pressure at the pinholes). After an overnight hybridization, all nonspecific binding is washed off. The microarray is dried and scanned in a special machine where a laser excites the dye and a detector measures its emission. The intensities of the features (several pixels make a feature) are quantified and normalized (see text). **B)** The output from a typical microarray experiment, a hierarchical clustering of cDNA microarray data obtained from 9 primary laryngeal tumors. Results were visualized using Tree View software, and include the dendrogram (clustering of samples) and the clustering of gene expression, based on genomic similarity. Tree View represents the 946 genes that best distinguish these 2 groups of samples. Genes whose expression is higher in the tumor sample relative to the reference sample are shown in red; those whose expression is lower than the reference sample are shown in green; and no change in gene expression is shown in black. (A) Reproduced with permission from Jacopo Werther/Wikimedia Common.; B) Used with permission from Patricia Reis and Shilpi Arora, the Ontario Cancer Institute and Princess Margaret Hospital, Toronto.)

Although the depth of coverage per cell is necessarily limited, larger patterns in tissue-specific or tumor-specific subtypes emerge after clustering analyses such as nearest-neighbor clustering or other types of unsupervised clustering (eg, Kiselev et al, 2019; see also Sec. 2.6). These methods have limitations, but when combined with other DNA sequencing data, they have helped to uncover fetal transcriptional programs that are retained in pediatric cerebellar tumors, and heterogeneity in tumors from a single patient, for example, in pediatric glioblastoma (Hoffman et al, 2019; Vladoiu et al, 2019).

2.2.13 Technologies for Studying Epigenetic Changes

Epigenetics relates to heritable changes in gene expression that are not encoded in the genome. These processes are mediated by the covalent attachment of chemical groups (eg, methyl or acetyl groups) to DNA and associated proteins, histones, and chromatin (Fig. 2–13). Examples of epigenetic effects include imprinting, gene silencing, X chromosome inactivation, position effect, reprogramming, and regulation of histone modifications and heterochromatin.

In general, cancer cells exhibit generalized, genome-wide hypomethylation and local hypermethylation of CpG islands associated with promoters (Novak, 2004). Hundreds to thousands of genes can be epigenetically silenced by DNA methylation during carcinogenesis. Epigenetic modifier drugs are in clinical use (Bates, 2020). Additionally, because tumor-derived DNA is present in various, easily accessible body fluids, tumor-specific epigenetic modifications could prove to be useful biomarkers for cancer prediction or prognosis (Woodson et al, 2008). Although the principles of epigenetics will be covered in a separate chapter (see Chap. 3), we will briefly outline techniques employed in the study of epigenetics below.

Epigenetic research uses a range of techniques to determine DNA–protein interactions, including chromatin immunoprecipitation (ChIP) (together with ChIP-on-chip and ChIP-seq), histone-specific antibodies, methylation-sensitive restriction enzymes, and bisulfite sequencing. Here, we focus on approaches for studying DNA methylation (Table 2–3). Sodium bisulfite converts unmethylated cytosines to uracil, whereas methylated cytosines (mC) remain unchanged (Fig. 2–14). This technique can reveal the methylation status of every cytosine residue, and it is amenable to massively parallel sequencing methods. Affinity-based methods using

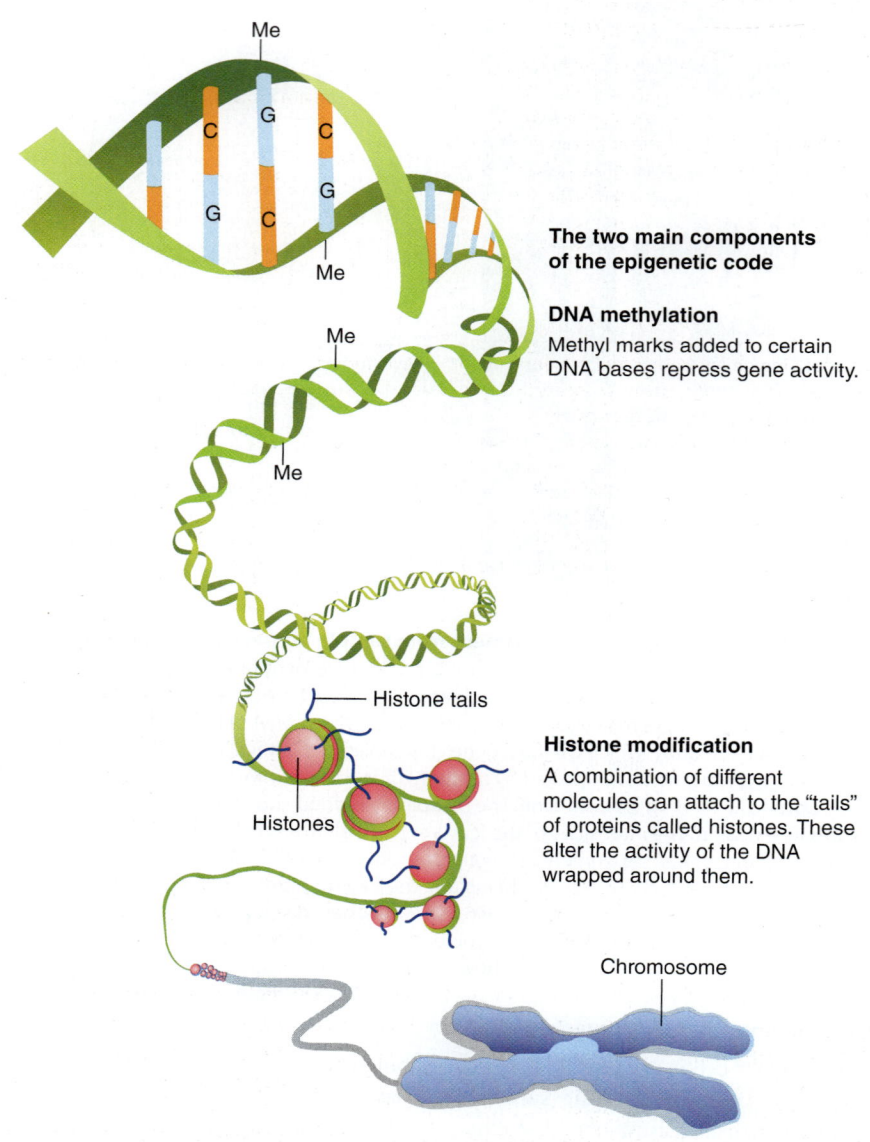

FIGURE 2–13 **An overview of the major epigenetic mechanisms that affect gene expression.** In addition, there are a number of varieties of histone modifications that are associated with alterations in gene expression or characteristic states, such as stem cells.

TABLE 2–3 Methods for analyzing DNA methylation.

Method	Description	Advantages	Disadvantages
Sodium bisulfite conversion	Treatment of denatured DNA (ie, single-stranded DNA) with sodium bisulfite leads to deamination of unmethylated cytosine residues to uracil, leaving 5-mC intact. The uracils are amplified as thymines, and 5-mC residues are amplified as cytosines in PCRs. Comparison of sequence information between the reference genome and bisulfite-treated DNA can provide single-nucleotide resolution information about cytosine methylation patterns.	Resolution at the nucleotide level Works on 5- methylated cytosines (mC)-containing DNA Automated analysis	Requires micrograms of DNA input Harsh chemical treatment of DNA can lead to its damage Potentially incomplete conversion of DNA Cannot distinguish 5-mC and 5-hmC Multistep protocol
Sequence-specific enzyme digestion	Restriction enzymes are used to generate DNA fragments for methylation analysis. Some restriction enzymes are methylation-sensitive (ie, digestion is impaired or blocked by methylated DNA). When used in conjunction with an isoschizomer that has the same recognition site but is methylation insensitive, information about methylation status can be obtained. Additionally, the use of methylation-dependent restriction enzymes (ie, requires methylated DNA for cleavage to occur) can be used to fragment DNA for sequencing analysis.	High enzyme turnover Well-studied Easy to use Availability of recombinant enzymes	Determination of methylation status is limited by the enzyme recognition site Overnight protocols Lower throughput
Methylated DNA	Fragmented genomic DNA (restriction enzyme digestion or sonication) is denatured and immunoprecipitated with antibodies specific for 5-mC. The enriched DNA fragments can be analyzed by PCR for locus-specific studies or by microarrays (MeDIP-chip) and massively parallel sequencing (MeDIP-seq) for whole genome studies.	Relatively fast Compatible with array-based analysis Applicable for high-throughput sequencing	Dependent on antibody specificity May require more than one 5-mC for antibody binding Requires DNA denaturation Resolution depends on the size of the immunoprecipitated DNA and for microarray experiments, depends on probe design Data from repeat sequences may be overrepresented
Methylated DNA-binding proteins	Instead of relying on antibodies for DNA enrichment, affinity-based assays use proteins that specifically bind methylated or unmethylated CpG sites in fragmented genomic DNA (restriction enzyme digestion or sonication). The enriched DNA fragments can be analyzed by PCR for locus-specific studies or by microarrays and massively parallel sequencing for whole genome studies.	Well-studied Does not require denaturation Compatible with array-based analysis Applicable for high-throughput sequencing	May require high DNA input May require a long protocol Requires salt elutions Does not give single-base methylation resolution data

Original DNA with methylated C^{m}pG ▶ G T T G C^m G C T C A C T G C C

DNA sequencing after CT conversion ▶ G T T G C G T T T A T T G T T

Positions: 1 2 3 4 5 6 7 8 9 10 11 12 13 14 15

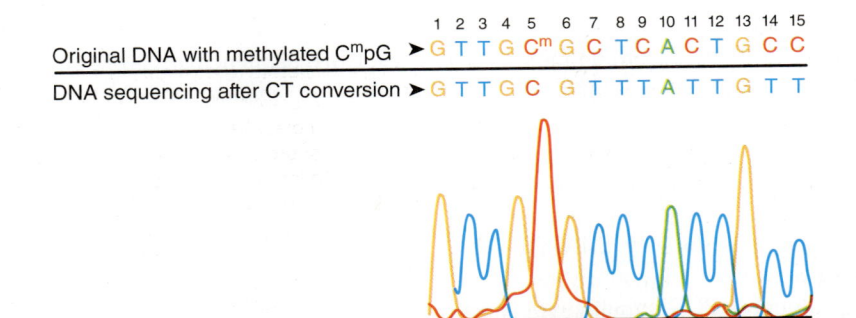

FIGURE 2–14 The most commonly used technique is sodium bisulfite conversion, the gold standard for methylation analysis. Incubation of the target DNA with sodium bisulfite results in conversion of all unmodified cytosines to uracils leaving the modified bases 5-methylcytosine or 5-hydroxymethylcytosine (5-mC or 5-hmC) intact. The most critical step in methylation analysis using bisulfite conversion is the complete conversion of unmodified cytosines. Generally, this is achieved by alternating cycles of thermal denaturation with incubation reactions. In this example, the DNA with methylated CpG at nucleotide position 5 was processed using a commercial kit. The recovered DNA was amplified by PCR and then sequenced directly. The methylated cytosine at position 5 remained intact, whereas the unmethylated cytosines at positions 7, 9, 11, 14, and 15 were completely converted into uracil following bisulfite treatment and detected as thymine following PCR.

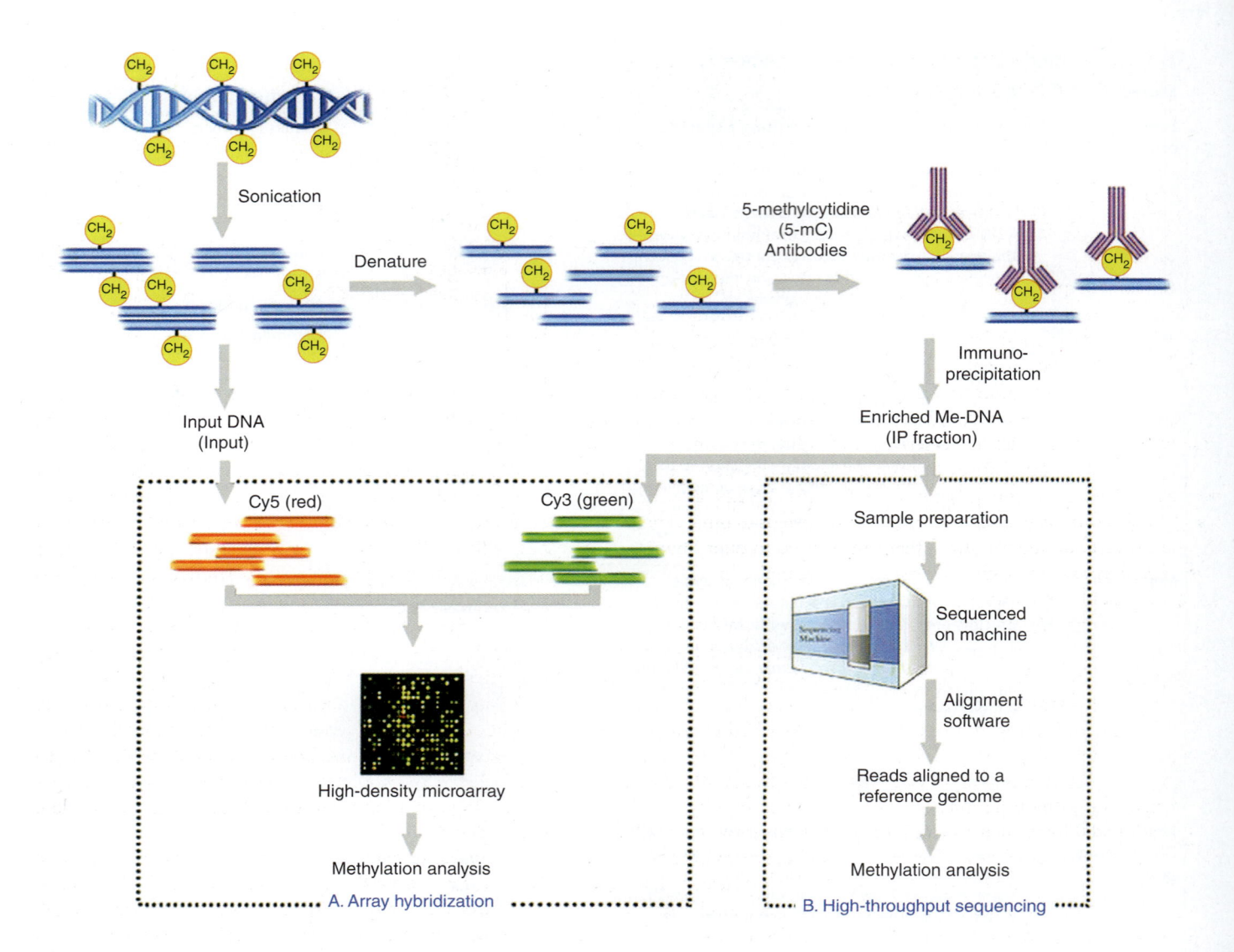

FIGURE 2-15 Schematic outline of MeDIP. Genomic DNA is sheared into approximately 400 to 700 bp using sonication and subsequently denatured. Incubation in 5-mC antibodies, along with standard immunoprecipitation (IP), enriches for fragments that are methylated (IP fraction). This IP fraction can become the input sample to 1 of 2 DNA detection methods: array hybridization using high-density microarrays (**A**) or high-throughput sequencing using the latest in sequencing technology (**B**). Output from these methods are then analyzed for methylation patterns to answer the biologic question. (Reproduced with permission from http://en.wikipedia.org/wiki/Methylated_DNA_immunoprecipitation.)

methyl-specific antibodies (MeDIP) are becoming more popular for whole-genome analyses as methyl-specific antibodies improve in sensitivity and specificity.

Analytical and enzymatic methods can be used to characterize isolated genomic DNA. High-performance liquid chromatography (HPLC) and matrix-assisted laser desorption/ionization–time of flight mass spectrometry (MALDI-TOF MS; see also Sec. 2.5) have been used to quantify modified bases in complex DNAs. Although HPLC is highly reproducible, it requires large amounts of DNA and is often unsuitable for high-throughput applications. In contrast, MALDI-TOF MS provides relative quantification and is amenable to high-throughput applications.

Other methods to detect methylation include real-time PCR, blotting, microarrays (eg, ChIP on chip), and sequencing (eg, ChIP-Sequencing [ChIP-Seq]). ChIP-Seq combines ChIP with massively parallel DNA sequencing to identify the binding sequences for proteins of interest. Both ChIP techniques require an antibody that recognizes an epigenetic modification of interest that is then used to "pull down" the associated DNA via crosslinking so it can be analyzed. Previously, ChIP-on-chip was the most common technique used to study protein-DNA relations. This technique also uses ChIP initially, but the selected DNA fragments are ultimately released ("reverse crosslinked") and the DNA is purified. After an amplification and denaturation step, the single-stranded DNA fragments are identified by labeling with a fluorescent tag such as Cy5 or Alexa 647 and poured over the surface of a DNA microarray, which is spotted with short, single-stranded sequences that cover the genomic portion of interest.

2.3 CREATING AND MANIPULATING MODEL SYSTEMS

2.3.1 Cell Culture/Cancer Cell Lines

Cells that are cultured directly from a patient are known as *primary cells*. With the exception of tumor-derived cells, most primary cell cultures have a limited life span. After a certain number of population doublings (called the *Hayflick limit*), cells undergo senescence and cease dividing although they generally retain viability. Some cell lines can proliferate indefinitely either because of random mutation or deliberate modification, such as enforced expression of the telomerase reverse transcriptase (see Chap. 9, Sec. 9.7). There are also numerous well-established cell lines derived from different cancer cell types such as LNCaP for hormone-sensitive prostate cancer; MCF-7 for hormone-sensitive breast cancer; LN229, a human glioblastoma cell line; and SaOS-2 for osteosarcoma. There are several online resources that can be used to query human cell lines and their characteristics, for example, https://www.coriell.org/1/NIGMS.

There are caveats that limit the validity of established cell lines to explore cancer biology: (1) The number of cells per volume of culture medium plays a critical role for some cell types. For example, a lower cell concentration makes granulosa cells undergo estrogen production, whereas a higher concentration makes them progesterone-producing theca lutein cells. (2) Cross-contamination of cell lines occurs frequently and is often caused by proximity (during culture) to rapidly proliferating cell lines such as HeLa cells. (3) Cells grow generally to fill the available area or volume, with accompanying nutrient depletion, accumulation of apoptotic/necrotic (dead) cells, and cell-to-cell contact, which leads to contact inhibition or senescence. Tumor cells grown continuously in culture may acquire further mutations and epigenetic alterations that can change their properties and may affect their ability to reinitiate tumor growth in vivo. (4) The extent to which cancer cell lines reflect the neoplasm from which they are derived is variable. For example, the prostate cancer cell line DU145 was derived from a brain metastasis, which is unusual in prostate cancer. Furthermore, the line does not express prostate-specific antigen and its hypotriploid karyotype is uncommon in prostate cancer. Increasing recognition of the genetic heterogeneity both between and within individual cancers (see Chap. 13) has raised concerns about how well individual cell lines represent the cancer type from which they were originally derived.

Many laboratories have adopted the use of 3-dimensional organoid model systems (Clevers, 2016), and they are increasingly prevalent as a model-of-choice for preclinical in vitro screens of potential anticancer drugs (Gerhards and Rottenberg, 2018). Organoid models have been established from many primary human tissues, including breast, lung, skin, kidney, gut, brain, and retina. These model systems more closely resemble the spatial organization and cellular heterogeneity observed in primary tissues. For example, the tissue architecture of 3D organoids promotes the correction of aberrant kinetochore attachments and thus may promote accurate chromosome segregation in polyploid tissues such as the liver (Knouse et al, 2018). Organoids (eg, multicellular tumor spheroids) can also be generated from tumor cells, and can be used for studying therapeutic effects of drugs or radiation against tumor cells in contact, which may differ from effects against cells in suspension (see Chap. 18, Sec. 18.4.7). However, organoids grown from cultured tumor cells do not contain the various "normal cell" populations that exist within human tumors and may also influence the therapeutic effects of drugs or radiation.

2.3.2 Manipulating Genes in Cells

The function of a gene can be studied by placing it into a cell different from the one from which it was isolated. For example, one may place a genetically altered oncogene, isolated from a tumor cell, into a normal cell to determine whether it causes malignant transformation. The process of introducing DNA plasmids into cells is termed *transfection*. Several transfection methods allow efficient introduction of foreign DNA into mammalian cells, including calcium phosphate or diethylaminoethyl (DEAE)-dextran precipitation, spheroplast fusion, lipofection, electroporation, and transfer using viral vectors. The efficiency of transfer must be high enough for easy detection, and it must be possible to recognize and select for cells containing the newly introduced gene. Control over the expression of introduced genes can be achieved by the use of inducible expression vectors. These vectors allow the manipulation of gene expression, most commonly when an exogenous, inducing agent (such as doxycycline), is added or taken away from culture media.

Some transfection methods require physical perturbation of cells (which may cause damage) to introduced DNA. Examples include electroporation (application of an electric charge), sonoporation (sonic pulses), and optical (laser) transfection. Particle-based methods, such as the gene gun (where the DNA is coupled to a nanoparticle of an inert solid and "shot" directly into the target cell), magnetofection (using magnetic forces to drive nucleic acid particle complexes into the target cell), and impalefection (impaling cells by elongated nanostructures such as carbon nanofibers or silicon nanowires that have been coated with plasmid DNA) are becoming less popular given the greater efficiency of viral transfection.

DNA can be introduced into cells using viruses as carriers; the technique is called *viral transduction*, and the cells are *transduced*. Retroviruses are very stable, as their cDNA integrates into the host mammalian DNA, but only relatively small pieces of DNA (up to 10 kbp) can be transferred. Adenoviral-based vectors can accommodate larger inserts (~36 kbp) and have a very high efficiency of transfer. With increasing frequency, lentiviruses (Fig. 2–16) are being used to introduce DNA into cells; they have the advantages of high-efficiency infection of dividing and nondividing cells, long-term stable expression of the transgene, and low immunogenicity.

Whichever method is used to introduce the DNA, it is usually necessary to select for retention of the transferred genes before assaying for expression. For this reason, a selectable

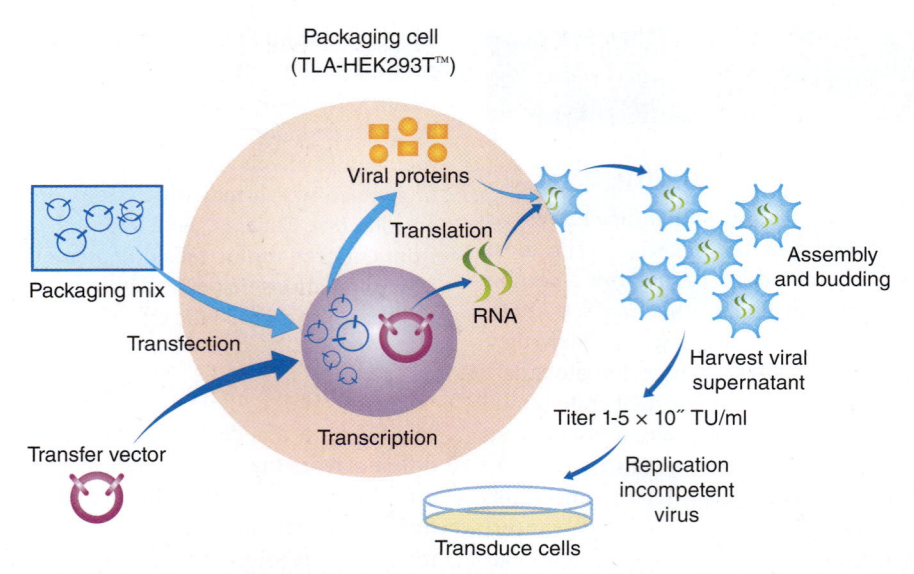

FIGURE 2–16 Schematic outlining the process of lentiviral transfection. Cotransfection of the packaging plasmids and transfer vector into the packaging cell line, HEK293T, allows efficient production of lentiviral supernatant. Virus can then be transduced into a wide range of cell types, including both dividing and nondividing mammalian cells. Note that the packaging mix is often separated into multiple plasmids, minimizing the threat of recombinant replication-competent virus production. Viral titers are measured in either transduction units (TU)/mL or multiplicity of infection (MOI), which is the number of transducing lentiviral particles per cell to which the following relationship applies under experimental conditions: (Total number of cells per well) × (Desired MOI) = Total TU needed (Total TU needed)/(TU/mL reported on certificate of authentication) = Total mL of lentiviral particles to add to each well.

gene, such as the gene encoding resistance to the antibiotics geneticin (G418), neomycin, or puromycin, can be introduced on the same plasmid that contains the gene of interest.

2.3.3 Micro-RNAs and RNA Interference

RNA interference (RNAi) is the process of mRNA degradation that is induced by double-stranded RNA in a sequence-specific manner. RNAi has been observed in all eukaryotes, from fission yeast to mammals. The power and utility of RNAi for silencing expression of any gene for which the sequence is available has driven its rapid adoption as a tool for genetic analysis.

RNAi is one of a larger set of sequence-specific cellular responses to RNA, collectively called *RNA silencing*. RNA silencing plays a critical role in regulation of cell growth and differentiation using endogenous small RNAs called *micro-RNAs*. These miRNAs also play a role in carcinogenesis. For example, miR-15a and miR-16-1 act as putative tumor suppressors by targeting the oncogene *BCL2*. The DNA codes for expression of these miRNAs occur in a cluster at the chromosomal region 13q14, which is frequently deleted in cancer and is down-regulated by genomic loss or mutations in CLL (Calin et al, 2005), prostate cancer (Bonci et al, 2008), and pituitary adenomas (Bottoni et al, 2005).

miRNAs are mostly transcribed from introns or other noncoding areas of the genome into primary transcripts of between 1 kb and 3 kb in length, called *pri-miRNAs* (Fig. 2–17). These transcripts are processed by the ribonucleases Drosha and DiGeorge Syndrome Critical Region gene 8 (DGCR8) complex in the nucleus, resulting in a hairpin-shaped intermediate of approximately 70 to 100 nucleotides, called precursor miRNA (pre-miRNA). The pre-miRNA is exported from the nucleus to the cytoplasm by exportin 5 (Perron and Provost, 2009). Once in the cytoplasm, the pre-miRNA is processed by Dicer, another ribonuclease, into a mature double-stranded miRNA of approximately 18 to 25 nucleotides. After strand separation, the guide strand or mature miRNA is incorporated into an RNA-induced silencing complex (RISC) and the passenger strand is usually degraded. The RISC complex is composed of miRNA, argonaute proteins, and other protein factors. The argonaute proteins have a crucial role in miRNA biogenesis, maturation, and miRNA effector functions (Gutbrod and Martienssen, 2020).

The discovery of the miRNAs suggested that RNAi might be triggered artificially in mammalian cells by synthetic genes that express mimics of endogenous triggers. Indeed, mimics of miRNAs in the form of short hairpin RNAs (shRNAs) have been invaluable in increasing our understanding of many biologic processes, including carcinogenesis. shRNAs contain a sense strand, antisense strand, and a short loop sequence between the sense and antisense fragments. Because of the complementarity of the sense and antisense fragments in their sequence, such RNA molecules tend to form hairpin-shaped dsRNA. shRNA can be cloned into a DNA expression vector and can be delivered to cells by transfection (see Sec. 2.3.2). These constructs then allow ectopic mRNA expression by an associated pol III–type promoter. The expressed shRNA is then exported into the cytoplasm where it is processed by Dicer into short-interference RNA (siRNA), which then get incorporated into the siRNA RISC. A number of transfection methods are suitable, including transient transfection, stable transfection, and delivery using viruses, with both constitutive and inducible promoter systems.

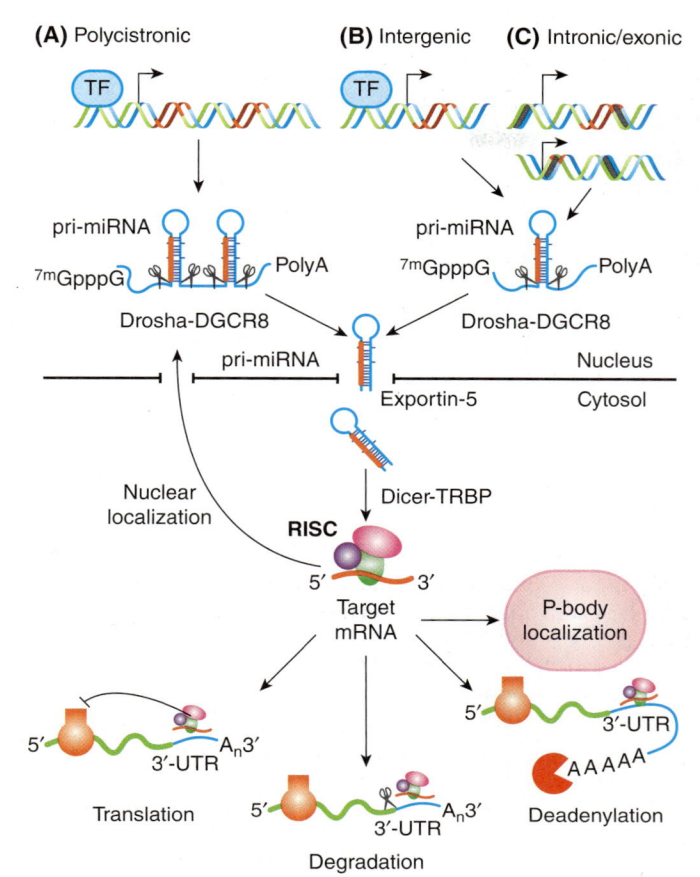

FIGURE 2–17 miRNA genomic organization, biogenesis, and function. Genomic distribution of miRNA genes. The sequence encoding miRNA is shown in red. *TF,* transcription factor. **A)** Clusters throughout the genome transcribed as polycistronic primary transcripts and subsequently cleaved into multiple miRNAs; **B)** intergenic regions transcribed as independent transcriptional units; and **C)** intronic sequences (in gray) of protein-coding or protein-noncoding transcription units or exonic sequences (black cylinders) of noncoding genes. pri-miRNAs are transcribed and transiently receive a 7-methylguanosine (7mGpppG) cap and a poly(A) tail. The pri-miRNA is processed into a precursor miRNA (pre-miRNA) stem-loop of approximately 60 nucleotides (nt) in length by the nuclear ribonuclease (RNase) III enzyme Drosha and its partner DiGeorge syndrome critical region gene 8 (DGCR8). Exportin-5 actively transports pre-miRNA into the cytosol, where it is processed by the Dicer RNase III enzyme, together with its partner TAR (HIV) RNA-binding protein (TRBP), into mature, 22 nt-long double-strand miRNAs. The RNA strand (in red) is recruited as a single-stranded molecule into the RNA-induced silencing (RISC) effector complex and assembled through processes that are dependent on Dicer and other double-strand RNA-binding domain proteins, as well as on members of the argonaute family. Mature miRNAs then guide the RISC complex to the 3′ untranslated regions (3′-UTRs) of the complementary mRNA targets and repress their expression by several mechanisms: repression of mRNA translation, destabilization of mRNA transcripts through cleavage, deadenylation, and localization in the processing body (P-body), where the miRNA-targeted mRNA can be sequestered from the translational machinery and degraded or stored for subsequent use. Nuclear localization of mature miRNAs has been described as a novel mechanism of action for miRNAs. *Scissors* indicate the cleavage on pri-miRNA or mRNA. (Reproduced with permission from Fazi F, Nervi C. MicroRNA: basic mechanisms and transcriptional regulatory networks for cell fate determination. *Cardiovasc Res* 2008 Sep 1;79(4):553-561.)

2.3.4 Site-Directed Mutagenesis

Following sequencing of the human genome (and that of other species), a plethora of genes has been identified without any knowledge of their function. Important clues concerning protein function may be provided through similarity in the amino acid sequence and secondary protein structure to other proteins or protein domains of known function. For example, many transcription factors have a characteristic motif through which DNA binding takes place (eg, leucine zipper or zinc finger domain; see Chap. 6, Sec. 6.2.6). One way of testing the putative function of a sequence is to see whether a mutation within the critical site causes loss of function. In the example of transcription factors, a single mutation might result in a protein that failed to bind DNA.

Site-directed mutagenesis permits the introduction of mutations at a precise point in a cloned gene, resulting in specific changes in the amino acid sequence. By site-directed mutagenesis, amino acids can be deleted, altered, or inserted, but for most experiments, the changes do not alter the reading frame and disrupt protein continuity. There are 2 classical methods of introducing a mutation into a cloned gene. The first method (Fig. 2–18A) relies on the chance occurrence of a restriction enzyme site in a region one wishes to alter. Typically, the gene is digested with the restriction endonuclease, and a few nucleotides may be inserted or deleted at this site by ligating a small oligonucleotide complementary to the cohesive DNA terminus that remains after enzyme digestion. The second method is more versatile but requires more manipulation (Fig. 2–18B) and takes advantage of the ability to introduce the desired mutation within a DNA template. The third method involves PCR to produce a fragment containing the desired mutation in sufficient quantity to be separated from the original, unmutated plasmid by gel electrophoresis. Following plasmid amplification (usually in *Escherichia coli*), commercially available kits (see Fig. 2–18C) can be used that involve a pair of complementary mutagenic primers that are used to amplify the entire plasmid DNA in a thermocycling reaction using a high-fidelity non–strand-displacing DNA polymerase. The reaction generates a nicked, circular DNA. The template DNA is eliminated by enzymatic digestion with a restriction enzyme such as *Dpn*I, which is specific for methylated DNA, as all the DNA produced from the *E coli* vector is methylated; the template plasmid that is biosynthesized in *E coli* will therefore be digested, whereas the mutated plasmid is unmethylated and left undigested. Site-directed mutagenesis has been considerably streamlined and simplified through the use of newer, more modular DNA assembly methods that involve cloning techniques such as Gibson Assembly, Golden Gate cloning, and ligase cycling reactions (Casini et al, 2015), and newer gene editing techniques using CRISPR-Cas9 technologies (see Sec. 2.3.6).

2.3.5 Transgenic and Knockout Mice

One way to investigate the effects of gene expression in specific cells on the function of the whole organism is to transfer genes into the germline and generate transgenic mice. For example,

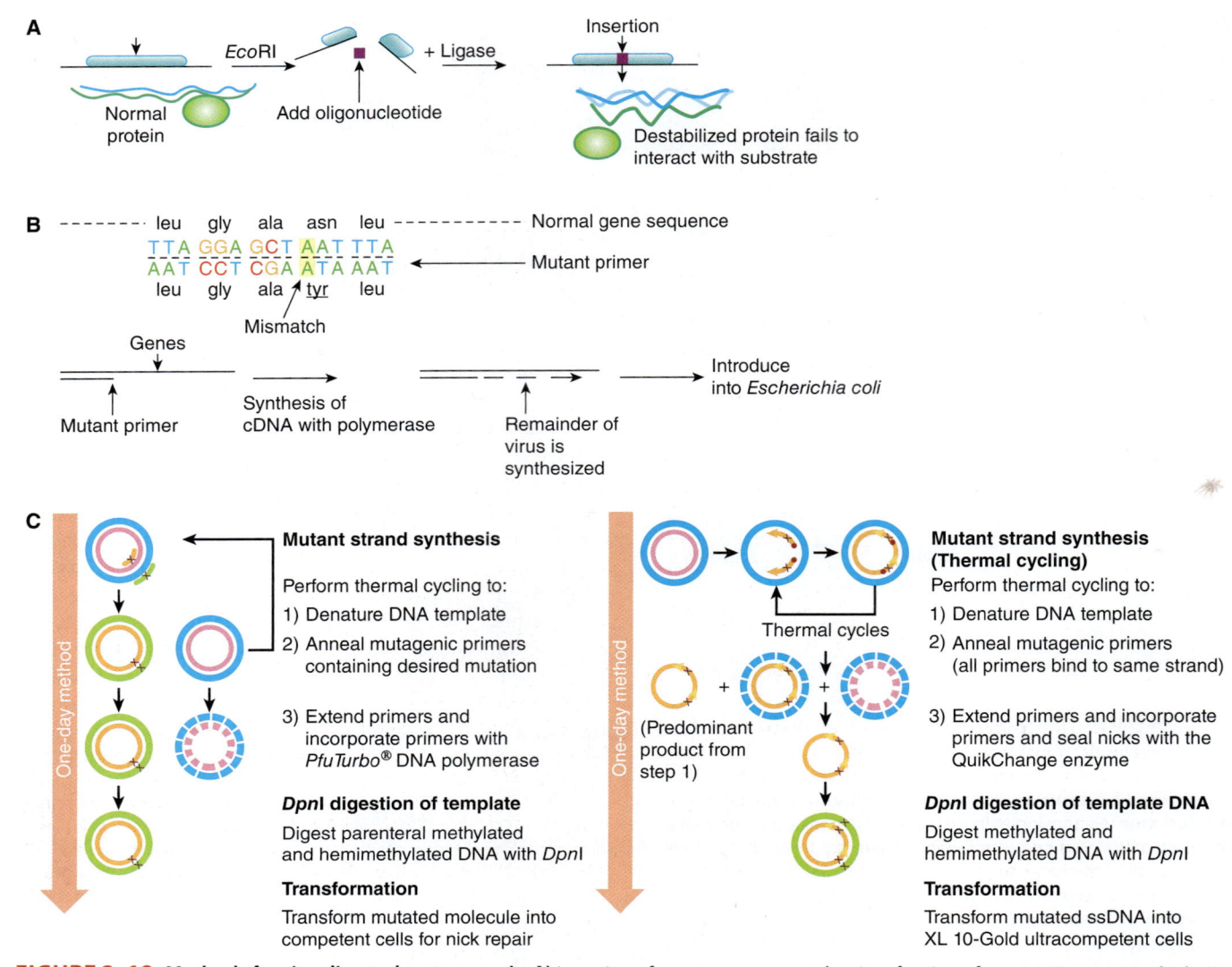

FIGURE 2–18 Methods for site-directed mutagenesis. **A)** Insertion of a new sequence at the site of action of a restriction enzyme by ligating a small oligonucleotide sequence within the reading frame of a gene. **B)** Use of a primer sequence that is synthesized to contain a mismatch at the desired site of mutagenesis. **C)** Outline of the PCR-based methodology.

inappropriate expression of an oncogene in a particular tissue can provide clues about the possible role of that oncogene in normal development and in malignant transformation. Usually, a cloned gene with the desired regulatory elements is microinjected into the male pro-nucleus of a single-cell embryo so that it can integrate into a host chromosome and become part of the genome. If the introduced gene is incorporated into the germline, the resulting animal will become a founder for breeding a line of mice, all of which carry the newly introduced gene. Such mice are called *transgenic mice*, and the inserted foreign gene is called a *transgene*. Its expression can be studied in different tissues of a whole animal. Each transgene will have a unique integration site in a host chromosome and will be transmitted to offspring in the same way as a naturally occurring gene. However, the site of integration often influences the expression of a transgene, possibly because of the activity of genes in adjacent chromatin. Sometimes the integration event also alters the expression of endogenous genes (insertional mutation); this observation led to the development of gene-targeting approaches, so that specific genes could be inactivated or "knocked out." The effect of the inserted or "knocked out" gene can then be studied for phenotypic effects in the animal (unless it turns out to be lethal in the embryo).

In vivo site-directed mutagenesis (Fig. 2–19) is the method by which a mutation is targeted to a specific endogenous gene. Instead of introducing a modified cloned gene at a random position as described above, a cloned gene fragment is targeted to a particular site in the genome by *homologous recombination* (a type of genetic recombination in which nucleotide sequences are exchanged between 2 similar or identical molecules of DNA). This process relies on the ability of a cloned mammalian gene or DNA fragment to undergo preferentially homologous recombination in a normal somatic cell at its naturally occurring chromosomal position, thereby replacing the endogenous gene. The intent is for the introduced mutation to disrupt expression of the endogenous gene, or to result in a

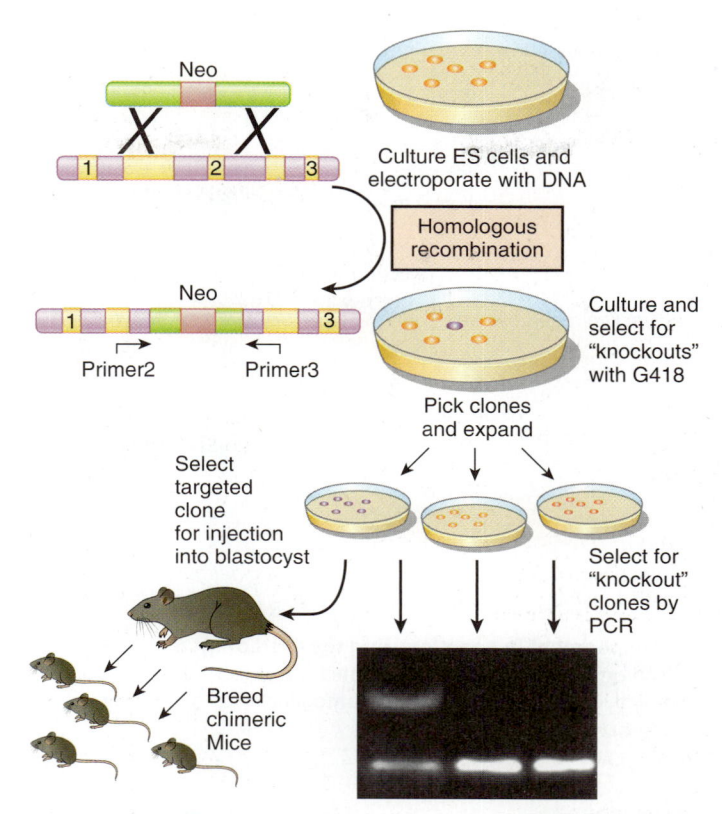

FIGURE 2–19 Disruption of a gene by homologous recombination in embryonic stem (ES) cells. Exogenous DNA is introduced into the ES cells by electroporation. The homologous region on the exogenous DNA is shown in gray, the selectable gene neomycin (*neo*) is speckled, and the target exons are black. The 2 recombination points are shown by Xs, and the exogenous DNA replaces some of the normal DNA of exon 2, thereby destroying its reading frame by inserting the small "neo" gene. ES cells that have undergone a successful homologous recombination are selected as colonies in G418 because of the stable presence of the neo gene. PCR primers for exons 2 and 3 are used to identify colonies in which a homologous recombination event has taken place. ES cells from such positive cells (*dark colony*) are injected into blastocysts, which are implanted into foster mothers (*white*). If germline transmission has been achieved, chimeric mice are bred to generate homozygotes for the "knocked out" gene.

prematurely truncated, nonfunctional protein product. In typical targeting experiments, a DNA construct is prepared with a gene encoding drug resistance (usually to G418) and the DNA of interest. Initially, the modified DNA is introduced into pluripotent stem cells derived from murine embryonic stem (ES) cells. The frequency of homologous recombination is low (less than 1 in a million cells), but is greatly influenced by factors such as the host vector, the method of DNA introduction, the length of the regions of homology, and whether the targeted gene is expressed in ES cells. ES cells that contain the correctly targeted gene disruption are selected by growth in medium containing G418, and these cells are cloned and tested with PCR for homologous recombination. Once an ES cell line with the desired modification has been isolated and purified, ES cells are injected into a normal embryo, where they often contribute to all the differentiated tissues of the chimeric adult mouse. If gametes are derived from the ES cells, then a *founder* line containing the modification of interest can be established.

Technologic advances in gene targeting by homologous recombination in mammalian systems have enabled the production of mutants in any desired gene. It is also possible to generate a *conditionally targeted mutation* within a mouse line using the *cre-loxP system*. This method takes advantage of the properties of the Cre recombinase enzyme first identified in P1 bacteriophage. Cre recognizes a 34-base pair DNA sequence (*loxP*). When 2 *loxP* sites are oriented in the same direction, the Cre recombinase will excise the intervening sequence; when they are oriented in the reverse direction, Cre will invert the intervening sequence. This system can be applied to the transgenic mouse in a number of ways (see Justice et al, 2011); for example, using homologous recombination, it is possible to replace a murine genomic sequence with the same sequence flanked by *loxP* sites. The resulting mice are normal, until the Cre recombinase is introduced. Introduction of the recombinase can be undertaken so that only a specific cell type may be affected, or only a particular phase of differentiation, or both, thus allowing for spatial and temporal control of mutation within the mouse genome. This system is advantageous in examining the role of essential genes in the mouse, particularly when knockout of the gene of interest is embryonic lethal. A conditional knockout mouse using the *cre-loxP* system may allow study of the effects of turning the gene on or off in a living animal. The *cre-loxP* system may also be used to generate chromosomal aberrations in a cell type–specific manner, which can improve understanding of the biology of some human diseases, particularly leukemias (Fig. 2–20).

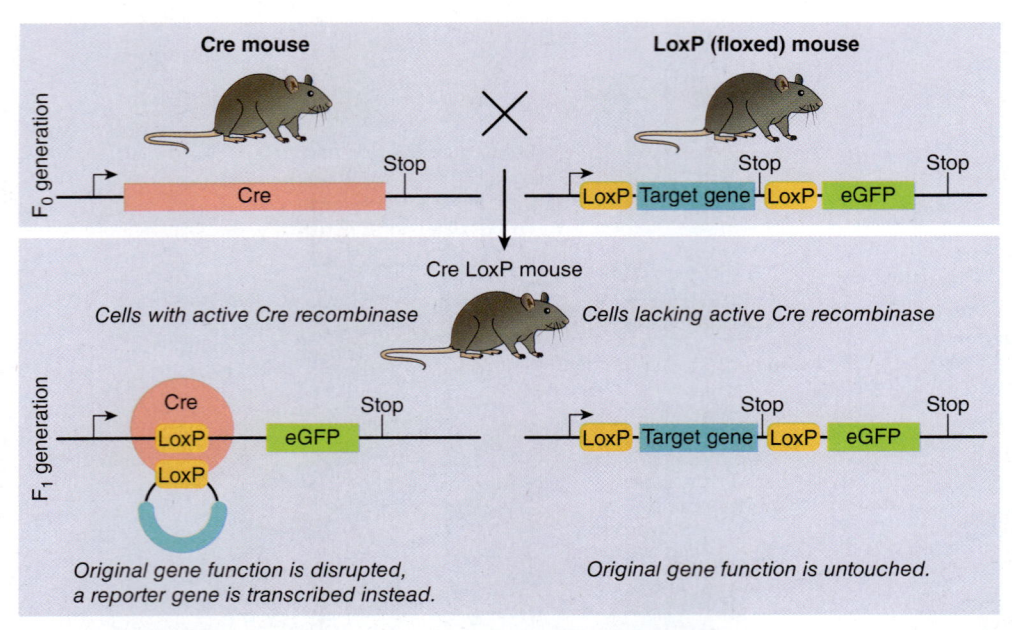

FIGURE 2–20 Illustration of a model experiment in genetics using the Cre-Lox system. The function of a target gene is disrupted by a conditional knockout. Typically, such an experiment would be performed with a tissue-specific promoter driving the expression of the Cre-recombinase (or with a promoter only active during a distinct time in ontogeny). (Reproduced with permission from Matthias Zepper/Wikipedia Commons http://en.wikipedia.org/wiki/File:CreLoxP_experiment.png.)

2.3.6 Other Methods of Gene Editing

Other means of targeting genes for manipulation in vivo include zinc finger nucleases and transcription activator-like effector nucleases (TALENs). Zinc finger nucleases (ZFNs) are synthetic proteins consisting of an engineered zinc finger DNA-binding domain (see Chap. 6, Sec. 6.2.6) fused to the cleavage domain of the FokI restriction endonuclease. ZFNs can be used to induce double-stranded breaks (DSBs) in specific DNA sequences and thereby promote site-specific homologous recombination and targeted manipulation of genomic loci in different cell types. G-rich sequences are the natural preference of zinc fingers, which is a limitation to their use. TALENs were discovered in plant pathogens but have been modified to contain a TALEN DNA binding domain for sequence-specific recognition fused to the catalytic domain of the Fok1 nuclease that introduces DSBs. The DNA-binding domain contains a highly conserved 33– to 34–amino acid sequence with the exception of the 12th and 13th amino acids. These 2 locations are highly variable (repeat variable di-residue [RVD]) and show a strong correlation with specific nucleotide recognition. This simple relationship between amino acid sequence and DNA recognition has allowed for the engineering of specific DNA-binding domains by selecting a combination of repeat segments containing the appropriate RVDs. Therefore, the DNA-binding domain of a TALEN can target a large recognition site (for instance, 17 bp) with high precision.

Gene editing capabilities have increased following the discovery of a site-specific DNA cleavage system called CRISPR-Cas (reviewed in Hsu et al, 2014). This system was discovered in bacteria as an acquired immunity to phage infection (Fig. 2–21), and is composed of Clustered, Regularly Inter-Spaced Palindromic Repeats (CRISPR) and their associated bacterial enzymes (Cas) (Lemay et al, 2017). After phage infection, double-stranded viral DNA is inserted into a CRISPR locus in the bacterial genome in the form of a protospacer. Adjacent to this protospacer are other DNA sequences (such as the PAM, protospacer adjacent motif) that play a key role in spacer insertion, and in later recognition of foreign DNA (see below). The CRISPR array is then transcribed and cleaved by various Cas enzymes or RNaseIII, depending on the species and the type of RNA-processing system they employ, into smaller RNAs called crRNAs. These crRNAs, which contain the complement of the CRISPR DNA sequence to be cleaved, are assembled into a ribonucleoprotein (RNP) complex along with specialized DNA nucleases. For example, in type II CRISPR, there are 2 crRNAs—one that contains a trans-activating small crRNA containing the CRISPR sequence (tracrRNA) and a longer crRNA containing more of the CRISPR array—that form a complex with the nuclease Cas9. This RNP uses the PAM sequence to target and cleave the corresponding CRISPR DNA within the phage.

The CRISPR system allows gene editing in many organisms not previously amenable to standard methods of homologous recombination-mediated gene manipulation, including various fungal, plant, and pathogen species. CRISPR-Cas also has promising applications in crop modification, and in the treatment of human disease, for example, to correct the underlying defect responsible for sickle cell disease (Demirci et al, 2019). In cancer, CRISPR-Cas has been used to map the genes essential for survival of different human cancer cell lines, and the genes whose deletion either sensitizes or confers resistance to various drug treatments (Gerhards and Rottenberg, 2018). Numerous online databases contain the wealth of data now

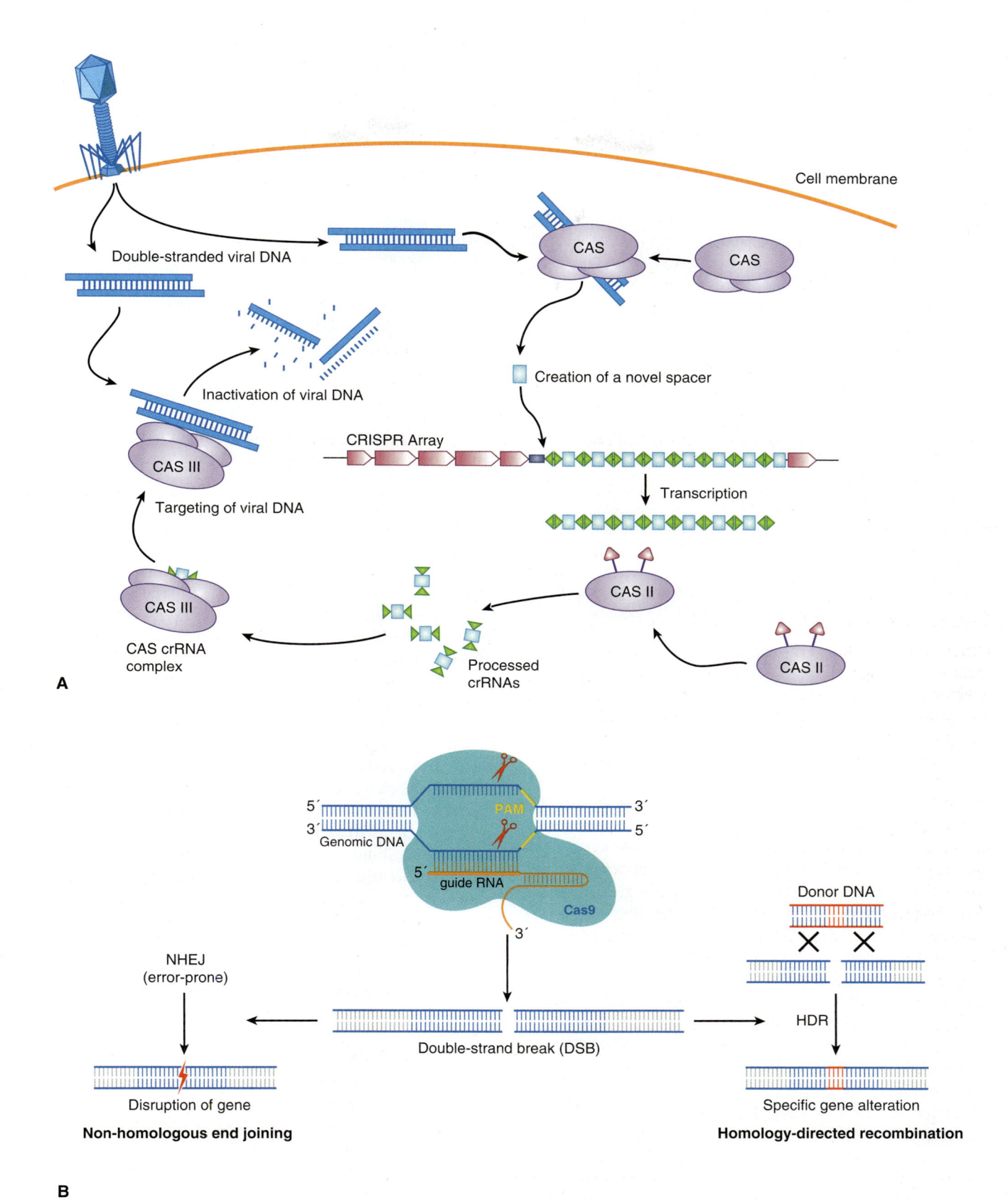

FIGURE 2–21 Schematic of the CRISPR-Cas system. The top panel depicts the stages of phage infection, in which the Cas enzymes process, integrate, transcribe, and incorporate crRNA in order to cleave invading phage DNA (adapted from James Atmos, CC BY-SA 3.0). The bottom panels depict the CRISPR-Cas complex bound to its target DNA. (Panel A Reproduced with permission from James Atmos/Wikimedia Commons https://commons.wikimedia.org/wiki/File:Crispr.png.)

available, including a repository of gene essentiality in human cell lines (https://depmap.org/portal/achilles/) and a repository containing all genome-wide CRISPR screens conducted to date (https://orcs.thebiogrid.org). In mouse genetics, CRISPR has increased the repertoire of possible gene mutations that can be introduced (Gurumurthy and Lloyd, 2019). For example, corrections of single point mutations can be made rapidly even in fertilized oocytes, and multiple genes can be altered simultaneously in a single injection experiment, obviating the need for lengthy breeding programs to study complex genetics.

Gene editing technology has been expanded to other types of bacterial enzymes with improved specificity and fewer potential off-target effects (eg, cleavage of sites other than the desired target), and to targeting of RNA as well as DNA (using Cas13) (Engreitz et al, 2019). In addition, the Cas enzymes have been exploited, through gene fusions, to direct DNA deaminases to specific genetic loci to generate multiple mutations, or to direct transcriptional activators, repressors, or other DNA-binding proteins to specific DNA loci (Engreitz et al, 2019). A natural inhibitory system to CRISPR-based cleavage, called anti-CRISPR, has also been discovered, and it has garnered promise as an "off-switch" for CRISPR and the mitigation of CRISPR off-target effects (Hwang and Maxwell, 2019).

2.4 PROTEOMICS

Proteomics refers to the systematic analysis of proteins in a biologic system. It uses a fusion of traditional protein biochemistry, analytical chemistry, and computer science to obtain a systems-wide understanding of biologic questions (summarized in Table 2–4).

TABLE 2–4 Types of Proteomics Studies.

Use	Application
Expression proteomics	Detection of all proteins present in a biological sample
Functional proteomics	Systematic detection of cellular protein–protein interactions
Quantitative proteomics	Quantify proteins on a relative or absolute scale
Posttranslational modification proteomics	Detection of the location of enzymatic and nonenzymatic posttranslational protein modifications (eg, phosphorylation, methylation, glycosylation, ubiquitination, sumoylation, oxidation, glycation, etc)
Chemical proteomics	Combining synthetic chemistry and proteomics to use defined chemical structures as molecular probes to isolate specific components of the proteome
Structural proteomics	Systematic determination of 3-dimensional structures for all proteins (ie, cryo-EM, x-ray or nuclear magnetic resonance based) and more recently crosslinking mass spectrometry and H/D-exchange mass spectrometry

Mass spectrometry (MS), x-ray crystallography, and nuclear magnetic resonance (NMR) spectroscopy are employed in the systematic analysis of protein-protein interactions, with high-throughput tools, such as protein and chemical microarrays, making an increasing contribution. Technologies such as cryo-electron microscopy (cryo-EM) and crosslinking mass spectrometry have also been used to study large protein complexes (Hampoelz et al, 2016; Hoelz et al, 2016; Kosinski et al, 2016). Other useful methods for interrogating protein-protein interactions that may be applied on a genome-wide scale, including the yeast 2-hybrid system (Colas and Brent, 1998; Fields, 2009), membrane 2-hybrid system (Snider et al, 2010) including its mammalian version MaMTH (Saraon et al, 2017) and protein complementation assays (PCAs) (Michnick et al, 2011). Each technique tends to enrich for specific types of protein interactions; for example, the yeast 2-hybrid system is highly sensitive, but assesses only direct interactions between bait protein (ie, the protein queried for interactions) and its interaction partner. Despite problems of signal-to-noise ratio, MS and other proteomic approaches can interrogate all detectable proteins that bind a bait protein, or can interrogate complex protein mixtures that have not been enriched for a particular protein.

BioID is another technological advance in the identification of protein-protein interactions (Roux et al, 2012; Gingras et al, 2019). This method uses proximity-dependent biotinylation to tag a protein-of-interest in cell culture, followed by capture of the tagged species via streptavidin linked to a solid-state support, followed by liquid chromatography MS. There are numerous biotin ligases that when fused to the "bait protein," will convert biotin to a reactive species, biotinoyl-AMP, that will then covalently modify nearby interacting proteins. This process can take several hours, but peroxidases can generate a bioreactive biotin "cloud" within minutes, thus enhancing the application to time-sensitive studies such as drug treatments, DNA damage, and other applications. Engineered versions of biotin ligases, such as TurboID and miniTurbo, lead to rapid biotin labeling in vivo with an enhanced signal-to-noise ratio. These techniques have been used successfully to study the dynamics of protein interactions during G-protein–coupled receptor signaling, and to uncover the very fine details of organellar composition based on protein proximity in living cells.

2.4.1 Mass Spectrometry

MS is an analytical tool used to determine the mass, structure, and/or elemental composition of a molecule. A mass spectrometer is a very sensitive "detector" that can be divided into 3 main components (Fig. 2–22): an *ion source*, used to transfer the molecules to be analyzed into the gaseous state (mass spectrometers are under high vacuum and therefore ions need to be transferred to the gas phase); a *mass analyzer*, used to measure the mass-to-charge ratio (m/z) of the generated ions (the elemental composition of analyzed ions results in specific m/z values used for identification); and a *detector*, used to register the intensity of the generated ions. A major development

Basic components of a mass spectrometer

Sample → Ion source → Mass analyzer → Detector

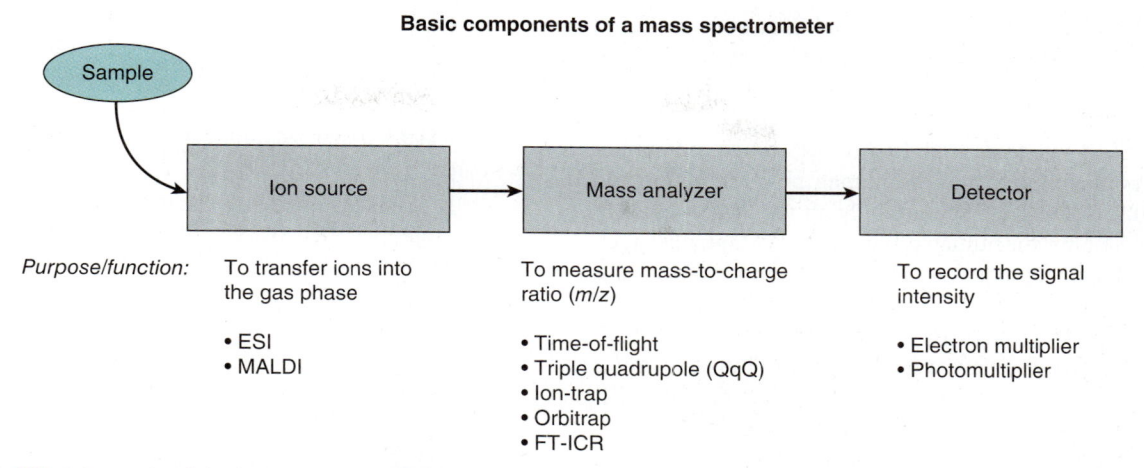

Purpose/function:
- Ion source: To transfer ions into the gas phase
  - ESI
  - MALDI
- Mass analyzer: To measure mass-to-charge ratio (m/z)
  - Time-of-flight
  - Triple quadrupole (QqQ)
  - Ion-trap
  - Orbitrap
  - FT-ICR
- Detector: To record the signal intensity
  - Electron multiplier
  - Photomultiplier

FIGURE 2–22 Schematic of the basic components of a mass spectrometer consisting of the ion source, the mass analyzer, and the detector. Individual examples for each component are listed in the figure. *ESI*, electrospray ionization; *FT-ICR*, Fourier transform–ion cyclotron resonance; *MALDI*, matrix-assisted laser desorption/ionization.

for MS-based proteomics was the introduction of mild ionization technologies (MALDI and ESI) capable of ionizing large, intact proteins or peptides.

In MALDI (*matrix-assisted laser desorption/ionization*), molecules to be analyzed (the analyte) are mixed with an energy-absorbing matrix consisting of organic aromatic acids (eg, sinapinic acid in a solvent mixture of water, acetonitrile, and matrix; ~1:1000) and spotted onto a stainless steel target plate, dried to generate a co-crystal of analyte and matrix molecules. Pulsed lasers are then fired onto the co-crystal; matrix molecules absorb most of the laser energy, thereby protecting from destruction the proteins and peptides being analyzed. The matrix molecules (organic acids) then transfer their charge to the peptide/protein molecules, resulting in mild ionization of these labile biomolecules (Fig. 2–23A).

Electrospray ionization (ESI) involves analyte molecules being dissolved in the liquid phase and ionized by the application of a high voltage (2-4 kV) applied directly to the solvent, resulting in a fine aerosol at the tip of a chromatography column. The solvents used in MS-based proteomics are polar, volatile solvents (ie, water/acetonitrile containing trace amounts of formic acid). This ionization is ideally suited for coupling

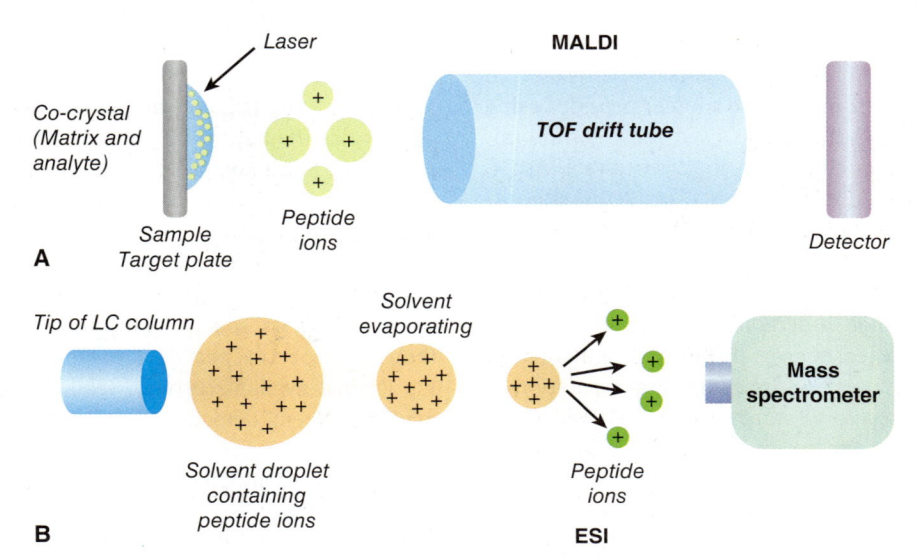

FIGURE 2–23 **Schematics of mild peptide ionizations used for proteomics analyses.** The 2 techniques used to ionize biologic materials include matrix-assisted laser desorption/ionization (MALDI) and electrospray ionization (ESI). Both are soft ionization techniques allowing for the ionization of biomolecules such as proteins and peptides. **A)** In MALDI, ionization is triggered by a laser beam (normally a nitrogen laser). A matrix is used to protect the biomolecule from being destroyed by direct contact with the laser beam. This matrix-analyte solution is spotted onto a metal plate (target). The solvent vaporizes, leaving only the recrystallized matrix with proteins spread throughout the crystals. The laser is fired at the cocrystals on the MALDI target. The matrix material absorbs the energy and transfers part of its charge to the analyte, thus ionizing them. **B)** In ESI, a volatile liquid containing the analyte is passed through a microcapillary (ie, chromatography column). As the liquid is passed out of the capillary it forms an aerosol of small droplets. As the small droplets evaporate, the charged analyte molecules are forced closer together and the droplets disperse. The ions continue along to the mass analyzer of a mass spectrometer.

with high-resolution separation technologies such as liquid chromatography or capillary electrophoresis and is the most commonly used method of ionization in MS-based proteomics (see Fig. 2–23B).

A major challenge for comprehensive MS-based proteomics is the extreme complexity of the human proteome (Cox and Mann, 2007). Although there are only about 20,000 genes in the human genome, the human proteome is substantially larger, as a result of splicing, posttranslational protein modifications, and/or protein processing. The number of protein variants (or *proteoforms*; Smith et al, 2013) is estimated to be more than 1 million. Proteins also have a large range of physicochemical properties, which complicates their extraction and/or solubilization. For example, membrane proteins have been underrepresented in proteomics studies as their solubility in polar, aqueous buffers is poor. Proteins in the human proteome span a wide range of concentrations, and the detection of low-abundance species in the presence of highly abundant proteins is a challenge even for modern, highly sensitive mass spectrometers. To overcome these problems, different analytical fractionations are used, aimed at minimizing sample complexity, thereby increasing the ability of the mass spectrometer to detect less abundant proteins. Fractionation methods can be applied to the intact protein (ie, chromatographic or electrophoretic), or proteins can first be digested and resulting peptides fractionated by liquid chromatography (either off-line as a prefractionation tool or directly coupled to the mass spectrometer). The MS is then used for detection and quantification, as described below.

2.4.2 Top-Down or Bottom-Up Proteomics

Conceptually, there are 2 different strategies for the MS-based analysis of proteins. In *bottom-up proteomics*, proteins or even complex proteomes are first digested to smaller peptides using sequence-specific enzymes (trypsin is used most commonly, but other proteases such as chymotrypsin, LysC, LysN, AspN, GluC, and ArgC are also used) (Swaney et al, 2010). Resulting peptides are then separated by liquid chromatography (LC) and analyzed by ESI-MS. This process is referred to as "LC-MS analysis" or shotgun proteomics. Parent or precursor ions (ie, ions that have not undergone any collision-induced fragmentation) are selected consecutively for fragmentation by the MS, depending on their intensity. Fragmentation is usually achieved using *collision-induced fragmentation* (CID) through collision with inert gas molecules such as helium. Alternative fragmentation mechanisms include *electron transfer dissociation* (ETD; Mikesh et al, 2006), *electron capture dissociation* (ECD; Appella and Anderson, 2007; Chowdhury et al, 2007), *higher-energy collisional dissociation* (HCD; Olsen et al, 2007) and *ultraviolet photodissociation fragmentation* (UVPD; Reilly, 2009; Fort et al, 2016). The resulting MS/MS spectra (ie, tandem mass spectra) contain information regarding the peptide amino acid sequence of the fragmented parent ions. The fragmentation of a parent/precursor peptide ion to a sequence-specific tandem mass spectrum used for detection is dependent on several parameters, including the energy used

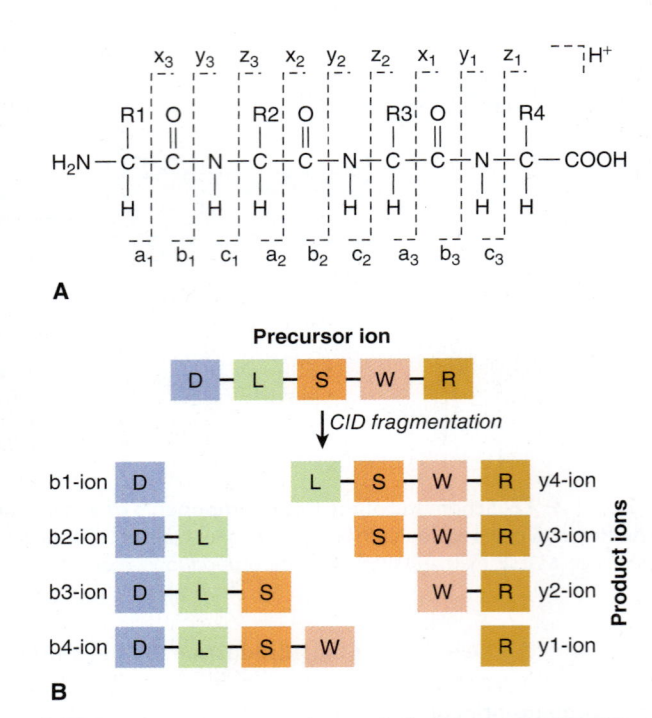

FIGURE 2–24 Schematic of peptide fragmentation by CID. **A)** Nomenclature of peptide fragments generated by CID. The cartoon shows a short peptide and possible breakpoints on fragmentations. Depending on if peptide fragment ions appear to extend from the N-terminus or the C-terminus of the parent peptide ion, different nomenclatures are used (b series, or y series). Under CID conditions, the most common breakpoint is the peptide bond (ie, at the amide bond). This results in b-ions (N-terminus) or y-ions (C-terminus). Additional possible fragment ions and their nomenclature are indicated in the figure. **B)** Cartoon of typical b- and y-type ions generated by CID fragmentation of a pentapeptide. CID, collision-induced.

for fragmentation, the fragmentation mechanism, and the amino acid sequence of the peptide. Resulting fragment ions can be classified according to a defined nomenclature (Roepstorff and Fohlman, 1984) (Fig. 2–24). Under conditions of CID fragmentation, *b-ions* and *y-ions* (ions generated from the N- or C-terminus of the peptide) are observed most commonly. Figure 2–25 is a schematic of an LC-MS analysis using data recorded on an LTQ-Orbitrap mass analyzer.

Modern mass spectrometers can record several hundred thousand spectra per day; computational spectral matching against available protein sequence databases is used for peptide/protein detection. To accomplish this task, several commercial or open-source algorithms are available and improved tools are constantly being developed. Careful interpretation of the results is crucial to ensure high data quality and minimize false-positive and false-negative detections. This process of automated spectral matching is dependent on the availability of well-annotated protein sequence databases that correlate experimentally recorded spectra to theoretically generated spectra from the protein sequence database. Any potential post-translational modification needs to be specified prior to database correlation. Algorithms for direct spectral searching, such as SpectraST, have been introduced in which experimental spectra are compared to accumulated

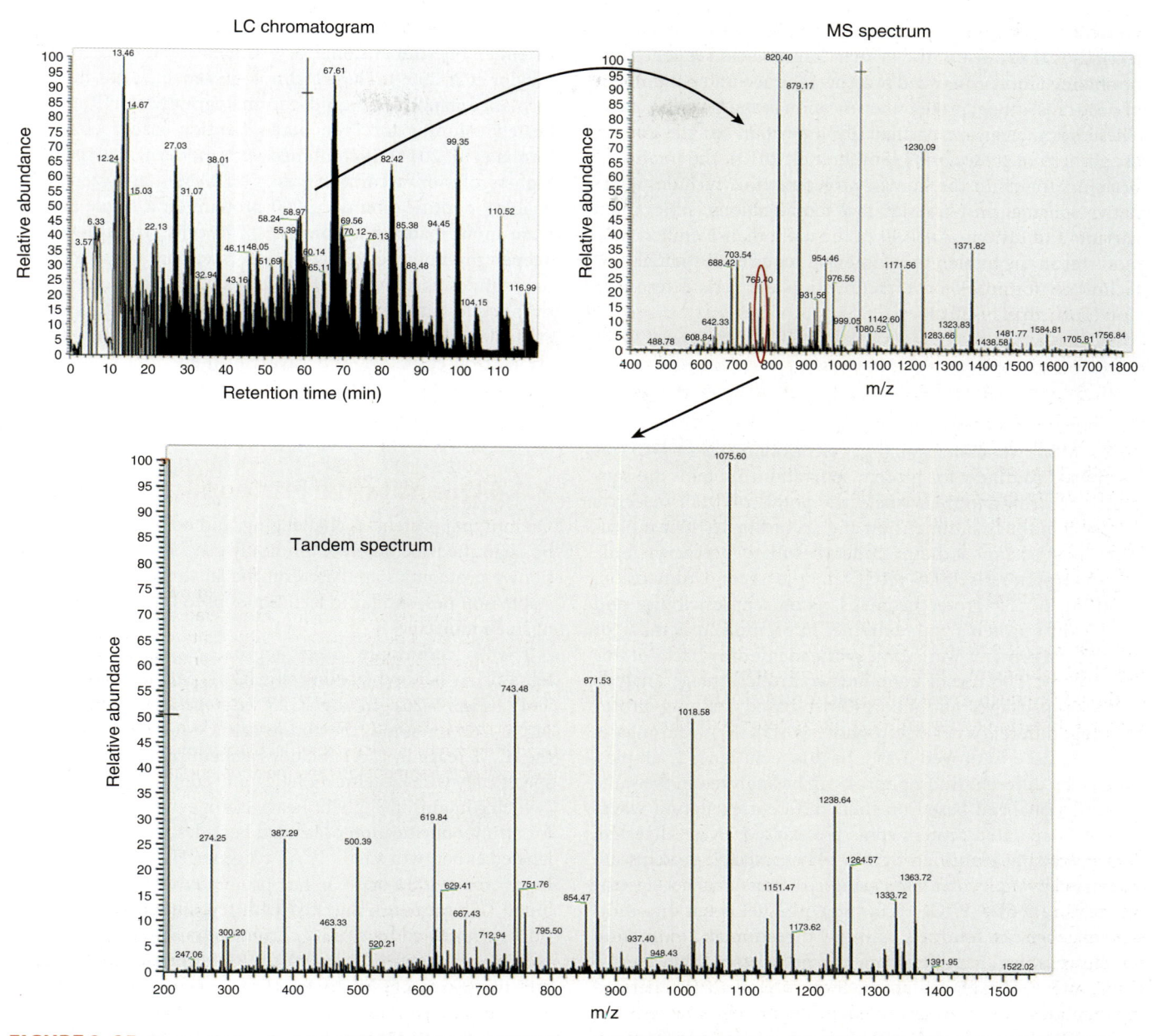

FIGURE 2-25 Screenshots of a typical "data-dependent" LC-MS experiment. Peptides are separated by nanoflow LC and analyzed by mass spectrometry in real-time. Briefly, as peptides are eluted from the chromatography column, they are ionized by electrospray ionization (ESI) and directly transferred into the mass spectrometer. The mass spectrometer performs a "full scan" to record the *m/z* ratios of all parent ions at that given time (ie, MS spectrum). An individual parent ion is then isolated by the mass analyzer and subjected to CID fragmentation resulting in a sequence-specific tandem mass spectrum (ie, MS/MS spectrum). In general, 1 to 10 parent ions are selected for subsequent fragmentation before the instrument performs another full scan. Peptide ions are generally selected based on intensity, and the most intense ions are preferentially fragmented at the expense of lower-intensity ions.

proteomics data. Large-scale synthetic peptide libraries have been generated for a substantial percentage of the human proteome (Marx et al, 2013; Zolg et al, 2017). These approaches enable the generation of high-quality consensus spectra covering much of the human proteome. An additional approach employs de novo sequencing. Here, mass spectra are interpreted without the use of protein sequence databases or spectral libraries either via manual (ie, interpreter evaluation) or more commonly via available algorithms (Biemann et al, 1966; Ma et al, 2003). This approach is useful for the sequencing of monoclonal antibodies where the genomic annotation is either sparse or not available (Tran et al, 2016).

Proteins can also be analyzed by *top-down proteomics* whereby intact proteins are ionized, fragmented by either ECD or ETD, and the resulting fragmentation pattern is used for protein detection (Kelleher, 2004). Although this strategy is less applicable to complex protein mixtures, and is used mainly for the analysis of purified/enriched proteins, major advances now enable top-down proteomics on a more "global" scale (Tran et al, 2011; Kellie et al, 2012; Catherman et al, 2013;

Fornelli et al, 2017). A potential advantage of top-down proteomics is that most of the primary amino acid sequence can be obtained for the analyzed proteins. The accurate assignment of posttranslational protein modification is another advantage. These advantages are particularly important for the correct assignment of *proteoforms* (Smith et al, 2013), the totality of protein variants in the human proteome; this includes alternative splicing, post-translational modifications, amino acid variants and fusions. Analysis of the more than 1 million proteoforms in the human proteome will require substantial new techniques for proteoform fractionation and mass determination (Fornelli et al, 2018).

2.4.3 Gel-Based or Gel-Free Approaches

Two approaches are available to fractionate samples just prior to LC-MS. Two-dimensional gel electrophoresis (2-DE) has been used routinely for protein separation. Proteins are separated according to their isoelectric point (pI) via isoelectric focusing in the first dimension and according to their molecular mass using sodium dodecyl sulfate–polyacrylamide gel electrophoresis (SDS-PAGE) in the second dimension, resulting in 2D proteome maps. Poor reproducibility and bias against proteins with extremes in pI, molecular mass, or membrane proteins were some of the major drawbacks of this technology. The use of computer-controlled image analysis software packages and fluorescence-based staining protocols (eg, difference gel electrophoresis [DIGE]) (Marouga et al, 2005) have improved 2-DE. In this technique, 2 samples, labeled by different fluorophores, can be analyzed in the same gel and visualized based on their different excitation wavelengths. Separated protein spots are excised, in-gel digested, and eventually identified by MS. Alternatively, proteins are separated by molecular mass using 1-dimensional gel electrophoresis (1D SDS-PAGE) and the entire gel is cut into individual *gel blocks*, followed by in-gel digestion and extraction of the resulting peptides from the gel matrix (Shevchenko et al, 1996). These resultant peptide mixtures are separated by LC and eluting peptides are identified by MS. This method is used routinely in modern proteomics laboratories and is termed *gel-enhanced LC-MS* or *GeLC-MS*.

Methods have been developed to eliminate the use of gel-based separation. In *gel-free* approaches, complex protein mixtures are first digested in-solution, resulting in highly complex peptide mixtures that are consecutively analyzed by LC-MS. In general, nano-bore LC columns are used for peptide separation (termed *shotgun proteomics*; Wolters et al, 2001) and separated ions are electrosprayed into the mass spectrometer.

An alternative gel-free approach relies on *multidimensional protein identification technology (MudPIT)* (Washburn et al, 2001; Wolters et al, 2001), which is similar to 2-DE, and separates peptides by 2 orthogonal chromatographic resins: strong cationic exchange (SCX) and reversed phase (RP18). This 2D shotgun proteomics approach enables better peptide separation, allowing the detection of lower abundance proteins. Substantial advances have been made in liquid chromatography (ie, liquid chromatography pumps that are able to deliver solvent flow-rates in the range of 50–400 nL/min) in either one-dimensional or 2-dimensional configurations (Taylor et al, 2009). These technologies enable ultra-high performance nano-flow liquid chromatography (UHPLC) with heated columns for even better peptide-based separations (Sinha et al, 2014). If combined with modern, fast-scanning, high-resolution/accurate mass (HRAM) analyzers, this enables identification of >5000 proteins in a single analysis from input material as low as 50,000 cells. To achieve even deeper proteome coverage, prior fractionation of proteins or peptides is required. This is achieved most commonly by peptide-based strong cationic exchange (SCX) (Marino et al, 2014; Binai et al, 2015) or basic reverse-phase fractionation (Doll et al, 2017). A caveat of these approaches is the increased analysis time and additional sample processing/handling, possibly introducing additional variation.

2.4.4 Quantitative Proteomics

Quantifying proteins is challenging, and not every protein can be quantified accurately. Commonly used strategies for quantitative proteomics are based on the labeling of proteins with stable isotopes, similar to techniques used for quantitative MS of small molecules.

The 3 commonly used approaches to quantify proteins using isotope labeling are ICAT, SILAC, and iTRAQ/TMT (Fig. 2–26). In the ICAT (*isotope-coded affinity tags*; Fig. 2–26A) method, the amino acid cysteine is modified by the ICAT reagent. ICAT includes a chemical group that reacts specifically with cysteine moieties, and contains a linker region (which contains the light or heavy isotopes) and a biotin group for affinity purification of labeled peptides. Protein lysates are labeled either with a light ICAT reagent (^{1}H or ^{12}C) or with the heavy analog (^{2}H or ^{13}C). The protein lysates are then combined (1:1 mixture), digested with trypsin, and labeled peptides are purified by affinity chromatography using the biotin moiety (ie, streptavidin column). Resulting peptide mixtures are analyzed by LC-MS to detect and quantify the relative levels of peptides/proteins in the mixture. Detection occurs as described above via correlation of the resulting MS/MS spectra against a protein sequence database using algorithms such as Sequest. Relative quantification is undertaken based on the intensity of parent ions, which differ in their mass based on the introduced light or heavy label.

SILAC (*stable isotope labeling with amino acids in cell culture*; Fig. 2–26B) involves the addition of an essential amino acid (ie, light or heavy isotope version of lysine) to the cell culture, resulting in its metabolic incorporation into newly synthesized proteins (Ong et al, 2002). After complete labeling of the cellular proteome (ie, keeping cells in culture for several divisions), cells are lysed, combined at a 1:1 ratio, and analyzed by MS as described above. Relative peptide quantification is accomplished by integration of the parent ion peak of either the light or heavy peptide ion. This procedure has been used for the relative quantification of tissue proteomes by metabolically labeling entire model organisms (Kruger et al, 2008). A variation of SILAC termed super-SILAC)

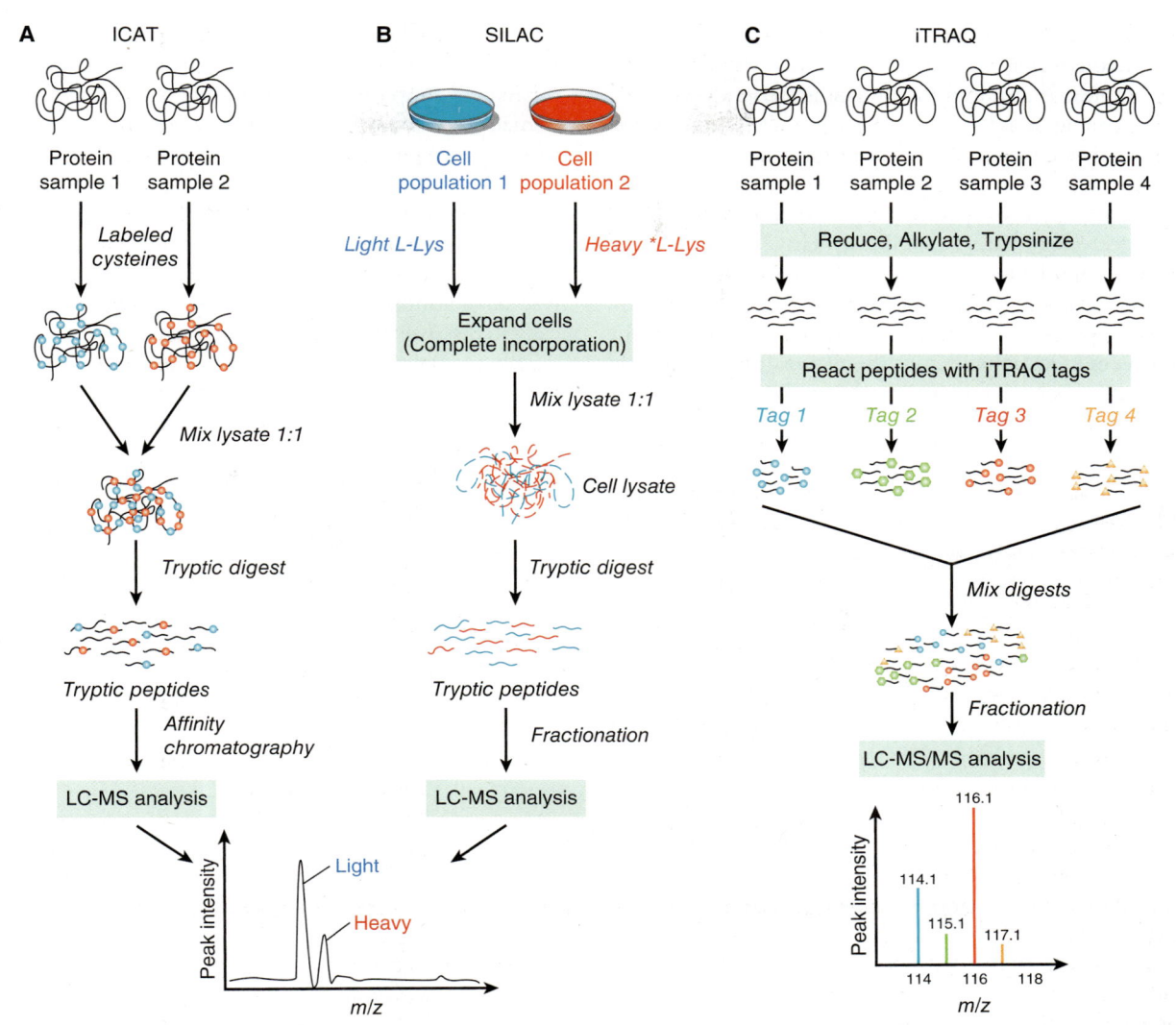

FIGURE 2–26 Graphic demonstration of the workflow of 3 proteomic methodologies developed to use stable isotope technology for quantitative protein profiling by mass spectrometry. **A)** ICAT can be used to label 2 protein samples with chemically identical tags that differ only in isotopic composition (heavy and light pairs). These tags contain a thiol-reactive group to covalently link to cysteine residues and a biotin moiety. The ICAT-labeled fragments can be separated, and quantified by LC-MS analysis. **B)** SILAC is a similar approach to quantify proteins in mammalian cells. Isotopic labels are incorporated into proteins by metabolic labeling in the cell culture. Cell samples to be compared are grown separately in media containing either a heavy (*red*) or light (*blue*) form on an essential amino acid such as L-lysine that cannot be synthesized by the cell. **C)** iTRAQ is a unique approach that can be used to label protein samples with 4 independent tag reagents of the same mass that can give rise to 4 unique reporter ions (m/z = 114 to 117) on fragmentation in MS/MS. This recorded data can be subsequently used to quantify the 4 different samples, respectively.

enables the analyses of human tumor tissues where the samples cannot be labeled in vivo with stable isotopes (Geiger et al, 2010). Instead, cancer cell lines are grown in SILAC media and added to a human tissue lysate prior to proteomic analysis. The labeled cancer cell lines enable normalization of all analyzed human samples.

iTRAQ (*isobaric tag for relative and absolute quantitation*; Fig. 2–26C) enables relative peptide quantification (Ross et al, 2004). Primary amines (lysine side chains and/or the N-terminus) are covalently labeled by the iTRAQ reagent. Tryptic peptide mixtures, from 4 or 8 different experimental conditions, are labeled individually, combined, and analyzed by LC-MS. In contrast to the ICAT reagent, the individual iTRAQ labels have the same mass. On fragmentation of a given parent ion via CID, the iTRAQ reagent releases a specific reporter ion for each experimental condition. The relative peak intensity of these reporter ions is used to quantify an individual peptide (Fig. 2–26). An analogous approach termed tandem mass tag (TMT) has recently been introduced. This technology has the potential for proteomic analysis of up to 11 samples at the same time (Zhang and Elias, 2017). This approach is useful for clinical proteomics, where clever "labeling strategies" have been applied to over 100 primary cancer tissues (Mertins et al, 2016; Zhang et al, 2016). By dedicating one of the TMT channels to a global pool of all analyzed tumor tissues (which serves as a global normalizing control), a defined number of samples can be analyzed concurrently, for example, 9 tumors in the case of the 10-plex reagent.

One drawback of label-based proteomics is the high cost of reagents and the complex labeling strategies to achieve analyses of large samples, as required for clinical proteomics. To overcome these problems, label-free peptide/protein quantification was developed using spectral counting and label-free peak integration. Spectral counting uses the total, combined number of tandem mass spectra (ie, spectral counts) recorded by MS/MS for each detected protein, as a semiquantitative measure of relative protein abundance (Liu et al, 2004) and is not limited by the number of analyzed samples. Label-free peak integration is conceptually similar to the peptide quantification used by isotope labeling technologies, but the major difference is that individual experimental conditions are not combined (ie, light and heavy isotope), but analyzed individually by LC-MS.

2.4.5 Challenges for Biomarker Discovery With Proteomics

MS-based proteomics can detect and quantify thousands of proteins in complex biologic samples and has been used extensively for biomarker discovery (Geyer et al, 2019; Huttenhain et al, 2019; Sinha et al, 2019; Sinha et al, 2019; Walloe et al, 2019). Nonetheless, few such studies have been validated biologically and introduced into clinical practice. Challenges to proteomics-based biomarker discovery include (1) extreme complexity of biologic samples; (2) heterogeneity of the disease and of the human population; (3) difficulty to obtain accurate quantification for all proteins in the course of a discovery proteomics experiment; (4) poor availability of adequate, well-annotated human samples (tissue or body fluids); and (5) the expensive and time-consuming process of proteomic analysis (Pepe et al, 2001). Also, most biomarker/clinical proteomics projects analyze small numbers of samples, which are not powered statistically to discover candidate biomarkers.

The combination of extensive discovery-based proteomics on patient samples, followed by the accurate quantification of putative biomarker candidates using targeted proteomics approaches (ie, multiple reaction monitoring [MRM-MS]) is a promising strategy (Fig. 2–27). The targeted proteomics approaches provide more precise quantification, most commonly through the use of a stable isotope–labeled standard. A goal is to perform rapid quantification of large numbers of candidate biomarkers in a multiplex manner to eliminate markers that do not perform according to preferred performance criteria. These "first stage" verification studies do not require antibodies for use in immune-assays, whose development is expensive and time consuming. Targeted proteomics provide

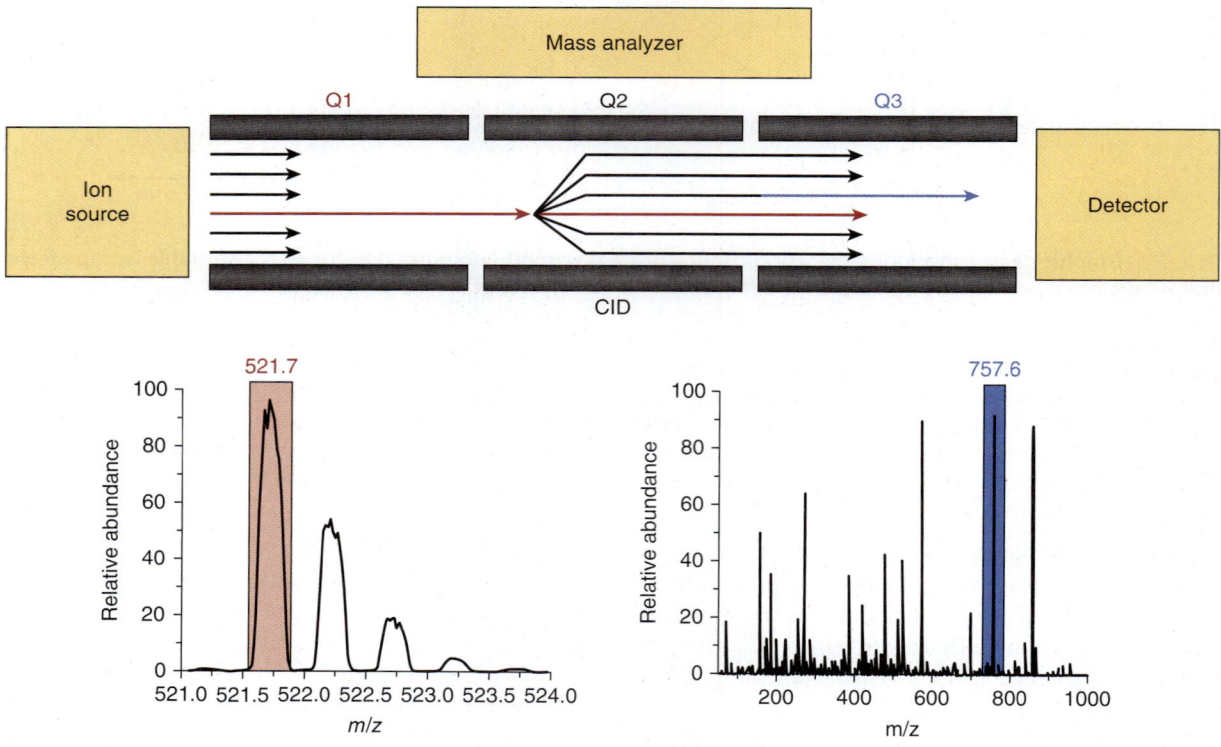

FIGURE 2–27 Schematic of a targeted proteomics experiment based on selected reaction monitoring-mass spectrometry (SRM-MS). Peptides that elute off an LC column are ionized by ESI and resulting ions are guided into the first quadrupole (*Q1*). This first quadrupole works as a mass filter and only allows predefined peptide ions of interest (based on a known *m/z* value) to pass to the second quadrupole (*Q2*), in which an inert gas induces fragmentation. All fragments, which are again known based on prior knowledge, are transferred to the third quadrupole (*Q3*), which, like Q1, acts as a mass filter, so that only preselected fragment ions will trigger a signal at the detector. In general 3-5 fragment ions per parent ion are allowed to pass. These parent-to-fragment ion pairs are called "transitions." The area under the curve of these ions can be used for quantification and, in general, stable isotope–labeled synthetic peptides are used for direct comparison and quantification.

therefore an analytical platform for the rapid evaluation (and triage) of a large number of candidate biomarkers. Promising candidates could then be further evaluated with immuneassays or through improvements of the targeted proteomics assays. Additional targeted (or semitargeted) approaches have been introduced. These include parallel reaction monitoring mass spectrometry (PRM-MS), a method that is similar to MRM-MS. Although data suggest that the sensitivity of PRM-MS is similar to MRM-MS, the advantages are the use of a high-resolution/accurate mass (HRAM) analyzer that reduces isobaric interference and allows recording of all peptide fragment ions, as compared to predefined fragment ions (or transitions) in MRM-MS; this facilitates post-analysis selection and removal of poor-performing fragment ions (Sinha et al, 2019).

A hybrid approach termed data-independent mass spectrometry (DIA; Venable et al, 2004) has been adapted and is often referred to as SWATH-MS (sequential window acquisition of all theoretical mass spectra) (Gillet et al, 2012). Here, the mass spectrometer selects large mass-to-charge segments for fragmentation, thereby generating complex co-fragments of multiple peptide ions at the same time. A potential advantage is that no peptide ions that elute off the liquid chromatography columns are lost. The caveat is that complex co-fragmentation spectra are not easily interpreted and their analysis requires spectral libraries and complex bioinformatics.

2.4.6 X-Ray Crystallography

In *X-ray crystallography*, a high-intensity x-ray beam is directed through the highly ordered crystalline phase of a pure protein. The crystalline protein diffracts the x-rays so that they give rise to a unique diffraction pattern (detected on an x-ray imaging screen or film). From the diffraction pattern, the distribution of electrons in the molecule is calculated, and a molecular model of the protein is then built progressively into the electron density map.

A critical step is the generation of crystals of the protein of interest, which is a trial-and-error procedure in which different solvent conditions are tested in multiple-well plates, with protein crystals almost always grown in solution. Crystal growth is characterized by 2 steps: nucleation of a microscopic crystallite (possibly having only 100 molecules), followed by growth of that crystallite, ideally to a diffraction-quality crystal (Chernov, 2003).

Favorable conditions are identified most often by screening: a large batch of the protein molecules is prepared, and a wide variety (up to thousands) of crystallization solutions are tested (Chayen, 2005). Thereafter, various conditions are used to lower the solubility of the molecule, including change in pH or temperature, adding salts or chemicals that lower the dielectric constant of the solution, or adding large polymers, such as polyethylene glycol, that drive the molecule out of solution. Because of the difficulty in obtaining large quantities (milligrams) of crystallization-grade protein, robots are used that can dispense accurately crystallization trial drops that are ~100 nL in volume (Stock et al, 2005). Pure protein (usually from recombinant sources) is divided into small drops of aqueous buffers that often contain 1 or more cosolvents or precipitants. The drop is left to evaporate or equilibrate with a reservoir solution (in the same well), and if conditions are favorable, the protein slowly comes out of solution in a crystalline form. This is the limiting step in crystallography, and it is currently impossible to predict a priori under which conditions, if any, a given protein will crystallize.

When a crystal is exposed to x-rays, it scatters them into a pattern that can be observed on a screen behind the crystal. The relative intensities of these spots provide information to determine the arrangement of molecules within the crystal in atomic detail. The recorded series of 2-dimensional diffraction patterns, each corresponding to a different crystal orientation, is converted into a 3-dimensional model of the electron density. Each spot corresponds to a different type of variation in the electron density; the crystallographer must determine which variation corresponds to which spot (indexing), the relative strengths of the spots in different images (merging and scaling), and how the variations should be combined to yield the total electron density (phasing).

The final step of fitting the atoms of the protein into the electron density map requires the use of interactive or semiautomated computer graphics programs. Initially, the electron density map contains many errors, but it can be improved through a process called *refinement* in which the atomic model is adjusted to improve the agreement with the measured diffraction data. The quality of an atomic model is judged through the standard crystallographic R-factor, which is a measure of how well the atomic model fits the experimental data.

High-resolution x-ray structures are useful in understanding the principles of molecular recognition in protein-ligand complexes. Determining the structure of imatinib bound to the *c-ABL* kinase domain is an example of the application of this approach. Imatinib was discovered by using high-throughput screening of compound libraries to identify the 2-phenylaminopyrimidine class of kinase inhibitors. The pharmaceutical properties of these compounds were then optimized through successive rounds of medicinal chemistry and evaluation of structure-activity relationships. Ultimately, the structural mechanism of the inhibition of *BCR-ABL* by imatinib was shown by x-ray crystallography to involve binding by the inhibitor to the inactive kinase structure of the enzyme. By virtue of its ability to bind this specific inactive enzyme conformation prior to substrate binding, imatinib semicompetitively blocks ATP binding and subsequent substrate recognition and phosphorylation. One advantage of imatinib is thus its conformational specificity for BCR-ABL; this fact also explains why bcr-abl mutations that are resistant to imatinib do so by shifting the enzyme equilibrium to a more open or active state (Schindler et al, 2000, Gambacorti-Passerini et al, 2003).

2.4.7 Nuclear Magnetic Resonance Spectroscopy

NMR spectroscopy takes advantage of nuclear spin (see Chap. 15, Sec. 15.3.2). When placed in a static magnetic field, nuclei with nonzero spin will align their magnetic dipoles with (low-energy state) or against (high-energy state) the magnetic field. Under normal circumstances, there is a small difference in the population distribution between the 2 energy states, thereby creating a net magnetization, which is then manipulated using multiple electromagnetic pulses (and recycle delays, which is the time period following the last acquisition time). Each nucleus absorbs energy from these pulses at a characteristic frequency that is dependent on its chemical properties and the surrounding environment. Structures of noncrystalline proteins in aqueous solution are derived from a series of NMR experiments that reveal interactions of nuclei that are close together in 3-dimensional space, even though they are distant within the protein's primary sequence. These data allow one to deduce protein conformations that satisfy a large number (hundreds to thousands) of experimental restraints: this necessitates extensive data collection (often more than 10 experiments lasting hours to days) and computer-assisted analysis of the spectra.

The main nucleus influencing NMR is that of hydrogen (^{1}H). However, proteins have hundreds to thousands of ^{1}H signals, many with the same resonance frequency. This problem is solved by the use of multidimensional NMR, in which protein samples are labeled with the NMR-active stable isotopes ^{15}N and ^{13}C. The incorporation of stable isotopes resolves the multiple signals in 2, 3, or 4 dimensions, each dimension corresponding to ^{1}H, ^{15}N, and/or ^{13}C resonance frequencies. Because of the poor signal-to-noise ratio of the NMR signals in large proteins, the size of proteins amenable to high-resolution NMR structural studies is limited to approximately 30 kilodaltons (kDa) or less. Larger molecules can be studied using partial or full deuteration (ie, incorporation of heavy hydrogen) in combination with special NMR techniques, but results in lower-resolution structural information. Samples need to be concentrated; this makes it difficult to study proteins with low solubility or those prone to aggregation or precipitation. Much time is devoted in optimizing the stability and solubility of a protein prior to the study by NMR spectroscopy.

2.4.8 Cryogenic Electron Microscopy

Protein structure determination by cryogenic electron microscopy (cryo-EM) involves imaging of samples embedded at low temperatures in a vitreous aqueous environment. Cryo-EM enables determination of the structure of large macromolecules, such as membrane-bound complexes, without the need for protein crystallization. Another powerful approach that allows visualization of complexes in their native environment is cryo-electron tomography (cryo-ET), whereby samples are imaged as they are tilted (Danev et al, 2019). These techniques show promise for therapeutic drug discovery; for example, cryo-EM has provided insights into the drug-ligand relationships of G-protein–coupled receptors (Garcia-Nafria and Tate, 2019).

2.4.9 Protein Arrays

A protein microarray allows characterization of multiple proteins in a biologic sample. There are 3 types of protein microarrays (2 of which are illustrated in Fig. 2–28). *Functional protein arrays* display folded and active proteins and are designed to assay functional properties (Hall et al, 2007). They are used for screening molecular interactions, studying protein pathways, identifying targets for protein-targeted molecules, and analyzing enzymatic activities. In *analytical* or *capture arrays*, affinity reagents (eg, antibodies) or antigens (that may be unfolded) are arrayed for profiling the expression of proteins (Sanchez-Carbayo et al, 2006) or for the quantification of antibodies in complex samples such as serum. Applications of antibody arrays include biomarker discovery and monitoring of protein quantities and activity states in signaling pathways (Sharon et al, 2010). Antigen arrays are applied for profiling antibody repertoires in autoimmunity, cancer, infection, or following vaccination. Moreover, antigen arrays are tools for controlling the specificity of antibodies and related affinity reagents. *Reverse-phase arrays* comprise cell lysates or serum samples. Replicates of the array can then be probed with different antibodies. Reverse-phase arrays are particularly useful for studying changes in the expression of specific proteins and protein modifications during disease progression and are applied primarily for biomarker discovery. Much of these findings are available publicly through the RPPA Society (Akbani et al, 2014; Nishizuka and Mills, 2016).

2.5 TRANSLATIONAL APPLICATIONS WITH CELLS AND TISSUES

Genetic or epigenetic analysis of primary human tumors (or other tissues) requires access to appropriately handled material. Generally, human tumor or tissue samples are fixed in formalin and then *embedded* in paraffin wax to preserve cell and tissue morphology for histologic analysis. Formalin fixation is an erratic process resulting often in unequal protein preservation. If tissues are snap-frozen after an operation (or biopsy) this improves preservation of cellular antigens or mRNA. Fixation limitations, as well as the presence of stroma, immune infiltrates, and secreted proteins, create difficulties for identifying genetic or epigenetic changes associated with tumor cells (or the stromal cell populations). It is relatively easy to retrieve the malignant cells from hematologic malignancies, but new techniques (such as laser capture microdissection; see below) have enhanced substantially the ability of scientists to isolate and analyze cells and tissue from solid tumors.

Although formalin crosslinks proteins, it has little effect on the structural integrity of DNA or miRNAs. Therefore, the ability to use FISH on paraffin-embedded archival specimens is dependent only on the accessibility of the target DNA within the cell nucleus and can be enhanced by pretreatment that increases the efficiency of hybridization. Such protocols are used routinely for the analysis of *HER2* in breast cancer tissues. miRNAs can also be retrieved from formalin-fixed tissue with reasonable success. There are protocols for extracting mRNA from archival formalin-fixed tissue, but its tendency to

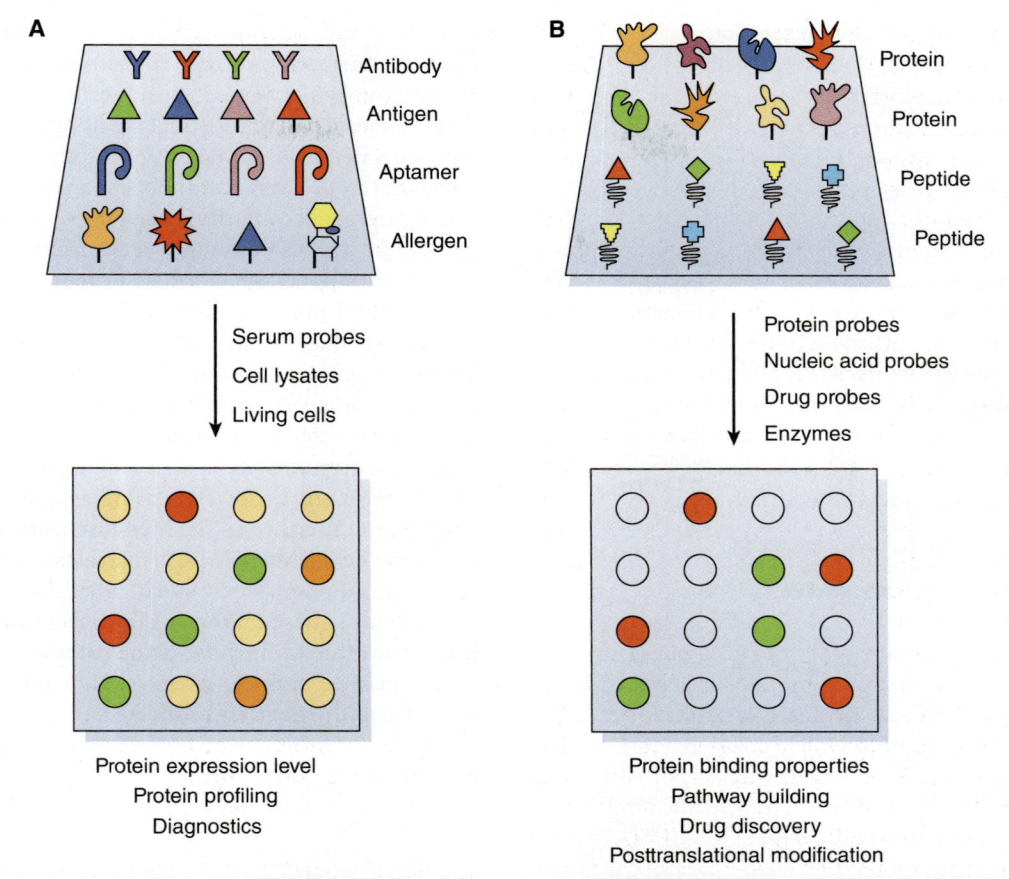

FIGURE 2–28 **A)** **Analytical protein microarray. Different types of ligands, including antibodies, antigens, DNA, or RNA aptamers (ie, short sequences that bind a specific target), carbohydrates, or small molecules, with high affinity and specificity, are spotted down.** These chips can be used for monitoring protein expression level, protein profiling, and clinical diagnostics. Similar to the procedure in DNA microarray experiments, protein samples from 2 biologic states to be compared are separately labeled with red or green fluorescent dyes, mixed, and incubated with the chips. Spots in red or green color identify an excess of proteins from one state over the other. **B)** Functional protein microarray. Native proteins or peptides are individually purified or synthesized using high-throughput approaches and arrayed onto a suitable surface to form the functional protein microarrays. These chips are used to analyze protein activities, binding properties, and posttranslational modifications. With the proper detection method, functional protein microarrays can be used to identify the substrates of enzymes of interest. Consequently, this class of chips is particularly useful in drug and drug-target identification and in building biologic networks. (Reproduced with permission from Phizicky E, Bastiaens PI, Zhu H, et al: Protein analysis on a proteomic scale. *Nature* 2003 Mar 13;422(6928):208-215.)

be degraded by ubiquitous RNases limits the performance of these assays.

2.5.1 Laser-Capture Microdissection

One problem associated with the molecular genetic analysis of small numbers of tumor cells is that associated normal cells can confound interpretation. Because stromal and other infiltrating cells are scattered throughout a tumor section, it is rarely possible to dissect a pure population of tumor cells cleanly. This problem has been circumvented by the use of laser capture microdissection, in which sections (usually from frozen tissue) are coated with a clear ethylene vinyl acetate (EVA) polymer prior to microscopic examination (Emmert-Buck et al, 1996). Tumor cells can be captured for subsequent analysis by briefly pulsing the area of interest with an infrared laser. The EVA film becomes adherent and attaches selectively to the tumor cells in the laser path. When sufficient cells have fused to the EVA film, it is placed into nucleic acid extraction buffers and used for PCR or other molecular analyses (Fig. 2–29). One application of laser capture microdissection is whole-genome amplification of captured cells, for example from a small number of tumor-derived cells. Several techniques including random PCR allow for the global amplification of all DNA sequences present in the microdissected samples, thereby increasing the amount of DNA for subsequent analysis. The method can also be adapted to generate representative amplification of the mRNA in a small number of cells. The technique has also been useful in providing DNA for molecular genetic studies using microdissected DNA from paraffin blocks, cDNA from single-cell RT-PCR reactions, and chromosome band–specific probes derived from microdissected chromosomal DNA.

2.5.2 Tissue Microarrays

Tissue microarrays (TMA) provide a method for relocating tissue from paraffin blocks so that tissue from multiple patients (or multiple blocks from the same patient) can be analyzed

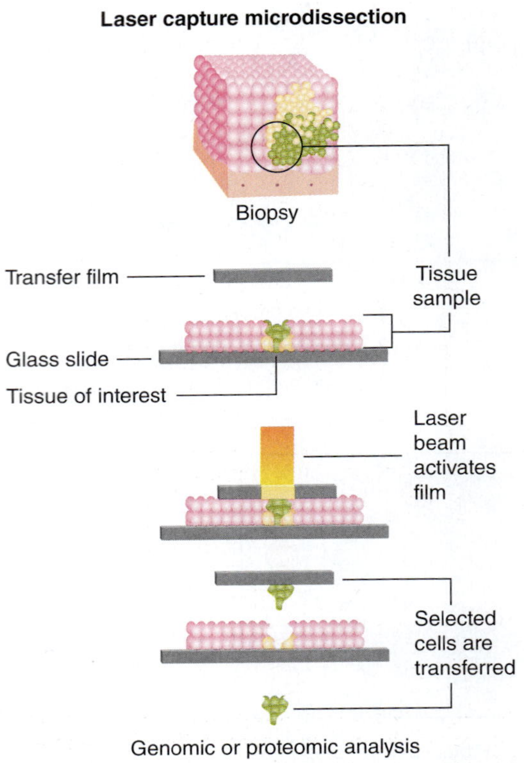

FIGURE 2–29 Outline of the process of laser-capture microdissection. Under a microscope–software interface, a tissue section (typically 5-50 μm thick) is assessed and cells are identified for the selection of targets for isolation. In general, collection technologies use an UV-pulsed laser for cutting the tissues directly, sometimes in combination with an infrared (IR) laser responsible for heating/melting a sticky polymer for cellular adhesion and isolation. After the collection, the tissue can be processed for protein, RNA, or DNA downstream analyses. (Reproduced with permission from National Cancer Institute at the National Institutes of Health.)

on the same slide. The microarray technique (Kononen et al, 1998) introduces a high-precision punching instrument that enables reproducible placement and relocation of distinct tissue samples. Construction of a TMA starts with the selection of suitable donor tissues and precise recording of the location of regions of interest. Needles with varying diameters of 0.6-2.0 mm are used to punch tissue cores from a predefined region of the tissue block. A hematoxylin and eosin stained slide arranged beside the donor block surface is used for orientation (Fig. 2–30). Tissue cores are transferred to a recipient paraffin wax block, into a ready-made hole, guided by a defined X–Y position. This technique minimizes tissue damage and allows sections to be cut from the donor paraffin wax block without loss of diagnostic details, even after the removal of multiple cores. The number of cores in the recipient paraffin block varies, with a maximum using a 0.6-mm needle of 600 to 2000 cores per standard glass microscope slide. Using this method, a cohort of samples (eg, from different patients) can be analyzed by staining just 1 or 2 master array slides, instead of staining hundreds of conventional slides. Each core on the array is similar to a conventional slide in that complete diagnostic and outcome information is maintained for each patient contributing to that core, so that rigorous statistical analysis can be performed when the arrays are analyzed.

A limitation of TMAs is that small punches of usually only a 0.6 mm diameter are taken from tumors with much larger diameter (up to several centimeters) and there may be considerable heterogeneity in the tissue sample. This problem can be reduced by analyzing multiple cores from each tissue sample. For example, the grading of breast cancer is dependent on the presence and number of mitoses. Because cell proliferation is higher at the periphery of the tumor, breast cancer arrays focusing on proliferation markers should be composed mainly of punches taken from the periphery of the tumor. Studies have shown that the frequency of prognostically significant gene amplifications in a series of invasive breast cancers, such as erbB2 or cyclin D1, is similar after TMA analysis to frequencies described in the literature using other techniques (Kononen et al, 1998). TMA is increasingly used for the identification and prognostic value of other cancer biomarkers, for example, for patients harboring the oncogenic BRAF mutation V600E, or in describing the tissue pathology that occurs during progressive multiple sclerosis (Giltnane and Rimm, 2004; Atak et al, 2016; Loveless et al, 2018).

2.5.3 Flow Cytometry

Flow cytometry enables the analysis of multiple properties of individual cells using a suspension of heterogeneous cells (Valihrach et al, 2018). The flow cytometer directs a beam of laser light of a single wavelength onto a hydrodynamically focused stream of saline solution, optimally of only 1 cell in diameter (Fig. 2–31A). Fluorescence detectors are aimed at the point where the stream passes through the light beam: one in line with the light beam (forward scatter) and several perpendicular to it (side scatter). Each suspended cell scatters the light as it passes through the beam. In addition, fluorescent molecules in the cell or attached to it may be excited and emit light at a longer wavelength than the light source. Forward scatter correlates with cell size and side scatter depends on the inner complexity or granularity of the cell (ie, shape of the nucleus, the amount and type of cytoplasmic granules, or the membrane roughness). Analysis of fluctuations in brightness at each detector (one for each fluorescent emission peak) provides information about the physical and chemical properties of individual cells. For example, fluorescently labeled antibodies can be applied to cells to quantify their ligands. Modern flow cytometers have multiple lasers and fluorescence detectors and can analyze multiple properties (using antibodies tagged with different fluorescent markers) of several thousand cells every second; they can separate, analyze, and isolate cells with specified properties. Acquisition of data is achieved by a computer using software that can adjust parameters (eg, voltage and compensation) for the sample being tested. Some instruments can take digital images of individual cells, allowing for analysis of location of the fluorescent signal within or on the surface of the cell.

Methods of Molecular Analysis 41

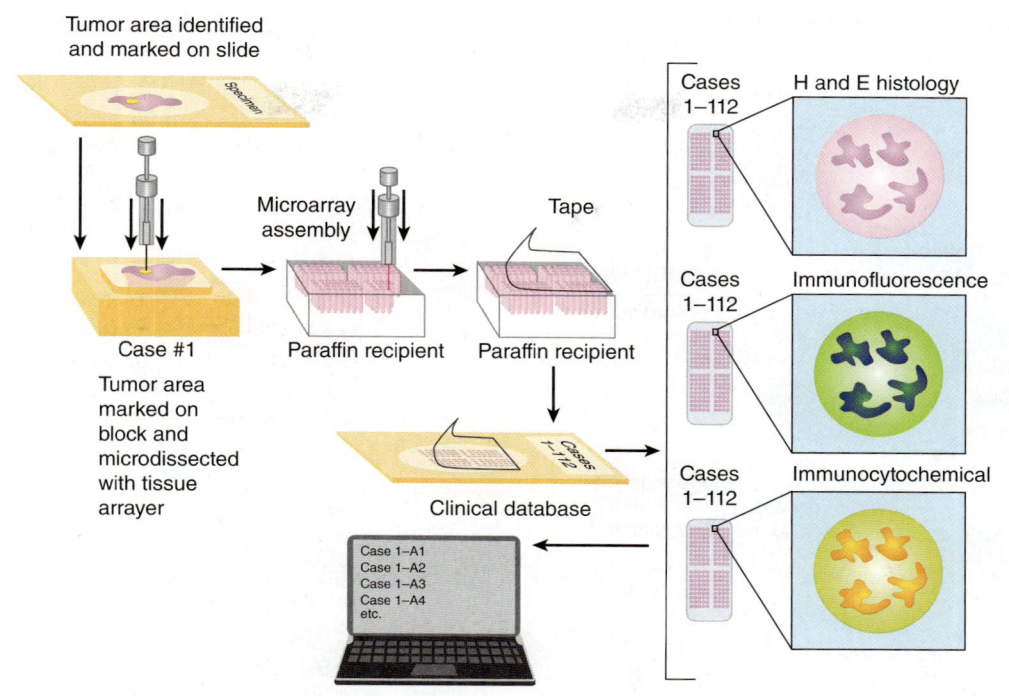

FIGURE 2–30 Outline of the process of TMA assembly. In the TMA technique, a hollow needle is used to remove tissue cores as small as 0.6 mm in diameter from regions of interest in paraffin-embedded tissues, such as clinical biopsies or tumor samples. These tissue cores are then inserted in a recipient paraffin block in a precisely spaced, array pattern, usually along with control samples. Sections from this block are cut using a microtome, mounted on a microscope slide, and then analyzed by any method of standard histologic analysis. Each microarray block can be cut into 100 to 500 sections, which can be subjected to independent tests. The number of spots on a single slide varies, depending on the array design, the current comfortable maximum with the 0.6-mm needle being about 600 spots per standard glass microscope slide. New technologies are under development that may allow as many as 2000 or more sections per slide. (Adapted with permission from http://apps.pathology.jhu.edu/blogs/pathology/wp-content/uploads/2010/05/Tissue_Microarray_Process.jpg.)

Applications of flow cytometry include analysis of the volume and morphologic complexity of cells; total DNA content and next-generation sequencing (NGS); total RNA content and sequencing (RNA-seq); microarray analysis or PCR; DNA copy number variation (by Flow-FISH); chromosome analysis and sorting (library construction, chromosome paints); protein expression and localization, western blotting and mass spectrometry including post-translation protein modifications; fluorescent protein detection; detection of cell surface antigens (cell differentiation [CD] markers); intracellular antigens (various cytokines, secondary mediators, etc); nuclear antigens; apoptosis (quantification, measurement of DNA degradation, mitochondrial membrane potential, permeability changes, caspase activity; see Chap. 8, Sec. 8.4); cell viability; and multidrug resistance (see Chap. 18) in cancer or stromal cells from the tumor cells.

Fluorescence-activated cell sorting is a specialized type of flow cytometry that allows a heterogeneous cell population to be sorted into 2 or more containers, based on the light-scattering and fluorescent properties of each cell (Fig. 2–31B). It uses a similar system of hydrodynamic focusing but with a large separation between cells relative to cell diameter. A vibrating mechanism causes the stream of cells to break into individual droplets with a low probability of more than 1 cell per droplet. Just before the stream breaks into droplets, the flow passes through a fluorescence-measuring station and an electrical charge is applied to the droplet, depending on the fluorescence-intensity measurement. The charged droplets then fall through an electrostatic deflection system that diverts droplets into different chambers based on their charge.

In mass spectroscopy or cyTOF (cytometry time-of-flight), antibodies are tagged with a heavy metal rather than a fluorophore, and the sample composition can be analyzed using TOF MS for up to 30 or more antibodies in a single experiment. This information can then be integrated with other high-throughput analysis of the sample (RNA-profiling, genome sequencing, etc.) to provide a comprehensive readout of dynamic and heterogeneous features of normal or tumor tissue sections (Bodenmiller, 2016).

2.6 BIOINFORMATICS AND OTHER TECHNIQUES OF DATA ANALYSIS

Bioinformatics employs a variety of computational techniques to analyze biologic data and to integrate the data with publicly available resources. The specific tools used to analyze large data sets depend on the specific method employed. This section outlines 4 considerations that are commonly encountered

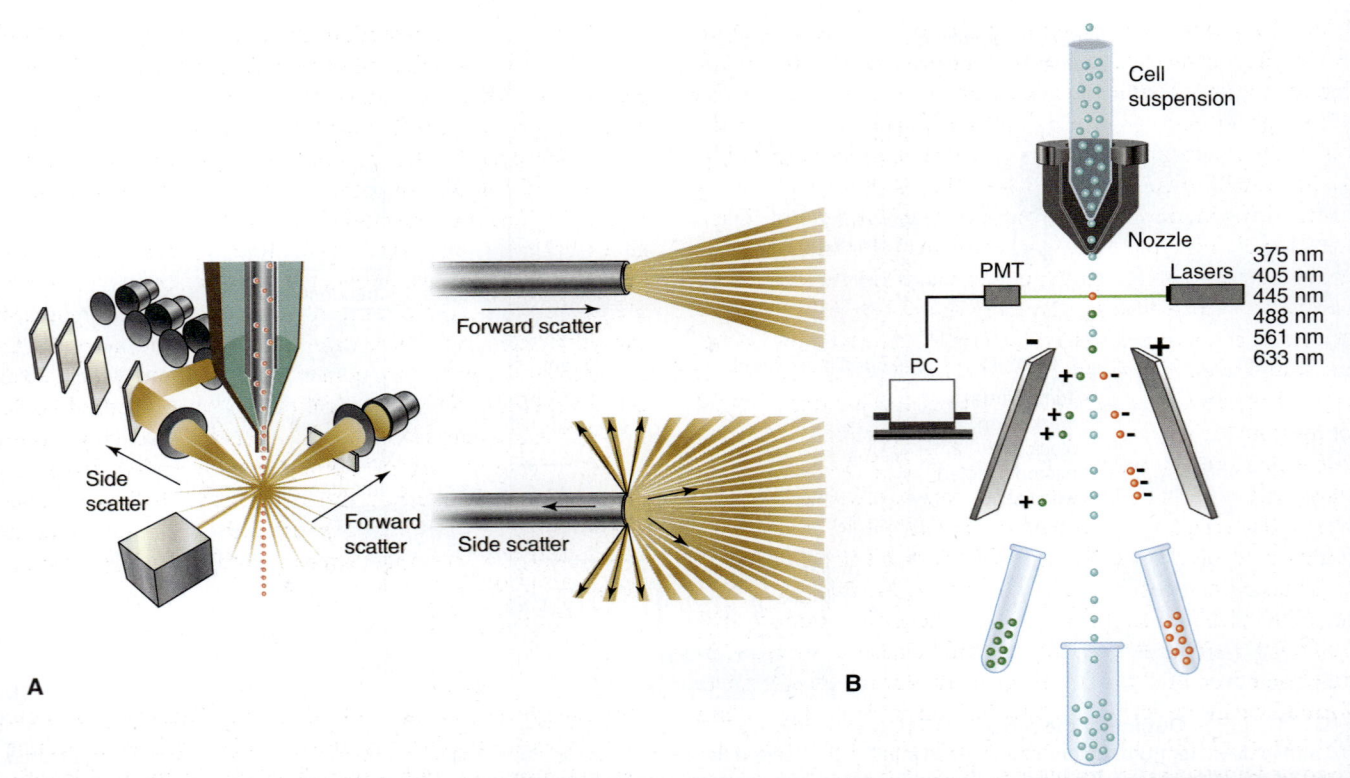

FIGURE 2–31 In flow cytometry, lenses are used to shape and focus the excitation beam from a laser, directing the beam through the hydrodynamically focused sample stream. **A)** Where the laser intersects the stream is the "interrogation zone," when the particle passes through the interrogation zone there is light scatter and possibly fluorescence; it is the detection and analysis of this light scatter and fluorescence that gives information about a particle. To detect the light scatter and fluorescent light, there are 2 detectors—one in line with the laser (to detect forward scatter) and one perpendicular to the laser (to detect side scatter). The intensity of the forward scatter is in relation to the particle size. The side scatter channel (SSC) detects light at a 90° angle to the laser source point; this scatter gives information on granularity and internal complexity. **B) Multiparametric flow cytometry.** Multiple lasers permit the fluorescence activation of numerous fluorochromes in the same sample, that can then be gated and sorted according to their particular properties. These sorted populations can then be harvested and analyzed via numerous applications, as mentioned in the text. (Part (B) Reproduced with permission from Hodne K, Weltzien FA. Single-Cell Isolation and Gene Analysis: Pitfalls and Possibilities. *Int J Mol Sci* 2015 Nov 10;16(11):26832-26849.)

in the analysis of large data sets, including statistical analysis, unsupervised clustering, gene signatures, and network analysis.

2.6.1 Statistical Analysis

A common question in the analysis of biologic data sets is whether 2 groups possess a statistically significant difference from each another. In statistics, the "null hypothesis" refers to the basal assumption that the 2 sample groups do not differ significantly. A statistical test is designed to query whether the null hypothesis can be rejected with a specified confidence level. In cancer research, for example, it is applied to situations involving different test situations that may include treatment/vehicle, case/control, and genetic-perturbation/wild-type comparisons. Several statistical tests have been evaluated to address 2-group comparisons, where it is common to apply t tests, for example, to compare the mean expression of a gene between 2 groups of samples. The t test assumes that the 2 groups have similar variability; in cancer studies, this assumption is often violated, as some tumor types are more heterogeneous than others, and there is usually more variability in tumors than normal tissues, but corrections can be applied.

The t test also assumes that the data are drawn (sampled) from a population with a normal distribution, and it is difficult to verify this assumption—tests for the normality of a distribution are insensitive. Finally, use of multiple t tests assumes that each test is independent of the others. For example, microarray data often violate this assumption, as the expression of RNA from different genes can be highly correlated.

Often, queries related to translational oncology involve assessment of patient survival or tumor recurrence as a function of time. The analysis of survival is usually performed using log-rank analysis (see Chap. 22, Sec. 22.3.6). An alternative, the Cox proportional hazards model, incorporates multiple regression and enables the difference between survival times of particular groups of patients to be tested while allowing for factors (covariates) that are likely to influence survival.

Independent of which statistical test is employed, the final set of P values must be considered carefully. A P value represents the chance of making a Type I (or α, false positive) error for testing a *single* hypothesis. Consider an experiment where 20 primary colon cancers are analyzed by microarray analysis to measure the mRNA abundance of 10,000 genes.

These 20 samples are randomly split into 2 groups of 10 each, where there is no expectation that the groups are actually different. A simple t test is used to compare the level of each of the 10,000 genes between groups, and a stringent P value threshold of .01 is applied. In this case, we predict that there will be $10,000 \times 0.01 = 100$ false-positives; that is, 100 genes will be found different between the 2 groups by chance alone. There are several "multiple testing adjustments" that help alleviate this problem. A stringent adjustment is called the *Bonferroni correction*, which involves dividing the threshold P value by the number of tests to be performed. In the example above, we would use a threshold of $P < .01/10,000$, or $P < 10^{-6}$. This type of adjustment is very conservative, as it assumes that all of the comparisons are independent (whereas many are often correlated) and suggests that, across all 10,000 tests, we will have only a 1% chance of finding even 1 false-positive. An alternative is called the *false-discovery rate* (FDR) adjustment, which controls the percentage of tests that will be expected to be false-positives. For example, if there are 100 genes with an FDR <0.1 (eg, an FDR of 10%), then we anticipate that $100 \times 0.1 = 10$ genes from this list will be false-positives. Calculation of the FDR for any experiment is complex but is performed easily in common statistical software packages, and the use of FDR-adjusted P values (also called q values) has become widespread in genomic studies.

2.6.2 Unsupervised Clustering

When analyzing large data sets across numerous samples, for example, the differentially expressed genes across the genome using RNA-seq, there remains the major challenge of interpreting their biologic relevance. A common technique is to group together similar patterns of change in gene expression. This approach may provide information about coregulation of genes, and coregulated genes are known to share biologic functions (Boutros and Okey, 2005). In this manner, patterns of similarity of differentially expressed genes might be used to inform disease etiology or mechanisms.

The next step is to select an appropriate method to classify patterns (eg, of gene expression). If the biologic question involves a characteristic of the samples—such as identifying novel tumor subtypes or predicting patient response—then supervised machine-learning methods (described below) are most appropriate. If the goal involves characteristics of individual genes, then an unsupervised method is more appropriate. These unsupervised methods are often called *clustering methods*, and available techniques are distinguished by their mathematical characteristics and the assumptions that they make. A commonly used method called *k-mean clustering* assumes that the number of "classes" of genes can be defined a priori but makes no other assumptions regarding the interrelationships between specific pairs of genes. Another common method, called *hierarchical clustering*, makes no assumptions regarding the number of classes of genes. Instead, it assumes that genes are related to each other in a hierarchical way, where certain gene pairs are more related than others (Duda et al, 2001).

A common misconception about unsupervised methods such as clustering is that all genes within a single group share a common mechanism. However, different genes may exhibit similar expression profiles, without sharing a common mechanism. For example, the p53 response might be abrogated in tumors by multiple mechanisms, each producing the same resulting expression profile. Many factors may lead to sets of genes being co-regulated, especially in genome-wide experiments where millions of gene-pairs are assessed. Clustering methods only identify genes that are correlated: hypotheses can be framed from these data, but there is no necessity for a single underlying mechanism (Boutros and Okey, 2005; Boutros, 2006). Newer applications of these methodologies include the analysis of single-cell RNA-sequencing, where specific clustering algorithms are recommended depending on whether the sequence reads represent shallow coverage over large numbers of cells, or whether the reads represent more in-depth coverage over a smaller cell population (Menon, 2018).

2.6.3 Gene Signatures

Increasingly microarray and other -omic data sets are being used to make predictions about clinical behavior. Features that are correlated with a specific clinical event are identified using an appropriate statistical methodology, and then merged to construct a multifeature predictive signature. Multivariable analysis, which is distinguished from multivariate analysis that refers to models with 2 or more dependent or outcome variables, is used to exclude factors that are correlated, thereby identifying independent predictors (Hidalgo and Goodman, 2013). This signature is then evaluated in independent groups of patients to test and demonstrate its robustness. This approach was first applied to demonstrate that acute myeloid and acute lymphoblastic leukemias could be distinguished on the basis of their mRNA expression profiles (Golub et al, 1999). Many studies extended this initial work to demonstrate that tumor subtypes could be distinguished and even discovered from microarray data (Bild et al, 2006; Chin et al, 2006; Neve et al, 2006).

A second major application of machine-learning techniques to -omic data has substantially changed clinical practice. Rather than defining tumor subtypes, investigators have sought to predict which patients might be under- or overtreated. The first major study identified a 70-gene signature that predicted survival of women with breast cancer (van't Veer et al, 2002). Subsequent external validations have helped this predictor to be developed into a tool that is used in clinical practice (Cardoso et al, 2016). Similar efforts have led to the development of prognostic signatures for other tumor types, including non–small cell lung carcinoma (Beer et al, 2002; Chen et al, 2007; Lau et al, 2007; Boutros et al, 2009) and serous ovarian cancers (Mok et al, 2009). Nevertheless, the field has come under critical review for the proliferation of poorly validated and described signatures (Shedden et al, 2008; Subramanian and Simon, 2010), with evidence that many studies are underpowered.

2.6.4 Network Analysis

Concurrently with the generation of large genome-wide data sets, researchers have developed a plethora of tools that enable not just the annotation of gene function, but the complex relationships between genes, RNA, and protein.

Gene ontology (GO) is a systematic attempt to organize and categorize what is known about gene function and localization. GO defines functions first in a general, nonspecific manner and is then refined into more specific statements. Each of these functions is given a specific GO identifier, and if a gene is assigned a specific function, it automatically "inherits" all less-specific functions (Consortium, 2001). Different genes possess varying degrees of GO annotation. Some well-characterized genes will be annotated with many different functions, whereas other less-characterized genes may possess little or no annotation. For example, a gene might first be described as involved in the general process of "metabolism," then the more specific process of "monosaccharide metabolism" (GO:0005996), then the more specific terms of "hexose metabolism" (GO:0019318), "fructose metabolism" (GO:0006000), and, ultimately, the most precise term, "fructose 1,6-bisphosphonate metabolism" (GO:0030388). The website geneontology.org contains a vast array of searchable GO-term data that can be queried for multiple parameters. There are also valuable online resources for protein localization, and even RNA or protein expression across all tissues within an organism (eg, see ebi.ac.uk; www.informatics.jax.org, and www.proteinatlas.org), and high-density mapping of proximal protein interactions within a human cell line (www.cell-map.org).

Multiple online tools associate each gene with its known GO annotation. These tools assign a statistical assessment of "GO enrichment": in other words, are there any specific GO terms that occur more often than expected by chance in this list of genes? Examples of newer databases that integrate genomics data with GO term enrichments include DepMap, which is the Cancer Dependency Map Project at the Broad Institute in Boston, MA (www.depmap.org). This online resource contains information about genetic dependency profiles across more than 500 human cell lines, genetic and pharmacologic properties of >1000 cell lines, genetic drivers of cancer, and other –omics data published or generated at the Broad Institute and elsewhere.

Complementary to these approaches are databases that contain annotated protein-protein interactions across a wide array of organisms and experimental conditions (see Sec. 2.5), including humans. Once a database of protein-protein interactions has been identified, a common approach is to superimpose a gene list on the overall network. Each gene in the list, along with its nearest neighbors (ie, the direct interactions), is then probed. The interaction network can be arranged in 2-dimensional space, and if the genes on the list are more proximal to one another than would be expected by chance alone, it is probable that they encode components of common functional pathways. This approach has identified critical characteristics of cancer cells, including opportunities to exploit synthetic lethal interactions, for example the exquisite sensitivity of BRCA-deficient cancers to PARP inhibition (O'Neil et al, 2017; Ashworth and Lord, 2018). The sophistication of these online data sets is ever-increasing. As one example, The BioGRID repository, which started as an initiative to map genetic and protein interaction networks in budding yeast, now includes more than 1.5 million biologic interactions across 71 species, including post-translational modifications, drug interactions, and CRISPR/Cas9 screen data (Oughtred et al, 2019) (www.thebiogrid.org).

Recent efforts in cancer research have focused on the integrated analysis of a large number of parameters; genetic, epigenetic, transcriptomics, and proteomics. These approaches have yielded insights regarding the molecular evolution of cancer, and the classification of tumor types into those with different prognostic outcomes or likelihood of treatment response. For example, in prostate cancer, the whole genome, transcriptome, and methylome of early-onset prostate cancers revealed age-related genomic alterations and a temporal regulation of mutational cancer evolution. These findings enabled researchers to identify 4 tumor subgroups, including an aggressive subgroup with recurrent genomic duplications (Gerhauser et al, 2018).

SUMMARY

- Cytogenetics and karyotyping inform tumor genomics and pathophysiology; increasingly, however, these techniques have been replaced by newer methods.
- There are an increasing array of methods to probe DNA, RNA, and proteins within cellular systems. These include standard techniques of Southern, northern, and western blots, respectively, as well as functional manipulations, including new methods of genome editing such as CRISPR-Cas. Ultimately, xenograft or mouse models can be manipulated to provide in vivo assessments of cancer initiation, progression, and therapeutics.
- PCR-based techniques allow the (1) amplification of small volumes of DNA and cDNA; (2) quantification, both relative and absolute, of particular DNA or RNA sequences; and (3) assistance in next-generation sequencing.
- High-throughput or "next-generation" sequencing approaches have become increasingly cost-effective and have provided startling new insights into cancer progression and diversity.
- Improved technologies have revealed the increasingly complex variation in the human genome at both the base-pair level (SNPs) and larger sequence levels (CNVs). The effect of these variations is being explored but is already known to influence cancer predisposition, progression, and response to treatment.
- Established techniques for the assessment of human tissue samples for translational research include TMA construction (with subsequent downstream analyses for immunohistochemistry, immunofluorescence, or FISH), laser capture microdissection (for gene expression), and

- flow cytometry (for a variety of applications such as surface protein assessments).
- ▶ Proteome research provides a comprehensive description of the proteins present in a biologic entity under specific conditions. With the recent advent of improved methods and the introduction of more sensitive and faster scanning mass spectrometers, the near-complete analyses of complex human proteomes is becoming feasible.
- ▶ Methodologic advances enable the accurate relative quantification of thousands of proteins using stable isotope technology.
- ▶ Targeted proteomics approaches based on selected reaction monitoring (SRM) are the most commonly used approach for multiplex quantification in biomarker verification experiments.
- ▶ Sophisticated bioinformatics approaches are quickly developing, and are invaluable in the analysis of large genomic (and other –omic) data sets.

ACKNOWLEDGMENTS

We also wish to thank previous authors of this chapter, namely Anthony Joshua, for his substantial contribution to the text.

REFERENCES

Akbani R, Becker KF, Carragher N, et al. Realizing the promise of reverse phase protein arrays for clinical, translational, and basic research: a workshop report: the RPPA (Reverse Phase Protein Array) society. *Mol Cell Proteomics* 2014;13(7):1625-1643.

Alkan C, Sajjadian S, Eichler EE. Limitations of next-generation genome sequence assembly. *Nat Methods* 2011;8(1):61-65.

Appella E, Anderson CW. New prospects for proteomics—electron-capture (ECD) and electron-transfer dissociation (ETD) fragmentation techniques and combined fractional diagonal chromatography (COFRADIC). *FEBS J* 2007;274(24):6255.

Ashworth A, Lord CJ. Synthetic lethal therapies for cancer: what's next after PARP inhibitors? *Nat Rev Clin Oncol* 2018;15(9):564-576.

Atak A, Mukherjee S, Jain R, et al. Protein microarray applications: autoantibody detection and posttranslational modification. *Proteomics* 2016;16(19):2557-2569.

Bailey P, Chang DK, Nones K, et al. Genomic analyses identify molecular subtypes of pancreatic cancer. *Nature* 2016;531(7592):47-52.

Bates SE. Epigenetic Therapies for Cancer. *N Engl J Med* 2020;383(7):650-663.

Beer DG, Kardia SL, Huang CC, et al. Gene-expression profiles predict survival of patients with lung adenocarcinoma. *Nat Med* 2002;8(8):816-824.

Biemann K, Cone C, Webster BR, Arsenault GP. Determination of the amino acid sequence in oligopeptides by computer interpretation of their high-resolution mass spectra. *J Am Chem Soc* 1966;88(23):5598-5606.

Bild AH, Yao G, Chang JT, et al. Oncogenic pathway signatures in human cancers as a guide to targeted therapies. *Nature* 2006;439(7074):353-357.

Binai NA, Marino F, Soendergaard P, Bache N, Mohammed S, Heck AJ. Rapid analyses of proteomes and interactomes using an integrated solid-phase extraction-liquid chromatography-MS/MS system. *J Proteome Res* 2015;14(2):977-985.

Bodenmiller B. Multiplexed epitope-based tissue imaging for discovery and healthcare applications. *Cell Syst* 2016;2(4):225-238.

Bohnert R, Vivas S, Jansen G. Comprehensive benchmarking of SNV callers for highly admixed tumor data. *PLoS One* 2017;12(10):e0186175.

Bonci D, Coppola V, Musumeci M, et al. The miR-15a-miR-16-1 cluster controls prostate cancer by targeting multiple oncogenic activities. *Nat Med* 2008;14(11):1271-1277.

Bottoni A, Piccin D, Tagliati F, Luchin A, Zatelli MC, degli Uberti EC. miR-15a and miR-16-1 down-regulation in pituitary adenomas. *J Cell Physiol* 2005;204(1):280-285.

Boutros PC. To cluster or not to cluster: the uses and misuses of clustering algorithms. *Hypothesis* 2006;4(1):28-32.

Boutros PC, Lau SK, Pintilie M, et al. Prognostic gene signatures for non-small-cell lung cancer. *Proc Natl Acad Sci U S A* 2009;106(8):2824-2828.

Boutros PC, Margolin AA, Stuart JM, Califano A, Stolovitzky G. Toward better benchmarking: challenge-based methods assessment in cancer genomics. *Genome Biol* 2014;15(9):462.

Boutros PC, Okey AB. Unsupervised pattern recognition: an introduction to the whys and wherefores of clustering microarray data. *Brief Bioinform* 2005;6(4):331-343.

Brothman AR, Persons DL, Shaffer LG. Nomenclature evolution: changes in the ISCN from the 2005 to the 2009 edition. *Cytogenet Genome Res* 2009;127(1):1-4.

Cai L, Yuan W, Zhang Z, He L, Chou KC. In-depth comparison of somatic point mutation callers based on different tumor next-generation sequencing depth data. *Sci Rep* 2016;6:36540.

Calin GA, Ferracin M, Cimmino A, et al. A MicroRNA signature associated with prognosis and progression in chronic lymphocytic leukemia. *N Engl J Med* 2005;353(17):1793-1801.

Cardoso F, van't Veer LJ, Bogaerts J, et al. 70-gene signature as an aid to treatment decisions in early-stage breast cancer. *N Engl J Med.* 2016;375(8):717-729.

Casini A, Storch M, Baldwin GS, Ellis T. Bricks and blueprints: methods and standards for DNA assembly. *Nat Rev Mol Cell Biol* 2015;16(9):568-576.

Catherman AD, Durbin KR, Ahlf DR, et al. Large-scale top-down proteomics of the human proteome: membrane proteins, mitochondria, and senescence. *Mol Cell Proteomics* 2013;12(12):3465-3473.

Catherman AD, Li M, Tran JC, et al. Top down proteomics of human membrane proteins from enriched mitochondrial fractions. *Anal Chem* 2013;85(3):1880-1888.

Cerami E, Demir E, Schultz N, Taylor BS, Sander C. Automated network analysis identifies core pathways in glioblastoma. *PLoS One* 2010;5(2):e8918.

Chayen NE. Methods for separating nucleation and growth in protein crystallisation. *Prog Biophys Mol Biol* 2005;88(3):329-337.

Chen HY, Yu SL, Chen CH, et al. A five-gene signature and clinical outcome in non-small-cell lung cancer. *N Engl J Med* 2007;356(1):11-20.

Cheng J, Demeulemeester J, Wedge DC, et al. Pan-cancer analysis of homozygous deletions in primary tumours uncovers rare tumour suppressors. *Nat Commun* 2017;8(1):1221.

Chernov AA. Protein crystals and their growth. *J Struct Biol* 2003;142(1):3-21.

Chin K, DeVries S, Fridlyand J, et al. Genomic and transcriptional aberrations linked to breast cancer pathophysiologies. *Cancer Cell* 2006;10(6):529-541.

Chowdhury SM, Munske GR, Ronald RC, Bruce JE. Evaluation of low energy CID and ECD fragmentation behavior of mono-oxidized thio-ether bonds in peptides. *J Am Soc Mass Spectrom* 2007;18(3):493-501.

Cieslik M, Chinnaiyan AM. Global genomics project unravels cancer's complexity at unprecedented scale. *Nature* 2020;578(7793):39-40.

Clevers H. Modeling development and disease with organoids. *Cell* 2016;165(7):1586-1597.

Colas P, Brent R. The impact of two-hybrid and related methods on biotechnology. *Trends Biotechnol* 1998;16(8):355-363.

Cox J, Mann M. Is proteomics the new genomics? *Cell* 2007;130(3):395-398.

Dalgleish JL, Wang Y, Zhu J, Meltzer PS. CNVScope: visually exploring copy number aberrations in cancer genomes. *Cancer Inform* 2019;18:1176935119890290.

Danev R, Yanagisawa H, Kikkawa M. Cryo-electron microscopy methodology: current aspects and future directions. *Trends Biochem Sci* 2019;44(10):837-848.

Demirci S, Leonard A, Haro-Mora JJ, Uchida N, Tisdale JF. CRISPR/Cas9 for sickle cell disease: applications, future possibilities, and challenges. *Adv Exp Med Biol* 2019;1144:37-52.

Diskin SJ, Hou C, Glessner JT, et al. Copy number variation at 1q21.1 associated with neuroblastoma. *Nature* 2009;459(7249):987-991.

Doll S, Dressen M, Geyer PE, et al. Region and cell-type resolved quantitative proteomic map of the human heart. *Nat Commun.* 2017;8(1):1469.

Duda RO, Hart PE, Stork DG. *Pattern classification*. 2nd ed. New York, NY: Wiley; 2001.

Emmert-Buck MR, Bonner RF, Smith PD, et al. Laser capture microdissection. *Science* 1996;274(5289):998-1001.

Engreitz J, Abudayyeh O, Gootenberg J, Zhang F. CRISPR tools for systematic studies of RNA regulation. *Cold Spring Harb Perspect Biol* 2019;11(8).

Ewing AD, Houlahan KE, Hu Y, et al. Combining tumor genome simulation with crowdsourcing to benchmark somatic single-nucleotide-variant detection. *Nat Methods* 2015;12(7):623-630.

Faria NR, Quick J, Claro IM, et al. Establishment and cryptic transmission of Zika virus in Brazil and the Americas. *Nature* 2017;546(7658):406-410.

Fields S. Interactive learning: lessons from two hybrids over two decades. *Proteomics* 2009;9(23):5209-5213.

Fornelli L, Durbin KR, Fellers RT, et al. Advancing top-down analysis of the human proteome using a benchtop quadrupole-orbitrap mass spectrometer. *J Proteome Res* 2017;16(2):609-618.

Fornelli L, Toby TK, Schachner LF, et al. Top-down proteomics: where we are, where we are going? *J Proteomics* 2018;175:3-4.

Fort KL, Dyachenko A, Potel CM, et al. Implementation of ultraviolet photodissociation on a benchtop Q exactive mass spectrometer and its application to phosphoproteomics. *Anal Chem* 2016;88(4):2303-2310.

Fraser M, Sabelnykova VY, Yamaguchi TN, et al. Genomic hallmarks of localized, non-indolent prostate cancer. *Nature* 2017;541(7637):359-364.

Fujimoto A, Furuta M, Totoki Y, et al. Whole-genome mutational landscape and characterization of noncoding and structural mutations in liver cancer. *Nat Genet* 2016;48(5):500-509.

Gambacorti-Passerini CB, Gunby RH, Piazza R, Galietta A, Rostagno R, Scapozza L. Molecular mechanisms of resistance to imatinib in Philadelphia-chromosome-positive leukaemias. *Lancet Oncol* 2003;4(2):75-85.

Garcia-Nafria J, Tate CG. Cryo-electron microscopy: moving beyond X-ray crystal structures for drug receptors and drug development. *Annu Rev Pharmacol Toxicol* 2020;60:51-71.

Geiger T, Cox J, Ostasiewicz P, Wisniewski JR, Mann M. Super-SILAC mix for quantitative proteomics of human tumor tissue. *Nat Methods* 2010;7(5):383-385.

Gerhards NM, Rottenberg S. New tools for old drugs: functional genetic screens to optimize current chemotherapy. *Drug Resist Updat* 2018;36:30-46.

Gerhauser C, Favero F, Risch T, et al. Molecular evolution of early-onset prostate cancer identifies molecular risk markers and clinical trajectories. *Cancer Cell* 2018;34(6):996-1011.e8.

Geyer PE, Voytik E, Treit PV, et al. Plasma proteome profiling to detect and avoid sample-related biases in biomarker studies. *EMBO Mol Med* 2019;11(11):e10427.

Ghosh R, Gilda JE, Gomes AV. The necessity of and strategies for improving confidence in the accuracy of western blots. *Expert Rev Proteomics* 2014;11(5):549-560.

Gillet LC, Navarro P, Tate S, et al. Targeted data extraction of the MS/MS spectra generated by data-independent acquisition: a new concept for consistent and accurate proteome analysis. *Mol Cell Proteomics* 2012;11(6):O111.016717.

Giltnane JM, Rimm DL. Technology insight: identification of biomarkers with tissue microarray technology. *Nat Clin Pract Oncol* 2004;1(2):104-111.

Gingras AC, Abe KT, Raught B. Getting to know the neighborhood: using proximity-dependent biotinylation to characterize protein complexes and map organelles. *Curr Opin Chem Biol* 2019;48:44-54.

Golub TR, Slonim DK, Tamayo P, et al. Molecular classification of cancer: class discovery and class prediction by gene expression monitoring. *Science* 1999;286(5439):531-537.

Gurumurthy CB, Lloyd KCK. Generating mouse models for biomedical research: technological advances. *Dis Model Mech* 2019;12(1):dmm029462.

Gutbrod MJ, Martienssen RA. Conserved chromosomal functions of RNA interference. *Nat Rev Genet* 2020;21:311-331.

Hall DA, Ptacek J, Snyder M. Protein microarray technology. *Mech Ageing Dev* 2007;128(1):161-167.

Hampoelz B, Mackmull MT, Machado P, et al. Pre-assembled nuclear pores insert into the nuclear envelope during early development. *Cell* 2016;166(3):664-678.

Hayward NK, Wilmott JS, Waddell N, et al. Whole-genome landscapes of major melanoma subtypes. *Nature* 2017;545(7653):175-180.

Hidalgo B, Goodman M. Multivariate or multivariable regression? *Am J Public Health*. 2013;103(1):39-40.

Hodne K, Weltzien FA. Single-cell isolation and gene analysis: pitfalls and possibilities. *Int J Mol Sci* 2015;16(11):26832-26849.

Hoelz A, Glavy JS, Beck M. Toward the atomic structure of the nuclear pore complex: when top down meets bottom up. *Nat Struct Mol Biol*. 2016;23(7):624-630.

Hoffman M, Gillmor AH, Kunz DJ, et al. Intratumoral genetic and functional heterogeneity in pediatric glioblastoma. *Cancer Res* 2019;79(9):2111-2123.

Hsu PD, Lander ES, Zhang F. Development and applications of CRISPR-Cas9 for genome engineering. *Cell* 2014;157(6):1262-1278.

Huttenhain R, Choi M, Martin de la Fuente L, et al. A targeted mass spectrometry strategy for developing proteomic biomarkers: a case study of epithelial ovarian cancer. *Mol Cell Proteomics* 2019;18(9):1836-1850.

Hwang S, Maxwell KL. Meet the anti-CRISPRs: widespread protein inhibitors of CRISPR-cas systems. *CRISPR J* 2019;2(1):23-30.

Ip CLC, Loose M, Tyson JR, et al. MinION analysis and reference consortium: phase 1 data release and analysis. *F1000Res* 2015;4:1075.

Justice MJ, Siracusa LD, Stewart AF. Technical approaches for mouse models of human disease. *Dis Model Mech* 2011;4(3):305-310.

Kelleher NL. Top-down proteomics. *Anal Chem* 2004;76(11):197A-203A.

Kellie JF, Catherman AD, Durbin KR, et al. Robust analysis of the yeast proteome under 50 kDa by molecular-mass-based fractionation and top-down mass spectrometry. *Anal Chem* 2012;84(1):209-215.

Kiselev VY, Andrews TS, Hemberg M. Challenges in unsupervised clustering of single-cell RNA-seq data. *Nat Rev Genet* 2019;20(5):273-282.

Knouse KA, Lopez KE, Bachofner M, Amon A. Chromosome segregation fidelity in epithelia requires tissue architecture. *Cell* 2018;175(1):200-211.e3.

Knudson AG Jr. Mutation and cancer: statistical study of retinoblastoma. *Proc Natl Acad Sci U S A* 1971;68(4):820-823.

Kononen J, Bubendorf L, Kallioniemi A, et al. Tissue microarrays for high-throughput molecular profiling of tumor specimens. *Nat Med* 1998;4(7):844-847.

Kosinski J, Mosalaganti S, von Appen A, et al. Molecular architecture of the inner ring scaffold of the human nuclear pore complex. *Science* 2016;352(6283):363-365.

Kruger M, Moser M, Ussar S, et al. SILAC mouse for quantitative proteomics uncovers kindlin-3 as an essential factor for red blood cell function. *Cell* 2008;134(2):353-364.

Lau SK, Boutros PC, Pintilie M, et al. Three-gene prognostic classifier for early-stage non small-cell lung cancer. *J Clin Oncol*. 2007;25(35):5562-5569.

Leary RJ, Lin JC, Cummins J, et al. Integrated analysis of homozygous deletions, focal amplifications, and sequence alterations in breast and colorectal cancers. *Proc Natl Acad Sci U S A* 2008;105(42):16224-16229.

Lemay ML, Horvath P, Moineau S. The CRISPR-Cas app goes viral. *Curr Opin Microbiol*. 2017;37:103-109.

Li H, Durbin R. Fast and accurate short read alignment with Burrows-Wheeler transform. *Bioinformatics*. 2009;25(14):1754-1760.

Liu H, Sadygov RG, Yates JR 3rd. A model for random sampling and estimation of relative protein abundance in shotgun proteomics. *Anal Chem* 2004;76(14):4193-4201.

Liu W, Sun J, Li G, et al. Association of a germ-line copy number variation at 2p24.3 and risk for aggressive prostate cancer. *Cancer Res* 2009;69(6):2176-2179.

Loman NJ, Quick J, Simpson JT. A complete bacterial genome assembled de novo using only nanopore sequencing data. *Nat Methods* 2015;12(8):733-735.

Loveless S, Neal JW, Howell OW, et al. Tissue microarray methodology identifies complement pathway activation and dysregulation in progressive multiple sclerosis. *Brain Pathol* 2018;28(4):507-520.

Ma B, Zhang K, Hendrie C, et al. PEAKS: powerful software for peptide de novo sequencing by tandem mass spectrometry. *Rapid Commun Mass Spectrom* 2003;17(20):2337-2342.

Marino F, Cristobal A, Binai NA, Bache N, Heck AJ, Mohammed S. Characterization and usage of the EASY-spray technology as part of an online 2D SCX-RP ultra-high pressure system. *Analyst* 2014;139(24):6520-6528.

Marouga R, David S, Hawkins E. The development of the DIGE system: 2D fluorescence difference gel analysis technology. *Anal Bioanal Chem* 2005;382(3):669-678.

Marx H, Lemeer S, Schliep JE, et al. A large synthetic peptide and phosphopeptide reference library for mass spectrometry-based proteomics. *Nat Biotechnol* 2013;31(6):557-564.

Menon V. Clustering single cells: a review of approaches on high-and low-depth single-cell RNA-seq data. *Brief Funct Genomics* 2018;17(4):240-245.

Mertins P, Mani DR, Ruggles KV, et al. Proteogenomics connects somatic mutations to signalling in breast cancer. *Nature* 2016;534(7605):55-62.

Metzker ML. Sequencing technologies—the next generation. *Nat Rev Genet* 2010;11(1):31-46.

Michnick SW, Ear PH, Landry C, Malleshaiah MK, Messier V. Protein-fragment complementation assays for large-scale analysis, functional dissection and dynamic studies of protein-protein interactions in living cells. *Methods Mol Biol* 2011;756:395-425.

Midha MK, Wu M, Chiu KP. Long-read sequencing in deciphering human genetics to a greater depth. *Hum Genet* 2019;138(11-12):1201-1215.

Mikesh LM, Ueberheide B, Chi A, et al. The utility of ETD mass spectrometry in proteomic analysis. *Biochim Biophys Acta* 2006;1764(12):1811-1822.

Mok SC, Bonome T, Vathipadiekal V, et al. A gene signature predictive for outcome in advanced ovarian cancer identifies a survival factor: microfibril-associated glycoprotein 2. *Cancer Cell* 2009;16(6):521-532.

Neve RM, Chin K, Fridlyand J, et al. A collection of breast cancer cell lines for the study of functionally distinct cancer subtypes. *Cancer Cell* 2006;10(6):515-527.

Nik-Zainal S, Davies H, Staaf J, et al. Landscape of somatic mutations in 560 breast cancer whole-genome sequences. *Nature* 2016;534(7605):47-54.

Nishizuka SS, Mills GB. New era of integrated cancer biomarker discovery using reverse-phase protein arrays. *Drug Metab Pharmacokinet* 2016;31(1):35-45.

Novak K. Epigenetics changes in cancer cells. *MedGenMed* 2004;6(4):17.

O'Neil NJ, Bailey ML, Hieter P. Synthetic lethality and cancer. *Nat Rev Genet* 2017;18(10):613-623.

Olsen JV, Macek B, Lange O, Makarov A, Horning S, Mann M. Higher-energy C-trap dissociation for peptide modification analysis. *Nat Methods* 2007;4(9):709-712.

Ong SE, Blagoev B, Kratchmarova I, et al. Stable isotope labeling by amino acids in cell culture, SILAC, as a simple and accurate approach to expression proteomics. *Mol Cell Proteomics* 2002;1(5):376-386.

Oughtred R, Stark C, Breitkreutz BJ, et al. The BioGRID interaction database: 2019 update. *Nucleic Acids Res* 2019;47(D1):D529-D541.

Pepe MS, Etzioni R, Feng Z, et al. Phases of biomarker development for early detection of cancer. *J Natl Cancer Inst* 2001;93(14):1054-1061.

Perron MP, Provost P. Protein components of the microRNA pathway and human diseases. *Methods Mol Biol* 2009;487:369-385.

Phizicky E, Bastiaens PI, Zhu H, Snyder M, Fields S. Protein analysis on a proteomic scale. *Nature* 2003;422(6928):208-215.

Puente XS, Bea S, Valdes-Mas R, et al. Non-coding recurrent mutations in chronic lymphocytic leukaemia. *Nature* 2015;526(7574):519-524.

Quick J, Loman NJ, Duraffour S, et al. Real-time, portable genome sequencing for Ebola surveillance. *Nature* 2016;530(7589):228-232.

Redon R, Ishikawa S, Fitch KR, et al. Global variation in copy number in the human genome. *Nature* 2006;444(7118):444-454.

Reilly JP. Ultraviolet photofragmentation of biomolecular ions. *Mass Spectrom Rev* 2009;28(3):425-447.

Roepstorff P, Fohlman J. Proposal for a common nomenclature for sequence ions in mass spectra of peptides. *Biomed Mass Spectrom* 1984;11(11):601.

Ross PL, Huang YN, Marchese JN, et al. Multiplexed protein quantitation in *Saccharomyces cerevisiae* using amine-reactive isobaric tagging reagents. *Mol Cell Proteomics* 2004;3(12):1154-1169.

Roux KJ, Kim DI, Raida M, Burke B. A promiscuous biotin ligase fusion protein identifies proximal and interacting proteins in mammalian cells. *J Cell Biol* 2012;196(6):801-810.

Sanchez-Carbayo M, Socci ND, Lozano JJ, Haab BB, Cordon-Cardo C. Profiling bladder cancer using targeted antibody arrays. *Am J Pathol* 2006;168(1):93-103.

Saraon P, Grozavu I, Lim SH, Snider J, Yao Z, Stagljar I. Detecting membrane protein-protein interactions using the mammalian membrane two-hybrid (MaMTH) assay. *Curr Protoc Chem Biol* 2017;9(1):38-54.

Scarpa A, Chang DK, Nones K, et al. Whole-genome landscape of pancreatic neuroendocrine tumours. *Nature* 2017;543(7643):65-71.

Schindler T, Bornmann W, Pellicena P, Miller WT, Clarkson B, Kuriyan J. Structural mechanism for STI-571 inhibition of abelson tyrosine kinase. *Science* 2000;289(5486):1938-1942.

Sharon D, Chen R, Snyder M. Systems biology approaches to disease marker discovery. *Dis Markers* 2010;28(4):209-224.

Sheer D, Squire J. Clinical applications of genetic rearrangements in cancer. *Semin Cancer Biol* 1996;7(1):25-32.

Shedden K, Taylor JM, Enkemann SA, et al. Gene expression-based survival prediction in lung adenocarcinoma: a multi-site, blinded validation study. *Nat Med* 2008;14(8):822-827.

Shevchenko A, Wilm M, Vorm O, Mann M. Mass spectrometric sequencing of proteins silver-stained polyacrylamide gels. *Anal Chem* 1996;68(5):850-858.

Sinha A, Huang V, Livingstone J, et al. The proteogenomic landscape of curable prostate cancer. *Cancer Cell* 2019;35(3):414-427.e6.

Sinha A, Hussain A, Ignatchenko V, et al. N-Glycoproteomics of patient-derived xenografts: a strategy to discover tumor-associated proteins in high-grade serous ovarian cancer. *Cell Syst* 2019;8(4):345-351.e4.

Sinha A, Ignatchenko V, Ignatchenko A, Mejia-Guerrero S, Kislinger T. In-depth proteomic analyses of ovarian cancer cell line exosomes reveals differential enrichment of functional categories compared to the NCI 60 proteome. *Biochem Biophys Res Commun* 2014;445(4):694-701.

Smith LM, Kelleher NL, Consortium for Top Down Proteomics. Proteoform: a single term describing protein complexity. *Nat Methods* 2013;10(3):186-187.

Snider J, Kittanakom S, Damjanovic D, Curak J, Wong V, Stagljar I. Detecting interactions with membrane proteins using a membrane two-hybrid assay in yeast. *Nat Protoc* 2010;5(7):1281-1293.

Speicher MR, Gwyn Ballard S, Ward DC. Karyotyping human chromosomes by combinatorial multi-fluor FISH. *Nat Genet* 1996;12(4):368-375.

Stock D, Perisic O, Lowe J. Robotic nanolitre protein crystallisation at the MRC laboratory of molecular biology. *Prog Biophys Mol Biol* 2005;88(3):311-327.

Subramanian J, Simon R. Gene expression-based prognostic signatures in lung cancer: ready for clinical use? *J Natl Cancer Inst* 2010;102(7):464-474.

Sudmant PH, Rausch T, Gardner EJ, et al. An integrated map of structural variation in 2,504 human genomes. *Nature* 2015;526(7571):75-81.

Swaney DL, Wenger CD, Coon JJ. Value of using multiple proteases for large-scale mass spectrometry-based proteomics. *J Proteome Res* 2010;9(3):1323-1329.

Taylor P, Nielsen PA, Trelle MB, et al. Automated 2D peptide separation on a 1D nano-LC-MS system. *J Proteome Res* 2009;8(3):1610-1616.

Tran JC, Zamdborg L, Ahlf DR, et al. Mapping intact protein isoforms in discovery mode using top-down proteomics. *Nature* 2011;480(7376):254-258.

Tran NH, Rahman MZ, He L, Xin L, Shan B, Li M. Complete de novo assembly of monoclonal antibody sequences. *Sci Rep* 2016;6:31730.

Uddin M, Thiruvahindrapuram B, Walker S, et al. A high-resolution copy-number variation resource for clinical and population genetics. *Genet Med* 2015;17(9):747-752.

Valihrach L, Androvic P, Kubista M. Platforms for single-cell collection and analysis. *Int J Mol Sci* 2018;19(3).

van't Veer LJ, Dai H, van de Vijver MJ, et al. Gene expression profiling predicts clinical outcome of breast cancer. *Nature* 2002;415(6871):530-536.

Veldman T, Vignon C, Schrock E, Rowley JD, Ried T. Hidden chromosome abnormalities in haematological malignancies detected by multicolour spectral karyotyping. *Nat Genet* 1997;15(4):406-410.

Venable JD, Dong MQ, Wohlschlegel J, Dillin A, Yates JR. Automated approach for quantitative analysis of complex peptide mixtures from tandem mass spectra. *Nat Methods* 2004;1(1):39-45.

Vladoiu MC, El-Hamamy I, Donovan LK, et al. Childhood cerebellar tumours mirror conserved fetal transcriptional programs. *Nature* 2019;572(7767):67-73.

Walloe L, Hjort NL, Thoresen M. Why results from Bayesian statistical analyses of clinical trials with a strong prior and small sample sizes may be misleading the case of the NICHD Neonatal Research Network Late Hypothermia Trial. *Acta Paediatr* 2019;108(7):1190-1191.

Wang Z, Gerstein M, Snyder M. RNA-Seq: a revolutionary tool for transcriptomics. *Nat Rev Genet* 2009;10(1):57-63.

Washburn MP, Wolters D, Yates JR 3rd. Large-scale analysis of the yeast proteome by multidimensional protein identification technology. *Nat Biotechnol* 2001;19(3):242-247.

Weir BA, Woo MS, Getz G, et al. Characterizing the cancer genome in lung adenocarcinoma. *Nature* 2007;450(7171):893-898.

Wolters DA, Washburn MP, Yates JR 3rd. An automated multidimensional protein identification technology for shotgun proteomics. *Anal Chem* 2001;73(23):5683-5690.

Woodson K, O'Reilly KJ, Hanson JC, Nelson D, Walk EL, Tangrea JA. The usefulness of the detection of GSTP1 methylation in urine as a biomarker in the diagnosis of prostate cancer. *J Urol* 2008;179(2):508-511; discussion 511-512.

Yoshimoto M, Bayani J, Nuin PA, Silva NS, Cavalheiro S, Stavale JN, Andrade JA, Zielenska M, Squire JA, de Toledo SR. Metaphase and array comparative genomic hybridization: unique copy number changes and gene amplification of medulloblastomas in South America. *Cancer Genet Cytogenet* 2006;170(1):40-47.

Zack TI, Schumacher SE, Carter SL, et al. Pan-cancer patterns of somatic copy number alteration. *Nat Genet* 2013;45(10):1134-1140.

Zhang H, Liu T, Zhang Z, et al. Integrated proteogenomic characterization of human high-grade serous ovarian cancer. *Cell* 2016;166(3):755-765.

Zhang L, Elias JE. Relative protein quantification using tandem mass tag mass spectrometry. *Methods Mol Biol* 2017;1550:185-198.

Zolg DP, Wilhelm M, Schnatbaum K, et al. Building ProteomeTools based on a complete synthetic human proteome. *Nat Methods* 2017;14(3):259-262.

Epigenetics

Kyaw Lwin Aung, Stanley Zhou, and Mathieu Lupien

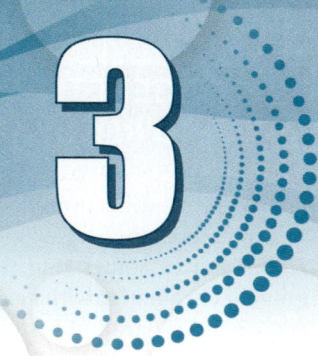

Chapter Outline

- 3.1 Introduction
- 3.2 Epigenetic Mechanisms and Regulation
  - 3.2.1 DNA Methylation
  - 3.2.2 Posttranslational Modifications of Histones
  - 3.2.3 Histone Variants
- 3.3 Epigenetic Variants in Cancer
  - 3.3.1 Epigenetic Variants at Gene Promoters
  - 3.3.2 Epigenetic Variants at Gene Enhancers
  - 3.3.3 Epigenetic Variants at Anchors of Chromatin Interactions
  - 3.3.4 Mutations in Chromatin Factors
  - 3.3.5 Epigenetics and Cancer Metabolism
- 3.4 Chromatin Factors as Drug Targets for the Treatment of Cancer
  - 3.4.1 DNA Methyltransferase Inhibitors
  - 3.4.2 Histone Deacetylase Inhibitors
  - 3.4.3 Lysine Methyltransferase and Demethylase Inhibitors
  - 3.4.4 Emerging Epigenetic Therapies
  - 3.4.5 Epigenetic Therapy in Combination With Other Cancer Therapies
- 3.5 Epigenetic Variants as Biomarkers for Precision Cancer Medicine
  - 3.5.1 Genetic Variants in Chromatin Factors
  - 3.5.2 Epigenetic Identity and Cancers of Unknown Primary
  - 3.5.3 Tracking Tumors Through Their Epigenetics in Liquid Biopsies
- Summary
- References

3.1 INTRODUCTION

The human genome found in each cell of the body consists of ~6 billion bases of DNA forming a sequence unique to each individual. This sequence contributes to differences in phenotypic traits among individuals, such as height, as well as risks of developing different diseases. However, the DNA sequence alone cannot account for the phenotypic identity that discriminates between different cell types and tissues of a human being, because (with few exceptions) the DNA sequence is largely identical in each cell. Thus, cell type–specific gene expression programs require an additional system of control to achieve this phenotypic diversity, a system commonly referred to as epigenetics.

Epigenetics relates to heritable changes that impact DNA templated processes, such as gene expression, that are not encoded in the primary linear DNA sequence. These processes are mediated by the covalent attachment of chemical groups (eg, methyl or acetyl groups) to DNA and associated proteins, histones and chromatin that together establish "chromatin states." Each state consists of a unique combination of DNA and histone modifications that demarcate DNA sequences with specific functions such as transcripts, silent genes, or *cis*-regulatory elements involved in modulating gene expression. Remarkably, through these layers of regulation, a single human genome, of which only ~1.5% encodes proteins, gives rise to hundreds of cell types with distinct gene expression patterns and functional phenotypes. Although the DNA and histone modifications that determine each chromatin state are conserved across cell types, the distribution of each state along the DNA varies from one cell type to another (Ernst et al, 2011) and is subject to change across development. Alterations to these chromatin states have been linked to the development and progression of various human disorders, including cancer (Feinberg, 2018). The sensitivity of chromatin states to cell-extrinsic factors also imparts an opportunity for therapeutic interventions aimed either to correct pathogenic alterations or to exploit vulnerabilities of the cancer cells (Pfister and Ashworth, 2017; Bates, 2020). In this chapter, the mechanisms of epigenetic regulation will be reviewed, with a focus on processes for which dysregulation contributes to malignancy and on opportunities to leverage modifiable chromatin states for anticancer therapy.

3.2 EPIGENETIC MECHANISMS AND REGULATION

Epigenetic modifications occur in the context of chromatin, a macromolecular complex composed of DNA bases wrapped around nucleosomes (Fig. 3–1). Nucleosomes are the basic units of chromatin, with each consisting of 147 base pairs of DNA winding around histone octamers that comprise pairs of the core H2A, H2B, H3, and H4 histone proteins. Although histone variants can replace these core proteins on the chromatin to delineate distinct chromatin states (Henikoff and Smith, 2015), the most commonly reported epigenetic modifications consist of DNA methylation and posttranslational modifications of histones. Chromatin is compacted to varying degrees to minimize the space needed to store the genetic information encoded within the human genome. Chromatin also needs to be accessible at discrete DNA sequences to allow the recruitment of DNA-binding proteins, such as transcription factors, and the protein complexes involved in DNA replication and repair (Fig. 3–1). Chromatin is described on the basis of its compaction either as heterochromatin or euchromatin: heterochromatin is compacted and it is transcriptionally inactive, whereas euchromatin underlies accessibility to the DNA, allowing DNA-templated processes to operate when needed.

3.2.1 DNA Methylation

DNA methylation is the covalent addition of a methyl group at position 5 of a cytosine (C) nucleotide (5mC), typically when it is positioned close to a guanine residue (G) (Fig. 3–2). This occurs mostly in regions dense in CpG dinucleotides (ie, adjacent C and G nucleotides) called CpG islands, which are found in approximately 70% of promoter regions of genes. Although methylation of promoter CpG islands has been considered as a relatively stable gene-silencing mechanism (Jones and Liang, 2009), its function is context-dependent. For instance, methylation at CpG islands in promoters can be associated with gene silencing, whereas methylation of CpG within gene bodies typifies transcribed genes (Guibert et al, 2009). DNA methylation is also observed near inactively transcribed genes, where it plays a critical role in maintaining genomic stability. Indeed, DNA methylation can keep silent repetitive sequences such as inserted retrotransposons, LINE (long interspersed elements) and/or SINE (short interspersed elements), thereby limiting their capacity to promote genomic instability (Bourque et al, 2018). Changes in DNA methylation patterns are also believed to play a role in cellular differentiation and in reprogramming cell behavior (De Carvalho et al, 2010).

Methylation of CpG dinucleotides is tightly regulated by a family of 3 DNA methyltransferases (DNMTs) that catalyze the transfer of a methyl group from the metabolite

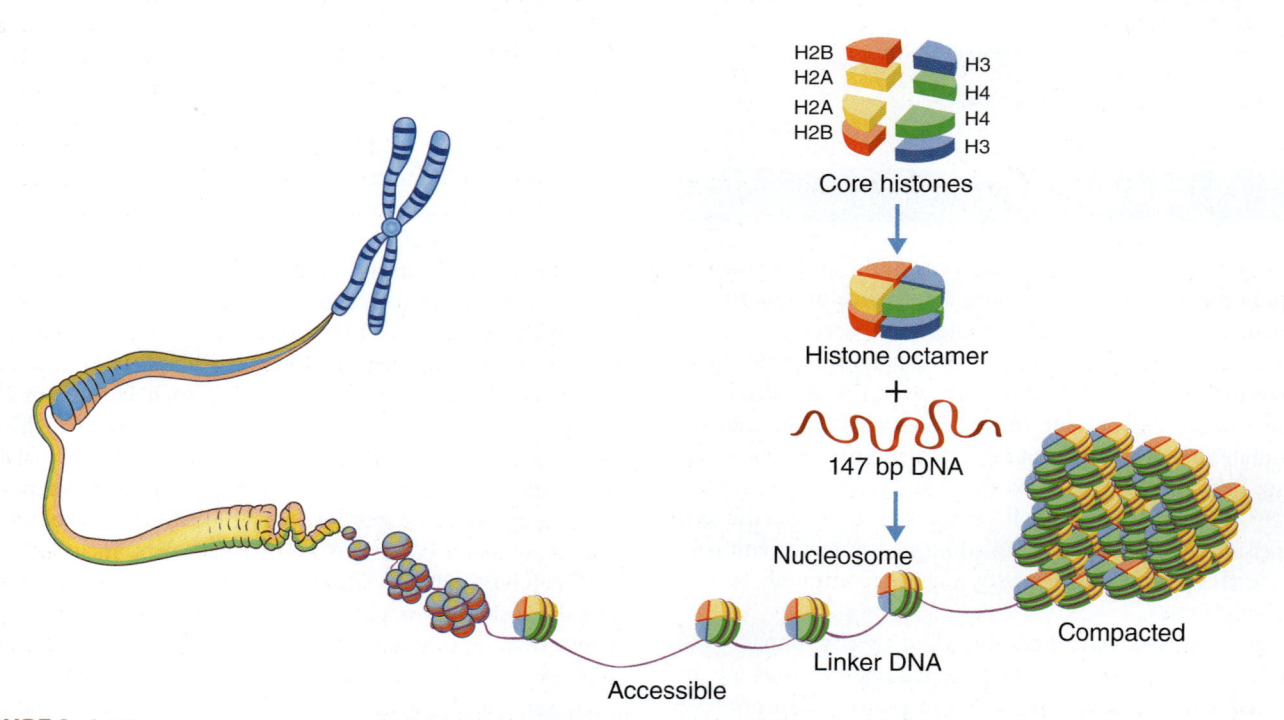

FIGURE 3–1 **The human genome is packaged into chromatin.** Stretches of 147 base pairs of DNA wrap around a protein octamer consisting of pairs of 4 core histone proteins, known as H2A, H2B, H3, and H4, to form a nucleosome, the basic unit of chromatin. Linker DNA stretches of different sizes lie between nucleosomes. Linker DNA serves as docking sites for proteins involved in transcriptional regulation, DNA repair, DNA replication, and other DNA templated processes. Nucleosome density along the genome varies from one region to another according to the cell and tissue type of origin. Nucleosome-dense regions define compacted chromatin known as heterochromatin, whereas regions low in nucleosomes and rich in linker DNA define accessible chromatin, known as euchromatin.

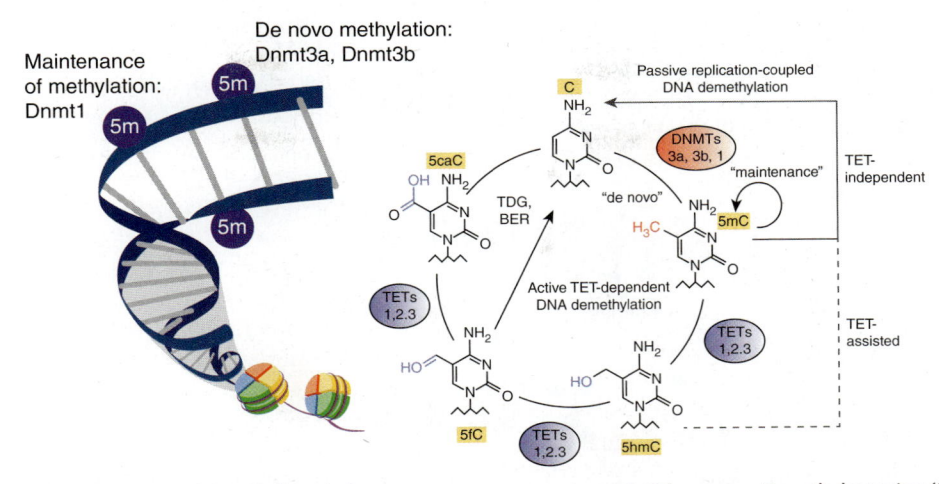

FIGURE 3-2 DNA methylation. The addition of methyl groups, most commonly on CpG known as 5-methylcytosine (5mC), is an epigenetic modification mediated by the DNA methyltransferases (DNMTs). Removal of methyl groups from the DNA involves a series of steps mediated by TET enzymes that first convert 5mC into 5-hydroxymethylcytosine (5hmC), then 5-formylcytosine (5fC), and finally 5-carboxylcytosine (5caC). (Adapted with permission from DNA methylation: a guide. Cambridge, UK: Abcam plc. https://www.abcam.com/epigenetics/dna-methylation-a-guide.)

S-adenosylmethionine (SAM). De novo DNA methylation patterns are established early in development by DNMT3A and DNMT3B, which are expressed throughout the cell cycle. When DNA is replicated before cell division, unmethylated daughter strands must be methylated to maintain the methylation patterns of the parental DNA. These modifications are catalyzed by "maintenance" methyltransferases, primarily via DNMT1 activity with contributions from DNMT3A and DNMT3B.

3.2.2 Posttranslational Modifications of Histones

The most studied posttranslational modifications of histones include acetylation, methylation, phosphorylation, sumoylation, and ubiquitination (Bannister and Kouzarides, 2011). Histone modifications occur predominantly in the amino terminus tails that protrude from the nucleosome (Fig. 3-3). Apart from playing a major role in transcription, histone modifications are associated with all DNA-related processes. Because of the great diversity of posttranslational modifications and their potential to coexist on any nucleosome, histone modifications provide a remarkable complexity reflected in various chromatin states. For instance, the co-occurrence of a trimethylated lysine 27 with trimethylated lysine 4 on histone 3 (H3K27me3 and H3K4me3) at gene promoters forms a "bivalent" chromatin state associated with genes poised for expression (Vastenhouw and Schier, 2012). The loss of either H3K27me3 or H3K4me3 over bivalent chromatin, such as observed during development, correlates with activation or repression of gene expression, respectively.

Acetylation neutralizes the positive charge of lysine residues on histone tails, weakening the interaction between histones and negatively charged DNA. Histone acetylation also serves as a recognition site for chromatin factors with their own ability to influence chromatin compaction. Histone acetylation is often associated with an accessible chromatin conformation, such as observed at active promoters or enhancers (Heintzman and Ren, 2007). Histone methylation is also a dynamic process that modulates the docking of chromatin-modifying enzymes, occurring on arginine, lysine, and histidine residues. Lysine residues can be mono- (me), di- (me2), or tri-methylated (me3). Depending on which lysine residue is modified, these specific histone methylation modifications are associated either with accessible and active chromatin (H3K4, H3K36, and H3K79) or with compacted and repressed chromatin (H3K9, H3K27, and H4K20). These methylation modifications are differentially localized throughout the genome. For example, whereas the H3K4me3 mark often accumulates at transcriptional start sites of actively transcribed genes, the H3K4me1 and me2 marks are mainly observed at enhancers permissive to transcription factor binding (Heintzman et al, 2007; Lupien et al, 2008).

Histone modifications and their functional effects are mediated by specific chromatin factors that can be classified as "writers," "readers," and "erasers." The "writer" proteins add modifications to histones, the "readers" are specialized proteins that recognize the modified histones through unique domains and the "eraser" proteins mediate the removal of modifications on histones (Arrowsmith et al, 2012). Well-characterized chromatin-modifying proteins (writers and erasers) include histone lysine acetyltransferases (HAT/KAT), histone lysine deacetylases (HDAC), histone lysine methyltransferases (KMT), and histone lysine demethylases (KDM), whereas readers of histone acetylation or methylation consist of proteins with bromodomains (BET) and tandem plant homeodomain (PHD) fingers or PWWP (Pro-Trp-Trp-Pro) domains, respectively.

3.2.3 Histone Variants

Histone variants are proteins with 1 or a few amino acid differences compared to their core histone counterparts, whose

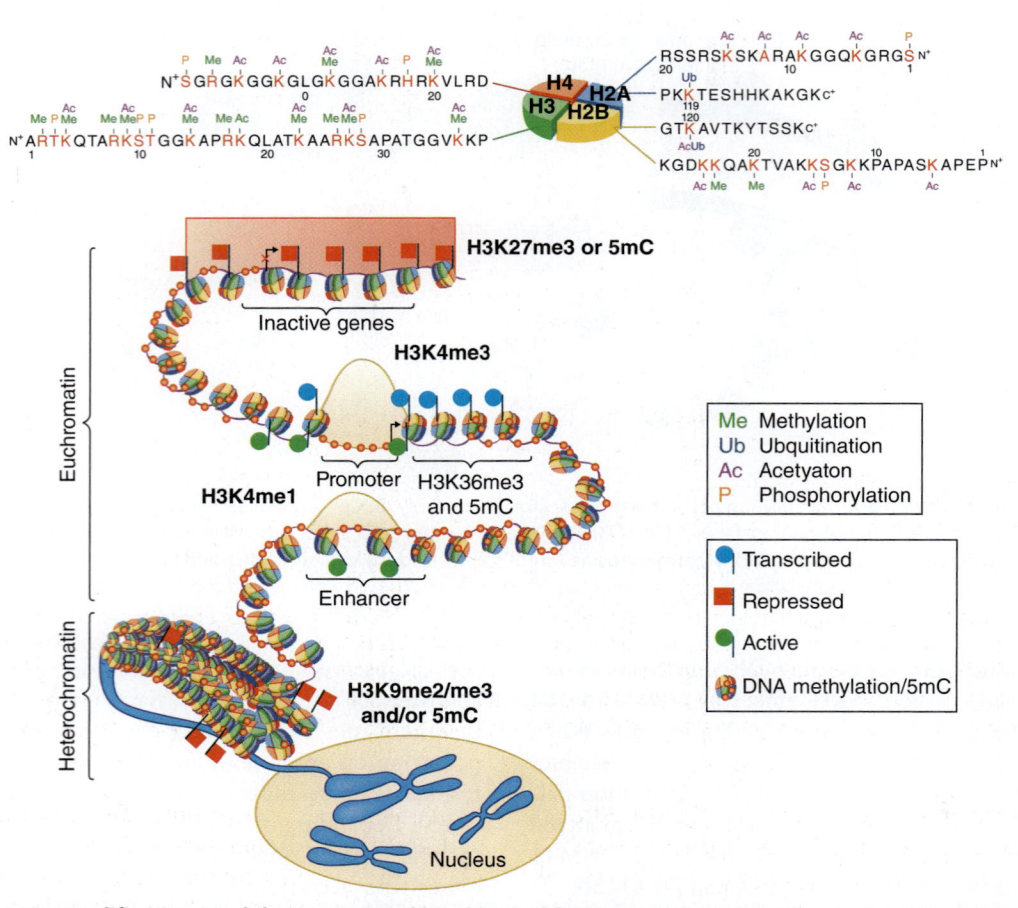

FIGURE 3–3 Histone modifications and their associated biochemical features. Nucleosomes can acquire epigenetic modifications through the posttranslational modification of their histones. Histone methylation, acetylation, ubiquitination, and phosphorylation are among the most common and well-studied epigenetic modifications that affect DNA templated processes. For instance, the addition of a methyl group to the lysine 4 residue of histone 3 (H3K4me1) is often found on nucleosomes in accessible chromatin, prone to recruiting transcription factors regulating gene expression from a distance. The addition of 3 methyl groups to the same residue (H3K4me3) is common on nucleosomes next to the promoter of expressed genes. Nucleosomes within the gene body of such expressed genes will commonly harbor H3K36me3 modifications. In contrast, silent genes will lie in compressed chromatin harboring nucleosome trimethylated on lysine 27 of histone 3 (H3K27me3) or other "repressive" histone modifications such as H3K9me2 or H3K9me3.

genes are separately encoded in DNA (Fig. 3–4) (Talbert et al, 2012). These variants have specific expression and distribution across the genome, conferring structural and functional properties on the nucleosome to affect chromatin compaction and histone posttranslational modifications (Buschbeck and Hake, 2017). Histone variants contribute to the diversity of chromatin states, and unlike canonical histones that are normally synthesized and deposited rapidly behind the replication forks during the S phase of the cell cycle (see Chap. 8, Sec. 8.2), histone variants are not cell cycle dependent (Henikoff and Smith, 2015). Of the four canonical histones (H1, H2A, H2B, and H3), variants are most prevalent for H2A and H3. The biologic significance of some of the variants, such as H2A.X, H2A.Z, H2A.B, macroH2A, cenH3, and H3.3 has been characterized (Buschbeck and Hake, 2017). Most contribute to differential control of transcription, whereas some have other key functional roles. For example, the serine residue of H2A.X (which comprises up to one-fourth of mammalian H2A) is a site for phosphorylation that serves as an early signaling event in DNA double-strand break repair (Morrison and Shen, 2009).

The cenH3 histone variant is a critical component of the eukaryotic centromere. CenH3 is inherited without requiring centromeric DNA sequences and is essential for the formation of kinetochore and for chromosome segregation.

3.3 EPIGENETIC VARIANTS IN CANCER

3.3.1 Epigenetic Variants at Gene Promoters

Differential methylation patterns that exist between cancers and their normal tissue counterparts have revealed changes in DNA methylation occurring throughout carcinogenesis (Fig. 3–5). Cancer cells display global hypomethylation coupled with local hypermethylation, typically found at promoters. As promoter methylation correlates with the reduced expression of their associated genes, hypermethylation is considered an avenue for silencing tumor suppressor genes during carcinogenesis (see Chap. 7, Sec. 7.4.2). The promoters of

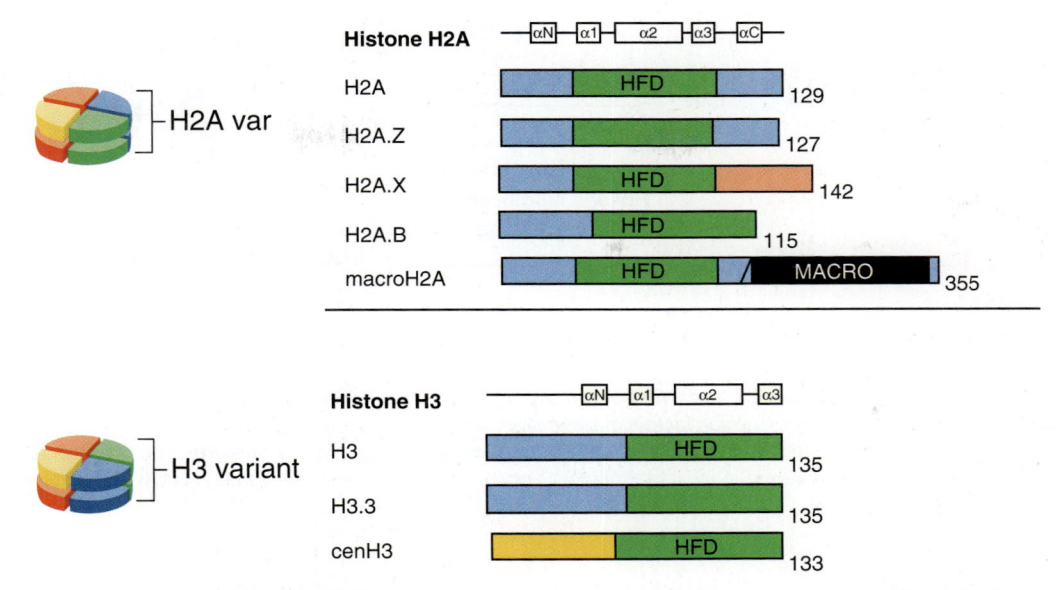

FIGURE 3-4 Histone variants. In addition to the core histones known as H2A, H2B, H3, and H4, nucleosomes can harbor histone variants. For example, the histone variants H2A.Z, H2A.X, H2A.B, or macroH2A can replace an H2A core histone in a nucleosome. Similarly, the H3 core histone can be replaced by the histone variants H3.3 or cenH3. These variants differ from core histone in their size or amino acid composition and associate with distinct functions that pertain to DNA-templated processes. (Reproduced with permission from Buschbeck M, Hake SB. Variants of core histones and their roles in cell fate decisions, development and cancer. *Nat Rev Mol Cell Biol* 2017 May;18(5):299-314.)

numerous tumor suppressor genes such as *RASSF1A*, *BRCA1*, *APC*, *MLH1*, and *p16* are observed to be hypermethylated in multiple epithelial and mesenchymal cancer types (Zhou et al, 2016). DNA demethylation also occurs at gene promoters during carcinogenesis. This phenomenon has been observed for genes encoding cancer testis antigens, whose expression is normally restricted to the testis. For example, demethylation at the *CTCFL/BORIS* promoter is associated with its overexpression in several cancers, where it appears to play a functional role in carcinogenesis, cancer progression, and the development of drug resistance (Debruyne et al, 2019). Promoter demethylation driving the aberrant expression of *uPA*, involved in tumor progression and metastasis (see Chap. 10, Sec. 10.2.2) is reported in invasive prostate cancer (Pakneshan et al, 2003). However, recent reports suggesting that DNA methylation in cancer serves mainly to block the expression of transposable elements is resulting in reappraisal of the principal roles of altered methylation in cancer (Roulois et al, 2015).

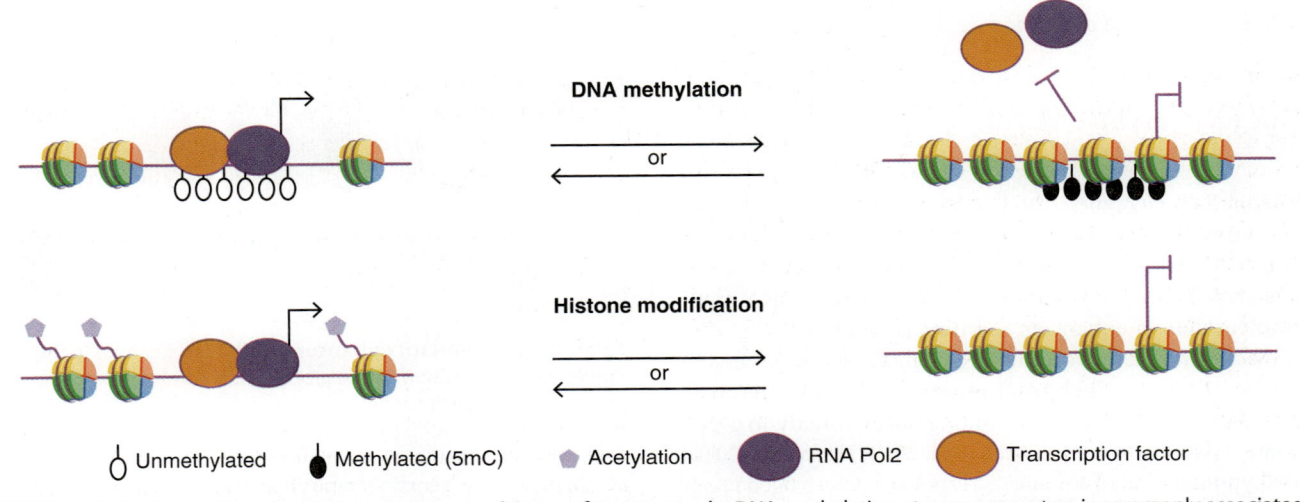

FIGURE 3-5 Epigenetic variants at promoters as drivers of oncogenesis. DNA methylation at gene promoters is commonly associated with gene repression. Acquisition of DNA methylation on the promoter of tumor suppressor genes or loss of DNA methylation on the promoter of oncogenes are epigenetic variants that can contribute to oncogenesis. Similarly, changes in the composition of histone modifications at promoters can impact the nature of promoters to increase or decrease expression of the associated gene. For instance, loss of histone acetylation is commonly associated with gene repression whereas gain in histone acetylation occur at the promoter of genes whose expression is increased. (Reproduced with permission from Zhou S, Treloar AE, Lupien M. Emergence of the Noncoding Cancer Genome: A Target of Genetic and Epigenetic Alterations. *Cancer Discov* 2016 Nov;6(11):1215-1229.)

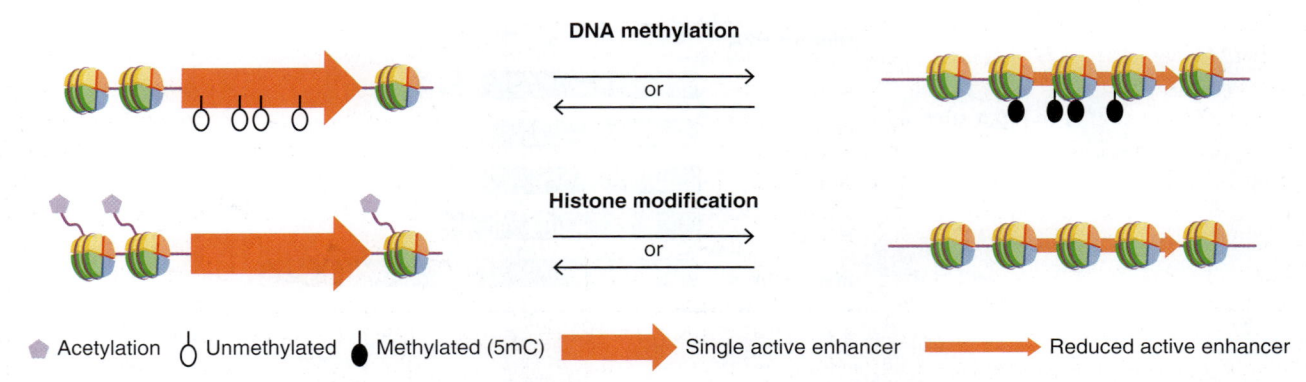

FIGURE 3-6 Epigenetic variants at enhancers as drivers of oncogenesis. Changes in DNA methylation or histone modifications at enhancers can modulate the interaction of transcription factors or other DNA-templated machinery to favor oncogenesis. These epigenetic variants can increase or decrease the transactivation potential of enhancers, thereby directly affecting the expression of associated gene(s). (Reproduced with permission from Zhou S, Treloar AE, Lupien M. Emergence of the Noncoding Cancer Genome: A Target of Genetic and Epigenetic Alterations. *Cancer Discov* 2016 Nov;6(11):1215-1229.)

Changes to the distribution of histone modifications across the genome also typify cancer development and progression. For instance, colorectal cancer initiation is characterized by gains and losses of the H3K4me3 modification at promoters that are associated with expression of differential genes (Akhtar-Zaidi et al, 2012). The loss of the H3K27me3 modification has also been linked to aberrant activation of oncogenic gene expression, including *MKI67* and *CD133*, a proliferation marker and a cancer stem cell marker, respectively (Hahn et al, 2014). Moreover, the loss of both H3K4me3 and H3K27me3 modifications is associated with aberrant gains in promoter methylation in colorectal cancer (Hahn et al, 2014). Apparent gains and losses of the H3K27me3 modification at promoters also discriminate androgen deprivation–resistant vs –sensitive prostate cancer cells, suggesting a role for epigenetic alterations at promoters during cancer progression (Xu et al, 2012). These observations imply that aberrant deposition of histone modifications plays a dynamic role in cancer processes.

3.3.2 Epigenetic Variants at Gene Enhancers

Cis-regulatory elements distal to genes, such as enhancers, are commonly altered in the course of cancer development, with direct consequences to the oncogenic process (Fig. 3–6) (Zhou et al, 2016). For instance, the acquisition of DNA methylation variants in enhancers can directly impact the binding of transcription factors on the DNA to alter gene expression. In colorectal cancer, the transcription factor FOXQ1 has been implicated in oncogenesis by binding preferentially to DNA-hypomethylated enhancers (Aran et al, 2013; Heyn et al, 2016). DNA-hypomethylated enhancers responsive to estrogen receptor alpha (ER) binding in breast cancer also contribute to the development of ER-positive breast cancer (Stone et al, 2015).

Enhancers are direct targets of oncogenic changes in histone modifications: in both normal and cancer cells, enhancers are commonly demarcated by nucleosomes mono- and dimethylated on lysine 4 of histone H3 (H3K4me1 and H3K4me2)

(Heintzman et al, 2009; He et al, 2010). Genome-wide profiling for H3K4me1 in both normal colon epithelia and colorectal cancer cells have revealed thousands of enhancer variants, termed variant enhancer loci (VELs) that are either lost or gained in colorectal cancer cells compared with normal colon crypts, suggestive of ectopic enhancer activity in the process of cancer initiation (Fig. 3–7). Although these VELs occur even in the absence of genetic alterations, they correspond to the decommissioning (lost VELs) or engagement (gained VELs) of new DNA sequences in colorectal cells that allow for differential expression of target genes in normal vs colon cancer cells (Akhtar-Zaidi et al, 2012). Enhancers, active in normal

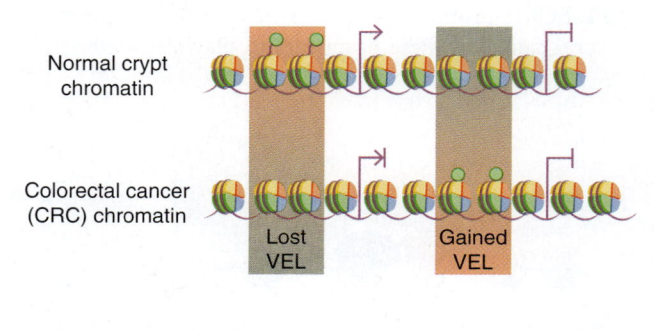

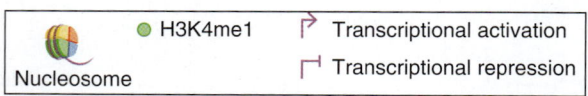

FIGURE 3-7 Variant enhancer loci (VELs). Changes in the epigenetic composition of enhancers that control the expression of genes from a distance define variant enhancer loci. These can be detected by comparing the epigenetic composition of the genome from normal tissue to that of a matched tumor sample. For instance, comparing the epigenetic composition of normal colon crypts to that of colorectal cancer cells reveals lost VELs based on losses in the monomethyl group on lysine 4 of histone 3 (H3K4me1) at specific genomic coordinates assigned to genes repressed in colorectal cancer compared with normal colon crypts. Similarly, gained VELs defined by the acquisition of H3K4me1 over specific genomic regions in colorectal cancer cells compared with normal crypts can be observed near genes overexpressed in colorectal cancer.

colon but inactive in colorectal cancer cells, are found near genes that are part of the normal colon gene expression profile; conversely, enhancers active in colorectal cancer cells but inactive in normal colon are associated with genes expressed in cancer cells. The presence of VEL also characterizes cancer progression. For example, many enhancers active in hormone-sensitive breast cancer cells are no longer active in hormone-resistant cells (Magnani et al, 2013). The presence of VELs reflects differences in the transcriptional machinery that underlie the identity of cancer cells and could inform alternative therapeutic strategies by serving as biomarkers of response, or by identifying therapeutic targets (Magnani et al, 2013; Kron et al, 2017).

3.3.3 Epigenetic Variants at Anchors of Chromatin Interactions

Distal *cis*-regulatory elements interact with the promoter of their target gene through physical contact, known as chromatin interactions (Fig. 3–8) (Schoenfelder and Fraser, 2019). These interactions are regulated through chromatin folding, bringing into close physical proximity 2 or more pieces of DNA that lie thousands to million base pairs apart from each other—a process regulated by proteins such as CTCF, ZNF143, and the cohesin complex (Zhou et al, 2016). A distinctive feature of CTCF-binding sites is the absence of DNA methylation (Ong and Corces, 2014), as the binding of CTCF to chromatin is negatively correlated with DNA methylation in all cell types. Consequently, cancer-associated changes to the DNA methylation profile at anchors of chromatin interactions can compromise CTCF binding and its activity. This was investigated in tumors exhibiting a CpG island methylator phenotype (CIMP), variably defined but loosely encompassing a hypermethylated phenotype exhibited by some tumors compared with others within cancer types (Jia et al, 2016). The CIMP phenotype has been reported in diverse cancer types, including leukemia, glioma, ependymoma, and colorectal cancer. In glioma, the CIMP phenotype can derive from mutations in the *IDH1* (isocitrate dehydrogenase) gene (see Section 3.3.5, and Chap. 12, Sec. 12.3.5), resulting in a discrete expression profile compared with non-CIMP glioma (Turcan et al, 2012; Flavahan et al, 2016). The expression differences between these subtypes can be partly explained by DNA hypermethylation over CTCF-binding sites, which blocks their ability to impose a specific organization to the chromatin at the *PDGFRA* (platelet-derived growth factor A) locus (Fig. 3–9) (Flavahan et al, 2016). This results in the aberrant expression of the *PDGFRA* oncogene. Although rare, the CIMP phenotype can also be observed in *IDH1* wild-type glioma (Turcan et al, 2012), implying the convergence of mechanisms to promote this phenotype.

3.3.4 Mutations in Chromatin Factors

Some of the most frequently mutated genes in cancer include those coding for chromatin factors (Fig. 3–10) (Shah et al, 2014). For instance, EZH2 is an H3K27me3 lysine methyltransferase involved in chromatin regulation, mutated in

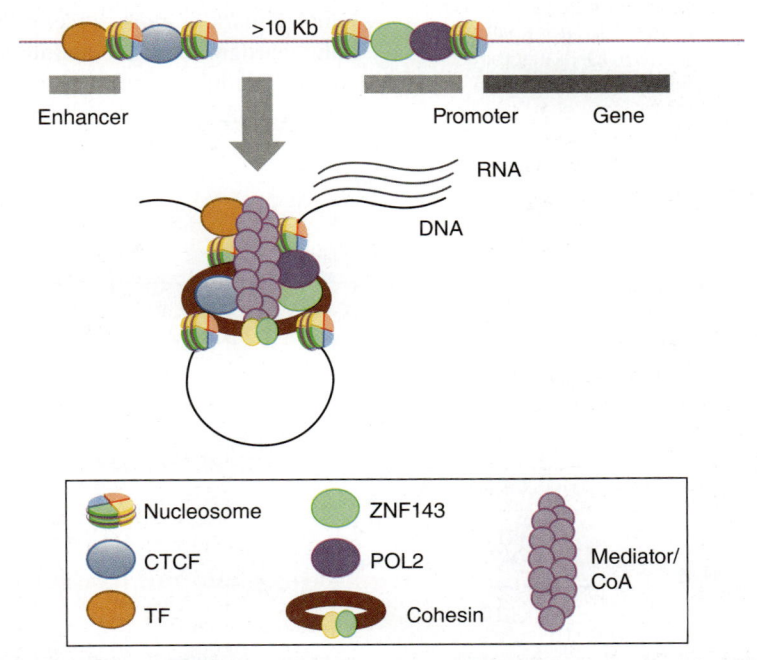

FIGURE 3–8 Three-dimensional organization of the genome. In addition to its different degrees of compaction, chromatin is organized in 3-dimensional space through chromatin interactions to bring into close proximity DNA sequences that are otherwise tens to thousands of kilobases apart. This process is regulated by discrete proteins, such as CTCF, the cohesin complex, and ZNF143 that bind DNA at the boundaries of chromatin interactions, known as anchors. One role for the 3-dimensional organization of the genome is to enable proteins recruited at enhancers to interact with other protein complexes recruited at promoters, potentiating the expression of target genes. (Reproduced with permission from Bailey SD, Zhang X, Desai K, et al. ZNF143 provides sequence specificity to secure chromatin interactions at gene promoters. *Nat Commun* 2015 Feb 3;2:6186.)

many tumors. Oncogenic gain-of-function mutations in this gene are found in melanoma and B-cell lymphoma (Kim and Roberts, 2016). In acute myeloid leukemia (AML), overexpression of wild-type *EZH2* and/or *EZH2* with gain-of-function mutations is thought to promote oncogenesis by suppressing differentiation programs in leukemic stem cells (Lund et al, 2014). Translocations in *MLL1*, a histone methyltransferase that methylates H3K4, are recognized as an important molecular event in both childhood acute lymphoblastic leukemia (ALL) and acute myeloid leukemia, as *MLL1* gene alterations are found in up to 70% of childhood ALL and AML (Li and Ernst, 2014). Mechanistically MLL fusion proteins recruit the DOT1L histone methyltransferase responsible for methylation of H3K79, leading to transcriptional deregulation (Bernt et al, 2011). *MLL2* and *MLL3* are also mutated in 18% of pediatric medulloblastomas, demonstrating the relevance of these alterations in nonhematologic cancers (Parsons et al, 2011).

Aberrant DNA methylation can result from mutations in both DNMT and DNA demethylases. This is best exemplified by loss-of-function mutations in *DNMT3A* and the demethylase encoding the *TET2* gene found in 20% and 25% of AML, respectively (Haladyna et al, 2015). Although studies in genetically engineered mouse models indicate that neither DNMT3A nor TET2 loss of function is sufficient to produce murine AML, the frequency of DNMT3A R882 and TET2 mutations implicate them in the pathogenesis of AML. They are also associated with poor survival in AML (Haladyna et al, 2015).

3.3.5 Epigenetics and Cancer Metabolism

One hallmark of most cancer cells is that they undergo metabolic reprogramming to maintain the high demand in energy and to produce enough biosynthetic precursors to sustain proliferation. Cancer cells experience a metabolic shift from

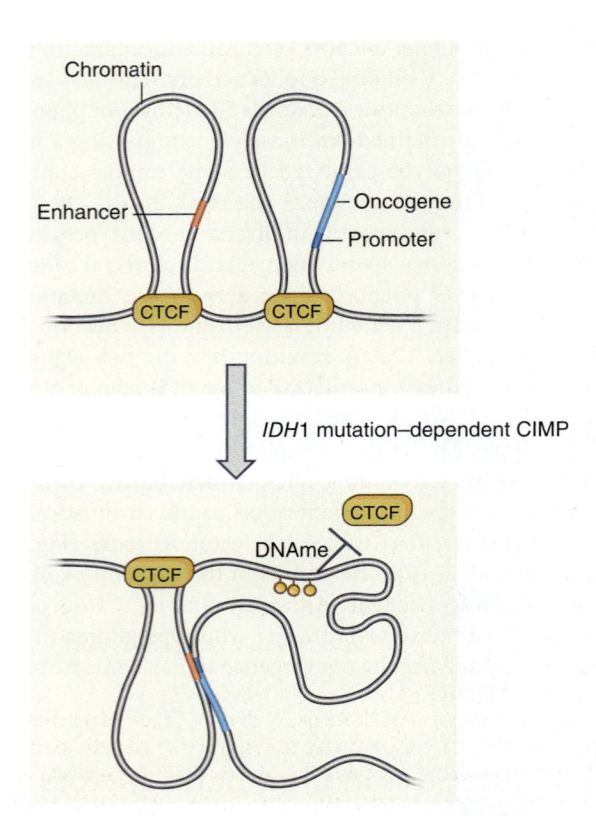

FIGURE 3-9 Epigenetic alterations at anchors of chromatin interactions as drivers of oncogenesis. The binding pattern of factors regulating the 3-dimensional genome organization can be impacted by epigenetic alterations. For instance, DNA methylation at anchors of chromatin interaction can restrict the recruitment of CTCF to alter chromatin interactions and downstream target gene expression, a phenomenon observed in CpG island methylator phenotype (CIMP) glioblastoma resulting from mutations in IDH1. (Reproduced with permission from Grimmer MR, Costello JF. Cancer: Oncogene brought into the loop. *Nature* 2016 Jan 7;529(7584):34-35.)

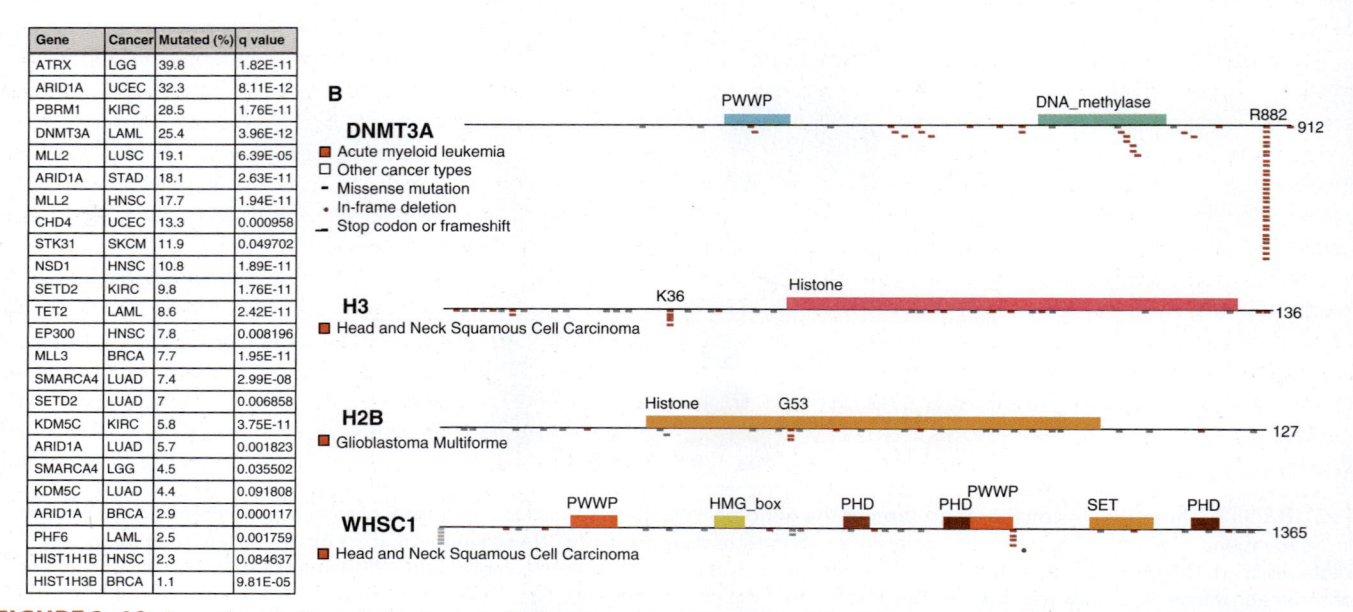

FIGURE 3-10 Somatic mutations and epigenetic factors. Genes encoding proteins relevant to epigenetic processes, including histones, epigenetic writers, erasers, and readers, are commonly mutated across diverse cancer types. (Reproduced with permission from Shah MA, Denton EL, Arrowsmith CH, Lupien M, Schapira M. A global assessment of cancer genomic alterations in epigenetic mechanisms. *Epigenetics Chromatin* 2014 Dec 4;7(1):29.)

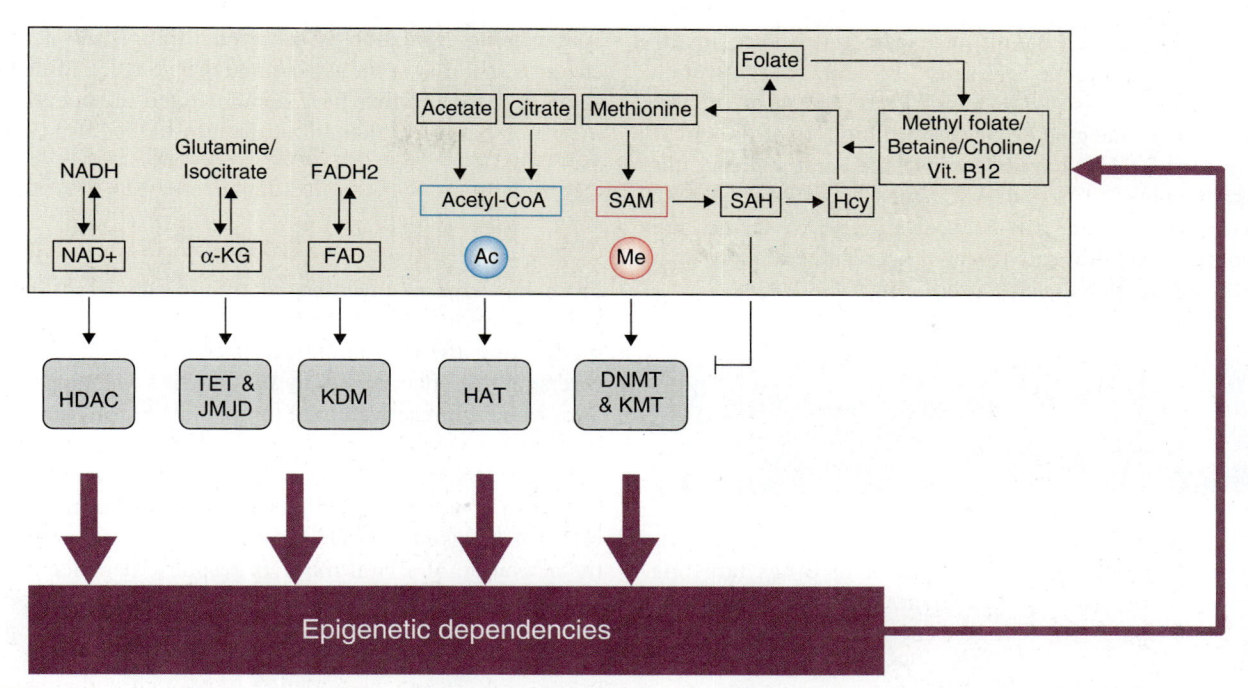

FIGURE 3–11 Interplay between epigenetic and metabolic processes. Epigenetic modifications are dependent on metabolites that serve as substrates or cofactors of epigenetic processes. For instance, histone and DNA methylation rely on S-adenosyl methionine (SAM) that serves as the universal methyl donor. Similarly, histone acetylation is dependent on the availability of acetyl-CoA. Fluctuations in the availability of these metabolites can directly impact epigenetic processes. Epigenetic dependencies are suggested to favor specific metabolic adaptation. (Adapted with permission from Tollefsbol TO: Medical Epigenetics. St. Louis, MO: Academic Press Elsevier; 2016.)

oxidative respiration to an energy-efficient aerobic glycolytic profile referred to as the Warburg effect (see Chap. 12, Sec. 12.3.1). They also preferentially convert pyruvate to lactate, diverting pyruvate from oxidative phosphorylation. Epigenetic mechanisms are linked to this switch in energy metabolism in cancer cells (Lu and Thompson, 2012), and the interplay between cancer metabolism and epigenetics is bidirectional (Fig. 3–11).

The epigenetic enzymatic machinery utilizes metabolite pools as cofactors that regulate their activity, as well as direct substrates for the methyl and acetyl moieties that are incorporated into DNA and histones (Johnson et al, 2015). A key metabolite for epigenetic reactions is SAM, which serves as the universal methyl donor for all methylation reactions occurring in cells. SAM is synthesized in the mitochondria and used as a substrate in the nucleus for DNA and histone methylation reactions. Donation of a methyl group from SAM releases SAH (S-adenosylhomocysteine), and the cellular ratio of SAM/SAH is a major determinant of chromatin methylation. An increase in the SAM/SAH ratio is associated with promoter hypermethylation at tumor suppressor genes in cancer. In contrast, decreased SAM/SAH is associated with promoter hypomethylation of oncogenes. Enzymatic methylation of histones by histone lysine methyltransferases also relies on SAM as the donor of the methyl group (Igarashi and Katoh, 2013). Disruption of these normally ordered processes can be affected by depletion of the SAM pool affected in other ways. For example, the aberrant production of nicotinamide N-methyltransferase, an enzyme that metabolizes SAM, has been observed in solid tumors, including lung, bladder, and colon cancers. This results in depletion of the donor methyl pool and is associated with reduced histone methylation level.

Acetyl–coenzyme A (acetyl-CoA), alpha-ketoglutarate (α-KG), succinate, SAH, nicotinamide (NAD), flavin adenine dinucleotide (FAD), and glucose are additional metabolites that contribute to maintaining the function of epigenetic enzymes (Johnson et al, 2015). For instance, acetyl-CoA is a by-product of the tricarboxylic acid cycle resulting from glucose and glutamine oxidation used as the donor for histone acetylation (Shi and Tu, 2015). The KDM1 class of lysine demethylases (KDM1A [also known as LSD1] and KDM1B) mediates the amine oxidation reaction using FAD as a cofactor (Hou and Yu, 2010). A second class, the Jumonji demethylases, also requires metabolic cofactors as their function depends on iron Fe(II) and α-KG as cofactors (Horton et al, 2011). Alteration of glutamine metabolism affects α-KG levels, and consequently impacts epigenetic profiles in cancer cells (Simpson et al, 2012). Of specific relevance to α-KG are recurrent mutations in the *IDH1* and *IDH2* genes identified in AML, gliomas, intrahepatic cholangiocarcinomas, and other cancers (Dang et al, 2016). *IDH1* and *IDH2* encode the metabolic enzymes that mediate the oxidative decarboxylation of isocitrate to α-KG in an NADP-dependent manner (see Chap. 12, Sec. 12.3.5). Oncogenic *IDH1* and *IDH2* mutations lead to aberrant enzymatic activity that results instead in the conversion of α-KG to 2-hydroxyglutarate (2-HG). The accumulation of 2-HG within cancer cells acts as a competitive inhibitor of α-KG–dependent dioxygenases such as the Jumonji class of demethylases and TET family of enzymes (involved in the demethylation of 5-methylcytosine) (Xu et al, 2011). Overall, this leads to an increase in DNA and histone methylation levels associated with malignancy. Selective inhibitors of the oncogenic mutant IDH1/2 have been developed and approved for the treatment of IDH-mutant AML (see Chap. 19, Sec. 19.6.3). Understanding the interplay between epigenetic enzymes and metabolite availability can reveal cancer vulnerabilities that occur through metabolic reprogramming.

3.4 CHROMATIN FACTORS AS DRUG TARGETS FOR THE TREATMENT OF CANCER

The progress made in understanding epigenetic mechanisms has ignited interest in the development of drugs targeting epigenetic alterations or dependencies in cancer (Bates SE, NEJM 2020) (Fig. 3–12). The concept of drugging the cancer epigenome is particularly attractive because of its reversibility. Emerging evidence suggests that epigenetic modifications play a role in tumor immune evasion, and epigenetic therapies might help overcome resistance to cancer immunotherapy (Yau et al, 2019).

Epigenetic regulation is achieved through the actions of enzymes that may serve as potential drug targets. Inhibitors of some of these enzymes have demonstrated therapeutic activity, which has led to their clinical approval (see also Chap. 19, Sec. 19.6.3).

3.4.1 DNA Methyltransferase Inhibitors

Promoter hypermethylation of tumor suppressor genes is found in multiple cancer types. DNMTs are responsible for methylating these promoter regions, and the possibility of reversing this effect makes them attractive as therapeutic targets. Although reactivation of tumor suppressor genes including *CDKN2A*, *MLH1*, and *RB* has been demonstrated through the use of DNMT inhibitors in laboratory models, the clinical relevance of this proposed mechanism is debated in light of recent findings linking DNMT inhibitor antitumor effects to the activation of a viral mimicry response dependent on the loss of DNA methylation at DNA repeat elements. Cytosine analogs and non-nucleoside agents have been developed as inhibitors of DNMT (Pfister and Ashworth, 2017). The cytosine analogs are incorporated into DNA and form covalent adducts with DNMT, making the enzyme unavailable for future replication cycles, resulting in DNA hypomethylation. Two nucleoside DNMT inhibitors, azacitidine and decitabine,

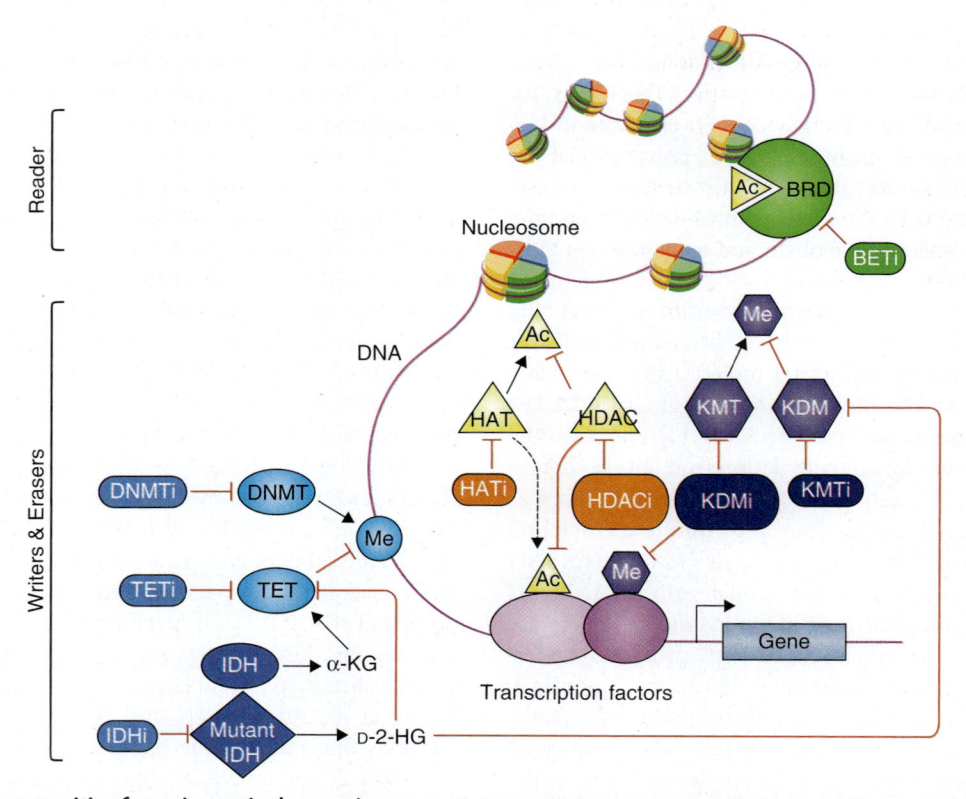

FIGURE 3–12 **Opportunities for epigenetic therapy in cancer.** Epigenetic enzymes are classified in one of 3 categories: readers, writers, or erasers. Each harbors unique domains compatible with the development of chemical probes to inhibit their function. Accordingly, a growing collection of chemical inhibitors are available against readers, including bromodomain inhibitors (BETi); writers, including lysine methyltransferase (KMTi), histone acetyltransferase (HATi), and DNA methyltransferase (DNMTi) inhibitors; and erasers histone deacetylase (HDACi), lysine demethylase (KDMi), and TET inhibitors (TETi). (Modified with permission from Morel D, Jeffery D, Aspeslagh S, Almouzni G, Postel-Vinay S. Combining epigenetic drugs with other therapies for solid tumours - past lessons and future promise. *Nat Rev Clin Oncol* 2020 Feb;17(2):91-107.)

have been approved for use in myelodysplastic syndrome. Non-nucleoside analog DNMT inhibitors have lacked potency and specificity and are no longer in development. Despite the perceived advantage that DNMT inhibitors may target multiple cancer pathways via global methylation, the nonspecific targeting of these inhibitors may produce undesirable effects. Indeed, these agents are associated with substantial toxicity, and DNMT inhibitors are used at low doses with the main purpose of reprogramming epigenetic function rather than producing cytotoxic effects. These agents have not shown activity against solid tumors when used alone, but there is some evidence that combining DNMT inhibitors with immune checkpoint blockade can induce antitumor immunity, and this is being evaluated in clinical trials (Yau et al, 2019).

3.4.2 Histone Deacetylase Inhibitors

Histone acetylation increases chromatin accessibility for gene transcription. HDACs are enzymes responsible for removing acetyl groups from histones making chromatin more compact and less accessible. Overexpression of HDACs is observed in multiple tumor types, indicating that they play an important role in tumorigenesis. HDAC inhibitors have been shown to induce tumor cell killing by multiple mechanisms including the induction of apoptosis, DNA damage, cell cycle arrest, inhibition of angiogenesis, and the generation of reactive oxygen species (Mottamal et al, 2015). The mechanisms underlying these observed effects are complex, as HDAC inhibition has genome-wide effects, including modulation of the activity of multiple transcription factors. To add to this complexity, there are 18 HDACs in humans and available HDAC inhibitors target classes as opposed to individual HDACs. Nonetheless, HDAC inhibitors (including vorinostat, belinostat, panobinostat, and romidepsin) have been approved for the treatment for several tumor types, including T-cell lymphomas and multiple myeloma (see Chap. 19, Sec. 19.6.3).

3.4.3 Lysine Methyltransferase and Demethylase Inhibitors

There are more than 60 different human lysine (symbol "K") MTs (Wagner and Jung, 2012). Each KMT is responsible for methylation of a limited number of specific lysine residues of the histone tail. Furthermore, different KMTs are typically responsible for the mono- or di-, vs trimethylation of a given residue. Thus, each KMT is associated with specific histone functions that are determined by both the site and level of methylation of lysine residues at the histone tails. This specificity of KMT activity allows more precise drug targeting, with the goal of developing epigenetic treatments tailored to individual cancers.

Two of the most promising classes of drugs are inhibitors of EZH2 and DOT1L. EZH2 is the catalytic subunit of the PRC2 complex that methylates the histone H3K27. PRC2 activity is linked to transcriptional silencing, and thus EZH2 inhibition is thought to promote the reexpression of silenced genes. *EZH2* overexpression, as well as gain-of-function mutations, have been detected in multiple cancers. Although overexpression is also found in solid tumors, gain-of-function mutations are found mainly in follicular lymphoma and diffuse large B-cell lymphoma (Morin et al, 2010). Loss-of-function *EZH2* alterations have also been reported, but these occur only in myeloid leukemias with chromosome 7q deletion (Ernst et al, 2010). EZH2 inhibition mainly causes growth inhibition in cells with *EZH2* overexpression or gain-of-function mutations. The first clinical evidence for antagonizing EZH2 as a therapeutic concept was achieved in early 2020, as tazemetostat, a competitive EZH2 inhibitor, was approved for use against epithelioid sarcoma with deletions in the *INI1/SMARCB1* gene.

DOT1L, an enzyme responsible for methylation of the histone H3K79, is essential for the maintenance and survival of leukemia cells with *MLL* translocations (Park et al, 2015). Multiple preclinical studies have demonstrated that DOT1L inhibitors selectively kill leukemia harboring *MLL* rearrangements (Winters and Bernt, 2017), supporting the development of specific inhibitors for cancers with these alterations. Although investigation of DOT1L inhibitors has largely been in hematopoietic malignancies, aberrant DOT1L has also been described in solid tumors, providing an additional rationale to evaluate inhibitors of this pathway.

Overexpression of lysine demethylases (KDMs) is observed in multiple tumor types, and the activity of these enzymes have been implicated in oncogenic processes, suggesting a role for therapeutic intervention (Jambhekar et al, 2017). The 2 distinct families of KDMs, the flavin-dependent KDM1 subfamily and the α-KG–dependent Jumonji C (JMJC) domain-containing subfamily, require different approaches to chemical inhibition but offer the potential opportunity to more precisely target their cellular functions. However, the structural conservation of the JMJC catalytic domains makes it difficult to target specifically individual members of the large JMJC domain-containing subfamily. Numerous reversible and irreversible inhibitors of KDM1A/LSD1 have been developed and in preclinical settings have shown promise in leukemic cell lines harboring MLL-AF9 fusion and small cell lung cancer cell lines with DNA hypomethylation (Harris et al, 2012). Clinical trials of LSD1 inhibitors are underway, and inhibitors of other KDMs including the JMJC-subfamily members KMD4A, KMD4B, and KMD5A are in development (Jambhekar et al, 2017).

3.4.4 Emerging Epigenetic Therapies

The BET (Bromodomain and extraterminal domain) family comprises bromodomain proteins BRD2, BRD3, BRD4, and BRDT. These proteins function as epigenetic "readers" and recognize epigenetic modifications as docking sites to recruit additional chromatin modifiers and/or remodeling enzymes. Translocations of BET proteins were found initially in a rare type of tumor, called NUT carcinoma where BRD4-NUTM1 or BRD3-NUTM1 fusion proteins upregulated *MYC* expression (French, 2016). Small-molecule BET inhibitors such as JQ1 and iBET have demonstrated preclinical activity across multiple cancer types both in cell lines and animal models (Stathis and Bertoni, 2018). Mechanisms leading to antitumor activity of BET inhibition in different cancers remain to be defined but are being explored in a number of clinical trials (Stathis and Bertoni, 2018). There is potential for BET inhibitors to synergize with other targeted therapies, which may be a consequence of blocking protective feedback mechanisms that often result from selective pathway inhibition. However, blocking protective feedback might also increase toxicity to normal tissues.

3.4.5 Epigenetic Therapy in Combination With Other Cancer Therapies

Given the genome-wide effects of epigenetic drugs and consequent broad changes elicited in gene expression, epigenetic modifying therapies have the potential to alter the tumor response to other treatment modalities. Particularly in solid tumors, where epigenetic agents can modify gene expression but have limited efficacy when used alone, combination strategies are worthy of study. Expansion in the number of available drugs targeting epigenetic proteins combined with an evolving understanding of the mechanisms that underlie resistance to conventional therapies will inform the design and implementation of such strategies.

As described in Chapter 21, cancer immunotherapy depends on the recognition of cancer cells as nonself by the immune system based on features such as viral or mutated protein expression (Ott et al, 2017), noncoding transcripts (Laumont et al, 2018), protein misfolding and expression of cancer testis antigens (Whitehurst, 2014), or repeat elements (Yau et al, 2019). Despite substantial survival benefits in responders to immunotherapy, overall response rates are often low and are biased toward certain cancer types over others (Sharma et al, 2017). Epigenetic repression of immunogenic proteins expressed in tumor cells, such as repeat elements and cancer testis antigens, contributes to immune evasion, suggesting a possible benefit to combining epigenetic therapy with immunotherapy (Fig. 3–13) (reviewed in Jones et al, 2019). Both clinical observations and preclinical evidence support the concept that disrupting epigenetically mediated immune evasion can create a more immunogenic state. For instance, DNMT inhibitors activate the viral mimicry immune response (associated with interferon activation) in both colorectal cancer and ovarian cancer models by inducing repeat element expression leading to double-stranded RNA (dsRNA) formation (Chiappinelli et al, 2015; Roulois et al, 2015) and can sensitize melanomas to anti-CTLA4 immune checkpoint blockade.

There is emerging evidence for the regulation of PD-L1 (a predictive biomarker of response to PD-1 and PD-L1 checkpoint blockade in some settings) by epigenetic mechanisms. Multiple epigenetic drugs, including DNMT inhibitors, HDAC inhibitors, and BET inhibitors, have been shown to regulate PD-L1 expression, and HDAC and DNMT inhibitors in combination with PD-1 blockade have been reported to suppress the growth of ovarian cancer in animal models (Stone et al, 2017). Response to anti-PD-1 therapies can also be improved when combined with ablation of the H3K4 demethylase LSD1 gene, which is associated with improved tumor T-cell infiltration in melanoma in animal models (Sheng et al, 2018). Based on these findings, clinical trials are evaluating combinations of epigenetic drugs with immune checkpoint blockade for various cancer types.

3.5 EPIGENETIC VARIANTS AS BIOMARKERS FOR PRECISION CANCER MEDICINE

3.5.1 Genetic Variants in Chromatin Factors

Targeted sequencing of DNA alterations has been incorporated rapidly into routine clinical care, where the identification of certain genomic alterations predicts benefit (or lack thereof) for a

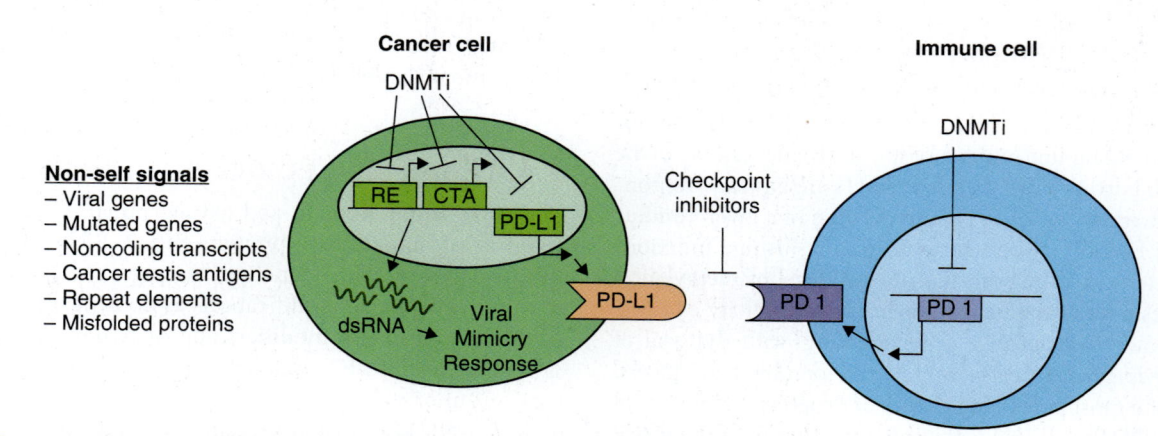

FIGURE 3–13 Epigenetic therapy and immunotherapy. Oncogenesis relies in part on the ability of cancer cells to be concealed from the immune system, preventing the detection of oncogenic "nonself" signals that arise from the expression of immunogenic elements such as viral elements, mutated genes, noncoding transcripts, misfolded proteins, cancer testis antigens, and DNA repeat elements. Immune evasion also benefits from blocking immune cell activation, such as through the expression of inhibitory checkpoints, such as PD-L1 in cancer cells. Because epigenetic drugs affect transcriptional processes, combination therapy relying on epigenetic drugs and immunotherapy are being considered for their value in promoting immune cell activation and/or increasing the expression of nonself signals.

range of targeted therapies (see Chap. 19, Sec. 19.8 and Chap. 22, Sec 22.3.2). Large-scale coordinated efforts, like those of the Cancer Genome Atlas Consortium, have revealed that mutation of genes encoding epigenetic machinery is commonly found across a range of solid and hematologic cancer types. Mutations in these genes impact enzymatic activity and thus have widespread effects on cellular gene expression. Mutations targeting these epigenetic-related genes are associated with cancer risk, pathogenesis, prognosis, and response to treatment.

Hematopoietic malignancies, where somatic alterations in epigenetic factors occur in up to 50% of patients, provide several examples of the clinical utility of targeted sequencing of epigenetic genes. Mutated *DNMT3A*, found in approximately 15% to 30% of cases of AML, is an independent predictor of shorter progression-free and overall survival (Patel et al, 2012), and is an indicator for treatment intensification for patients with intermediate-risk AML (Saygin et al, 2018). Mutations in *IDH1* and *IDH2* alter DNA methylation through their metabolic effects (see Section 3.3.5), and whereas the prognostic effects of IDH mutations in established AML remain uncertain, detection of *IDH1/2* mutations in apparently healthy individuals are associated with increased risk of developing leukemia (Desai et al, 2018). The availability of specific inhibitors of IDH1/2 enzymes (eg, ivosidenib, enasidenib) enables directed therapy for individuals with IDH-mutated AML and might offer future opportunities for screening and prevention of AML for individuals with detectable premalignant states. Loss-of-function mutations in *TET2* are recurrent in myelodysplastic syndrome and AML. TET2 enzymes are dependent on ascorbate as a cofactor for optimal activity, suggesting the possibility of administration of vitamin C to enhance TET2 function either through the remaining wild-type allele or restoration of the mutant proteins–targeted prevention or therapy (Das et al, 2019), an approach also proposed to counter the effects of IDH1 mutations in AML (Mingay et al, 2018).

Epigenetic factors also have prognostic and therapeutic relevance for solid tumors. In glioma, *IDH1/2* mutations are independently associated with better prognosis (Cohen et al, 2013), and noninvasive diagnosis and monitoring through use of molecular imaging or biochemical detection might be used to detect 2-HG produced by mutant IDH. In addition to the potential for targeting these cancers with mutant IDH inhibitors, the presence of these alterations appears to influence sensitivity to conventional therapies, including the chemotherapy temozolomide. This is likely mediated in part by promoter methylation and epigenetic silencing of *MGMT*, which functions in alkylator-induced DNA repair. Alterations in other epigenetic factors involved in tumorigenesis have also been implicated in sensitivity to different classes of DNA-damaging therapies. For example, mutations in the SWI/SNF chromatin remodeling complex subunit *ARID1A*, observed commonly in ovarian clear cell carcinoma, endometrial cancer, and at lower frequencies in many solid tumor types, impair the DNA damage checkpoint and confer sensitivity to PARP inhibitors (see Chap. 19, Sec. 19.6.2) and radiation in preclinical models (Shen et al, 2015).

As efforts to characterize the biologic consequences of cancer-associated epigenetic alterations and the clinical features of these molecularly defined cancers mature, opportunities to leverage molecular profiling to inform the application of standard and targeted therapies will expand.

3.5.2 Epigenetic Identity and Cancers of Unknown Primary

Accounting for 3% to 5% of all metastatic human tumors, cancers of unknown primary (CUP) are histologically diagnosed metastases for which the origin of the primary tumor is unknown. These cancers are generally treated with cytotoxic combination chemotherapy but have poor outcome (Varadhachary and Raber, 2014). The identification of the primary tumor origin is a major goal in the evaluation of patients presenting with CUP because it affects treatment strategies. The use of molecular tools to assess tissue of origin in CUP has focused initially on gene expression profiling, which could succeed in 60% to 90% of patients (Handorf et al, 2013). However, the clinical utility of these tests has been limited, and their dependence on RNA demands adequate tissue sampling, which is often difficult or impossible. Emerging evidence suggests that DNA methylation may permit the accurate characterization of unknown primary tumors (Fig. 3–14) (Conway et al, 2019).

The large number of epigenetic features that can be assessed has enabled the development of accurate molecular classifiers, which perform better than gene expression–based platforms. For example, a microarray-based DNA methylation signature (EPICUP) trained from 2790 tumor samples of 38 cancer types identified the primary tumor origin in an independent validation set of 7691 known tumor samples with 97.7% sensitivity and 99.6% specificity (Moran et al, 2016). Application of this DNA methylation–based classifier predicted a primary of origin in nearly 90% of 216 patients with unknown primary, and those patients who received a tumor type–specific therapy had improved overall survival relative to those who did not (Moran et al, 2016). Chromatin accessibility profiles represent an alternative epigenetic characteristic to discriminate individual tumors according to their tissue of origin, as exemplified by the study of such profiles generated across 410 tumor samples collected from 23 different cancer types (Corces et al, 2018). Collectively, these results illustrate the potential for epigenetic profiling to contribute to cancer diagnostics and clinical management.

Improved methods for processing and preserving tumor samples for epigenetic assays are being used in the clinical setting, and technical progress is allowing epigenetic assays to be applied to small amounts of biological material. Epigenetic assays can thus be integrated into molecular profiling algorithms to evaluate and inform patient management.

3.5.3 Tracking Tumors Through Their Epigenetics in Liquid Biopsies

Liquid biopsy, which characterizes circulating tumor cells or cell-free circulating tumor DNA (ctDNA) in the peripheral

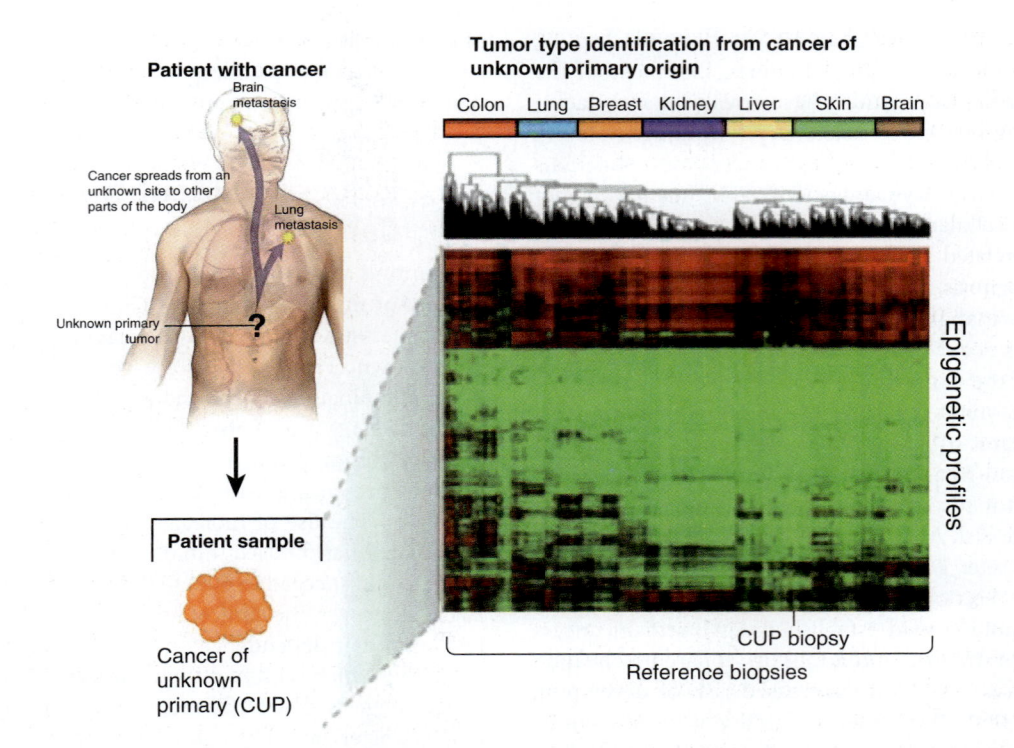

FIGURE 3–14 **Epigenetic identity for cancers of unknown primary.** Each tissue type and cancers arising from these harbor unique epigenetic identities. These epigenetic features also serve to distinguish different cancer subtypes. Collectively, this allows for assigning cancer of unknown primary to their tissue of origin and to their cancer type/subtype, which may have a role in diagnosis or treatment selection. (Reproduced with permission from PDQ® Adult Treatment Editorial Board. PDQ Carcinoma of Unknown Primary Treatment. Bethesda, MD: *National Cancer Institute*. Updated October 23, 2019. Available at: https://www.cancer.gov/types/unknown-primary/patient/unknown-primary-treatment-pdq. Accessed 07/31/2020)

blood, has rapidly emerged as a diagnostic technology in oncology (Fig. 3–15). Although clinical applications of liquid biopsy have focused on identifying somatic point mutations in ctDNA to permit delivery of matched targeted therapy (eg, EGFR inhibitors for EGFR mutant non–small cell lung cancer), a role for epigenetic profiling of ctDNA is emerging.

The characteristic epigenetic patterns in tumors and their similarities with their tissue of origin are largely retained in cell-free DNA, in both their DNA methylation as well as chromatin accessibility patterns (Snyder et al, 2016; Shen et al, 2018). Because DNA methylation profiles in tumors consist of tens to hundreds of thousands of discriminating sites across the genome in comparison to a handful to a hundred recurrent somatic genetic alterations, DNA methylation profiling of cell-free DNA ensures a high sensitivity to detect and characterize small quantities of ctDNA (Locke et al, 2019). The

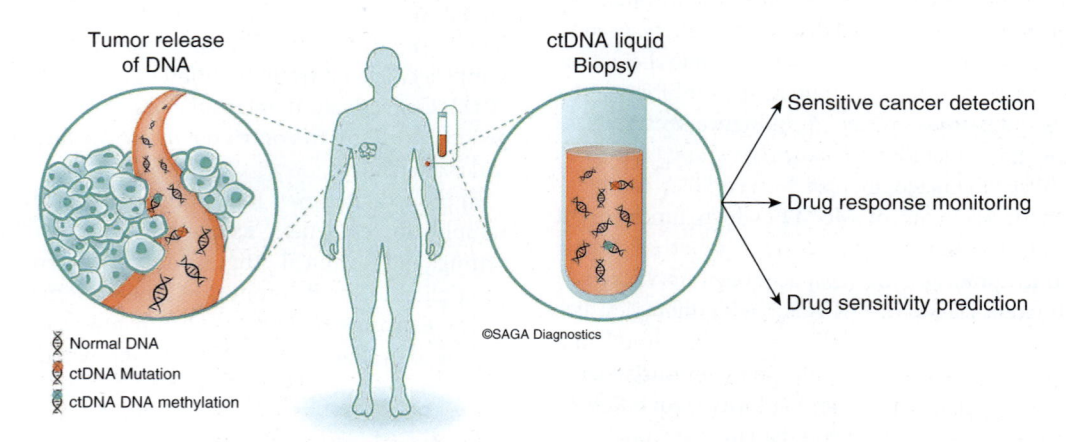

FIGURE 3–15 **Cancer monitoring based on the epigenetics of liquid biopsies.** Tumors naturally shed their DNA into the bloodstream, where it can be detected and is known as circulating tumor DNA (ctDNA). Profiling the DNA methylation of ctDNA and comparing it to the unique DNA methylation pattern of tumors from different tissues offers an avenue for the early detection of tumors, prediction of drug sensitivity to inform treatment selection, or for the monitoring of response to treatment. (Reproduced with permission from ©SAGA Diagnostics https://sagadiagnostics.com/science)

first liquid biopsy ctDNA test approved for cancer screening in healthy individuals targets methylation of a specific locus—the *SEPT9* (*Septin9*) promoter (Lamb and Dhillon, 2017). Following demonstration that colorectal cancer exhibits increased *SEPT9* promoter methylation compared with normal tissues, development and clinical evaluation of a PCR-based peripheral blood assay achieved sensitivity of >75% (including 60% of early-stage cancers) with high specificity (>97.5%).

Evaluation of a single locus limits the application of a given test to a specific diagnostic question. Efforts to develop single- or pan-cancer blood-based screening or detection tests have converged around broader evaluation of differentially methylated regions. One example is the development of a ctDNA-targeted sequencing assay incorporating detection of somatic variants, methylation alterations, and other epigenetic variations at transcription factor–binding sites associated with colorectal cancer. Compared with detection of somatic mutations alone, the assay increased sensitivity from 56% to more than 90%, including for those with early-stage disease, while maintaining high specificity (Kim et al, 2019). Adopting a pure epigenetic approach using targeted bisulfite sequencing to assess DNA methylation, the largest commercial effort to develop a pan-cancer screening test has demonstrated the ability to detect disease and assign tissue of origin reliably in more than 20 tumor types (Liu et al, 2020). Reflecting the very high specificity required for a test intended for application in a healthy population, this approach has lower sensitivity for any given cancer type but illustrates the high content of biologic information encoded in DNA methylation. Ongoing trials are evaluating the clinical utility of such approaches in large populations, both for primary cancer screening and markers of persisting "molecular residual disease" following definitive therapy for early-stage cancer.

Although DNA methylation tests are predicted to be more useful than genetic tests, studies are needed to evaluate their clinical utility and cost effectiveness relative to other screening methods and/or to favor their inclusion in multimodal testing (Wang et al, 2014). In contrast to tissue biopsies, the ease of access and noninvasive nature of liquid biopsies offers an opportunity to track the patient's status, monitor treatment response, and to detect early recurrence.

SUMMARY

- Epigenetics relates to heritable changes in gene expression that are not encoded in the primary DNA sequence and is responsible for generation of different cell types with distinct gene expression patterns and functional phenotypes.
- Epigenetic changes influence the structure of chromatin, which contributes to the development and progression of various human disorders, including cancers.
- The characteristics of chromatin are determined mainly by the presence of DNA methylation and/or posttranslational modifications of histones and the presence of histone variants.
- Recurrent mutations in genes that regulate chromatin are common and are responsible for aberrant DNA methylation, histone posttranslational modifications, and dysregulation of histone variants that are implicated in cancer initiation, progression, and resistance to treatment.
- Epigenetic alterations are labile and reversible, thereby providing opportunities for anticancer drug development.
- A pleiotropic genome-wide effect induced by targeting epigenetic effectors could be exploited for reprogramming cancer cells for therapeutic advantage.
- Epigenetic profiles can discriminate cancer types and track tumor evolution in liquid biopsies. They may have a role in screening healthy individuals for cancer.

REFERENCES

Akhtar-Zaidi B, Cowper-Sal-lari R, Corradin O, et al. Epigenomic enhancer profiling defines a signature of colon cancer. *Science* 2012;336(6082):736-739.

Aran D, Sabato S, Hellman A. DNA methylation of distal regulatory sites characterizes dysregulation of cancer genes. *Genome Biol* 2013;14:R21.

Arrowsmith CH, Bountra C, Fish PV, Lee K, Schapira M. Epigenetic protein families: a new frontier for drug discovery. *Nat Rev Drug Discov* 2012;11(5):384-400.

Bannister AJ, Kouzarides T. Regulation of chromatin by histone modifications. *Cell Res* 2011;21(3):381-395.

Bates SE. Epigenetic Therapies for Cancer. *N Engl J Med* 2020;383:650-663.

Bernt KM, Zhu N, Sinha AU, et al. MLL-rearranged leukemia is dependent on aberrant H3K79 methylation by DOT1L. *Cancer Cell* 2011;20(1):66-78.

Bourque G, Burns KH, Gehring M, et al. Ten things you should know about transposable elements. *Genome Biol* 2018;19(1):199.

Buschbeck M, Hake SB. Variants of core histones and their roles in cell fate decisions, development and cancer. *Nat Rev Mol Cell Biol* 2017;18(5):299-314.

Chiappinelli KB, Strissel PL, Desrichard A, et al. Inhibiting DNA methylation causes an interferon response in cancer via dsRNA including endogenous retroviruses. *Cell* 2015;162(5):974-986.

Cohen AL, Holmen SL, Colman H. IDH1 and IDH2 mutations in gliomas. *Curr Neurol Neurosci Rep* 2013;13(5):345.

Conway AM, Mitchell C, Kilgour E, Brady G, Dive C, Cook N. Molecular characterisation and liquid biomarkers in Carcinoma of Unknown Primary (CUP): taking the "U" out of "CUP." *Br J Cancer.* 2019;120(2):141-153.

Corces MR, Granja JM, Shams S, et al. The chromatin accessibility landscape of primary human cancers. *Science* 2018;362(6413).

Dang L, Yen K, Attar EC. IDH mutations in cancer and progress toward development of targeted therapeutics. *Ann Oncol.* 2016;27(4):599-608.

Das AB, Kakadia PM, Wojcik D, et al. Clinical remission following ascorbate treatment in a case of acute myeloid leukemia with mutations in TET2 and WT1. *Blood Cancer J* 2019;9(10):82.

Debruyne DN, Dries R, Sengupta S, et al. BORIS promotes chromatin regulatory interactions in treatment-resistant cancer cells. *Nature.* 2019;572(7771):676-680.

De Carvalho DD, You JS, Jones PA. DNA methylation and cellular reprogramming. *Trends Cell Biol* 2010;20(10):609-617.

Desai P, Mencia-Trinchant N, Savenkov O, et al. Somatic mutations precede acute myeloid leukemia years before diagnosis. *Nat Med* 2018;24(7):1015-1023.

Ernst J, Kheradpour P, Mikkelsen TS, et al. Mapping and analysis of chromatin state dynamics in nine human cell types. *Nature* 2011;473(7345):43-49.

Ernst T, Chase AJ, Score J, et al. Inactivating mutations of the histone methyltransferase gene EZH2 in myeloid disorders. *Nat Genet* 2010;42(8):722-726.

Feinberg AP. The key role of epigenetics in human disease prevention and mitigation. *N Engl J Med* 2018;378(14):1323-1334.

Flavahan WA, Drier Y, Liau BB, et al. Insulator dysfunction and oncogene activation in IDH mutant gliomas. *Nature* 2016;529(7584):110-114.

French CA. Small-molecule targeting of BET proteins in cancer. *Adv Cancer Res* 2016;131:21-58.

Guibert S, Forné T, Weber M. Dynamic regulation of DNA methylation during mammalian development. *Epigenomics* 2009;1(1):81-98.

Hahn MA, Li AX, Wu X, et al. Loss of the polycomb mark from bivalent promoters leads to activation of cancer-promoting genes in colorectal tumors. *Cancer Res* 2014;74(13):3617-3629.

Haladyna JN, Yamauchi T, Neff T, Bernt KM. Epigenetic modifiers in normal and malignant hematopoiesis. *Epigenomics* 2015;7(2):301-320.

Handorf CR, Kulkarni A, Grenert JP, et al. A multicenter study directly comparing the diagnostic accuracy of gene expression profiling and immunohistochemistry for primary site identification in metastatic tumors. *Am J Surg Pathol* 2013;37(7):1067-1075.

Harris WJ, Huang X, Lynch JT, et al. The histone demethylase KDM1A sustains the oncogenic potential of MLL-AF9 leukemia stem cells. *Cancer Cell* 2012;21(4):473-487.

He HH, Meyer CA, Shin H, et al. Nucleosome dynamics define transcriptional enhancers. *Nat Genet* 2010;42(4):343-347.

Heintzman ND, Hon GC, Hawkins RD, et al. Histone modifications at human enhancers reflect global cell-type-specific gene expression. *Nature* 2009;459(7243):108-112.

Heintzman ND, Ren B. The gateway to transcription: identifying, characterizing and understanding promoters in the eukaryotic genome. *Cell Mol Life Sci* 2007;64(4):386-400.

Heintzman ND, Stuart RK, Hon G, et al. Distinct and predictive chromatin signatures of transcriptional promoters and enhancers in the human genome. *Nat Genet* 2007;39(3):311-318.

Henikoff S, Smith MM. Histone variants and epigenetics. *Cold Spring Harb Perspect Biol* 2015;7(1):a019364.

Heyn H, Vidal E, Ferreira HJ, et al. Epigenomic analysis detects aberrant super-enhancer DNA methylation in human cancer. *Genome Biol* 2016;17:11.

Horton JR, Upadhyay AK, Hashimoto H, Zhang X, Cheng X. Structural basis for human PHF2 Jumonji domain interaction with metal ions. *J Mol Biol* 2011;406:1-8.

Hou H, Yu H. Structural insights into histone lysine demethylation. *Curr Opin Struct Biol* 2010;20(6):739-748.

Igarashi K, Katoh Y. Metabolic aspects of epigenome: coupling of S-adenosylmethionine synthesis and gene regulation on chromatin by SAMIT module. *Subcell Biochem* 2013;61:105-118.

Jambhekar A, Anastas JN, Shi Y. Histone lysine demethylase inhibitors. *Cold Spring Harb Perspect Med* 2017;7(1):a026484.

Jia M, Gao X, Zhang Y, Hoffmeister M, Brenner H. Different definitions of CpG island methylator phenotype and outcomes of colorectal cancer: a systematic review. *Clin Epigenetics* 2016;8:25.

Johnson C, Warmoes MO, Shen X, Locasale JW. Epigenetics and cancer metabolism. *Cancer Lett* 2015;356(2 Pt A):309-314.

Jones PA, Liang G. Rethinking how DNA methylation patterns are maintained. *Nat Rev Genet* 2009;10(11):805-811.

Jones PA, Ohtani H, Chakravarthy A, De Carvalho DD. Epigenetic therapy in immune-oncology. *Nat Rev Cancer* 2019;19(3):151-161.

Kim KH, Roberts CWM. Targeting EZH2 in cancer. *Nat Med* 2016;22(2):128-134.

Kim ST, Raymond VM, Park JO, et al. Abstract 916: Combined genomic and epigenomic assessment of cell-free circulating tumor DNA (ctDNA) improves assay sensitivity in early-stage colorectal cancer (CRC). *Cancer Res* 2019;79:916-916.

Kron KJ, Murison A, Zhou S, et al. TMPRSS2-ERG fusion co-opts master transcription factors and activates NOTCH signaling in primary prostate cancer. *Nat Genet* 2017;49(9):1336-1345.

Lamb YN, Dhillon S. Epi proColon® 2.0 CE: a blood-based screening test for colorectal cancer. *Mol Diagn Ther* 2017;21(2):225-232.

Laumont CM, Vincent K, Hesnard L, et al. Noncoding regions are the main source of targetable tumor-specific antigens. *Sci Transl Med* 2018;10(470):eaau5516.

Li BE, Ernst P. Two decades of leukemia oncoprotein epistasis: the MLL1 paradigm for epigenetic deregulation in leukemia. *Exp Hematol* 2014;42(12):995-1012.

Liu MC, Oxnard GR, Klein EA, et al. Sensitive and specific multi-cancer detection and localization using methylation signatures in cell-free DNA. *Ann Oncol.* 2020;31:745-759.

Locke WJ, Guanzon D, Ma C, et al. DNA methylation cancer biomarkers: translation to the clinic. *Front Genet.* 2019;10:1150.

Lu C, Thompson CB. Metabolic regulation of epigenetics. *Cell Metab* 2012;16:9-17.

Lund K, Adams PD, Copland M. EZH2 in normal and malignant hematopoiesis. *Leukemia* 2014;28(1):44-49.

Lupien M, Eeckhoute J, Meyer CA, et al. FoxA1 translates epigenetic signatures into enhancer-driven lineage-specific transcription. *Cell* 2008;132(6):958-970.

Magnani L, Stoeck A, Zhang X, et al. Genome-wide reprogramming of the chromatin landscape underlies endocrine therapy resistance in breast cancer. *Proc Natl Acad Sci U S A* 2013;110(16):E1490-E1499.

Mingay M, Chaturvedi A, Bilenky M, et al. Vitamin C-induced epigenomic remodelling in IDH1 mutant acute myeloid leukaemia. *Leukemia* 2018;32(1):11-20.

Moran S, Martínez-Cardús A, Sayols S, et al. Epigenetic profiling to classify cancer of unknown primary: a multicentre, retrospective analysis. *Lancet Oncol* 2016;17(10):1386-1395.

Morin RD, Johnson NA, Severson TM, et al. Somatic mutations altering EZH2 (Tyr641) in follicular and diffuse large B-cell lymphomas of germinal-center origin. *Nat Genet* 2010;42(2):181-185.

Morrison AJ, Shen X. Chromatin remodelling beyond transcription: the INO80 and SWR1 complexes. *Nat Rev Mol Cell Biol* 2009;10(6):373-384.

Mottamal M, Zheng S, Huang TL, Wang G. Histone deacetylase inhibitors in clinical studies as templates for new anticancer agents. *Molecules* 2015;20(3):3898-3941.

Ong CT, Corces VG. CTCF: an architectural protein bridging genome topology and function. *Nat Rev Genet* 2014;15(4):234-246.

Ott PA, Hu Z, Keskin DB, et al. An immunogenic personal neoantigen vaccine for patients with melanoma. *Nature* 2017;547(7662):217-221.

Pakneshan P, Xing RH, Rabbani SA. Methylation status of uPA promoter as a molecular mechanism regulating prostate cancer invasion and growth in vitro and in vivo. *FASEB J* 2003;17(9):1081-1088.

Park JW, Kim KB, Kim JY, Chae YC, Jeong OS, Seo SB. RE-IIBP methylates H3K79 and induces MEIS1-mediated apoptosis via H2BK120 ubiquitination by RNF20. *Sci Rep* 2015;5:12485.

Parsons DW, Li M, Zhang X, et al. The genetic landscape of the childhood cancer medulloblastoma. *Science* 2011;331:435-439.

Patel JP, Gönen M, Figueroa ME, et al. Prognostic relevance of integrated genetic profiling in acute myeloid leukemia. *N Engl J Med* 2012;366(12):1079-1089.

Pfister SX, Ashworth A. Marked for death: targeting epigenetic changes in cancer. *Nat Rev Drug Discov* 2017;16(4):241-263.

Roulois D, Loo Yau H, Singhania R, et al. DNA-demethylating agents target colorectal cancer cells by inducing viral mimicry by endogenous transcripts. *Cell* 2015;162(5):961-973.

Saygin C, Hirsch C, Przychodzen B, et al. Mutations in DNMT3A, U2AF1, and EZH2 identify intermediate-risk acute myeloid leukemia patients with poor outcome after CR1. *Blood Cancer J* 2018;8(1):4.

Schoenfelder S, Fraser P. Long-range enhancer–promoter contacts in gene expression control. *Nat Rev Genet* 2019;20(8):437-455.

Shah MA, Denton EL, Arrowsmith CH, Lupien M, Schapira M. A global assessment of cancer genomic alterations in epigenetic mechanisms. *Epigenet Chroma* 2014;7(1):29.

Sharma P, Hu-Lieskovan S, Wargo JA, Ribas A. Primary, adaptive, and acquired resistance to cancer immunotherapy. *Cell* 2017;168(4):707-723.

Shen J, Peng Y, Wei L, et al. ARID1A deficiency impairs the DNA damage checkpoint and sensitizes cells to PARP inhibitors. *Cancer Discov* 2015;5(7):752-767.

Shen SY, Singhania R, Fehringer G, et al. Sensitive tumour detection and classification using plasma cell-free DNA methylomes. *Nature* 2018;563(7732):579-583.

Sheng W, LaFleur MW, Nguyen TH, et al. LSD1 ablation stimulates anti-tumor immunity and enables checkpoint blockade. *Cell* 2018;174(3):549-563.e19.

Shi L, Tu BP. Acetyl-CoA and the regulation of metabolism: mechanisms and consequences. *Curr Opin Cell Biol* 2015;33:125-131.

Simpson NE, Tryndyak VP, Pogribna M, Beland FA, Pogribny IP. Modifying metabolically sensitive histone marks by inhibiting glutamine metabolism affects gene expression and alters cancer cell phenotype. *Epigenetics* 2012;7(12):1413-1420.

Snyder MW, Kircher M, Hill AJ, Daza RM, Shendure J. Cell-free DNA comprises an in vivo nucleosome footprint that informs its tissues-of-origin. *Cell* 2016;164(1-2):57-68.

Stathis A, Bertoni F. BET proteins as targets for anticancer treatment. *Cancer Discov* 2018;8(1):24-36.

Stone A, Zotenko E, Locke WJ, et al. DNA methylation of oestrogen-regulated enhancers defines endocrine sensitivity in breast cancer. *Nat Commun* 2015;6:7758.

Stone ML, Chiappinelli KB, Li H, et al. Epigenetic therapy activates type I interferon signaling in murine ovarian cancer to reduce immunosuppression and tumor burden. *Proc Natl Acad Sci U S A* 2017;114(51):E10981-E10990.

Talbert PB, Ahmad K, Almouzni G, et al. A unified phylogeny-based nomenclature for histone variants. *Epigenet Chroma* 2012;5:7.

Turcan S, Rohle D, Goenka A, et al. IDH1 mutation is sufficient to establish the glioma hypermethylator phenotype. *Nature* 2012;483(7390):479-483.

Varadhachary GR, Raber MN. Cancer of unknown primary site. *N Engl J Med* 2014;371(8):757-765.

Vastenhouw NL, Schier AF. Bivalent histone modifications in early embryogenesis. *Curr Opin Cell Biol* 2012;24(3):374-386.

Wagner T, Jung M. New lysine methyltransferase drug targets in cancer. *Nat Biotechnol* 2012;30(7):622-623.

Wang B, Mezlini AM, Demir F, et al. Similarity network fusion for aggregating data types on a genomic scale. *Nat Methods* 2014;11(3):333-337.

Whitehurst AW. Cause and consequence of cancer/testis antigen activation in cancer. *Annu Rev Pharmacol Toxicol* 2014;54:251-272.

Winters AC, Bernt KM. MLL-rearranged leukemias—an update on science and clinical approaches. *Front Pediatr* 2017;5:691.

Xu K, Wu ZJ, Groner AC, et al. EZH2 oncogenic activity in castration-resistant prostate cancer cells is polycomb-independent. *Science* 2012;338(6113):1465-1469.

Xu W, Yang H, Liu Y, et al. Oncometabolite 2-hydroxyglutarate is a competitive inhibitor of α-ketoglutarate-dependent dioxygenases. *Cancer Cell* 2011;19(1):17-30.

Yau HL, Ettayebi I, De Carvalho DD. The cancer epigenome: exploiting its vulnerabilities for immunotherapy. *Trends Cell Biol* 2019;29:31-43.

Zhou S, Treloar AE, Lupien M. Emergence of the noncoding cancer genome: a target of genetic and epigenetic alterations. *Cancer Discov* 2016;6(11):1215-1229.

Cancer Epidemiology

Matthew T. Warkentin, Lidija Latifovic, Geoffrey Liu, and Rayjean J. Hung

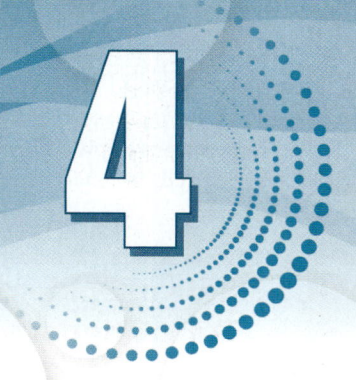

Chapter Outline

4.1 Introduction and Terminology
    4.1.1 Epidemiology: Definition and Scope
    4.1.2 General Approach
    4.1.3 Role of Epidemiology in Translational Medicine

4.2 Descriptive Epidemiology
    4.2.1 Incidence, Mortality, Case Fatality, and Age-Standardized Incidence Rates
    4.2.2 Prevalence
    4.2.3 The Role of Sampling
    4.2.4 Geographic Variation
    4.2.5 Time Trends

4.3 Analytic Epidemiology Study Designs and Considerations
    4.3.1 Ecologic Design
    4.3.2 Case-Control Design
    4.3.3 Cohort Design
    4.3.4 Cross-Sectional Design
    4.3.5 Familial Design
    4.3.6 Random Error and Bias

4.4 Analytic Epidemiology
    4.4.1 Basic Comparative Approaches: Relative Risk, Odds Ratio
    4.4.2 Probability, Distributions, and Tests of Association
    4.4.3 Regression Approaches
    4.4.4 Interaction

4.5 Cancer Epidemiology in Action: Success Stories
    4.5.1 Infection and Cancer
    4.5.2 Tobacco and Cancer
    4.5.3 Alcohol and Head and Neck Cancer

4.6 Emerging Areas in Epidemiology
    4.6.1 Genomic Epidemiology
    4.6.2 Genomic Risk Studies Based on Mechanistic Principles: Alcohol, Alcohol Dehydrogenase, and Head and Neck Cancer:
    4.6.3 Pharmacogenomic Epidemiology and Pharmacoepidemiology

4.7 Issues and Challenges in Cancer Epidemiology
    4.7.1 Observational Studies vs Clinical Trials, Predictive vs Prognostic Biomarkers
    4.7.2 Exposure Misclassifications: The Example of Diet and Occupation
    4.7.3 High-Dimensionality Data and Multiple Comparisons
    4.7.4 Analyses Across Multiple Studies

Summary

References

4.1 INTRODUCTION AND TERMINOLOGY

4.1.1 Epidemiology: Definition and Scope

Epidemiology is the study of distribution and determinants of disease and disease outcomes in human populations. The primary research question for epidemiologists is why individuals, or different populations, have different risks of disease or disease outcomes. Epidemiology is broadly focused, examining a full spectrum of disease determinants. These encompass biologic, environmental (including lifestyle), social, and economic factors. Consequently, concepts and methods from other disciplines, such as biological sciences and sociology, are critical to the design, conduct, and analysis of epidemiologic studies. Important contributions are also made from the field of statistics. Epidemiology provides a critical link between clinical or laboratory results and observed health effects in populations. An observational approach is often the only way to examine risk between disease and a specific risk factor because, for example, it is unethical to assign individuals to an arm of a randomized trial that exposes them to a suspected carcinogen.

4.1.2 General Approach

Epidemiology is often dichotomized into two disciplines: descriptive and analytic. Descriptive epidemiology primarily describes rates of disease in populations, either over time or across geographic areas or demographic subgroups. Analytic epidemiology focuses on individuals in a population, comparing diseased to nondiseased members to determine which factors increase risk for disease. Measures commonly used in descriptive epidemiology are described in Section 4.2. Measures used in analytic epidemiology are described in Section 4.3.

4.1.3 Role of Epidemiology in Translational Medicine

Whereas in vitro and in vivo studies using cell lines and animal models can control for a multitude of experimental conditions, this is difficult in human studies. Ethical and feasibility considerations prevent deliberate repeated exposures of known carcinogens to human subjects and randomization of human groups to receive either inferior therapies or environmental exposures; further, the genetic background of individuals cannot be manipulated ethically or logistically for experimental purposes even in this new era of organism-wide genome editing technologies such as CRISPR/Cas9 (Zhang et al, 2014). Although some experiments in humans may utilize intermediate subclinical end points that are reversible following brief exposure to a potential carcinogen, these intermediate end points are often not a replacement for the clinical outcome of interest. An example of this type of intermediate end point is the measurement of carcinogen-adduct formation in humans after a single exposure to a putative carcinogen. Such results may support the role of such a carcinogen, but do not provide evidence of increased rates of cancer in individuals exposed to the putative carcinogen. In general, the process of translating basic science discoveries into the clinical setting requires studies of humans, their biologic specimens, and associated clinical data. Such studies require consideration of many factors that can affect the development of disease or its outcome. This is particularly important in the omics era (eg, genomics, proteomics, epigenomics, metabolomics, transcriptomics, and more), where a large number of biologic parameters can be considered alongside classical clinical and epidemiologic factors, all of which could affect risk of the disease or outcome of interest.

In the face of such analyses, epidemiologic principles become important. The majority of epidemiologic studies involve observational data (whether aggregate or individual data) where, by definition, the investigator can only observe the characteristics of the population of interest, and cannot intervene to standardize exposures and other factors (such as confounders; see Sec. 4.3.6) that may affect the outcomes of interest. Thus, a key feature of epidemiology has been the development of methodologic designs and tools to account for such confounders. These same tools must be adapted when analyzing human observational studies involving biologic parameters.

Epidemiologic studies can serve not only to validate biologic principles and translate findings into the clinical setting, but their findings can lead to new avenues of basic research. For example, long before the existence of an activating epidermal growth factor receptor (EGFR) mutation was found to drive certain lung tumors that are sensitive to small molecular inhibitors (see Chap. 7, Sec. 7.5.3), there were clinical and epidemiologic clues to the existence of a biologically distinct subset of such patients. Patients with tumors that were highly sensitive to EGFR inhibitor drugs were more likely to be lifetime never-smokers, of Asian descent, had developed the histologic subtype of adenocarcinoma, and were often female (Coate et al, 2009). In another example, there has been a dramatic increase since 2000 in the incidence of oropharyngeal cancers, an anatomic subset of head and neck squamous cancers. The patients in this subset were more likely to be younger, lifetime never-smokers, have lower rates of alcohol use, and be of higher socioeconomic status when compared to the traditional head and neck cancer patient. As time went on, these oropharyngeal cancers were found to be associated with human papillomavirus infection (see Chap. 7, Sec. 7.4.4; Chung and Gillison, 2009). The relationship between human papilloma virus (HPV), alcohol, and head and neck cancer is discussed in more detail in Sections 4.5.1 and 4.5.3.

4.2 DESCRIPTIVE EPIDEMIOLOGY

4.2.1 Incidence, Mortality, Case Fatality, and Age-Standardized Incidence Rates

An *incidence rate* refers to the number of new cases of a disease observed over a specific time period in a defined population, whereas *mortality rate* refers to the number of *deaths* during a specific time period in a defined population. *Cause-specific mortality rates* are mortality rates where only specific causes of death (eg, death due to lung cancer) are considered. The denominator of incidence and mortality rates is the total person-time at risk, defined as the product of the number of individuals in the population and the time period of observation. For example, in a town with a population of 40,000, the number of new cases of cancer in a single year is divided by 40,000 to give the rate per person-year with the assumption of complete follow-up (births, deaths, and migration during the year are ignored). Similarly, the cancer mortality rate per person-year would be calculated as the number of deaths from cancer in a year divided by 40,000.

A direct calculation of an incidence rate, as determined in the above example, is termed the *crude incidence rate*, because the calculation is performed without consideration of important factors that may differ across populations. A major factor in the comparison of different populations is the difference in age distribution. Both cancer incidence and mortality increase markedly with age, and comparisons using crude rates for populations with different age distributions can be misleading. Reducing the effect of age in the calculation of the incidence of cancer (or of any other disease) allows comparison of cancer incidence across diverse communities or geographical regions that have different age distributions. The procedure requires adjusting (or *standardizing*) rates so that they are representative of the age distribution of some reference population. Typically, the reference population is chosen to be the age distribution at a particular census date of the relevant country (eg, Canada year 2016 census). Different *age-standardized* rates can then

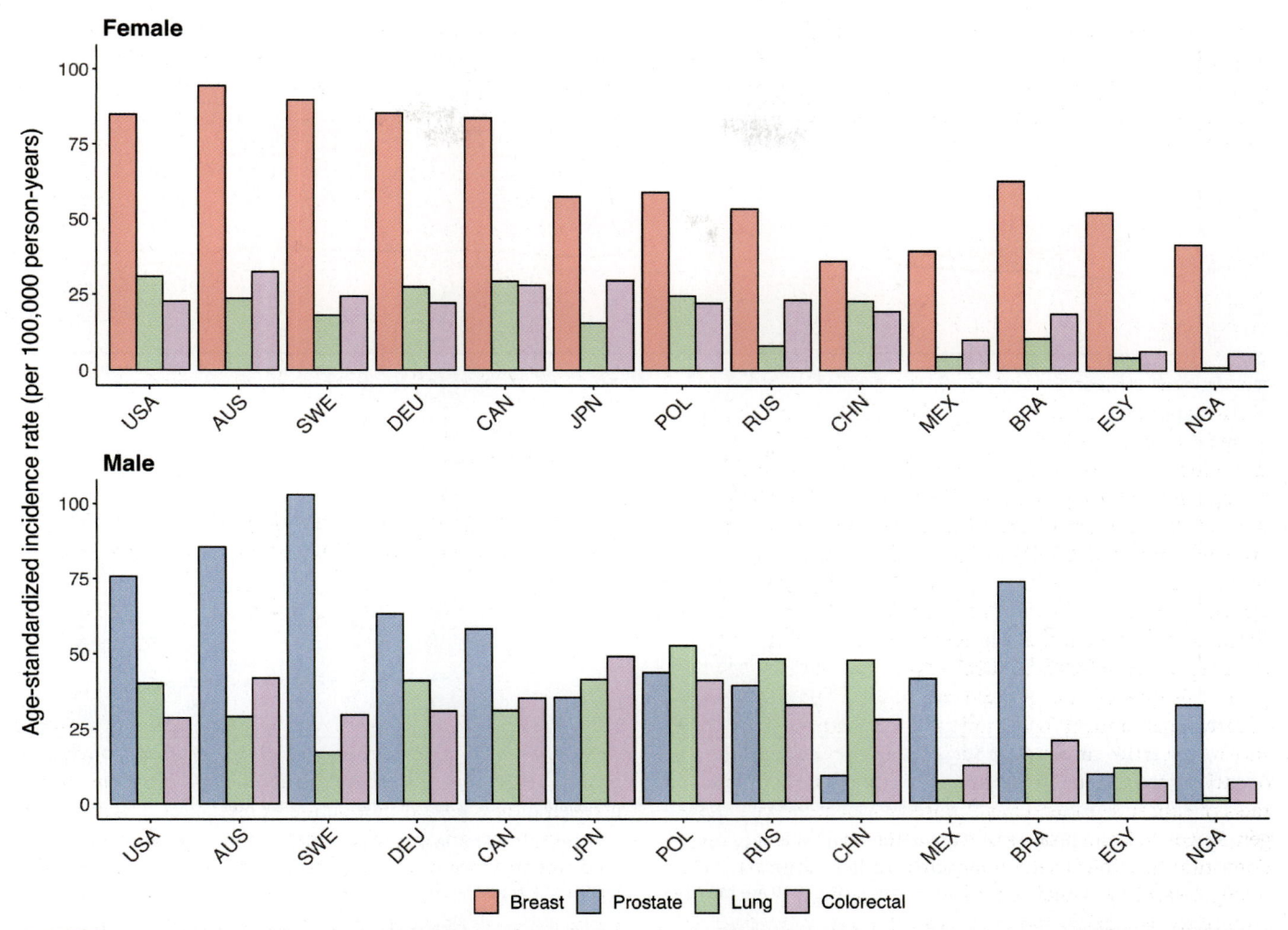

FIGURE 4–1 Age-standardized incidence rates (per 100,000 person-years) by sex for select geographical regions and cancers from 2018. Countries on the X-axis are ordered according to decreasing GDP per capita (USD) in 2018 (data obtained from the World Bank). Incidence rates were obtained from the Global Cancer Observatory. The country codes correspond to the International Organization for Standardization 3166-1 alpha-3 codes (https://unstats.un.org/unsd/tradekb/knowledgebase/country-code). (Data from Bray et al, 2018; Ferlay et al, 2018; Ferlay et al, 2019.)

be compared to each other, if they are adjusted to the same reference standard. Figures 4–1 and 4–2 show examples of age-standardized cancer incidence.

The age-standardized rate is commonly presented in publications as it accounts for differences in age distributions between populations or changes in age within populations over time. However, adjusted rates should be viewed as relative indices rather than actual measures of occurrence. Rates can also be compared within age groups, most often using 5-year age bands (0–4, 5–9, 10–14, etc). This method is informative about the disease pattern over the life course, and a comparison across populations can be made within age groups.

The *case fatality rate* or the *case fatality ratio* is the probability of dying from a disease and is estimated as the number of deaths caused by a specific disease in a defined population divided by the number of individuals who have been diagnosed with that particular disease, in a certain time period. In other words, the case fatality rate can be viewed as the ratio of the cause-specific mortality rate and cause-specific incidence rate. For example, the case fatality rate for breast cancer in the Western world is currently around 25 individuals per 100, or 25%. This means that for every 100 breast cancer diagnoses, 25 of these individuals will eventually die as a result of breast cancer. Contrast this result with pancreatic cancer, where the case fatality rate is more than 95%.

4.2.2 Prevalence

Prevalence is defined as the proportion of a population that has a disease at a specific time point (*point prevalence*) or the average proportion over a time period (*period prevalence*), and usually includes both new cases and previously diagnosed cases that are still alive. Including all people with a previous diagnosis assumes (often incorrectly) that the disease is never cured; it raises the question as to whether long-term survivors of cancer should be included in the prevalent group. Decisions should be made to ensure that prevalence reflects the actual burden of disease in the population, whereby one might consider excluding cases who are alive and free of disease beyond a specified time period after diagnosis. For example,

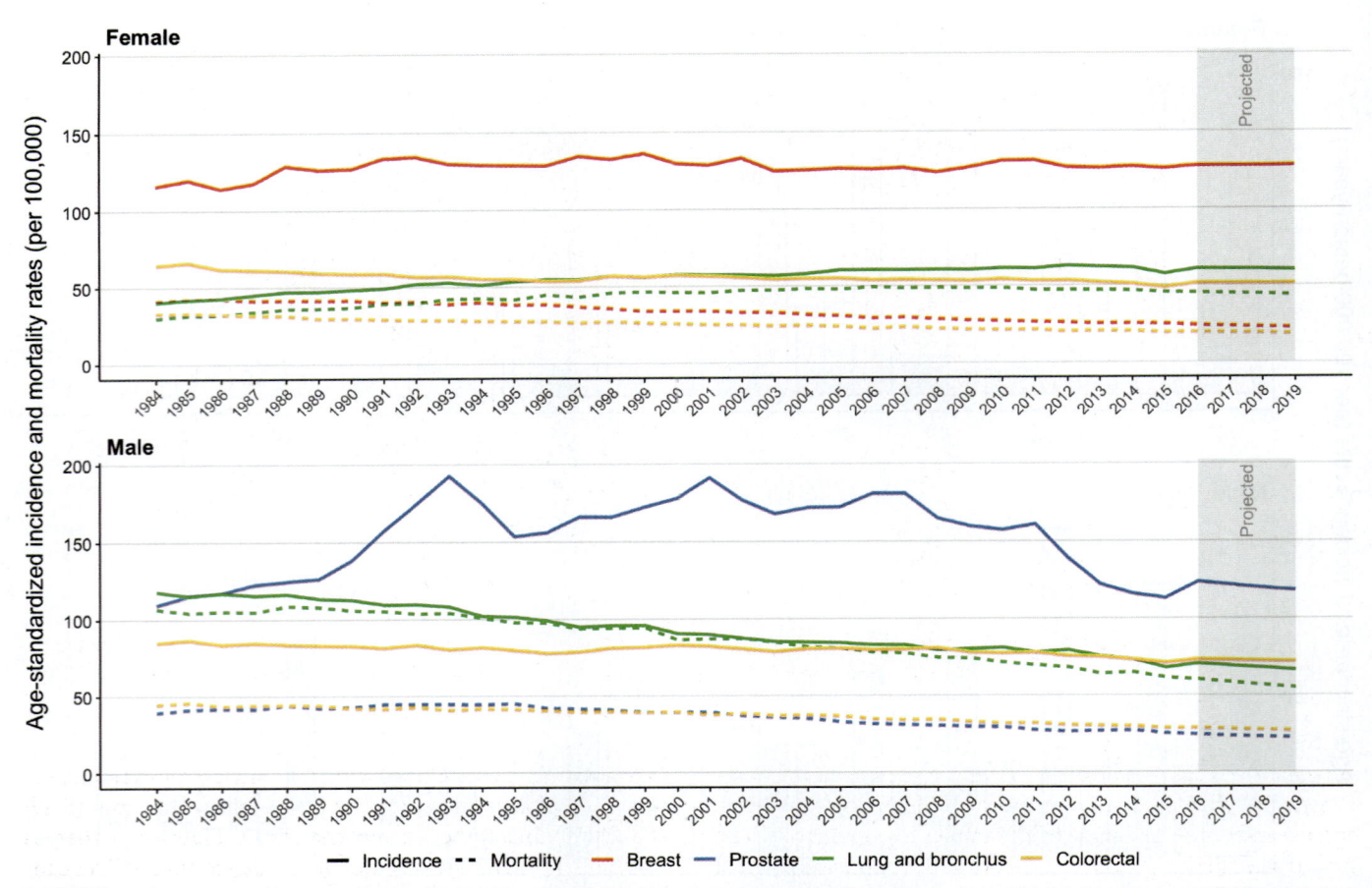

FIGURE 4–2 Age-standardized incidence and mortality rates across 35 years in Canada. Age-standardized incidence (*solid lines*) and mortality (*dashed lines*) rates for lung (*green*), colorectal (*yellow*), breast (*red*), and prostate cancer (*blue*) in Canada, per 100,000 people for years 1984 to 2019. Incidence and mortality rates for 2016–2019 are based on projections. (Data from *Canadian Cancer Statistics*, 2019.)

people with resected localized disease who are alive and well at 5 years should not be included for most sites (eg, colon cancer), whereas those with ER+ breast cancer can never be considered cured. Both cancer incidence and cancer prevalence are important measures. Cancer incidence reflects how commonly cancer develops in a population and the impact of preventive measures and health service utilization. In contrast, cancer prevalence is important when considering the overall burden of a cancer on a global health system, and planning health care services for longer-term survivors.

Prevalence is a function of both cancer incidence and cancer survivorship. Figure 4–2 shows the relationship between incidence, mortality, and prevalence. For prostate, breast and colorectal cancers, the age-standardized incidence rates (solid line) are substantially higher than their corresponding morality rates (dashed lines), as a result of higher survival rates (all greater than 40%). This leads to a higher prevalence. In contrast, for lung cancer, the mortality rate is very close to the incidence rate, which represents a low survival rate (of approximately 10–20%). This leads to a relatively lower prevalence in comparison, as a high proportion of lung cancer patients die rapidly from their diseases, resulting in few long-term survivors.

Incidence, and especially prevalence, can depend heavily on whether there is widespread application of screening. For example, prostate-specific antigen (PSA) screening for prostate cancer (and, to a lesser extent, mammographic screening for breast cancer) leads to "overdiagnosis," or detection of latent or indolent cancers that are destined never to become clinically apparent (see Chap. 22, Sec. 22.4.3). This effect is much less likely for other types of cancer such as lung and colorectal cancer. Variable use of screening in different geographical areas can explain marked differences in disease prevalence and confound the use of such information to plan health services.

4.2.3 The Role of Sampling

A major focus of epidemiology is to identify associations that are true for an entire population under study. Optimally, one would collect information from every member of the population of interest regarding their exposure to a putative risk factor that may be implicated in disease causation. In the real world, it is usually not feasible to collect data from an entire population, and only subsets of the population can be studied. Even the most comprehensive data from countries with a mandatory census will have noncompliant individuals. Because of cost and feasibility, basic census data are collected from as many individuals as possible, while detailed comprehensive

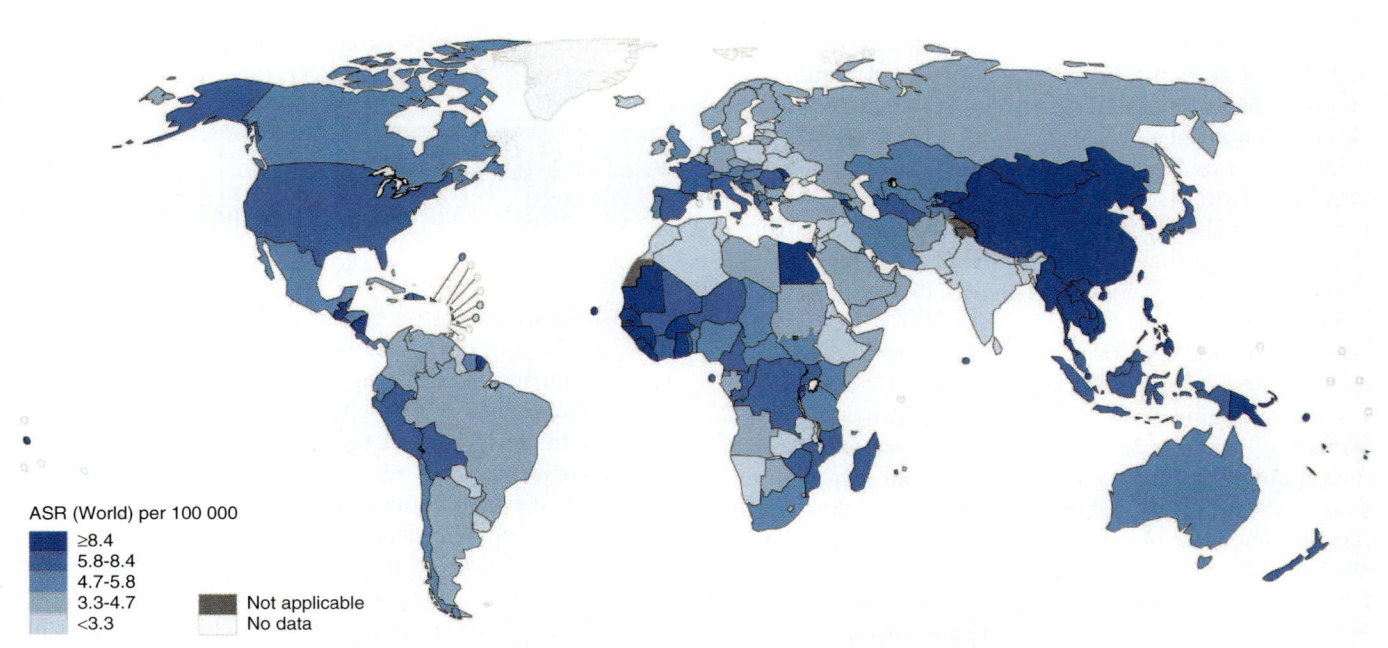

FIGURE 4–3 **Global variation in incidence of liver cancer.** Age-standardized incidence rates (ASR) of liver cancer for 2018, per 100,000 person-years, across different countries. The heatmap was obtained from the Global Cancer Observatory. (Data from Bray et al, 2018; Ferlay et al, 2018; Ferlay et al, 2019.)

information is collected from a subset of the population. Sampling is therefore a key component of epidemiologic analyses, because inferences are made from samples to populations. The goal of sampling is to collect a subset of the population where the exposure and/or disease status information is representative of the underlying population of interest. Representative samples are critically important in descriptive epidemiology for producing the types of statistics described in the previous section (incidence, mortality, prevalence, etc). For example, one might be interested in the prevalence of a specific exposure (eg, smoking rates) or the burden of a specific cancer (eg, esophageal cancer) in a population. However, in some scenarios, representative samples may not be necessary for the objectives of the research or for good scientific inference, and decisions to seek representative samples should be considered critically (Ebrahim and Smith, 2013; Rothman et al, 2013). Ideally, the results found in a sample should reflect true associations in the underlying population. When the results are different, bias and measurement errors may explain these discrepancies (see Sec. 4.3.6).

4.2.4 Geographic Variation

Geographic variations in cancer incidence can be a result of differences in prevalence of the underlying causes including environmental and racial (ie, genetic) differences, or to differences in diagnostic criteria. In addition, geographic comparison can be complicated by differences in screening, which, by detecting occult disease, usually has a much larger effect on the incidence of disease than on mortality (see Chap. 22, Sec. 22.4.3). Figure 4–1 shows age-standardized incidence rates by sex, across different countries and for selected cancer sites. Some large variations can be observed across countries, and there may also be large variations within countries: for example, the rate of esophageal cancer varies by 10-fold within Iran (Saidi et al, 2000). In another example, shown in Figure 4–3, there is substantial geographic variation in incidence rates of liver cancer (Bray et al, 2018). The highest incidence rates are observed in several countries in Northern and Western Africa, including Egypt, the Gambia, Guinea, and Eastern and Southeastern Asia including Mongolia, Cambodia, and Vietnam. Lower rates are observed in Northern America, Eastern Europe, Western Asia, and South Central Asia. This variation is partially accounted for by the prevalence of chronic infection with hepatitis B and C virus (HBV and HCV), which are causally associated with 80% to 95% of liver (hepatocellular) cancer (Maupas and Melnick, 1981), exposure to Alfatoxin B1, and alcohol-related cirrhosis (Wong et al, 2017). Obesity, diabetes, and metabolic syndrome are other well-documented risk factors for liver cancer in more-developed countries and increasingly in developing countries (Wong et al, 2017). Similarly, the variation of cervical cancer can be accounted for partially by the prevalence of HPV, as cervical cancer is strongly associated with a few of the oncogenic genotypes of HPV (Munoz et al, 2003). Infection and cancer is described in more detail in Section 4.5.1.

4.2.5 Time Trends

Figure 4–2 shows the age-standardized incidence rate (ASR) of the most common cancer sites in Canada for males and females in the last 35 years. Lung cancer incidence rates in men have been decreasing steadily since the mid-1980s from approximately 117.8 to 67.4 per 100,000 males in 2015, whereas the lung cancer incidence rate in women continues to rise from approximately 40.1 per 100,000 in 1984 to 57 per

100,000 females in 2015 (Canadian Cancer Society, 2019). The long-term projection suggests that this trend is beginning to level off. This pattern corresponds to the patterns of tobacco consumption in men and women with a lag time of approximately 20 years. In contrast, colorectal cancer rates have remained relatively stable over the same period. Breast cancer incidence has slightly increased during this period. Changes over time for prostate cancer incidence rates have already been highlighted in Section 4.2.2 and are further discussed in Section 4.3.6.4.

Worldwide, the incidence rate of stomach cancer in men has been decreasing in the last 30–40 years. Regardless of this steady decline, based on the number of new cases and deaths worldwide for 2018, stomach cancer was still the sixth most common incident cancer following cancer of the lung, breast, prostate, colon, and nonmelanoma of the skin and the third leading cause of cancer death after lung and colorectal (Bray et al, 2018). In contrast, the incidence of thyroid cancer is increasing most rapidly among all cancers and it has doubled in women in the last 10 years, in both Northern America (particularly in Canada), Australia/New Zealand and Eastern Asia (Lundgren et al, 2003; Davies and Welch, 2006; Bray et al, 2018). The increase in incidence of thyroid cancer is mainly observed for papillary thyroid cancer, and it may be a result of a change in morphologic recognition of this tumor (Lundgren et al, 2003). More frequent use of medical imaging may also contribute to the increased detection of early-stage, asymptomatic cancers. The mortality due to thyroid cancer did not increase during the same period of time.

Overall, the incidence rates of many common cancers are decreasing in developed countries as a result of initiatives to decrease the prevalence of known risk factors. However, geographic variations in cancer rates demonstrate the complex contribution of societal, economic, and lifestyle factors in shaping the cancer burden profiles of different regions. Tobacco use, infections, high body mass index, and ultraviolet radiation remain important risk factors for cancer worldwide. A lack of access to diagnosis and treatment and necessary data to inform cancer policy are also common (Torre et al, 2016; Bray et al, 2018).

Publications based on the Automated Cancer Information System (ACIS), an authoritative source of European data on cancer incidence and survival of children and adolescents, have provided detailed statistics of major childhood cancer in Europe between 1978 and 1997 (Kaatsch et al, 2006). This analysis, based on 33 cancer registries in 15 European countries, showed an increased rate of childhood cancer in all regions for the majority of tumor types, including soft-tissue sarcoma (annual rate of increase 1.8%), brain tumors, tumors of the sympathetic nervous system, germ cell tumors, and leukemias (annual rate of increase 0.6%). Diagnostic methods can only partially explain these upward trends, and factors such as changing lifestyle and environmental exposures may be important. Ionizing radiation and prior chemotherapy are accepted risk factors and birth weight, parental age, maternal occupational exposure to pesticides, and congenital anomalies as well as common genetic variation are consistently associated with most types of childhood cancers (Spector et al, 2015).

4.3 ANALYTIC EPIDEMIOLOGY STUDY DESIGNS AND CONSIDERATIONS

4.3.1 Ecologic Design

Ecologic studies focus on groups of individuals (or populations) as the unit of observation. These groups may include people living in a defined geographic area, or people from different schools or workplaces. The outcome in these studies is generally the incidence rate (eg, of cancer). Distinct from the descriptive methods described above (Sec. 4.2) is that analytic ecologic studies seek to move beyond simply estimating disease prevalence and incidence and identify the factors that produce the prevalence and incidence rates observed in defined populations. For example, an ecologic study may look at the association between use of alcohol and incidence of liver cancer in different countries. Measures of exposure to potential disease-related factors can be classified into three subgroups:

1. Aggregate measures—characteristics of a group summarized as a mean or median of some putative exposure or the proportion exposed for the group (eg, median or mean income, proportion of smokers, alcohol sales figures).
2. Environmental measures—physical characteristics of the defined area of interest (eg, measures of air pollution, urban neighborhood green index).
3. Global measures—characteristics of groups or locations for which there is no analog at the individual level (eg, laws or regulations that reduce exposure to secondhand smoke, health care coverage).

Relative to other study designs, ecologic studies are generally inexpensive as data are often readily available. The availability of data can often permit comparisons where exposure differs markedly across populations, such as data representing intake of some foods or nutrients across countries, which may be critical in finding associations.

The most important bias related to ecologic studies is known as the *ecologic fallacy*, where associations between aggregate measures of exposure and disease may not represent associations at the individual level. Ecologic studies generally assume that all members of a group exhibit characteristics of the group as a whole. When this assumption does not hold, the association for the ecologic exposure measure will be flawed and can even be in the opposite direction than that of the individual measure. A commonly cited example is an ecologic study that identified suicide rates to be positively correlated with the proportion of Protestants in Prussian communities. However, it cannot be concluded that a greater proportion of Protestants were committing suicide: an alternative explanation is that differences in suicide rates between communities might be explained by other groups, such as Catholics, having a higher suicide rate in Protestant communities, perhaps because of social isolation (Szklo and Nieto, 2007). An ecologic design does not allow one to distinguish between these two opposing explanations because individual-level measures (in this example, information on faith and cause of death for each of the study subjects) are not available.

Although ecologic studies are economical and are useful for exploratory analysis, causal inference is not usually possible given the lack of temporality and inability to attribute group level effects to individuals. This is because ecologic studies are done at the aggregate level and there is no way to confirm that the exposed individuals are the ones who also developed the outcome under study or that the exposure occurred before the outcome. In addition, the availability of information to adjust for confounding is often limited. Ecologic studies are often best suited to the evaluation of population-level factors such as the infrastructure, vaccination programs, or community socioeconomic status, or for assessing large contrasts in exposure, in large populations with disease rates that are stable over time.

4.3.2 Case-Control Design

In contrast to a cohort study (see Sec. 4.3.3) where incidence of disease is compared amongst differently exposed groups, case-control studies take the opposite approach and recruit newly diagnosed cases (case series) and compare these to controls (control series) with respect to their exposure to a potential disease-related factor (Fig. 4–4). The recruitment of incident cases means that there is no need to wait for disease to occur. This greatly reduces costs relative to cohort studies, particularly for rare diseases, because there is no need to recruit large number of subjects and wait for disease occurrence.

Various sampling strategies are employed for selecting the cases and controls for case-control studies. In hospital-based studies, patients diagnosed with the disease of interest may be recruited as cases for an analysis of cancer risk, or as the basis of a nested study for other disease-related outcomes. For studies of patients who have already developed a disease (eg, cancer), a case-control study might compare patients with the presence or absence of other important outcomes (eg, patients in remission vs patients who have relapsed from disease; patients with significant treatment toxicities vs those without toxicities). When all newly diagnosed cases over a defined period of time are recruited in a case-control study, this is known as *cumulative incidence sampling*.

In hospital-based studies, controls can be obtained from groups of patients whose reason for attendance at an outpatient clinic or less frequently, admission to hospital, are expected to be unrelated to the potential disease-related factors of interest. Bias by confounding and selection can occur if clinic visits or hospitalization of controls are associated with the disease-related factors (eg, Berkson's bias), or the cases and controls originate from geographic areas that do not entirely overlap (see Sec. 4.3.6 and Table 4–2). An example of this is if patients with cancer travel great distances to attend a hospital because of its reputation, whereas controls attend the hospital because it is the nearest to their residence. Selecting cancer cases and controls from a well-defined population, referred to as a *population-based case-control study*, addresses this bias. This can be accomplished by using cancer registries that register all cancers in a geographic region and by randomly recruiting control subjects from the same region.

Two other types of case-control studies are the *nested case-control* and *case-cohort* designs, in which patients who were

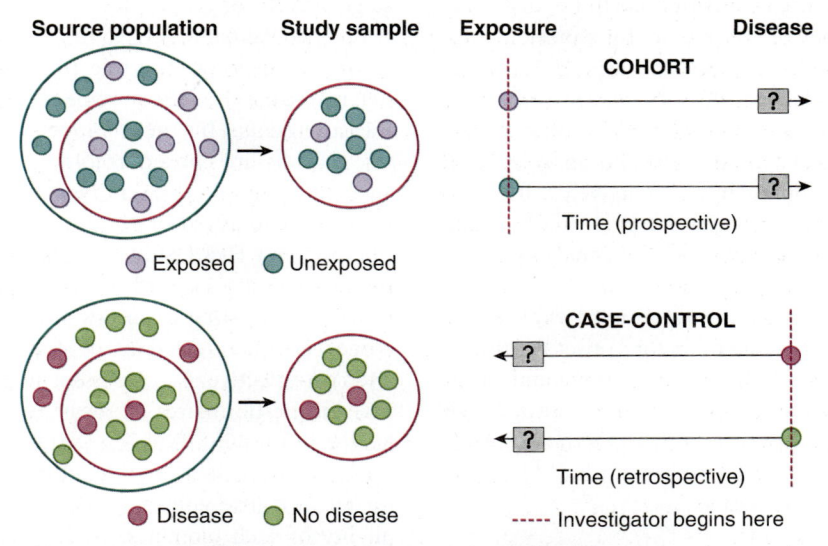

FIGURE 4–4. The cohort and case-control study designs are common in epidemiology. In a cohort study, an outcome or disease-free source population is defined, and participants are recruited based on whether they were exposed to the factor or event under study and followed in time to determine whether the outcome of interest occurs. The investigator compares the difference in incidence of the outcome in the exposed and unexposed groups. In case-control studies, participants are selected from a defined population based on whether they have the disease or outcome under study (cases) and are asked to retrospectively provide information on whether they were exposed to the factor of interest. The investigator compares the odds of exposure to the factor of interest among cases relative to those without the outcome under study (controls).

originally assembled as a cohort, are analyzed as if the study was of a case-control design. The word *nested* refers to performing a case-control analysis "nested" within a larger cohort study. In a *nested case-control* study, cases that occurred in a defined cohort are identified, whereas controls, matched for the most important confounding variables (eg, age and sex), are selected from among those in the cohort who have not developed the disease but have been followed for the same amount of time as cases. This is known as *incidence-density sampling*. In *case-cohort* studies, all cases are identified, and a random sample of the entire cohort at baseline is selected to serve as the control series (note: some participants who were originally assigned to the control group may later become cases). Using these designs, the odds ratio can estimate relative risk without the rare disease assumption (see Sec. 4.4.1). The case-cohort design has the added benefit that a single control series can be used for multiple different case groups. Relative risks cannot be estimated directly within a case-control analysis but are estimated using the odds ratio, and can approximate relative risks under certain conditions (Sec. 4.4.1 and Table 4–4).

The Framingham Heart Study and the Nurses' Health Study are seminal examples of long-term cohort studies that originally recruited healthy individuals and followed them for a prolonged time period (Mahmood et al, 2014; Colditz et al, 2016). Participants of these cohorts completed questionnaires that included detailed information about smoking exposures, medication use (eg, aspirin and metformin use), exercise patterns, and diet. During the follow-up of these studies, a number of cancer outcomes were reported. These well-defined cohorts can be used to select cases and controls for studies alternative to the original study objectives. The odds of exposure for cases and controls can be compared as in a case-control study. These cohorts have been used extensively as the basis for case-control studies that have made seminal contributions to the discovery and validation of a number of risk factors for cancer including smoking, diet, exercise, energy balance, aspirin and other medication use, and many others.

For many research questions, nested designs offer reductions in cost and effort of data collection and analysis compared with the full cohort approach, with relatively minor loss in statistical efficiency. These designs are particularly useful when biologic materials are being analyzed (analysis of the biologic material is expensive). Selection from a defined cohort has additional advantages, in that information on exposure to the disease-related factor is collected before onset of disease instead of after diagnosis as in a population- or hospital-based case-control study. This removes potential bias resulting from diseased subjects reporting exposures differently than controls (recall bias, Table 4–2), or blood-based measures of biomarkers being influenced by disease onset.

4.3.3 Cohort Design

A cohort study follows a group of people over time comparing those exposed to a factor that may influence risk or outcome of disease to those not exposed to the factor. Individuals typically enter into a cohort because they meet clear-cut criteria using a defined sampling protocol. Cohorts can be prospective or retrospective (historical). In a prospective cohort, individual study subjects are recruited at a specific point or range in time. Measurements of potential disease-related factors (baseline measures) are made as individuals are recruited into the cohort, and study subjects are then followed over time with further measurements possible. Because exposed and nonexposed individuals within the study are followed over time, relative risk can be calculated directly (see Sec. 4.4.1 and Table 4–3). A retrospective cohort makes use of existing databases for information about disease (usually identifying incident cases or deaths) and the disease-related factor of interest. In specific circumstances, biologic samples are also available for translational experiments from these retrospective cohorts, either because they were collected as part of a parallel biobanking process or because such samples were stored long-term following original diagnostic biopsies. The quality of preservation, the quantity of usable material, and the completeness of collection across the entire cohort should be assessed critically, as should the quality of retrospectively collected clinical and epidemiologic information.

Although a typical epidemiologic cohort study begins with a healthy population (where risk of disease is the outcome being assessed), a growing number of observational cohorts follow individuals with disease (such as cancer), where the outcomes being assessed are treatment-related responses or toxicity, rates of disease relapse and progression, course of disease over time, and/or overall survival (see Chap. 22, Sec. 22.3). Sometimes, these disease-specific cohorts are labeled *case series*. Case series may involve carefully collected sets of patients, but they may also consist of a convenient, haphazardly collected set of available cases. Use of the term *cohort* implies a well-defined set of patients adhering to specific entry criteria, such as stage-specific or geographic-specific sets of individuals.

Prospective cohorts have the advantage of allowing investigators to control subject selection, ascertainment of events, to determine baseline measurements, and follow-up for repeated measurements. In most modern large-scale cohort studies, subjects are chosen according to some defining criteria, such as occupation (eg, nurses in the Nurses' Health Study; Colditz et al, 2016) or residing in a particular area (eg, the Framingham Heart Study; Mahmood et al, 2014). Generally, incidence of disease is the outcome of interest. Often, multiple diseases (including a variety of cancers and noncancer outcomes) are investigated in one study, to maximize its efficiency and cost-effectiveness. Assessments may involve interviews or mailed questionnaires or measures made at a clinic such as height and weight. Biologic samples may be taken and stored for later assessment of molecular and genetic biomarkers. As for retrospective cohort studies, it is important to ensure the quality of such biomaterials. In analyses of disease risk, the advantage of prospective cohort studies over observational approaches is that exposure to a disease-related factor is measured prior to development of disease; this property makes cohort studies important for determining causality and for early detection of molecular risk factors in translational science. Assessing exposure after development of disease can lead to bias. For example, biomarker levels in blood could be influenced by the presence of disease; thus, obtaining specimens well before diagnosis can lessen (but does not rule out) the presence of disease at the time of sampling; stage of disease at diagnosis can be a factor affecting the appropriate time of sampling prior to diagnosis.

Ascertainment of outcome is critical in a cohort study. When the outcome is the development of cancer, a pathology report from a cancer registry is often used to identify the case and confirm the diagnosis. An accurate date of diagnosis is required so that prevalent cases are not counted, and it is essential when one of the outcomes is survivorship after diagnosis. When the outcome of interest is response to treatment, toxicity, recurrence, and/or survival, careful standardization for measuring each outcome must take place, usually with systematic repeated evaluations (eg, standardizing a follow-up schedule). Many subjects can be lost to follow-up despite extensive efforts to track them. Losing subjects to follow-up can introduce bias if these losses are differential with respect to either the potential disease-related factor or the outcome of interest. Linkage to cancer registries and mortality databases can permit tracking of individuals so that disease occurrence and vital status can be ascertained even if subjects are lost to routine follow-up. Although overall survival is a hard outcome measure (alive or dead), loss of subjects to follow-up still requires clinical interpretation. Other outcomes, such as disease-free survival and cancer-specific mortality, are subject to greater error and bias (see Chap. 22, Sec. 22.3).

Prospective cohort studies designed to evaluate risk of disease are very expensive. For a disease such as cancer, many individuals would have to be recruited to ensure that a sufficient number of incident cases will occur for meaningful analyses. In studies where the cohort is defined based on a specific risk exposure with a long latency period, researchers may have to wait for many years after recruitment before sufficient numbers of cases are available for analysis.

Cohort studies of clinical outcome after cancer diagnosis are also expensive, because of the need to perform accurate and careful patient follow-up. Heterogeneity in treatment and patient management can be a substantial source of confounding in such studies. Thus, unlike cohort studies of disease risk, it is easier to analyze and interpret single-institution cohort studies or cohort studies involving a small number of institutions that follow similar treatment plans, compared with those studies in which treatments are heterogeneous. Yet, single-institution studies can suffer because of inclusion of a highly selected subset of patients, limiting generalizability. In contrast, the analysis of cancer registry data for a geographic region has the advantage of providing an analysis of what is expected in the real world, but may suffer from wide variability in patient management (eg, therapy, monitoring, and follow-up). Finally, randomized controlled trials offer the opportunity to have well-defined, homogenous treatments and well-characterized outcomes, mostly in multinational and multi-institutional setting; however, the treatments are fixed as part of the trial, and therefore only specific therapies can be studied in this context.

In summary, the advantages of the cohort study design are that it overcomes some of the limitations associated with the ecologic and case-control study designs (see Sec. 4.3.1–4.3.2). Temporality can be established and information bias is reduced compared to case-control studies, as differential reporting relative to the outcome is less likely when data are collected before the development of disease. However, loss to follow-up can have an impact on the internal validity of cohort studies and can result in selection bias when it is related to both exposure and outcome.

4.3.4 Cross-Sectional Design

In a cross-sectional study, sampling and surveying of individuals from an underlying population to determine disease status and exposure takes place at a specific time point. For example, we are interested in learning about the prevalence of diabetes in women with breast cancer. We randomly sample 10,000 women from an underlying population and find that 300 individuals have received a diagnosis of breast cancer by the date of sampling. We then find that 2000 women from our sample have a diagnosis of diabetes by the date of sampling. Table 4–1 presents the data from this hypothetical study: the odds ratio of diabetes as a risk factor for breast cancer is AD/BC = (120/380)/(1880/7620) ≈ 1.28.

Because cases may include subjects who have had their disease for many years, cross-sectional studies are sometimes referred to as prevalence studies. The main drawback for this design is survival (or prevalence) bias. A factor found to be more prevalent in cases than controls may not be causally related to the onset of disease but instead may be related to living with the disease, its survival, its treatment, or other factors after diagnosis. In the example above, it is likely that having a diagnosis of breast cancer results in increased physical and emotional stress (eg, from surgical procedures, psychosocial stress, or stress that leads to poor eating habits). Subclinical or borderline diabetic patients might become fully diabetic as a result of these stressors. Second, women diagnosed with breast cancer have more tests, including standard blood work, which can increase the detection of diabetes. Third, chemotherapy for breast cancer is administered commonly with corticosteroids (either to prevent anaphylactoid reactions or as an antiemetic), which can convert subclinical to clinically apparent diabetes.

In another example of potential bias in a cross-sectional study, emphysema may appear to protect against development

TABLE 4–1 Results of a hypothetical cross-sectional study evaluating the relationship between the prevalence of diabetes and breast cancer.

		Breast Cancer Yes	Breast Cancer No	Total
Diabetes	Yes	120 (a)	1880 (b)	2,000
	No	380 (c)	7620 (d)	8,000
	Total	500	9500	10,000

of early-stage lung cancer. The reason for this unexpected finding may be a result of emphysema patients dying earlier after diagnosis of lung cancer, or they may receive suboptimal therapy because of poor tolerance of surgery. Thus, a substantial proportion of individuals who have lung cancer with severe emphysema may have died by the time of the cross-sectional sampling and thereby distort the relationship between lung cancer and emphysema; this is known as survival bias (see Table 4–2). Other study designs, such as case-control or cohort, which restrict cases to those who are newly diagnosed are more appropriate.

Cross-sectional study designs are most useful when studying prevalence questions, such as with health and economic policy research (eg, How commonly are prostate cancer and dementia found together? What proportion of breast cancer survivors is overweight?). Many cross-sectional studies utilize information routinely collected for other reasons (eg, census data) and thus it can be of low cost to perform such secondary analyses. Prospectively designed cross-sectional studies of cancer are uncommon, primarily because of the potential for the biases listed above, and the relatively large numbers of individuals (and associated expense) required for completing such a study.

4.3.5 Familial Design

Familial studies are used to examine the association of genetic factors with risk of disease (Thomas, 2004). Early family-based studies involved sibling pairs (eg, twin studies) with 1 affected and 1 unaffected sibling, which could be analyzed using methods similar to those used in case-control studies. Other studies identified a single affected offspring and 2 unaffected parents; these can be analyzed using the *transmission disequilibrium test*, which compares parental alleles to those of the diseased offspring (case) and determines if there is excess transmission of specific alleles to the offspring. Newer statistical methods allow for analyses using families with affected individuals and 1 or more siblings, parents, or combinations of both (Thomas, 2004). The advantage of family-based designs over a case-control design is that they are not subject to bias because of the presence of a systematic difference in allele frequencies between subpopulations as a result of different ancestry (known as *population stratification*). Bias occurs when such a systematic difference goes unrecognized, leading to potential genetic associations that are thought to be related to the disease of interest, but are, in reality, associated with genetic differences arising from individuals having different ethnic backgrounds.

A major difficulty for family-based studies is recruitment of controls. If the diseased subject is older, parents may be deceased or not well enough to join a study. Recruitment of siblings can also be difficult as a subject must have a sibling willing to enroll in the study. For these reasons, familial study designs are rarely employed in cancer outside of pediatric populations. Instead, study designs in adult cancers generally rely on case-control studies where controls are matched to cases for racial group and/or ethnicity, and statistical methods are employed to control for population stratification.

4.3.6 Random Error and Biases

The study designs described above employ different strategies to select an appropriate sample from which to estimate the effect of an exposure on an outcome in the target population. However, any selected sample is just one of many hypothetical samples that could have been selected from the population and the accuracy of the estimate of the association between the exposure and disease status in the selected sample is affected by both random and systematic error. Random error, which can arise because of random variability in the selection of the sample or random errors inherent in measurement tools, affects the precision of the study results and can be quantified using statistics such as the standard error. Generally, as the sample size increases, the standard error decreases; therefore, small effects observed based on small sample sizes are likely due to random error rather than real phenomena. Uncertainties in the estimates made about the population parameters from the sample are typically presented as the confidence interval and *P* value. Bias—a result of systematic errors in sample selection and measurement—affects the validity of the estimates, is not reduced by increases in sample size, and is typically harder to quantify.

4.3.6.1 Random Error *Random error*, the deviation that arises by chance between the observed value (in the sample) and its true value (in the underlying population), can distort the results of epidemiologic studies.

Assessment of cancer diagnosis should be reasonably accurate as diagnosis is generally verified with a pathology report. However, the determination of cause of death can be more problematic if death certificates are used. For example, any person diagnosed with cancer will often be assumed to have died as a result of it, and other common causes of death such as cardiovascular disease may be ignored. Assessment of exposure is problematic, and misclassification of subjects with respect to their exposure can be extensive. Recall of past exposures, such as diet, may show both random error and recall bias (see Sec. 4.3.6.3). Error in the measurement of biomarkers depends not only on the accuracy of the bioassay but on how well a single measurement may reflect long-term levels of the biomarker. The latency period for cancer can be many years and a single measurement of a biomarker during an individual's lifetime may not represent long-term levels.

4.3.6.2 Bias Due to Confounding Bias can be related to the identification of cases, measurement of exposure, or systematic errors in data collection or improper analysis of the data. Many different kinds of biases have been described (Sackett, 1979; Szklo and Nieto, 2007; Rothman et al, 2008). We describe the main types of bias found in observational studies, including confounding, selection, and information bias.

Confounding is defined as the distortion of the effect of an exposure on risk (of disease or outcome) that arises because of an association with other factors that affect such a risk. Confounding can lead to spurious associations, mask associations that are real, or distort the strength of an association. A variable is considered to be a confounder if it is associated with the potential disease-related factor under investigation (either

A
Tooth loss - Lung cancer
           ↖   ↗
              Smoking (confounder)

B
Smoking ——→ Bronchial dysplasia ——→ Lung cancer
                  (nonconfounder)

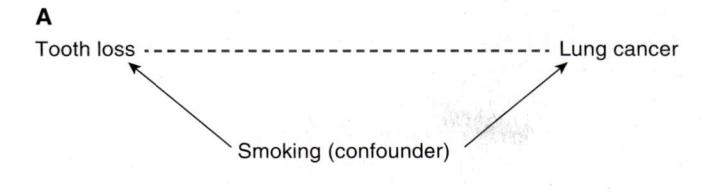

FIGURE 4–5 Confounding in epidemiologic studies. The confounder is related to both the exposure of interest and to either disease or outcome. Example **A** reflects confounding by smoking. Example **B** is not an example of confounding because bronchial dysplasia lies in the causal pathway leading to lung cancer.

causally or noncausally) and is causally related to the outcome of interest (either risk of disease or its outcome). An example of a confounder is smoking in lung cancer (Fig. 4–5A). Suppose we are studying the association between tooth loss and lung cancer risk. Tooth loss, a marker of poor hygiene, is associated strongly with heavy smoking. We may, therefore, find an association between tooth loss and lung cancer because both are associated with heavy smoking. In reality, tooth loss does not lead to lung cancer: the true association is between smoking and lung cancer.

A variable is not considered to be a confounder if it lies in the same causal pathway as the potential disease-related factor under investigation. For example, bronchial dysplasia is an intermediary in the pathway between smoking and lung cancer, and is thus not a confounder (see Fig. 4–5B).

In summary, there are 3 criteria for a variable to be a confounder:

1. a confounding factor must be a risk factor for the disease;
2. a confounding factor must be associated with the exposure under study in the source population; and
3. a confounding factor should *not* be an intermediate factor in a causal path between exposure and disease.

The degree of confounding depends on the magnitude of the association between the confounder and the outcome of interest (eg, smoking–lung cancer), the magnitude of the association between the confounder and the exposure (eg, tooth loss–smoking) and the prevalence of the confounder among those who are not exposed and do not have the outcome (eg, smoking prevalence among lung cancer-free population). Confounding can be dealt with in different ways. Individuals who have a disease (eg, cancer cases) and those without disease (eg, healthy controls) can be matched on potential confounding variables (eg, age and sex are commonly matched in a case-control study) to reduce or eliminate confounding by these variables, or data can be analyzed within specific strata of the confounding variable (eg, analyses stratified by ethnic group). Referring to the tooth loss and smoking example, studying the association between tooth loss and lung cancer among never-smokers only would minimize the confounding effect by smoking. In addition, one can control for confounding using multiple regression analysis, which is discussed in Section 4.4.3.

4.3.6.3 Selection and Information Bias
Selection (or Sampling) bias refers to systematic differences between those who are selected to participate or are retained in a study vs those who are eligible for the study but do not participate or are lost to follow-up. An example of sampling bias results from recruiting cases from a surgical clinic to represent the entire population of stomach cancer. Because surgeons generally see operable patients, the study population will be skewed toward earlier-stage patients with localized disease rather than the entire population of patients with stomach cancer. The selection of a comparison group (controls) that is not representative of the population from where the cases originated in case-control studies (see Sec. 4.3.2) can also produce selection bias. For example, if a hospital-based case-control study aiming to study the relation between alcohol consumption and liver cancer risk recruits the comparison group from the trauma ward, the alcohol consumption (exposure) distribution of the recruited controls might not be representative of the general population where the cases arise from, which would lead to bias in the effect estimation. Similarly, refusal to participate or nonresponse that is related to either the exposure or the outcome of interests can also produce selection bias. In the cohort study setting, differential loss to follow-up between exposed and unexposed individuals (see Sec. 4.3.3), refusal to participate or nonresponse that is related either to the exposure or the outcome of interest, or differential referral or diagnosis of participants can all produce selection bias.

Information bias occurs as a consequence of errors in obtaining the needed information, which is often termed *misclassification*. Misclassification can lead to results from studies that do not represent true associations in the underlying population. An example of information bias occurs if lung cancer patients overestimate their exposure to asbestos (compared with healthy controls) while underestimating their cigarette smoking history (perhaps as a means of reducing their own culpability in developing this disease). The observed effect is a smaller-than-true risk associated with cumulative smoking, and an exaggerated risk associated with asbestos. This bias particularly affects case-control studies (see Sec. 4.3.2) where cases are recruited after their diagnosis, and is referred to as *recall bias*. Such a bias would be absent if individuals were asked for their exposure status prior to developing their cancer (as in cohort studies; see Sec. 4.3.3).

Generally, nondifferential misclassification of a dichotomous (ie, positive or negative) exposure will lead to a bias toward the null (relative risk estimates will indicate a weaker association than actually exists or indicate no association when a true association is present). For example, when evaluating the association between smoking and lung cancer, if never-smokers are sometimes misclassified as ever-smokers, and vice versa, this will mask the true effect toward the null (no association), and in the extreme situation where the majority of individuals are misclassified, the effect can switch directions so that it appears as if smoking prevents lung cancer. However, misclassification of a multilevel exposure may result in bias toward or away from the null.

Misclassification can also be differential: for example, assuming a molecular test is being evaluated for its ability to discriminate groups with and without cancer; however, the samples from the cancer and noncancer groups are handled in systematically different ways. This error can occur during specimen collection, handling, and storage or during laboratory analysis, leading to misclassification of the lab results that is differential by their disease status. The resultant error is directional in nature (ie, nonrandom) and biases the results of the study.

Efforts to increase the accuracy of assessment of exposure or use of large samples that can detect the attenuated associations are the best ways to address this problem. We discuss some other strategies in Section 4.7.2. Table 4–2 defines and describes other common examples of selection and information biases.

4.3.6.4 Bias in Cancer Screening

Two special causes of bias are related to cancer screening and affect incidence, prevalence, mortality, and survival rates. Figure 4–2 shows that prostate cancer had 2 peaks of incidence in 1993 and 2001. Each peak was related to the clinical adoption of a screening test based on the serum levels of PSA. The first peak followed initial adoption of the PSA test, whereas the second peak may be explained by increased PSA testing related to increased awareness of the test (Canadian Cancer Society, 2010). Screening results in individuals with subclinical cancer being diagnosed and such men would either have been detected clinically at a later date, or more frequently not at all, because latent prostate cancer is very common in elderly men and only progresses to clinical disease in a small subset. Overdiagnosis bias and lead-time bias probably accounted for these peaks in Figure 4–2.

Overdiagnosis bias refers to the detection of subclinical or indolent cases of cancer that would never have become clinically diagnosed in individuals who would have eventually died from an unrelated cause. Because overdiagnosis results in an increase in cancer incidence, and apparent prolonged survival after diagnosis, it increases prevalence of the disease, but of subclinical disease that has no real clinical relevance.

Lead-time bias refers to the longer survival after diagnosis that results from diagnosis at an earlier time during the course of the disease, rather than to improved survival as a result of treatment (Figure 4–6). This effect will increase the apparent prevalence of disease. *Length-time bias* occurs when screened subjects with better prognosis are detected by a screening program. This can result from more rapidly growing (and more lethal) cancers being diagnosed outside of the

TABLE 4–2 Types of selection and information biases in epidemiologic studies.

Bias*	Study Design	Description
Selection Bias		
Survival bias	Cross-sectional studies, case-control studies of rapidly fatal cancers	Survival of cases is related to exposure. Exposed cases may be over- or underrepresented in sample.
Detection bias	Case-control studies, cohort studies	Detection of cases is related to exposure to potential disease-related factors, with cases in the exposed group over- or underrepresented.
Self-selection bias	All types	A common form of selection bias, which occurs when study participants who agreed to participate in the study are different from source population regarding the exposure of interests. One of the known examples is healthy-worker effect.
Sampling or ascertainment bias	All types	Some members of the population may be less likely to be included than others, resulting in a nonrandom sample. This includes the biases resulted from differential catchment areas between cases and controls.
Differential loss to follow-up	Cohort studies, survival analyses	Subjects with exposure are either more or less likely to be lost to follow-up (losses can be a result of mortality, migration, or refusal to continue with study).
Lead-time bias	Cohort studies, survival analyses	The appearance of prolonged survival as a result of earlier diagnoses because of earlier detection of the disease, without affecting the actual outcome of treating the disease.
Overdiagnosis bias	All types	The appearance of increase in early-stage disease with improved survival, because of new detection technologies that identify previously undiagnosed subclinical disease that would otherwise never have required treatment.
Berkson's bias	Hospital-based case-control studies	A factor that is affected by both exposure of interest and disease is termed a *collider*. In this scenario, the possibilities of admission into hospitals are affected by exposures of interest and disease condition. Therefore when hospitalization is the condition of study recruitment, it becomes a *collider* and can introduce bias. The bias can be in either directions.
Information Bias		
Recall bias	Case-control studies (with interview/questionnaires)	Cases recall exposure differently than controls, either over- or underreporting exposure relative to controls.
Interviewer or experimenter's bias	Case-control studies	Interviewer/experimenter knows disease status of study subjects and over- or underreports exposure, either consciously or unconsciously affecting the results.

*All biases listed may lead to over- or underestimated risk estimates.

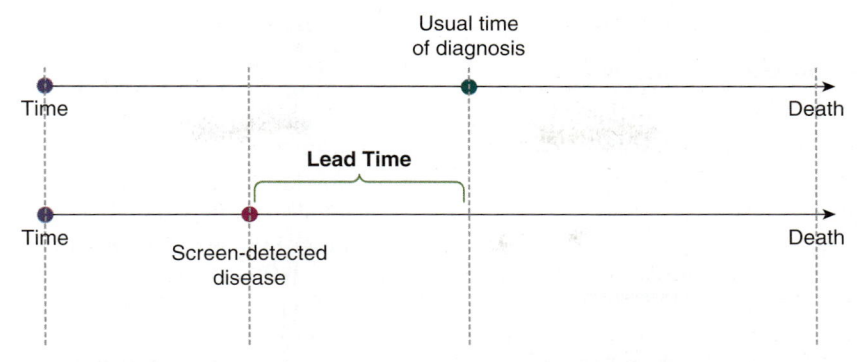

FIGURE 4–6 Lead-time bias. Lead time bias occurs if a screening test increases the perceived survival time without affecting the course of the disease.

screening program (interval-detected cancers), thus leading to an impression of better survival among screened subjects. These topics are discussed in more detail in Chapter 22, Section 22.4.3, and Figures 22–9 and 22–10.

4.4 ANALYTIC EPIDEMIOLOGY

4.4.1 Basic Comparative Approaches: Relative Risk, Odds Ratio

The *relative risk* measures the risk in a group either exposed or having a greater exposure to a potential disease-related factor and compares it to the risk in a group that is not exposed or has lower exposure to the factor. The risk itself may be related to the development of a specific cancer, its precursor, its subsequent complications, or to a specific cancer outcome such as response to therapy, toxicity to treatment, prognosis, or survival of the patient. In a population-based study of cancer/precancer risk, individuals who develop cancer/precancer and those who do not are classified into exposed and nonexposed groups according to their baseline measures, which are taken well before any individuals have developed cancer/precancer. In a population study of cancer outcome, individuals who develop a specific outcome (eg, alive/dead at a specific reference time point, response or toxicity to therapy, or presence/absence of cancer complications) and those who do not are classified into exposed and nonexposed groups. Other outcomes such as time-to-event survival analyses are covered elsewhere (Chap. 22, Sec. 22.3.6). In either example, the relative risk can then be calculated by dividing the risk of disease (or outcome) in the exposed group by the risk of disease (or outcome) in the unexposed group, as shown in Table 4–3. Another related measure of relative risk is the *rate ratio*. It can be calculated when disease (eg, incidence) rates (Sec. 4.2.1) are available by dividing the rate of a disease in a group exposed to a specific factor by the rate in a group that is unexposed or has lower exposure to the same factor. The rate ratio is useful in comparing populations in defined geographic areas with different exposures (eg, cigarette smoking or industrial pollution).

A relative risk of 1 (or more precisely, a relative risk not statistically different than 1) indicates that there is no detectable increased risk of disease (or outcome) in the exposed group. A relative risk significantly greater than 1 indicates that risk is increased among the exposed, and a relative risk significantly less than 1 indicates lower risk in the exposed group, when compared to the unexposed groups. The farther away the value is from 1 (either very large numbers or very small numbers), the stronger the association.

Within either the entire population or a representative subset, the relative risk can be directly calculated because the size of both the exposed and unexposed groups from which cancer cases arose is known. In contrast, if a study selects cases from a population and then compares them to a selected set of controls, the size of the underlying exposed and unexposed groups in the population, and therefore the relative risk, cannot be directly calculated. Instead, the *odds ratio* must be calculated as outlined in Table 4–4.

The odds ratio is generally presented as an approximate measure of relative risk. This approximation is valid if the prevalence of the disease is relatively low in the population, typically less than 10%. Although prevalence of all cancers together is relatively high in most Western populations, the prevalence of each individual cancer is quite low. This approximation can be demonstrated by starting with Equation 4.1 (below) for the calculation of relative risk as defined in Table 4–3. If the disease is rare, then only a small change to the resulting estimate will be seen if both A (subjects with exposure and disease) and C (subjects with no exposure and disease) are removed from the denominator of the first and second parts of the equation (Eq. 4.2). The resulting equation can be rearranged so that

TABLE 4–3 Calculation of relative risk of disease.

		Diseased	Nondiseased	Total
Exposure classification	Exposed	a	b	E^+
	Unexposed	c	d	E^-
	Total	D^+	D^-	

The letters a, b, c, and d are counts of the number of subjects in each group.

1. Risk of disease among exposed = $a/(a+b) = a/E^+$
2. Risk of disease among exposed = $c/(c+d) = c/E^-$
3. Relative risk as a result of exposure = $\dfrac{a/(a+b)}{c/(c+d)} = \dfrac{a/E^+}{c/E^-}$

TABLE 4-4 Calculation of the odds ratio.

		Disease Classification		
		Diseased (cases)	Nondiseased (controls)	Total
Exposure classification	Exposed	a	b	E⁺
	Unexposed	c	d	E⁻
	Total	D⁺	D⁻	

The letters a, b, c, and d are counts of the number of subjects in each group.
1. Odds of exposure in cases = a/c
2. Odds of exposure in controls = b/d
3. Odds ratio = $\dfrac{a/c}{b/d} = \dfrac{ad}{bc}$

it is identical to the equation for the odds ratio (Eq. 4.3) in Table 4-4.

Relative Risk = $a/(a+b) \div c/(c+d)$ [Eq. 4.1]

$\approx a/b \div c/d$ [a and c are removed from denominator] [Eq. 4.2]

$\approx a/c \div b/d$ or ad/bc [Eq. 4.3]

The relative risk and odds ratio are relative measures of effect and quantify the strength of an association between biomarkers, clinical, or epidemiologic factors and disease.

4.4.2 Probability, Distributions, and Tests of Association

Let us assume that in the South Pacific there are exactly 1000 adult islanders (age 18 years and older) living on a remote atoll (Island A). On this island, 400 individuals have high blood pressure. If we are allowed to check for high blood pressure in 100 islanders (ie, sampling the population), we may obtain 40 with hypertension, but we may by chance also obtain 39, 38, 37, or 41, 42, 43 individuals with high blood pressure, but it would be highly unlikely to obtain either no individuals with high blood pressure or all 100 individuals. If we repeated the experiment a million times, each time sampling 100 individuals randomly, the most frequent result will be 40 individuals with high blood pressure, with other results farther away from 40 (in either direction) being less frequent. These results, if plotted, will form a shape similar to a normal distribution or a probability curve (*Note:* with 2 possible outcomes, hypertensive or not hypertensive, the distribution is in fact binomial but approximately equal to the normal distribution given the large number of data, thus leading to a bell-shaped curve; see Fig. 4-7). If we obtain a value from a sample that falls outside a certain range of values, then we might conclude it is highly unlikely that the value comes from a population similar to the Island A population. This range is conventionally chosen to be the 95% confidence interval, in which case the top and bottom 2.5% of values are considered to be too different to be likely to have come from a population like Island A. Under different circumstances and depending on the experimental design of each study, different distributions or curves may be more appropriate, as would different ranges of confidence intervals.

If on a sister island (Island B) with 1000 people, we sample 100 individuals once and find that 29 of them have hypertension (Fig. 4-7, yellow bar), are the individuals on Island B similar to those on Island A? From Figure 4-7, the chance of this

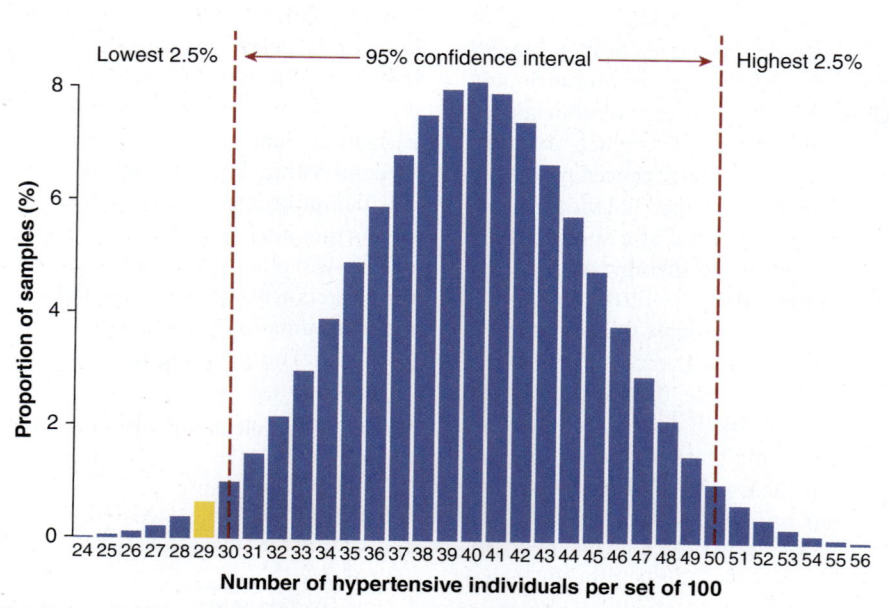

FIGURE 4-7 Normal distribution approximation of binomial distribution for a 100-patient sample for a 40% proportion. Assume that an underlying adult population has a 40% prevalence of hypertension. Researchers repeatedly and randomly sampled 100 individuals from this population (Island A) and reported the prevalence of hypertension in each sample. The X-axis shows the number of hypertensive individuals in each set of 100. The Y-axis shows the proportion of samples with that number of hypertensive individuals. The 95% confidence interval (within which 95% of these samples fall, around the median of 40) is shown in between the red dotted lines. The yellow bar represents the probability a sample of 29 hypertensive patients (Island B) would occur if drawn from a population like Island A (less than 2.5%).

happening if the populations of the 2 sets of islanders have the same risk of hypertension is found to be outside of the 95% confidence interval. We conclude that Island B's population has a different risk of hypertension than Island A's population.

A chi-squared (χ^2) and t test are different tests for association. Each is based on an underlying distribution and compares the result of one group with that of another. The tests are considered significant when the 2 groups are thought to be too different from each other for the variable of interest to have come from the same underlying population. *Chi-squared tests* evaluate variables that are discrete categorical values (eg, ex-smoker, current smoker, never smoker; or male, female), whereas *t tests* evaluate continuous variables (eg, hormone levels, age). An extension of the *t* test to compare 3 or more groups of a continuous variable is the analysis of variance, abbreviated as ANOVA.

Because *t* tests and ANOVAs assume that the underlying distribution of the continuous variable is normally distributed, their use is less appropriate when the underlying distribution deviates from a bell-shaped normally distributed curve. Tests that depend on an underlying distribution of variables are known as parametric tests. An example of a situation where a parametric test may not be appropriate occurs in a patient population that has a continuous variable of interest with 2 widely separated modes or peaks in its distribution, similar to 2 humps of a camel, instead of a bell-shaped curve. A sample containing a mix of both males and females may have a bimodal distribution for height or weight due to natural differences in these traits. When the assumption of normal distribution no longer holds, either some form of data transformation is needed to change the distribution back into a bell-shaped curve or alternative tests of association should be considered. If the distribution curves are skewed in one direction or another, one common transformation is to analyze the logarithm of the original variable. For a 2-humped camel distribution, no amount of variable transformation can render the shape of the underlying population back into one that is bell-shaped. In this setting, using an alternative test consists of ranking the values of the continuous variable from 1, 2, 3, through to the last value. For example, if we want to compare the values of Group A with 43 individuals to Group B with 57 individuals, we simply rank the values of both groups combined from 1 through 100, where 1 is the lowest value and 100 is the highest value. When values are tied, the ranks are averaged and tied values are then given these averaged ranks. The ranks for each group are summed and averaged, and these averages are then compared to each other to determine if the average ranks are similar between groups. By avoiding analysis of the actual values but instead using the ranks, we no longer assume any specific distribution of values in the underlying continuous variable; these tests are termed nonparametric tests. To compare 2 groups, the Wilcoxon rank-sum test (also known as the Mann-Whitney *U* test) is used (Neuhäuser, 2011; Rey and Neuhäuser, 2011). To compare 3 or more groups, the extended test is the Kruskal-Wallis test (Kruskal and Wallis, 1952). In general, when parametric assumptions hold, nonparametric tests reduce the power of a study to detect a difference as compared to using a parametric test, but they are more appropriate when the underlying continuous variable deviates greatly from a bell-shaped normally distributed curve.

4.4.3 Regression Approaches

Sometimes, one wants to evaluate the association of more than 1 variable or factor (also known as a predictor or independent variable) with disease risk or outcome (the dependent variable) simultaneously. Chi-squared and *t* tests can only evaluate 1 variable at a time. Regression techniques are statistical methods to examine the association of multiple potential disease-related factors with disease or disease outcome. Multivariate regression analysis permits simultaneous inclusion of many covariates (ie, factors) that are essential in controlling for confounding (see Sec. 4.3.6.2); this allows for consideration (and adjustment) of multiple factors in the same analysis. Including multiple variables in the same model is the equivalent of asking what the true association of the factor of interest is when many other predictor variables are considered simultaneously. In biomarker and biospecimen analyses, such factors of interest can involve protein levels, immunohistochemical staining patterns, serologic levels, germline variation, somatic alterations, and epigenetic markers, whereas clinicoepidemiologic factors may include, age, gender, patient comorbidities and general state of health, tumor grade and histologic subtype, disease stage at diagnosis, and treatment.

Regression models generally follow a common pattern. Equation 4.4 represents a univariate analysis where x represents the value of the independent (predictor) variable, whereas y represents the dependent (outcome) variable. β_0 is a nominal constant, whereas β_1 represents the association between x and y in the model, and its value is a constant that is generated as part of the regression analysis. The more the value of β_1 deviates from 0 (whether a large positive or large negative value), the stronger the magnitude of association between x and y.

$$y = \beta_0 + \beta_1 x \quad \text{[Eq. 4.4]}$$

In Equation 4.5, a single model now incorporates multiple (n) independent variables as predictors of the outcome, y. This type of model is useful if all n variables are of interest as predictors of outcome, y. At other times, one is only interested in the association between y and a single predictor variable, x_1, whereas the other variables $x_2, \ldots, x_n$, represent potential confounders; however, a statistical model does not discriminate between confounders and predictors of interest. It is the role of the researcher to draw appropriate conclusions from the data. Data for each study participant (ie, values for x_1 through x_n and for y) are placed into the regression analysis, and values for β_0 through β_n are generated as part of the regression model.

$$y = \beta_0 + \beta_1 x_1 + \beta_2 x_2 + \beta_3 x_3 + \beta_4 x_4 + \ldots + \beta_n x_n \quad \text{[Eq. 4.5]}$$

Table 4–5 describes the various formats in which to incorporate the independent predictors, x_n, into a regression model. Table 4–6 summarizes the format of the outcome variable, y, which determines the type of regression.

TABLE 4-5 Different formats for the independent variable, x_n.

Types of Independent Variable, x_n	Examples of How Variable x_n Can Be Incorporated Into a Regression Model
Dichotomized (ie, two-level) (eg, gender)	Male = 0; Female = 1

Categorized (eg, smoking status)	Indicator Variables:
	  Current smoker: Current = 1, Former = 0, Never = 0
	  Former smoker: Current = 0, Former = 1, Never = 0
	  Never smoker: Current = 0, Former = 0, Never = 1

Ordinal (ranked order) (eg, quartiles of intake of fruit, disease stages at diagnosis, germline variation)	Ordinal Categories (where Q1 to Q4 represents quartiles 1 to 4)
	  Lowest quartile: Q1 = 0
	  Second quartile: Q2 = 1
	  Third quartile: Q3 = 2
	  Highest quartile: Q4 = 3
	Indicator Variables:
	  Lowest quartile: Q1 = 1, Q2 = 0, Q3 = 0, Q4 = 0
	  Second quartile: Q1 = 0, Q2 = 1, Q3 = 0, Q4 = 0
	  Third quartile: Q1 = 0, Q2 = 0, Q3 = 1, Q4 = 0
	  Highest quartile: Q1 = 0, Q2 = 0, Q3 = 0, Q4 = 1

Continuous (eg, age, weight)	Continuous: value (V) can range from 0 to infinity
	Dichotomized at median:
	  Below median, V = 0
	  Median or above, V = 1
	Divided into tertiles (T):
	  Lowest tertile: T = 0
	  Second lowest tertile: T = 1
	  Highest tertile: T = 2

TABLE 4-6 The relationship between type of outcome variable and regression model.

Type of Outcome Variable (y)	Type of Regression Model
Continuous variable (eg, hormone levels; weight loss)	Linear regression
Dichotomous variable (eg, toxicity/no toxicity) Disease (case)/no disease (control)	Logistic regression
Ordinal variable (eg, nonsmoker, mild smoker, heavy smoker; disease response, disease stability, disease progression)	Polytomous ordinal logistic regression (3 or more nominal categories)
Survival outcome or time-to-event (with censoring) (see Chap. 22, Sec. 22.4.1)	Cox proportional hazards regression

The process of building a statistical model and model selection among candidate models is a crucial part of analytic epidemiology and involves consideration of many different aspects. A thorough description of these considerations is beyond the scope of this single chapter. There are entire textbooks dedicated to best practices for model building strategies (for details, see Rothman et al, 2008 chap. 21; Royston and Sauerbrei, 2008 ; Harrell, 2015). One may ask why not simply include all covariates into a model. In addition to the increased model complexity and the difficulty in providing meaningful interpretation, if too many predictors are included for estimation, model coefficients can become unstable in small data sets or data sets where few events of interest have occurred. Before moving on to multivariable methods, univariate associations for each predictor with the outcome are typically examined. The process for selecting covariates for inclusion in a multivariable model can vary and several different approaches exist for these purposes, such as forward, backward, or stepwise variable selection. However, these methods have been criticized for being too data driven, reliant only on statistical significance, and ignore important biologic or clinical relevance (Greenland 1989; Greenland et al, 2016). Other approaches for variable selection can be based on a priori knowledge, the use of causal diagrams such as *directed acyclic graphs* (DAG) (Greenland, 1989; Shrier and Platt, 2008), or through the use of more complex statistical approaches that are beyond the scope of this chapter (eg, penalized regression) (Walter and Tiemeier, 2009).

All regression analyses make assumptions about the nature of their underlying variables x_n and y. For instance, linear regression analyses assume that a continuous, independent x_n variable will have a linear relationship with the y outcome variable. If this is not true, then the x_n variable may need to be transformed to a format where a linear relationship between x_n and y exists; these may include taking the square root or taking the logarithmic function of x_n. In another example, the association between average adult weight and cancer risk may be the result of a threshold effect, in which case, dichotomizing weight at the threshold (rather than treating the variable as a continuous variable) would be more appropriate. In the case of a Cox proportional hazards model, the assumption is that the ratio of hazards (defined as the rate of dying or other event in a short period of time) between the comparator arms remain constant. Many survival curves violate this assumption, most obviously when they cross each other. It is therefore critical that assumptions behind each of these models are checked, and any deviations from these assumptions lead to disclosure and use of alternative methods of analyses (see Chap. 22, Sec. 22.3.6).

A useful property of the logistic regression function is that the β estimates generated in the model are mathematically related to an odds ratio. This relationship is as follows:

$$\text{Odds ratio of variable } x_n = e^{\beta n}, \text{ where } \beta_n \text{ is derived from an equation similar to Eq. 4.5} \quad [\text{Eq. 4.6}]$$

4.4.4 Interaction

The term *interaction* has been used in the context of statistical, biologic, and public health concepts. In general, interaction

Cancer Epidemiology

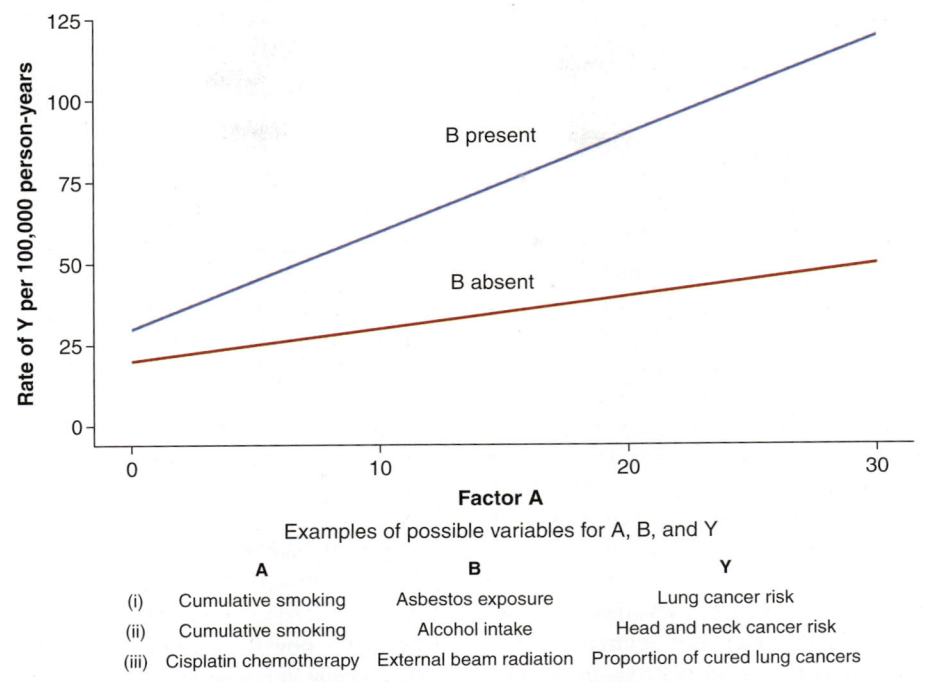

Examples of possible variables for A, B, and Y

	A	B	Y
(i)	Cumulative smoking	Asbestos exposure	Lung cancer risk
(ii)	Cumulative smoking	Alcohol intake	Head and neck cancer risk
(iii)	Cisplatin chemotherapy	External beam radiation	Proportion of cured lung cancers

FIGURE 4–8 Interaction between 2 independent predictors of disease or outcome. In the example, an increase from 0 to 30 units for the factor of interest, A, results in the disease rate increasing from 20 per 1000 to 50 per 1000 when factor B is absent. In the presence of factor B the same increase in factor A results in a much greater increase in disease rate: from 30 per 1000 to 120 per 1000. Factor A interacts with factor B as factor A has a stronger effect on disease rates in the presence of factor B. Note that the examples in the table are not associated with the values given in the graph, which is presented for illustrative purposes.

refers to 2 or more factors modifying the effect of one another with respect to outcome. Epidemiologists often refer to this as *effect modification*. An interaction may arise when considering the relationship among multiple variables and describes a situation in which the simultaneous influence of 2 variables on a third is synergistic or antagonistic. A classic example is the interaction between smoking and asbestos exposure. Each factor individually increases lung cancer risk, but exposure to asbestos increases the cancer risk in smokers much more than simply adding the 2 risks together.

In cancer, interaction analyses often focus on gene–environment interactions, where the goal has been to identify environmental factors that, in the presence of the right combination of genetic or host factors, substantially modify (typically increase) the risk of developing certain cancers. In pharmacogenetics and biomarker research, interaction analyses are increasingly important (see Sec. 4.7.1).

Interaction should not be confused with *confounding*. A confounder has a stable effect on the relationship of the exposure-to-risk and disease-to-outcome variables; proper analysis will "correct" such a confounder effect and produce an accurate estimate of risk for a potential disease-related factor. In an interaction, the risk estimate for the factor changes with different levels of the variable it interacts with, as illustrated in Figure 4–8. Interaction can be explored using regression techniques through the inclusion of a cross-product term in a regression model (see eq. 4.7). Statistical significance of the interaction term suggests significant interaction is present.

$$y = \beta_0 + \beta_1 x_1 + \beta_2 x_2 + \beta_3 x_3 + \beta_4 x_1 * x_3 \quad [\text{Eq. 4.7}]$$

In general, confounders are considered a nuisance, and their inclusion in regression models is solely for adjustment to obtain unbiased estimates for the association of interest. However, significant interactions are important findings that should be reported and investigated further.

4.5 CANCER EPIDEMIOLOGY IN ACTION: SUCCESS STORIES

4.5.1 Infection and Cancer

There has been increasing recognition of the role of infection in cancer etiology. Specific examples include schistosomal infestations and bladder cancer, hepatitis viruses and hepatocellular carcinoma (HCC), and HPVs and cervical, anal, and head and neck cancer (see Chap. 7, Sec. 7.4.4). It has been estimated that attributable risk of all cancers worldwide to infections is approximately 15%, and that by reducing the effects of these infectious agents (through improved hygiene and public health measures, vaccination, and sometimes screening), cancer incidence might decrease by up to 5% in Western countries and up to 50% in some developing countries (eg, those in sub-Saharan Africa) (Plummer et al, 2016). Despite the advent of hepatitis B vaccinations and antibiotic treatment of *Helicobacter pylori*, the most important carcinogenic infections remain *H pylori*, HPV, hepatitis B and C infections, and Epstein-Barr virus (EBV). In sub-Saharan Africa, HIV and Human Herpesvirus type 8 (HHV-8) have contributed to the high rates of Kaposi sarcoma.

One of the most successful applications of analytic epidemiology is the research that helped establish a role for EBV in the etiology of Burkitt lymphoma (see Chap. 7, Sec. 7.4.4). Endemic Burkitt lymphoma occurs in children, primarily in equatorial Africa and Papua New Guinea, and the most frequent presentation of the tumor is a distinctive lesion of the jaw. In early ecologic studies, this information was circulated to medical units in Africa and presence of the lesion was mapped to geographic location. Results indicated an association between the presence of Burkitt lymphoma and low-lying areas in tropical Africa (Burkitt, 1962a,b), suggesting that a virus transmitted by an insect vector might play a role in the etiology of this cancer. Laboratory-based studies by Epstein, Achong, and Barr implicated EBV as an etiologic agent, and following further research, EBV became the first virus to be implicated in the development of a human cancer (Thompson and Kurzrock, 2004). Additional research indicates that malarial infections, which correlate with the incidence of Burkitt lymphoma, may interact with EBV to increase risk of Burkitt lymphoma (Brady et al, 2007).

The evidence associating HBV and HCC was first observed in ecologic studies, where a high prevalence of serum hepatitis B surface antigen (HBsAg) positivity was correlated with the high prevalence of HCC (Maupas and Melnick, 1981). Cohort studies also showed that populations receiving vaccination for HBV have much lower risk of developing HCC than those without vaccination (Lee et al, 1998). HCV was also identified as an etiologic factor, both as a cofactor and an independent risk factor for HCC (Yu et al, 2005). Nowadays, HBV vaccination is administered routinely in high-prevalence regions, and has reduced the incidence of HCC by ~75% in school-age children in the last several decades (Chien et al, 2006).

The association between HPV and cervical cancer was proposed by zur Hausen when he found HPV DNA in cervical cancer tissues (zur Hausen, 1977). A subsequent large cross-sectional study by the International Agency for Research on Cancer (IARC) reported HPV DNA, predominately HPV types 16 and 18, in 93% of cervical tumor samples, thus providing strong epidemiologic evidence of the association (Bosch et al, 1995). Now HPV is accepted as a necessary cause of cervical cancer; however, only a small proportion of HPV carriers develop cervical cancer, suggesting that other etiologic factors are involved (Munoz et al, 2003). In 2006, the first HPV vaccine was approved by the US Food and Drug Administration (FDA) (Markowitz et al, 2007) and HPV vaccine is now recommended in North America and Europe for school-age children of both sexes to prevent both cervical and oropharyngeal cancers (see Chap. 7, Sec. 7.4.4). A recent Cochrane review found the vaccines safe, with efficacy demonstrated at reducing the precancerous lesions of the cervix (Arbyn and Xu, 2018); it will take a number of additional years of follow-up to document significant decreases in cervical cancer rates because of its long latency.

There is a rising incidence of oropharyngeal squamous cell carcinoma in the developed world, particularly with a unique pattern involving the base of the tongue and tonsillar bed in younger men, despite decreasing use of alcohol and tobacco and decreasing incidence of other subtypes of head and neck squamous cell carcinomas (Shiboski et al, 2005). This increase in incidence is so striking that one study extrapolated that by 2020, oropharyngeal cancers could overtake the incidence of cervical cancer in the United States (Chaturvedi et al, 2011). Research has identified HPV as a potentially important etiologic factor (Gillison et al, 2001). Unlike the heavy smoker and alcohol user, these HPV-associated oropharyngeal cancers typically occurred in individuals of higher socioeconomic status, often in married, light or never smoking, younger individuals but in still male-predominant cohorts, and in individuals with a history of multiple sexual partners. Although more likely to be diagnosed with extensive nodal disease, treatment responses and relapse-free and survival outcomes are better in these individuals than in those with tumors not associated with HPV. As a result, ongoing clinical trials are focusing on deescalating the aggressive multimodality therapies that had been the standard of practice. The identification of the unique clinicoepidemiologic characteristics of HPV-associated oropharyngeal carcinomas has also led to a new staging system (Lydiatt et al, 2017), Within a decade, the way clinicians think about oropharyngeal carcinoma, how it is treated, and how it is staged has changed dramatically in Europe and North America, as a result of identification of a paradoxical rise in incidence in this subset of head and neck squamous cell cancers, coincident with a fall in smoking-related HPV-negative oropharyngeal carcinoma rates due to dropping smoking rates in the same regions.

4.5.2 Tobacco and Cancer

Tobacco consumption is the most recognized risk factor for human cancer in Western countries. Annually it accounts for approximately 29% of cancer deaths in the United States (CDC, 2008), and approximately 6 million deaths worldwide (WHO, 2015). Epidemiologic studies have identified numerous detrimental health effects of tobacco consumption over the last 60 years, with the most striking example being Sir Richard Doll's British studies that established the association between tobacco smoking and lung cancer (Doll et al, 2004). Since then, numerous epidemiologic studies have been conducted for different cancer sites. In 2012, an IARC monograph stated that there is sufficient evidence to conclude that, in humans, tobacco smoking causes cancer of the lung, head and neck (including oral cavity, oropharynx, and larynx), esophagus, stomach, colorectum, pancreas, liver, kidney, bladder, cervix, and myeloid leukemia (Fig. 4–9) (IARC, 2012). In addition to adult cancers, parental tobacco smoking in the time period just before conception or during pregnancy is associated with a higher risk of hepatoblastoma in the offspring (Secretan et al, 2009).

Data for lung cancer are overwhelming: 84% of male lung cancer and 81% of female lung cancer is attributable to tobacco use (USDHHS 2014 Surgeon General's Report). The proportion of lung cancers due to tobacco smoking is declining in developed countries but continues to rise in developing countries (Torre et al, 2016). Increasing intensity of cigarette smoking (ie, number of cigarettes per day) and increasing duration of smoking (ie, years) are both associated with increasing risk of lung cancer; increasing number of years since smoking

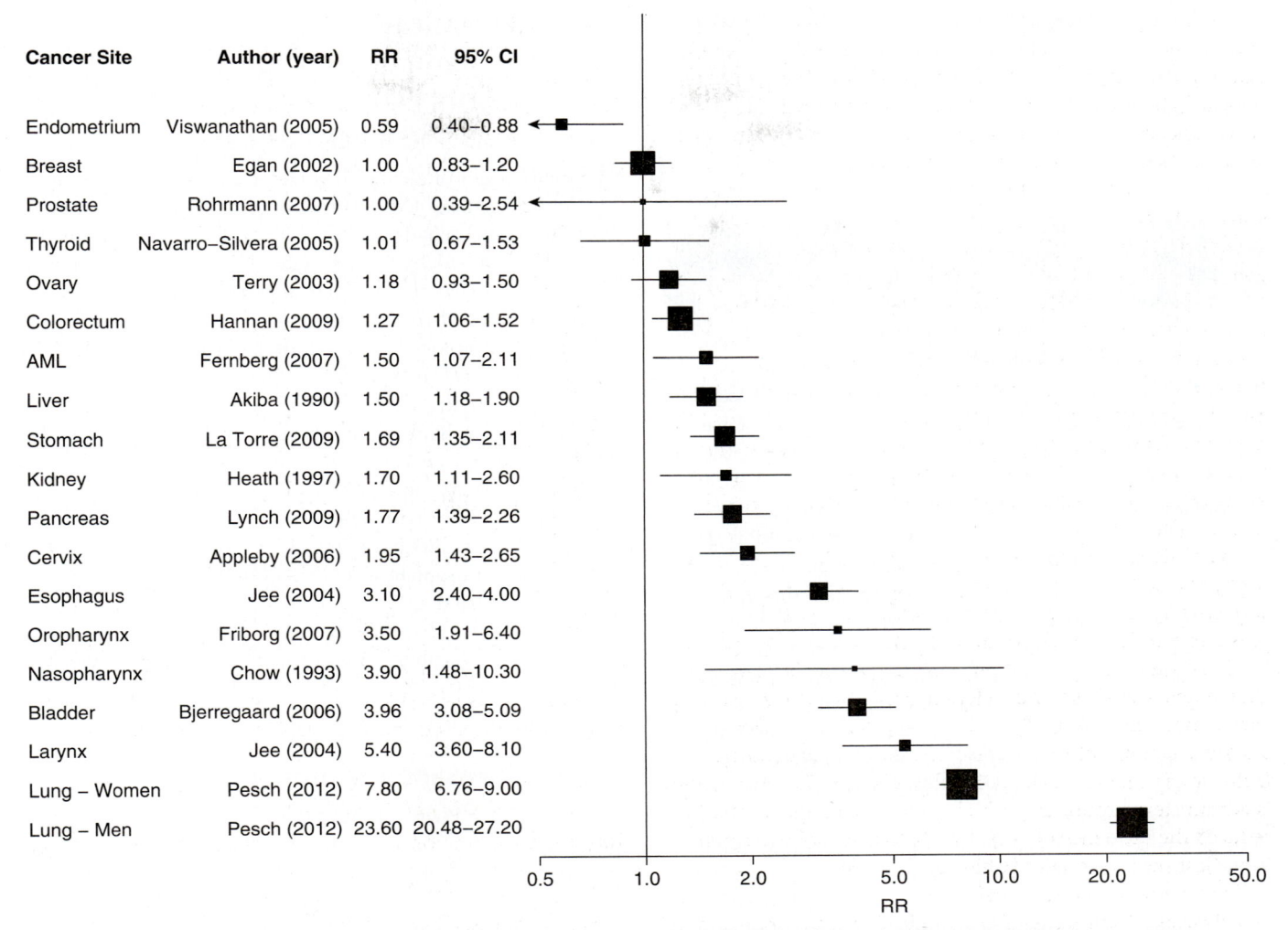

Cancer Site	Author (year)	RR	95% CI
Endometrium	Viswanathan (2005)	0.59	0.40–0.88
Breast	Egan (2002)	1.00	0.83–1.20
Prostate	Rohrmann (2007)	1.00	0.39–2.54
Thyroid	Navarro–Silvera (2005)	1.01	0.67–1.53
Ovary	Terry (2003)	1.18	0.93–1.50
Colorectum	Hannan (2009)	1.27	1.06–1.52
AML	Fernberg (2007)	1.50	1.07–2.11
Liver	Akiba (1990)	1.50	1.18–1.90
Stomach	La Torre (2009)	1.69	1.35–2.11
Kidney	Heath (1997)	1.70	1.11–2.60
Pancreas	Lynch (2009)	1.77	1.39–2.26
Cervix	Appleby (2006)	1.95	1.43–2.65
Esophagus	Jee (2004)	3.10	2.40–4.00
Oropharynx	Friborg (2007)	3.50	1.91–6.40
Nasopharynx	Chow (1993)	3.90	1.48–10.30
Bladder	Bjerregaard (2006)	3.96	3.08–5.09
Larynx	Jee (2004)	5.40	3.60–8.10
Lung – Women	Pesch (2012)	7.80	6.76–9.00
Lung – Men	Pesch (2012)	23.60	20.48–27.20

FIGURE 4–9 Relative risks of cigarette smoking for various cancers. The relative risks (RRs) and 95% confidence intervals (CIs) for developing various cancers, comparing current smokers to never smokers. All estimates except for lung are from selected key studies from the tables of published studies reviewed by the International Agency for Research on Cancer (IARC). The Y-axis indicates various primary cancer sites. The X-axis is the relative risk. Data for men and women were considered together, where applicable. *AML*, acute myeloid leukemia. (Data from IARC Monographs on Tobacco and Involuntary Smoking, 2004 and Tobacco Smoking, 2012, based on selected representative large cohort or population-based studies, or meta or pooled analysis, when available; lung cancer estimates were from *Pesch* et al., 2012.)

cessation is associated with a fall in risk. Similar dose-dependent findings have been found for the risk of bladder, oral cavity, and other solid tumors. There have been more than 50 studies of secondhand smoking and lung cancer risk, many in lifetime never-smoking spouses. Most, especially those associated with higher secondhand smoking exposures, have shown significant increased lung cancer risks associated with inhaling smoke from others (IARC, 2004).

Understanding of the association between tobacco use and cancer risk (in addition to associations between tobacco use and nonmalignant diseases such as cardiovascular disease) through epidemiologic studies have helped governments to implement policy for tobacco control, including banning smoking in public buildings, increasing tobacco taxes, and placing warning labels on packaging. Government intervention and control policy have helped to reduce tobacco consumption at the population level substantially, and to reduce cancer deaths related to tobacco consumption (Chaloupka et al, 2011; Thun and Freedman, 2018).

4.5.3 Alcohol and Head and Neck Cancer

Epidemiologic studies have described associations between alcohol consumption and cancer risk at various sites, including cancers of the oral cavity, pharynx, larynx, esophagus, liver, female breast, and colorectum (Baan et al, 2007; IARC, 2010). Studies have also investigated the dose–response relationship between alcohol consumption and cancer risk, and the synergism between alcohol and tobacco smoking. Because alcohol is often consumed concurrently with tobacco products, there was a need to take tobacco smoking into account either by study design or statistical analysis to address potential confounding. The dose–response relationship between alcohol and non-HPV associated head and neck cancers was shown to be linear with an approximately 2- to 3-fold increased risk per 50 g of alcohol per day, depending on the cancer site (IARC, 2010). The effect of smoking and alcohol consumption appear to be multiplicative for non–HPV-associated head and neck cancer, showing a synergistic interaction between these 2 factors (see Fig. 4–8).

4.6 EMERGING AREAS IN EPIDEMIOLOGY

4.6.1 Genomic Epidemiology

4.6.1.1 Genome-Wide Association Studies of Cancer Risk
Genome-wide association studies (GWAS; see Chap. 2, Sec. 2.11) aim to investigate the majority of genetic variations across the genome, and do not require prior knowledge of the functional significance of the variants studied. They have been used extensively to identify potential susceptibility genes in various health research domains. Genome-wide scans for many tumor types have been completed, and this approach has been successful in identifying cancer susceptibility loci. A catalog of published GWAS with complete references is maintained by the National Human Genome Research Institute and European Bioinformatics Institute (available at http://www.ebi.ac.uk/gwas/). Examples of how genetic studies have contributed to the understanding of cancer etiologies are given below, although as yet, few of the findings from GWAS is of strong enough magnitude to translate into the clinical setting. Hence, GWAS is still predominately research tool used to identify novel biological pathways for further basic and translational research. In addition to genomic analysis, the field of molecular epidemiology of cancer has expanded to include epigenomics, transcriptomics, proteomics, metabolomics, and more. The advances and applications of some of these various newly emerging fields are described in later chapters.

4.6.1.2 Addiction to Nicotine, and Risk of Lung Cancer
A previous linkage analysis of 52 high-risk pedigrees identified a lung cancer susceptibility locus at chromosome 6q23-25 (Bailey-Wilson et al, 2004), but specific susceptibility genes that influence lung cancer susceptibility were not defined until the GWAS findings were reported in 2008, when researchers identified susceptibility loci at 15q25 and 5p15 (Hung et al, 2008). The Ch15q25 region is composed of several nicotinic acetylcholine receptor genes and the 5p15 region includes the genes *hTERT* (human telomerase reverse transcriptase) (see Chap. 9, Sec. 9.7) and *CLPTM1L* (cleft lip and palate transmembrane protein 1–like protein), both of which play a role in apoptotic resistance. The *hTERT* gene is the most likely candidate in this region. The Ch15q25 region was also shown to be associated with nicotine addiction and smoking behaviors (Thorgeirsson et al, 2008; Hancock et al, 2015), although the association between 15q25 and smoking is not sufficient to explain its strong association with risk of lung cancer. Recently, a large consortium analysis demonstrated the substantial heterogeneity in genetic architectures across lung cancer histologic subtypes (McKay et al, 2017).

4.6.2 Genomic Risk Studies Based on Mechanistic Principles: Alcohol, Alcohol Dehydrogenase, and Head and Neck Cancer

The metabolism of alcohol involves 2 families of genes: alcohol dehydrogenases (*ADHs*) that oxidize ethanol to acetaldehyde, and acetaldehyde dehydrogenases (*ALDHs*) that further metabolize acetaldehyde to acetate. The genetic variation of *ADHs* and *ALDHs* that influences enzyme activity has been investigated for their association with head and neck cancer in several epidemiologic studies (IARC, 2010). *ADH1B* (*1/*1, where 1/1 is a genotype designation) and *ADH1C* are associated with increased risk of head and neck cancers, although the mechanism has not been elucidated. The *ALDH2 Glu487Lys* allele (rs671, also known as *2 variant allele) encodes an inactive form of the enzyme, and this Lys variant is prevalent in approximately 30% of Asian populations. The heterozygous carriers have approximately 10% enzyme activity, and they accumulate acetaldehyde and have increased risks for alcohol-related esophageal and head and neck cancers compared with individuals with the common alleles. These findings have contributed to the understanding of alcohol as a carcinogen (IARC, 2010).

4.6.3 Pharmacogenomic Epidemiology and Pharmacoepidemiology

Pharmacogenomic epidemiology is focused on personalizing medicine through the evaluation of tumor and germline (heritable) genetic and genomic factors to select appropriate and individualized therapies. These factors, or biomarkers, are assessed for their association with pharmacokinetic and pharmacodynamic roles in affecting treatment response, recurrence, disease progression and survival, and toxicity of treatment (see Chap. 18, Sec. 18.2.3, and Chap. 22, Sec. 22.3.2). The field is both promising and challenging simultaneously.

The classical example of the difficulties in moving pharmacogenomic biomarker discoveries into clinical practice has been the genetic disorder that results in the absence of functional dihydropyrimidine dehydrogenase (DPD), or DPD deficiency, and the resultant severe hematologic and gastrointestinal toxicities that affect such patients who receive fluoropyrimidines such as 5-fluorouracil (Chap. 18, Sec. 18.3.2). The original identification of this extreme toxicity came from observational reports, which detected a potential toxicity signal in a small proportion of patients; the field of epidemiology research focused on identifying rare extreme toxicity signals in observational populations is known as pharmacovigilance. Though some pharmacovigilance analyses rely on passive reporting of unusual adverse events by health professionals and patients, an active form of a pharmacovigilance study is the phase IV study, which is a formal observational study often required by regulatory bodies such as the Food and Drug Administration in the United States, Health Canada, or the European Medicines Agency to study the longer-term safety

TABLE 4–7 Examples of cancer pharmacogenetic studies that evaluated the combined influence of genetic polymorphisms (host factor) with systemic drug (environmental factor) interaction on adverse events of the drug.

Drug Adverse Event	Targeted Genes or GWAS	Environmental (Drug) Agent	Genetic Polymorphism (Gene)	Strength of Genetic Association with Adverse Event When Exposed to the Drug	Reference (n Cases/n Controls)
Hearing loss in children	Targeted genes (220 drug-metabolism genes) with replication study	Cisplatin	rs12201199 (TPMT) rs9332377 (COMT)	OR = 17 OR = 5.5	Ross et al, 2009 (discovery 33/20; replication 112 total)
Hearing loss in children	GWAS and replication study	Cisplatin	rs1872328, (ACYP2)	OR = 4.5	Xu et al, 2015 (GWAS 93/145, replication 19/49)
Hearing loss in adults	Targeted genes (220 drug-metabolism genes) with replication study	Cisplatin	rs4788863 (SLC16A5)	OR = 17	Drögemöller et al, 2017 (discovery 23/73; replication 14/78)
Cardiotoxicity in children	Targeted genes (220 drug-metabolism genes) with replication study	Anthracycline	rs7853758 (SLC28A3)	OR = 2.9	Visscher et al, 2012 (discovery 38/118; replication 40/148)
Cardiotoxicity in children	Targeted genes with replication study	Anthracycline	rs2229774 (RARG)	OR = 4.7	Aminkeng et al, 2015 (discovery 280 total; replication 176 total)
Musculoskeletal adverse events in adults	GWAS	Aromatase inhibitors	rs11849538 (TCL1A)	OR = 2.1	Ingle et al, 2010 (292/585)
Peripheral neuropathy in adults	GWAS with replication study	Paclitaxel	rs10771973 (FGD4)	OR = 1.6	Baldwin et al, 2012 (discovery 855 total; replication 271 total)

GWAS, Genome-wide association studies; OR, odds ratio.
Codes for genetic polymorphisms (rs followed by number) are established reference identification numbers for each polymorphism.

and rare adverse events of newly approved drugs. It is through pharmacovigilance reports of these rare but extreme toxicities of 5-fluorouracil that a deficiency in an enzyme along the catabolic pathway of 5-fluorouacul was first discovered. DPD is the enzyme responsible for more than 85% of the inactivation and metabolism of 5-fluorouracil. Though initial genetic evaluations identified a few genetic variants that led to such toxicity, broader evaluations suggest that this rare syndrome of DPD deficiency appears to be multifactorial, including multiple functional genetic variants within the DPD gene, and genetic and epigenetic regulation of other genes that secondarily alter DPD function. Pharmacologic factors (drug-drug interactions) are also being evaluated. Thus, the original single defect in one gene leading to a single phenotype is too simplistic a model to explain sensitivity to fluoropyrimidines. Additional factors also explain the low positive predictive value of currently available tests; as such, routine clinical testing is generally not recommended yet.

Several newer pharmacogenetic studies have identified promising associations between heritable genetic variations and either toxicity or efficacy of drugs (Table 4–7). Each of these studies has either used observational methods or involved secondary analyses of randomized clinical trials. Some have selected candidate polymorphisms (eg, of genes known to be important in metabolism of anticancer drugs), whereas others have used GWAS approach without a primary hypothesis to study the effect of genes on adverse effects of specific drugs. These studies have led to the discovery of unexpected genetic variants that have a biologic rationale for their association with the pharmacogenetic effects (Ingle, 2010). Validation studies are ongoing.

In addition to heritable genetic associations with drug therapy, molecular epidemiologic studies and secondary analyses of randomized controlled trials have demonstrated well-known associations between tumor markers and treatment outcomes. Examples include estrogen receptor/progesterone receptor status and benefit from antiestrogen therapy in breast cancer (see Chap. 20, Sec. 20.4); KRAS mutation predicts lack of efficacy of monoclonal antibody therapy targeting EGFR in colorectal cancer (Chap. 19, Sec. 19.4.1). In contrast, other markers were studied primarily through prospectively designed trials, even if there were initial observational data suggesting a relationship: Her2/neu overamplification predicts efficacy of monoclonal antibody therapy targeting Her2/neu in breast cancer (Chap. 19, Sec. 19.4.2); and ROS1 mutations and ALK translocations predict for response to small molecule inhibitors of their associated targets of ROS1 and ALK in non–small cell lung cancer (Chap. 19, Sec. 19.6.4). In the case of EGFR-sensitizing mutations and response to EGFR tyrosine kinase inhibitors in lung cancer, some of the drugs were evaluated through secondary analyses of trials whereas other drugs were studied through prospective trials (Chap. 19, Sec. 19.4.1).

4.7 ISSUES AND CHALLENGES IN CANCER EPIDEMIOLOGY

4.7.1 Observational Studies vs Clinical Trials, Predictive vs Prognostic Biomarkers

Observational studies are the most common way to study the risk of disease and can also provide useful data for certain outcomes analyses. In contrast, randomized clinical trials are primarily designed to compare 2 or more categories of a specific variable. Typically, these categories are interventional therapies such as drug therapy, radiotherapy, or surgery; the intervention is assigned randomly to minimize selection and other biases between the groups, as randomization controls for both known and unknown confounders (see Chap. 22, Sec. 22.3.4). After the completion of a randomized clinical trial, the data collected can be used to evaluate many other parameters than the original randomized variable. Further, many trials now collect biospecimens in addition to clinical and outcome variables and can be used for secondary analyses to relate these variables to outcomes of the trial. A randomized clinical trial can therefore be treated as a specialized form of cohort study.

When molecular factors are evaluated that might predict response, toxicity, or outcome related to the therapy used in a randomized trial, a secondary analysis can determine whether the pharmacogenomic factor is predictive of response to treatment or simply prognostic, independent of the treatment received (see Chap. 22, Sec. 22.5). A prognostic risk factor may stratify patients into high- or low-risk categories, which can lead to differential interventional approaches: a patient at high risk for relapse may be offered more aggressive therapy, whereas a patient at low risk for relapse may be offered less aggressive and less toxic therapy.

One of the formal statistical methods for determining whether a marker is predictive is to identify an interaction between a biomarker and a treatment arm, implying that the biomarker has a different effect in the presence of the treatment than in the absence of treatment. Although observational studies may occasionally be used to study such interactions (Bradbury et al, 2009), randomized trials offer the best method, partly because the choice of therapy is less confounded by other key prognostic variables such as patient comorbidity.

Table 4–8 compares the use of randomized trials with observational studies. A randomized trial of the right set of patients may not be available (wrong patient subgroup, wrong therapy, rare cancer type where no such randomized trials are being conducted) and also has the limitation that patients are highly selected to participate, usually those without comorbidity and with high performance status. An observational study may be the only option to answer a specific research question and can give information about patients in a real-world environment (see also Chap. 22, Sec. 22.3.10). Thus, both types of studies will continue to be important for epidemiologic and translational research. Figure 4–10 details the long journey from biomarker discovery through to clinical adoption. Epidemiologic studies are key to several of the steps in the biomarker development pipeline.

4.7.2 Exposure Misclassifications: The Example of Diet and Occupation

As discussed briefly in Section 4.3.6.3, misclassification of exposure has been a challenge for cancer epidemiology, and specific examples include assessment of dietary and occupational exposures. The general hypotheses are that certain micronutrients or specific chemical agents related to

TABLE 4–8 Comparing the advantages and disadvantages of using randomized trials (RCTs) vs observational studies as sources of epidemiologic analyses.

Randomized Trials	Observational Studies
Advantages	**Advantages**
• Designed to measure survival differences, so good resource for secondary analyses of factors related to disease outcome (clinicoepidemiologic and biologic)	• Standard source for epidemiologic studies of disease risk
• Collect detailed treatment toxicity data	• Evaluate rare and long-term toxicities
• Randomization should ensure equal distribution of confounding variables	• Large, diverse populations
• Accessible specimens for translational research	• Follow-up can be extensive
• Can incorporate collection of epidemiologic data in study design	• Large number of drugs and drug combinations
• Efficient use of resources by tagging epidemiologic study onto trial	• Include a wide range of comorbidities and past medication history
Disadvantages	• Can be utilized in rarer cancers where randomized trials are not available
• Not a good source for analyses of disease risk (because of highly selected case-entry criteria and lack of concurrent healthy controls in study)	• Can study standard, approved drugs where no randomized trial data exist
• The highly selected populations of RCTs with rigid exclusion and inclusion criteria may limit generalizability of effects to the broader patient population	**Disadvantages**
	• Prone to selection and confounding bias
• Either the experimental or standard arm will become obsolete; thus, at least 1 arm may become irrelevant to clinical practice	

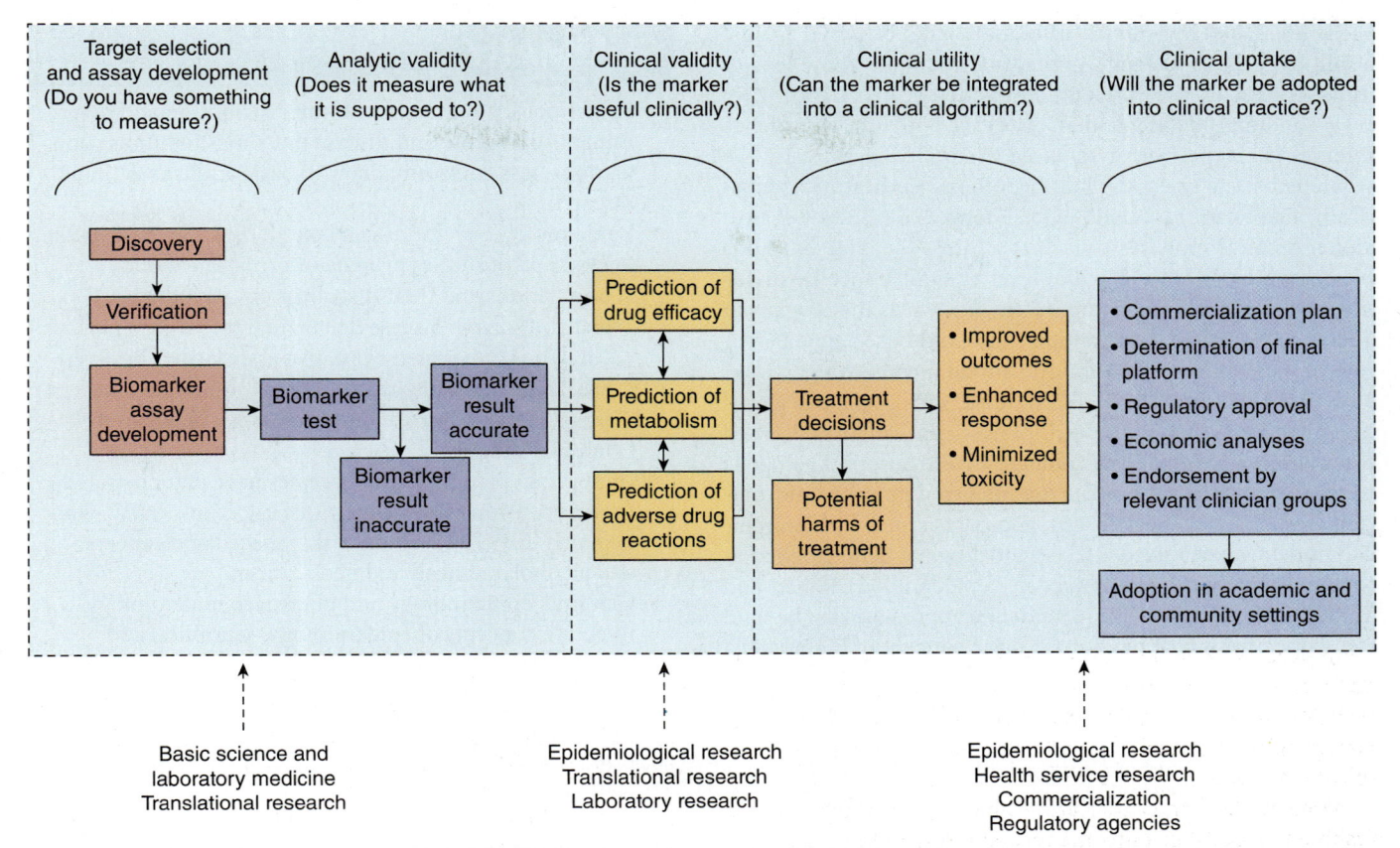

FIGURE 4–10 The long road from biomarker discovery to clinical use, and where epidemiologic studies play a key role.

occupations can affect cancer risk. Proper assessment of these exposures requires a comprehensive study protocol, thorough validation, and substantial resources.

For dietary exposures, specific instruments, such as 24-hour recall and the food frequency questionnaire (FFQ), have been developed to assist the validation of the self-reported dietary history. To validate a specific dietary exposure, biochemical indicators (if available) might be measured, such as serum level of vitamin B or folate. This approach, however, is subject to biomarker instability, laboratory measurement error, and when repeated samples are not available, the measurement at one point in time may not reflect the long-term exposure history. Nevertheless, biomarkers can provide qualitative information regarding the validity of information obtained from questionnaires.

A major problem arises with highly correlated exposures, where the challenge is to distinguish the independent effect of specific nutrients or foods, when food items are typically consumed in groups, and patterns of consumption are reflective of general lifestyle and socioeconomic status. To complicate matters, the same nutrients may exhibit different properties in different foods (eg, nitrates in smoked meat vs in green leafy vegetables). Yet, analysis based on a specific nutrient can be related more directly to a biologic mechanism and avoid the issues of interrelated dietary behavior patterns (eg, the tendency to eat certain foods together, such as milk and cereal, or certain habits together such as alcohol and tobacco consumption). In general, maximum information can be obtained when analyses are performed using all of the data, including nutrient levels, food items, and food groups.

Mendelian randomization has been proposed to address the issues of complex exposures (Smith and Ebrahim, 2003). The basic concept of Mendelian randomization is to analyze variants in genes (both as single genes or multiple genes) that determine metabolism of nutrients as instrumental (ie, surrogate) variables for the specific nutrients of interest, as genetic alleles are randomly assorted in the population based on Mendel's laws and their assortments are unrelated to other factors such as lifestyles or other food intake (ie, they are unconfounded). Specific examples include ALDH (for alcohol consumption) and cardiovascular disease, or lactase persistence genotype (for milk consumption) and cancer (Smith and Ebrahim, 2003). The ideal instrumental variable needs to have very strong and specific correlations with the nutrient of interest, but for some nutrients, such an instrumental variable may not be available. Nevertheless, it provides a potential alternative solution to the issues of misclassification and high correlation in nutritional epidemiology.

4.7.3 High-Dimensionality Data and Multiple Comparisons

Biologic and genetic data from cancer epidemiologic studies typically involve tens or hundreds of thousands of variables related to genetics or biomarkers to be tested against a null hypothesis. Genetic imputation methods allow tens of millions of sequence variants to be tested (Chap. 2, Sec. 2.6). If we conduct 100 independent tests each with 95% confidence interval (5% type I error rate, see Chap. 22, Sec. 22.5.2), we would expect to reject the null hypothesis (indicating a statistically significant association) for 5 tests as a result of chance alone. A conventional approach to address the issue of multiple comparisons is to alter the level of significance by dividing it by the number of comparisons, known as the *Bonferroni* adjustment method. For example, one would use a type I error rate of 0.05/100 = 0.0005 for 100 simultaneous comparisons. However, this approach has limitations, such as a naïve global null hypothesis that ignores prior knowledge, and it is deemed too conservative for epidemiologic investigation. Analogous to Bayesian statistical models that incorporate prior information (see Chap. 22, Sec. 22.4.5), approaches such as hierarchical modeling and mixed effects modeling are being applied to the field of genomic and molecular epidemiology (Chen and Witte, 2007). Details of these modeling approaches are beyond the scope of this chapter, but the basic concept of hierarchical modeling is to incorporate prior knowledge of markers into analysis through a prior matrix of quantitative weighting factors (Brenner et al, 2013; Poirier et al, 2015). These weighted factors are used to "adjust" for the biologic and genetic results, thereby improving the potential for finding true positive associations.

4.7.4 Analyses Across Multiple Studies

To integrate evidence from multiple studies, approaches such as pooled analysis and meta-analysis (see Chap. 22, Sec. 22.3.8) are being applied in cancer epidemiology. Meta-analysis based on published results is susceptible to publication bias, and it is difficult to conduct detailed analysis for specific subgroups using meta-analysis based on published data. Although meta-regression has been used to evaluate the influence of clinicoepidemiologic variables on study effect size, its utility has been limited to improving parameter estimates, and it has not been able to evaluate multiple, potentially interacting or modifying clinicoepidemiologic and biologic factors on outcomes. For detailed analyses, researchers have addressed the above limitations by combining individual-level data from different studies, analogous to patient-based meta-analysis of therapeutic trials. The methodology of meta-analysis and pooled analysis is described elsewhere (van Houwelingen et al, 2002). To facilitate this type of pooled analysis, several cancer consortia have emerged, including the International Lung Cancer Consortium, the Breast Cancer Association Consortium, and the Pancreatic Cancer Case-Control Consortium (Ioannidis et al, 2005; see http://epi.grants.cancer.gov/Consortia/). The website lists consortia publications that replicate initial findings in the post-GWAS era, showing that such consortia are an efficient way to replicate an initial finding and provide further evidence for supporting or disputing an observed association.

SUMMARY

▶ Epidemiology is the study of the distribution and determinants of disease and disease outcomes in human populations. It is complementary to basic and translational research.
▶ Epidemiologic methods can be descriptive or analytic:
  • Descriptive studies provide information about populations and their distributions, including distributions of disease determinants.
  • Analytic studies assess putative associations between risk factors and disease and disease outcomes and include case-control, cohort, cross-sectional, and familial designs.
▶ Important epidemiologic successes have demonstrated the relationships between various infections (HPV, viral hepatitis, EBV) and cancer risk, tobacco and cancers, and alcohol and head and neck cancer.
▶ Genomic epidemiology and pharmacoepidemiology integrate concepts of epidemiology, genomics, and clinical trials/drug development.
▶ Opportunities and challenges for the future include
  • utilizing secondary analyses of clinical trials,
  • novel analytic approaches to handle exposure misclassifications, and
  • high-dimensional data and multiple comparisons, and multi-omics analyses.

REFERENCES

Aminkeng F, Bhavsar AP, Visscher H, et al. A coding variant in RARG confers susceptibility to anthracycline-induced cardiotoxicity in childhood cancer. *Nat Genet* 2015;47(9):1079-1084.

Arbyn M, Xu L, Simoens C, Martin-Hirsch PPL. Prophylactic vaccination against human papillomavirus to prevent cervical cancer and its precursors. *Cochrane Database Syst Rev* 2018;5:CD009069.

Baan R, Straif K, Grosse Y, et al. Carcinogenicity of alcoholic beverages. *Lancet Oncol* 2007;8(4):292-293.

Bailey-Wilson JE, Amos CI, Pinney SM, et al. A major lung cancer susceptibility locus maps to chromosome 6q23-25. *Am J Hum Genet* 2004;75:460-474.

Baldwin RM, Owzar K, Zembutsu H, et al. A genome-wide association study identifies novel loci for paclitaxel-induced sensory peripheral neuropathy in CALGB 40101. *Clin Cancer Res* 2012;18(18):5099-5109.

Bosch FX, Manos MM, Munoz N, et al. Prevalence of human papillomavirus in cervical cancer: a worldwide perspective. International biological study on cervical cancer (IBSCC) Study Group. *J Natl Cancer Inst* 1995;87:796-802.

Bradbury PA, Kulke MH, Heist RS, et al. Cisplatin pharmacogenetics, DNA repair polymorphisms, and esophageal cancer outcomes. *Pharmacogenet Genomics* 2009;19:613-625.

Brady G, MacArthur GJ, Farrell PJ. Epstein-Barr virus and Burkitt lymphoma. *J Clin Pathol* 2007;602:1397-1402.

Bray F, Ferlay J, Soerjomataram I, Siegel RL, Torre LA, Jemal A. Global Cancer Statistics 2018: GLOBOCAN estimates of incidence and mortality worldwide for 36 cancer in 185 countries. *CA Cancer J Clin* 2018; 68:394-424.

Brenner DR, Brennan P, Boffetta P, et al. Hierarchical modeling identifies novel lung cancer susceptibility variants in inflammation pathways among 10,140 cases and 11,012 controls. *Hum Genet* 2013;132(5):579-589.

Burkitt D. A "tumour safari" in East and Central Africa. *Br J Cancer* 1962a;16:379-386.

Burkitt D. Determining the climatic limitations of a children's cancer common in Africa. *Br Med J* 1962b;2:1019-1022.

Canadian Cancer Society. *Canadian Cancer Statistics 2010*. Toronto, Canada: Canadian Cancer Society; 2010.

Canadian Cancer Society's Advisory Committee on Cancer Statistics. *Canadian Cancer Statistics 2017*. Toronto, ON: Canadian Cancer Society; 2017.

Canadian Cancer Society's Advisory Committee on Cancer Statistics. *Canadian Cancer Statistics 2019*. Toronto, ON: Canadian Cancer Society; 2019.

Centers for Disease Control and Prevention (CDC). Smoking-attributable mortality, years of potential life lost, and productivity losses—United States, 2000-2004. *MMWR Morbid Mortal Wkly Rep* 2008;57(45):1226-1228.

Chaloupka FJ, Straif K, Leon ME. Effectiveness of tax and price policies in tobacco control. *Tobacco Control* 2011; 20(3):235-238.

Chaturvedi AK, Engels EA, Pfeiffer RM, et al. Human papillomavirus and rising oropharyngeal cancer incidence in the United States. *J Clin Oncol* 2011;29(32):4294-4301.

Chen GK, Witte JS. Enriching the analysis of genomewide association studies with hierarchical modeling. *Am J Hum Genet* 2007;81:397-404.

Chien YC, Jan CF, Kuo HS, et al. Nationwide hepatitis B vaccination program in Taiwan: effectiveness in the 20 years after it was launched. *Epidemiol Rev* 2006;28:126-135.

Chung CH, Gillison ML. Human papillomavirus in head and neck cancer: its role in pathogenesis and clinical implications. *Clin Cancer Res* 2009;15:6758-6762.

Coate LE, John T, Tsao MS, Shepherd FA. Molecular predictive and prognostic markers in non-small-cell lung cancer. *Lancet Oncol* 2009;10:1001-1010.

Colditz GA, Philpott SE, Hankinson SE. The impact of the nurses' health study on population health: prevention, translation, and control. *Am J Public Health* 2016;106(9): 1540-1545.

Davies L, Welch HG. Increasing incidence of thyroid cancer in the United States, 1973-2002. *JAMA* 2006;295: 2164-2167.

Doll R, Peto R, Boreham J, Sutherland I. Mortality in relation to smoking: 50 years' observations on male British doctors. *BMJ* 2004;328:1519.

Drögemöller BI, Monzon JG, Bhavsar AP, et al. Association between slc16a5 genetic variation and cisplatin-induced ototoxic effects in adult patients with testicular cancer. *JAMA Oncol* 2017;3(11):1558-1562.

Ebrahim S, Smith DG. Commentary: should we always deliberately be non-representative? *Int J Epidemiol* 2013;42(4): 1022-1026.

Ferlay J, Colombet M, Soerjomataram I, et al. Estimating the global cancer incidence and mortality in 2018: GLOBOCAN sources and methods. *Int J Cancer* 2019;144(8):1941-1953.

Ferlay J, Ervik M, Lam F, et al. *Global Cancer Observatory: Cancer Today*. Lyon, France: International Agency for Research on Cancer; 2018.

Gillison ML, Koch WM, Capone RB, et al. Evidence for a causal association between human papillomavirus and a subset of head and neck cancers. *J Natl Cancer Inst* 2001; 92(9):709-720.

Greenland S. Modeling and variable selection in epidemiologic analysis. *Am J Public Health* 1989;79(3):340-349.

Greenland S, Daniel R, Pearce N. Outcome modelling strategies in epidemiology: traditional methods and basic alternatives. *Int Journal Epidemiol* 2016;45(2):565–575.

Hancock DB, Reginsson GW, Gaddis NC, et al. Genome-wide meta-analysis reveals common splice site acceptor variant in CHRNA4 associated with nicotine dependence. *Transl Psychiatry* 2015;5:e651.

Harrell FE. *Regression Modeling Strategies: With Applications to Linear Models, Logistic and Ordinal Regression, and Survival Analysis*. 2nd ed. Heidelberg: Springer.

Hung RJ, McKay JD, Gaborieau V, et al. A susceptibility locus for lung cancer maps to nicotinic acetylcholine receptor subunit genes on 15q25. *Nature* 2008;452:633-637.

Ingle JN, Schaid DJ, Goss PE, et al. Genome-wide associations and functional genomic studies of musculoskeletal adverse events in women receiving aromatase inhibitors. *J Clin Oncol* 2010;28:4674-4682.

International Agency of Research on Cancer (IARC). *Alcohol Consumption and Ethyl Carbamate. IARC Monographs on the Evaluation of the Carcinogenic Risk of Chemicals to Humans*. Lyon, France: IARC; 2010.

International Agency of Research on Cancer (IARC). *Tobacco Smoking. IARC Monographs on the Evaluation of the Carcinogenic Risk of Chemicals to Humans*. Lyon, France: IARC; 2012.

International Agency of Research on Cancer (IARC). *Tobacco Smoke and Involuntary Smoking. IARC Monographs on the Evaluation of the Carcinogenic Risk of Chemicals to Humans*. Vol. 83. Lyon, France: IARC; 2004.

Ioannidis JP, Bernstein J, Boffetta P, et al. A network of investigator networks in human genome epidemiology. *Am J Epidemiol* 2005;162:302-304.

Kaatsch P, Steliarova-Foucher E, Crocetti E, et al. Time trends of cancer incidence in European children (1978-1997): report from the Automated Childhood Cancer Information System project. *Eur J Cancer* 2006;42:1961-1971.

Kruskal WH, Wallis WA. Use of ranks in one-criterion variance analysis. *J Am Stat Assoc* 1952;47(260):583-621.

Lee MS, Kim DH, Kim H, et al. Hepatitis B vaccination and reduced risk of primary liver cancer among male adults: a cohort study in Korea. *Int J Epidemiol* 1998;27:316-319.

Lundgren CI, Hall P, Ekbom A, et al. Incidence and survival of Swedish patients with differentiated thyroid cancer. *Int J Cancer* 2003;106:569-573.

Lydiatt WM, Patel SG, O'Sullivan B, et al. Head and neck cancers—major changes in the American Joint Committee on Cancer eighth edition cancer staging manual. *CA Cancer J Clin* 2017;67(2):122-137.

Mahmood SS, Levy D, Vasan RS, Wang TJ. The Framingham Heart Study and the epidemiology of cardiovascular disease: a historical perspective. *Lancet* 2014;383(9921):999-1008.

Markowitz LE, Dunne EF, Saraiya M, et al. Quadrivalent human papillomavirus vaccine: recommendations of the Advisory Committee on Immunization Practices (ACIP). *MMWR Recomm Rep* 2007;56:1-24.

Maupas P, Melnick JL. Hepatitis B infection and primary liver cancer. *Prog Med Virol* 1981;27:1-5.

McKay JD, Hung RJ, Han Y, et al. Large-scale association analysis identifies new lung cancer susceptibility loci and heterogeneity in genetic susceptibility across histological subtypes. *Nat Genet* 2017;49(7):1126-1132.

Munoz N, Bosch FX, de Sanjose S, et al. Epidemiologic classification of human papillomavirus types associated with cervical cancer. *N Engl J Med* 2003;348:518-527.

Neuhäuser M. Wilcoxon-Mann-Whitney Test. In: Lovric M, ed. *International Encyclopedia of Statistical Science*. Berlin: Springer; 2011.

Pesch B, Kendzia B, Gustavsson P, et al. Cigarette smoking and lung cancer—relative risk estimates for the major histological types from a pooled analysis of case–control studies. *Int J Cancer* 2012;131(5):1210-1219.

Plummer M, de Martel C, Vignat J, et al. Global burden of cancers attributable to infections in 2012: a synthetic analysis. *Lancet Global Health* 2016;4(9):e609-e616.

Poirier JG, Brennan P, McKay JD, et al. Informed genome-wide association analysis with family history as a secondary phenotype identifies novel loci of lung cancer. *Genet Epidemiol* 2015;39(3):197-206.

Rey D, Neuhäuser M. Wilcoxon-signed-rank test. In: Lovric M, ed. *International Encyclopedia of Statistical Science*. Berlin: Springer; 2011.

Ross CJ, Katzov-Eckert H, Dubé MP, et al. Genetic variants in TPMT and COMT are associated with hearing loss in children receiving cisplatin chemotherapy. *Nat Genet* 2009;41:1345-1349.

Rothman KJ, Gallacher JE, Hatch EE. Why representativeness should be avoided. *Int J Epidemiol* 2013;42(4):1012-1014.

Rothman K, Greenland S, Lash TL. *Modern Epidemiology*. 3rd ed. Philadelphia, PA: Lippincott Williams & Wilkins; 2008.

Royston P, Sauerbrei W. *Multivariable Model-building: A pragmatic Approach to Regression Analysis Based on Fractional Polynomials for Modelling Continuous Variables*. Chichester, UK: John Wiley & Sons Ltd; 2008.

Sackett DL. Bias in analytic research. *J Chronic Dis* 1979;32:51-63.

Saidi F, Sepehr A, Fahimi S, et al. Oesophageal cancer among the Turkomans of northeast Iran. *Br J Cancer* 2000;83:1249-1254.

Secretan B, Straif K, Baan R, et al. A review of human carcinogens—part E: tobacco, areca nut, alcohol, coal smoke, and salted fish. *Lancet Oncol* 2009;10:1033-1034.

Shiboski CH, Schmidt BL, Jordan RC. Tongue and tonsil carcinoma: increasing trends in the U.S. population ages 20-44 years. *Cancer* 2005;103(9):1843-1849.

Shrier I, Platt RW. Reducing bias through directed acyclic graphs. *BMC Med Res Methodol* 2008;8:70.

Smith GD, Ebrahim S. "Mendelian randomization": can genetic epidemiology contribute to understanding environmental determinants of disease? *Int J Epidemiol* 2003;32:1-2.

Spector LG, Pankrats N, Marcotte EL. Genetic and nongenetic risk factors for childhood cancer. *Pediatr Clin North Am* 2015;62(1):11-25.

Szklo M, Nieto FJ. *Epidemiology: Beyond the Basics*. 2nd ed. Sudbury, MA: Jones and Bartlett; 2007.

Thomas DC. *Statistical Methods in Genetic Epidemiology*. New York, NY: Oxford University Press; 2004.

Thompson MP, Kurzrock R. Epstein-Barr virus and cancer. *Clin Cancer Res* 2004;10:803-821.

Thorgeirsson TE, Geller F, Sulem P, et al. A variant associated with nicotine dependence, lung cancer and peripheral arterial disease. *Nature* 2008;452:638-642.

Thun MJ, Freedman ND. Chapter 11. Tobacco. In: Thun MJ, Linet MS, Cerhan JJR, Haiman CA, Schottenfeld D, eds. *Cancer Epidemiology and Prevention*. 4th ed. New York: Oxford University Press; 2018.

Torre LA, Siegel RL, Ward EM, et al. Global cancer incidence and mortality rates and trends—an update. *Cancer Epidemiol Biomarkers Prev* 2016;25(1):16.

US Department of Health and Human Services (USDHHS). 2014 Surgeon General's Report: The Health Consequences of Smoking-50 Years of Progress. Chapter 12: Smoking-Attributable Morbidity, Mortality and Economic Costs. P647-699. Atlanta, GA: US Department of Health and Human Services, Centers for Disease Control and Prevention, National Center for Chronic Disease Prevention and Health Promotion, Office on Smoking and Health; 2014

van Houwelingen HC, Arends LR, Stijnen T. Advanced methods in meta-analysis: multivariate approach and meta-regression. *Stat Med* 2002;21:589-624.

Visscher H, Ross CJ, Rassekh SR, et al. Pharmacogenomic prediction of anthracycline-induced cardiotoxicity in children. *J Clin Oncol* 2012;30(13):1422-1428.

Walter S, Tiemeier H. Variable selection: current practice in epidemiological studies. *Eur J Epidemiol* 2009;24(12):733-736.

Wong MC, Jiang JY, Goggins WB, et al. International incidence and mortality trends of liver cancer: a global profile. *Sci Rep* 2017;7:45846.

World Bank, World Development Indicators. (2018). *GDP per capita (current US$)* [Data file]. https://data.worldbank.org/indicator/ny.gdp.pcap.cd.

World Health Organization. *WHO Report on the Global Tobacco Epidemic 2015: Raising Taxes on Tobacco*. Geneva: World Health Organization; 2015.

Xu H, Robinson GW, Huang J, et al. Common variants in ACYP2 influence susceptibility to cisplatin-induced hearing loss. *Nat Genet* 2015;47(3):263-266.

Yu MW, Yeh SH, Chen PJ, et al. Hepatitis B virus genotype and DNA level and hepatocellular carcinoma: a prospective study in men. *J Natl Cancer Inst* 2005;97:265-272.

Zhang F, Wen Y, Guo X. CRISPR/Cas9 for genome editing: progress, implications and challenges. *Hum Mol Genet* 2014;23(R1):R40-R46.

zur Hausen H. Human papillomaviruses and their possible role in squamous cell carcinomas. *Curr Top Microbiol Immunol* 1977;78:1-30.

Carcinogenesis

Denis M. Grant

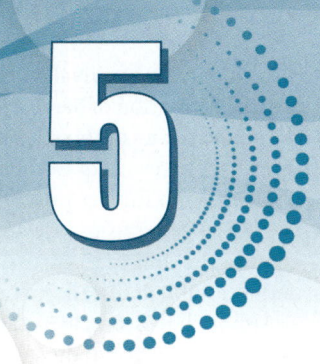

Chapter Outline

5.1 Models of Carcinogenesis
    5.1.1 Tumor Initiation, Promotion, and Progression
    5.1.2 Genetic Instability and the Hallmarks of Cancer

5.2 Chemical Carcinogenesis
    5.2.1 Genotoxic Carcinogens, Metabolic Activation, and DNA-Damaging Species
    5.2.2 Nature and Consequences of DNA Damage
    5.2.3 Exogenous vs Endogenous Chemical Carcinogens
    5.2.4 Chemicals as Modifiers of Cell Proliferation, Cell Death, and Inflammation

5.3 Assessment of Carcinogenic Risk
    5.3.1 Population Epidemiology of Carcinogens
    5.3.2 Short-term Assays
    5.3.3 Cellular Transformation Assays
    5.3.4 Animal Bioassays

5.4 Molecular Epidemiology of Carcinogenesis
    5.4.1 Biomarkers for Assessment of Carcinogen Exposure
    5.4.2 Genetic Variation in Risk From Carcinogen Exposure
    5.4.3 "Omics" Technologies and Molecular Signatures of Exposure and Risk

5.5 Cancer Chemoprevention

Summary

References

5.1 MODELS OF CARCINOGENESIS

Cancer is a disease that results from cumulative genetic changes. Sporadic mutations take place in all cells of the body and may lead eventually to a cell that is transformed and whose progeny develop into a cancer. Any agent or process that increases genetic changes will increase the probability of a cancer developing, so that minimizing the incidence of cancer requires identification of and avoidance of exogenous agents (ie, carcinogens) that can cause it (Okey and Harper, 2007; Loeb and Harris, 2008). Carcinogens include chemical agents (Wogan, 2004), many of which are known to be mutagenic (described in Section 5.2), ionizing and ultraviolet radiation (Chap. 9, Sec. 9.2.2 and Chap. 15, Sec. 15.4.1), and some viruses, which can introduce oncogenes into the human genome (Chap. 7, Sec. 7.4.4). Although the mechanisms that lead to cancer differ following exposure to these different types of exposure, there are some common properties.

5.1.1 Tumor Initiation, Promotion, and Progression

Both epidemiologic and experimental studies have confirmed that a latent period (often decades in humans) exists between the exposure to a carcinogenic agent and the appearance of cancer. This knowledge led to the formulation of a sequential model that divided the carcinogenic process into 3 stages, termed tumor initiation, tumor promotion, and tumor progression.

Tumor initiation is the process by which a carcinogenic agent interacts with DNA to produce damage that, if not repaired before the next cell division, could lead to error-prone DNA replication, resulting in fixation of mutations within the genome of individual cells. The efficiency and fidelity of DNA repair (see Chap. 9, Sec. 9.3) and the balance of cell proliferation and cell death are important in determining if this process leads to cancer. If a mutation disrupts the function of a gene whose product plays a role in maintaining the terminally differentiated function of the cell, the cell may acquire an altered (usually less differentiated) phenotype. Although initiation is irreversible, not all initiated cells will go on to establish a tumor, as many of these cells may die by apoptosis (see Chap. 8, Sec. 8.4), and further proliferation-enhancing signals are required for initiated cells to progress along the pathway to autonomous (cancerous) growth.

Tumor promotion involves the clonal expansion of an initiated cell as a consequence of events that alter gene expression, so as to provide the cell with a selective proliferative advantage. Although there is no single unifying mechanistic feature of tumor-promoting agents, they tend to be nongenotoxic and to cause cells to divide but not to differentiate terminally or die, resulting in the survival and proliferation of preneoplastic cells and the formation of benign lesions such as papillomas, nodules, or polyps. Many of these lesions may regress spontaneously, but a few cells may acquire additional mutations over time that allow them to further progress to a malignant neoplasm.

Tumor progression describes the stage whereby lesions acquire the ability to further grow, to invade adjacent tissues, and to establish distant metastases.

Although this simple 3-stage model has been a useful conceptual framework for understanding carcinogenesis, the distinction between genotoxic carcinogens as tumor initiators and nongenotoxic carcinogens as tumor promoters is overly simplistic. DNA damage in key genes may occur—and for most cancers is likely required—also at later stages of tumor development: multiple sequential mutations in combination with epigenetic changes and prolonged alterations in the cellular microenvironment are usually required to convert a normal cell into a malignant tumor.

5.1.2 Genetic Instability and the Hallmarks of Cancer

Increased genetic instability and alterations in karyotype are often observed in tumor cells (see Chap. 9, Sec. 9.2). Inherited or acquired mutations in genes such as p53, retinoblastoma (Rb) or DNA mismatch repair genes can create a "mutator phenotype" of enhanced random mutation that accelerates the accumulation of further DNA damage that may be required for the development of cancer. This concept underlines the potential importance of DNA-damaging agents not only at the initiation stage but also at later stages of the carcinogenic process.

We now conceptualize the process and features of carcinogenesis as a more complex, temporally fluid, and intertwined set of phenotypic features that may be displayed by cancerous cells and tissues (Hanahan and Weinberg, 2011). The 8 hallmarks of cancer include sustaining proliferative signaling; evading growth suppressors; avoiding immune destruction; enabling replicative immortality; activating invasion and metastasis; inducing angiogenesis; resisting cell death; and deregulating cellular energetics. In addition, 2 "enabling characteristics" for tumor growth are genome instability and mutations, and tumor-promoting inflammation. Acquisition of any of these characteristics may be driven by both genetic and epigenetic changes. These hallmarks are also mechanistically related to 5 overlapping models of carcinogenesis: mutational, genomic instability, nongenotoxic clonal expansion, cell selection, and microenvironment (Vineis et al, 2010). Exogenous chemicals, radiation, and carcinogenic viruses may each contribute to the genetic, epigenetic, and microenvironmental alterations that are required for the acquisition of such characteristics that allow tumor growth to proceed.

5.2 CHEMICAL CARCINOGENESIS

Epidemiologic evidence that chemicals can cause human cancer dates to 1775 when Percival Pott observed a correlation between scrotal cancer and soot exposure in English chimney sweeps, and Butlin later suggested that the better hygiene practices of European sweeps reduced their cancer risk. In 1895, Rehn reported a high rate of bladder cancer in German factory workers who were exposed to aniline-based azo dyes. The 20th century saw the association of specific chemicals with increased cancer risk, and the development of methods to identify cellular and molecular targets of the causative agents and to elucidate mechanisms involved in the conversion of normal cells into tumor-producing cells. Yamagiwa's production of skin tumors in rabbits by the direct application of coal tar in 1915 led to the isolation, identification, synthesis, and biologic testing of polycyclic aromatic hydrocarbons (PAHs) as chemical carcinogens, including dibenz[*a,h*]anthracene and benzo[*a*]pyrene (Fig. 5–1). Subsequent research demonstrated that the aromatic amine β-naphthylamine (Fig. 5–1), a reagent used in manufacturing azo dyes, caused bladder tumors in dogs.

Although it has been estimated that exposure to environmental chemical pollutants accounts for no more than 1% to 3% of all human cancers (Klaunig and Kamendulis, 2008), such estimates do not include workplace chemical exposures (5% of all cancers) or cigarette smoke (30% of all cancers), and they tend to focus primarily on genotoxic chemicals as causative agents. They may also underestimate the importance of the interplay between the tumor-initiating effects of low-level genotoxic exposure, the additional effects of nongenotoxic chemicals, and the potentially reversible modulating effects of diet, exercise, and other lifestyle factors on tumor growth.

Carcinogen-induced DNA damage leading to fixed mutations that could be transmitted to progeny cells is a key event in the process by which exposure to carcinogens leads to uncontrolled cell division and tumor growth. That many carcinogens require enzymatic bioactivation into electrophilic metabolites that bind covalently with DNA was established by the Millers in the 1960s. This research was followed by identification of specific DNA adducts of various chemicals including benzo[*a*]pyrene and aflatoxin B_1, and demonstration of their binding to human tissues. Key target genes for carcinogens (oncogenes and tumor suppressor genes; see Chap. 7) were identified subsequently, whose functionally altered products are key to the initiation, promotion, or progression of tumor growth.

5.2.1 Genotoxic Carcinogens, Metabolic Activation, and DNA-Damaging Species

Chemicals can contribute to the carcinogenic process either through their ability to damage DNA and produce somatic mutations in cells or as a consequence of their ability to establish a cellular microenvironment that provides initiated cells with a growth advantage via metabolic changes, local vascular alterations, and/or the ability to evade apoptosis, terminal differentiation, and contact inhibition.

Genotoxic carcinogens have a wide diversity of chemical structures (see Fig. 5–1) but they share the property of either being directly electrophilic (electron-seeking) or of being

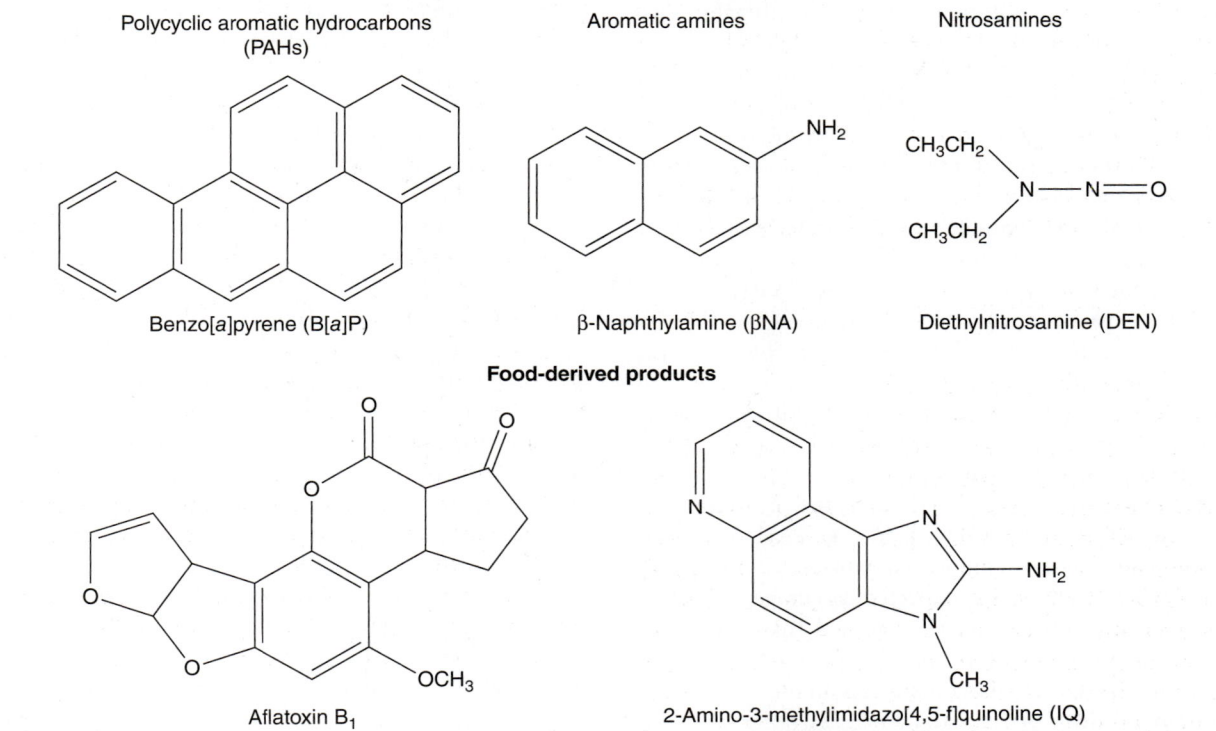

FIGURE 5–1 Structures of some direct-acting carcinogens and procarcinogens that require metabolic activation.

capable of conversion to electrophiles. These reactive electrophiles interact with nucleophilic (electron-rich) groups on intracellular molecules such as DNA and proteins, forming either covalent adducts or oxidative damage. If this damage to DNA is not repaired before the next cycle of DNA replication, it may lead to errors in replication and hence to fixation of the damage as nucleotide substitutions. Damage to key cellular proteins may also result in cell death, which may trigger the development of an inflammatory microenvironment that promotes the proliferation of any surviving initiated cells (see Sec. 5.2.4).

Some genotoxic carcinogens, including carbamoyl halides, lactones and mustards (see Fig. 5–1), are direct-acting because they are either already electrophilic or are spontaneously hydrolyzed into electrophiles. However, most genotoxic carcinogens require enzymatic bioactivation to electrophilic or electrophile-generating metabolites in order to damage DNA (Guengerich, 2001). These reactions are catalyzed largely by drug-metabolizing enzymes whose normal physiological role is protective, converting lipophilic chemicals into water-soluble metabolites that can be more readily eliminated from the body via the urine or bile. Drug-metabolizing enzymes have evolved both multiplicity and catalytic promiscuity to ensure that most potentially harmful environmental chemicals will undergo biotransformation, inactivation, and elimination. However, they may also lead to inadvertent biotransformation of some chemicals into reactive electrophiles with the potential to damage DNA. Because biotransformation can produce many metabolites from a single chemical via cooperating and competing pathways, the net effect of exposure to a carcinogen in a particular individual will depend on the balance of activating vs detoxifying pathways.

The cytochrome P450 (CYP) mixed-function monooxygenase superfamily are the drug-metabolizing enzymes that have been studied most intensively. These phase I enzymes catalyze the hydroxylation of carbon, nitrogen, and sulfur atoms on chemical molecules to produce metabolites that are more polar and either stable and excreted, reactive (eg, epoxides, nitroso compounds), or possess structures that make them suitable substrates for further metabolism by phase II conjugating enzymes (see below). Procarcinogen bioactivation may also be catalyzed by non-CYP phase I enzymes such as nicotinamide adenine dinucleotide phosphate (NAD(P)H) quinone oxidoreductase, aldo-keto reductase, and various peroxidases (Shimada, 2006).

Phase II conjugating enzymes such as the uridine diphosphate (UDP)-glucuronosyltransferases (UGTs), sulfotransferases (SULTs), arylamine *N*-acetyltransferases (NATs), and glutathione *S*-transferases (GSTs) can produce either stable conjugated metabolites or unstable conjugates that decompose spontaneously to reactive electrophiles. The likelihood of either protection against, or enhancement of, the DNA-damaging potential by the activity of phase I and phase II enzymes depends on the structure of the particular chemical, the chemical reactivity of the metabolites produced, and the relative levels of expression of the various enzymes that may compete or collaborate in activation and detoxification in a given tissue. For example, potential carcinogen-bioactivating oxidases such as CYP1A2 show liver-selective expression, while others, such as CYP1A1 and cyclooxygenase, are present at high levels in the lung and bladder, respectively.

Three extensively studied classes of chemical carcinogens that require metabolic activation are the PAHs, such as benzo[*a*]pyrene (B[*a*]P; Fig. 5–2); the aromatic amines, such as β-naphthylamine (βNF; Fig. 5–3); and the nitrosamines, such as diethylnitrosamine (DEN; Fig. 5–4). PAHs, aromatic amines, and nitrosamines comprise a substantial fraction of the total number of known or suspected carcinogenic chemicals in humans according to the US National Toxicology Program (NTP) *14th Report on Carcinogens* (National Toxicology Program, 2016). Although many chemicals on the NTP list are reagents or by-products of industrial processes, others are present in food or in the natural environment. Examples include aflatoxin B$_1$, a potent liver carcinogen produced by *Aspergillus* fungi that contaminates improperly stored grains and nuts, and heterocyclic amines such as 2-amino-3-methylimidazo[4,5-*f*]quinoline (IQ), produced by the reaction of amino acids with creatine during high-temperature cooking of meat (see Fig. 5–1). The single-step metabolic activation pathway of aflatoxin B$_1$ is shown in Figure 5–5.

The pathways shown in Figures 5–2 to 5–5 illustrate the following 3 principles of metabolic activation: (1) oxidative metabolism—often mediated by 1 or more CYP isozymes—in initiating activation; (2) participation of multiple enzymes that either act sequentially or catalyze the same reaction; and (3) nonenzymatic, spontaneous chemical decomposition of unstable metabolites. These pathways represent only a subset of those that contribute to metabolic activation and do not include competing pathways that can produce stable, excretable metabolites and are thus protective.

The structures of the ultimate reactive electrophilic species that are produced by metabolic activation of carcinogens vary widely. DNA damage may arise from the covalent interaction of its nucleotide bases with at least 11 different types of carbon, nitrogen, and sulfur electrophiles on carcinogen molecules (Klaunig and Kamendulis, 2008). Of these, key examples

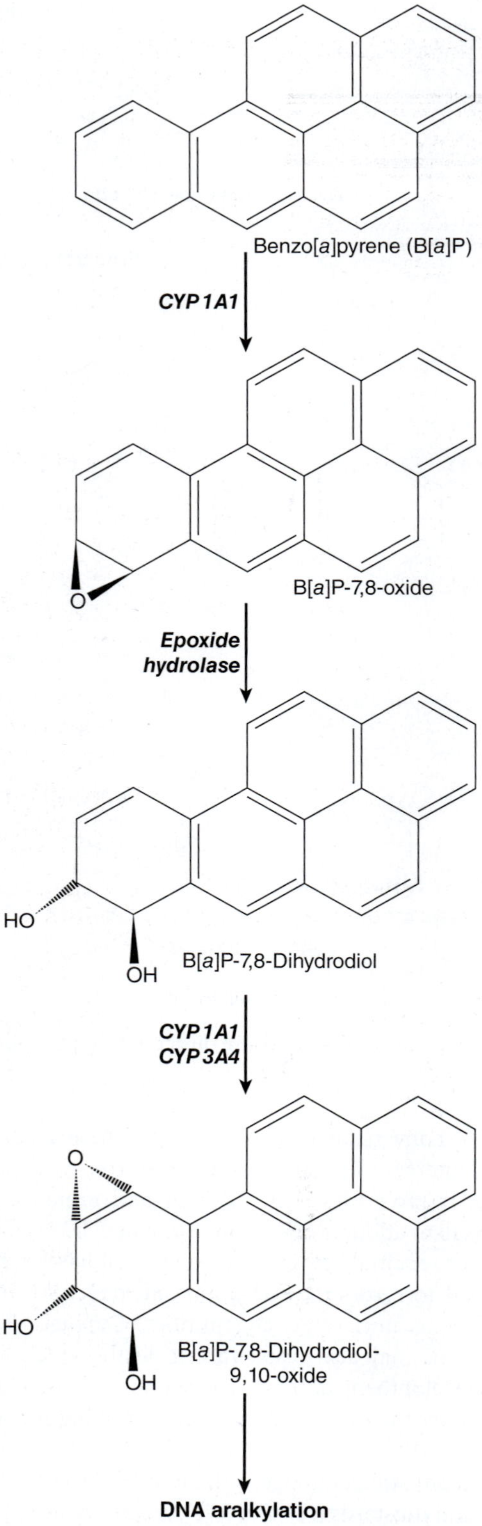

FIGURE 5–2 A proposed metabolic activation pathway for the polycyclic aromatic hydrocarbon benzo[*a*]pyrene (B[*a*]P).

are epoxides produced from the PAHs (see Fig. 5–2) and aflatoxin B$_1$ (see Fig. 5–5), nitrenium ions derived from aromatic amines (see Fig. 5–3), and carbonium ions derived from nitrosamines (see Fig. 5–4).

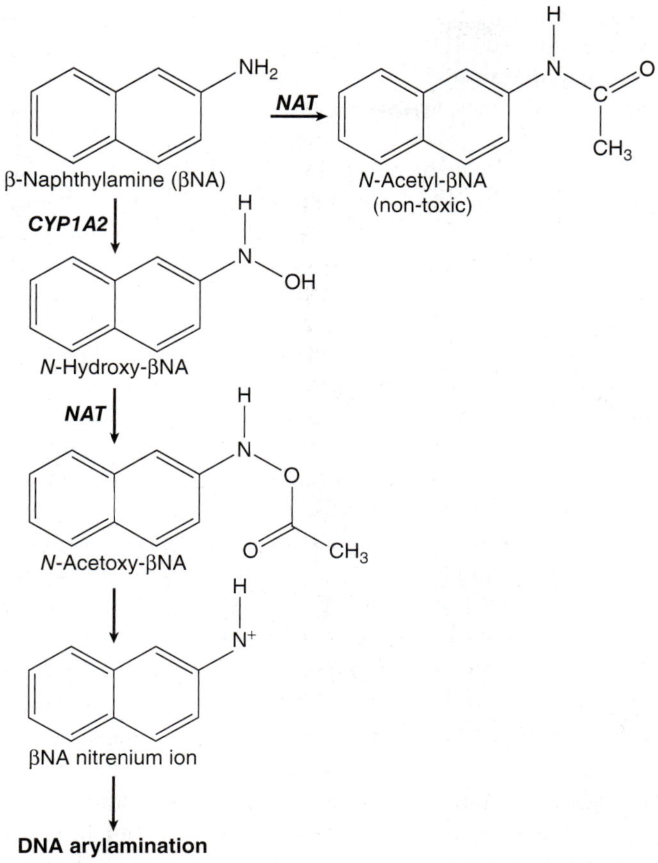

FIGURE 5-3 Proposed metabolic activation and detoxification pathways for the aromatic amine β-naphthylamine.

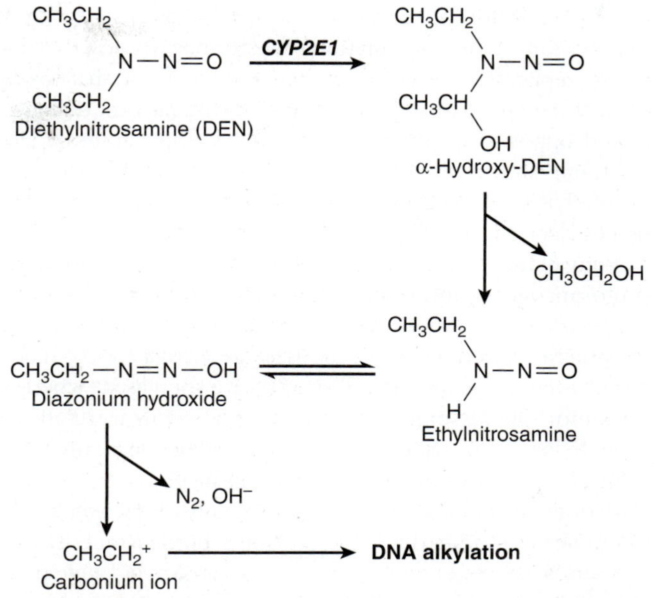

FIGURE 5-4 A proposed metabolic activation pathway for diethylnitrosamine.

5.2.2 Nature and Consequences of DNA Damage

Different types of DNA-damaging chemicals produce distinctive patterns of damage on the individual bases of DNA. In general, damage can consist of either a carcinogen adduct covalently bound to DNA, or of oxidative DNA damage. The site and type of adduct depend on the strength (charge) of the electrophile, the availability of nucleophilic sites (the unpaired O: and N: atoms) on DNA bases or the phosphodiester backbone, and the size of the adduct. Strong electrophiles can bind to many nucleophilic targets, whereas weaker electrophiles can only bind to strong nucleophiles. Thus, distinct chemical-selective patterns of nucleotide damage and resulting mutations (see below) may be observed. The persistence of particular adducts in specific genes is important in predicting carcinogenic risk, and the identification of these genes is important in monitoring DNA mutation profiles as biomarkers of either carcinogen exposure or cancer risk.

There are a large number of possible oxidized forms of each of the 4 bases of DNA, but 8-*oxo*-deoxyguanosine is abundant and has been used as a sensitive marker of overall oxidative DNA damage. Oxidative DNA damage can result from increased intracellular levels of reactive oxygen species (ROS), including superoxide anion radicals, hydrogen peroxide, and hydroxyl radicals. ROS can be produced both by exogenous chemicals, often as a by-product of CYP metabolism, and by endogenous processes. The latter include oxidative phosphorylation and inflammatory cell activation (Sec. 5.2.4).

Once DNA damage has occurred, there are 2 possible cellular outcomes. Most probable is repair of the damage by DNA repair enzymes (see Chap. 9, Sec. 9.3). If DNA repair has not

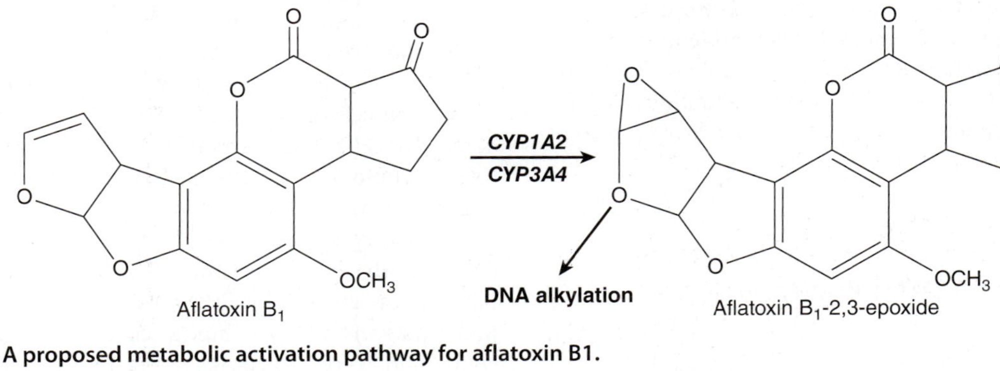

FIGURE 5-5 A proposed metabolic activation pathway for aflatoxin B1.

taken place before the next cycle of DNA replication prior to cell division, 3 types of mutational events may occur: (a) error-prone replication resulting in incorporation of the wrong complementary base (often adenine) in the nascent daughter strand opposite an adducted, apurinic, or apyrimidinic site; (b) frame-shift mutations (most commonly single-base deletions) that tend to occur when a carcinogen adduct is bound to a nucleotide base; and (c) DNA strand breaks.

Many of the relevant gene targets for cancer development are proto-oncogenes and tumor suppressor genes, and mutations at specific sites in these genes have been detected in tumors. In general, when proto-oncogenes are activated by mutational events, signals for cell growth are increased, whereas, for tumor suppressor genes, which normally downregulate cell growth, loss of function abolishes this negative regulation (see Chap. 7). For example, in chemically induced rodent tumors, mutations commonly activate the *ras* family of oncogenes. Rat mammary tumors induced by exposure to nitrosomethylurea contain H-*ras* genes that have been activated by a single point mutation in codon 12 of the gene, whereas in mouse skin papillomas induced by 7,12-dimethylbenz[a]anthracene, an activating mutation occurs in codon 61 of the same gene. The reasons for DNA site selectivity may include localized DNA accessibility in the context of chromatin packing, the nucleophilicity of particular bases within the exposed DNA region, the structure of the bioactivated chemical relative to the topography of the exposed DNA region, and the efficiencies (both substrate affinity and turnover rates) of DNA repair enzymes expressed within a given target tissue.

It has been estimated that mutations in the tumor suppressor gene *p53* are present in more than 50% of human tumors. The sites of mutation are not random but occur at discrete "hotspots" (see Chap. 7, Sec. 7.6.1), and some of them may occur during tumor promotion and progression. Different carcinogens may leave distinct mutational signatures in *p53* and other genes. Lung tumors that develop in nonsmokers contain a different spectrum of *p53* mutations than those in smokers, whereas tumors in ex-smokers retain the smokers' pattern, indicating the persistence of molecular lesions that underlie the development of cancer (Hainaut and Pfeifer, 2001). More than 50% of the liver tumors from aflatoxin B_1-exposed populations in Africa and China have a G-to-T transition at codon 249 of the *p53* gene, which is not present in tumors from patients with low aflatoxin B_1 exposure (Shen and Ong, 1996). This mutation produces an amino acid change from arginine to serine that alters the binding properties of the p53 protein to a hepatitis B viral antigen and confers a subtle growth advantage to initiated cells. Thus the codon 249 mutation in *p53* is a molecular signature linking aflatoxin B_1 exposure and viral infection in the eventual development of hepatocellular carcinoma.

5.2.3 Exogenous vs Endogenous Chemical Carcinogens

It is important to place DNA damage produced by foreign electrophiles in the context of substantial damage that occurs within cells in the absence of exogenous chemical exposure. More than 10,000 DNA-damaging events occur in every cell each day due to ambient ionizing radiation and to reactive oxygen and nitrogen species and products of lipid peroxidation that are generated by normal endogenous oxidative metabolism. Much of this high "background" damage may also be caused by exposure to low levels of the many natural and synthetic toxic chemicals and food constituents that enter the human body. The massive scale of this damage emphasizes the role of cellular DNA repair pathways that ensure high efficiency, redundancy, and fidelity of repair for a broad range of DNA damage (see Chap. 9, Sec. 9.3). DNA damage that is detectable as a result of exposure to exogenous chemicals must produce a signal above this high level of endogenous damage and very efficient repair. As discussed in Section 5.3, this has important implications for the interpretation of dose-response relationships and thresholds for chemical exposure, as many tests for carcinogen potency assume that cancer risk at low doses may be predicted by linear extrapolation from experimental administration of high doses. Also, DNA damage may be necessary but not sufficient for tumor formation, and additional tumor-promoting effects of chemicals on cellular homeostasis and the microenvironment of DNA-damaged cells contribute strongly to tumor formation.

5.2.4 Chemicals as Modifiers of Cell Proliferation, Cell Death, and Inflammation

Relative to normal cells, cancerous cells have impaired ability to control cell division, to age, and to undergo apoptotic (programmed) cell death. Any chemical agent that triggers or contributes to the impairment of these processes could promote progression to malignancy, tumor growth, and metastasis, especially with chronic exposure. The nongenotoxic tumor promoters shown in Figure 5–6 are thought to function in this manner. Tetradecanoyl phorbol acetate (TPA) acts as a proinflammatory agent and inducer of oxidative stress to provide a microenvironment that favors the proliferation of initiated cells. 2,3,7,8-Tetrachlorodibenzo-*p*-dioxin (TCDD) functions by inhibiting the apoptosis of initiated cells (Schrenk et al, 2004) and by influencing the expression of T helper cells that play a role in cancer cell immune surveillance (see Chap. 21, Sec. 21.4.3). Phenobarbital influences both cellular proliferation and apoptosis by altering patterns of DNA methylation, thus modifying epigenetic control of gene expression (see Chap. 3, Sec. 3.1.1) in cancer cells (Phillips and Goodman, 2009). Chemicals may also promote the growth of initiated cells indirectly; for example, by causing the death of nearby cells that triggers the establishment of a chronic tumor-promoting inflammatory environment.

Epidemiologic and experimental evidence indicates that inflammatory cells play pivotal roles in carcinogenesis by facilitating both tumor-initiating and tumor-promoting events (Grennikov, 2010). Consistent associations between chronic inflammation and risk of human cancer include those between colitis and colon cancer, gastric acid reflux and esophageal

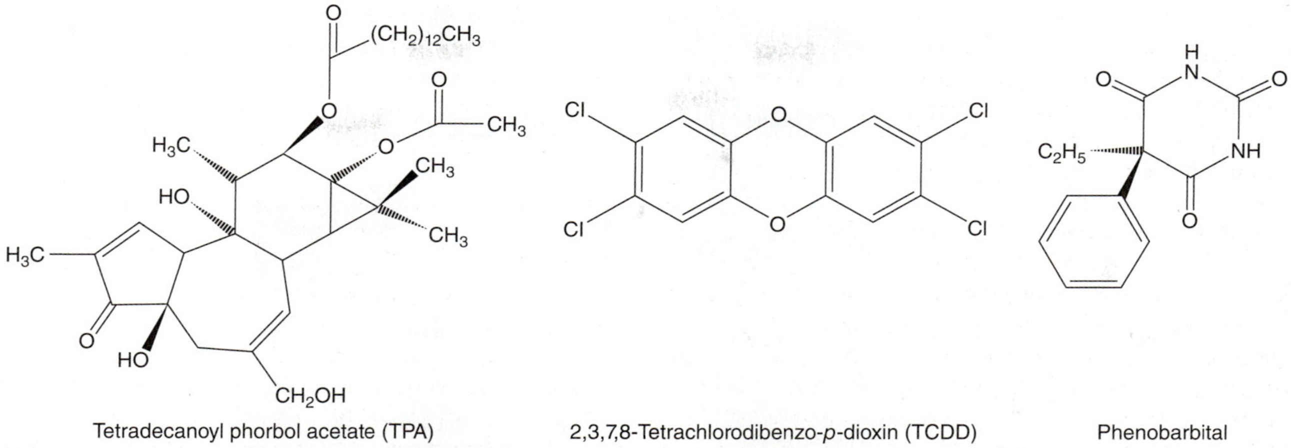

FIGURE 5-6 Structures of some established tumor promoters.

cancer, hepatitis B or C infection and liver cancer, papillomavirus infection and cervical and head and neck cancer, and schistosomiasis infection and urinary bladder cancer. Inflammation is recognized as an enabling hallmark of cancer (Hanahan and Weinberg, 2011).

Acute inflammatory responses may be elicited by infections, metabolic stress, generation of ROS, hypoxia or tissue injury, which can produce necrotic or autophagic cell death as opposed to the generally noninflammatory apoptotic cell death (see Chap. 8, Sec. 8.4). With the exception of infection, exogenous chemicals may trigger any of the events listed above. Contents released from dead cells, such as the chromatin-associated protein high mobility group box 1 (HMGB1) (Campana et al, 2008), can trigger the activation of nearby resident macrophages to release proinflammatory cytokines such as interleukin-6 (IL-6) and tumor necrosis factor alpha (TNF-α), as well as oxidant-generating enzymes such as NADPH oxidase (NOX) in a transient "respiratory burst" that produces high levels of free radicals and other reactive oxygen and nitrogen species. Although designed to quickly kill invading pathogens, the respiratory burst can damage the DNA, RNA, proteins, and lipids of neighboring cells (Ohshima et al, 2003) and activate proinflammatory transcription factors such as nuclear factor-κB (NF-κB), which drive the expression of genes whose products can result in chronic inflammation (Karin and Greten, 2005).

Some chemicals may increase cancer risk by more than one mechanism. For example, diethylnitrosamine (DEN; see Figs. 5-1 and 5-4) is a potent liver carcinogen that produces not only liver DNA damage in mice, but also acute hepatic necrosis associated with increased levels of reactive oxygen species (ROS) and release of intracellular damage-associated molecular pattern molecules (DAMPs); the net effect is an elevation in proinflammatory IL-6 and TNF-α levels, subsequent activation of NF-κB, and compensatory cellular proliferation that promotes tumor growth. Thus, DEN can act as a "complete carcinogen" because it serves both tumor-initiating and tumor-promoting functions (Maeda et al, 2005; Naugler et al, 2007). Administration of the antioxidant butylated hydroxyanisole to DEN-treated mice reduces tumorigenicity by preventing the accumulation of ROS that can both damage DNA and activate *jun* kinase-mediated cellular proliferation pathways.

5.3 ASSESSMENT OF CARCINOGENIC RISK

Establishing that an agent is a human carcinogen is a challenging and protracted process (Grad, 2008). Humans are exposed to chemicals, viruses, and radiation in foods, medicines, and the environment, and there is a long latent period between exposure and tumor appearance. The most productive approach has involved astute clinical observation together with epidemiologic and laboratory studies in vitro and in vivo. Reduction of risk first requires that the factors contributing to risk be identified. These factors may be external or they may be intrinsic to the population at risk. A systematic, stepwise approach is employed by governmental regulatory agencies which, in order to reliably determine risk, must integrate the multiple factors that interact in human carcinogenesis (Fig. 5-7). Risk assessment relies heavily on data from laboratory animals despite the caveats that apply in extrapolating data on carcinogenesis from animals to humans. The US Environmental Protection Agency (EPA) 2005 *Guidelines for Carcinogen Risk Assessment* uses the following set of criteria to categorize chemicals according to their risk: (1) carcinogenic to humans; (2) likely to be carcinogenic to humans; (3) suggestive evidence of carcinogenic potential; (4) inadequate information to assess carcinogenic potential; and (5) not likely to be carcinogenic in humans. A "mode of action framework" takes into account the chemical's hypothesized mode of action and biologic plausibility; identification of key events; the strength, specificity, and consistency of epidemiologic associations; dose-response and temporal relationships; consideration of other modes of action; support for the proposed mode of action in laboratory animals; relevance of the mode of action to humans; and subgroups that may be particularly susceptible. Table 5-1 lists some of the methods that are used to determine the carcinogenicity of chemicals, which are described in further detail below.

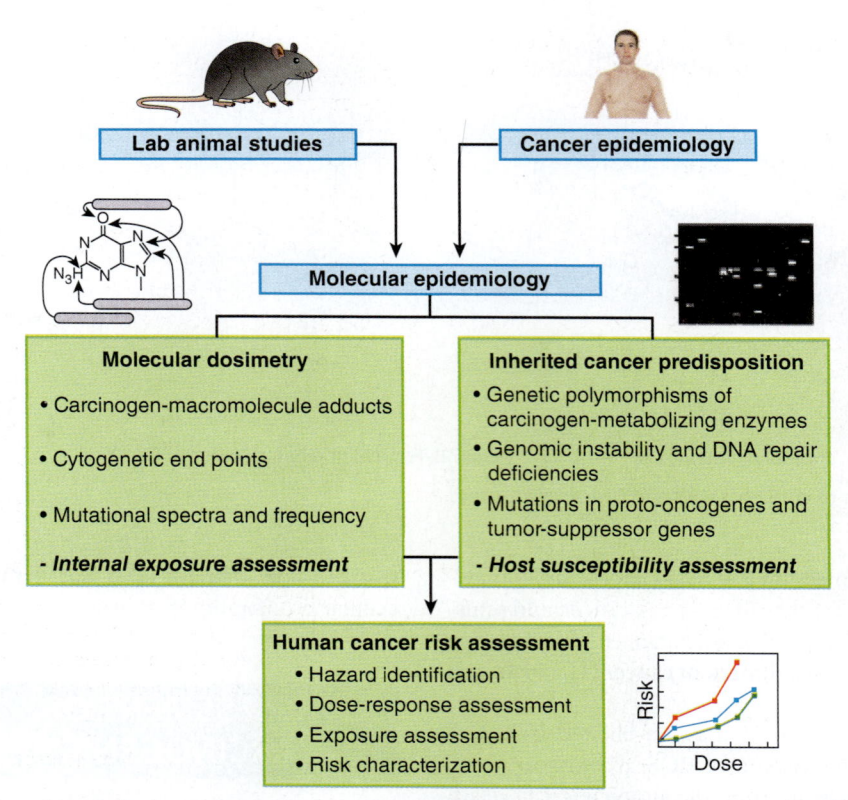

FIGURE 5–7 Strategy for using multiple approaches to assess chemical carcinogens for their risk of causing human cancer. (Adapted with permission from Harris CC: p53: at the crossroads of molecular carcinogenesis and risk assessment. *Science* 1993 Dec 24;262(5142):1980-1981.)

5.3.1 Population Epidemiology of Carcinogens

Epidemiologic observations provide the cornerstone for identifying cancer risk (see Chap. 4). Earliest observations were of associations between exposure to chemicals in industrial settings and the incidence of cancers at a variety of tissue sites. The early associations were often striking because the exposure levels to particular chemicals were so high and led to drastic improvements in industrial practices. Examples include the increased incidence of bladder cancer in workers exposed to azo dyes or benzidine, and associations between lung cancer risk and occupational exposure to asbestos, radon, and ionizing radiation. Fortunately, such exposures and cancer clusters occur very rarely today. It is more challenging to establish unequivocally a causal association between cancer risk and exposure to chemicals at the low levels that occur in the environment or the cleaner workplace. Nonetheless, epidemiologic evidence for a chemical-cancer association should prompt the conduct of dose-response and mechanistic studies using the experimental methods outlined below. These studies are then used to inform regulatory action that is designed to reduce exposure and risk where appropriate.

Even when epidemiologic studies suggest that a particular agent is carcinogenic, and it is shown to be DNA-damaging or mutagenic in laboratory animals or in vitro tests, several features of carcinogens make it a challenge to establish unequivocally that they do or do not cause cancer in humans. These are outlined in Table 5–2.

5.3.2 Short-term Assays

The main advantages of using in vitro assays to predict the carcinogenic activity of chemicals lie in the drastically shortened

TABLE 5–1 Assays for carcinogens.

Long-term assays
Clinical observation and epidemiology
Bioassays in laboratory animals, principally rodents
Short-term assays
Detection of DNA damage
Covalent adducts of the test compound with DNA after metabolic activation
DNA strand breakage
Detection of chromosomal damage
Chromosomal abnormalities by cytogenetics
Sister chromatid exchange
Micronucleus frequency
Sperm abnormalities
Detection of mutational events
Bacterial mutagenesis (Ames *Salmonella* assay, etc)
Sex-linked mutations and reciprocal translocations in *Drosophila*
Mutational spectra in transgenic mice
Unscheduled DNA synthesis in cells in culture
Neoplastic transformation of mammalian cells in culture

TABLE 5–2 Features of chemical carcinogens that cause difficulty in deciding that a chemical does or does not cause cancer in humans.

1. The time interval between exposure to a potential carcinogen and the clinical detection of a tumor may be 20 years or more in humans. This long latent period for many cancers makes it difficult to link current disease to exposures that may have occurred decades earlier.
2. The degree of cancer risk is driven by the level of carcinogen exposure, but it is often difficult to quantify the amount and type of exposure, especially when it may have occurred decades earlier. The use of biomarkers of exposure has limited utility as most have limited persistence after exposure ends.
3. Humans are exposed to a multitude of chemicals and other potentially carcinogenic agents (viruses, ionizing radiation, etc). These complex exposure patterns confound attempts to attribute the disease to a particular agent.
4. Individuals may vary widely from one another in their susceptibility to carcinogens as a result of genetic variation at key loci, such as those governing DNA repair capacity or pathways of carcinogen activation and detoxification.
5. Because of the generally low levels of exposure encountered today, the statistical power for detecting carcinogens is low unless the population studied is very large or unless there is a dramatic increase in tumor incidence at a particular site.

time to obtain results and reduced cost compared to animal testing. Table 5–1 lists several commonly used classes of short-term assays.

The covalent binding of carcinogenic chemicals to DNA may be measured by several techniques. One still widely used method involves exposure of cultured cells or living animals to a carcinogen, isolation of DNA, radioactive postlabeling of adducted DNA species, and their separation by silica gel chromatography. This method allows for the identification and quantification of multiple specific adducts but involves the use of potentially hazardous radioactivity. DNA-carcinogen adducts are increasingly being identified and quantified, even in DNA isolated from humans exposed to carcinogens in the environment, using liquid chromatography coupled with mass spectrometry (see Chap. 2, Sec. 2.4). Finally, antibodies that recognize particular DNA-adducted carcinogens can be used in an immunoassay or with immunohistochemistry following exposure of animals or cultured cells to the carcinogen.

Other types of DNA damage may also be measured in short-term assays. Oxidative DNA damage following carcinogen exposure may be monitored by quantifying 8-*oxo*-deoxyguanosine using either liquid chromatography or an immunoassay. The comet assay provides a general measure of overall DNA damage in individual cells using single-cell agarose gel electrophoresis of cell nuclei to visualize fragmented DNA (see Chap. 9, Sec. 9.6). Indirect methods for monitoring levels of DNA damage include immunoblotting and immunohistochemical assays for the phosphorylated histone protein H2AX (γ-H2AX; see Chap. 9, Fig. 9-11), which is produced after a variety of different types of DNA damage, and an assay for unscheduled DNA synthesis, which is a marker for DNA repair occurring subsequent to carcinogen-induced DNA damage. Newer, high-throughput methods can assess the extent of carcinogen-induced DNA damage throughout the genome. For example, a technique called HS-Damage-Seq can generate genome-wide "damage maps" after exposure to UV irradiation (Hu et al, 2017). Such methods are more likely to be capable of identifying causal mutations rather than those that provide general damage biomarkers. It is also important to note that the carcinogen-induced mutational load observed in nuclear DNA may not be seen in mitochondrial DNA, as has been shown using mice that are deficient in mitochondrial import of the DNA repair enzymes OGG1 and MUTYH (Kauppila et al, 2018).

Cytogenetic methods are used for detecting gross chromosomal abnormalities caused by carcinogen exposure. These include breaks, terminal deletions, rearrangements, and translocations; quantitation of damage-induced sister chromatid exchanges of differentially stained chromatids; and the frequency of micronuclei arising as a result of disruption of DNA distribution into nuclei during cell replication.

Many of the methods for detecting DNA damage assume that DNA damage is correlated with DNA mutation—an assumption that does not take into account DNA repair. For this reason, methods have evolved to measure the frequency of carcinogen-induced mutations in bacteria, mammalian cells, and whole animals. The Ames test (Fig. 5–8) uses strains

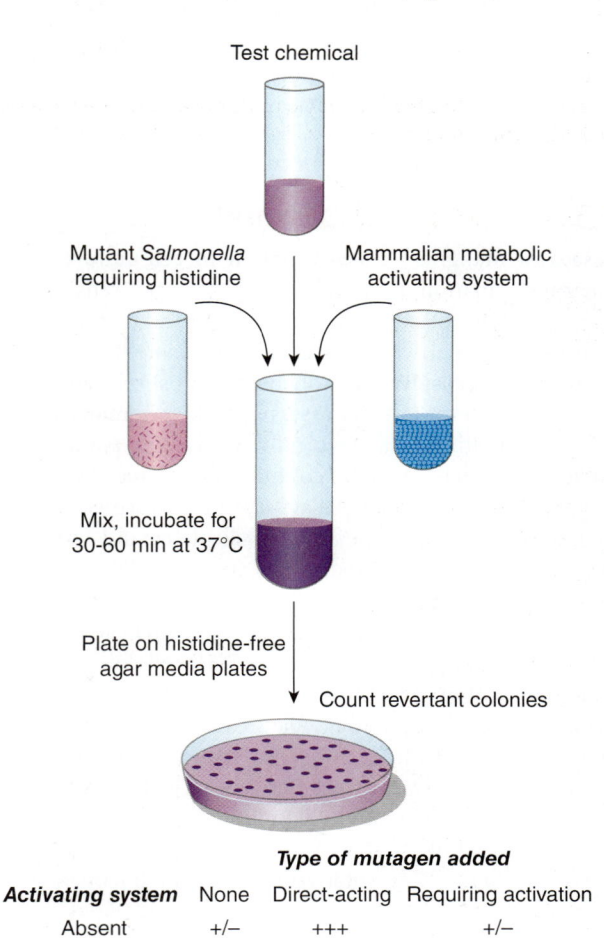

Activating system	None	Direct-acting	Requiring activation
Absent	+/–	+++	+/–
Present	+/–	+++	+++

FIGURE 5–8 Detection of mutagenic chemicals in *Salmonella typhimurium* (**Ames test**). (Data from Cohen SM, Ellwein LB. Genetic errors, cell proliferation, and carcinogenesis. *Cancer Res* 1991 Dec 15;51(24):6493-505.)

of *Salmonella typhimurium* that have a mutation preventing them from synthesizing the amino acid histidine; thus, they will grow only if histidine is added to the growth medium. Exposure of these bacteria to a mutagen can result in reversion of the mutation back to histidine-independent growth in some bacteria, which can then grow on histidine-deficient agar plates. The number of revertant colonies that grow on these plates is a measure of the mutagenic potency of the test compound. Because most chemicals must be activated to be mutagenic or carcinogenic, these assays are usually conducted in the presence of drug-metabolizing enzymes to generate the relevant reactive electrophile, or strains of *Salmonella* expressing recombinant human drug-metabolizing enzymes may be employed. An analogous method using mammalian splenic T cells monitors chemical-induced mutations in the endogenous hypoxanthine phosphoribosyltransferase (*Hprt*) gene.

The above assays to detect potential carcinogens make the assumption that rates of mutation are predictive of rates of tumor formation. Although most of the agents that are carcinogenic in humans are also mutagenic in bacteria and cause cytogenetic changes in rodent bone marrow, some chemicals that test positive in short-term assays or even in chronic rodent studies have not been shown to be carcinogenic in humans. Assessment of the carcinogenic potential of nongenotoxic carcinogens is even more challenging because there is no mechanism on which to base large-scale in vitro screening assays for them.

5.3.3 Cellular Transformation Assays

Assays of malignant transformation in cell culture monitor the transformation of normal or immortalized cells into those that are capable of extensive proliferation and that have tumor-forming potential when injected into recipient animals. Cell transformation assays are probably the most relevant and predictive short-term tests for assessing risk of human cancer.

Transformation assays typically involve the plating of cells on soft agar plates and the counting of colonies that are able to grow after 3-4 weeks. Assays can be performed in as little as 1 week with the use of microwell plates and intracellular dyes that permit automated colony counting. The Syrian hamster embryo (SHE) assay is still used widely (Ahmadzai et al, 2015), and it is the only cell culture assay that can exhibit features of multistage transformation. SHE cell colonies with an altered phenotype are counted 7-8 days after carcinogen exposure, based on morphologic features such as cell piling, randomly oriented 3-dimensional growth, cell crisscrossing, and decreased cytoplasm/nucleus ratios. SHE cells can be cryopreserved and they maintain metabolic capabilities that eliminate the need for addition of an exogenous source of bioactivating enzymes when testing putative genotoxicant chemicals.

5.3.4 Animal Bioassays

In vivo carcinogenicity assays in rodents involve either chronic repeated administration of high doses of a potential carcinogen, or administration of the chemical at a sensitive developmental stage. Genetically modified strains of mice that have been made either more or less susceptible to carcinogens because of altered procarcinogen bioactivation (Matsumoto et al, 2007; Sugamori et al, 2012) or DNA repair (Wijnhoven and Van Steeg, 2003) have also been utilized to better define mechanisms of bioactivation, DNA damage and repair in tumor development, as well as to provide more rapid, robust, and economically practical in vivo test systems. For instance, genetic deficiency in the oxidative DNA damage repair enzyme OGG1 enhances the lung tumorigenicity of the tobacco smoke-derived nitrosamine NNK in female mice but not in males, suggesting a sex hormone effect on sensitivity or response to oxidative DNA damage (Igarashi et al, 2009).

Transgenic animals carrying retrievable target genes (eg, genes of viruses that infect bacteria—known as bacteriophages) are also used for in vivo testing of putative mutagens (Long et al, 2016). After in vivo exposure of the transgenic animal to a carcinogen and subsequent isolation of genomic DNA from any tissue of interest, the phage carrying the target transgene (such as the *lacZ* gene of a bacteriophage lambda) are retrieved from the mammalian host's genome. Bacteria are then exposed to the bacteriophages under conditions that select for growth of only those bacteria infected by viruses harboring mutated target transgenes. Thus, the mutation frequency in the carcinogen-exposed animal is proportional to the number of bacteriophage plaques observed on agar plates. Such systems can provide valuable information regarding mutation potential and tissue specificity, but the assay is expensive and used more commonly following a primary screen in microorganisms.

Because testing of putative carcinogens in animals is time-consuming, expensive, and requires large numbers of animals to obtain valid results, it is generally used to confirm results obtained from the above-described short-term tests in bacteria or cell culture. Studies in rodents are also criticized because they usually employ doses of suspected carcinogens far in excess of the probable human exposure for economic reasons. At high doses, acute cytotoxicity of an agent can cause necrosis, inflammation, and compensatory proliferation that contribute to tumor growth, and this phenomenon may not occur at lower exposure levels. However, most carcinogens that induce a high frequency of tumors at high doses will also induce some tumors at lower doses in studies using large numbers of animals. High doses are used for the practical reason of reducing the number of animals required, but such designs require the assumption that the dose-response relationship allows for valid extrapolation of risk from high to low doses. Study designs for most animal bioassays can detect a tumor incidence of approximately 5% but not as low as 1%, whereas in humans a tumor incidence of 1% would be unacceptably high.

The incidence of cancer caused by chemical agents generally increases with dose in both rodents and humans, but carcinogenic potency can differ between closely related compounds. Based on rodent studies, the following generalizations concerning the quantitative relationship between exposure and response to carcinogens can be made:

1. A single exposure to some carcinogens may induce tumors in a high proportion of animals. For example, a single dose of a polycyclic aromatic hydrocarbon (PAH) can induce mammary carcinomas in more than 90% of female rats if the compound is administered as they are approaching sexual maturity. Similarly, 1 or 2 doses of diethylnitrosamine or 4-aminobiphenyl can produce a high incidence of liver tumors in adult mice if they are administered between days 8 and 15 after birth, when the liver is still actively proliferating.

2. Tumor production is often enhanced and the latency period reduced if chemical exposure is repeated. Repeated exposures either enhance the likelihood of mutations in key genes, or produce changes in the microenvironment that promote the growth of initiated cells.

3. Tumor susceptibility varies widely among animal species and even between strains of the same species. For example, rats are much more susceptible to aflatoxin B_1-induced liver tumors than mice, and some hybrid offspring of inbred strains of mice are more susceptible to tumors than their inbred parents after exposure to many different chemicals.

4. Dose-response curves for carcinogenicity may vary in different tissues even within the same animals. For example, Figure 5–9 shows dose-response relationships for the carcinogen 2-acetylaminofluorene. At lower doses, liver tumors predominate, whereas at higher doses bladder tumors are more common, and the shapes of the dose-response curves differ markedly. The difference in tissue response is not related to differences in carcinogen pharmacokinetics, metabolism, or resultant DNA damage and mutation, but rather to increased rates of cell proliferation in bladder at higher doses of the chemical.

5. There is a very broad range of potency among different chemical carcinogens. As shown in Figure 5–10, less than 1 µg/d of aflatoxin B_1 is sufficient to produce tumors in 50% of rats after a lifetime of exposure, whereas trichloroethylene or saccharin require more than 1 g/d to produce the same incidence of tumors. Moreover, saccharin produces

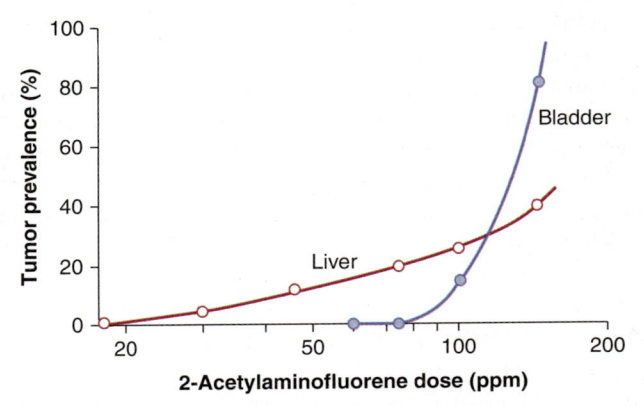

FIGURE 5–9 Dose-response curves for the production of liver and bladder tumors in female mice treated with 2-acetylaminofluorene. Tumors were observed after treatment for 18-33 months. *PPM*, parts per million. (Modified with permission from Maugh TH 2nd: Chemical carcinogens: how dangerous are low doses? *Science* 1978 Oct 6;202(4363):37-41.)

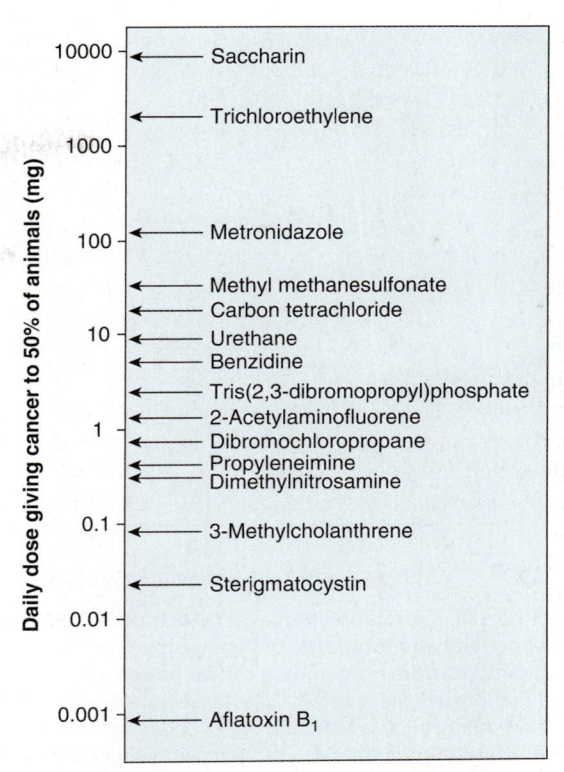

FIGURE 5–10 Range of carcinogenic potencies for various chemicals.

tumors in rodents not because of its DNA-damaging ability but rather because at such high doses the chemical precipitates in the urine and the crystals elicit a chronic tumor-promoting inflammation of the bladder lumen. It is therefore important to relate tumor-producing doses of chemicals with the expected daily or lifetime exposures to the chemicals in humans.

5.4 MOLECULAR EPIDEMIOLOGY OF CARCINOGENESIS

Molecular epidemiology makes use of molecular markers that may relate quantitatively to either carcinogen exposure or to predisposition to cancer in human populations (see Fig. 5–7 and Chap. 4, Sec. 4.6). In estimating risk, molecular techniques allow for studies of human cancer incidence to be supplemented by surrogate markers and biologic endpoints rather than only by cancer outcomes.

5.4.1 Biomarkers for Assessment of Carcinogen Exposure

The carcinogen dose received by individuals may be quantified by measuring biomarkers of exposure, such as carcinogen-DNA adduct levels, DNA damage levels, or mutation frequencies in accessible cells. For example, Figure 5–11 illustrates that the level of B[*a*]P adducts in DNA samples from lungs of smokers was highly correlated with the activity of a

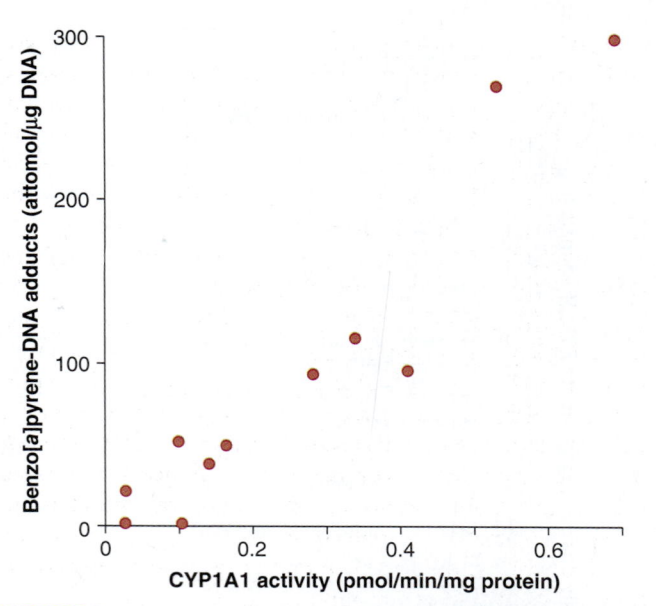

FIGURE 5-11 Correlation between cytochrome P450 isoform CYP1A1 activity and formation of benzo[*a*]pyrene DNA adducts in lung samples from human lung cancer patients. (Reproduced with permission from Alexandrov K, Rojas M, Geneste O, et al. An improved fluorometric assay for dosimetry of benzo(a)pyrene diol-epoxide-DNA adducts in smokers' lung: comparisons with total bulky adducts and aryl hydrocarbon hydroxylase activity. *Cancer Res* 1992 Nov 15;52(22):6248-6253.)

key bioactivating enzyme, CYP1A1 (Alexandrov et al, 1992). CYP1A1 not only bioactivates B[*a*]P but its expression is also induced by it. CYP1A1 activity is also correlated with the level of exposure to cigarette smoke, a major source of B[*a*]P. Thus, an increase in CYP1A1 activity might be expected to associate with an increase in subsequent risk of lung cancer. More recent studies have indicated that aldehydes rather than CYP1A1-bioactivated B[*a*]P produce most of the lung DNA damage that is observed after inhalation of cigarette smoke, and aldehydes actually inhibit the DNA-damaging effects of B[*a*]P and other tobacco smoke carcinogens (Weng et al, 2018). Although these types of studies are informative, they are often limited by the requirement for lung biopsies to obtain tissue for analysis. In the Physicians Health Study, white blood cells were used as an accessible surrogate for lung tissue (Tang et al, 2001): current smokers who displayed elevated levels of carcinogen-DNA adducts in their white blood cells were more likely to be diagnosed with lung cancer within 13 years than smokers who had lower adduct levels. Thus, adduct levels in white blood cells of smokers may provide a predictive biomarker for risk of lung cancer, although the identities of the causative adducts remain to be definitively established.

5.4.2 Genetic Variation in Risk From Carcinogen Exposure

In populations where all members are exposed to the same carcinogens, some individuals develop cancer and others do not. For example, although cigarette smoking is a strong risk factor for lung cancer, some smokers develop lung cancer and a large number do not. One potential reason for this interindividual variation in risk is related to differences in the activities of the drug-metabolizing enzymes responsible for either detoxifying or activating procarcinogenic chemicals. Many epidemiologic studies have shown that genetic polymorphisms in drug-metabolizing enzymes may be associated (although usually weakly) with altered susceptibility to chemical carcinogens. For example, variations in the activity of arylamine *N*-acetyltransferase 2 (NAT2), which can play roles in either the detoxification or the metabolic activation of aromatic amines (see Fig. 5–3), are associated with altered risk for bladder cancer in populations that have been exposed to these agents (Hein et al, 2000). However, such associations are often inconsistent from study to study. For example, in one study, individuals with an Ile[462]Val mutation in the PAH-metabolizing enzyme CYP1A1 were shown to have a 4.5-fold higher risk of lung cancer than those with the wild-type enzyme (San Jose et al, 2010), whereas other studies have shown no association between this variant and elevated risk of lung cancer. Particular combinations of polymorphisms can act additively or synergistically to increase risk. For example, one study found no significant associations between risk for lung cancer and allelic variants in any of 10 postulated lung cancer susceptibility genes when considered individually, whereas a particular combination of 5 of these variants produced a 5.2-fold increase in overall risk and an even higher 18-fold increased risk in females (Klinchid et al, 2009).

Genetic variations in DNA repair enzymes are often associated with drastically increased predisposition to cancer. Any defect in the ability to repair DNA damage will result in the accumulation of mutations and hence drive its phenotype toward malignant growth. Examples of genetic defects in DNA repair that can significantly increase sensitivity to any DNA-damaging stimulus, including carcinogenic chemicals, include breast cancer susceptibility genes (BRCA1/2), xeroderma pigmentosum (XP), Werner syndrome, ataxia-telangiectasis mutated (ATM), and Turcot syndrome (see also Chap. 9, Sec. 9.5).

A major goal of molecular epidemiology is to identify individuals and populations with elevated cancer risk because of heritable predisposing factors so that preventive strategies can be implemented. Mutation in tumor suppressor genes, such as the retinoblastoma gene, *RB*, confer a very high cancer risk in individuals who carry them (see Chap. 7, Sec. 7.6.4), but such mutations are rare and do not constitute a major attributable risk to the population.

5.4.3 "Omics" Technologies and Molecular Signatures of Exposure and Risk

High-throughput screening (see Chap. 2) can be used to study the structure and function of the genome (DNA sequences), the transcriptome (mRNA expression levels), the proteome (proteins encoded by genes and transcripts), and the metabolome (small-molecule chemical fingerprints of intracellular processes) as they respond to toxic substances. The goal of such studies is to elucidate molecular mechanisms of toxicity and to derive molecular expression patterns that may better predict toxic events. Carcinogenesis is amenable to all of these approaches. Research has identified mutational signatures that associate with different human tumors (Alexandrov et al, 2020), as well as carcinogen-induced somatic mutations that are associated with tumor growth (Rose et al, 2020). Current research is studying the effects of exposures of experimental animals to genotoxic and nongenotoxic carcinogens on global gene expression profiles, protein expression patterns, epigenetic changes, and metabolic variables, and their consequences. For example, chronic exposure of rats to the genotoxic carcinogen *N*-nitrosomorpholine demonstrated a concordance among altered gene, protein, and histopathologic expression profiles for 8 candidate proteins in liver (Oberemm et al, 2009). Other proof-of-principle studies have compared the gene expression profiles of known carcinogens to identify predictive multigene expression signatures for each class of chemical, as well as to distinguish between chemicals that act to facilitate tumor growth by genotoxic and nongenotoxic modes of action (Moffat et al, 2015). Integrated systems biology that uses computational modeling will be required to analyze the vast amount of data that can be generated by these techniques and will contribute ultimately to enhancing our understanding of the complex impact of carcinogens on the human genome and the cellular processes that it encodes.

With the advent of high-throughput DNA and RNA sequencing, novel roles for both coding and noncoding RNA and DNA regions as drivers of carcinogenesis are being identified (Caiment et al, 2015; Rheinbay et al, 2020). Although there is considerable evidence from tumor genome analyses that the original cell type in which initiating events occur, or "cell of origin," plays a key role in determining eventual tumorigenic outcomes and phenotypes (Wang et al, 2013; Hoadley et al, 2018; Bolen et al, 2019), these and other studies also suggest that the nature of the oncogenic mutational events occurring in these cells also plays a significant role (Bhagirath et al, 2015; ICGC/TCGA Consortium, 2020). Advanced proteomics techniques are also furthering our understanding of tumor initiation and progression mechanisms and allowing for the identification of novel tumor biomarkers that could guide focused therapies (Kondo, 2019). For example, a combination of RNA transcriptome sequencing (RNAseq) and proteomic analysis has revealed new candidate pathways and factors that may control HPV-mediated oncogenic transformation and therefore deserve further study (Yang et al, 2019).

5.5 CANCER CHEMOPREVENTION

Because carcinogenesis is complex and multistage, chemopreventive agents could act by a variety of mechanisms. However, any potential chemical to prevent cancer must pose a very low health risk, because it would require long-term administration. Candidates for chemopreventive therapy fall into 2 main categories: (1) the general population and (2) those at elevated risk because of genetic predisposition or heightened levels of carcinogen exposure. Specific chemical interventions have been investigated and some have been approved for individuals at higher risk of malignancy. These may be aimed either at preventing DNA damage or at reducing the likelihood that DNA-damaged cells will proliferate to form a malignancy.

As described earlier, many procarcinogens are bioactivated to their DNA-binding metabolites by isozymes of the CYP superfamily. Chemicals that inhibit particular CYPs and/or induce the phase II conjugating enzymes that facilitate excretion of CYP-produced oxidized metabolites could reduce metabolic activation of carcinogens. There is support for this concept from the association between intake of fruits and vegetables, many of which contain enzyme inducers, and cancer risk: in experimental animals, certain chemicals found in cruciferous vegetables can reduce the metabolism and covalent binding of carcinogens to DNA and subsequent tumorigenesis (Srinivasan et al, 2008; Takemura et al, 2010).

However, indiscriminate inhibition of CYP enzymes would not be a safe chemopreventive strategy because CYP enzymes facilitate elimination of many potentially harmful chemicals, as well as enabling the clearance of therapeutically administered drugs. Moreover, the catalytic promiscuity of CYPs is such that even isoform-selective inhibition is likely to alter the disposition of many chemicals entering the body, including therapeutically useful drugs. Finally, a particular CYP isoform may play competing roles in both carcinogen activation and carcinogen elimination that may not be apparent from in vitro investigations. For example, CYP1A2 catalyzes the first step in the bioactivation of aromatic amines into DNA-binding electrophiles (see Fig. 5–3), including those from the cigarette smoke component 4-aminobiphenyl, with subsequent covalent DNA binding of these metabolites, production of DNA mutations, and transformation of cultured cells. However, in mice, the absence of CYP1A2 (achieved by gene knockout) does not protect against either DNA damage or the formation of liver tumors following 4-aminobiphenyl exposure. It is presumed that the protective effect resulting from CYP1A2's contribution to the efficient in vivo elimination of this chemical outweighs its ability to produce DNA-damaging metabolites (Nebert et al, 2004). Moreover, other CYP isoforms such as CYP2E1 are now known to play equally important roles in the bioactivation of 4-aminobiphenyl (Wang et al, 2015).

A strategy of inducing expression of metabolizing enzymes to increase carcinogen elimination has similar challenges. High levels of phase II drug-conjugating enzymes were thought to protect from chemical carcinogenesis. However, inhibition of a given phase II enzyme may either be protective by preventing formation of an unstable metabolite (eg, acetylating, glucuronidating, and sulfonating enzymes can all produce unstable oxyester metabolites of aromatic amines), or may be risk-enhancing if the enzyme's predominant function in vivo is to produce a stable and readily excretable metabolite.

Whether either phase I or phase II drug-metabolizing enzyme induction or inhibition is beneficial or harmful depends on which chemical agent is the main threat.

Unfortunately, exposure often occurs to complex mixtures of structurally unrelated chemicals (cigarette smoke contains several different PAHs, aromatic amines, nitrosamines, and aldehydes), and manipulations that protect from one class of carcinogen might increase the risk from another chemical class, or even between individual chemicals of the same class.

Chemicals that reduce either the levels of reactive oxygen species, inflammatory mediators or inflammation-inducing pathogens also have potential to protect against the development of tumors. Effective antioxidants, such as flavonoids, polyphenols, isothiocyanates, and phytoalexins found in foods, may reduce cellular oxidant burden and thus the levels of oxidative DNA and protein damage. Agents that inhibit inflammation, such as nonsteroidal anti-inflammatory drugs that inhibit prostaglandin synthesis by blocking cyclooxygenase (COX) enzymes, have also been studied as potential cancer chemopreventive agents (Das et al, 2007; Lee et al, 2008). Results of these studies have been equivocal, and the possible cardiovascular side effects associated with large-scale use of these compounds also limit their practical utility.

Reducing the incidence of infection as a result of pathogens that cause chronic inflammatory conditions via immunization, such as papillomavirus vaccines for cervical cancer and hepatitis B/C virus vaccines for liver cancer, is effective in reducing cancer risk. However, it remains to be determined to what extent the reduced cancer risk is due to reduced infection-associated chronic inflammation vs a reduction in direct viral oncogenic mechanisms.

Other chemoprevention strategies aim to reduce or delay the proliferation of initiated cells. The selective estrogen receptor modulator (SERM) tamoxifen was approved over 2 decades ago for the prevention of estrogen receptor (ER)–positive breast cancer in female relatives of ER-positive breast cancer patients, and the second-generation SERM raloxifene was approved 10 years later based on the results of the STAR trial showing a similar efficacy to tamoxifen with fewer side effects (Vogel, 2009). However, the use of both of these agents is low and decreasing, largely because of real and perceived risks of serious proliferative side effects in other tissues with little perceived benefit by patients (Nichols et al, 2015; Pinsky et al, 2018). The dihydrotestosterone synthesis inhibitor finasteride has been tested for the chemoprevention of prostate cancer, and although it shows a modest reduction in the occurrence of low-grade tumors, the risk for aggressive tumors is increased and overall survival is unchanged (Thompson et al, 2013). The SELECT trial to test a combination of selenium supplements plus vitamin E for prostate cancer prevention was also negative (Lippman et al, 2009), as was a study to test 13-cis-retinoic acid for the prevention of lung cancer in high-risk individuals (Kelly et al, 2009).

Thus, the relationships between exogenous chemicals, endogenous hormonal signaling pathways, and dietary/lifestyle factors with cancer risk and prevention are complex. Tumor production in rodents by potent genotoxic carcinogens such as aflatoxin B_1 may be reduced, even after initiation has occurred, by dietary manipulations such as reducing the percentage or the source (ie, animal vs plant) of dietary protein. Epidemiologic studies show consistently that diets rich in fruits and vegetables, which contain high levels of antioxidants, reduce risk for cancers at many sites. Also, increasing evidence suggests that obesity resembles a chronic inflammatory state, which is known to be tumor-promoting (Longo and Fontana, 2010). Thus, for the general population, the most logical chemoprevention strategy is to encourage a healthy lifestyle that includes exercise and caloric moderation to maintain a healthy body weight, the intake of diets that are rich in fruits and vegetables, and avoidance of carcinogen exposure.

SUMMARY

- Many chemical carcinogens form adducts with bases in DNA either directly or, more often, after metabolic activation.
- Cancers arise from multiple sequential unrepaired lesions that tend to accumulate at specific sites in oncogenes or tumor-suppressor genes that regulate cell cycle, proliferation, and cellular microenvironment.
- Genetic variation in the capacity to activate or detoxify carcinogens or to repair DNA damage alters cancer risk.
- Many short-term methods to identify carcinogens rely on the assumption that most carcinogens are genotoxic, although this is now known to be overly simplistic.
- Nongenotoxic carcinogens may contribute to the provision of a selective growth advantage to DNA-damaged and initiated cells by a variety of mechanisms.
- Emerging toxicogenomic technologies allow for a better understanding of the mechanisms of contribution to cancer risk by both genotoxic and nongenotoxic chemicals.
- Based on knowledge of the mechanisms by which chemical carcinogens act, it may be possible to manipulate biochemical or cellular defense systems to reduce cancer risk, and clinical trials of chemoprevention have been completed or are underway, with mixed results.
- The most effective method to reduce the human cancer burden is likely to be through reduction of exposure to known carcinogens, especially to high-risk agents such as cigarette smoke, and by dietary and lifestyle interventions.

REFERENCES

Ahmadzai AA, Trevisan J, Pang W, et al. Classification of agents using Syrian hamster embryo (SHE) cell transformation assay (CTA) with ATR-FTIR spectroscopy and multivariate analysis. *Mutagenesis* 2015;30(5):603-612.

Alexandrov K, Rojas M, Geneste O, et al. An improved fluorometric assay for dosimetry of benzo(a)pyrene diol-epoxide-DNA adducts in smokers' lung: comparisons with total bulky adducts and aryl hydrocarbon hydroxylase activity. *Cancer Res* 1992;52(22):6248-6253.

Alexandrov LB, Kim J, Haradhvala NJ, et al. The repertoire of mutational signatures in human cancer. *Nature* 2020;578(7793):94-101.

Bhagirath D, Zhao X, West WW, Qiu F, Band H, Band V. Cell type of origin as well as genetic alterations contribute to breast cancer phenotypes. *Oncotarget* 2015;6(11):9018-9030.

Bolen CR, Klanova M, Trneny M, et al. Prognostic impact of somatic mutations in diffuse large B-cell lymphoma and relationship to cell-of-origin: data from the phase III GOYA study. Haematologica 2019.

Caiment F, Gaj S, Claessen S, Kleinjans J. High-throughput data integration of RNA-miRNA-circRNA reveals novel insights into mechanisms of benzo[a]pyrene-induced carcinogenicity. *Nucleic Acids Res* 2015;43(5):2525-2534.

Campana L, Bosurgi L, Rovere-Querini P. HMGB1: a two-headed signal regulating tumor progression and immunity. *Curr Opin Immunol* 2008;20(5):518-523.

Das D, Arber N, Jankowski JA. Chemoprevention of colorectal cancer. *Digestion* 2007;76(1):51-67.

Gad SC. Carcinogenicity studies. In: Gad SC, ed. *Preclinical Development Handbook: Toxicology*. Hoboken, NJ: Wiley-Interscience; 2008;423-458.

Grivennikov SI, Greten FR, Karin M. Immunity, inflammation, and cancer. *Cell* 2010;140(6):883-899.

Guengerich FP. Forging the links between metabolism and carcinogenesis. *Mutat Res* 2001;488(3):195-209.

Hainaut P, Pfeifer GP. Patterns of p53 G-->T transversions in lung cancers reflect the primary mutagenic signature of DNA-damage by tobacco smoke. *Carcinogenesis* 2001;22(3):367-374.

Hanahan D, Weinberg RA. Hallmarks of cancer: the next generation. *Cell* 2011;144(5):646-674.

Hein DW, Doll MA, Fretland AJ, et al. Molecular genetics and epidemiology of the NAT1 and NAT2 acetylation polymorphisms. *Cancer Epidemiol Biomarkers Prev* 2000;9(1):29-42.

Hoadley KA, Yau C, Hinoue T, et al. Cell-of-origin patterns dominate the molecular classification of 10,000 tumors from 33 types of cancer. *Cell* 2018;173(2):291-304 e296.

Hu J, Adebali O, Adar S, Sancar A. Dynamic maps of UV damage formation and repair for the human genome. *Proc Natl Acad Sci U S A* 2017;114(26):6758-6763.

ICGC/TCGA Consortium. Pan-cancer analysis of whole genomes. *Nature* 2020;578(7793):82-93.

Igarashi M, Watanabe M, Yoshida M, et al. Enhancement of lung carcinogenesis initiated with 4-(N-hydroxymethylnitrosamino)-1-(3-pyridyl)-1-butanone by Ogg1 gene deficiency in female, but not male, mice. *J Toxicol Sci* 2009;34(2):163-174.

Karin M, Greten FR. NF-kappaB: linking inflammation and immunity to cancer development and progression. *Nat Rev Immunol* 2005;5(10):749-759.

Kauppila JHK, Bonekamp NA, Mourier A, et al. Base-excision repair deficiency alone or combined with increased oxidative stress does not increase mtDNA point mutations in mice. *Nucleic Acids Res* 2018;46(13):6642-6669.

Kelly K, Kittelson J, Franklin WA, et al. A randomized phase II chemoprevention trial of 13-CIS retinoic acid with or without alpha tocopherol or observation in subjects at high risk for lung cancer. *Cancer Prev Res* 2009;2(5):440-449.

Klaunig JE, Kamendulis LM. Chemical carcinogenesis. In: Klaassen CD, ed. *Casarett and Doull's Toxicology - The Basic Science of Poisons*. New York, NY: McGraw-Hill; 2008:329-379.

Klinchid J, Chewaskulyoung B, Saeteng S, Lertprasertsuke N, Kasinrerk W, Cressey R. Effect of combined genetic polymorphisms on lung cancer risk in northern Thai women. *Cancer Genet Cytogenet* 2009;195(2):143-149.

Kondo T. Cancer biomarker development and two-dimensional difference gel electrophoresis (2D-DIGE). *Biochim Biophys Acta* 2019;1867(1):2-8.

Lee JM, Yanagawa J, Peebles KA, Sharma S, Mao JT, Dubinett SM. Inflammation in lung carcinogenesis: new targets for lung cancer chemoprevention and treatment. *CRC Crit Rev Oncol Hematol* 2008;66(3):208-217.

Lippman SM, Klein EA, Goodman PJ, et al. Effect of selenium and vitamin E on risk of prostate cancer and other cancers: the Selenium and Vitamin E Cancer Prevention Trial (SELECT). *JAMA* 2009;301(1):39-51.

Loeb LA, Harris CC. Advances in chemical carcinogenesis: a historical review and prospective. *Cancer Res* 2008;68(17):6863-6872.

Long AS, Lemieux CL, Arlt VM, White PA. Tissue-specific in vivo genetic toxicity of nine polycyclic aromatic hydrocarbons assessed using the MutaMouse transgenic rodent assay. *Toxicol Appl Pharmacol* 2016;290:31-42.

Longo VD, Fontana L. Calorie restriction and cancer prevention: metabolic and molecular mechanisms. *Trends Pharmacol Sci* 2010;31(2):89-98.

Maeda S, Kamata H, Luo JL, Leffert H, Karin M. IKKbeta couples hepatocyte death to cytokine-driven compensatory proliferation that promotes chemical hepatocarcinogenesis. *Cell* 2005;121(7):977-990.

Matsumoto Y, Ide F, Kishi R, et al. Aryl hydrocarbon receptor plays a significant role in mediating airborne particulate-induced carcinogenesis in mice. *Environ Sci Technol* 2007;41(10):3775-3780.

Moffat I, Chepelev N, Labib S, et al. Comparison of toxicogenomics and traditional approaches to inform mode of action and points of departure in human health risk assessment of benzo[a]pyrene in drinking water. *CRC Crit Rev Toxicol* 2015;45(1):1-43.

National Toxicology Program. 14th Report on Carcinogens. https://ntp.niehs.nih.gov/whatwestudy/assessments/cancer/roc/index.html. Published 2016.

Naugler WE, Sakurai T, Kim S, et al. Gender disparity in liver cancer due to sex differences in MyD88-dependent IL-6 production. *Science* 2007;317(5834):121-124.

Nebert DW, Dalton TP, Okey AB, Gonzalez FJ. Role of aryl hydrocarbon receptor-mediated induction of the CYP1 enzymes in environmental toxicity and cancer. *J Biol Chem* 2004;279(23):23847-23850.

Nichols HB, Deroo LA, Scharf DR, Sandler DP. Risk-benefit profiles of women using tamoxifen for chemoprevention. *J Natl Cancer Inst* 2015;107(1):354.

Okey AB, Harper PA. Chemical carcinogenesis. In: Kalant H, Grant DM, Mitchell J, eds. *Principles of Medical*

Pharmacology, 7th ed. Toronto, Canada: Elsevier Canada; 2007:900-911.

Oberemm A, Ahr HJ, Bannasch P, et al. Toxicogenomic analysis of *N*-nitrosomorpholine induced changes in rat liver: comparison of genomic and proteomic responses and anchoring to histopathological parameters. *Toxicol Appl Pharmacol* 2009;241(2):230-245.

Ohshima H, Tatemichi M, Sawa T. Chemical basis of inflammation-induced carcinogenesis. *Arch Biochem Biophys* 2003;417(1):3-11.

Phillips JM, Goodman JI. Multiple genes exhibit phenobarbital-induced constitutive active/androstane receptor-mediated DNA methylation changes during liver tumorigenesis and in liver tumors. *Toxicol Sci* 2009;108(2):273-289.

Pinsky PF, Miller E, Heckman-Stoddard B, Minasian L. Use of raloxifene and tamoxifen by breast cancer risk level in a Medicare-eligible cohort. *Am J Obstet Gynecol* 2018;218:606 e601-606 e609.

Rheinbay E, Nielsen MM, Abascal F, et al. Analyses of non-coding somatic drivers in 2,658 cancer whole genomes. *Nature* 2020;578(7793):102-111.

Rose Y, Halliwill KD, Adams CJ, et al. Mutational signatures in tumours induced by high and low energy radiation in Trp53 deficient mice. *Nat Commun* 2020;11(1):394.

San Jose C, Cabanillas A, Benitez J, Carrillo JA, Jimenez M, Gervasini G. CYP1A1 gene polymorphisms increase lung cancer risk in a high-incidence region of Spain: a case control study. *BMC Cancer* 2010;10:463.

Schrenk D, Schmitz HJ, Bohnenberger S, Wagner B, Worner W. Tumor promoters as inhibitors of apoptosis in rat hepatocytes. *Toxicol Lett* 2004;149(1-3):43-50.

Shen HM, Ong CN. Mutations of the p53 tumor suppressor gene and ras oncogenes in aflatoxin hepatocarcinogenesis. *Mutat Res* 1996;366(1):23-44.

Shimada T. Xenobiotic-metabolizing enzymes involved in activation and detoxification of carcinogenic polycyclic aromatic hydrocarbons. *Drug Metab Pharmacokinet* 2006;21(4):257-276.

Srinivasan P, Suchalatha S, Babu PV, Devi RS, Narayan S, Sabitha KE, Shyamala Devi CS. Chemopreventive and therapeutic modulation of green tea polyphenols on drug metabolizing enzymes in 4-nitroquinoline 1-oxide induced oral cancer. *Chem Biol Interact* 2008;172(3):224-234.

Sugamori KS, Brenneman D, Sanchez O, et al. Reduced 4-aminobiphenyl-induced liver tumorigenicity but not DNA damage in arylamine *N*-acetyltransferase null mice. *Cancer Lett* 2012;318(2):206-213.

Takemura H, Nagayoshi H, Matsuda T, et al. Inhibitory effects of chrysoeriol on DNA adduct formation with benzo[a]pyrene in MCF-7 breast cancer cells. *Toxicology* 2010;274(1-3):42-48.

Tang D, Phillips DH, Stampfer M, et al. Association between carcinogen-DNA adducts in white blood cells and lung cancer risk in the physicians health study. *Cancer Res* 2001;61(18):6708-6712.

Thompson IM Jr, Goodman PJ, Tangen CM, et al. Long-term survival of participants in the prostate cancer prevention trial. *N Engl J Med* 2013;369(7):603-610.

Vineis P, Schatzkin A, Potter JD. Models of carcinogenesis: an overview. *Carcinogenesis* 2010;31(10):1703-1709.

Vogel VG. The NSABP Study of Tamoxifen and Raloxifene (STAR) trial. *Expert Rev Anticancer Ther* 2009;9(1): 51-60.

Wang S, Bott D, Tung A, Sugamori KS, Grant DM. Relative contributions of CYP1A2 and CYP2E1 to the bioactivation and clearance of 4-aminobiphenyl in adult mice. *Drug Metab Dispos* 2015;43(7):916-921.

Wang ZA, Mitrofanova A, Bergren SK, et al. Lineage analysis of basal epithelial cells reveals their unexpected plasticity and supports a cell-of-origin model for prostate cancer heterogeneity. *Nat Cell Biol* 2013;15(3):274-283.

Weng MW, Lee HW, Park SH, et al. Aldehydes are the predominant forces inducing DNA damage and inhibiting DNA repair in tobacco smoke carcinogenesis. *Proc Natl Acad Sci U S A* 2018;115(27):E6152-E6161.

Wijnhoven SW, Van Steeg H. Transgenic and knockout mice for DNA repair functions in carcinogenesis and mutagenesis. *Toxicology* 2003;193(1-2):171-187.

Wogan GN, Hecht SS, Felton JS, Conney AH, Loeb LA. Environmental and chemical carcinogenesis. *Semin Cancer Biol* 2004;14(6):473-486.

Yang R, Klimentova J, Gockel-Krzikalla E, et al. Combined transcriptome and proteome analysis of immortalized human keratinocytes expressing human papillomavirus 16 (HPV16) oncogenes reveals novel key factors and networks in HPV-induced carcinogenesis. *mSphere* 2019;4(2).

Cellular Signaling

Lea A. Harrington

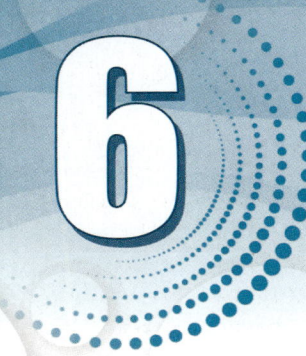

Chapter Outline

- 6.1 Introduction
- 6.2 Growth Factor Signaling
  - 6.2.1 Extracellular Growth Factors and Receptor Tyrosine Kinases
  - 6.2.2 Formation of Multiprotein Complexes and Signal Transmission
  - 6.2.3 RAS Proteins
  - 6.2.4 Mitogen-Activated Protein Kinase Signaling
  - 6.2.5 Phosphoinositide Signaling
  - 6.2.6 Transcriptional Response to Signaling
  - 6.2.7 Biological Outcomes of Growth Factor Signaling
  - 6.2.8 Suppression of Growth Factor Signaling via Protein Phosphatases
- 6.3 Cytoplasmic Tyrosine Kinase Signaling
  - 6.3.1 Cytokine Signaling
  - 6.3.2 Integrin Signaling
- 6.4 Developmental Signaling
  - 6.4.1 WNT Signaling
  - 6.4.2 NOTCH Signaling
  - 6.4.3 Hedgehog Signaling
  - 6.4.4 Signal Transduction by the Transforming Growth Factor–β Superfamily
- 6.5 The Role of Ubiquitin in Cell Signaling
  - 6.5.1 The Ubiquitin Proteasome System
  - 6.5.2 The Ubiquitin Code
  - 6.5.3 Clinical Implications of the UPS and Proteostasis in Oncology
- Summary
- References

6.1 INTRODUCTION

The perturbation and conscription of normal cellular signaling processes is one of the defining features in the development of cancer (Hanahan and Weinberg, 2011). A major challenge in the development of therapeutics against signaling networks is the ability to target these perturbations without interfering with the ability of normal cells and tissues to receive and respond to extracellular signals. The ability to respond to extracellular signals is essential to our ability to respond to our physical or chemical environment, and to initiate the necessary modifications of cell metabolism, morphology, movement, and proliferation. These responses are brought about by elaborate networks of intracellular signals transmitted by changes in protein phosphorylation and enzymatic activity, localization, and the formation of protein-protein complexes. In turn, cellular responses are triggered by the recognition of extracellular signals at the cell surface, resulting in the activation of cytoplasmic enzymes that trigger biochemical cascades in the cytoplasm and nucleus. These signal transduction networks are critical to numerous cellular processes that range from the generalized control of cell proliferation and survival, to specialized functions such as the immune response and angiogenesis. This chapter will focus on how the dysregulation of networks involved in normal growth, adhesion, and development contribute to malignant transformation in human cells, and how these perturbations can be exploited to develop new cancer therapeutics.

6.2 GROWTH FACTOR SIGNALING

6.2.1 Extracellular Growth Factors and Receptor Tyrosine Kinases

Cells communicate with the external environment in myriad ways that include binding of small molecules to the cell surface, antigen stimulation through their interaction with immune cells, or via interactions with other cells and the extracellular matrix. In this chapter, the focus is on secreted polypeptide molecules called growth factors or cytokines, and how their recognition by membrane-bound receptors results

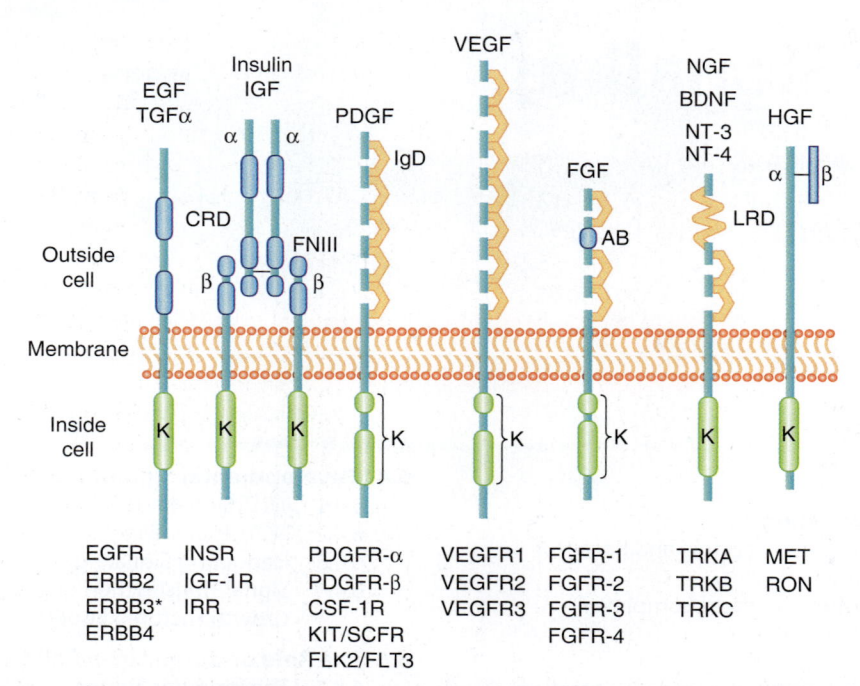

FIGURE 6–1 The receptor protein tyrosine kinases. Representative molecules from selected RPTK families of receptors ("R") are shown below and representative ligands above. *EGF*, epidermal growth factor; *FGF*, fibroblast growth factor; *HGF*, hepatocyte growth factor; *NGF*, nerve growth factor; *PDGF*, platelet-derived growth factor; *VEGF*, vascular endothelial growth factor. All members have a conserved intracellular kinase domain (K). Some of the common structural elements found in the extracellular ligand binding domain include the CRD (cysteine-rich domain), FNIII (fibronectin type III repeats), IgD (immunoglobulin-like domain), AB (acid-rich box), and LRD (leucine-rich domain); *TGF-α*, transforming growth factor-alpha; *IGF*, insulin-like growth factor; *BDNF*, brain derived neurotrophic factor; *NT-3*, neurotrophin 3; *NT-4*, neurotrophin 4.

in intracellular biochemical signaling responses that control cellular properties including cell proliferation.

There are at least 7 types of growth factor receptors with known roles in cancer development (Fig. 6–1). These receptor "families" are composed of a polypeptide (often monomeric or dimeric) that contains a transmembrane domain and an associated intracellular kinase domain. These receptors can be grouped according to the types of polypeptides that bind to them, and by the architecture of the receptor itself; for example, transmembrane-spanning polypeptides that contain a ligand-binding domain and an intracellular tyrosine kinase domain (eg, epidermal growth factor receptor [EGFR]), or serine/threonine kinase domain (eg, transforming growth factor–β receptor [TGFβRI/II]), tyrosine kinase receptors that are linked to extracellular "alpha-chain" extracellular ligand-binding domains (eg, insulin growth factor receptor 1 [IGF1R]), or tyrosine kinase–associated polypeptides whose extracellular domain contains 3, 5, or up to 7 Ig-like ligand-binding domains, for example, vascular endothelial growth factor (VEGF), platelet-derived growth factor receptor (PDGFRα/β), or fibroblast growth factor receptor (FGFR1-4), respectively (Tiash and Chowdhury, 2015).

As discussed below, mutations in these receptor complexes often accompany malignant transformation, which results in the constitutive activation of the growth factor receptor signaling network, which is then rendered refractory to the normal feedback mechanisms that limit receptor activity.

A defining event on growth factor binding to its cognate receptor is the phosphorylation of numerous endogenous proteins, and the regulation of this process is often subverted in cancer. Most growth factor receptors contain intracellular protein kinase domains that are linked to the extracellular domain via a short, single, hydrophobic helix transmembrane component. Examples are the receptor protein tyrosine kinases (RPTKs), which phosphorylate substrates on tyrosine, and which contain evolutionarily conserved core catalytic domains approximately 260 residues in length. Not only do these kinases phosphorylate key intracellular protein substrates, but they also phosphorylate residues within and adjacent to the catalytic domain (juxtamembrane region) that play important roles in receptor regulation. Members of the PDGFR and VEGFR families of receptors are further distinguished by a split kinase domain in which important autophosphorylation sites are present on a kinase insert within the catalytic domain. Another distinguishing feature among RPTK subgroups resides in the extracellular growth factor–binding domains, which are grouped by sequence homology, or by the presence of sequence motifs also found in other functionally unrelated molecules such as EGF repeats, immunoglobulin repeats, or fibronectin type III repeats (see Fig. 6–1). These extracellular domains of RPTKs are also commonly posttranslationally modified by glycosylation.

The signaling cascade is initiated by binding of the growth factor or ligand to the receptor, which induces conformational changes in the extracellular domain to facilitate dimerization (Fig. 6–2) or membrane clustering (Mugler et al, 2012). Some ligands, such as PDGF, are themselves dimeric forms of a single subunit and naturally induce a symmetric ligand/receptor

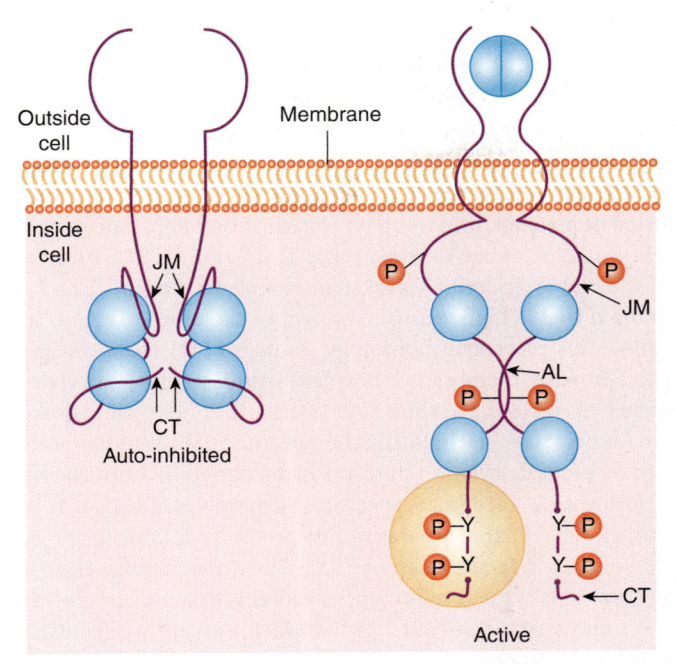

FIGURE 6-2 Growth factor receptor dimerization and activation. In the absence of ligand (eg, EGF) binding, the intracellular kinase domain is inactive, held in a repressed conformation by intramolecular interactions involving the juxtamembrane region (JM), carboxyterminal tail (CT), and activation loop (AL). Ligand binding induces receptor dimerization, relief of inhibitory constraints, and autophosphorylation of the intracellular domains on tyrosine residues. These autophosphorylation sites function to both enhance the catalytic activity and serve as docking sites for intracellular signaling molecules that bind to phosphotyrosine. *P*, phosphate; *Y*, tyrosine.

dimer. Structural studies have revealed how other ligands that exist as monomers, such as EGF, induce receptor dimerization through receptor-receptor interactions. These studies revealed that binding of EGF to EGFR (encoded by *ERBB1*) induces a conformation change that exposes a dimerization loop that mediates association of neighboring, ligand-occupied receptors. Similar dimerization loops are found in the other members of the EGFR family (ERBB2, ERBB3, and ERBB4), allowing the formation of heterodimers between different members of the ERBB family. Such structural studies are informing possible mechanisms by which drug resistance arises against targeted EGFR inhibitors (Goyal et al, 2017).

Receptor dimerization is often an obligate step in the signaling cascade, as it permits the juxtaposition of 2 catalytic domains that act on one another in *trans* (called transphosphorylation) at key tyrosine residues within the catalytic domain and in the noncatalytic regulatory regions of the cytoplasmic domain. For example, phosphorylation of the kinase activation loop induces a conformation change that opens the catalytic site to adenosine triphosphate (ATP) binding and substrate recognition. Outside the catalytic site, phosphorylation of other residues is needed to create binding sites for downstream signaling molecules (see Fig. 6-2) (Pawson and Nash, 2003; Lemmon and Schlessinger, 2010).

The importance of receptor dimerization in the regulation of downstream signaling is not restricted to the catalytic site.

Other dimerization-dependent conformational changes occur within the cytoplasmic domain and are required for full catalytic activity. Intermolecular interactions are also required to limit the access of RPTKs to their protein substrates and block the enzyme active site. As 2 examples, the juxtamembrane region of receptors from the PDGFR family represses the activity of the kinase domain and this repression is relieved by phosphorylation of tyrosine residues in the juxtamembrane region (Lemmon and Schlessinger, 2010). Similarly, the carboxyterminal tail of the angiopoietin receptor Tie2 blocks the active site of the kinase domain, thus preventing substrate access (Barton et al, 2014).

There are multiple RPTKs for which small molecule inhibitors are in clinical use against cancer. For the EGFR-associated receptors, which are frequently mutated in cancer, clinically approved small molecule inhibitors, that include gefitinib and erlotinib, bind the ATP-binding site and inhibit tyrosine phosphorylation (see also Chap. 19, Sec. 19.4.1). For the VEGFR1-3, PDGFR, and FGFR RPTKs, inhibitors that act against one or a subset of this class of RPTKs are approved for metastatic renal cell carcinoma and other types of cancer (see Chap. 11, Sec. 11.7.1, and Chap. 19, Sec. 19.3). Humanized antibodies against RPTKs that inhibit other aspects of receptor activation or downstream signaling are also used clinically; their targets include ERBB1/2 (cetuximab, panitumumab, trastuzumab), IGF1R (ganitumab), and VEGFR2 (ramucirumab) (see Chap. 19) (Tiash and Chowdhury, 2015; Goyal et al, 2017).

6.2.2 Formation of Multiprotein Complexes and Signal Transmission

Protein phosphorylation evolved as a communication signal between proteins because it is a reversible, dynamic, and temporally adaptable modification that can form hydrogen bonds or salt bridges, intra or inter-molecularly, in a manner that is stronger than either aspartate or glutamate (Hunter, 2012). Concomitant with the evolution of protein kinases were modular protein domains that are recognized and bound to phosphorylated serine/threonine or tyrosine motifs. These phospho-specific recognition motifs are replete across nature. Most often, they recognize very short domains (less than 10 a.a.) of a conserved peptide motif, often via recognition of phosphorylated residues within the motif, for example, phosphothreonine for forkhead-associated (FHA) domains, or tyrosine for Src Homology 2 (SH2) domains or phosphotyrosine–binding (PTB) domains (see Figs. 6-2 and 6-3) (Wagner et al, 2013; Almawi et al, 2017).

The SH2 domain was identified as a conserved region containing approximately 100 amino acids found outside the catalytic domain of the Sarcoma (SRC) family of cytoplasmic tyrosine kinases (DeClue et al, 1987; Koch et al, 1989; Moran et al, 1990). The specificity of SH2 domain recognition is determined both by the requirement for phosphotyrosine, common to almost all SH2 domains, and by 3 to 4 amino acids (often termed the +1, +2, and +3 "X" residues relative to the phosphotyrosine) on the carboxyterminal side of the tyrosine residue (Fig. 6-3). Determination of the crystal structure of SRC

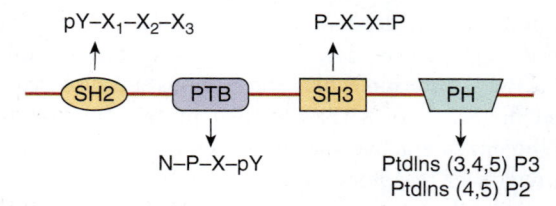

FIGURE 6-3 Examples of modular interaction domains. Representation of the protein modules commonly found in intracellular signaling proteins that are linked to growth factor receptor signaling cascades. Each is shown with its consensus peptide or phospholipid binding target. *N*, Asparagine; *P*, proline; *X*, any amino acid; *Y*, tyrosine. The domains are represented as if linked together on a single polypeptide to illustrate how the presence of multiple domains within signaling molecules would facilitate the assembly of larger signaling complexes. *SH2*, Src homology 2; *SH3*, Src homology 3; *PTB*, phosphotyrosine binding; *PH*, pleckstrin homology.

kinases was instrumental in defining the role of SH2 domains in catalysis and protein substrate recognition. Individual SH2 domains bind selectively to distinct phosphopeptide motifs, and the preferred consensus binding sequences for most SH2 domains have been defined. PTB domains can also specifically bind phosphotyrosine-containing peptides but, in contrast to SH2 domains, PTB domains recognize phosphotyrosine within a sequence motif that includes amino acids on the aminoterminal side of the tyrosine residue (Fig. 6-3) (Blaikie et al, 1994; Forman-Kay and Pawson, 1999).

Activation of growth factor receptors results in the autophosphorylation of the receptor at multiple tyrosine residues, leading to the creation of docking sites for cytoplasmic proteins that contain SH2 or PTB domains. Docking sites can also be created by the phosphorylation of cytoplasmic molecules, such as insulin receptor substrate-1 (IRS-1) by the insulin receptor, which becomes a docking site for SH2 domain–containing proteins. In this way, SH2 and PTB domains play a crucial role in linking external signals received by a membrane receptor to cytoplasmic signaling networks.

Since the original description of the SH2 domain, many additional protein modules have been identified, and their 3-dimensional structures have been described and distinct target specificities defined. These interaction modules represent independently folding domains with amino and carboxy termini in close proximity to a discrete surface ligand–binding interface, even when incorporated into a larger polypeptide (Sicheri and Kuriyan, 1997; Barford and Neel, 1998). In addition to the tyrosine-phosphorylated peptides described above, the specific binding partners for protein modules include phosphoserine- or phosphothreonine-containing peptides, proline-rich peptides, carboxyterminal motifs, and membrane phospholipids.

Two additional protein interaction domains commonly found in signaling molecules downstream of RPTKs are the SH3 (SRC homology 3) and PH (pleckstrin homology) domains (Fig. 6-3). SH3 domains are approximately 60 amino acids in length and are commonly found in signaling proteins in combination with other interaction molecules. These modules often bind to proline-based motifs in target proteins, and the interaction is not dependent on changes induced by phosphorylation. SH3 domains are known to function both in the assembly of multiprotein complexes and as regulatory domains in intramolecular interactions. One of the first protein phospho-dependent modules identified was purified as a 47-kDa protein that became phosphorylated during degranulation of platelets, and was later shown to be a substrate of protein kinase C (Imaoka et al, 1983; Tyers et al, 1987). Cloning of the cDNA encoding pleckstrin revealed a novel, ~120-a.a. domain that is highly conserved across evolution (Tyers et al, 1988); this pleckstrin homology domain (PH) interacts specifically with membrane phosphoinositides (phosphorylated forms of phosphatidylinositol [PtdIns]). Phosphoinositides are found at low levels within the cell and can be rapidly modified by phosphorylation in response to signaling. Importantly, PH domains recognize specific phosphoinositides such as PtdIns(3,4,5)P3 that are transiently produced following activation of growth factor receptors. Thus, an important function of PH domains is the recruitment of proteins to the membrane in the vicinity of an activated growth factor receptor (Scheffzek and Welti, 2012).

There is an additional class of signaling proteins that have no catalytic function (eg, NCK [non-catalytic region of tyrosine adaptor protein 1], CRK [CT10 regulator of kinase], and GRB2 [growth factor receptor bound-2]) and are composed entirely of SH2 and SH3 domains (Reebye et al, 2012). These molecules are adaptor proteins that function by interacting with signaling enzymes that do not contain SH2 domains (or other phosphotyrosine-containing modules such as PTB domains), thereby coupling them to a tyrosine kinase signaling complex. Each of these adaptor molecules has a different capacity to form protein complexes because of the binding specificity of its SH2 and SH3 domains, and the result is an organized but complex network of protein-protein interactions essential to coordinate an appropriate cellular response.

Figure 6-4 illustrates 2 examples of how protein modules function to activate growth factor receptor signal transduction. The SH2 and SH3 domain–containing adaptor protein GRB2 plays a critical role in the activation of the small guanosine triphosphatase (GTPase) protein, RAS, a central transducer of growth factor receptor signals. As described below, RAS proteins are membrane-associated molecules that actively signal when bound to the guanine triphosphate nucleotide GTP. The SH2 domain of GRB2 associates with activated growth factor receptors, whereas its SH3 domains are bound to proline-based motifs in SOS (son-of-sevenless), a guanine nucleotide exchange protein that activates RAS. Consequently, receptor activation leads to the recruitment of the GRB2-SOS complex close to its target, RAS, leading to its activation and downstream signaling (Lemmon and Schlessinger, 2010).

Activation of growth factor receptors also results in the activation of phosphoinositide kinases that phosphorylate the 3′ hydroxyl group of the inositol ring. Phosphatidylinositol-3-kinase (PI3K) is a heterodimer made up of a catalytic subunit, p110, and a regulatory subunit, p85, that contains 2 SH2 domains. Following receptor activation, the PI3K is recruited

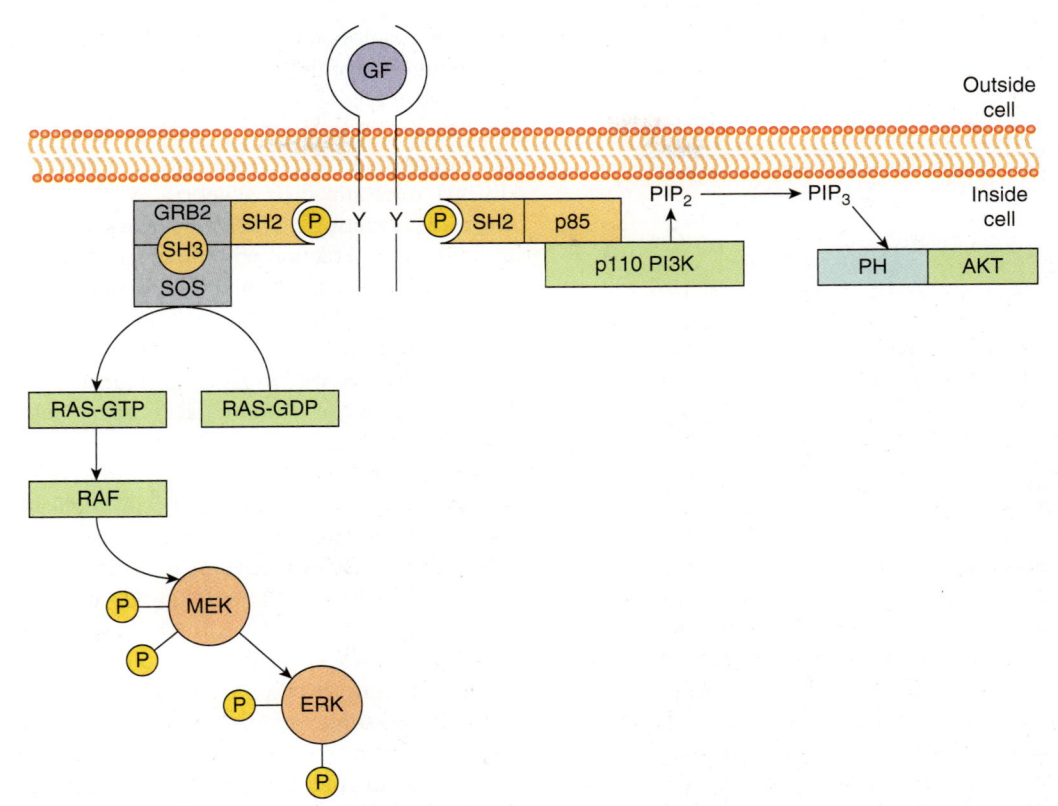

FIGURE 6–4 Recruitment of cytoplasmic signaling molecules by receptor protein tyrosine kinases. Binding of a receptor to a growth factor (GF) leads to phosphorylation of the intracellular domain on tyrosine (Y) residues; this interaction allows the SH2 domain–mediated association of enzymes and adaptor molecules such as GRB2 and p85. GRB2 is associated with the guanine nucleotide exchange factor SOS (son-of-sevenless). SOS recruited to activated receptor complexes then catalyzes the exchange of guanosine diphosphate (GDP) for guanosine triphosphate (GTP) on RAS. GTP-bound RAS binds the protein kinase RAF and activates a kinase cascade including MEK and ERK (see Sec. 6.2.4). The heterodimeric phosphoinositide kinase, phosphatidylinositol-3-kinase (PI3K), is composed of a catalytic subunit, p110, and an adaptor or regulatory subunit, called p85 that contains 2 SH2 domains. Binding of the p85/p110 complex to activated growth factor receptors via the p85 SH2 domain activates catalytic activity of p110, which phosphorylates phosphatidylinositol-4,5-bisphosphate (PIP$_2$). The product of this reaction, phosphatidylinositol-3,4,5-triphosphate (PIP$_3$), serves as a membrane anchoring site for PH domain–containing proteins such as AKT. See text for additional details.

to the activated receptor by the p85 SH2 domains, which binds to specific phosphotyrosine interaction motifs, leading to activation of the p110 catalytic subunit and the production of PtdIns(3,4,5)P3 (described in Sec. 6.2.5) (Lemmon and Schlessinger, 2010).

6.2.3 RAS Proteins

RAS proteins control signaling networks that regulate normal cell growth and malignant transformation. Three human *RAS* genes encode the proteins, H-RAS, K-RAS, and N-RAS, and are part of a large family of low-molecular-weight GTP-binding proteins. RAS proteins have a molecular weight of 21 kDa and share 85% sequence homology: they are GTPases that cycle between an active GTP-bound "on" and an inactive guanosine diphosphate (GDP)–bound "off" configuration in response to extracellular signals, essentially functioning as a molecular binary switch (Fig. 6–5). RAS is activated by guanine nucleotide exchange factors (GEFs), such as SOS described above, that releases RAS-bound GDP and allows GTP binding to RAS (Buday and Downward, 2008).

RAS activation is a key signaling event in the development of several types of cancer (Li et al, 2018). For example, the chemical induction of skin or mammary tumors in the rat is consistently accompanied by the acquisition of activating mutations in RAS (see Chap. 5, Sec. 5.2.2). Whole exome sequencing also supports a role of activating RAS mutations early in the development of human cancers, such as pancreatic ductal adenocarcinoma and non–small cell lung cancer, although the genetic alterations tend to differ between different tumor types (Li et al, 2018). Thus, research has focused on the mechanisms by which RAS is activated (ie, converted to the active, GTP-bound form), and the downstream effectors that lead to activation of downstream signaling cascades. A well-characterized effector is the protein kinase RAF. RAS-GTP binding to RAF activates its kinase activity, and consequently activates a downstream cascade of protein kinases that include MEK and ERK (see Fig. 6–4). Additional RAS-GTP effectors include the exchange factor for another small GTPase RAL (RALGDS), and the p110 catalytic subunit of PI3K (see Fig. 6–5). Through these diverse effectors, RAS proteins regulate cell cycle progression, cell survival, and cytoskeletal organization.

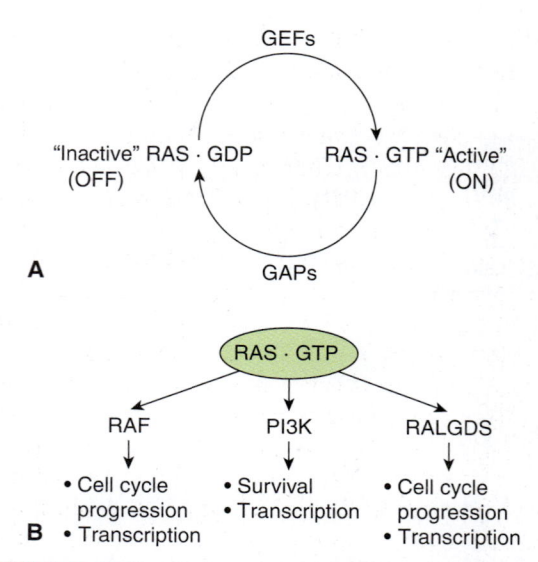

FIGURE 6–5 RAS protein activation and downstream signaling. **A)** The small GTPase RAS cycles between an inactive GDP-bound state and the active GTP-bound state. RAS activation is regulated by guanine nucleotide exchange factors (GEFs) that promote exchange of GDP for GTP. GTP hydrolysis requires GTPase-activating proteins (GAPs) that enhance the weak intrinsic GTPase activity of RAS proteins. **B)** Once in its active GTP-bound form, RAS interacts with different families of effector proteins including RAF protein kinases, PI3Ks and RAL GDS, a GEF for the RAS-related protein RAL. Activation of these downstream pathways leads to cellular responses including gene transcription, cell cycle progression, and survival.

Termination of RAS activity occurs through a feedback loop that involves hydrolysis of GTP, converting it to GDP by action of GTPase-activating proteins (GAPs) that promote the intrinsic GTPase activity of the RAS proteins themselves (Fig. 6–5). Therefore, a balance between the activities of GEFs and GAPs determines the activity of normal RAS proteins. For example, when GAPs are inactivated, the balance tips to RAS activation. Both the GEFs and several of the GAP family members, which are often represented by p120^{GAP}, are themselves regulated by receptor tyrosine kinase signaling cascades.

The normal function of RAS proteins requires posttranslational modification. Newly synthesized RAS proteins are modified by the addition of a lipid chain to a cysteine residue in the carboxy terminus of RAS proteins. This covalently linked lipid is either a farnesyl or geranylgeranyl group (collectively termed *prenylation*) and is required for RAS association with intracellular membranes. Prenylation is important for the oncogenic activity of RAS proteins. Both H-RAS and N-RAS are also subsequently modified by the addition of 2 palmitoyl long-chain fatty acids that are important for the correct localization of these proteins to specific parts of the membrane. RAS proteins are activated and signal from specific microdomains within the plasma membrane, as well as distinct subcellular compartments such as the Golgi and endosomes.

Abnormalities in RAS protein activity have been identified in greater than 30% of human malignancies, either via genetic alterations (most commonly in K-RAS) that lock RAS in an active GTP-bound state, or via deregulated signaling from upstream components (see Chap. 7, Sec. 7.5.5). Although most common oncogenic RAS mutations (eg, at RAS glycine residues that include G12, G13, and G16) act to impede GAP-mediated GTP hydrolysis and thus render RAS preferentially GTP-bound and active, each of these residues serves slightly distinct roles and their genetic alteration elicits distinct biochemical alterations. These alterations, in turn, affect activity cycling and interaction with downstream partners; for example, the point substitution at G13 to glutamate (G13D) potentiates GEF-mediated exchange but the G12 point substitution to valine (G12V) does not (Li et al, 2018).

RAS proteins are essential for normal cell function, but the specificity of tumor-specific isoforms of RAS have made targeting activated RAS an intensive focus for anticancer therapeutics. Statins, which are used widely to lower serum cholesterol, have also been implicated in lowering incidence and mortality of several types of human cancer (Demierre et al, 2005; Nielsen et al, 2012). Statins inhibit the enzyme 3-hydroxy-3-methylglutaryl coenzyme A reductase (HMGCR), which catalyzes the conversion of HMG-CoA to mevalonate (MVA), a precursor to geranylgeranyl pyrophosphate and farnesyl pyrophosphate. These 2 end products are essential substrates of protein farnesyl transferase or geranylgeranyl transferase that lead to protein prenylation, which is required for membrane localization of all proteins in the RAS-GTPase superfamily. Inhibitors of these enzymes were developed as potential inhibitors of oncogenic RAS activity in cancer treatment, with limited success (Berndt et al, 2011). The efficacy of farnesyl transferase inhibitors (FTIs) does not necessarily depend on the presence of activating RAS mutations, and may affect any number of the hundreds of other proteins that are modified by prenylation. The (limited) ability of statins to inhibit cancer cell proliferation has also been shown to act independently of RAS protein prenylation (Yu et al, 2018). Other mediators of protein prenylation may be targets in cancer therapy; for example, RHEB, an activator of TORC1 (described in Sec. 6.2.5), may affect FTI activity in tumors. The FTI lonafarnib has been approved for the treatment of progeria, a disease characterized by accelerated aging, increased cancer risk, and early mortality. Akin to the impact of FTIs on RAS, lonafarnib inhibits the prenylation of the defective lamin A protein (called progerin) in Hutchinson-Gilford progeria syndrome patients, thus mitigating disease phenotypes and leading to a lower mortality rate (Gordon et al, 2018).

6.2.4 Mitogen-Activated Protein Kinase Signaling

Mitogen-activated protein kinases (MAPKs) control highly conserved signaling pathways that regulate all eukaryotic cells. Mammalian cells contain multiple distinct MAPK pathways that respond to divergent signals including growth factors and environmental stresses such as osmotic stress and ionizing radiation. All MAPK pathways include a core 3-tiered signaling unit, in which MAPKs are activated by the sequential activation of linked serine/threonine kinases (Fig. 6–6).

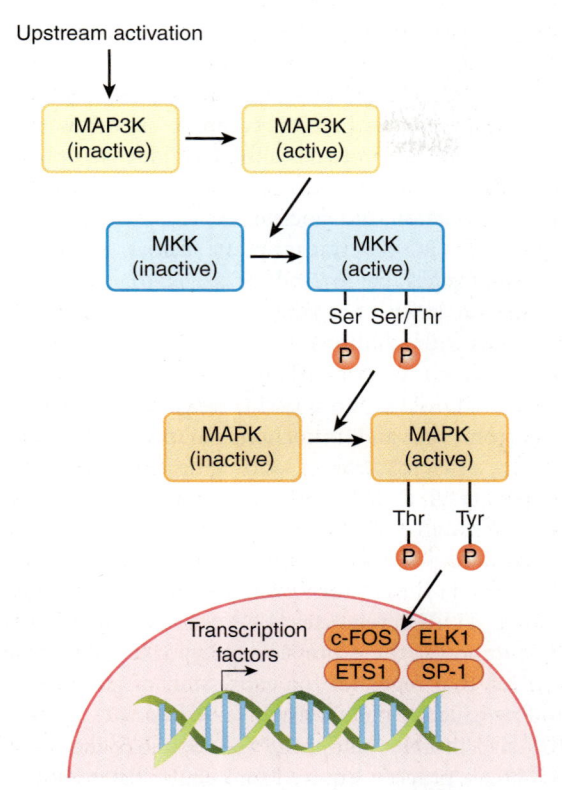

FIGURE 6–6 The MAPK core signaling module. All MAPK pathways include a core 3-tiered signaling unit, in which MAPKs are activated by the sequential activation of linked serine/threonine kinases. The MKKs are unique dual specificity kinases that phosphorylate both tyrosine (Y) and threonine (T) residues within an activation motif found in the MAPKs. P, phosphate. Transcription factors that are regulated by MAPK signaling include c-FOS (which is complexed with JUN to form AP-1), ETS1, ELK1, and SP-1.

The MAPK pathway is activated by phosphorylation of threonine and tyrosine residues in a T-X-Y (T = threonine, X = any amino acid, Y = tyrosine) motif in the kinase activation loop. This phosphorylation is achieved by a family of dual-specificity kinases referred to as MEKs or MKKs (MAPK-kinase). MEK (mitogen-activated protein [MAP] / extracellular signal-related kinase [ERK] kinase) activity is regulated by serine and threonine phosphorylation catalyzed by kinases called MAP3Ks (MAPK-kinase-kinase). Several distinct families of MAP3Ks are activated by diverse upstream stimuli that link the activation of the MAPK signaling unit to extracellular signals. These structurally related pathways are controlled by stimuli that elicit very distinct physiological consequences (eg, mitogenesis or the stress response). Within each pathway, specificity is determined by scaffold molecules that link specific core components. Similarly, although all MAPKs phosphorylate very similar consensus motifs in their target substrates, specificity of protein substrate selection is ensured by docking domains that mediate binding of specific kinases to their substrates (Cargnello and Roux, 2011).

Three distinct MAPK pathways have been characterized in mammalian cells: the extracellular signal regulated kinase 1 and 2 (ERK1/2), the c-JUN N-terminal kinase or stress-activated protein kinase (JNK/SAPK), and p38. As described in Section 6.2.3, activation of RAS proteins causes the activation of RAF, a MAP3K upstream of ERK1/2. ERK kinase activation is a final signaling step that is shared among several pathways stimulated by growth factor receptors, such as those for EGF, PDGF, FGF (see Chap. 7, Sec. 7.5.3), and by more diverse stimuli from cytokine receptors and antigen receptors (Cargnello and Roux, 2011). RAF directly activates MEK-1/2 by phosphorylating it on serine residues, which enhances the availability of the catalytic site to potential substrates. One hallmark of RAF that is shared with other serine/threonine protein kinases in the MAPK signaling network is their trans-activation via side-by-side dimerization of homotypic (same) or heterotypic (different) kinases (Lavoie et al, 2014). Knowledge of the crystal structures of the active RAF complex has led to new strategies for drug development, including dabrafenib and vemurafenib (see below, and Chap. 19, Sec. 19.5.3), and other second-generation inhibitors that limit RAF dimerization and signaling activation (Brummer and McInnes, 2020).

Activated MEK-1/2 is a dual-specificity kinase that phosphorylates the ERK kinases. MEK-induced phosphorylation of ERK occurs on threonine and tyrosine residues in the activation loop, which induces catalytic activation of ERK and phosphorylation of both cytoplasmic and nuclear protein substrates that regulate cell migration, proliferation, and differentiation. In the cytoplasm, activated ERK phosphorylates cytoskeletal proteins as well as the 90-kDa ribosomal S6 kinase (RSK) family of protein kinases. Activated RSK kinases regulate translation, transcription, and survival signaling through phosphorylation of both nuclear and cytoplasmic substrates (Houles and Roux, 2018). Activation of ERK also induces its translocation to the nucleus where it phosphorylates and activates transcription factors (see Sec. 6.2.6), including SP1 (Specificity Protein 1), ETS1 (v-ets erythroblastosis virus E26 oncogene homolog 1), ELK1 (ETS-like 1), and cFOS (Finkel–Biskis–Jinkins murine osteogenic sarcoma; c-FOS exists in a heterodimer with JUN/AP-1) (Fig. 6–6).

Dysregulation of MAPK signaling has been implicated in malignant transformation. Increased levels of activated ERKs are frequently found in human tumors, and often are attributable to the presence of mutations in RAS or other upstream components in growth factor signaling cascades. Mutations in the RAS-MAPK signaling cascade are found in about 80% of melanomas (where *RAS* and *BRAF* mutations are mutually exclusive), and in 67% of T-cell precursor acute lymphoblastic leukemia, 55% colon/rectal cancers, and a substantial fraction of lung adenocarcinomas (Li et al, 2018). Key downstream MAPKs in cancer are the RAF serine/threonine kinases, ARAF, BRAF, and RAF1 (CRAF). Activating mutations in the RAF family member BRAF occur in at least 50% of malignant melanomas and at lower frequency in a wide range of other human tumors (see also Chap. 7, Sec. 7.5.5) (Li et al, 2018). The most common alteration in BRAF are point substitutions at Valine 600 (V600), which is a residue located within the activation loop of the kinase domain and leads to constitutive activation (Proietti et al, 2020). The selective BRAF inhibitors vemurafenib, dabrafenib, and encorafenib are used widely in patients with advanced melanoma that harbor a BRAF V600 alteration (see also Chap. 19, Sec. 19.5.3). Vemurafenib has selective activity against major sites of genetic alteration in BRAF that incude V600E, V600D, and V600R; dabrafenib has selective activity against these aforementioned variants and V600K; whereas encorafenib targets V600E, V600K, and, to some extent, wild-type BRAF.

6.2.5 Phosphoinositide Signaling

Phosphoinositides are rare phospholipids of cell membranes that are dynamically regulated in response to growth factor signaling. They contribute to signal propagation by 2 main mechanisms; by serving as precursors of the second messengers diacylglycerol (DAG) and inositol triphosphate (Ins(1,4,5)P3) and Ca^{2+}, or by binding to signaling proteins that contain specific phosphoinositide-binding modules. Figure 6–7 illustrates some of the important phospholipid products that function in growth factor signal transduction. Phosphoinositides can be phosphorylated or dephosphorylated by lipid kinases and phosphatases at distinct positions on the inositol ring in response to growth factor signaling. Activation of PI3K (described in Sec. 6.2.2), which specifically phosphorylates the 3′ position, leads to the rapid production of PtdIns(3,4,5)P3. PtdIns(3,4,5)P3 levels are tightly controlled by the action of inositol phosphatases. Phosphatase and tensin homolog (PTEN) is a 3′-phosphoinositide phosphatase that dephosphorylates the 3′ position of PtdIns(3,4,5)P3 and PtdIns(3,4)P2 and, therefore, functions as a major negative regulator of PI3K signaling (see Chap. 7, Sec. 7.6.2).

The production of PtdIns(3,4,5)P3 leads to the recruitment of the PH-domain–containing protein serine/threonine kinases PDK1 and AKT. AKT is activated by conformational changes evoked by phospholipid binding, and phosphorylation by PDK1 at threonine 308. Full activation of AKT requires phosphorylation at a second site (S473) by the serine kinase complex mTOR Complex 2 (TORC2) (Hoxhaj and Manning, 2020). Numerous important substrates for activated AKT have been identified that fall into 2 main classes, as regulators of cell survival or regulators of cell proliferation (see Chap. 8, Sec. 8.2.4). AKT phosphorylates substrates that, in turn, lead to the activation of TORC1, the serine/threonine kinase mammalian target of rapamycin (mTOR) complex (see below) involved in the regulation of protein translation, glucose uptake, and glycolysis. Activated AKT also controls cell survival through the phosphorylation and nuclear exclusion of the Forkhead Box class "O" (FOXO) transcription factors, preventing the expression of genes that can induce cell death.

Mammalian target of rapamycin (mTOR) is an S/T kinase that interacts with additional proteins to form 2 distinct functional complexes, termed mTOR Complex 1 (TORC1) and 2 (TORC2). TORC1 controls a wide range of cellular processes ranging from cell and mitochondrial metabolism, protein translation, cell proliferation, and aging (Morita et al, 2015; Papadopoli et al, 2019). For example, it stimulates protein synthesis through the phosphorylation of eukaryotic translation initiation factor–binding protein (4E-BP1) and S6 kinase 1 (S6K1) that in turn promote cap-dependent protein translation. TORC1 regulates ATP production and metabolism by promoting the expression of hypoxia-inducible factor 1α (HIF1α) that regulates the expression of glycolytic genes controlling glucose metabolism (see Chap. 12, Sec. 12.2.3). TORC1 also inhibits autophagy (see Sec. 6.5 and Chap. 12, Sec. 12.3.6), a process required for cellular catabolism under nutrient starvation, by phosphorylation and inhibition of the activity of autophagy-related gene 13 (ATG13), which forms part of a kinase complex required to initiate autophagy. Less is known about the functions of TORC2, but its activity also promotes cell growth through activation of protein kinases AKT (described above), serum- and glucocorticoid-induced kinase (SGK1), and protein kinase C-α (PKCα). The SGK1 kinase is activated by TORC2 and regulates ion transport and cell proliferation. TORC2 can also regulate actin cytoskeleton dynamics through the phosphorylation and activation of protein kinase C alpha (PKCα).

Human malignancies are frequently associated with inactivating mutations in the PTEN gene (see Chap. 7, Sec. 7.6.2). Loss of PTEN leads to accumulation of 3′-phosphoinositides,

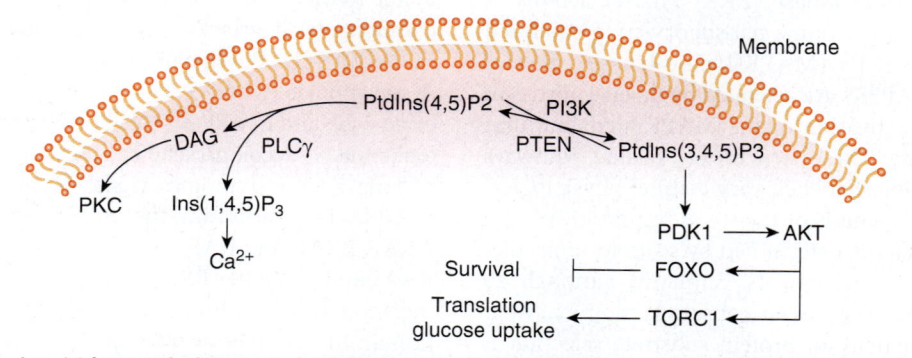

FIGURE 6–7 Phosphoinositide metabolism in growth factor signaling. The positions in the inositol ring that are modified by phosphorylation are numbered. PtdIns(4,5)P2 is hydrolyzed by phospholipase Cγ (PLCγ) to produce second messengers DAG (diacylglycerol) and inositol triphosphate (Ins(1,4,5)P3) that result in activation of protein kinase C (PKC) and release of calcium (Ca^{2+}) from intracellular stores. Lipid kinases (PI3K) and phosphatases (PTEN) positively or negatively regulate the phosphorylation of the inositol 3′ position and the production of PtdIns(3,4,5)P3. PtdIns(3,4,5) signals downstream to activate PDK1 and AKT and the activation of metabolic and survival pathways (see text for details).

causing deregulated AKT activity and malignant transformation. PTEN also plays a role in chromatin organization and the DNA damage response; it is found as an early genetic perturbation in mismatch repair (MMR) deficiency (Lopez et al, 2020). PTEN loss is also thought to contribute to tumorigenesis via perturbations in genome stability, for example, via effects on checkpoint control, including increased AKT-mediated cytoplasmic sequestration of the checkpoint kinase 1, CHK1 (see Chap. 8, Sec 8.3.1, and Chap. 9, Sec. 9.4) (Fusco et al, 2020). PTEN loss also influences the tumor microenvironment, and downregulation of PTEN-targeted microRNAs stimulates tumor invasiveness (Bronisz et al, 2011).

Variations in PI3K are one of the most frequently reported sequence alterations in cancer, and across all human cancers, PIK3-CA is the most frequently mutated oncogene (Vasan et al, 2019). Inhibitors against PI3K have generally been found to be toxic, and although some drugs such as the PI3Kα inhibitor alpelisib have been approved by the FDA after a large phase III clinical trial showed improved progression-free survival in patients harboring ER+, PIK3CA-mutant metastatic breast cancer (Andre et al, 2019). Inhibition of mTOR (TORC1) and its downstream inhibitor, PTEN, have also shown promise as a therapeutic strategy against cancer (Fusco et al, 2020). Loss of PTEN is often accompanied by microsatellite instability and other hypermutated phenotypes, and PTEN-deficient tumors are being investigated for their response to the immune checkpoint inhibitor, pembrolizumab. PTEN loss or inactivation may promote resistance to other agents including the CDK4/6 inhibitor ribociclib and the aromatase inhibitor letrozole (Fusco et al, 2020). PTEN alterations are also associated with resistance in patients treated with PI3Kα inhibitors (Juric et al, 2015; Costa et al, 2020; Razavi et al, 2020), and PTEN is of interest as a biomarker of breast cancers that are proficient in mismatch repair (Lopez et al, 2020). The mTOR inhibitors sirolimus (rapamycin) and its analogs, temsirolimus and everolimus, are used as immune suppressors in organ transplants, and also have limited activity as anticancer agents (see Chap. 19, Sec. 19.5.2).

6.2.6 Transcriptional Response to Signaling

One important consequence of growth factor signaling is the transcription of genes that coordinate cell growth, cellular differentiation, cell death, and other biological effects. Transcription of genes is catalyzed by the enzyme RNA polymerase II and is regulated by supporting molecules, collectively termed *transcription factors*. Transcription factors can activate or repress gene expression by binding to specific DNA recognition sequences, typically 6 to 8 base pairs in length, that are found in the promoter regions at the 5′ (proximal) end of genes. The formation of RNA transcripts is influenced by the interaction of these gene-specific factors with elements of a common core of molecules regulating the activity of RNA polymerase II. The activity of transcription factors can be modified, frequently by phosphorylation, through the activity of many of the signaling pathways described above, including the MAPK and PI3K pathways. Even mTOR, which was previously thought to act primarily in the cytoplasm, can modulate transcription, histone modifications, and chromatin remodeling in the nucleus (Laribee and Weisman, 2020).

Transcription factors are modular, consisting of a specific DNA-binding region that binds to specific DNA sequences, and an activation or repression domain, which interacts with other proteins to stimulate or repress transcription from a nearby promoter. Based on the structure of their DNA-binding domains, transcription factors can be placed into homeodomain (sometimes called *helix-turn-helix*), zinc-finger, or leucine-zipper, and helix-loop-helix (HLH), families (Fig. 6–8).

The homeodomain factors contain a 60–amino acid DNA-binding domain called a *homeobox*: the name is derived from the *Drosophila* homeotic genes that determine body structure identity. In vertebrates, homeodomain proteins have similar properties and function as master regulators during development. The homeodomain contains 3 helical regions. The third helical region, as well as amino acids at the amino-terminal end of the homeodomain, directly contact DNA.

Zinc-finger (ZNF) transcription factors contain a sequence of 20 to 30 amino acids with 2 paired cysteine or histidine residues that are coordinated by a zinc ion. Binding of the zinc ion folds these polypeptide sequences into compact domains with α helices that insert into the DNA (see Fig. 6–8).

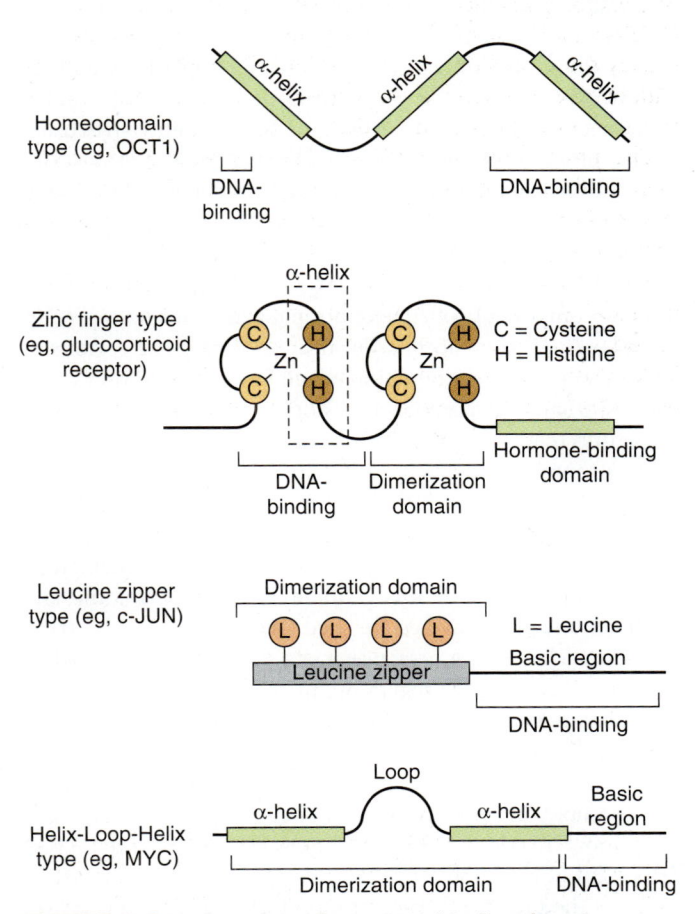

FIGURE 6–8 Transcription factor DNA-binding domain classes. The general structure of the 4 major classes of DNA-binding domains found in modular transcription factors.

Many ZNF factors also contain a SCAN domain, and these so-called ZSCAN proteins (there are more than 50 members in humans) play numerous roles in differentiation and growth, and in the development of cancers. For example, copy number variations in one ZSCAN gene, *MZF1*, are seen in breast, lung, bladder, glioma, and colon cancer, and other ZSCAN members are implicated in numerous cancers (Huang et al, 2019).

Leucine-zipper transcription factors contain helical regions with leucine residues occurring at every seventh amino acid, which all protrude from the same side of the α-helix. These leucines form a hydrophobic interaction surface with leucine zippers of similar proteins. Additional members of this family contain other hydrophobic amino acids in the α-helices that comprise the dimerization domain. The DNA-binding regions of the α-helices contain basic amino acids that interact with the DNA backbone. These factors, also referred to as *basic zipper proteins*, bind to DNA as homo- or heterodimers, and include the FOS/JUN pair (also called the AP-1 transcription factor), which becomes activated by cellular stress. Members of this group also tend to become activated by proliferative and developmental stimuli.

Basic helix-loop-helix factors share similarities with the basic zipper factors described above but include a loop region that separates the 2 α-helical regions of the polypeptide. The carboxyterminal α-helix mediates formation of homo- or heterodimers that contact DNA with basic amino acids found in the aminoterminal helix.

Transcriptional activation and repression domains are structurally diverse regions, ranging from the random coil conformation of acidic activation domains to the highly structured ligand-binding domains of hormone receptors. Both transcription activators and repressors exert their effects by binding to multisubunit coactivators or corepressors that act to modify chromatin structure and assembly of RNA Pol II complexes. Enzymes that regulate histone acetylation and phosphorylation are key components of transcriptional activator and repressor complexes. Histone acetylation near the promoter regions of genes facilitates the interaction of the DNA with transcription factors, whereas deacetylation results in condensed chromatin structures that inhibit assembly of the transcription machinery at the promoter (see Chap. 3, Sec. 3.1.2).

Alteration in transcription factor (TF) function, which can cause unregulated activation or repression of gene expression, can lead to transformation and is well documented in human cancers. Numerous genome-wide transcriptome and epigenetic studies have established that changes in the transcriptional landscape of cancer cells promote their transformation. Major master regulators of these transitions include cancer-associated transcription factors such as MYC and p53, and the aberrant reacquisition of developmentally regulated factors can also influence cancer progression (Patra, 2020). For example, in glioblastoma, the neurodevelopmental transcriptional regulators POU3F2, SOX2, SALL2, and OLIG2 are essential for glioblastoma propagation (Suva et al, 2014), whereas the proneural transcription factor ASCL1 suppresses glioblastoma via the reestablishment of responsiveness to differentiation (Park et al, 2017).

6.2.7 Biological Outcomes of Growth Factor Signaling

Growth factor signaling results in changes in gene expression that influence myriad physiological responses such as cell cycle progression, cellular differentiation, cell growth, survival, or apoptosis. Changes in gene expression downstream of growth factor signaling proceed in 2 stages. Expression of immediate early genes, which often encode transcription factors, does not require new protein synthesis. Immediate early gene expression is followed by expression of other genes, sometimes called *delayed response genes*, which are often the products of the transcription induced by the immediate early genes.

Cells in the G1 phase of the cell cycle respond to external stimuli by either withdrawing from the cell cycle (G0) or advancing through the restriction point (see Chap. 8, Sec. 8.2.1) toward cell division. Progression through G1 and entry into S phase normally requires stimulation by mitogens, such as growth factors. For example, the D-type cyclins are expressed as part of the delayed early response to stimulation of growth factor signaling cascades. These D-type cyclins assemble with cyclin-dependent kinases, and the active complex phosphorylates and inactivates the retinoblastoma (Rb) protein, releasing the E2F transcription factor family that in turn activates the transcription of genes required for S-phase entry (see Chap. 8, Sec. 8.2.3). A common property of cancer cells is their ability to undergo G1-phase progression in the absence of external mitogenic stimuli. Activating mutations in any of the growth factor signaling components upstream of G1 checkpoint control can uncouple these transcriptional regulatory networks, and lead to precocious S-phase entry and cell cycle progression.

A second important consequence of growth factor signaling is cell survival. Normal cells require continuous exposure to survival factors, such as soluble growth factors, or cell matrix interactions, to suppress apoptosis. Tissue homeostasis is maintained through the limited supply or spatial restriction of these factors that limit cell expansion. Evasion of this control mechanism is another common feature of tumor cells. As discussed above (Sec. 6.2.5), activating mutations in survival pathways, such as activating mutations in the PI3K pathway or loss of function mutations in PTEN, can confer resistance to apoptotic signals that would normally limit deregulated cell proliferation.

6.2.8 Suppression of Growth Factor Signaling via Protein Phosphatases

Signaling from activated growth factor receptors is tightly regulated both temporally and spatially, and often involves coordinated regulation through protein phosphatases. Protein phosphatases can be broadly defined as lipid phosphatases (eg, PTEN and phosphoinositol phosphatases) that attenuate or antagonize lipid-directed protein kinase activation (eg, PI3K-AKT), protein tyrosine phosphatases (referred to as the PTP superfamily), and protein serine/threonine phosphatases.

More than 100 PTP family members have been identified in humans (Hatzihristidis et al, 2014). Whether they recognize phosphotyrosine (pY) solely or a combination of phosphorylated tyrosine/serine/threonine (Y/S/T) residues, the catalytic core contains a conserved catalytic domain of ~200 to 240 amino acids, and a signature motif that is critical for enzymatic activity (Tonks, 2006). For almost every RTK, there is a PTP associated with the complex that attenuates its activity and that is corecruited to active receptor complexes, for example, through interactions with SH2, PTB, or TKB domains. For example, the opposing action of protein tyrosine phosphatases can eliminate docking sites for proteins containing SH2 domains or inhibit tyrosine kinase activity by dephosphorylation of regulatory phosphorylation sites in the kinase activation loop. PTPs also play a critical role in the immune response, and the inhibition of specific PTPs such as PTB1B or TC-PTP (which inhibit the JAK-STAT [Janus-activated kinase-signal transducers and activators of transcription] complex, among other targets) have been proposed as a means to promote T-cell differentiation and thus enhance CAR-T–mediated responses (see Chap. 21, Sec. 21.5.5) (Penafuerte et al, 2017). Genetic alterations in one tyrosine phosphatase, SHP2 (encoded by *PTPN11*), are found in humans with Noonan syndrome who have a higher prevalence of certain cancers, and alterations in PTPN11 are found in a subset of acute myeloid lymphoma (AML) patients (Mohi and Neel, 2007). Allosteric inhibitors of SHP2 have been found to inhibit tumor growth in vitro and in mouse tumor xenograft models (Chen et al, 2016; Garcia Fortanet et al, 2016).

The Ser/Thr (S/T) phosphatases play important roles in normal and cancer cell proliferation. There are 2 broad classes of S/T phosphatases: type I (PP1) and type II (PP2). PP1 contains 3 isoforms—α, β, and γ—that each localize to different subcellular compartments. The PP2 group are further divided into 3 groups: metal-independent members such as PP2A, PP4, PP5, and PP6, Ca^{2+}-dependent members such as PP2B and PP7, and Mg^{2+}/Mn^{2+}-dependent members such as PP2C. These enzymes typically exist as heterodimers or heterotrimers. For example, PP2A is composed of a catalytic subunit (PP2Ac; with 2 isoforms in humans) and 2 structural subunits (PP2A A; also with 2 isoforms in humans), and several regulatory subunit families; B, B′, B″, and B‴ that influence localization and substrate specificity. PP2A enzymes play key roles in the cell cycle and the DNA damage response (Peng and Maller, 2010), as well as WNT signaling (see Sec. 6.4.1), stem cell function, and cancer (Grech et al, 2016; Thompson and Williams, 2018). Biochemical and clinical evidence points to PP2A as a tumor suppressor, thus underscoring its importance in attenuating cell signaling involved in cancer. It regulates signaling via β-catenin and, depending on the context, can positively or negatively regulate WNT signaling. A role of PP2A-PR61α has also been established in stem cell renewal via effects on c-Myc dephosphorylation (Thompson and Williams, 2018). Other PP2A targets include TP53, CDC25, PI3K/AKT, RAF/MAPK/ERK, p70 S6K, mTOR, FOXM1, and BCL-2/Caspase-3 (Grech et al, 2016). For these reasons, approaches to selectively activate PP2A function (alone, or in combination with other protein kinase inhibitors) are considered potential strategies for the treatment of cancer (Westermarck, 2018).

6.3 CYTOPLASMIC TYROSINE KINASE SIGNALING

Tyrosine kinases (TKs) also play a central role in the transmission of signals from distinct classes of cell surface receptors that themselves do not possess intrinsic TK activity. Cytoplasmic TKs are recruited to cell surface molecules following receptor activation, and many of the intracellular events that occur resemble those evoked by receptor TKs as described in Section 6.2. Figure 6–9 depicts a schematic showing selected cytoplasmic TKs. A feature of these cytoplasmic TKs is the presence of conserved protein modules, such as SH2 and SH3 domains. These protein modules function to regulate kinase activity and serve to couple these molecules to extracellular receptors. Some of the features of receptor signaling pathways that utilize cytoplasmic TKs are described below.

6.3.1 Cytokine Signaling

Cytokines regulate the proliferation, differentiation, and activity of hematopoietic cell lineages through interaction with structurally and functionally related receptors of the cytokine receptor superfamily. These receptors do not contain intrinsic TK activity but rather transmit intracellular signals through the association with the Janus kinase (JAK) family of kinases (Martin, 2003; Hosseini et al, 2020). With some exceptions, for example, the receptors for granulocyte colony-stimulating factor (G-CSF) and erythropoietin (see Chap. 17, Sec. 17.5.2), most cytokine receptors are multisubunit complexes and contain a unique ligand-binding subunit and a common or shared signaling subunit. There are 4 distinct signaling chains: the gp130 subunit (interleukin [IL]-6Rβc, where "c" denotes the chain, is common to other cytokine receptors), and the IL-3Rβc, IL-2Rβc, and IL-2Rγc chains that can transmit signals from many different ligands.

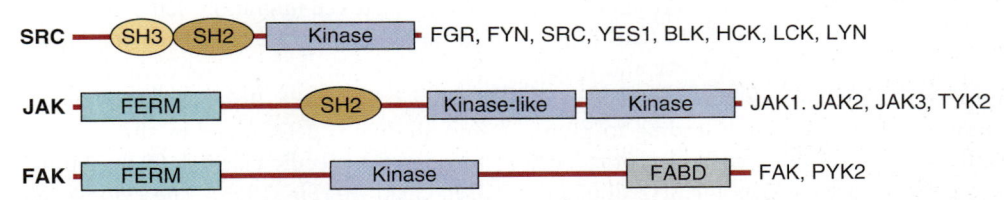

FIGURE 6–9 Cytoplasmic protein TKs. The general structure of several cytoplasmic protein TK families is illustrated. Members of each family are listed beside each diagram.

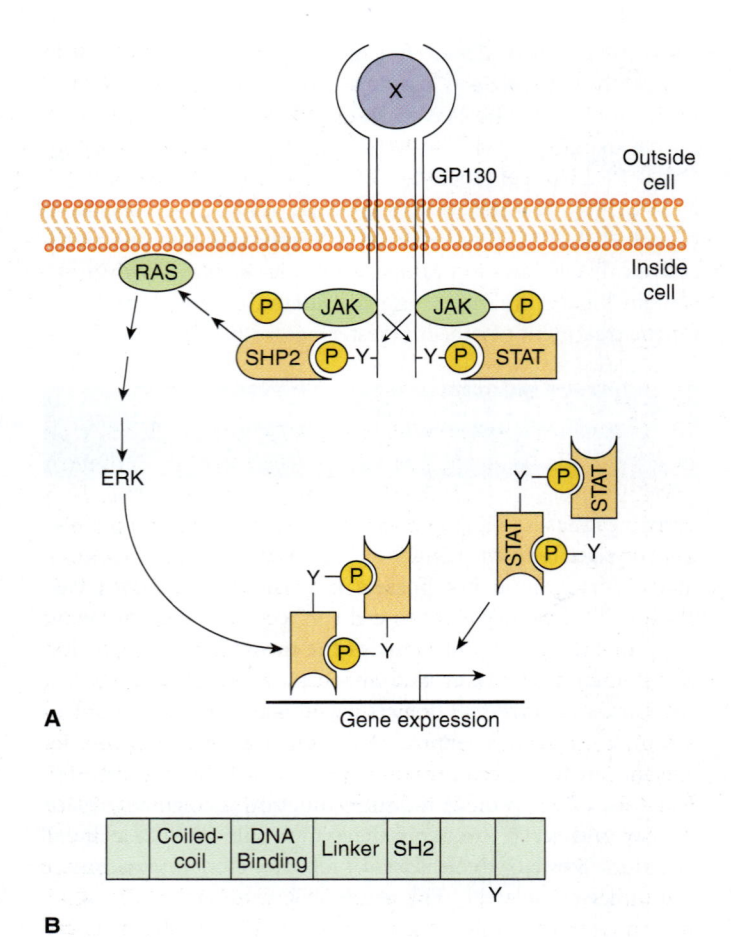

FIGURE 6–10 Cytokine receptor signaling. **A)** Cytokine (X) binding induces receptor dimerization resulting in JAK activation and phosphorylation of the GBP130 receptor subunit. STATs then bind the phosphorylated receptor and are subsequently phosphorylated, inducing dimerization and transport to the nucleus, where they activate downstream target genes. GBP130 phosphorylation also results in recruitment of tyrosine phosphatase SHP2, which in turn leads to RAS activation. **B)** Structure of the STATs. STATs contain a DNA-binding domain, an SH2 domain, and a conserved tyrosine residue in the carboxy terminus.

Similar to the signaling cascade observed with other receptor types, cytokine binding leads to initiation of downstream signaling events (Fig. 6–10). As the cytoplasmic domains of the common receptor subunits do not possess intrinsic TK activity, noncovalent association with the JAK family of cytoplasmic TKs is required for signal transmission. The JAKs contain a FERM domain ([Four] 4.1 protein, Ezrin, Radixin, Moesin), an SH2 domain, a functional TK domain, and a kinase-like domain (or pseudokinase domain) that can exert autoinhibitory activity on the kinase domain (Fig. 6–9). The FERM domain functions to regulate JAK kinase activity and mediate association with receptors. Upon cytokine binding, JAKs are tyrosine phosphorylated and activated, leading to phosphorylation of specific tyrosine residues on the receptor. This activated complex generates docking sites for SH2 domain–containing proteins such as the STAT family of transcription factors (Fig. 6–10) as well as GRB2 and PI3K (described in

Sec. 6.2). STATs are tyrosine phosphorylated, inducing homo- or heterodimerization and subsequent transport to the nucleus where they regulate gene expression. STATs contain a conserved amino-terminal DNA–binding domain that is specific to the STAT family of proteins, a conserved SH2 domain, and a carboxyterminal tyrosine residue that mediates dimerization. In addition to tyrosine phosphorylation, STATs can be phosphorylated by serine/threonine kinases such as ERK and mTOR (see Sec. 6.2), and serine phosphorylation of STAT regulates its ability to activate transcription.

Both gene translocations and activating point mutations in JAK2 have been identified in myeloproliferative disorders and leukemia. A common feature of the translocations is a protein product that fuses the kinase domain of JAK2 with a dimerization or oligomerization domain of the fusion partner leading to constitutive kinase activation. JAK2 point substitutions, such as V617F, are found frequently in myeloproliferative diseases. The V617F variant is thought to disrupt the autoinhibitory interaction between the pseudokinase and catalytic kinase domains. Several JAK2 kinase inhibitors have been developed and assessed in clinical trials. For example, ruxolitinib is a JAK2 kinase inhibitor that is FDA approved for the treatment of myelofibrosis. Several other JAK/STAT inhibitors have been FDA approved for autoimmune diseases, and others are being evaluated in clinical trials for treatment of cancer (Hosseini et al, 2020).

6.3.2 Integrin Signaling

Mammalian cells express cell adhesion molecules that mediate their attachment to the extracellular matrix (ECM) and/or their interaction with the same or different cell types (see Chap. 10, Sec. 10.2). Most adhesion molecules are transmembrane proteins, but some are anchored in the plasma membrane by a C-terminal glycophosphatidyl-inositol moiety. Interactions between cells and the ECM are essential for cell survival and cell proliferation, and can regulate differentiation. Loss of interactions between the cell and ECM results in induction of apoptosis in both epithelial and endothelial cells. However, a common property of malignant cells is that they continue to survive and proliferate in the absence of interactions with the ECM.

Integrins are transmembrane cell surface receptors expressed in all cell types that serve as the primary physical link between the ECM and the actin cytoskeleton, and they enable direct communication across the plasma membrane. Integrins recognize and bind to specific ECM ligands (such as collagen, laminin, and fibronectin) and transduce signals leading to the activation of intracellular signaling networks that regulate cell migration, cell polarity, cell proliferation, and survival. Integrins are composed of membrane spanning α and β subunits that associate noncovalently to form a heterodimer on the cell surface. Receptor diversity and versatility in ligand binding is determined by the extracellular domains, and through the specific pairing of 9 β subunits and 16 α subunits (see Chap. 10, Fig. 10–5). The cytoplasmic domains of both α- and β-integrin subunits are conserved among vertebrate species and *Drosophila*, and serve as a binding platform for both actin cytoskeleton binding proteins, such as α-actinin, paxillin, tensin and talin, and intracellular signaling components, such as cytoplasmic TKs, Focal Adhesion Kinase (FAK) and SRC families (Fig. 6–9) (Cooper and Giancotti, 2019).

The binding of integrins to ECM ligands induces integrin clustering and subsequent recruitment of actin filaments and signaling proteins to the integrin cytoplasmic domain (see Chap. 10, Fig. 10–5). These large transmembrane adhesion complexes composed of the ECM and intracellular signaling components are called focal adhesions (FAs). The dynamic formation and remodeling of FAs assures cell adhesion to the ECM in addition to the targeted localization of actin filaments and signaling components necessary for the establishment of cell polarity, directed cell migration, and maintenance of cell proliferation and survival. In addition to providing a physical link between the ECM and the cytoskeleton, binding of integrins to their ligands elicits a variety of intracellular signaling events. For example, integrin signaling regulates the formation of filopodia, lamellipodia, and stress fibers through the RHO family of small GTPases CDC42, RAC, and RHO. It can also stimulate tyrosine phosphorylation and subsequent activation of cellular proteins, including the FAK and SRC cytoplasmic TKs that regulate remodeling of FAs (Fig. 6–9). Furthermore, activation of the RAS family of GTPases by integrins is important for the activation of serine-threonine kinases such as ERK, PAK, and JNK that regulate gene expression and cell cycle progression.

Alterations in integrin levels have been observed during tumor progression, and these changes appear to be tumor- and integrin-specific (Cooper and Giancotti, 2019). Loss of integrin $\alpha_2\beta_1$ is observed in some tumors, whereas other integrins such as $\alpha_v\beta_3$, $\alpha_v\beta_6$, and $\alpha_5\beta_1$ are upregulated in epithelial tumors and associated with disease progression, metastasis, and/or tumor-induced migration of vascular endothelial cells (see Chap. 10, Sec. 10.2.3). As one example, FAK is amplified or overexpressed in approximately 40% of ovarian cancers, 25% of invasive breast cancers, and in metastatic prostate cancer (Cooper and Giancotti, 2019). Alterations in FAK can occur in the context of other oncogenic mutations, for example, in PTEN-deficient T-ALL cells, and can sensitize these cells to PI3K/AKT/mTOR inhibition (You et al, 2015). Monoclonal antibodies and RGD (arginylglycylaspartic acid) peptides that block integrin ligand binding or function have been investigated as potential cancer therapeutics, for example, via the integrin-blocking peptide cilengitide in glioblastoma, but phase III trials failed to show improvement in overall survival (Cooper and Giancotti, 2019). Combination therapies may prove more effective, and preclinical studies have shown that cilengitide and verapamil together reduced tumor growth and metastasis in murine models of lung and pancreatic cancer (Wong et al, 2015).

6.4 DEVELOPMENTAL SIGNALING

Cell–cell signaling is a fundamental aspect of early development that is required to generate the functional and morphological diversity of cell types and patterns found in most animals. These signaling networks include WNT, Hedgehog, TGF-β, NOTCH, JAK/STAT, and nuclear hormone pathways. Depending on the cellular context, these networks activate specific target genes and produce a spectrum of cellular signals, resulting in numerous effects on cellular physiology and embryonic development. Predictably, abnormal activation of these crucial pathways is observed in disease states such as cancer, and understanding their dysregulation is central to our knowledge of cancer etiology and in the development of targeted therapies.

6.4.1 WNT Signaling

The WNT proteins (Int/Wingless = WNT; first found in mice as integration 1 and then as Wingless in flies), are intimately involved in the multicellular development of organisms. They consist of secreted glycoproteins with 19 known human members that are highly conserved throughout evolution (Nusse and Clevers, 2017). WNT proteins bind to the Frizzled (FZ) family of transmembrane receptors, of which 10 members have been identified (Fig. 6–11). Together with their coreceptors, low-density lipoprotein receptor–related proteins LRP5 and LRP6, ligand-bound FZ receptors initiate signaling to downstream intracellular targets. The affinity of FZ receptors for specific ligands determines the activation of 3 alternate intracellular pathways: (1) the WNT pathway, which leads to regulation of gene expression through β-catenin; (2) the WNT/planar cell polarity pathway, which activates cytoskeleton reorganization through RHO (RAS Homolog) and JNK; and (3) the WNT/Ca^{2+} pathway, which involves the activation of phospholipase C and protein kinase C. WNT signaling is also regulated via protein turnover, and signaling is attenuated via the transmembrane E3 ligases RNF43 (Ring finger protein 43) and its homolog ZNRF3 that target membrane-bound WNT and promote FZD receptor turnover (see Sec. 6.5). R-spondins counteract this WNT attenuation by binding to LGR4/5 and RNF43/ZNRF3 extracellular domains, leading to ubiquitination and clearance of RNF43/ZNRF3 (Krishnamurthy and Kurzrock, 2018).

A key mediator of WNT signaling is β-catenin. In the absence of WNT, β-catenin is degraded through a series of phosphorylation and ubiquitination steps mediated by the Ubiquitin Proteasome System (UPS) (see Sec. 6.5). In the absence of β-catenin, T-cell factor (TCF) together with corepressors such as histone deacetylase (HDAC) and Groucho/transducin-like-enhancer of split (TLE) repress the transcription of WNT target genes. Upon WNT activation, the destruction complex is inactivated, allowing β-catenin accumulation and entry into the nucleus where it interacts with the lymphoid enhanced transcription factor (LEF) and the TCF family of transcription factors to regulate transcription of specific target genes. These transcription factors bind directly to DNA but are incapable of activating gene transcription independently of β-catenin. Known target genes include *MYC*, *CCND1* (cyclin D1), and *MMP7* (metalloproteinase 7).

Constitutive activation of the WNT pathway has been observed in many cancers including colorectal carcinoma (CRC). Adenomatous polyposis coli (APC) is a tumor suppressor that forms part of the destruction complex and is encoded

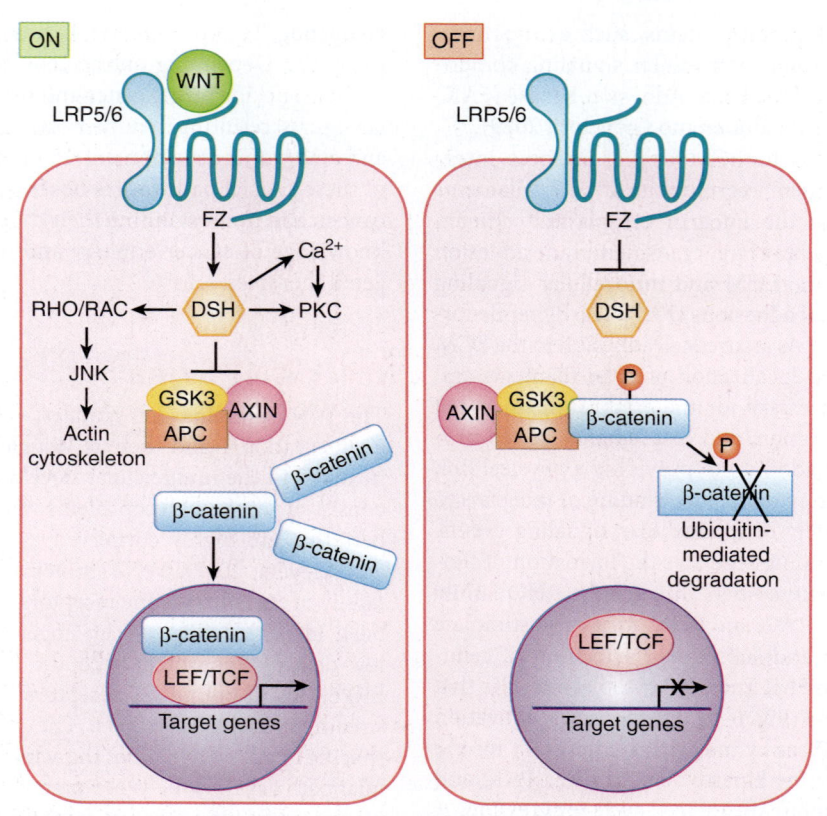

FIGURE 6-11 **WNT signaling.** *ON:* In the canonical WNT signaling pathway, WNT binding to Frizzled (FZ) LRP5/6 complex on the target cell results in recruitment of Dishevelled (DSH) to FZ. This interaction results in inactivation of the kinase glycogen synthase kinase 3 (GSK3), thereby stabilizing β-catenin. β-Catenin accumulates in the cytoplasm and shuttles to the nucleus, where it functions as a cotranscriptional activator with LEF/TFC to regulate transcription of target genes. *OFF:* In the absence of WNT, β-catenin is phosphorylated and exists within a destruction complex (together with APC, GSK3, and AXIN) and is targeted for ubiquitin-dependent proteasomal degradation. The noncanonical WNT pathways include WNT/Ca^{2+} and WNT/Planar cell polarity pathways (see text).

by the gene responsible for the onset of familial adenomatous polyposis (FAP), an autosomal dominant, inherited disease that predisposes patients to multiple colorectal polyps and cancers. In this disease, mutations in the APC gene result in ineffective β-catenin degradation and constitutive activation of β-catenin/TCF target genes. Consistent with this observation, in 50% of cases of sporadic CRC, mutations that protect β-catenin from degradation have been observed (Nusse and Clevers, 2017). Activating mutations in β-catenin or in other components of the WNT pathway are also observed in a wide variety of human malignancies. For example, WNT activation is evident in more than half of all breast cancers, and it is associated with poorer overall survival. Other genetic alterations that lead to WNT activation in cancer include RNF43 loss-of-function alterations, which are found in more than 18% of colorectal and endometrial cancers. WNT activation is also found in cancers of the lung, breast, cervix, stomach, pancreas, ovary, prostate, hepatocellular carcinoma (HCC), blood, and medulloblastoma (Polakis, 2007; Krishnamurthy and Kurzrock, 2018).

Antagonists of WNT signaling have been investigated for their activity against various cancers. Small molecule antagonists of TCF/β-catenin interaction inhibit proliferation of CRC, HCC, and multiple myeloma cells. Furthermore, inhibition of the WNT target COX-2 with nonsteroidal anti-inflammatory drugs in patients with FAP or in a human FAP mouse model significantly reduces the number of intestinal polyps (Oshima et al, 1996; Steinbach et al, 2000). Inhibitors of porcupine (PORCN), a membrane-bound O-acetyltransferase that promotes WNT ligand secretion include LGK974 and ETC-159. LGK974 blocks WNT signaling and inhibits tumor growth, especially in cancer lines that harbor activated NOTCH1, and they are in Phase I/II clinical trials as potential treatments for metastatic colorectal cancer or head and neck cancers (Krishnamurthy and Kurzrock, 2018). Several other WNT inhibitors are in clinical trial, including vantictumab, an antibody that targets 5 of 10 FZD receptors, and ipafricept, a recombinant fusion protein that blocks WNT signaling via interaction with WNT ligands. Other inhibitors that interfere with β-catenin destruction are also under development. These inhibitors target tankyrase, a poly (ADP-ribose) polymerase, the FZD-interactor disheveled (DVL), the β-catenin transcriptional co-activator TCF, and other WNT coactivators such as the transcriptional coactivator CBP (CREB-binding protein) (Nusse and Clevers, 2017).

Compounds that target the other 2 pathways, WNT/Planar cell polarity or WNT/Ca^{2+}, are also under development. Small molecule–mediated inhibition of RAC, a downstream effector of the WNT/PCP pathway, can suppress the growth and invasion of prostate cancer cells and leukemia cells under experimental conditions. Inhibition of PKC (protein kinase C), a WNT/Ca^{2+} pathway effector (Kikkawa, 2019), has demonstrated limited success in a number of malignancies including melanoma, non-Hodgkin lymphoma, and ovarian cancer. FOXY-5, an agonist of the WNT tumor suppressor, WNT5a, can eradicate breast cancer in a mouse model (Safholm et al, 2008). Other WNT pathway inhibitors are in clinical trials, including the PORCN inhibitors and LGR5 antibody-drug candidates, which inhibit several types of WNT signaling (Katoh, 2017). Monoclonal antibodies and CAR-T cells have also been developed against the membrane-bound, orphan tyrosine kinase receptors ROR1/ROR2, which are also targets of WNT activation. These approaches are in early clinical trials for chronic lymphocytic leukemia and breast, pancreatic, liver, ovarian, and solid tumors (Katoh and Katoh, 2017).

6.4.2 NOTCH Signaling

The NOTCH signaling cascade is highly conserved and plays a crucial role in stem cell self-renewal (see Chap. 13, Sec. 13.3.2 and 13.4.3), cell fate determination, epithelial cell polarity/adhesion, cell division, and apoptosis. NOTCH is a ligand-activated cell surface receptor initially identified in *Drosophila*, and subsequently identified in *Caenorhabditis elegans* and vertebrates. Mammals possess 4 NOTCH proteins (NOTCH1-4) that function as receptors for 5 NOTCH ligands (DELTA-LIKE1, -3, -4 and JAGGED1, -2) (Fig. 6–12). Glycosylation by FRINGE glycosyltransferases (LUNATIC, MANIC, and RADICAL FRINGE) modifies the specificity of ligand-receptor interactions. The NOTCH receptor is a large, single-pass transmembrane protein that contains several conserved protein-protein interaction motifs (Fig. 6–12). The large extracellular domain contains multiple EGF-like repeats involved in ligand binding, and 3 cysteine-rich LIN12/NOTCH repeat (LNR) regions thought to play an inhibitory role in receptor activation. This region is followed by a single transmembrane domain, an intracellular domain composed of a sequence N-terminal to the ankyrin repeats (called RAM23) that interacts with proteins from the CSL (CBF1/SU[H]/LAG1) family of transcription factors, 6 tandem ankyrin repeats involved in mediating protein-protein interactions with regulators of the receptor, and a proline, glutamine, serine, and threonine-rich (PEST) sequence associated with high rates of protein turnover.

NOTCH signaling involves complex cleavage events that occur during receptor maturation and transmission of the NOTCH signal. During its maturation, NOTCH is first processed into 2 distinct fragments that interact to form a heterodimer on the cell surface (see Fig. 6–12*B*). In this heterodimeric form, NOTCH binds to transmembrane ligands presented on neighboring cells. NOTCH ligand-receptor interaction leads to 2 proteolytic cleavages of the receptor. The first cleavage event, mediated by metalloproteases of the ADAM (a disintegrin and metalloproteinase) family, releases the NOTCH extracellular domain. The second cleavage, executed by a presenilin-protease (γ-secretase) complex, releases the cytoplasmic domain fragment of intracellular NOTCH (NIC) from the plasma membrane. NIC enters the nucleus and modulates the expression of target genes predominantly by converting the CSL repressor, a conserved transcriptional factor named

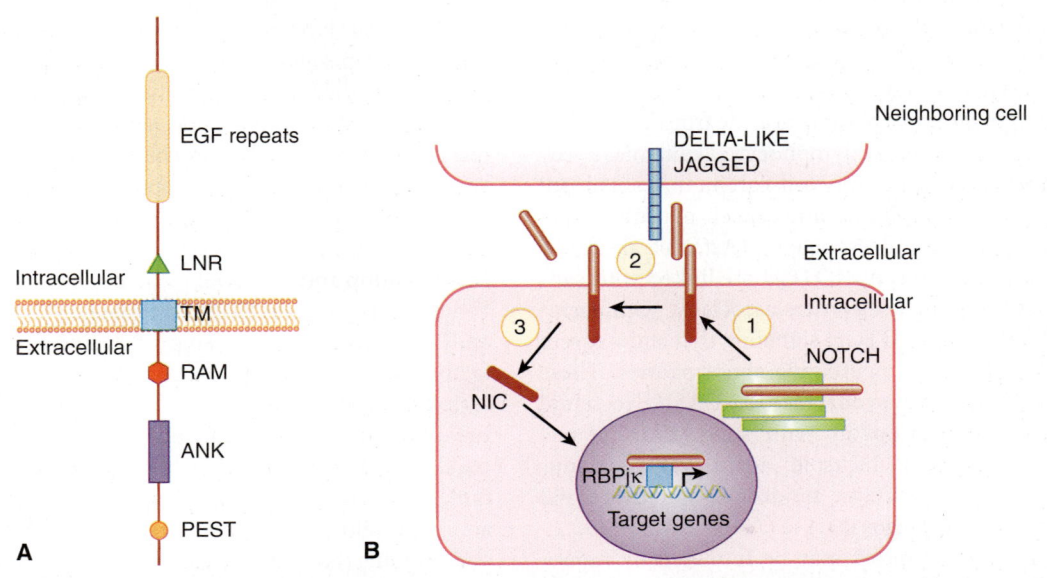

FIGURE 6–12 NOTCH receptor signaling. **A)** Schematic of the NOTCH receptor. *EGF*, epidermal growth factor–like repeats; *LNR*, Lin12/NOTCH repeat region (that is contained within the NOTCH negative regulatory region [NRR]); *TM*, transmembrane domain; *RAM*, RAM23 domain; *ANK*, ankyrin repeats; *PEST*, proline, glutamate, serine, threonine-rich region. **B)** Model of NOTCH pathway. (1) NOTCH is first processed in the trans-Golgi network into a heterodimer that is found on the cell surface. (2) Ligand (DELTA-LIKE, JAGGED) presented on neighboring cells causes a second cleavage event that releases the extracellular domain of NOTCH. (3) This triggers a final cleavage event mediated by the γ-secretase complex, releasing the active intracellular domain of NOTCH (NIC). NIC translocates to the nucleus where it functions as a cotransactivator with the CSL family of transcription factors (such as RBP-Jκ) to regulate target genes that include HES and HEY.

for its orthologs in mammals (CBF-1/RBG-Jκ), flies (Suppressor of hairless) and *C elegans* (Lag-1), to an activator of transcription. In humans, downstream targets of this complex, mediated by CBF-1 (C-repeat/DRE binding factor 1), include members of the HES and HEY families, which encode basic helix-loop-helix transcriptional regulatory proteins.

NOTCH activation has been strongly linked to human cancers, most notably T-cell acute lymphoblastic leukemia (T-ALL), where a recurrent t(7;9)(q34;q34.3) chromosomal translocation results in a dominantly active NOTCH1 receptor. NOTCH and WNT also cooperate to promote glioblastoma, and inhibition of both pathways impairs glioblastoma stem cell proliferation through the upregulation of Achaete-Scute Family Basic HLH Transcription Factor 1(ASCL1) and the induction of differentiation (Rajakulendran et al, 2019). Aberrant NOTCH signaling can also contribute to the development of other solid malignancies such as breast cancer. The *Notch4* locus was identified as a common proviral integration site in mouse mammary tumor virus (MMTV)–induced mammary adenocarcinomas in mice, leading to overexpression of NIC protein (Gallahan and Callahan, 1987). In human breast cancer, high-level expression of JAGGED1 and/or NOTCH1 correlates with and is an independent prognostic indicator of poor outcome (Reedijk et al, 2005). NOTCH affects multiple cellular processes, and aberrant NOTCH activity influences breast cancer progression through the maintenance of tumor-initiating cells and by promoting proliferation, motility, and survival of cancer cells. Genome-wide sequencing of cancers has revealed that NOTCH signaling is perturbed in at least 3 distinct ways. In T-ALL, in which NOTCH1 alterations are observed in 50% to 60% of cases, these alterations include chromosomal translocations, point substitutions, and in-frame insertions/deletions that lead to NOTCH activation, via alterations specific to the negative regulatory region (NRR, which encompasses the LNR [Lin 12/NOTCH repeat] region) within NOTCH. Genetic alterations in NOTCH 1, 2, 3 have been identified in many types of cancers aside from T-ALL and breast cancer including chronic lymphocytic leukemia, B-cell and T-cell lymphomas, squamous cell carcinoma, small cell lung carcinoma, low-grade glioma, and cancers of the adenoid, glomus, urothelial tract, and esophagus (Aster et al, 2017). Although somatic mutations in NOTCH are linked with cancer, there are several human disorders associated with germline genetic alterations in NOTCH signaling that show severe vascular, cardiovascular, or neurologic abnormalities. These disorders include Alagille syndrome, CADASIL (cerebral autosomal-dominant arteriopathy with subcortical infarcts and leukoencephalopathy), bicuspid aortic valve, Hajdu-Cheney syndrome, Adams-Oliver syndrome, spondylocostal dysostosis, and Dowling-Degos disease (Aster, 2014).

NOTCH ligands or receptors may be inhibited by monoclonal antibodies, RNA interference, soluble ligands, or receptor decoys. Inhibition of enzymes involved in glycosylation or cleavage of receptors, such as γ-secretase inhibitors (GSIs) or ADAM inhibitors, are also potential approaches to target NOTCH therapeutically. Among NOTCH pathway inhibitors, potent GSIs were developed originally to inhibit the γ-secretase complex that plays a role in plaque formation in Alzheimer disease (Golde et al, 2013). The discovery of γ-secretase–dependent NOTCH1 mutations in T-ALL accelerated the evaluation of GSIs in preclinical studies, where induction of apoptosis and reduced cell proliferation was demonstrated in several human cancer models. GSI treatment also blocks NOTCH signaling and growth of human breast cancer xenografts and tumors in an HER-2 transgenic breast cancer mouse model. Therapeutic strategies to block NOTCH signaling are under development for multiple cancer types, including the desmoid and adenoid cystic carcinomas in patients harboring NOTCH genetic alterations. Clinical trials are ongoing with at least 4 small molecule GSIs (RO492907, LY3039478, PF-03084014, and BMS-906024); monoclonal antibodies directed against NOTCH (brontictuzumab, tarextumab) and the Delta-Like Ligand 4 receptor DLL-4 (demcizumab, enoticumab), and a molecule that blocks NOTCH transcriptional activation (CB-201) (Moore et al, 2020).

6.4.3 Hedgehog Signaling

Hedgehog (HH) proteins act as key mediators of fundamental processes in embryonic development, and serve broad roles in the proliferation, migration, and differentiation of target cells that, in turn, impinge on the maintenance of stem cell populations and in cancer cell signaling (Niyaz et al, 2019). HH signaling is essential to the growth, patterning, and morphogenesis of many different tissues and organs including the skin, brain, gut, lung, and bone, and HH proteins play a role in hematopoiesis. The HH signaling pathway is highly conserved throughout evolution, and much of what is known about signaling in vertebrates has been inferred from studies in *Drosophila* (Niyaz et al, 2019). In humans, there are 3 homologs of the *Drosophila Hh* gene; sonic hedgehog (*SHH*), desert hedgehog (*DHH*), and Indian hedgehog (*IHH*). The *Hh* gene products encode ligands that signal through a membrane–receptor complex including the Patched (PTC1 and PTC2) and Smoothened (SMO) receptors, which together form a molecular switch controlling activation of downstream target genes (Fig. 6–13). In the absence of ligand, PTC inhibits SMO accumulation and activation, whereas the interaction between HH and PTC releases SMO. Activated SMO allows expression and/or proteolytic processing of 3 zinc-finger transcription factors (see Sec. 6.2.6; GLI1, 2, and 3) and ultimately to transcription of HH target genes through direct interaction with the consensus binding sequence 5′-TGGGTGGTA-3′. Several regulators of HH signaling have been identified, including molecules that modify the ligand, such as Hedgehog interacting protein (HIP) and Hedgehog acyltransferase (HHAT), and proteins that function downstream of SMO, including the serine/threonine protein kinase Fused (FU) and the Suppressor of Fused (SU[FU]) (Skoda et al, 2018).

Given its critical role in development, disturbances in HH signaling can result in disease states. Inactivation of the HH signaling pathway during development results in an

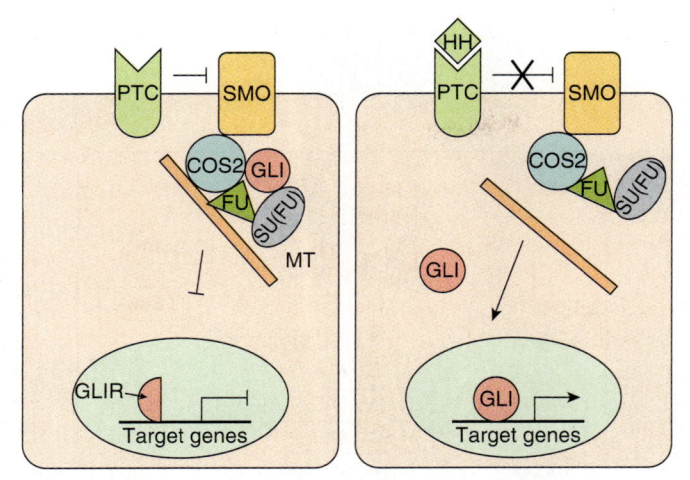

FIGURE 6–13 Hedgehog signaling. In the absence of HH, PTC silences SMO, the key signal transducer of the HH pathway. Binding of HH to PTC prevents SMO inhibition and results in nuclear translocation of activated GLI. Release of SMO inhibition results in nuclear translocation of activated GLI transcription factors and HH target gene expression. GLI is found in a complex with Fused (FU), Costal2 (COS2), and Suppressor of Fused (SU[FU]) bound to microtubules (MT). On activation of SMO, this complex is disassembled, releasing GLI and allowing nuclear translocation and upregulation of downstream target genes. Target genes include WNT, bone morphogenetic protein (BMP), and PTC itself.

abnormality in which the embryonic forebrain fails to develop into 2 hemispheres, whereas abnormal activation of this pathway has been implicated in the development of malignancy. Aberrant HH pathway activation in cancer is thought to occur via at least 3 mechanisms: cell-autonomous and ligand-dependent, ligand-dependent via autocrine/juxtacrine signaling, and ligand-dependent via paracrine or reverse paracrine signaling (Skoda et al, 2018). As an example of the first mechanism, *PTC1* loss-of-function or *SMO* gain-of-function mutations have been observed in sporadic basal cell carcinoma (BCC) and medulloblastoma. Consistent with these observations, Gorlin (basal cell nevus) syndrome, which results from *PTC1* genetic abnormalities, leads to a predisposition to BCC, medulloblastoma, and rhabdomyosarcoma. These findings have been recapitulated in mouse models of SMO activation or PTC inactivation, where animals frequently develop BCC or medulloblastoma.

GLI activation can also result in malignancy (Jetten, 2019). This propensity may occur via *K-RAS* activating mutations that increase GLI transcriptional activity or through alterations within the *GLI* genes themselves; both mechanisms of HH activation have been observed in pancreatic carcinoma. Mutations in *SU(FU)* have been identified in patients with medulloblastomas. HH signaling in malignancy can also be induced by pathways that are commonly activated in human cancer, such as PI3K/AKT and MEK (see Sec. 6.2.4).

Related to the second and third mechanisms, aberrant HH activation may also occur through ligand-mediated mechanisms in an autocrine or paracrine manner (reviewed in Skoda et al., 2018). In multiple malignancies, including small cell lung cancer (SCLC), pancreatic adenocarcinoma, colon cancer, prostate cancer, glioblastoma, and malignant melanoma, tumor cells synthesize and respond to HH ligand. In B-cell lymphoma and multiple myeloma, stromal production of HH ligand in the spleen, lymph nodes, and bone marrow supports the growth of tumor cells. Conversely, tumor production of HH ligand can stimulate HH signaling in stromal cells of the tumor microenvironment, resulting in the expression of HH target genes in those cells to increase the stromal content of tumors.

A role for HH signaling in the maintenance of tumor-initiating cells (TICs) has been reported for multiple tumor types, including breast and pancreatic cancer, glioblastoma, multiple myeloma, and chronic myeloid leukemia (Skoda et al, 2018). Analogous to normal tissue stem cells, TICs are defined by their capacity to self-renew and to regenerate tumors containing differentiated progeny similar to the original tumor (see Chap. 13, Sec. 13.3.2).

Emerging evidence also implicates HH signaling in tumor invasion and metastases. In primary colon cancer, HH signaling is upregulated in the TIC compartment and is accompanied by elevated expression of SNAIL (encoded by *SNAI1*), which is involved in the epithelial-to-mesenchymal transition (EMT) and metastasis (see Chap. 10, Sec. 10.5.5) (Yao et al, 2018). For example, growth and metastases of primary colon cancer in a xenograft model requires active HH signaling and induction of EMT (Varnat et al, 2009).

Several HH antagonists are undergoing clinical testing in a wide range of malignancies, including BCC. An early encouraging report of the SMO antagonist GDC-0449 demonstrated a 55% clinical response rate, including 2 complete remissions in 33 patients with advanced BCC (Skoda et al, 2018). More than 50 HH signaling pathway inhibitors (HPIs) have been identified to date that include antibodies and small molecules against HH ligand, SMO antagonists, GLI inhibitors, and others. For example, there are at least 6 SMO inhibitors in clinical trials and 2 inhibitors that have received FDA approval (vismodegib and sonidegib). Sonidegib has shown promising results against BCC and is also being explored in the treatment of medulloblastoma, carcinomas of the ovary, pancreas, lung and kidney, and blood cancers, including myeloid leukemia and lymphoma (Skoda et al, 2018).

6.4.4 Signal Transduction by the Transforming Growth Factor–β Superfamily

Members of the TGF-β superfamily regulate a number of developmental and homeostatic processes, such as cell proliferation, differentiation, apoptosis, cell adhesion, and migration (Mullen and Wrana, 2017). They constitute a conserved family of proteins with at least 32 vertebrate members and over a dozen structurally and functionally related proteins found in invertebrates including *C. elegans* and *Drosophila*. There are 2 general branches of this superfamily, including a

TGF-β/activin/nodal branch and a bone morphogenic protein (BMP) branch whose members have diverse, but often complementary, effects. Some members are widely expressed during embryogenesis and in adult tissues, whereas others are expressed in only a few cell types and for restricted periods during development. TGF-β is an immunosuppressive cytokine that plays a prominent role in the generation and effector function of T cells, including Treg cells, dendritic cells, and natural killer cells (Batlle and Massague, 2019) (see Chap. 21, Sec. 21.4).

TGF-β, the prototypic member of this superfamily, is a secreted growth factor synthesized as an inactive precursor and is proteolytically processed into a mature secreted ligand. On dimerization, TGF-β becomes biologically active and binds to a cell surface receptor complex consisting of 2 distinct single-pass transmembrane proteins known as the type I and type II receptors, both of which contain an intracellular serine-threonine kinase domain (Fig. 6–14) (Mullen and Wrana, 2017). Ligand binding induces association of the type I and type II receptors into a heterotetrameric complex. This association leads to unidirectional phosphorylation and subsequent activation of the kinase domain of the type I receptor by the type II receptor. The activated type I receptor then signals to the SMAD (for Sma and Mad proteins from *C. elegans* and *Drosophila*, respectively) family of intracellular mediators, which function to carry the signal from the cell surface directly to the nucleus. There are 3 distinct classes of SMADs: receptor-regulated or R-SMADs (SMADs 1, 2, 3, 5, and 8), common mediator or Co-SMAD4, and inhibitory SMADs 6 and 7 (called I-SMADs) (Fig. 6–14). The activated type I receptor directly phosphorylates and activates the R-SMADs leading to interaction with Co-SMAD4. The inhibitory SMADs counteract the effects of R-SMADs and antagonize TGF-β signaling. An additional level of regulation of TGF-β signaling occurs with SMAD Ubiquitin Regulator Factors SMURF1 and SMURF2. These proteins are E3 ubiquitin-protein ligases that regulate SMAD levels (see Sec. 6.5). SMURFs orchestrate ubiquitin transfer to the R-SMADs causing their ubiquitination and subsequent proteasomal degradation.

The biological output of TGF-β signaling is primarily driven via the type I receptor. In vertebrates, there are 7 distinct type I receptors that interact with 1 of 5 type II receptors. The signal from the type I receptor is funneled through 1 of 2 groups of SMAD proteins. Specific R-SMADs recognize different DNA-binding proteins and regulate distinct target genes, thereby generating diverse biological responses. For example, phosphorylation and activation of R-SMADs SMAD2 and SMAD3 transduce a TGF-β–like signal, whereas activation of R-SMADs SMAD1, SMAD5, and SMAD8 transduce signals initiated by bone morphologic proteins. There is also evidence that TGF-β can signal through SMAD independent processes by activation of RHO-A, RAS, and TGF-β activated kinase I (TAK1).

Mutations in the TGF-β family of ligands are responsible for a variety of human diseases, including cancer, hereditary chondrodysplasias, and pulmonary hypertension (Batlle and Massague, 2019). TGF-β signaling is an important mediator of immune tolerance, and mutations in Tgf-β1 in mice lead to multiorgan inflammation and death shortly after birth. In humans, aberrant TGF-β signaling is associated with the inflammatory bowel disorders called Crohn's disease and ulcerative colitis. This role in inflammation is one means by which TGF-β signaling influences cancer progression where, depending on the context, it can function as both a tumor suppressor and as a tumor promoter. For example, in colon cancer, TGF-β can switch from an inhibitor of primary tumor growth to a stimulator of proliferation in metastatic cells. The immunohistochemical staining intensity of TGF-β is an independent marker of colon cancer progression to metastases (Picon et al, 1998). Mutations in the TGF-β receptors have been identified in several human cancers, with a recent meta-analysis demonstrating that the TGF-β type I 6A polymorphic allele (containing a deletion of 3 alanine residues from the N-terminus) is associated with increased cancer risk (Batlle and Massague, 2019).

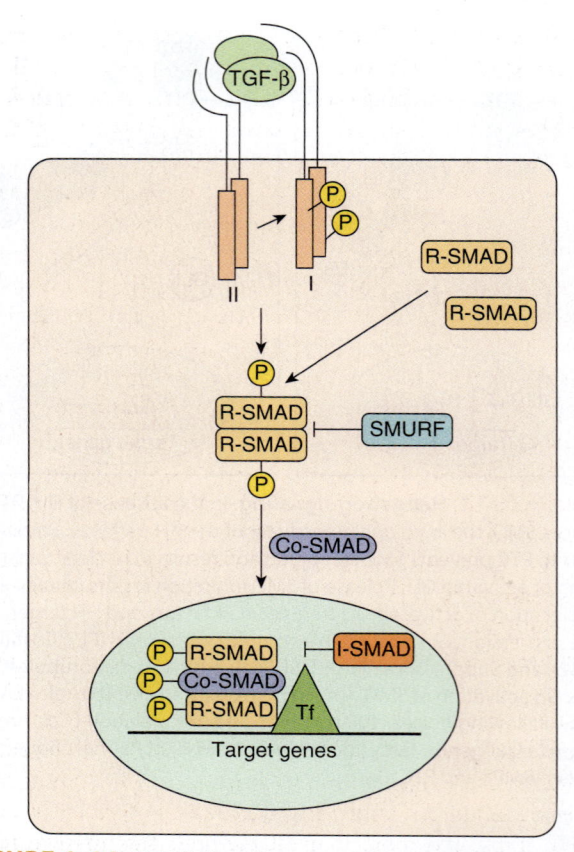

FIGURE 6–14 TGF-β signaling. TGF-β ligand binding induces the association of type II and type I receptor heterodimers into a heterotetrameric complex. This results in phosphorylation and subsequent activation of the type I receptor that then phosphorylates a member of the R-SMAD class of proteins (SMADs 1, 2, 3, 5, or 8). Phosphorylated R-SMADs interact with the Co-SMAD, SMAD4, and this complex then accumulates in the nucleus. SMURFs are E3 ubiquitin-protein ligases that orchestrate ubiquitin transfer to the R-SMADs, causing their ubiquitination and subsequent proteasomal degradation. In the nucleus, the activated SMAD complex associates with DNA-binding cofactors, coactivators, and corepressors that regulate transcription of target genes. *Tf*, Transcription factors. Inhibitory SMADS (SMAD 6, 7; I-SMADs) attenuate signaling by binding with and competing with R-SMAD function.

Mutations in SMAD2 are found in colorectal and lung cancers, and SMAD4 mutations are found in several types of colorectal, pancreatic, and lung cancers. These point mutations in the SMAD proteins lead to loss of phosphorylation of SMAD2 and subsequent loss of association with SMAD4.

TGF-β signaling is thought to promote the later stages of cancer development by facilitating a tumor microenvironment (TME) that promotes immune suppression and other changes in the stroma that contribute to tumor development. Not only do cancer cells themselves secrete TGF-β but so do other cells in the TME including Tregs, fibroblasts, macrophages, and platelets. The net effect is to provide an environment whereby cancer cells can evade immune recognition and destruction (Batlle and Massague, 2019).

Genetic alterations in TGF-β or SMAD are frequently observed in cancer, including 25% to 50% of colorectal or pancreatic adenocarcinomas, and in 10% to 20% of adenocarcinomas of the head and neck, bladder and endometrium, and squamous carcinomas of the lung and cervix (Batlle and Massague, 2019). Agents that target TGF-β signaling are being developed, including TGF-β–neutralizing antibodies, soluble TGF-βR:Fc fusion proteins (which contain the TGF-βR extracellular domain and compete for ligand binding), antisense oligonucleotides, and other inhibitors of TGF-β receptors. Several of these agents are in clinical trials, including small molecule inhibitors, antibodies against TGF-β, receptor-based TGF-β traps, and more indirect methods that involve adoptive cell transfer of T cells that target TGF-β (see Chap. 21, Sec. 21.5.5). These trials encompass several cancer types and the agents are often combined with approved drugs such as paclitaxel, or with chemoradiation, or stereotactic ablative radiotherapy. Given its role in immune function, several trials are underway to examine if TGF-β blockade with drugs can promote immunotherapy treatments. An example is galunisertib, a small molecule that inhibits TGFBR1 activity that has shown promise against hepatocellular carcinoma and is being explored as an adjunct therapy in combination with PD-1 checkpoint inhibitors for several cancer types (Batlle and Massague, 2019).

6.5 THE ROLE OF UBIQUITIN IN CELL SIGNALING

6.5.1 The Ubiquitin Proteasome System

The *ubiquitin proteasome system* (UPS) is a major contributor to the dynamic control of the stability, interactions, and activity of most of the proteome (Yau and Rape, 2016) (for further discussion of the proteome, see Chap. 2, Sec. 2.4). Studies of ATP-dependent proteolysis in the 1960s led to the discovery that a small highly conserved protein called ubiquitin is covalently conjugated to a myriad of cellular proteins (Hershko and Ciechanover, 1998). The covalent attachment of ubiquitin serves as a tag that marks substrate proteins for rapid degradation and other fates (Fig. 6–15). A hierarchical enzyme cascade mediates protein ubiquitination, also termed ubiquitylation. Ubiquitin is first activated as a thioester linkage to an E1 activating enzyme in an ATP-dependent fashion, then transferred to an intermediary E2 conjugating enzyme also as a thioester, and finally conjugated as a stable isopeptide bond to a substrate lysine residue by an E3 ligase enzyme. Reiteration of the catalytic cycle generates a polyubiquitin chain on the substrate that is thereby targeted to a large compartmentalized protease complex called the 26S proteasome that rapidly degrades ubiquitinated proteins. The 26S proteasome is composed of a regulatory 19S cap subunit that binds and unfolds ubiquitinated substrates, which are then fed into a 20S core particle that forms a barrel-like structure with a multitude of inward-facing proteases that rapidly degrade the substrate into short peptides. Ubiquitin conjugates can be disassembled by a plethora of deubiquitinating enzymes, such that ubiquitination can be dynamically tuned according to the physiological needs of the cell. The 26S proteasome also plays a key role in innate immunity and antigen presentation, and in this unique functional setting it is called the *immunoproteasome* (see Chap. 21, Sec. 21.2.1).

Substrate recognition by the UPS is dictated by specific protein interactions between the substrate and its cognate E3 enzyme (Fig. 6–15). Often, these interactions are mediated

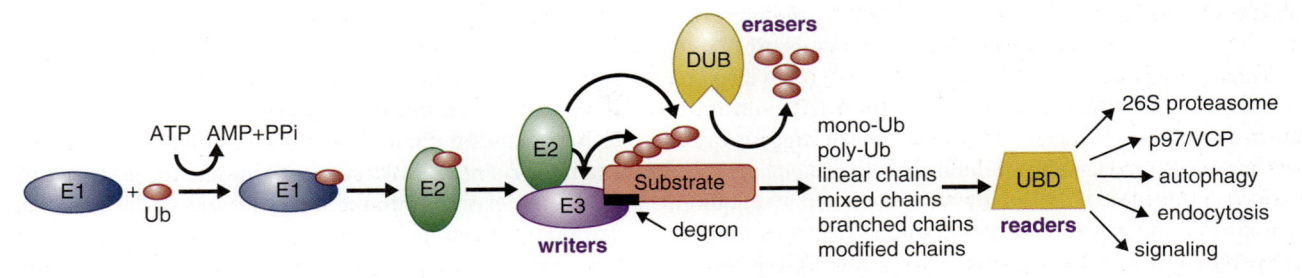

FIGURE 6–15 The ubiquitin proteasome system. The ubiquitin proteasome system (UPS) is a multistep process by which proteins are tagged and degraded. A free ubiquitin moiety is first thioesterified to a ubiquitin-activating enzyme (E1) and subsequently transferred to a ubiquitin-conjugating enzyme (E2), which, in partnership with an ubiquitin ligase (E3), transfers ubiquitin either directly to the specific protein substrate or via a thioester intermediate on the E3. De-ubiquitinating enzymes (DUBs) catalyze the removal of ubiquitin. The large variety of binding sites that E3 ligases use to recognize substrates are called degrons. There are multiple types of ubiquitin chains, which are recognized by ubiquitin readers via ubiquitin binding domains (UBDs) and targeted for degradation via the 26S proteasome or directed to other fates as indicated. (Reproduced with permission from Chatr-Aryamontri A, van der Sloot A, Tyers M. At Long Last, a C-Terminal Bookend for the Ubiquitin Code. *Mol Cell* 2018 May 17;70(4):568-571.)

by short peptide motifs termed *degrons*, which are bound by specific recognition domains in the E3. The first degrons discovered were mapped to the N-terminal amino acid of the substrate, termed the *N-end rule pathway* (Bachmair et al, 1986). Recently, a corresponding set of degrons has been discovered at substrate C-termini (Koren et al, 2018; Lin et al, 2018). A multitude of other degrons have also been identified and are typically short linear motifs that occur in disordered protein regions (Lucas and Ciulli, 2017). Degrons can be degenerate and are often combinatorial in nature, such that multiple signals can be integrated during substrate recognition. Many degrons depend on post-translation modifications, such as phosphorylation, thereby coupling cellular signaling to ubiquitin-mediated degradation. However, the precise mechanisms by which most of the thousands of documented UPS substrates are recognized remain to be elucidated.

Examples of ubiquitin-mediated degradation relevant to cell signaling in oncology include: cell cycle–targeted degradation of cyclins via the APC/C complex; degradation of the CDK2 inhibitor p27 via the SCF-SKP2 complex (see Chap. 8, Fig. 8–10); oxygen-dependent degradation of the HIF1α transcription factor via the CRL2-VHL complex (see Chap. 7, Table 7–1, and Chap. 11, Sec. 11.5.6); regulation of DNA damage/repair and DNA replication; and control of the mitotic spindle checkpoint (see Chap. 9, Secs. 9.3.6, 9.4.1, and 9.4.2). The stability and activity of many oncogenes and tumor suppressors are also regulated by the UPS, including MYC, p53, and PTEN (see Chap. 7, Secs. 7.5.2, 7.6.1, and 7.6.2). Perturbed ubiquitination of other signaling receptors such as RPTKs can result in prolonged activation and oncogenic signaling. An example is the mutation of c-CBL (named after cellular Castitas B Lymphoma), which is an E3 ligase that regulates the ubiquitination and activity of several RPTKs including T-cell receptors and TAMs (named for their prototypical RPTKs TYRO3, AXL, and MERTK members) (Paolino and Penninger, 2016). Another CBL family member, CBL-b, is recruited to activated RPTKs through its phosphotyrosine-binding TKB domain, and in turn promotes receptor ubiquitination (Kales et al, 2010). Ablation or inactivation of CBL-b activity has uncovered critical roles for this E3 ligase in cancer and metastasis. For example, loss of CBL-b function increases the ability to reject tumors in vivo (Chiang et al, 2007; Loeser et al, 2007; Paolino et al, 2011), and promotes the ability of natural killer (NK) cells to spontaneously target metastatic cancers in mice (Paolino et al, 2014) (see Chap. 21, Sec. 21.2.3). A small molecule that binds CBL-b TAM substrates leads to a reduction in metastatic tumors, which suggests drug-based approaches to facilitate NK killing are, in principle, feasible (Paolino et al, 2014). c-CBL activity is not restricted to ubiquitin, and it also promotes the conjugation of another ubiquitin-like moiety, NEDD8, to substrates that include the TGF-β type II receptor and c-SRC (Katzav and Schmitz, 2015).

6.5.2 The Ubiquitin Code

The diversity and specificity of the UPS in humans arises from the combinatorial possibilities afforded by 2 human E1 enzymes, 38 E2 enzymes, and more than 800 E3 enzymes, each of which recognizes a selected set of substrate proteins. Specificity in ubiquitin conjugation is controlled largely at the level of E3 enzymes, which fall into 3 major classes that have distinct enzymatic mechanisms. The HECT domain enzymes, for Homologous to the E6-AP Carboxyl Terminus, bear a catalytic cysteine residue that accepts ubiquitin from the E2 as a thioester prior to transfer to the substrate. In contrast, RING domain E3 ligases (such as the CBL-b, SCF or APC/C enzymes) directly bridge the E2 to the substrate and do not form a catalytic intermediate. The RING domain is a zinc-binding motif that serves as the E2 docking site and can also occur as a structural variant called the U-box that acts similarly but does not complex with zinc. RING E3s can be monomeric or multimeric in nature. The cullin-RING ligases or CRLs comprise the largest class of E3 in humans and constitute a modular architecture whereby a host of substrate-specific adaptor subunits recruit substrates to a core complex composed of the cullin and RING protein subunits. The archetypal CRL family (also called SCF enzymes) recruits substrates via some 70 different adapters called F-box proteins. A third class of E3 ligases, called the RING between RING (RBR) E3 enzymes, contain 2 RING domains, one of which binds the E2, while the other mediates ubiquitin transfer via a catalytic cysteine. E3 enzymes themselves can be regulated by subunit assembly and posttranslational modification. For example, activation of the CRL enzymes requires modification by a ubiquitin-related modifier called NEDD8, which itself is activated by dedicated E1 and E2 enzymes (Rulina et al, 2016; Liu et al, 2018). Each E3 may operate in conjunction with different E2 enzymes in different contexts; for example, some E2s can only add an initial priming ubiquitin to a substrate, with subsequent chain extension dependent on a different E2 (Hill et al, 2019). Finally, E3 enzymes often physically associate with deubiquitinating (DUB) enzymes of which more than 100 are known in humans (Harrigan et al, 2018), thereby allowing dynamic local control of the extent of substrate ubiquitination.

Ubiquitin can mark substrates in different configurations, either as an extended ubiquitin chain or individual ubiquitin moieties. Ubiquitin chains are formed by the covalent attachment of ubiquitin to itself by reiterative catalytic cycles of the E3 enzyme. Because ubiquitin contains 7 different lysine residues, these chains occur in different linkage formats, which in turn mark the substrate for different fates. The originally discovered and predominant linkage occurs at lysine 48 of ubiquitin and serves to direct substrates to the 26S proteasome. Other ubiquitin chain linkages serve different functions; for example, lysine 63 links chains to initiate the assembly of protein complexes in immune signaling and in the DNA damage response. Mixed linkage and branched ubiquitin chains have also been discovered. Attachment of single ubiquitin moieties by yet other E3s directs proteins to different subcellular compartments for cargo sorting, for example, during receptor internalization. These different substrate fates are determined by a host of modular ubiquitin binding domains that recognize the different configurations of ubiquitin linkages.

An intricate ubiquitin code is controlled by writers (E3 enzymes), erasers (DUB enzymes), and readers (UBDs), analogous to the codes imparted by protein phosphorylation or histone modification systems (Yau and Rape, 2016) (Fig. 6–15). The ubiquitin code is complex in part because most E3s can target more than 1 substrate and, conversely, many substrates are targeted by more than 1 E3. Of the many thousands of substrate-ubiquitin conjugates identified by mass spectrometry, only a small fraction has been assigned to a particular E3 enzyme. Moreover, each E3 can interact with more than 1 E2 enzyme, and any given substrate can be deubiquitinated by multiple DUB enzymes. Further complexity is conferred by the different types of ubiquitin chains themselves, which range from monoubiquitination through polyubiquitin chains (Kwon and Ciechanover, 2017). Polyubiquitin chains can also be extended and modified by conjugation to other ubiquitin-like modifiers such as NEDD8 and SUMO, which further diversify the ubiquitin code (Ciechanover, 2015). Although SUMO conjugation is catalyzed by a unique E1 and E2 enzyme, and just a few E3 enzymes, more than 1000 proteins are substrates for SUMOylation. Like ubiquitin, SUMO moieties can be removed via SUMO isopeptidases (called ULP, SENP, or SUSP) (Bekes et al, 2011). SUMOylation is an important regulator of numerous cellular processes; examples include the DNA damage response (Chap. 9, Sec. 9.4), tumor suppression (eg, via PTEN SUMO regulation; see Chap. 7, Fig. 7–15), β-catenin degradation (Nishida et al, 2001), as well as chromatin regulation and the transcriptional response to stress (Srikumar et al, 2013; Lewicki et al, 2015). SUMO-targeted ubiquitin ligases (STUBLs) can also generate hybrid chains in which ubiquitin is added to SUMO chains (Kwon and Ciechanover, 2017).

6.5.3 Clinical Implications of the UPS and Proteostasis in Oncology

Protein homeostasis, or *proteostasis*, refers to all of the mechanisms by which the ~10,000 proteins specific to each cell type, produced by complex transcriptional and translational programs, are assembled and maintained in a properly folded state and held at appropriate levels for normal physiological function. Defects in proteostasis are found in aging, cancer, and in other diseases such as cystic fibrosis. In cancer, perturbations in proteostasis can occur as a result of aneuploidy and other genetic and epigenetic alterations that affect protein copy number and/or protein folding/degradation (Oromendia and Amon, 2014). Three of the major processes that ensure normal proteostasis are translational control via the ribosome, protein complex assembly and folding via molecular chaperones, and regulated protein degradation. The UPS is integrated with other mechanisms of protein degradation. For example, misfolded proteins in the endoplasmic reticulum (ER) are sensed by the unfolded protein response (UPR) and removed by the ER-associated degradation (ERAD) system, which is composed of a specific set of E2 and E3 enzymes. A dedicated degradation system, termed *autophagy*, operates in close conjunction with the UPS to degrade large macromolecular aggregates, cytoplasmic constituents and entire organelles in response to nutrient stress or various forms of damage (Kwon and Ciechanover, 2017). Autophagy entails the envelopment of substrates by double membrane vesicles that subsequently fuse with the lysosome, leading to degradation by a host of lytic enzymes within the lysosome. The formation of autophagic membranes is triggered by the conjugation of the ubiquitin-like modifier LC3 to the lipid phosphatidylethanolamine (PE) by a dedicated E1-E2-E3 enzyme cascade. Substrates of the autophagy system may be targeted by ubiquitin-dependent or -independent mechanisms (Pohl and Dikic, 2019). The role of autophagy in cancer is complex but it may represent a therapeutic target in some contexts (Levy et al, 2017) (see Chap. 8, Sec. 8.4.6, Chap. 12, Sec. 12.3.6).

Protein misfolding or aggregation due to aneuploidy, mutations or other forms of proteotoxic stress activates a complex protein chaperone system, originally termed the heat shock response due to its induction by high temperature. A cohort of protein chaperones, notably HSP70 and HSP90, recognize denatured proteins through a suite of specific adaptor proteins. The HSPs undergo an ATP-driven conformational cycle that refolds client proteins to restore normal structure and function. The HSP chaperone system is under tight homeostatic control by the heat shock transcription factors (HSFs), which themselves are substrates of the system. Proteins that fail to be refolded by HSP chaperones are re-directed to the UPS for degradation, thus linking these two main proteostasis systems. Given that proteostatic stress that is an intrinsic feature of cancer cells, the HSP chaperone system promotes cancer cell survival (Dai and Sampson, 2016).

Multiple approaches that modulate protein degradation by small molecules are under investigation as cancer therapeutics (Bondeson and Crews, 2017; Gatel et al, 2020). Small molecule inhibitors of the 20S peptidase activity of the 26S proteasome include bortezomib, the next-generation inhibitors carfilzomib, and orally available ixazomib, all of which are used to treat multiple myeloma and mantle cell lymphoma (see Chap. 19, Sec. 19.7.1) (Gupta et al, 2019). An inhibitor of CRL enzyme activation called MLN4924 (also called Pevonedistat) is in clinical development against AML and other cancers (Zhou and Jia, 2020). In human xenograft models, there is evidence that MNL4924 may be an effective therapy against retinoblastoma (Aubry et al, 2020). Multiple inhibitors of HSP90 have been developed and are in various stages of clinical evaluation (Yuno et al, 2018; Shimomura et al, 2019). Proteostasis may also impact drug resistance, as there is increasing evidence that autophagy may mediate drug resistance (see Chap. 18, Sec. 18.4.6). For example, in breast cancer, inhibition of autophagy restores sensitivity to tamoxifen (see Chap. 21, Sec. 21.4.3.3).

Genetic alterations of the UPS system may yield therapeutic opportunities for cancer treatment. FBXW7 is an F-box protein that associates with the SCF core complex to control the degradation of oncogenic proteins that include cyclin E, MYC, mTOR, JUN, and NOTCH. FBXW7 is one of the most commonly mutated UPS genes in cancer, and is located in a genomic region (4q32) that is deleted in more than 30% of all human cancers (Davis et al, 2014; Yeh et al, 2018). There are at least 8 other F-box proteins implicated in cancer for which small molecule inhibitors are in development, including agents that inhibit SKP2 expression or substrate recognition (Liu and Mallampalli, 2016). In myeloid cancers, genetic alterations in CBL-b are also common: point substitutions in the cytoplasmic phosphotyrosine-containing domain within colony stimulating factor receptor (CSF-1R) that binds CBL-b are found in children with secondary myelodysplasia or AML, and oncogenic mutations in CBL-b have been identified in AML and other myeloid cancers (Katzav and Schmitz, 2015). Moreover, higher levels of expression of the *CBL-b* gene are associated with better overall survival of women with breast cancer (Liu et al, 2020). TAMs are important substrates for CBL-b in cancer, and one small molecule TAM inhibitor (BMS-777607) was found to enhance the efficacy of anti-PD1 antibody treatment in a mouse model of triple negative breast cancer (Kasikara et al, 2019).

Finally, an innovative new strategy exploits the UPS to enable the programmed elimination of cancer-associated proteins by small molecules termed protein degraders (Schapira et al, 2019). One such class of compounds, referred to as molecular glues, is represented by the immunomodulatory imide drugs (IMiDs) lenalidomide and pomalidomide, which are derivatives of thalidomide. The IMiDs recruit non-native (neo) substrates such as the transcription factors Ikaros and Aiolos to cereblon (CRBN), a substrate recruitment factor for a CRL-based E3 ligase, by engaging a joint binding pocket formed between the substrate and the E3. The IMiDs are clinically approved for relapsed/refractory multiple myeloma and myeloid dysplastic syndromes associated with 5q cytogenetic abnormalities (Richardson et al, 2019). Other IMiDs, such as iberdomide (CC-220), are in development against lenalidomide- and pomalidomide-resistant multiple myeloma (Bjorklund et al, 2020). A related class of protein degradation-inducing compounds called proteolysis-targeted chimeras (PROTACs) are also in development against many targets in cancer. A PROTAC consists of two covalently linked moieties: one that engages an E3 ligase and the other that binds to the desired target protein, which is thereby recruited for ubiquitination and degradation (Schapira et al, 2019). Small molecule ligands for several E3s, notably CRBN and VHL, have been used to construct PROTACs. This approach has demonstrated preclinical efficacy against BET domain epigenetic readers such as BRD2 (Chap. 3, Sec. 3.4.4), the androgen receptor (Chap. 20), MDM2 (Chap. 9, Sec. 9.4.1), BRAF-V600E (Chap. 6, Sec. 6.2.4) and other cancer-associated targets (Li and Song, 2020). These novel proteostasis modulators represent an exciting frontier of cancer drug discovery.

SUMMARY

- Cell signaling typically involves ligand binding to an extracellular receptor that initiates a signaling cascade via receptor dimerization events that are homotypic (between the same 2 receptors) or heterotypic (between different types of receptors)
- Cell-surface receptors often contain, or complex with, protein kinase modules that carry out protein phosphorylation on tyrosine, serine or threonine residues of substrates. These post-translational modifications confer an extraordinary diversity and specificity of modular interactions that dictate numerous cellular responses.
- Many of these receptor kinase complexes undergo somatic alterations in cancer to generate an activated or sustained signaling response that is oncogenic. Examples of such activated signaling cascades include RAS and its associated kinase effector RAF, receptor protein tyrosine kinases (RPTKs), and mitogen-activated protein kinases (MAPKs)
- Secreted cytokines and polypeptides play key roles in driving cancer but are also important during normal early development. Critical ligands include WNT (Int/Wingless), NOTCH, HEDGEHOG, and transforming growth factor–beta (TGF-β)
- Phosphoinositide signaling, in which the phosphoinositide (PI) lipids themselves are substrates important for cancer metabolism by lipid kinases or phosphatases (such as Phosphatase and Tensin homolog PTEN), or that activate lipid-bound kinases such as AKT
- Other phosphatase classes play key roles in early development and cancer and include the protein tyrosine phosphatases (PTP superfamily) and serine-threonine (S/T) phosphatases. Often these signaling events serve to attenuate cell signals by removing phosphate and, thus, play a tumor-suppressive role in cancer development
- Normal cellular physiology relies on the appropriate abundance and conformation of myriad signaling factors. The multifaceted proteostasis network - including the ubiquitin proteasome system, autophagy and protein chaperones - is frequently perturbed in cancer cells

ACKNOWLEDGMENTS

We thank Mike Tyers for suggestions to Section 6.5, and C. Jane McGlade and Michael Reedijk who were the authors of this chapter in the fifth edition.

REFERENCES

Almawi AW, Matthews LA, Guarne A. FHA domains: phosphopeptide binding and beyond. *Prog Biophys Mol Biol* 2017;127:105-110.

Andre F, Mills D, Taran T. Alpelisib for PIK3CA-mutated advanced breast cancer. Reply. *N Engl J Med* 2019;381(7):687.

Aster JC. In brief: notch signalling in health and disease. *J Pathol* 2014;232(1):1-3.

Aster JC, Pear WS, Blacklow SC. The varied roles of notch in cancer. *Annu Rev Pathol* 2017;12:245-275.

Aubry A, Yu T, Bremner R. Preclinical studies reveal MLN4924 is a promising new retinoblastoma therapy. *Cell Death Discov* 2020;6:2.

Bachmair A, Finley D, Varshavsky A. In vivo half-life of a protein is a function of its amino-terminal residue. *Science* 1986;234(4773):179-186.

Barford D, Neel BG. Revealing mechanisms for SH2 domain mediated regulation of the protein tyrosine phosphatase SHP-2. *Structure* 1998;6(3):249-254.

Barton WA, Dalton AC, Seegar TC, Himanen JP, Nikolov DB. Tie2 and Eph receptor tyrosine kinase activation and signaling. *Cold Spring Harb Perspect Biol* 2014;6(3):a009142.

Batlle E, Massague J. Transforming growth factor-beta signaling in immunity and cancer. *Immunity* 2019;50(4):924-940.

Bekes M, Prudden J, Srikumar T, Raught B, Boddy MN, Salvesen GS. The dynamics and mechanism of SUMO chain deconjugation by SUMO-specific proteases. *J Biol Chem* 2011;286(12):10238-10247.

Berndt N, Hamilton AD, Sebti SM. Targeting protein prenylation for cancer therapy. *Nat Rev Cancer* 2011;11(11):775-791.

Bjorklund CC, Kang J, Amatangelo M, et al. Iberdomide (CC-220) is a potent cereblon E3 ligase modulator with antitumor and immunostimulatory activities in lenalidomide- and pomalidomide-resistant multiple myeloma cells with dysregulated CRBN. *Leukemia* 2020;34(4):1197-1201.

Blaikie P, Immanuel D, Wu J, Li N, Yajnik V, Margolis B. A region in Shc distinct from the SH2 domain can bind tyrosine-phosphorylated growth factor receptors. *J Biol Chem* 1994;269:32031-32034.

Bondeson DP, Crews CM. Targeted protein degradation by small molecules. *Annu Rev Pharmacol Toxicol* 2017;57:107-123.

Bronisz A, Godlewski J, Wallace JA, et al. Reprogramming of the tumour microenvironment by stromal PTEN-regulated miR-320. *Nat Cell Biol* 2011;14(2):159-167.

Brummer T, McInnes C. RAF kinase dimerization: implications for drug discovery and clinical outcomes. *Oncogene* 2020;39(21):4155-4169.

Buday L, Downward J. Many faces of Ras activation. *Biochim Biophys Acta* 2008;1786:178-187.

Cargnello M, Roux PP. Activation and function of the MAPKs and their substrates, the MAPK-activated protein kinases. *Microbiol Mol Biol Rev* 2011;75(1):50-83.

Chatr-Aryamontri A, van der Sloot A, Tyers M. At long last, a C-terminal bookend for the ubiquitin code. *Mol Cell* 2018;70(4):568-571.

Chen YN, LaMarche MJ, Chan HM, et al. Allosteric inhibition of SHP2 phosphatase inhibits cancers driven by receptor tyrosine kinases. *Nature* 2016;535(7610):148-152.

Chiang JY, Jang IK, Hodes R, Gu H. Ablation of Cbl-b provides protection against transplanted and spontaneous tumors. *J Clin Invest* 2007;117(4):1029-1036.

Ciechanover A. The unravelling of the ubiquitin system. *Nat Rev Mol Cell Biol* 2015;16(5):322-324.

Cooper J, Giancotti FG. Integrin signaling in cancer: mechanotransduction, stemness, epithelial plasticity, and therapeutic resistance. *Cancer Cell* 2019;35(3):347-367.

Costa C, Wang Y, Ly A, et al. PTEN loss mediates clinical cross-resistance to CDK4/6 and PI3kalpha inhibitors in breast cancer. *Cancer Discov* 2020;10(1):72-85.

Dai C, Sampson SB. HSF1: guardian of proteostasis in cancer. *Trends Cell Biol* 2016;26(1):17-28.

Davis RJ, Welcker M, Clurman BE. Tumor suppression by the Fbw7 ubiquitin ligase: mechanisms and opportunities. *Cancer Cell* 2014;26(4):455-464.

DeClue JE, Sadowski I, Martin GS, Pawson T. A conserved domain regulates interactions of the v-fps protein-tyrosine kinase with the host cell. *Proc Natl Acad Sci U S A* 1987;84(24):9064-9068.

Demierre MF, Higgins PD, Gruber SB, Hawk E, Lippman SM. Statins and cancer prevention. *Nat Rev Cancer* 2005;5(12):930-942.

Forman-Kay JD, Pawson T. Diversity in protein recognition by PTB domains. *Curr Opin Struct Biol* 1999;9:690-695.

Fusco N, Sajjadi E, Venetis K, et al. PTEN Alterations and their role in cancer management: are we making headway on precision medicine? *Genes (Basel)* 2020;11(7):719.

Gallahan D, Callahan R. Mammary tumorigenesis in feral mice: identification of a new int locus in mouse mammary tumor virus (Czech II)-induced mammary tumors. *J Virol* 1987;61:66-74.

Garcia Fortanet J, Chen CH, Chen YN, et al. Allosteric inhibition of SHP2: identification of a potent, selective, and orally efficacious phosphatase inhibitor. *J Med Chem* 2016;59(17):7773-7782.

Gatel P, Piechaczyk M, Bossis G. Ubiquitin, SUMO, and Nedd8 as therapeutic targets in cancer. *Adv Exp Med Biol* 2020;1233:29-54.

Golde TE, Koo EH, Felsenstein KM, Osborne BA, Miele L. gamma-Secretase inhibitors and modulators. *Biochim Biophys Acta* 2013;1828(12):2898-2907.

Gordon LB, Shappell H, Massaro J, et al. Association of lonafarnib treatment vs no treatment with mortality rate in patients with hutchinson-gilford progeria syndrome. *JAMA* 2018;319(16):1687-1695.

Goyal S, Jamal S, Shanker A, Grover A. Structural basis for drug resistance mechanisms against EGFR. *Curr Top Med Chem* 2017;17(22):2509-2521.

Grech G, Baldacchino S, Saliba C, et al. Deregulation of the protein phosphatase 2A, PP2A in cancer: complexity and therapeutic options. *Tumour Biol* 2016;37(9):11691-11700.

Gupta N, Hanley MJ, Xia C, Labotka R, Harvey RD, Venkatakrishnan K. Clinical pharmacology of ixazomib: the first oral proteasome inhibitor. *Clin Pharmacokinet* 2019;58(4):431-449.

Hanahan D, Weinberg RA. Hallmarks of cancer: the next generation. *Cell* 2011;144(5):646-674.

Harrigan JA, Jacq X, Martin NM, Jackson SP. Deubiquitylating enzymes and drug discovery: emerging opportunities. *Nat Rev Med* 2018;17(1):57-78.

Hatzihristidis T, Liu S, Pryszcz L, et al. PTP-central: a comprehensive resource of protein tyrosine phosphatases in eukaryotic genomes. *Methods* 2014;65(2):156-164.

Hershko A, Ciechanover A. The ubiquitin system. *Annu Rev Biochem* 1998;67:425-479.

Hill S, Reichermeier K, Scott DC, et al. Robust cullin-RING ligase function is established by a multiplicity of polyubiquitylation pathways. *eLife* 2019;8:e51163.

Hosseini A, Gharibi T, Marofi F, Javadian M, Babaloo Z, Baradaran B. Janus kinase inhibitors: a therapeutic strategy for cancer and autoimmune diseases. *J Cell Physiol* 2020;235(9):5903-5924.

Houles T, Roux PP. Defining the role of the RSK isoforms in cancer. *Semin Cancer Biol* 2018;48:53-61.

Hoxhaj G, Manning BD. The PI3K-AKT network at the interface of oncogenic signalling and cancer metabolism. *Nat Rev Cancer* 2020;20(2):74-88.

Huang M, Chen Y, Han D, Lei Z, Chu X. Role of the zinc finger and SCAN domain-containing transcription factors in cancer. *Am J Cancer Res* 2019;9(5):816-836.

Hunter T. Why nature chose phosphate to modify proteins. *Philos Trans R Soc Lond B Biol Sci* 2012;367(1602):2513-2516.

Imaoka T, Lynham JA, Haslam RJ. Purification and characterization of the 47,000-dalton protein phosphorylated during degranulation of human platelets. *J Biol Chem* 1983;258(18):11404-11414.

Jetten AM. Emerging roles of GLI-similar kruppel-like zinc finger transcription factors in leukemia and other cancers. *Trends Cancer* 2019;5(9):547-557.

Juric D, Castel P, Griffith M, et al. Convergent loss of PTEN leads to clinical resistance to a PI(3)Kalpha inhibitor. *Nature* 2015;518(7538):240-244.

Kales SC, Ryan PE, Nau MM, Lipkowitz S. Cbl and human myeloid neoplasms: the Cbl oncogene comes of age. *Cancer Res* 2010;70:4789-4794.

Kasikara C, Davra V, Calianese D, et al. Pan-TAM tyrosine kinase inhibitor BMS-777607 enhances anti-PD-1 mAb efficacy in a murine model of triple-negative breast cancer. *Cancer Res* 2019;79(10):2669-2683.

Katoh M. Canonical and non-canonical WNT signaling in cancer stem cells and their niches: cellular heterogeneity, omics reprogramming, targeted therapy and tumor plasticity (Review). *Int J Oncol* 2017;51(5):1357-1369.

Katoh M, Katoh M. Molecular genetics and targeted therapy of WNT-related human diseases (review). *Int J Mol Med* 2017;40(3):587-606.

Katzav S, Schmitz ML. Mutations of c-Cbl in myeloid malignancies. *Oncotarget* 2015;6(13):10689-10696.

Kikkawa U. The story of PKC: a discovery marked by unexpected twists and turns. *IUBMB Life* 2019;71(6):697-705.

Koch CA, Moran M, Sadowski I, Pawson T. The common src homology region 2 domain of cytoplasmic signaling proteins is a positive effector of v-fps tyrosine kinase function. *Mol Cell Biol* 1989;9(10):4131-4140.

Koren I, Timms RT, Kula T, Xu Q, Li MZ, Elledge SJ. The eukaryotic proteome is shaped by E3 ubiquitin ligases targeting C-terminal degrons. *Cell* 2018;173(7):1622-1635.e14.

Krishnamurthy N, Kurzrock R. Targeting the Wnt/beta-catenin pathway in cancer: update on effectors and inhibitors. *Cancer Treat Rev* 2018;62:50-60.

Kwon YT, Ciechanover A. The ubiquitin code in the ubiquitin-proteasome system and autophagy. *Trends Biochem Sci* 2017;42(11):873-886.

Laribee RN, Weisman R. Nuclear functions of TOR: impact on transcription and the epigenome. *Genes (Basel)* 2020;11(6):641.

Lavoie H, Li JJ, Thevakumaran N, Therrien M, Sicheri F. Dimerization-induced allostery in protein kinase regulation. *Trends Biochem Sci* 2014;39(10):475-486.

Lemmon MA, Schlessinger J. Cell signaling by receptor tyrosine kinases. *Cell* 2010;141:1117-1134.

Levy JMM, Towers CG, Thorburn A. Targeting autophagy in cancer. *Nat Rev Cancer* 2017;17(9):528-542.

Lewicki MC, Srikumar T, Johnson E, Raught B. The S. cerevisiae SUMO stress response is a conjugation-deconjugation cycle that targets the transcription machinery. *J Proteomics* 2015;118:39-48.

Li S, Balmain A, Counter CM. A model for RAS mutation patterns in cancers: finding the sweet spot. *Nat Rev Cancer* 2018;18(12):767-777.

Li X, Song Y. Proteolysis-targeting chimera (PROTAC) for targeted protein degradation and cancer therapy. *J Hematol Oncol* 2020;13(1):50.

Lin HC, Yeh CW, Chen YF, et al. C-Terminal end-directed protein elimination by CRL2 ubiquitin ligases. *Mol Cell* 2018;70(4):602-613.e3.

Liu S, Wan J, Kong Y, Zhang Y, Wan L, Zhang Z. Inhibition of CRL-NEDD8 pathway as a new approach to enhance ATRA-induced differentiation of acute promyelocytic leukemia cells. *Int J Med Sci* 2018;15(7):674-681.

Liu X, Teng Y, Wu X, et al. The E3 ubiquitin ligase Cbl-b predicts favorable prognosis in breast cancer. *Front Oncol* 2020;10:695.

Liu Y, Mallampalli RK. Small molecule therapeutics targeting F-box proteins in cancer. *Semin Cancer Biol* 2016;36:105-119.

Loeser S, Loser K, Bijker MS, et al. Spontaneous tumor rejection by cbl-b-deficient CD8+ T cells. *J Exp Med* 2007;204(4):879-891.

Lopez G, Noale M, Corti C, et al. PTEN expression as a complementary biomarker for mismatch repair testing in breast cancer. *Int J Mol Sci.* 2020;21(4):1461.

Lucas X, Ciulli A. Recognition of substrate degrons by E3 ubiquitin ligases and modulation by small-molecule mimicry strategies. *Curr Opin Struct Biol* 2017;44:101-110.

Martin GS. Cell signaling and cancer. *Cancer Cell* 2003;4(3):167-174.

Mohi MG, Neel BG. The role of Shp2 (PTPN11) in cancer. *Curr Opin Genet Dev* 2007;17(1):23-30.

Moore G, Annett S, McClements L, Robson T. Top notch targeting strategies in cancer: a detailed overview of recent insights and current perspectives. *Cells* 2020;9(6):1503.

Moran MF, Koch CA, Anderson D, et al. Src homology region 2 domains direct protein-protein interactions in signal transduction. *Proc Natl Acad Sci U S A* 1990;87(21):8622-8626.

Morita M, Gravel SP, Hulea L, et al. mTOR coordinates protein synthesis, mitochondrial activity and proliferation. *Cell Cycle* 2015;14(4):473-480.

Mugler A, Bailey AG, Takahashi K, ten Wolde PR. Membrane clustering and the role of rebinding in biochemical signaling. *Biophys J* 2012;102(5):1069-1078.

Mullen AC, Wrana JL. TGF-beta family signaling in embryonic and somatic stem-cell renewal and differentiation. *Cold Spring Harb Perspect Biol* 2017;9(7):a022186.

Nielsen SF, Nordestgaard BG, Bojesen SE. Statin use and reduced cancer-related mortality. *N Engl J Med* 2012;367(19):1792-1802.

Nishida T, Kaneko F, Kitagawa M, Yasuda H. Characterization of a novel mammalian SUMO-1/Smt3-specific isopeptidase, a homologue of rat axam, which is an axin-binding protein promoting beta-catenin degradation. *J Biol Chem* 2001;276(42):39060-39066.

Niyaz M, Khan MS, Mudassar S. Hedgehog signaling: an Achilles' heel in cancer. *Transl Oncol* 2019;12(10):1334-1344.

Nusse R, Clevers H. Wnt/beta-catenin signaling, disease, and emerging therapeutic modalities. *Cell* 2017;169(6):985-999.

Oromendia AB, Amon A. Aneuploidy: implications for protein homeostasis and disease. *Dis Model Mech* 2014;7(1):15-20.

Oshima M, Dinchuk JE, Kargman SL, et al. Suppression of intestinal polyposis in Apc delta716 knockout mice by inhibition of cyclooxygenase 2 (COX-2). *Cell* 1996;87(5):803-809.

Paolino M, Choidas A, Wallner S, et al. The E3 ligase Cbl-b and TAM receptors regulate cancer metastasis via natural killer cells. *Nature* 2014;507(7493):508-512.

Paolino M, Penninger JM. The role of TAM family receptors in immune cell function: implications for cancer therapy. *Cancers (Basel)* 2016;8(10):97.

Paolino M, Thien CB, Gruber T, et al. Essential role of E3 ubiquitin ligase activity in Cbl-b-regulated T cell functions. *J Immunol* 2011;186(4):2138-2147.

Papadopoli D, Boulay K, Kazak L, et al. mTOR as a central regulator of lifespan and aging. *F1000Res* 2019;8.

Park NI, Guilhamon P, Desai K, et al. ASCL1 reorganizes chromatin to direct neuronal fate and suppress tumorigenicity of glioblastoma stem cells. *Cell Stem Cell* 2017;21(2):209-224.e7.

Patra SK. Roles of OCT4 in pathways of embryonic development and cancer progression. *Mech Ageing Dev* 2020;189:111286.

Pawson T, Nash P. Assembly of cell regulatory systems through protein interaction domains. *Science* 2003;300:445-452.

Penafuerte C, Perez-Quintero LA, Vinette V, Hatzihristidis T, Tremblay ML. Mining the complex family of protein tyrosine phosphatases for checkpoint regulators in immunity. *Curr Top Microbiol Immunol* 2017;410:191-214.

Peng A, Maller JL. Serine/threonine phosphatases in the DNA damage response and cancer. *Oncogene* 2010;29(45):5977-5988.

Picon A, Gold LI, Wang J, Cohen A, Friedman E. A subset of metastatic human colon cancers expresses elevated levels of transforming growth factor beta1. *Cancer Epidemiol Biomarkers Prev* 1998;7(6):497-504.

Pohl C, Dikic I. Cellular quality control by the ubiquitin-proteasome system and autophagy. *Science* 2019;366:818-822.

Polakis P. The many ways of Wnt in cancer. *Curr Opin Genet Dev* 2007;17:45-51.

Proietti I, Skroza N, Michelini S, et al. BRAF inhibitors: molecular targeting and immunomodulatory actions. *Cancers (Basel)* 2020;12(7):1823.

Rajakulendran N, Rowland KJ, Selvadurai HJ, et al. Wnt and Notch signaling govern self-renewal and differentiation in a subset of human glioblastoma stem cells. *Genes Dev* 2019;33(9-10):498-510.

Razavi P, Dickler MN, Shah PD, et al. Alterations in PTEN and ESR1 promote clinical resistance to aleplisib plus aromatase inhibitors. *Nat Cancer* 2020;1:382-393.

Reebye V, Frilling A, Hajitou A, Nicholls JP, Habib NA, Mintz PJ. A perspective on non-catalytic Src homology (SH) adaptor signalling proteins. *Cell Signal* 2012;24(2):388-392.

Reedijk M, Odorcic S, Chang L, et al. High-level coexpression of JAG1 and NOTCH1 is observed in human breast cancer and is associated with poor overall survival. *Cancer Res* 2005;65(18):8530-8537.

Richardson PG, Oriol A, Beksac M, et al. Pomalidomide, bortezomib, and dexamethasone for patients with relapsed or refractory multiple myeloma previously treated with lenalidomide (OPTIMISMM): a randomised, open-label, phase 3 trial. *Lancet Oncol* 2019;20(6):781-794.

Rulina AV, Mittler F, Obeid P, et al. Distinct outcomes of CRL-Nedd8 pathway inhibition reveal cancer cell plasticity. *Cell Death Dis* 2016;7(12):e2505.

Safholm A, Tuomela J, Rosenkvist J, Dejmek J, Harkonen P, Andersson T. The Wnt-5a-derived hexapeptide Foxy-5 inhibits breast cancer metastasis in vivo by targeting cell motility. *Clin Cancer Res* 2008;14:6556-6563.

Schapira M, Calabrese M, Bullock AN, Crews CM. Targeted protein degradation: expanding the toolbox. *Nat Rev Drug Disc* 2019;18(12):949-963.

Scheffzek K, Welti S. Pleckstrin homology (PH) like domains—versatile modules in protein-protein interaction platforms. *FEBS Lett* 2012;586(17):2662-2673.

Shimomura A, Yamamoto N, Kondo S, et al. First-in-human phase I study of an oral HSP90 inhibitor, TAS-116, in patients with advanced solid tumors. *Mol Cancer Ther* 2019;18(3):531-540.

Sicheri F, Kuriyan J. Structures of Src-family tyrosine kinases. *Curr Opin Struct Biol* 1997;7(6):777-785.

Skoda AM, Simovic D, Karin V, Kardum V, Vranic S, Serman L. The role of the Hedgehog signaling pathway in cancer: a comprehensive review. *Bosn J Basic Med Sci* 2018;18(1):8-20.

Srikumar T, Lewicki MC, Costanzo M, et al. Global analysis of SUMO chain function reveals multiple roles in chromatin regulation. *J Cell Biol* 2013;201(1):145-163.

Steinbach G, Lynch PM, Phillips RK, et al. The effect of celecoxib, a cyclooxygenase-2 inhibitor in familial adenomatous polyposis. *N Engl J Med* 2000;342(26):1946-1952.

Suva ML, Rheinbay E, Gillespie SM, et al. Reconstructing and reprogramming the tumor-propagating potential of glioblastoma stem-like cells. *Cell* 2014;157(3):580-594.

Thompson JJ, Williams CS. Protein phosphatase 2A in the regulation of Wnt signaling, stem cells, and cancer. *Genes (Basel)* 2018;9(3):121.

Tiash S, Chowdhury EH. Growth factor receptors: promising drug targets in cancer. *J Cancer Metastasis Treat* 2015;1:19-200.

Tonks NK. Protein tyrosine phosphatases: from genes, to function, to disease. *Nat Rev Mol Cell Biol* 2006;7(11):833-846.

Tyers M, Rachubinski RA, Sartori CS, Harley CB, Haslam RJ. Induction of the 47 kDa platelet substrate of protein kinase C during differentiation of HL-60 cells. *Biochem J* 1987;243(1):249-253.

Tyers M, Rachubinski RA, Stewart MI, et al. Molecular cloning and expression of the major protein kinase C substrate of platelets. *Nature* 1988;333(6172):470-473.

Varnat F, Duquet A, Malerba M, et al. Human colon cancer epithelial cells harbour active HEDGEHOG-GLI signalling that is essential for tumour growth, recurrence, metastasis and stem cell survival and expansion. *EMBO Mol Med* 2009;1:338-351.

Vasan N, Razavi P, Johnson JL, et al. Double PIK3CA mutations in cis increase oncogenicity and sensitivity to PI3Kalpha inhibitors. *Science* 2019;366(6466):714-723.

Wagner MJ, Stacey MM, Liu BA, Pawson T. Molecular mechanisms of SH2- and PTB-domain-containing proteins in receptor tyrosine kinase signaling. *Cold Spring Harb Perspect Biol* 2013;5(12):a008987.

Westermarck J. Targeted therapies don't work for a reason; the neglected tumor suppressor phosphatase PP2A strikes back. *FEBS J* 2018;285(22):4139-4145.

Wong PP, Demircioglu F, Ghazaly E, et al. Dual-action combination therapy enhances angiogenesis while reducing tumor growth and spread. *Cancer Cell* 2015;27(1):123-137.

Yao Z, Han L, Chen Y, et al. Hedgehog signalling in the tumourigenesis and metastasis of osteosarcoma, and its potential value in the clinical therapy of osteosarcoma. *Cell Death Dis* 2018;9(6):701.

Yau R, Rape M. The increasing complexity of the ubiquitin code. *Nat Cell Biol* 2016;18(6):579-586.

Yeh CH, Bellon M, Nicot C. FBXW7: a critical tumor suppressor of human cancers. *Mol Cancer* 2018;17(1):115.

You D, Xin J, Volk A, et al. FAK mediates a compensatory survival signal parallel to PI3K-AKT in PTEN-null T-ALL cells. *Cell Rep* 2015;10(12):2055-2068.

Yu R, Longo J, van Leeuwen JE, et al. Statin-induced cancer cell death can be mechanistically uncoupled from prenylation of RAS family proteins. *Cancer Res* 2018;78(5):1347-1357.

Yuno A, Lee MJ, Lee S, et al. Clinical evaluation and biomarker profiling of Hsp90 inhibitors. *Methods Mol Biol* 2018;1709:423-441.

Zhou L, Jia L. Targeting protein neddylation for cancer therapy. *Adv Exp Med Biol* 2020;1217:297-315.

Oncogenes and Tumor-Suppressor Genes

Previn Dutt and Vuk Stambolic

Chapter Outline

7.1 Introduction
7.2 Discovering the Genetic Basis of Cancer
    7.2.1 Historical Perspective
    7.2.2 Transforming Retroviruses and the Discovery of Oncogenes
    7.2.3 Isolation of the First Tumor Suppressor
    7.2.4 The Genomics Age and Beyond
7.3 The Properties of Neoplastic Cells
7.4 The Basis of Tumorigenesis
    7.4.1 Changes at the Genetic Level
    7.4.2 Changes at the Epigenetic Level
    7.4.3 Changes at the RNA Level
    7.4.4 Viruses and Changes at the Protein Level
7.5 Gain of Function Events
    7.5.1 BCR-ABL
    7.5.2 MYC
    7.5.3 EGFR/ERBB2
    7.5.4 PI3 Kinase
    7.5.5 RAS and RAF
    7.5.6 IDH
7.6 Loss-of-Function Events
    7.6.1 p53
    7.6.2 PTEN
    7.6.3 BRCA1 and BRCA2
    7.6.4 Retinoblastoma Protein
7.7 Therapeutic Strategies Guided by Cancer Genetics
Summary
References

7.1 INTRODUCTION

Cancer is fundamentally driven by genetic changes in normal cells that result in the acquisition of transformative malignant properties. These mutations permit the uncontrolled replication of the transformed cancer cells, a small fraction of which ultimately gains the ability to leave their tissue of origin and invade distant parts of the body where metastatic lesions are established. The second half of the 20th century witnessed a steady stream of breakthroughs in the field of cancer research, largely spurred by an explosion of technologies facilitating the analysis of tumors at a molecular level. Recent advances in low-cost high-throughput sequencing of cancer genomes (Chap. 2) are enabling a detailed mapping of the genetic events associated with the transformation of nonmalignant cells to metastatic cancer cells.

Comprehensive surveys of cancer genomes have highlighted the complexity of the disease and are also guiding the development of targeted anticancer treatments based on discrete molecular features (see Chap. 19). These efforts are revealing the extreme genetic heterogeneity that exists among tumors originating in the same tissue and, conversely, the similarities occasionally found in cancers arising in different tissues (see Chap. 13). Although a given tumor may harbor hundreds of mutations, only a few can truly be regarded as "driver" mutations that confer a selective growth advantage to transformed cells. The remaining "passenger" mutations result from the genetic instability of cancer cells without contributing actively to oncogenesis. Distinguishing between the driver and passenger mutations is critical for the identification of therapeutic targets and the development of tailored treatment regimens designed to maximize anti-cancer activity while minimizing side effects (Fig. 7–1) (Pon and Marra, 2015).

7.2 DISCOVERING THE GENETIC BASIS OF CANCER

7.2.1 Historical Perspective

The pronounced age dependence of cancer onset, coupled with the more limited life expectancies of premodern times, meant that cancer was a less prevalent killer than other diseases until comparatively recently. As a result, although humans have been

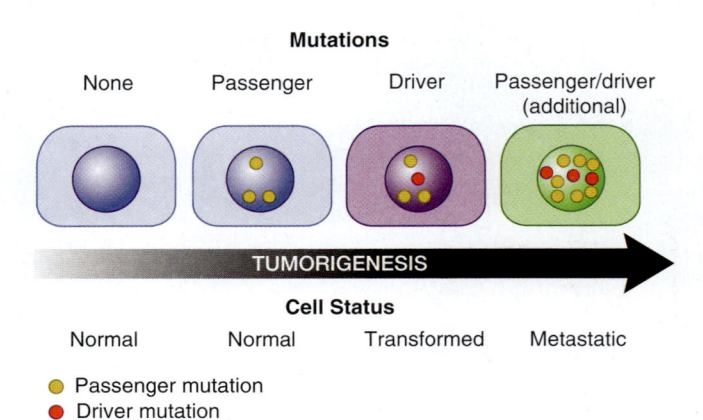

FIGURE 7-1 Passenger and driver mutations. Recent tumor sequencing efforts have revealed that transformed cells acquire a genetic landscape marked by the accumulation of numerous mutations. Among these genetic changes, however, are a much more limited subset of driver mutations that actively impart oncogenic properties, with the remaining passenger mutations representing inert changes that are neither selected for or against during tumorigenesis. Distinguishing between driver and passenger mutations is a critical research objective as the former represent potential therapeutic targets.

afflicted by the disease since the beginning, references to cancer in the historical sources are scarce, and a proper understanding of its nature has long proved elusive. Hippocrates attributed the disease to an excess of "black bile," one of the 4 constituent fluids the ancient Greeks believed made up the human body. Remarkably, this humoral theory persisted as the dominant explanation for cancer for nearly 2 millennia thereafter.

The genesis of understanding cancer as a genetic disease can be traced to experiments carried out more than a century ago, the implications of which would go largely unappreciated for decades. In 1902, the German biologist Theodor Boveri manipulated the structure of sea urchin chromosomes and uncovered an association between malignant cellular growth and genomic abnormalities (Hansford and Huntsman, 2014). Based on these findings, he speculated presciently on the existence of cell-cycle checkpoints as well as oncogenes and tumor suppressors, which are now known actors in oncogenesis. However, the first definitive correlation between chromosomal defects and cancer in humans was not reported until 1960, with the discovery of the chronic myeloid leukemia (CML)–associated Philadelphia chromosome, generated by a gene translocation event (Mughal et al, 2016).

7.2.2 Transforming Retroviruses and the Discovery of Oncogenes

Although retroviruses have not been linked widely to human cancers, they can transform rodent and chicken cells, and much of the pioneering work leading to the identification of the first oncogenes was carried out in these model systems. In 1911, Peyton Rous demonstrated that cell-free filtrates isolated from chicken sarcomas, later determined to contain retroviruses, were capable of inducing tumor growth when introduced into healthy birds (Rous, 1911). He also documented the various characteristics which these tumors shared with the original sarcomas, such as morphologic appearance as well as the capacity to metastasize and invade distant tissues.

These seminal experiments led ultimately to the isolation of viral oncogenes from several transforming tumor viruses. In 1976, Bishop and Varmus isolated the oncogenic region of the Rous sarcoma virus, containing the *v-src* gene, by comparing the genetic content of a transformation-defective version of the virus with that of its highly transforming counterpart (Stehelin et al, 1976). They discovered that the normal avian DNA contained a nearly identical version of the *v-src* gene and proposed that oncogenes were altered versions of normal cellular genes, which they termed *proto-oncogenes*. Moreover, their findings suggested correctly that other oncogenes might be found in the genomes of other transforming retroviruses. Similarly, *v-myc* was identified in the MC29 avian myelocytomatosis virus, *v-erbb* in the avian erythroblastosis virus, whereas *v-h-ras* and *v-k-ras* were found in murine leukemia viruses.

Attention increasingly shifted toward the identification of human oncogenes. In 1982, the first somatically mutated cellular oncogenes were isolated in various laboratories by employing strategies that involved introducing DNA isolated from human cancer cell lines into mouse fibroblasts, which were then monitored for transformation. Isolation of individual genes from the transformed fibroblasts led to the identification of the activated mutant versions of the *H-RAS* and *K-RAS* oncogenes, derived from human bladder and lung carcinoma cell lines, respectively (Der et al, 1982). A year later, mutant *N-RAS* was similarly isolated from a neuroblastoma cell line (Shimizu et al, 1983).

7.2.3 Isolation of the First Tumor Suppressor

Although the prevailing view in the 1970s was that neoplastic transformation resulted from activating mutations in oncogenes, it was during this period that Alfred Knudson proposed his "two-hit" hypothesis to explain multistage cancer progression, that would ultimately lead to the discovery of inactivating mutations in tumor-suppressor genes (Knudson, 1971). His argument was premised on the suggestion that the mutational requirements of cancer progression could be delineated by comparing the incidence rates of inherited and sporadic forms of retinoblastoma. Individuals who had inherited one mutant allele presented the disease at a frequency consistent with a single somatic mutation, whereas individuals who had not inherited a mutant allele exhibited an age-onset pattern consistent with 2 mutations. It soon became clear that the onset of hereditary retinoblastoma could be explained by loss of heterozygosity (LOH) at a tumor-suppressor locus. In the inherited heterozygous state, sufficient functional tumor suppressor is expressed from the wild-type allele to compensate for the inactive protein produced by the mutant allele and prevent tumorigenesis. Disease progression is contingent on the loss of the heterozygous state through inactivation of the wild-type allele, which ablates expression of the tumor-suppressor activity.

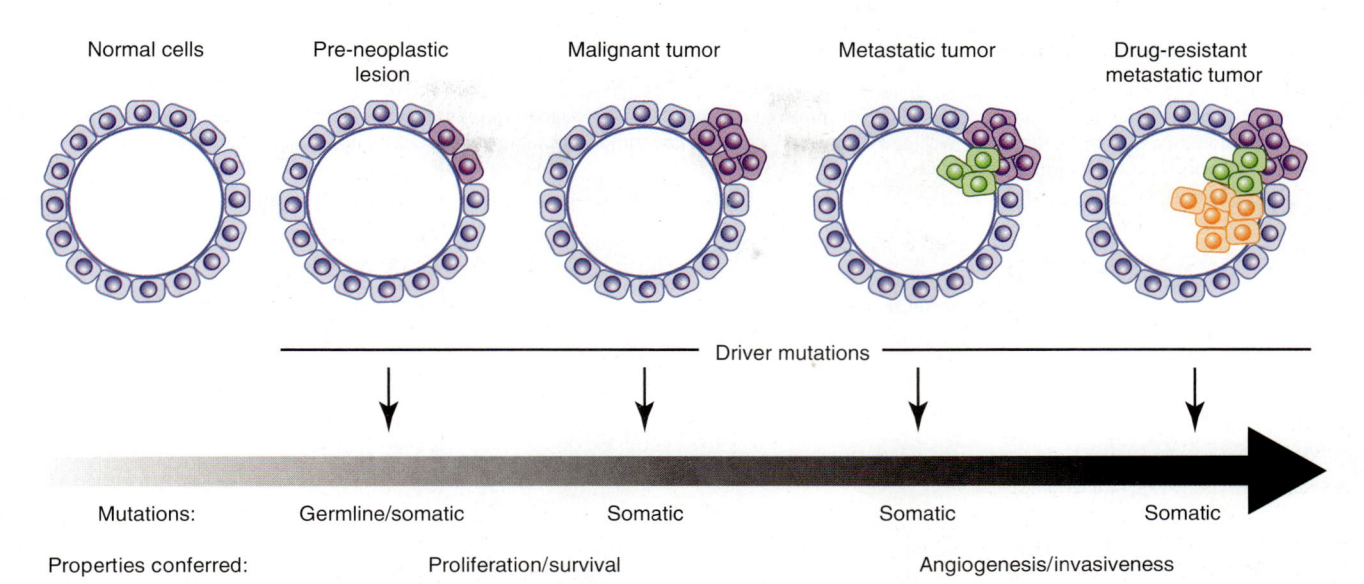

FIGURE 7-2 Multistage oncogenesis. During oncogenesis, a tumor progressively acquires a set of abnormal properties that enable it to support the growing mass of cells and ultimately metastasize to distant sites. It has long been recognized that this constitutes a multistep process involving a series of oncogenic hits, potentially occurring at both the germline (inherited) or somatic level. More recently, it has been appreciated that, in addition to genetic mutations, these hits can entail changes at the epigenetic, transcriptomic, proteomic, and metabolic levels. Moreover, these tumorigenic programs can be driven by different sets of oncogenic hits and progress at different rates. In the final stage, novel mutations enable tumor cells to become resistant to therapeutic intervention.

During the 1980s, the molecular basis for the Knudson model was revealed with the mapping of the retinoblastoma (*Rb1*) locus to a chromosomal region containing homozygous deletions, in both inherited and sporadic retinoblastomas (Cavenee et al, 1983). In 1986, a complementary DNA (cDNA) fragment mapping to the *Rb1* locus was isolated and found to be at least partially deleted in retinoblastomas (Friend et al, 1986). The following year, 2 groups cloned the Rb cDNA and reported that the transcript was either expressed in a truncated form or was entirely undetectable in tumors (Fung et al, 1987; Lee et al, 1987). Collectively, these results demonstrated the existence of a recessively acting cancer gene, with the homozygous loss of the wild-type *Rb1* locus correlating with retinoblastoma development, as predicted by Knudson's theoretical work 15 years earlier (see also Sec. 7.6.4).

7.2.4 The Genomics Age and Beyond

By the beginning of the 1990s, a clearer picture of the genetic changes accompanying cancer progression led to the realization that cancer is a disease involving a combination of either inherited or somatic mutations, resulting in the activation of oncogenes or inactivation of tumor-suppressor genes (Fig. 7–2). Since then, additional putative oncogenes and tumor suppressors have been cataloged using both classical methods as well as novel high-throughput sequencing (Table 7–1; see Chap. 2, for techniques). Functional characterization of proteins encoded by oncogenes and tumor-suppressor genes has led to an improved understanding of the processes responsible for tumorigenesis. A more complete understanding of cancer must include consideration of epigenetic factors and other disease-associated changes beyond the genomic level, which influence normal and malignant cellular behavior (see Chap. 3).

Comprehensive analyses of genomic, epigenetic, transcriptomic, proteomic, and metabolic states have been rendered practical by the advent of these new high-throughput technologies. A clearer picture delineating the cellular events occurring at each stage of cancer progression is becoming available. This, in turn, is encouraging the reclassification of cancers by molecular alterations rather than tissue of origin, as well as promoting the identification of novel drug targets, and the development of prognostic tools capable of predicting metastatic propensity, therapeutic response, and survival (Fig. 7–3).

7.3 THE PROPERTIES OF NEOPLASTIC CELLS

The various tissues of the human body have evolved tightly regulated homeostatic mechanisms and lineage differentiation pathways that govern their function and regeneration capacity. Tumorigenesis is initiated when small populations of cells acquire genetic mutations that enable them to circumvent the homeostatic programs specific to their tissue microenvironment. The subsequent survival and expansion of the tumor mass is contingent on the acquisition of additional neoplastic properties. Ultimately, tumor cells gain metastatic potential, involving the capacity to migrate from their tissue of origin and invade distant sites to establish secondary malignancies (see Chap. 10).

Hanahan and Weinberg proposed that virtually all cancer cells exhibit certain hallmark properties: self-sufficiency in

TABLE 7–1 Oncogenes and tumor-suppressor genes.

Tumor initiation, expansion, and metastasis are driven by a combination of oncogene gain-of-function and tumor-suppressor loss-of-function mutagenic events, which confer neoplastic properties on the population of cancer cells. These aberrations may occur at the genetic, epigenetic, transcriptomic, proteomic, or metabolic levels. Some well-characterized oncogenes and tumor suppressors are listed, along with the tumors they are commonly associated with and approved targeted therapies.

Oncogene	Cancer	Targeted Therapy
p110α	breast, prostate, endometrial, colorectal, cervical, head and neck, gastric, lung	
EGFR	lung, glioma, colorectal, ovarian, breast	gefitinib, erlotinib, cetuximab, afatinib, osimertinib
ERBB2 (HER2)	breast, gastric, ovarian, bladder	trastuzumab, lapatinib, neratinib, pertuzumab
B-RAF	melanoma, thyroid, colorectal, ovarian	vemurafenib, dabrafenib
K-RAS	pancreatic, lung, colorectal, endometrial, ovarian	
H-RAS	bladder	
N-RAS	melanoma, AML	
MYC	lymphomas, colorectal, breast, prostate, melanoma, neuroblastoma, ovarian	
BCR-ABL	CML, ALL, AML	imatinib, dasatinib, nilotinib, ponatinib, bosutinib
IDH1	glioblastoma, AML	
IDH2	glioblastoma, AML	enasidenib
JAK2	CML, ALL	
KIT	gastrointestinal stromal tumors, AML, melanoma	
MET	kidney, gastric, lung, head and neck, colorectal	
FLT-3	AML	midostaurin
ALK	lung	alectinib, brigatinib, ceritinib, crizotinib
ROS1	lung	crizotinib
NTRK	various solid tumors	entrectinib
Tumor Suppressor	**Cancer**	**Targeted Therapy**
p53	lung, colorectal, bladder, ovarian, head and neck, gastric, breast, prostate	
PTEN	glioblastoma, melanoma, prostate, breast, endometrial, thyroid, lung, colorectal, AML, CLL	
p16^{INK4A}	melanoma, pancreatic, lung, bladder, head and neck, colorectal, breast	
p14^{ARF}	lung, bladder, head and neck, colorectal, breast	
BRCA1	breast, ovarian	olaparib
BRCA2	breast, ovarian	olaparib
LKB1	lung, gastrointestinal, pancreatic, cervical, melanoma	
VHL	kidney, adrenal, hemangioblastoma	
APC	colorectal, gastric	
FBXW7	ALL, bile duct, colorectal, gastric, endometrial, lung, pancreatic, prostate, ovarian	
Rb	retinoblastoma, lung, bladder, esophageal, osteosarcoma, glioma, liver, CML, prostate, breast	
NF1	neurofibroma, neuroblastoma, glioma, colorectal	
NF2	meningioma, schwannoma, glioma	

Abbreviations: *ALL*, acute lymphoblastic leukemia; *AML*, acute myelogenous leukemia; *CML*, chronic myeloid leukemia; *CLL*, chronic lymphocytic leukemia

growth signals, insensitivity to antigrowth signals, evasion of apoptosis, limitless replicative potential, sustained angiogenesis, genomic instability, deregulated metabolism, the capacity for invasion and metastasis, as well as the ability to circumvent immune clearance and stimulate tumor-promoting inflammation (Hanahan and Weinberg, 2000; Hanahan and Weinberg, 2011). Although a disproportionate number of cancer-associated mutations are found in a small group of critical regulatory genes, each of these characteristics can be acquired through distinct sets of mutations, and the extreme

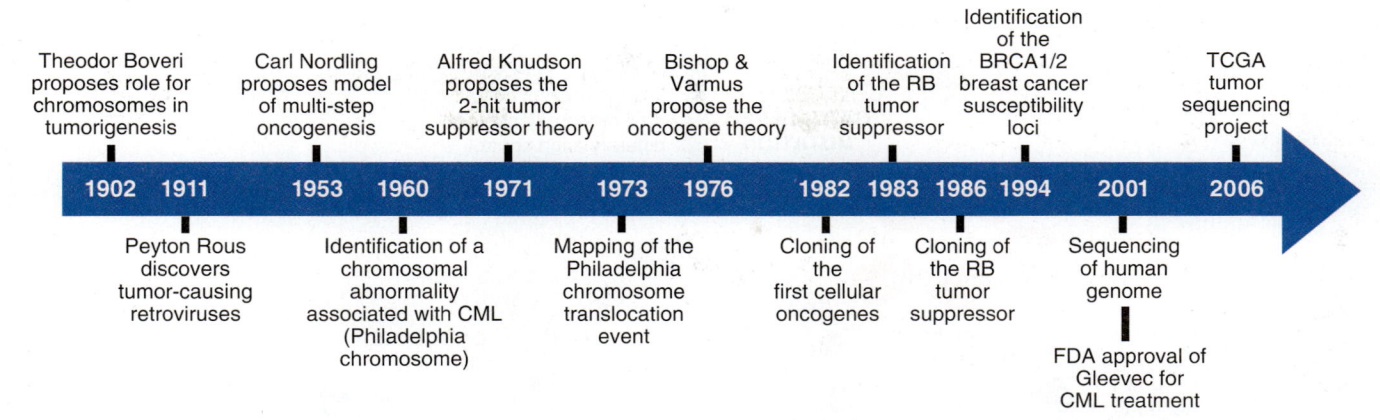

FIGURE 7-3 Timeline of cancer discoveries. For much of the past 2 millennia, our understanding of cancer remained relatively static. Beginning in the middle of the 19th century technologic improvements have revolutionized our capacity to study the disease and led to a number of paradigm-shifting discoveries. This process has accelerated in recent decades such that individual tumors can now be comprehensively analyzed and, in some cases, personalized therapies designed to target the appropriate oncogenic mechanisms.

genetic heterogeneity of cancer cells serves as a platform for the selection of tumor-promoting properties. Aberrant autocrine growth signaling, as well as hyperactivation of transmembrane receptors or intracellular signal transducers, can engender self-sufficiency in growth signals (Chap. 6). Acquired insensitivity to antigrowth signals often involves inactivation of the Rb protein or inhibition of terminal differentiation (Sec. 7.6.4). Resistance to apoptotic death is frequently associated with loss of the p53 tumor suppressor (Sec. 7.6.1), as well as the upregulation of antiapoptotic proteins such as BCL2 (Chap. 8, Sec. 8.4.1). The replicative potential of normal cells is limited by the progressive attrition of telomeres at chromosome ends, a tendency counteracted in malignant cells through activation of the telomerase enzyme (Chap. 9, Sec. 9.7). The nutrient requirements of expanding tumors necessitate the de novo formation of blood vessels, triggered by a combination of upregulated proangiogenic factors, such as vascular endothelial growth factor (VEGF), and downregulation of inhibitory factors like thrombospondin-1 (Chap. 11). The spread of tumor cells to secondary sites requires the disruption of cell-cell and cell–extracellular matrix (ECM) contacts, as well as the capacity to penetrate tissue compartments, often through upregulation of extracellular protease activity (see Chap. 10).

Although the reductionist approach of characterizing tumors by autonomous molecular changes in their cells can be beneficial, it is also important to conceptualize tumors within their tissue contexts. Solid tumors in particular are heterotypic collections of cells that include stromal compartments supporting the growth of the malignant cells (Chap. 12, Sec. 12.2). This idea was encapsulated in a model of oncogenesis advocated by Kinzler and Vogelstein, who classified cancer-associated genetic changes as gatekeeper, caretaker, and landscaper mutations (Kinzler and Vogelstein, 1998; Fig. 7-4). The gatekeepers are generally tumor suppressors that normally constrain growth by regulating cell-cycle progression and activating apoptotic mechanisms as required. The caretakers, often DNA repair proteins, impede oncogenesis by preventing the genetic instability that favors the creation of tumorigenic mutations (Chap. 9, Sec. 9.3). Alterations in stromal cells, which promote tumorigenesis, were termed landscaper mutations. One noteworthy example is represented by the presence of senescent cells within tumors. Both normal and malignant cells can enter into a growth-arrested senescent state either because of intrinsic stress or therapeutic intervention. Though senescent cells, by definition, cannot contribute to tumor growth through their own proliferation, they can support tumorigenesis through the secretion of cytokines, growth factors, and proteases, a phenomenon known as the senescence-associated secretory phenotype (SASP) (Rao and Jackson, 2016). Although senescence has generally been thought of as a tumor-suppressive mechanism, it now appears that cells can acquire the capacity to secrete factors that promote, for instance, an immunosuppressive environment amenable to tumor expansion.

7.4 THE BASIS OF TUMORIGENESIS

Although cancer cells are defined at the cellular level by a handful of hallmark properties, changes at the molecular level are numerous, diverse, and complex. Mutagenic processes arise both intrinsically, for instance from errors associated with DNA replication, as well as from extrinsic sources such as chemical toxins or tumor viruses. The genetic mutations that are responsible for cancer initiation are accompanied by additional alterations at the epigenetic, transcript, and protein levels (Fig. 7-5). Deregulation at any one of these levels may induce a cascade of additional mutagenic effects, creating the molecular basis for tumor expansion through clonal selection. In addition to point mutations, which can result in changes to amino acid sequences, other mutagenic events include gene amplification, deletions and insertions, as well as chromosomal translocations. The expression levels of cancer-associated genes can also be modulated epigenetically through

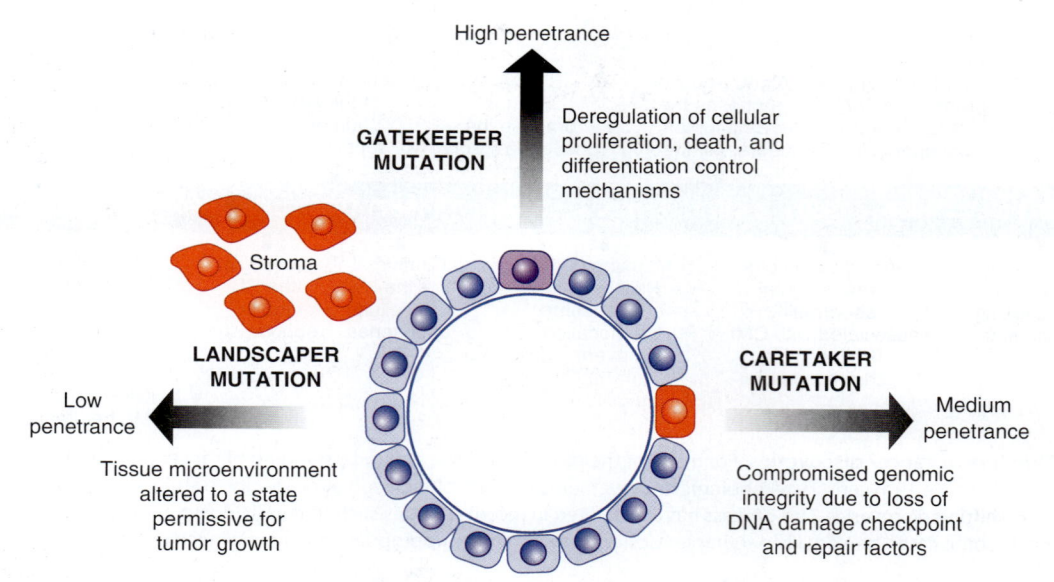

FIGURE 7–4 Gatekeeper, caretaker, and landscaper mutations. In the late 1990s, Kenneth Kinzler and Bert Vogelstein proposed a model of tumorigenesis based on their observations of the oncogenic mechanisms underlying hereditary colorectal cancer. Tumor-promoting genes were classified as gatekeepers, caretakers, and landscapers according to their function. Gatekeeper genes encode proteins that regulate cell fate, be it proliferation, growth, arrest, death, or differentiation. Because a deregulation in these mechanisms is likely to lead directly to abnormal growth, mutations in these genes correlate with the highest risk of cancer. Caretaker genes encode proteins that are responsible for guarding the integrity of the genome, with loss of function increasing the risk of acquiring mutations, for instance in gatekeeper genes, that would lead to oncogenic growth. Mutations occurring in cells of the surrounding tissue stroma can create a microenvironment that is more permissive for tumorigenesis, and the associated genes were categorized as landscapers. As the functions of these genes are primarily supportive, in isolation, these mutations are much less penetrant.

promoter methylation, as well as the methylation, acetylation, and phosphorylation of histones (Chap. 3). Additional changes in the expression levels of proteins arise due to the modulation of transcriptional rates and messenger RNA (mRNA) stability, often involving the actions of small noncoding RNAs (Chap. 2, Sec. 2.3.3). Viral proteins can transform infected cells by directly interacting with and modifying the behavior of critical regulatory proteins in the host. Ultimately, the deregulation of oncogenic targets, through an array of mutagenic mechanisms, is the means through which tumorigenesis confers the hallmark properties of cancer on transformed cells.

Specific oncogenes and tumor-suppressor genes are mutated in some types of cancers but not others, even varying among tumor subtypes that arise within the same tissue. Understanding why certain mutations or combinations of mutations occur preferentially in specific tumors is important, but remains speculative. The specific mutations capable of conferring neoplastic properties are dictated by the specific regulatory mechanisms that normally control these processes in the given tumor cell progenitor. Multiple, partially redundant, regulatory networks regulate most cellular functions. Because these networks have varying influence in different cell types, the severity of the effects caused by their disruption will also vary, and mutations in specific cancer genes will be subject to different selective pressures, depending on the cellular context in which they occur. Mutations that confer a selective advantage in one cell type may have little effect or even compromise the viability of another cell type. Factors likely to govern the effect of a specific mutation include the expression level of the gene, the existence of compensatory mechanisms, developmental stage, as well as the modifying effects of other mutations.

7.4.1 Changes at the Genetic Level

The human genome is subject to a wide array of mutations, ranging from point mutations affecting single nucleotides to large-scale rearrangements involving megabases of DNA (Fig. 7–6). Thousands of nucleotide variations have been cataloged by genome sequencing, with many causing changes in the amino acid sequences of the encoded proteins, sometimes resulting in hyperactivation of oncoproteins or inactivation of tumor suppressors.

Although gene amplification and deletion have long been recognized as oncogenic events, the prevalence of such cancer-associated rearrangements in the human genome has probably been underappreciated. Since the discovery of the translocation event resulting in the generation of the oncogenic *BCR-ABL* fusion gene (Sec. 7.5.1), additional cancer-associated gene fusions have been identified in a wide array of tumors (Table 7–2) (Kumar-Sinha et al, 2015; Mertens et al, 2015; Schram et al, 2017). The search for gene fusions has been aided by the advent of RNAseq methodologies (Chap 2, Sec. 2.2.12) which, when combined with bioinformatic analytic tools, can identify these events (Yoshihara et al, 2015).

Gene fusions result from intra- or inter-chromosomal translocations, as well as deletions, inversions, and tandem duplications (see Fig. 7–6). The expression of one of the genes

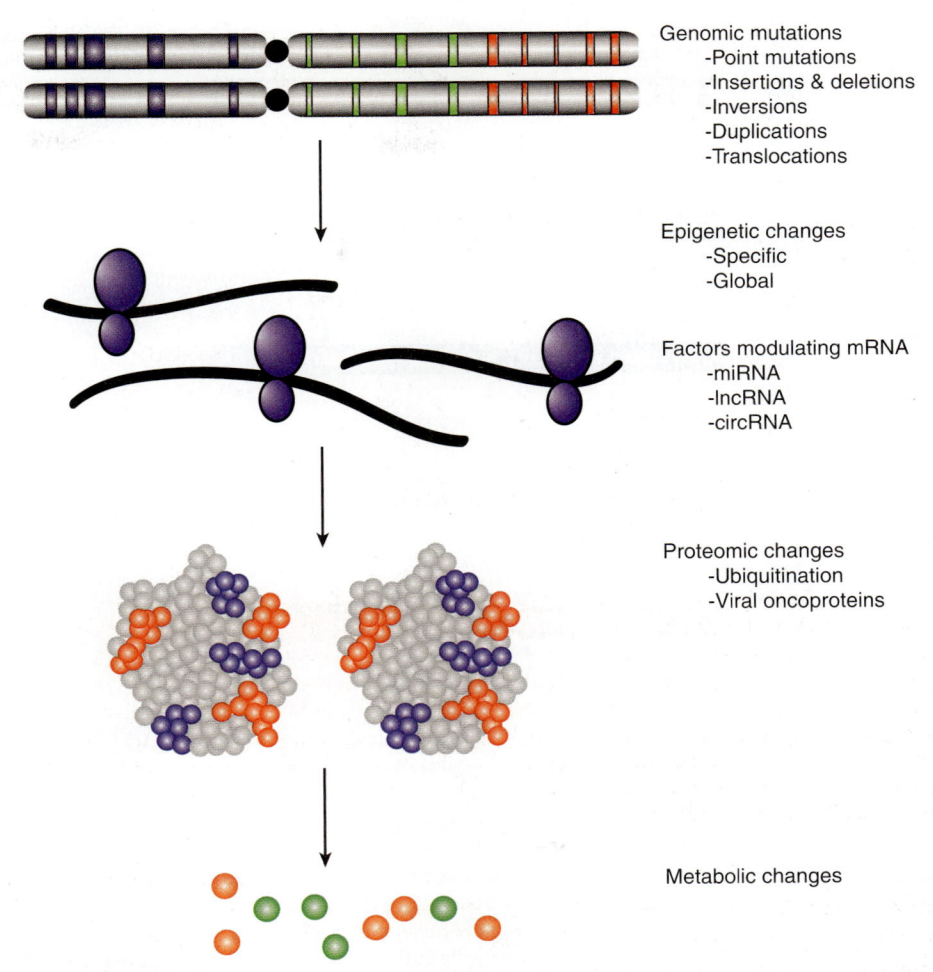

FIGURE 7–5 Cancer targets multiple regulatory levels. Cancer has long been said to be a genetic disease, and large chromosomal abnormalities along with much smaller mutations have been cataloged since the 1960s. Previously, these might have been assumed to affect the function or expression of 1 or 2 proteins. More recently, broader changes affecting the epigenome, transcriptome, proteome, as well as the metabolic status of cells have also been associated with tumorigenesis. New oncogenic actors, such as microRNAs (miRNAs) and oncometabolites, continue to emerge and contribute to a much more textured picture of the transformed phenotype. Moreover, oncogenic hits at any of these regulatory levels tend to engender further hits at other levels, synergistically promoting carcinogenesis.

Cancer-related changes at a given regulatory level beget changes at other levels, collectively contributing to the oncogenic state

Genomic mutations
- Point mutations
- Insertions & deletions
- Inversions
- Duplications
- Translocations

Epigenetic changes
- Specific
- Global

Factors modulating mRNA
- miRNA
- lncRNA
- circRNA

Proteomic changes
- Ubiquitination
- Viral oncoproteins

Metabolic changes

may be altered as a result of its juxtaposition with the transcriptional regulatory elements of the second gene (see Fig. 7–7). For instance, some follicular lymphomas feature translocation events between chromosomes 14 and 18 that bring the *BCL2* gene, encoding the antiapoptotic BCL2 protein, under the control of the immunoglobulin (Ig) heavy-chain gene enhancer, rendering the cells resistant to cell death signals (Chap. 8, Sec. 8.4). Gene fusions that result in the addition or deletion of regulatory domains can cause constitutive activation of the affected protein, forced multimerization, differential subcellular localization, or altered protein-protein interactions. For example, recombination between chromosomes 9 and 12 is found in leukemic cells of CML and acute lymphoblastic leukemia (ALL), resulting in production of the constitutively active TEL-JAK fusion tyrosine kinases that regulate cell proliferation, survival, and differentiation.

More than half of all prostate cancers harbor a *TMPRSS2-ERG* fusion event, caused by an intra-chromosomal deletion on chromosome 21, in which the gene encoding the ERG transcription factor is brought under the control of the androgen-dependent regulatory elements of the *TMPRSS2* gene promoter, leading to its aberrant expression (Adamo and Ladomery, 2016). Some non–small cell lung cancers feature a fusion between the *EML4* gene and the *ALK* tyrosine kinase gene, which results in forced oligomerization and constitutive activation of the kinase (Bayliss et al, 2016).

Gene amplification events produce regions of DNA (amplicons) containing multiple copies of oncogenes, such as the breast cancer–associated *ERBB2* (*HER2*) or *MYC*, and thereby stimulate oncogenic pathways by increasing oncogene dosage. The deletion of regulatory modules, such as the epidermal growth factor receptor (*EGFR*) ligand-binding domain, can also result in oncogenic deregulation of proteins. Conversely, the deletion of tumor-suppressor genes, such as *PTEN*, is also a common oncogenic event (Sec. 7.6.2). Point mutations can affect enzymatic activity, regulatory post-translational modification sites, protein-protein interactions, protein stability, and subcellular localization. Moreover, many of the oncoproteins

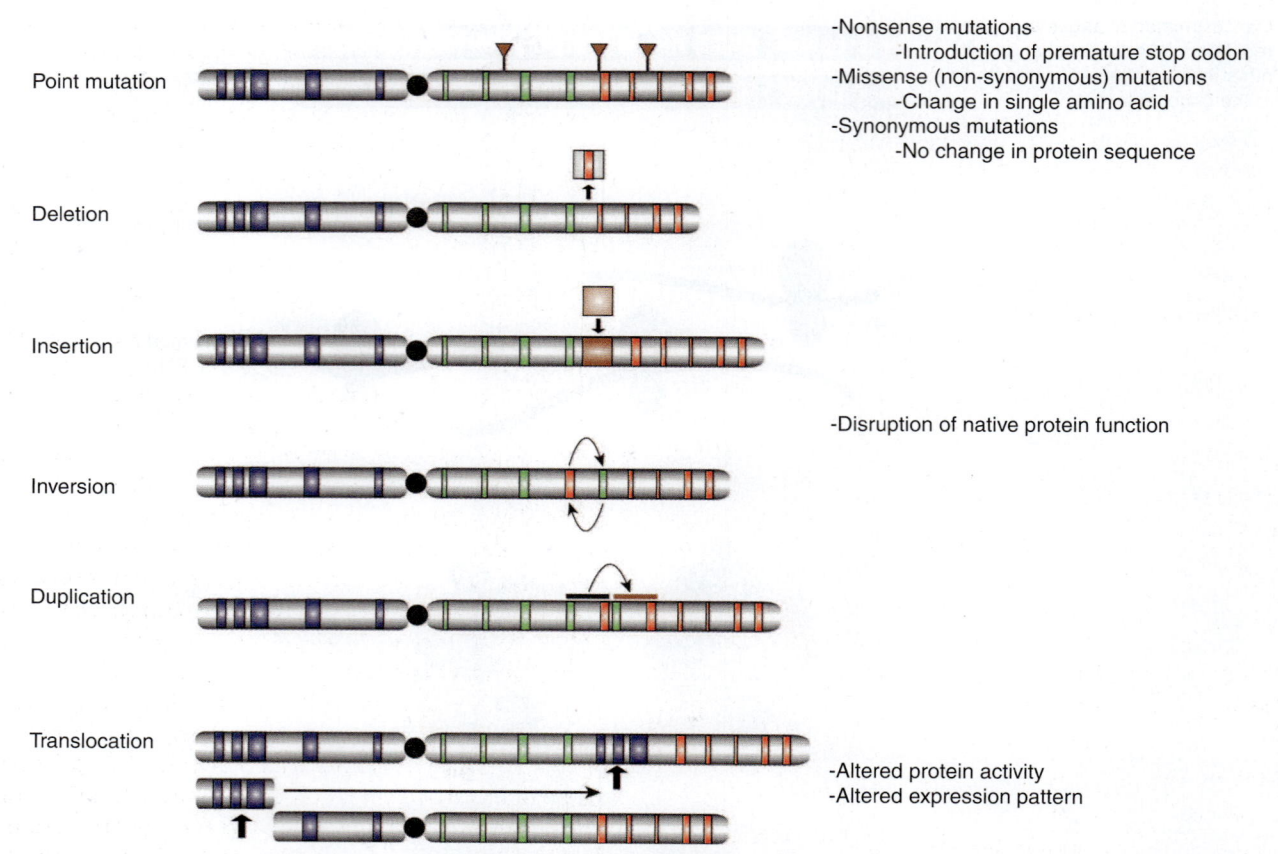

FIGURE 7-6 Classes of genetic mutations. The role of chromosome abnormalities in oncogenesis has been suspected for more than a century, and specific genetic mutations have been identified since the 1960s. Whereas the available technologies once severely limited our capacity to characterize mutations in a timely fashion, with new-generation sequencing techniques it is now possible to develop a list of the entire set of genetic abnormalities in a given tumor cell in a relatively cost-effective manner. It is clear that the volume of genetic mutations in a given cancer cell is far greater than once suspected, encompassing point mutations affecting single nucleotides, deletions, insertions, inversions, duplications, as well as intra- and interchromosomal translocations, all of varying sizes. Some mutations are functionally inert, whereas others can dramatically alter the activity and/or expression pattern of the affected protein(s).

that are initially sensitive to a given therapeutic agent often acquire secondary mutations that render them refractory to the drug (Chap. 19).

7.4.2 Changes at the Epigenetic Level

Epigenetic effects entail heritable changes in gene expression that are not the result of alterations in the primary DNA sequence (see Chap. 3, Sec. 2.X). Because these can also influence oncogenic progression, epigenetic changes may also represent targets for therapeutic intervention (Fig. 7–8).

The preeminent epigenetic factors are the pattern of DNA methylation, as well as the so-called *histone code* created by the patterns of acetylation, methylation, and phosphorylation of the DNA-associated histone proteins. The methylation pattern of the cellular genome, whereby DNA methyltransferases attach methyl groups to cytosines within CpG dinucleotides, specifies which genes are transcribed or silenced. The CpG dinucleotides are enriched within CpG islands that span the 5′ ends of some genes, typically including the promoter and first exon (Esteller, 2008). In mammals, the majority of genes have promoters containing CpG islands, and promoter methylation results in the silencing of the associated gene(s). Histone modifications alter localized chromatin structure, rendering regions either amenable or resistant to transcription. The various histone modifications do not occur independently, but rather entail a complicated interplay that controls gene expression collectively.

Tumorigenesis frequently appears to coincide with both global and local epigenetic changes (Bennett and Licht, 2018; Nebbioso et al, 2018). At a global level, the genome typically becomes hypomethylated during oncogenic progression. A sizable portion of the human genome consists of repetitive stretches of identical or similar sequences, a subset of which are transposable DNA elements that have the capacity to alter their genomic location. The methylation of these repetitive sequences is thought to block the activation and movement of transposable elements and, therefore, prevent chromosomal instability (Anwar et al, 2017). Thus, global hypomethylation of the genome may contribute to the genomic instability that is a prominent feature of transformed cells (see Chap. 3, Sec. 3.1 and 3.3).

Changes in promoter methylation patterns of critical cancer-associated genes also feature prominently during

TABLE 7–2 Cancer-associated gene fusions.

Numerous examples of tumor-promoting gene fusions have now been identified and characterized in a broad range of cancers. Some of the most prominent cancer-associated fusion genes are listed. Tumor genomic and RNA sequencing has led to the discovery of novel gene fusions which could not be readily detected using older technologies.

Fusion Gene	Cancer
BCR-ABL	CML, ALL, AML
BRAF-SND1	pancreas, prostate
CCDC6-RET	lung, thyroid
CD74-ROS1	lung
EGFR-SEPT14	glioblastoma
EML4-ALK	lung
ERG-EWSR1	bone
ETV1-TMPRSS2	prostate
ETV6-NTRK3	salivary gland, thyroid, colon
EZR-ROS1	lung
FGFR3-TACC3	glioblastoma, lung, bladder, cervical, glioma, head and neck, liver
FLI1-EWSR1	bone
IGH-BCL2	lymphoma
IGH-MYC	Burkitt lymphoma
MLL-ENL	AML, ALL
MLL-AF9	AML, ALL
NPM1-ALK	T-cell lymphoma
PML-RARA	AML
RET-KIF5B	lung
ROS1-SDC4	lung
TEL-JAK	CML, ALL
TMPRSS2-ERG	prostate
WT1-EWSR1	soft tissue

Abbreviations: ALL, acute lymphoblastic leukemia; AML, acute myelogenous leukemia; CML, chronic myeloid leukemia.

tumorigenesis, with hypermethylation-associated silencing of tumor-suppressor genes and hypomethylation-mediated activation of oncogenes (Pfeifer, 2018). Cancer-associated hypermethylation of the *Rb1* tumor-suppressor gene promoter was noted in the 1980s, and similar epigenetic targeting of other tumor-suppressor promoters, including those for *BRCA1* and *PTEN*, has since been reported (see Sec. 7.6). A detailed understanding of the role of epigenetics in neoplastic transformation remains a work in progress. For instance, the evolving tumor microenvironment, notably hypoxia, is now understood to affect epigenetic patterns, because several epigenetic processes are oxygen dependent (see Chap. 12, Sec. 12.4).

7.4.3 Changes at the RNA Level

For decades, the central dogma of molecular biology conceptualized a cellular landscape in which functions were carried out mostly by proteins, encoded by the genome, with RNA confined to mediating the flow of information between the genome and proteome. Confounding this view was the realization that only 1% to 2% of the human genome encodes protein sequences, leaving a mystery as to the purpose of the remaining "junk" DNA. This paradox has increasingly been resolved with growing revelations into the variety of roles that noncoding RNAs (ncRNA) play in the cell, acting not only at the transcriptional level but also at the genomic and proteomic levels as well.

The most widely studied of these noncoding RNAs are microRNAs (miRNAs), 20- to 30-nucleotide molecules, generated by defined posttranscriptional maturation steps, that hybridize to complementary sequences in target mRNA transcripts to block gene expression (Olive et al, 2015; Drusco and Croce, 2017) (see Chap. 2, Sec. 2.3.3). This inhibition may be accomplished either by promoting transcript degradation or by interfering with the translation process. MicroRNAs control many cellular processes, regulating at least one-third of all human genes, rendering them key modulators of tumorigenesis. MicroRNAs that normally suppress transformation by targeting oncogenic transcripts are downregulated in some cancers, whereas those targeting tumor-suppressor transcripts are sometimes overexpressed (Svoronos et al, 2016).

Genes encoding microRNAs, no less than protein-encoding genes, are subject to mutations and epigenetic regulation resulting in altered function (Ferreira and Esteller, 2018). MicroRNA expression can also be affected by oncogenic changes occurring at any of the posttranscriptional steps whereby the immature RNA molecule is processed into the mature microRNA form. Deletions in the 13q14 chromosomal region are common abnormalities associated with chronic lymphocytic leukemia (CLL). The underlying molecular cause was previously uncertain as no protein-coding tumor-suppressor gene could be identified in the region. The nature of the oncogenic mechanism only became clear when the miR-15/miR-16 microRNA gene cluster was localized to this segment and found to target the antiapoptotic BCL2 protein (Chap. 8, Sec. 8.4.1), which is found at elevated levels in CLL samples (Cimmino et al, 2006). The LET-7 microRNA family members, which target the *RAS* and *MYC* oncogenes, are downregulated in many cancers, including lung, breast, and colon tumors (Johnson et al, 2005; Sampson et al, 2007). Interestingly, genes encoding epigenetic regulators have been found to be subject to miRNA regulation, creating the potential for influencing oncogenesis through global epigenetic effects. One notable example is miR-29, a microRNA found to be deregulated in cancers, which has been shown to target the DNMT3A and DNMT3B methyltransferases, thereby affecting global methylation levels (Fabbri et al, 2007). MicroRNAs are attractive therapeutic focal points because individual molecules regulate dozens to hundreds of targets, theoretically affecting several oncogenic pathways simultaneously. On the other hand, ascribing effects to a given miRNA can be challenging due to this promiscuity of targets while, conversely, a given transcript can be affected by multiple miRNAs. Indeed, some miRNAs have been shown to be oncogenic in one context and tumor suppressive in another (Svoronos et al, 2016).

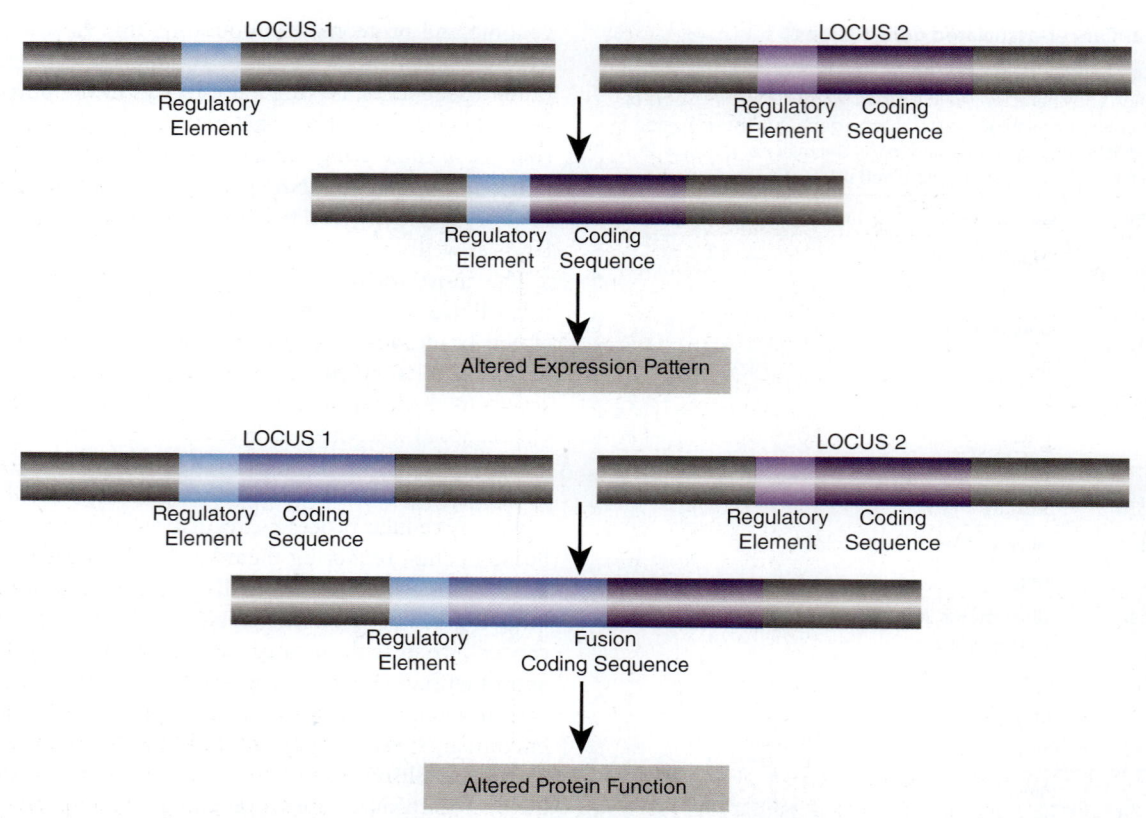

FIGURE 7-7 Effects of translocations. The first observed cancer-associated chromosomal abnormality was a reciprocal translocation between chromosomes 9 and 22, resulting in the so-called Philadelphia chromosome, identified in chronic myeloid leukemia (CML) patients. The functional result of this genetic event is the creation of the BCR-ABL fusion protein that causes the constitutive activation of the ABL kinase. This represents an example of a chromosomal translocation that alters the activity of the affected protein(s). In other translocations, it is the expression pattern of the protein that is altered, rather than its structure or direct function. One such example is the juxtaposition of the *MYC* gene with the powerful IgH transcriptional regulatory elements observed, for instance, in Burkitt lymphoma that results in a dramatic upregulation of the MYC transcription factor.

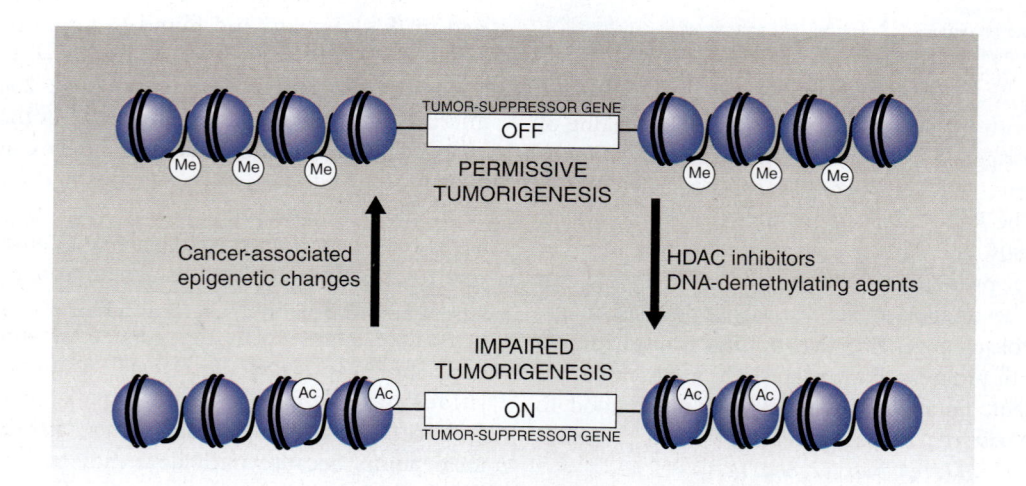

FIGURE 7-8 Epigenetic therapy. Global changes in the cellular epigenome frequently accompany transformation, and the epigenetic silencing of tumor-suppressor genes or activation of oncogenes is now a recognized tumorigenic mechanism. Clinical testing suggests that the tumor-suppressor genes can be reactivated through the application of DNA methyltransferase inhibitors (eg, azacitidine), to reduce the methylation of promoter regions, and histone deacetylase (HDAC) inhibitors (eg, entinostat) that activate gene loci through chromatin remodeling. It is anticipated that epigenetic therapies will be most effective in a combinatorial setting, enhancing the response of other anticancer agents.

Beyond miRNAs, the 2 most notable classes of regulatory RNAs are long noncoding RNAs (lncRNAs), by convention those exceeding 200 nucleotides, and covalently closed circular RNAs (circRNA) often generated by back splicing of transcripts. lncRNAs are a heterogeneous collection of molecules, some of which affect the transcription and translation of target mRNAs, while others carry out an array of emerging functions. These include serving as structural platforms for higher-order complexes and as targeting guides for other functional actors. Though the precise roles of circRNA remain to be fully delineated, it appears that they too affect cell functions at multiple regulatory levels. One intriguing functional aspect of lncRNAs and circRNAs is their ability to regulate the activity of miRNAs. In these scenarios, the noncoding RNAs act as sponges, competitively interacting with the miRNAs thereby blocking their ability to bind their target transcripts. The capacity of these noncoding RNAs to affect each other in addition to the targeted transcripts, creating so-called microRNA axes, adds an additional layer of regulatory complexity (Anastasiadou et al, 2018).

7.4.4 Viruses and Changes at the Protein Level

Virally encoded oncoproteins often trigger tumorigenic programs by directly interacting with critical host cell regulatory proteins and signaling pathways. The first identified human tumor virus, the Epstein-Barr virus (EBV), was discovered in the 1960s when Joseph Epstein detected viral particles in Burkitt lymphoma biopsies (Young et al, 2016). Several human tumor viruses have since been identified, with roughly 20% of all cancers thought to have at least some viral etiology.

Beyond lymphomas, there is a very strong association between EBV infection and undifferentiated nasopharyngeal carcinoma (NPC), in certain populations, with additional evidence linking it to some gastric carcinomas. Although more than 90% of the human population becomes infected with EBV before the age of 20 years, a causative role for the virus in oncogenesis exists at much lower rates (Rickinson and Kieff, 2007). The interplay between viral, genetic, and environmental factors is an important consideration in assessing the contribution of EBV and other viruses to cancer.

EBV contains a double-stranded DNA genome that codes for immediate-early, early, and late gene products. The B lymphocyte is the preferred target of EBV, resulting in latent and then lytic infection stages that are marked by the expression of distinct sets of gene products. Latency is characterized by the synthesis of 6 EBV nuclear antigens (EBNA-LP, EBNA-1, EBNA-2, EBNA-3A, EBNA-3B, and EBNA-3C) and 3 membrane proteins (LMP1, LMP2A, and LMP2B). EBNA-LP and EBNA-2 activate transcription from viral and cellular genes including *c-MYC* (see Sec. 7.5.2). LMP1 has transforming effects in rodent fibroblast cell lines, enabling them to grow under low serum conditions, generate colonies in soft agar, and form tumors in nude mice (Li and Chang, 2003). It protects cells from apoptosis through induction of Bcl-2 (see Chap. 8, Sec. 8.4) and constitutively activates NF-κB, p38/MAPK, Jun kinase (JNK), JAK3, and PI3K (see Chap. 6, Sec. 6.2). Upregulation of these protein kinase pathways can promote tumorigenesis by stimulating production of the vascular endothelial growth factor (VEGF), interleukin (IL)-6, IL-8, CD40, fibroblast growth factor (FGF), EGFR, phosphorylation of p53, activation of AKT/PKB, and expression of DNA methyltransferase and telomerase (Soni et al, 2007; Kung et al, 2011). LMP2 contributes to oncogenesis, at least partly, through an association with Src family tyrosine kinases. In EBV-linked gastric carcinomas, the LMP2 protein also enhances STAT3 activation, resulting in transcription of the DNMT1 methyltransferase, ultimately leading to CpG island methylation in the PTEN promoter and loss of PTEN expression.

Human papillomaviruses (HPVs) are non-enveloped DNA viruses that are linked strongly to cervical cancer, the third most common cancer in women worldwide (Harden and Munger, 2017; Mittal and Banks, 2017). There has also been increasing recognition of HPV involvement in head and neck cancers, with approximately 60% to 70% of oropharyngeal squamous cell carcinomas now diagnosed in North America being linked to HPV (Chung and Gillison, 2009; Gillison et al, 2015). Presently, there are 3 FDA-approved HPV vaccines targeting somewhat different spectra of HPV types, but crucially sharing efficacy against the high-risk HPV16 and HPV18 viruses. Clinical studies evaluating the impact of vaccination programs have confirmed significant reductions in HPV infections and associated precancerous lesions, although studies to assess the effect on invasive cervical cancer rates are still ongoing (de Sanjose et al, 2019).

Papillomaviruses contain a single molecule of circular double-stranded DNA, which encodes 8 "early" genes (*E1* to *E8*) and 2 "late" genes (*L1* and *L2*). A comparison of high-risk and low-risk viruses has allowed the mapping of transformation properties to the *E5*, *E6*, and *E7* genes. The E5 protein can dimerize with growth factor receptors, such as EGFR, leading to activation of the MAPK pathway and cell proliferation. In malignant cells, HPV DNA is integrated randomly into various chromosomes, resulting in substantial deletions or disruption of the viral genome, particularly the *E2* gene, which has a negative regulatory effect on the expression of the HPV proteins E6 and E7. These latter 2 proteins are always retained and consistently expressed in cervical tumor tissue and cell lines, suggesting that one or both of these proteins may be required for transformation by HPV. In order to facilitate viral replication, the E7 oncoprotein forces the host cell into a replicative cell cycle phase by promoting degradation of the pRb tumor-suppressor, whereas the E6 protein blocks ensuing cell death by inactivating the p53 tumor suppressor. This intervention into the host cell cycle induces a state of replicative stress that would normally result in cell cycle arrest or death through mechanisms that are in turn disabled by the E7 protein. Thus, the E7 protein both induces replicative stress and permits host cell tolerance of this state, resulting in the genomic instability that causes oncogenesis (Moody, 2019).

7.5 GAIN OF FUNCTION EVENTS

7.5.1 BCR-ABL

The Philadelphia chromosome was initially described as a minute chromosome and assumed to be the product of a loss of genetic material from chromosome 22. Improvements in cytogenetics showed that the deletion in chromosome 22 was matched by a comparable insertion in chromosome 9 (Rowley, 1973). By 1985, it had been determined that cells of most CML patients feature reciprocal translocation events between the long arms of the 2 chromosomes, resulting in the creation of a *BCR-ABL* hybrid gene (see Fig. 7–7). The same translocation event has been found to occur in 25% to 30% of adult and 2% to 10% of pediatric ALL, and occasionally in cases of acute myelogenous leukemia (AML).

The ABL kinase is the human homolog of the transforming sequence found in the Abelson murine leukemia virus. Whereas the protein normally shuttles between the nucleus and cytoplasm, the product of the *BCR-ABL* fusion gene is a constitutively active tyrosine kinase localized permanently in the cytoplasm. The addition of the BCR gene product appears to promote extensive multimerization of the fusion protein, facilitating self-activation by trans-autophosphorylation. During the chronic phase of CML, the BCR-ABL kinase activates pathways while also increasing genomic instability. In the absence of therapeutic intervention, additional genomic aberrations ultimately lead to a transition from the chronic to the advanced CML phase known as blast crisis that is more difficult to treat. The blast phase is marked by increased proliferation accompanied by impaired apoptosis and differentiation, which together increase the population of blast progenitors.

The correlation of a disease state with a specific genetic lesion offered the possibility for targeted therapeutic intervention. The subsequent development and successful application of imatinib, which binds near the adenosine triphosphate (ATP)–binding site and locks BCR-ABL in an inhibited conformation, is a major achievement of targeted cancer therapy (Chap. 19, Sec. 19.6.4.1).

7.5.2 MYC

MYC family members are global transcription factors that activate some target genes while repressing others, thereby affecting numerous cellular processes including proliferation, growth, apoptosis, angiogenesis, metabolism, and immune surveillance (Fig. 7–9) (Tu et al, 2015). This central regulatory role renders MYC one of the most potent oncogenic drivers in human cancer. Because roughly 15% of all human genes are regulated by MYC, it can be difficult to identify the specific MYC targets that are impactful in a particular oncogenic program. Rather, MYC overexpression results in pleiotropic downstream effects that collectively promote oncogenic transformation. For example, MYC contributes to cell-cycle progression by downregulation of CDK inhibitors and upregulation of CYCLIN D1, CDK4, CDC25A, and E2F transcription factors (Chap. 8, Sec. 8.2.2). Paradoxically, MYC upregulation, by itself, can also trigger apoptosis in some cells, and additional oncogenic mutations capable of blocking cell death are required for transformation (Gabay et al, 2014). MYC deregulation also correlates with general chromosomal instability, resulting from oxidative stress, proliferation-associated replication stress, and impaired DNA damage response (Kuzyk and Mai, 2014; Kumari et al, 2017). The precise effect of MYC activation on cell fate is highly dependent on cell type and developmental stage, as well as its genetic and epigenetic context.

MYC upregulation is a frequent occurrence in cancer cells, driven either by oncogenic mutations in signaling pathways that control MYC expression and stability or via mutations in the MYC gene itself. Gene amplification, involving whole genome doubling or tandem duplications, is the most common mechanism of MYC deregulation and is observed in virtually all cancer types (Kalkat et al, 2017). The *MYCN* gene, which is normally expressed during development, has been found amplified in neuroblastomas, and increased copy numbers of the related MYCL1 gene have been observed in several cancers, including ovarian tumors.

MYC expression can also be elevated through translocation events that bring the MYC gene under the control of highly active transcriptional enhancers. Noteworthy examples are found in Burkitt lymphomas, as well as other human B-cell lymphomas, which frequently feature chromosome translocation events between chromosome 8, where the *MYC* gene is located, and chromosomes 14, 2, or 22, where the Ig heavy- and light-chain genes reside. These rearrangements have the effect of bringing the *MYC* gene under the transcriptional control of *Ig* gene enhancer elements, leading to its overexpression. This mechanism of *MYC* upregulation is mimicked in some mouse plasmacytomas that feature recombination events between the MYC and immunoglobin (*Ig*) heavy-chain genes.

In human cancers, elevation of *MYC* transcription is sometimes achieved through mutations or epigenetic effects in the endogenous *MYC* gene promoter region. A comparable paradigm is found in the ability of some transforming viruses to direct oncogenesis through proviral DNA integration in the proximity of proto-oncogenes or tumor-suppressor genes, leading to altered expression or splicing. One specific example is the mechanism of chicken B-cell lymphogenesis by the slowly transforming avian leukosis virus (ALV). Analysis of lymphomas from independently infected birds revealed proviral integration at specific sites, giving rise to similar viral-host hybrid RNAs. The viral coding segments were often altered in ways that precluded viral protein expression, indicating that they were dispensable for transformation. The hybrid RNAs, driven by the more potent viral promoter, were found to include cellular *MYC* coding sequences leading to increased expression of MYC protein, suggesting that proviral integration promoted oncogenesis through upregulation of MYC levels. This constituted the first observation

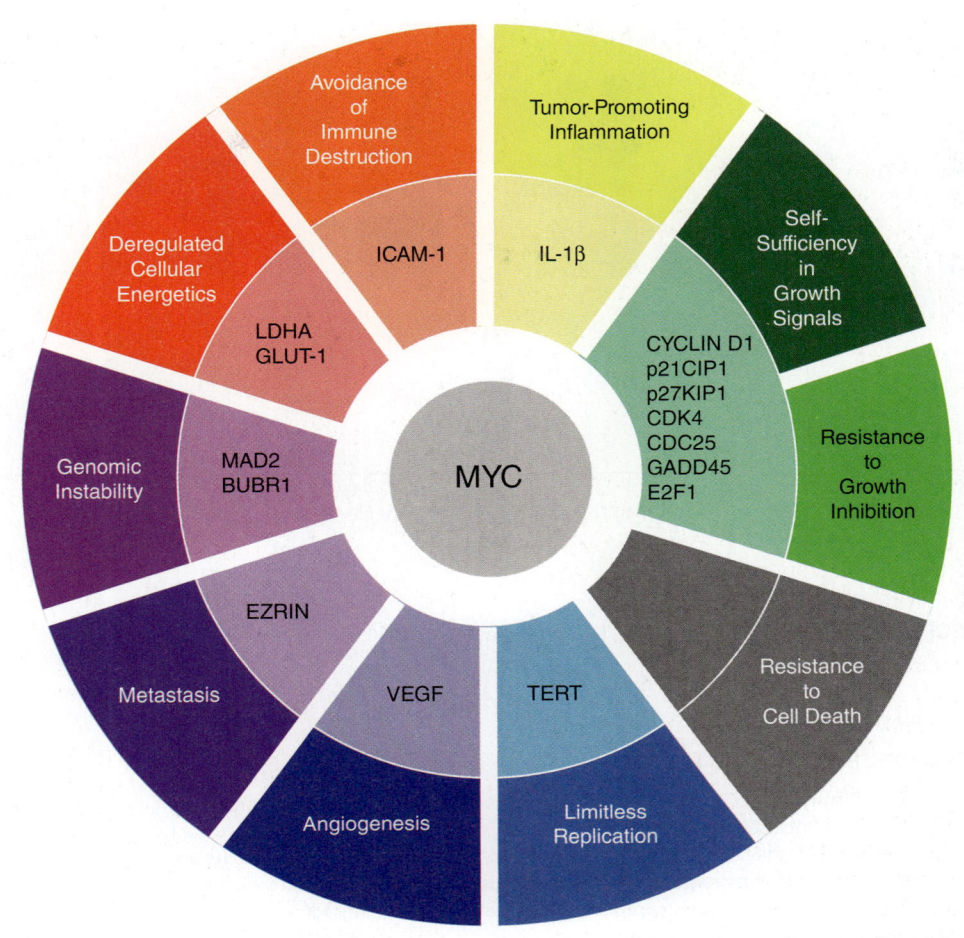

FIGURE 7–9 MYC targets and promotion of tumorigenesis. The MYC transcription factor is thought to regulate the expression of roughly 15% of all human genes and is frequently upregulated in a variety of cancers. MYC upregulates the expression of some genes while repressing the expression of other targets. Unsurprisingly, given the number of genes affected by MYC, its deregulation contributes to the acquisition of many of the characteristic properties of cancer cells, as defined by Douglas Hanahan and Robert Weinberg. One notable exception is the paradoxical induction of apoptosis by MYC overexpression, necessitating the disengagement of cell death pathway(s) by additional oncogenic hits in order to foster transformation. Some of the MYC-regulated genes involved in tumorigenesis are denoted, though the particular MYC targets critical to oncogenesis will undoubtedly vary in different tumors.

of neoplastic transformation caused by the upregulation of a nonmutated cellular gene.

7.5.3 EGFR/ERBB2

The epidermal growth factor (EGF) family is composed of 11 related ligands that stimulate intracellular signaling by binding to the EGF receptors, ERBB1 (EGFR), ERBB3, and ERBB4 (Yarden and Pines, 2012). A fourth member of the EGF receptor family, ERBB2 (HER2), cannot bind ligands itself, but is activated by dimerization with other family members (see also Chap. 6, Sec. 6.2). The EGF receptors are transmembrane proteins consisting of an N-terminal extracellular ligand-binding ectodomain, an intracellular kinase domain, and a C-terminal regulatory tail that contains docking sites for a number of downstream effectors. Ligand binding to the ectodomain induces receptor dimerization, transmitting conformational changes that promote kinase activation. Both homodimers and some heterodimer combinations can form active receptor signaling complexes. The ERBB3 receptor binds ligands but has an inactive kinase domain and therefore can only transmit the EGF signal as part of a heterodimer with an active family member (Fig. 7–10). Specific ligands can promote different dimer conformations, affecting dimer stability and generating variations in downstream signaling and cell fate. Collectively, the ligands and their receptors influence an array of cell functions including growth, proliferation, survival, migration, and adhesion.

All 3 portions of the ERBB1 receptor are subject to oncogenic mutations (Arteaga and Engelman, 2014). Ligand-independent dimerization is enabled by point mutations or, more commonly, deletions within the ectodomain that leave the receptors in a constitutively activated conformation. Many such deletion mutants have been characterized, with one notable example being the variant III mutant, which is particularly common in gliomas, and much less frequently observed in lung, breast, ovarian, and other cancers (Gan et al, 2013). These deletion mutants

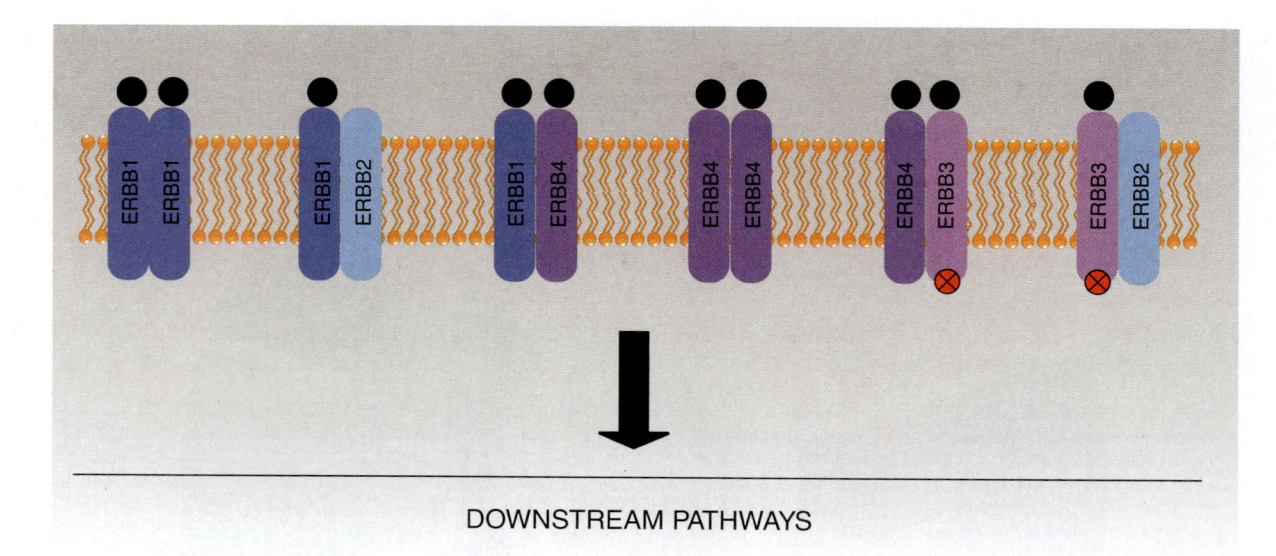

EGF FAMILY LIGANDS:

ERBB1: EGF, Amphiregulin, TGFα, Epiregulin, Epigen, Betacellulin, HB-EGF

ERBB2: ---

ERBB3: Neuregulin 1, Neuregulin 2

ERBB4: Epiregulin, Betacellulin, HB-EGF, Neuregulin 1, Neuregulin 2, Neuregulin 3, Neuregulin 4

FIGURE 7–10 EGF receptor family. The EGF receptor family consists of four transmembrane proteins that couple a ligand-binding domain that responds to external stimuli with intracellular tyrosine kinase domains responsible for signal transduction. ERBB1 (EGFR), ERBB3, and ERBB4 each respond to a particular set of EGF family ligands, with some overlap, whereas ERBB2 appears to be an orphan receptor which must dimerize with ERBB1 or ERBB3 in order to engage downstream pathways. In addition, ERBB3 has an inactive kinase domain and transmits signals by dimerizing with ERBB2 or ERBB4. Collectively, these receptors regulate pathways that impact a number of cell processes, and are prominently deregulated in a number of cancers.

mimic the avian erythroblastosis virus v-ErbB oncoprotein, from which the EGFR family members took their names. Numerous point mutations are also found in the kinase domain, especially in non–small cell lung cancers, which promote constitutive activation, even in the absence of ligand-induced dimerization. Indeed, kinase domain mutations are predictive of therapeutic sensitivity to tyrosine kinase inhibitors (TKIs) such as gefitinib and erlotinib (see Chap. 19, Sec. 19.4) (Stewart et al, 2015). The effects of the point mutations are also closely replicated by small insertions and deletions within the kinase domain.

Activation of the EGFR receptor results in phosphorylation of tyrosine residues in the C-terminal tail, which serve as docking sites for the recruitment of downstream effectors (see Chap. 6, Sec. 6.2.1). Activating point mutations result in the receptor tail attaining a phosphorylation status intermediate between that of unstimulated and growth factor–stimulated wild-type receptors. Whereas stimulated wild-type EGFRs activate several downstream pathways, the mutant receptors tend to activate mitogen-activated protein (MAP) kinase and phosphatidylinositol-3 (PI3) kinase signaling at the expense of the other pathways. Normally, EGF signaling is attenuated by a feedback mechanism that involves the removal of the receptors from the cell membrane by endocytosis, followed by lysosomal degradation or recycling. Some point mutations disrupt this regulatory mechanism, resulting in hyperactivation of the EGF pathway (Tomas et al, 2014).

EGF signaling has an important physiological role in mammary development, and deregulation of downstream pathways feature prominently in many breast tumors (Schmitt, 2009). The ERBB2/ERBB3 heterodimeric receptor complex is a potent signal transducer, particularly of the PI3 kinase pathway, because the ERBB3 receptor recruits the PI3 kinase directly rather than through intermediary adaptor proteins. The *ERBB2(HER-2)* gene is amplified or overexpressed in roughly one-quarter of all human breast cancers, as well as a smaller percentage of ovarian and gastric cancers. Overexpression of the ERBB2 receptor has also been correlated with elevated ERBB3 levels. Although *ERBB2* somatic mutations have now been identified in a number of cancers, gene amplification is the most common mechanism for oncogenic upregulation of the receptor. Amplification of the *ERBB2* gene is generally an early event in breast cancer progression and is associated with poor prognosis in breast and gastric cancers. Targeting it with drugs such as trastuzumab has improved the prognosis of individuals with these tumors (Chap. 19, Sec. 19.4).

7.5.4 PI3 Kinase

In response to specific upstream signals, the PI3 kinases phosphorylate the 3′ hydroxyl group of phosphatidylinositols,

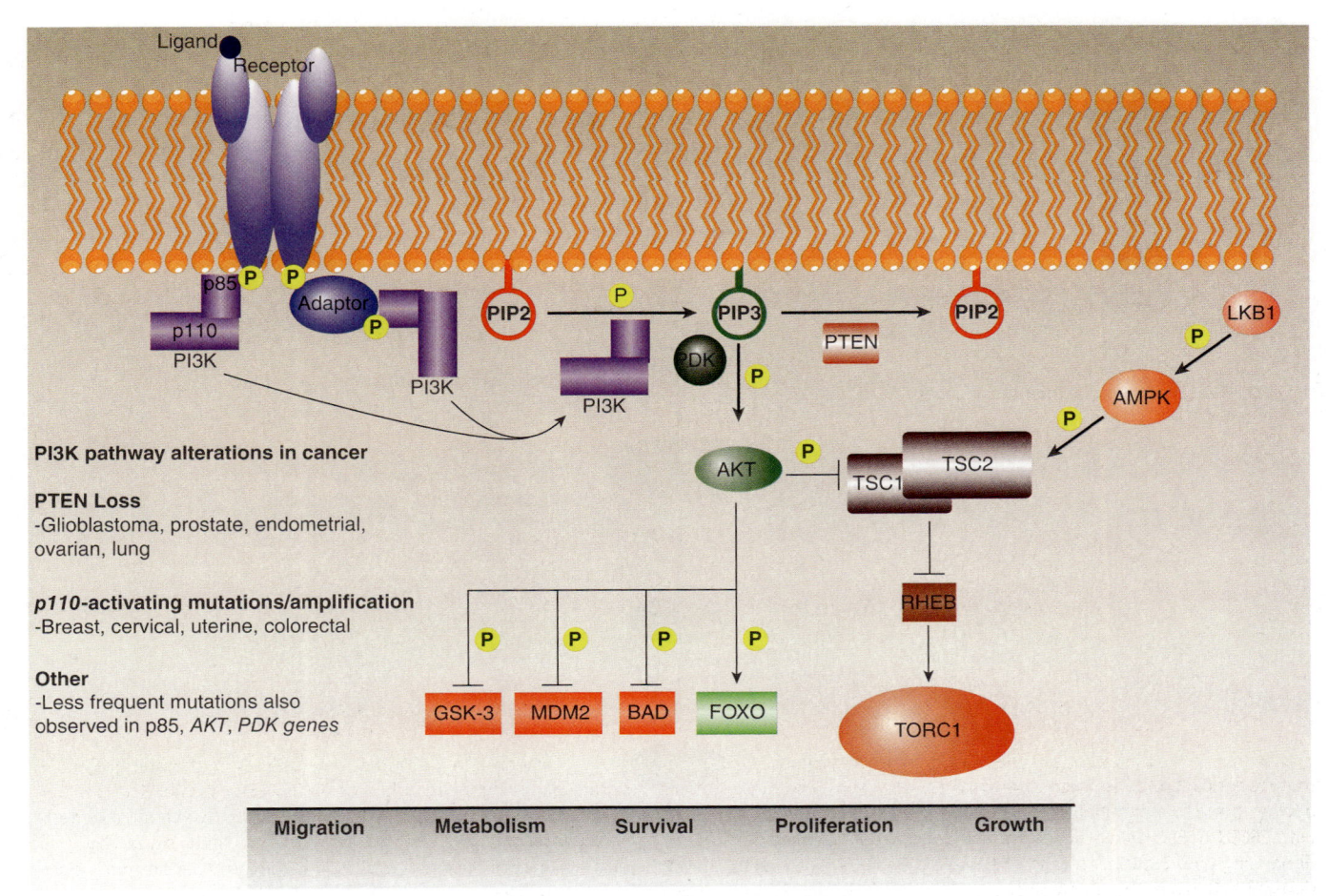

FIGURE 7–11 PI3 kinase pathway. The PI3 kinase pathway regulates a variety of cell functions including migration, metabolism, survival, proliferation, and growth. It is frequently deregulated in human cancers at various points. In response to external stimuli, activated receptor tyrosine kinases recruit PI3 kinase via its p85 regulatory subunit, either directly or mediated by an adaptor protein such as IRS-1. On recruitment, activated PI3 kinase converts PIP$_2$ (phosphatidylinositol 4,5-bisphosphate) to PIP$_3$ (phosphatidylinositol 3,4,5-triphosphate). This reaction is antagonized by the lipid phosphatase, PTEN, which therefore acts as a brake on the pathway. PH-domain proteins, such as the PDK1 and AKT kinases, are recruited to the plasma membrane by PIP$_3$, whereupon PDK1 contributes to the activation of AKT, which then transmits the signal downstream by phosphorylating a range of targets. AKT also modulates the RHEB GTPase-TORC1 signaling axis by downregulating the TSC1-TSC2 complex, which is modulated by a number of upstream signals, including activation by LKB1-AMPK in response to energy deprivation. The PI3 kinase pathway is generally overstimulated in cancers through aberrant activation of the receptors, activating mutations in the PI3 kinase catalytic subunit (p110α), and through the loss of PTEN.

generating membrane-embedded lipid secondary messengers that activate downstream pathways (Fig. 7–11; see also Chap. 6, Sec. 6.2.5) (Fruman et al, 2017; Manning and Toker, 2017). Although the superfamily includes several isoforms, most research has focused on the Class IA PI3 kinases, which consist of p110 catalytic and p85 regulatory subunits. These preferentially convert phosphatidylinositol 4,5-bisphosphate (PIP$_2$) to phosphatidylinositol 3,4,5-triphosphate (PIP$_3$), which recruits Pleckstrin homology (PH) domain-containing proteins, such as the PDK1 and PKB/AKT serine/threonine kinases, to the membrane for activation.

PI3 kinase signaling is one of the most commonly activated pathways in human cancers, with mutations observed at various nodes. Most common are activating mutations in the *PIK3CA* gene, encoding the p110α subunit, found in various tumors, especially breast, cervical, uterine, and colorectal cancers (Zhang et al, 2017; Janku et al, 2018). These mutations result in constitutive activation of the kinase in the absence of upstream signaling, a buildup of PIP$_3$, and increased mobilization of downstream pathways that regulate cellular growth, proliferation, survival, migration, and glucose metabolism. Remarkably, approximately 80% of all somatic PI3 kinase mutations occur at 3 hotspot residues: E542K and E545K within the helical domain, and H1047R in the kinase domain. All 3 mutations have been found to increase the in vitro activity of the kinase as well as PI3 kinase signaling in cells and tissues bearing the mutations. Amplifications of the *PIK3CA* gene are often observed in lung, ovarian, cervical, esophageal, as well as head and neck cancers. The effects on PKB/AKT function vary from tumor to tumor; however, on the whole, point mutations in the *PIK3CA* gene tend to be more predictive of pathway activation than gene amplification (Zhang et al, 2017). Less frequent cancer-associated mutations have also been identified in the *PIK3R* gene, encoding the p85 subunit, as well as

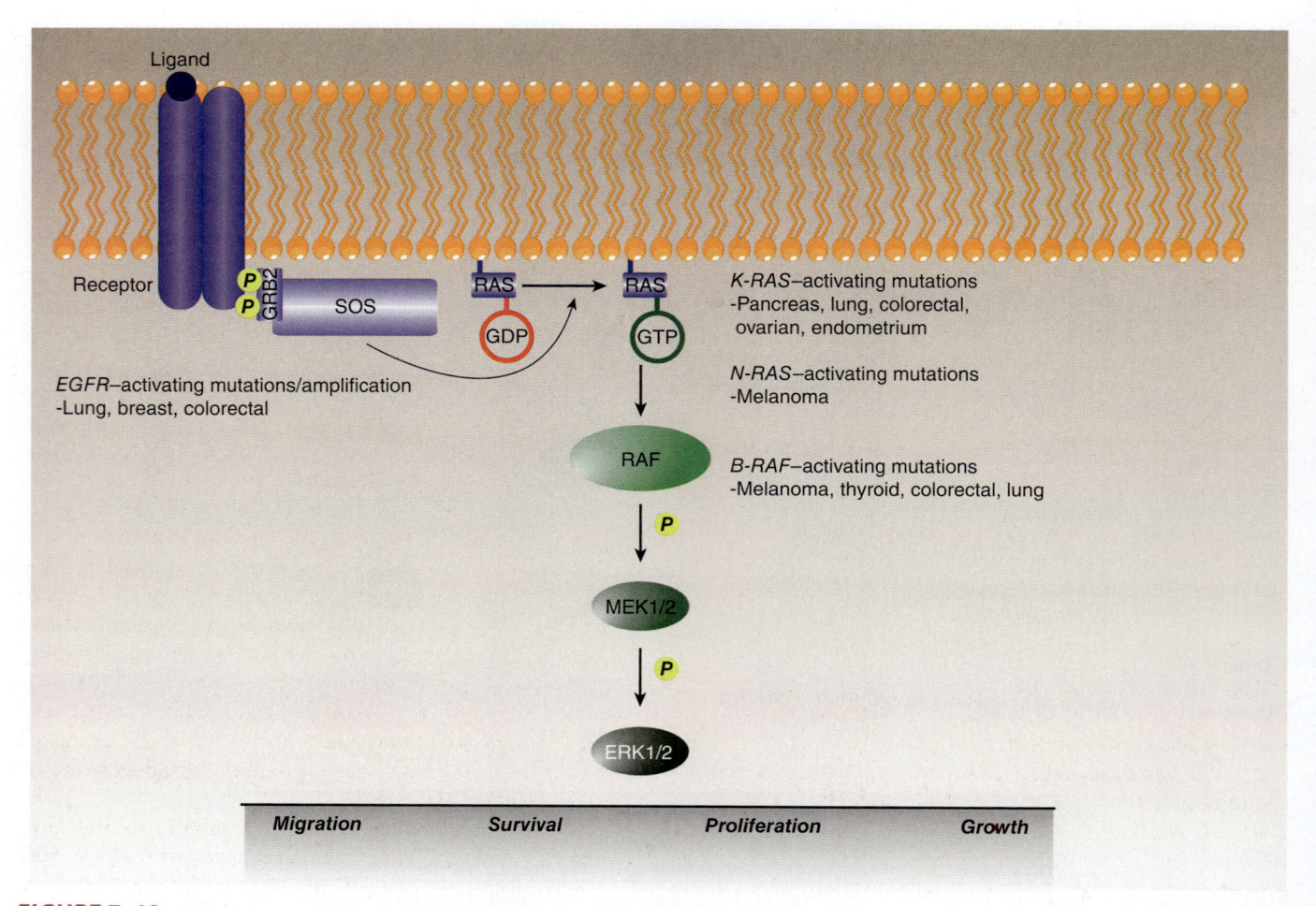

FIGURE 7-12 MAP kinase pathway. The MAPK/ERK pathway is frequently deregulated during oncogenesis. The canonical pathway is stimulated by ligand binding to their cognate receptors, ultimately resulting in activation of the ERK1/2 kinase. Activated receptors recruit adaptors, such as GRB2, and guanine nucleotide exchange factors (GEFs), such as SOS, which promotes the GTP loading of RAS. RAF is then activated by RAS-GTP, triggering a kinase cascade resulting in the sequential activation of MEK1/2 and ERK1/2, whose downstream targets regulate a number of cell functions including migration, survival, proliferation, and growth. Overactivation of the pathway through activating mutations or amplification of receptors, as well as activating mutations in various RAS isoforms or B-RAF, is commonly observed in human cancers.

the *AKT* genes, encoding the most prominent downstream effectors of PI3 kinase signaling.

7.5.5 RAS and RAF

The importance of MAP kinase signaling in neoplastic transformation is evident from the frequency of oncogenic mutations affecting multiple proteins in the pathway, including growth factor receptors, RAS guanosine triphosphatase (GTPase), and its immediate target, RAF (Fig. 7–12) (Karreth and Tuveson, 2009). The pathway modulates many cellular processes, including proliferation, growth, survival, differentiation, and migration, albeit in a tissue-dependent manner (Chap. 6, Sec. 6.2.3). RAS genes are among the most commonly mutated genes in human cancer, with aberrations detected in 25% to 30% of all tumors (Simanshu et al, 2017). Among the 3 RAS genes, most mutations are observed in the K-RAS gene, especially in pancreatic, lung, colon, and endometrial tumors. Mutations in the N-RAS gene are most commonly observed in melanomas with H-RAS mutations found in cancers of the adrenal gland and thymus.

RAS acts as a membrane-bound binary signaling switch, alternating between inactive GDP-bound and active GTP-bound states, with the GDP-to-GTP exchange driven by upstream signals. The most common RAS mutations are gain-of-function substitutions in codons 12, 13, and 61, which impair RAS-GTP hydrolysis, thereby locking the protein into an activated state and resulting in upregulation of its downstream effectors.

The primary downstream effectors of RAS are the 3 RAF family serine/threonine kinases. Activated RAS recruits RAF monomers and promotes the formation of active RAF homo- and heterodimers. B-RAF is the most frequently mutated RAF family member with approximately 8% of all human cancers exhibiting B-RAF mutations, including 50% of melanomas, as well as thyroid, colon, and lung cancers (Karoulia et al, 2017). The V600E substitution accounts for roughly 80% to 90% of all B-RAF mutations, with less common mutations at V600 and non-V600 positions, B-RAF fusions, and in-frame deletions accounting for the remaining mutations. B-RAF mutants can be broadly classified based on their activation status, dependency on upstream RAS activation, and dimerization requirement (Yao et al, 2017). The V600 mutants signal as activated monomers in the absence of RAS signaling, whereas the non-V600 mutants signal as dimers either independently of RAS, in the case of activating mutations, or contingent on RAS activity. The precise nature of the mutation is an important consideration guiding therapeutic approaches targeting B-RAF. For instance, vemurafenib, a drug that specifically targets V600E monomers, has led to marked improvement in outcome in treating melanomas expressing this mutant. By contrast, tumors expressing B-RAF mutants that signal as dimers are insensitive to vemurafenib. It should be noted that tumors harboring V600E mutations in other tissues, such as colorectal cancers, have generally proven to be refractory to vemurafenib treatment, demonstrating that proper consideration must also be given to the precise signaling mechanisms engaged by the mutant protein.

7.5.6 IDH

Extensive genomewide sequencing has identified surprisingly few novel oncogenes and tumor-suppressor genes. The *IDH1* and *IDH2* genes, encoding 2 isocitrate dehydrogenase metabolic enzymes, are the most prominent examples of cancer genes discovered by this method (see also Chap. 12, Sec. 12.3.5). Exon sequencing carried out on human glioblastoma multiforme, as well as other cancers, revealed somatic mutations in IDH1 and IDH2 at homologous arginine positions in some of the sampled tumors (Parsons et al, 2008; Yan et al, 2009). Functional characterization of the mutant proteins indicated that the amino acid substitutions destroyed their ability to convert isocitrate into α-ketoglutarate (αKG), suggesting that these were novel tumor suppressors. However, there was no evidence of an LOH at the *IDH* loci in human tumors, indicating that they did not conform to Knudson's 2-hit tumor-suppressor model. An alternative explanation arose from the observation that cells harboring the tumor-associated *IDH1* mutation exhibit an accumulation of the 2-hydroxyglutarate (2-HG) metabolite (Dang et al, 2009). An analysis of the effects of the mutation on the IDH1 structure suggested that although the active site of the mutant enzyme failed to interact with isocitrate, its normal substrate, it could interact with αKG and convert it to 2-HG. Thus, the arginine substitution represents a neomorphic mutation that destroys the normal enzymatic activity while creating a novel one. The prevailing evidence suggests that 2-HG promotes oncogenesis by inhibiting histone and DNA demethylation, altering cellular epigenetics in a manner that favors proliferation over terminal differentiation (Waitkus et al, 2018). In addition to gliomas, *IDH1* and especially *IDH2* mutations have also been detected in AML genomes, similarly leading to an accumulation of 2-HG (Ward et al, 2010). Indeed, elevated serum 2-HG levels have now been suggested as a noninvasive test for IDH mutations. Importantly, knockdown of *IDH1* and *IDH2* reduced the growth of cultured glioma cells, consistent with their roles as oncogenes rather than tumor-suppressor genes (Ward et al, 2010).

7.6 LOSS-OF-FUNCTION EVENTS

7.6.1 p53

The most extensively studied tumor-suppressor gene is the p53 transcription factor, the so-called guardian of the genome, discovered in 1979 as an interacting partner of the SV40 viral T-antigen (Kastenhuber and Lowe, 2017). In response to cellular stresses, a variety of mechanisms converge on p53 leading to its stabilization and accumulation. Contingent on the nature of the stress and the cellular context, p53 then activates the expression of genes leading to DNA repair and growth arrest on the one hand and apoptotic cell death on the other (Fig. 7–13). In the absence of p53, cells are impaired in their ability to respond appropriately to oncogenic mutations and stresses, leading to proliferation, growth, and marked genetic instability. In addition to these canonical functions, p53 is now understood to control the expression of sets of genes involved in other roles, including autophagy, metabolism, inflammation, and cell plasticity. Like the pleiotropic effects of Myc activation, the relative importance of the different p53-mediated functions in a given oncogenic program vary depending on the particular cellular context.

The *TP53* gene, encoding the p53 protein, is the most commonly mutated gene in human cancers, with 40% to 50% of all tumors presenting p53 mutations. These are found at wildly varying frequencies in different cancer types, ranging from roughly 10% in some leukemias to more than 90% in ovarian serous carcinomas. In addition to somatic changes, germline p53 mutations lead to Li-Fraumeni syndrome, a rare but highly penetrant autosomal dominant disorder that leads to a wide spectrum of cancers, notably osteosarcomas, soft tissue sarcomas, adrenocortical carcinomas, as well as breast and brain cancers (Bougeard et al, 2015). For both somatic and germline mutations, oncogenic progression almost always involves LOH through deletions at the second p53 locus.

Although thousands of p53 mutations have been cataloged, more than 80% of these cluster within the region encoding the central DNA-binding domain, with more than a quarter of all mutations localized to one of 6 "hotspot" residues. Two of these mutations, R248Q and R273H, interfere directly with the contact between p53 and DNA, whereas the other mutations, R249S, G245S, R175H, and R282W, cause varying degrees of structural disruption that also impinge on the DNA-binding ability of the protein (Sabapathy and Lane, 2018). The traditional models of p53 function, in relation to oncogenesis, involve a combination of loss-of-function and dominant-negative effects, the latter mediated by dimerization of mutant p53 with wild-type p53 (thereby inhibiting normal p53 function), prior to LOH. The inability of mutant p53 to bind DNA results in reduced expression of p53 targets, including the gene that encodes the MDM2 ubiquitin ligase, which influences the turnover of p53 itself.

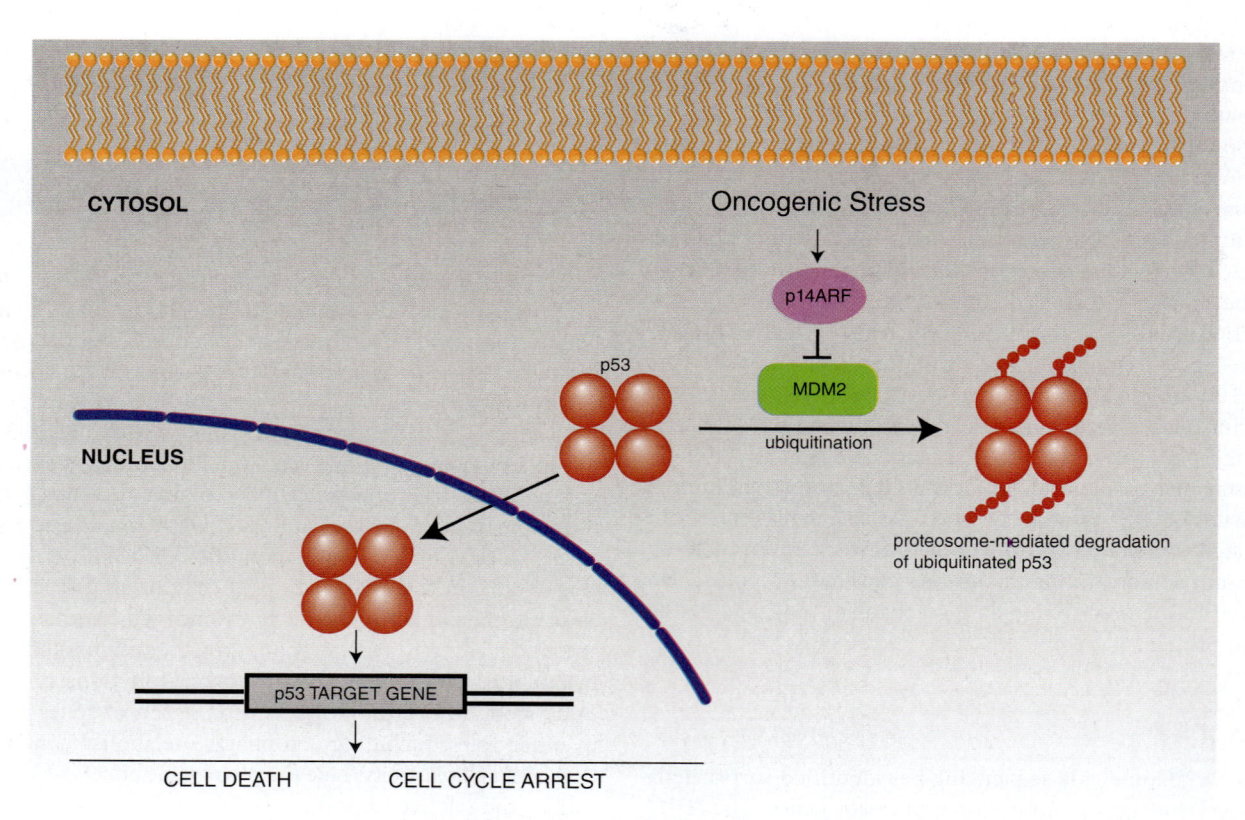

FIGURE 7–13 p53 and cell fate determination. The p53 tumor suppressor represents a critical regulatory node for cell fate determination and is the most frequently mutated gene in human cancers. The levels of p53 are normally constrained, primarily by the action of MDM2, which promotes the ubiquitination and proteasomal degradation of the protein. In response to cellular stresses, p53 is stabilized and translocates to the nucleus and regulates gene expression. Depending on the level of stress, p53 can promote different cellular outcomes, notably cell cycle arrest to permit the alleviation of the particular stress or, in irretrievable cases, cell death. Because oncogenic stresses can inhibit MDM2, through the activity of p14^{ARF}, tumorigenic progression requires either the circumvention or loss of p53 activity.

Consequently, mutant p53 levels are frequently elevated in tumors, enhancing the dominant-negative effect.

7.6.2 PTEN

Identified during the 1990s as the major tumor suppressor at chromosome 10q23, PTEN was found to directly counter PI3 kinase signaling by acting as a lipid phosphatase for PIP$_3$, the product of PI3 kinase activity (see Fig. 7–11) (Chalhoub and Baker, 2009; Hollander et al, 2011; Manning and Toker, 2017). Downregulation of PTEN is associated with increased PIP$_3$ levels and hyperactivation of downstream PKB/AKT-mediated signaling. Although reported initially to be a cytoplasmic enzyme, nuclear PTEN pools have since been identified in several cell types, an intriguing finding given that PTEN loss is associated with genomic instability (Bassi et al, 2013). At least in part, this is attributable to the involvement of nuclear PTEN in double-strand break repair. Nuclear localization of PTEN is achieved through the covalent attachment of small ubiquitin-like modifier (SUMO) proteins to specific lysine residues in the protein (ie, sumoylation). PTEN structure consists of a short N-terminal lipid-binding domain followed by the phosphatase domain, a membrane-binding C2 domain, and a C-terminal tail that influences stability and subcellular localization. In addition to its established lipid phosphatase activity, PTEN is also capable of acting as a protein phosphatase in vitro, though not all of these putative substrates have been validated in vivo.

Germline *PTEN* mutations are causal in the related Cowden, Bannayan-Riley-Ruvalcaba, Proteus, and Proteus-like hamartoma syndromes, collectively known as PTHS (PTEN hamartoma tumor syndromes). These clinically distinct conditions are marked by small benign growths and, in Cowden syndrome, carry an enhanced risk for developing breast, thyroid, and endometrial cancers. Progression from benign to malignant tumor growth, in Cowden syndrome, coincides with LOH at the *PTEN* locus.

Somatic PTEN loss of function at the genomic, epigenomic, transcriptional, or protein levels is found in a wide array of cancers, especially glioblastoma, prostate, endometrial, ovarian, and lung tumors. Chromosomal deletions at the 10q23 locus are the most common mechanism of PTEN loss (Alvarez-Garcia et al, 2019). In addition, missense and nonsense point substitutions have been observed, as well as frameshift mutations yielding truncations that disrupt the phosphatase and/or C2 domains, hence compromising catalytic activity. Tumors harboring a single mutated PTEN allele have frequently been found to lack PTEN immunostaining, suggesting additional mechanisms of PTEN loss. It has since become evident that

PTEN expression can be silenced by methylation of the *PTEN* promoter, which has been found in lung, breast, colorectal, endometrial, and ovarian cancers, in particular.

Beyond genomic and epigenomic disruptions, PTEN is also downregulated at the transcript level by miRNAs. For example, the miR-21 microRNA, which promotes tumorigenesis by targeting the PTEN transcript, is overexpressed in a wide array of cancers, including hematologic malignancies such as AML and CLL, along with solid tumors such as glioblastomas, breast, colon, and lung cancers (Leslie and Foti, 2011). The miR-124, miR-22, miR-26a, miR-19a, and miR-17-92 cluster are also thought to affect PTEN levels in various cancers. The stability of PTEN is further modulated at the protein level through the concerted action of ubiquitination, sumoylation, and phosphorylation of regulatory sites. The critical role played by PTEN in suppressing tumorigenesis in many tissues is underscored by the variety of means through which its function is controlled (see Fig. 7–14).

7.6.3 BRCA1 and BRCA2

In 1994, linkage analysis studies correlated the *BRCA1* and *BRCA2* genes with hereditary breast cancer, and thousands of germline and somatic mutations have since been identified in both genes (Narod and Foulkes, 2004). *BRCA1* mutations associate with high-grade infiltrating ductal carcinomas, frequently exhibiting a basal, triple-negative phenotype (ie, without expression of hormone receptors or HER-2/ERBB2; see Chap. 20, Sec. 20.3), whereas *BRCA2* mutations do not correlate with a particular tumor histopathology (Tung and Garber, 2018). *BRCA1* and *BRCA2* carriers have a heightened risk for developing ovarian tumors, and male carriers of *BRCA2* have an increased risk of prostate cancer.

The BRCA1/2 tumor suppressors play central roles in the maintenance of genomic integrity (Roy et al, 2011; George et al, 2017). The BRCA1 structure consists of an N-terminal RING domain, a central DNA-binding region

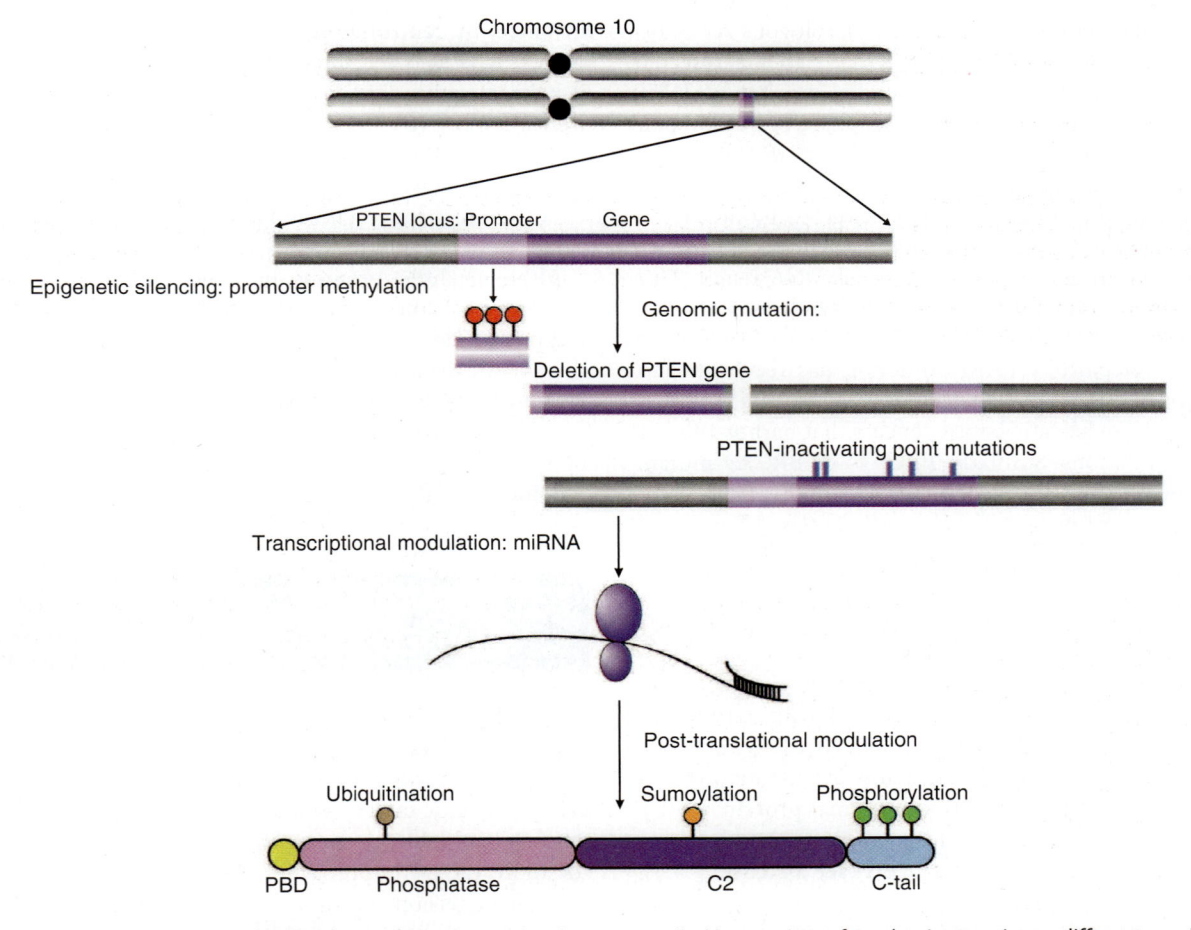

FIGURE 7–14 **Mechanisms of PTEN deregulation.** PTEN levels are controlled by a variety of mechanisms acting at different regulatory levels. Deletions in the 10q23 chromosomal region were frequently observed in certain cancers and subsequently led to the identification of the PTEN tumor-suppressor locus. The absence of PTEN immunostaining in tumors harboring deletion of a single copy of the PTEN gene suggested the existence of additional mechanisms of PTEN loss. It is now clear that silencing of PTEN expression through methylation of the PTEN promoter as well as post-transcriptional inhibition mediated by miRNAs represent prominent oncogenic mechanisms. Though less common, inactivating point mutations in the PTEN gene have also been cataloged. PTEN protein stability is modulated by a number of factors, including ubiquitination, sumoylation, and phosphorylation. Because tumor progression is sensitive to changes in PTEN levels, perturbation in any of these regulatory inputs will influence the course of tumorigenesis.

including the coiled-coil domain, and a C-terminal BRCT (BRCA1 C-terminus) domain, all of which mediate interactions critical to the functions of the protein in the realms of DNA repair, cell-cycle checkpoint control, chromatin remodeling, and ubiquitination. The RING domain, which interacts with the BARD1 protein to create an E3 ubiquitin ligase holoenzyme, is a common target for oncogenic mutations as are the DNA-binding and BRCT domains. BRCA1 is involved in the resection step of DNA double-strand break repair by homologous recombination, via its interaction with the MRN endonuclease complex (see Chap. 9, Sec. 9.X). Moreover, BRCA1 also appears to modulate DNA damage–triggered cell-cycle checkpoints by regulating activation of the Chk1 kinase (see Chap. 9, Sec. 9.4.1).

BRCA2 is a large protein containing several regions known to mediate interactions, notably 8 central BRCT repeats that bind RAD51, a key protein involved in DNA repair, (see Chap 9, Sec. 9.3.4) and C-terminal nucleic acid recognition sequences (known as OB folds) that interact with single-stranded DNA (ssDNA). The primary function of the protein is to facilitate DNA repair by homologous recombination through the recruitment of RAD51 to the resected single-stranded DNA stretches generated at sites of DNA damage. BRCA1 is also involved in this phase of DNA repair via its interaction with BRCA2. Tumors that lack functional BRCA1 or BRCA2 are therefore deficient in homologous recombination and can be selectively targeted by inhibition of poly(adenosine diphosphate-ribose) polymerase (PARP), which provides an alternative pathway for DNA repair. This is the prototype example of the use of "synthetic lethality" in the treatment of cancer (see Chap. 19, Sec. 19.6.2). In recent years, olaparib, a PARP inhibitor, has received FDA approval for treatment of advanced ovarian cancers as well as HER2-negative metastatic breast cancers that harbor BRCA1 or BRCA2 mutations. Similarly, BRCA1- or BRCA2-mutant tumors appear to be sensitized to the crosslinking DNA damage induced by platinum-based chemotherapies.

7.6.4 Retinoblastoma Protein

The RB1 gene, the first tumor-suppressor locus to be identified, is now known to be inactivated in many human cancers, beyond this historic association with retinoblastoma (see also Sec. 7.2.3) (Dick et al, 2018). Direct RB1 mutation, or disruptions in the pathways regulating the functions of the encoded retinoblastoma protein (pRb), are widespread in cancer, including most breast and lung tumors, as well as HPV-related cancers (see also Sec. 7.4.4). The best-understood pRb function is its role as a cofactor interacting with and regulating the activity of transcription factors, notably those of the E2F family. Originally, the tumor-suppressor function of pRb was attributed largely to its role in constraining cell-cycle progression, at the G1 to S phase transition, by influencing the expression of genes under the control of E2F transcription factors (Chap. 8, Sec. 8.3.4). In its hypophosphorylated form, pRb binds E2F proteins and prevents them from activating target genes required for cell-cycle progression. In response to proliferative signals, Cyclin D-Cdk4/6 complexes phosphorylate pRb, resulting in its dissociation, thereby liberating the E2F proteins to activate the appropriate gene expression program. pRb is now known to influence the expression of transcriptional targets that impact a wide array of cellular processes encompassing inflammation, metabolism, autophagy, adhesion, differentiation, and cell death. Deregulation of any of these through RB1 inactivation has the potential to promote various stages of tumorigenesis, although the precise pRb contribution likely varies in different tumors.

pRb interacts with as many as 200 proteins, many of which have functions unrelated to direct transcriptional regulation. Notably, pRb serves as an adaptor for the recruitment of epigenetic regulators such as histone modifiers, DNA methyltransferases, and SWI/SNF chromatin remodeling complexes, impacting chromatin status both at specific loci and at a global level, thereby affecting genomic stability as well. In this context, pRb acts to preserve chromosomal integrity by silencing repetitive DNA sequences found, for instance, in centromeres, telomeres, and transposable elements. It is also recruited to sites of DNA damage, where it interacts with elements of the DNA repair machinery as well as SWI/SNF complexes, in order to facilitate repair. pRb also helps maintain chromosomal integrity and cell ploidy by interacting with condensin proteins at centromeres, contributing to proper chromosomal segregation during the G2/M cell cycle phase.

Although little progress has been made in developing E2F-targeted compounds, the loss of pRb function affects responsiveness to chemotherapy and can therefore inform therapeutic decisions. Cells that are deficient in pRb function are sensitized to DNA-damaging agents owing to the aforementioned DNA repair defect. By contrast, agents that act by blocking proliferation, such as CDK4/6 inhibitors, tend to require pRb action and are therefore less effective.

7.7 THERAPEUTIC STRATEGIES GUIDED BY CANCER GENETICS

The treatment of cancers with radiation and chemotherapy leads to the killing of both malignant and untransformed cells, resulting in varying levels of toxicity. The reliance of cancer cells on specific molecular alterations and signaling pathways, where identifiable, presents oncologists with an opportunity for more targeted approaches. The concept of personalized medicine envisions profiling all of the aberrations in individual tumors, through genomic and RNA sequencing, and then tailoring treatments to maximize the killing of cancer cells while reducing attendant side effects (see Table 7–1). Several notable successes highlight the attractiveness of this approach (Hyman et al, 2017). It has become routine to test for common recurrent mutations, including translocations or gene amplifications, for *BCR-ABL* in CML, *EGFR* and *ALK* in non–small cell lung cancer, *BRAF* in melanoma, as well as *HER2* in breast and stomach cancer, and to target these tumors with appropriate agents. These treatments are discussed in detail in Chapter 19.

On this basis, next-generation sequencing to detect and target other genes has become popular and is marketed to patients and their physicians. Unfortunately, the aforementioned examples notwithstanding, multiple published trials have collectively shown that this approach has not yet made a substantial impact on outcome, with response rates of <5% of the patients with advanced cancer who undergo genetic sequencing (Tannock and Hickman, 2019). The reasons for this minimal influence on outcome are multiple but include:

1. Disease progression during the time between molecular profiling and selection of a matching drug, compromising the suitability of the chosen treatment.
2. Lack of availability of a matched targeted agent.
3. An inability to combine targeted agents at optimal concentrations because of toxicity, thereby restricting the therapeutic window.
4. Poor response to a targeted agent despite matching. This may be due to incomplete pathway inhibition or an insufficient understanding of the regulation of the function of the targeted protein, as well as tumor-specific variables impacting its progression.
5. Intra- or intertumor heterogeneity, such that the molecular profile represents only one part of the biopsied tumor while inadequately capturing the genetic variance at spatially distinct regions of the same tumor or metastatic growths (see Chap. 13, Sec. 13.4).
6. Difficulties in identifying the genuine drivers of individual tumors. For instance, in some cases, changes in common cancer genes are observed in normal tissue and may not actually drive a subsequent malignancy. As a consequence, targeting these genes would be futile.

Although some of these limitations might be overcome with further study and the advent of novel technologies, the heterogeneity of tumors in both space and time, along with the adaptability of cancer cells brought about by their genetic instability, may represent a fundamental barrier to purely targeted therapeutic approaches. These issues are discussed further in Chapters 13, 19, and 22.

SUMMARY

- Advances in technology have allowed cancer biologists to develop a comprehensive picture of the genetic events underlying tumorigenesis. They facilitate the identification of oncogenic events in a given cancer in a cost-effective and high-throughput manner.
- Cancers are very heterogeneous and should be viewed as a series of mutagenic alterations, occurring not only at the genomic, but also at the epigenomic, transcriptomic, proteomic, and metabolic levels.
- Genetic changes confer a selective advantage that constitutes the transformed phenotype, encompassing properties that are particular to cancer cells. These include self-sufficiency in growth signals, insensitivity to antigrowth signals, resistance to cell death, limitless replicative potential, angiogenesis, genomic instability, deregulated metabolism, the capacity for invasion and metastasis, as well as the ability to circumvent immune clearance and generate tumorigenic inflammation.
- A critical challenge is to sift among the long list of changes occurring during transformation, so as to identify the indispensable oncogenic processes, which may then be targeted therapeutically (see Table 7–1).
- Acquiring such an understanding requires a confluence of efforts in many fields including bioinformatics, bioengineering, and pharmacology, as well as basic biologic and translational research.
- Comprehensive efforts promise to reveal novel cancer genes, such as *IDH1* and *IDH2*, while confirming the importance of more established oncogenes, like *BCR-ABL*, *MYC*, *EGFR*, *ERBB2*, *PIK3CA*, *RAS*, and *RAF*, along with the *TP53*, *PTEN*, *BRCA1*, *BRCA2*, and *RB1* tumor-suppressor genes.
- A clearer understanding of the oncogenic processes underlying specific cancers could enable personalized therapeutic approaches, presumably leading to more effective clinical outcomes.

REFERENCES

Adamo P, Ladomery MR. The oncogene ERG: a key factor in prostate cancer. *Oncogene* 2016;35(4):403-414.

Alvarez-Garcia V, Tawil Y, Wise HM, Leslie NR. Mechanisms of Pten loss in cancer: it's all about diversity. *Semin Cancer Biol* 2019;59:66-79.

Anastasiadou E, Jacob LS, Slack FJ. Non-coding RNA networks in cancer. *Nat Rev Cancer* 2018;18(1):5-18.

Anwar SL, Wulaningsih W, Lehmann U. Transposable elements in human cancer: causes and consequences of deregulation. *Int J Mol Sci* 2017;18(5):974.

Arteaga CL, Engelman JA. ERBB receptors: from oncogene discovery to basic science to mechanism-based cancer therapeutics. *Cancer Cell* 2014;25(3):282-303.

Bassi C, Ho J, Dowling RJ, et al. Nuclear PTEN controls DNA repair and sensitivity to genotoxic stress. *Science* 2013;341(6144):395-399.

Bayliss R, Choi J, Fennel DA, et al. Molecular mechanisms that underpin EML4-ALK driven cancers and their responses to targeted drugs. *Cell Mol Life Sci* 2016;73(6):1209-1224.

Bennett RL, Licht JD. Targeting epigenetics in cancer. *Annu Rev Pharmacol Toxicol* 2018;58:187-207.

Bougeard G, Renaux-Petel M, Flaman JM, et al. Revisiting Li-Fraumeni syndrome from TP53 mutation carriers. *J Clin Oncol* 2015;33(21):2345-2352.

Cavenee W, Dryja T, Phillips R, et al. Expression of recessive alleles by chromosomal mechanisms in retinoblastoma. *Nature* 1983;305(5937):779-784.

Chalhoub N, Baker SJ. PTEN and the PI3-kinase pathway in cancer. *Annu Rev Pathol* 2009;4:127-150.

Chung CH, Gillison ML. Human papillomavirus in head and neck cancer: its role in pathogenesis and clinical implications. *Clin Cancer Res* 2009;15(22):6758-6762.

Cimmino A, Calin GA, Fabbri M, et al. miR-15 and miR-16 induce apoptosis by targeting BCL2. *Proc Natl Acad Sci U S A* 2006;102(39):13944-13949.

Dang L, White DW, Gross S, et al. Cancer-associated IDH1 mutations produce 2-hydroxyglutarate. *Nature* 2009;462(7274):739-744.

De Sanjose S, Brotons M, LaMontagne DS, Bruni L. Human papillomavirus vaccine disease impact beyond expectations. *Curr Opin Virol* 2019;39:16-22.

Der CJ, Krontiris TG, Cooper GM. Transforming genes of human bladder and lung carcinoma cell lines are homologous to the ras genes of Harvey and Kirsten sarcoma viruses. *Proc Natl Acad Sci U S A* 1982;79(11):3637-3640.

Dick FA, Goodrich DW, Sage J, Dyson NJ. Non-canonical functions of the Rb protein in cancer. *Nat Rev Cancer* 2018;18(7):442-451.

Drusco A, Croce CM. MicroRNAs and cancer: A long story for short RNAs. *Adv Cancer Res* 2017;135:1-24.

Esteller M. Epigenetics in cancer. *N Engl J Med* 2008;358(11):1148-1159.

Fabbri M, Garzon R, Cimmino A, et al. MicroRNA-29 family reverts aberrant methylation in lung cancer by targeting DNA methyltransferases 3A and 3B. *Proc Natl Acad Sci U S A* 2007;104(40):15805-15810.

Ferreira HJ, Esteller M. Non-coding RNAs, epigenetics, and cancer: tying it all together. *Cancer Metastasis Rev* 2018;37(1):55-73.

Friend S, Bernards R, Rogelj S, et al. A human DNA segment with properties of the gene that predisposes to retinoblastoma and osteosarcoma. *Nature* 1986;323(6089):643-646.

Fruman DA, Chiu H, Hopkins BD, et al. The PI3K pathway in human disease. *Cell* 2017;170(4):605-635.

Fung Y, Murphree A, T'Ang A, et al. Structural evidence for the authenticity of the human retinoblastoma gene. *Science* 1987;236(4809):1657-1661.

Gabay M, Li Y, Felsher DW. MYC activation is a hallmark of cancer initiation and maintenance. *Cold Spring Harb Perspect Med* 2014;4(6):a014241.

Gan HK, Cvrljevic AN, Johns TG. The epidermal growth factor receptor variant III (EGFRvIII) where wild things are altered. *FEBS J* 2013;280(21):5350-5370.

George A, Kaye S, Banerjee S. Delivering widespread BRCA testing and PARP inhibition to patients with ovarian cancer. *Nat Rev Clin Oncol* 2017;14(5):284-296.

Gillison ML, Chaturvedi AK, Anderson WF, Fakhry C. Epidemiology of human papillomavirus-positive head and neck squamous cell carcinoma. *J Clin Oncol* 2015;33(29):3235-3242.

Hanahan D, Weinberg RA. The hallmarks of cancer. *Cell* 2000;100(1):57-70.

Hanahan D, Weinberg RA. Hallmarks of cancer: the next generation. *Cell* 2011;144(5):646-674.

Hansford S, Huntsman DG. Boveri at 100: Theodor Boveri and genetic predisposition to cancer. *J Pathol* 2014;234(2):142-145.

Harden ME, Munger K. Human papillomavirus molecular biology. *Mutat Res Rev Mutat Res* 2017;772:3-12.

Hollander MC, Blumenthal GM, Dennis PA. PTEN loss in the continuum of common cancers, rare syndromes and mouse models. *Nat Rev Cancer* 2011;11(4):289-301.

Hyman DM, Taylor BS, Baselga J. Implementing genome-driven oncology. *Cell* 2017;168(4):584-599.

Janku F, Yap TA, Meric-Bernstam F. Targeting the PI3K pathway in cancer: are we making headway. *Nat Rev Clin Oncol* 2018;15(5):273-291.

Johnson SM, Grosshans H, Shingara J, et al. RAS is regulated by the let-7 microRNA family. *Cell* 2005;120(5):635-647.

Kalkat M, De Melo J, Hickman KA, et al. MYC deregulation in primary human cancers. *Genes* 2017;8(6):151.

Karoulia Z, Gavathiotis E, Poulikakos PI. New perspectives for targeting RAF kinases in human cancer. *Nat Rev Cancer* 2017;17(11):676-691.

Karreth FA, Tuveson DA. Modelling oncogenic Ras/Raf signalling in the mouse. *Curr Opin Genet Dev* 2009;19(1):4-11.

Kastenhuber ER, Lowe SW. Putting p53 in context. *Cell* 2017;170(6):1062-1078.

Kinzler KW, Vogelstein B. Landscaping the cancer terrain. *Science* 1998;280(5366):1036-1037.

Knudson AG. Mutation and cancer: statistical study of retinoblastoma. *Proc Natl Acad Sci U S A* 1971;68(4):820-823.

Kumar-Sinha C, Kalyana-Sundaram S, Chinnaiyan AM. Landscape of gene fusions in epithelial cancers: seq and ye shall find. *Genome Med* 2015;7:129.

Kumari A, Folk WP, Sakamuro D. The dual roles of MYC in genomic instability and cancer chemoresistance. *Genes* 2017;8(6):158.

Kung CP, Meckes DG, Raab-Traub N. Epstein-Barr virus LMP1 activates EGFR, STAT3, and ER through effects of PKCδ. *J Virol* 2011;85(9):4399-4308.

Kuzyk A, Mai S. c-MYC-induced genomic instability. *Cold Spring Harb Perspect Med* 2014;4(4):a014373.

Lee W, Bookstein R, Hong F, et al. Human retinoblastoma susceptibility gene: cloning, identification, and sequence. *Science* 1987;235(4794):1394-1399.

Leslie NR, Foti M. Non-genomic loss of PTEN function in cancer: not in my genes. *Trends Pharmacol Sci* 2011;32(3):131-140.

Li HP, Chang YS. Epstein-Barr virus latent membrane protein 1: structure and functions. *J Biomed Sci* 2003;10(5):490-504.

Manning BD, Toker A. AKT/PKB signaling: navigating the network. *Cell* 2017;169(3):381-405.

Mertens F, Johansson B, Fioretos T, et al. The emerging complexity of gene fusions in cancer. *Nat Rev Cancer* 2015;15(6):371-381.

Mittal S, Banks L. Molecular mechanisms underlying human papillomavirus E6 and E7 oncoprotein induced cell transformation. *Mutat Res Rev Mutat Res* 2017;772:23-35.

Moody CA. Impact of replication stress in human papillomavirus pathogenesis. *J Virol* 2019;93(2):e01012-e01017.

Mughal TI, Radich JP, Deininger MW, et al. Chronic myeloid leukemia: reminiscences and dreams. *Haematologica* 2016;101(5):541-558.

Narod SA, Foulkes WD. BRCA1 and BRCA2: 1994 and beyond. *Nat Rev Cancer* 2004;4(9):665-676.

Nebbioso A, Tambaro FP, Dell'Aversana C, Altucci L. Cancer epigenetics: moving forward. *PLoS Genet* 2018;14(6):e1007362.

Olive V, Minella AC, He L. Outside the coding genome, mammalian microRNAs confer structural and functional complexity. *Sci Signal* 2015;8(368):re2.

Parsons DW, Jones S, Zhang X, et al. An integrated genomic analysis of human glioblastoma multiforme. *Science* 2008;321(5897):1807-1812.

Pfeifer GP. Defining driver DNA methylation changes in human cancer. *Int J Mol Sci* 2018;19(4):1166.

Pon JR, Marra MA. Driver and passenger mutations in cancer. *Annu Rev Pathol* 2015;10:25-50.

Rao SG, Jackson JG. SASP: tumor suppressor or promoter? Yes! *Trends Cancer* 2016;2(11):676-687.

Rickinson AB, Kieff E. Epstein-Barr virus and its replication. In: Knipe DM, Howley PM, eds. *Field's Virology*. Philadelphia, PA: Lippincott, Williams & Wilkins; 2007:2603-2654.

Rous P. Transmission of a malignant new growth by means of a cell-free filtrate. *JAMA* 1911;56:198.

Rowley JD. A new consistent chromosomal abnormality in chronic myelogenous leukaemia identified by quinacrine fluorescence and Giemsa staining. *Nature* 1973;243(5405):290-293.

Roy R, Chun J, Powell SN. BRCA1 and BRCA2: different roles in a common pathway of genome protection. *Nat Rev Cancer* 2011;12(1):68-78.

Sabapathy K, Lane DP. Therapeutic targeting of p53: all mutants are equal, but some mutants are more equal than others. *Nat Rev Clin Oncol* 2018;15(1):13-30.

Sampson VB, Rong NH, Han J, et al. MicroRNA let-7a down-regulates MYC and reverts MYC-induced growth in Burkitt lymphoma cells. *Cancer Res* 2007;67(20):9762-9770.

Schmitt F. HER2+ breast cancer: how to evaluate? *Adv Ther* 2009;26(suppl 1):S1-S8.

Schram AM, Chang MT, Jonsson P, et al. Fusions in solid tumours: diagnostic strategies, targeted therapy, and acquired resistance. *Nat Rev Clin Oncol* 2017;14(12):735-748.

Shimizu K, Goldfarb M, Suard Y, et al. Three human transforming genes are related to the viral ras oncogenes. *Proc Natl Acad Sci U S A* 1983;80(8):2112-2116.

Simanshu D, Nissley DV, McCormick F. RAS proteins and their regulators in human disease. *Cell* 2017;170(1):17-33.

Soni V, Cahir-McFarland E, Kieff E. LMP1 trafficking activates growth and survival pathways. *Adv Exp Med Biol* 2007;597:173-187.

Stehelin D, Varmus H, Bishop J, et al. DNA related to the transforming gene(s) of avian sarcoma viruses is present in normal avian DNA. *Nature* 1976;260(5547):170-173.

Stewart EL, Tan SZ, Liu G, Tsao MS. Known and putative mechanisms of resistance to EGFR targeted therapies in NSCLC patients with EGFR mutations—a review. *Transl Lung Cancer Res* 2015;4(1):67-81.

Svoronos AA, Engelman DM, Slack FJ. OncomiR or tumor suppressor? The duplicity of microRNAs in cancer. *Cancer Res* 2016;76(13):3666-3670.

Tannock IF, Hickman JA. Molecular screening to select therapy for advanced cancer. *Ann Oncol* 2019;30(5):661-663.

Tomas A, Futter CE, Eden ER. EGF receptor trafficking: consequences for signaling and cancer. *Trends Cell Biol* 2014;24(1):26-34.

Tu WB, Helander S, Pilstal R, et al. Myc and its interactors take shape. *Biochim Biophys Acta* 2015;1849(5):469-483.

Tung NM, Garber JE. BRCA1/2 testing: therapeutic implications for breast cancer management. *Br J Cancer* 2018;119(2):141-152.

Waitkus MS, Diplas BH, Yan H. Biological role and therapeutic potential of IDH mutations in cancer. *Cancer Cell* 2018;34(2):186-195.

Ward PS, Patel J, Wise DR, et al. The common feature of leukemia-associated IDH1 and IDH2 mutations is a neomorphic enzyme activity converting alpha-ketoglutarate to 2-hydroxyglutarate. *Cancer Cell* 2010;17(3):225-234.

Yan H, Parsons DW, Jin G, et al. IDH1 and IDH2 mutations in gliomas. *N Engl J Med* 2009;360(8):765-773.

Yao Z, Yaeger R, Rodrik VS, et al. Tumours with class 3 BRAF mutants are sensitive to the inhibition of activated RAS. *Nature* 2017;548(7666):234-238.

Yarden Y, Pines G. The ERBB network: at last, cancer therapy meets systems biology. *Nat Rev Cancer* 2012;12(8):553-563.

Yoshihara K, Wang C, Torres-Garcia W, et al. The landscape and therapeutic relevance of cancer-associated transcript fusions. *Oncogene* 2015;34(37):4845-4854.

Young LS, Yap LF, Murray PG. Epstein-Barr virus: more than 50 years old and still providing surprises. *Nat Rev Cancer* 2016;16(12):789-802.

Zhang Y, Kwok-Shing Ng P, Kucherlapati M, et al. A pan-cancer proteogenomic atlas of PI3K/AKT/mTor pathway alterations. *Cancer Cell* 2017;31(6):820-832.

Cell Proliferation and Death

Kelsie L. Thu, David W. Cescon, and Razqallah Hakem

Chapter Outline

- 8.1 Introduction
- 8.2 Molecular Control of Cell Proliferation
  - 8.2.1 The Mammalian Cell Cycle
  - 8.2.2 Primary Effectors of Cell-Cycle Control
  - 8.2.3 Molecular Mechanisms Regulating Progression Through the Cell Cycle
  - 8.2.4 Cell Growth
  - 8.2.5 Modifications to Control of Cell Proliferation in Cancer
  - 8.2.6 Therapeutic Targeting of Cell Proliferation and Growth in Cancer
- 8.3 Genomic Instability and Checkpoint Pathways
  - 8.3.1 The DNA Damage Checkpoints
  - 8.3.2 The Spindle Assembly Checkpoint
  - 8.3.3 Mitotic Errors and Aneuploidy
  - 8.3.4 Modifications of Cell-Cycle Checkpoints in Cancer
  - 8.3.5 Targeting Genomic Instability and Cell-Cycle Checkpoints for Cancer Therapy
- 8.4 Cell Death
  - 8.4.1 Mechanisms of Apoptosis
  - 8.4.2 The Mitochondrial Apoptotic Pathway
  - 8.4.3 The Death Receptor Apoptotic Pathway
  - 8.4.4 Apoptosis, Developmental Defects, and Disease
  - 8.4.5 Mechanisms Leading to Necrosis
  - 8.4.6 Additional Mechanisms Associated With Cell Death
  - 8.4.7 Modifications to Control of Cell Death in Cancer
- Summary
- References

8.1 INTRODUCTION

Our cells are continuously proliferating and dying. Development from a single-celled egg into adults with approximately 10^{14} cells requires massive cell proliferation. However, selective cell death is also essential for development, for example, to prune excess neurons in the brain and to sculpt the fingers. As adults, most of our organs exist in a dynamic steady state, being constantly renewed by cell proliferation and death. For example, more than a million blood and intestinal cells are turned over *every second*. In the extreme, cells live for only a few days before dying, as is the case for neutrophils and the cells that line the small intestine. In the midst of this continual and profuse cell renewal lies the constant threat of cancer. Cancerous cells invariably contain alterations to genes encoding regulators of cell proliferation and cell death and are generally thought to arise from actively proliferating cell types.

This chapter discusses the molecular control of the cell cycle and of the processes that lead to cell death, many of which are modified in the processes of malignant transformation and tumor progression. Chapter 12 discusses the growth of tumors and the patterns of cell proliferation and cell death that influence tumor growth, together with the tumor microenvironment and metabolism with which they are closely linked. Chapter 13 discusses the properties of tumor stem cells with high proliferative potential.

8.2 MOLECULAR CONTROL OF CELL PROLIFERATION

Cell proliferation is perhaps best viewed as a combination of 2 distinct processes: the cell cycle, which replicates and segregates the genome, and cell growth, which doubles all other components of the cell. The cell cycle and cell growth are intertwined in most normal and cancerous cells, but the 2 processes can be uncoupled, both in the laboratory and as part of normal development.

8.2.1 The Mammalian Cell Cycle

The cell cycle is partitioned into 4 phases: G_1, S, G_2, and M. This organization reflects the 2 primary goals of the cell cycle: to replicate the genome of the mother cell during DNA synthesis or S phase and to segregate the replicated genome into 2 daughter cells during mitosis or M phase (Fig. 8–1). Two gap

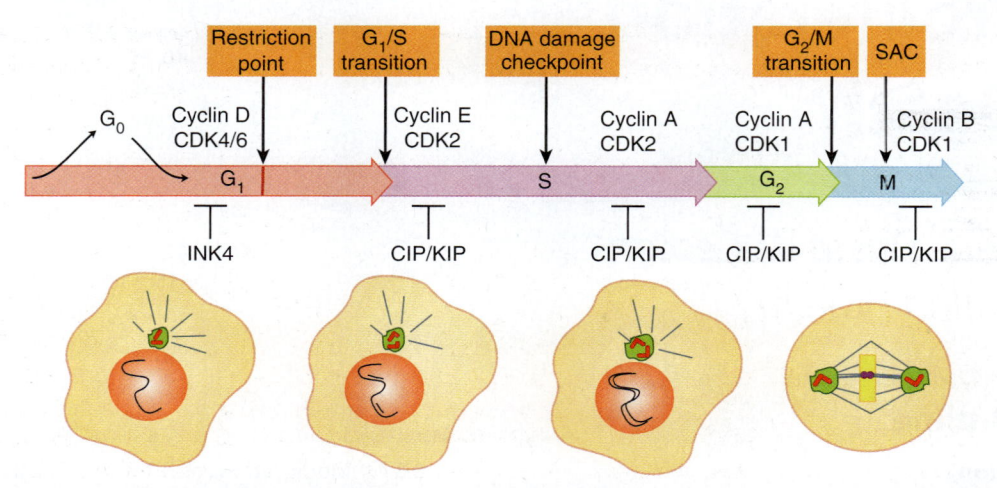

FIGURE 8-1 **The key events of the cell cycle.** In cells, the nucleus (orange) contains chromosomes (black). The centrosomes (green) are centered around centrioles (red). Most microtubules (blue) project from the centrosome. Chromosome and centrosome duplication begin at the start of S phase. During mitosis, chromosomes (yellow) condense and the 2 sister chromatids become apparent, remaining joined at the centromeres, which is also the location of the kinetochores (purple) that bind the sister chromatids to bundles of microtubules from opposing poles. Cell structures are not drawn to scale. Throughout the cell cycle, multiple checkpoints exist and CDK inhibitor proteins (CKIs) act to ensure the fidelity of genome duplication and cell division. *SAC*, spindle assembly checkpoint.

phases (G_1, G_2) separate these fundamental events. The combined G_1, S, and G_2 phases are frequently referred to as interphase. When cells cease proliferating because of insufficient nutrients, lack of growth factors, or on differentiation, they exit the cell cycle from G_1 phase and enter a quiescent state called G_0. Most cells in the body are in the G_0 state. If cells in G_0 are instructed to start proliferating, they must transition back into G_1 phase before starting another cell cycle.

8.2.1.1 The Genome Is Duplicated During S Phase

Replicating the genome is the first of the cell cycle's 2 primary objectives. Each of the more than 6 billion base pairs in the DNA of a human cell must be replicated exactly once per cell cycle. To replicate so many base pairs, DNA synthesis is initiated at thousands of replication origins scattered throughout the genome (Fig. 8–2A, B; Fragkos et al, 2015). At each replication origin, double-stranded DNA (dsDNA) is unwound into 2 single strands and large protein complexes containing DNA polymerase load onto the single-stranded DNA (ssDNA) (Fig. 8–2C). As they begin to replicate the ssDNA, these protein complexes progress away from the origin, unwinding the dsDNA in front of them and leaving 2 copies of dsDNA in their wake, thereby creating a structure called a replication fork (Fig. 8–2C; Burgers and Kunkel, 2017). When replication forks progressing away from neighboring origins of replication collide, replication stops, the DNA replication complexes are removed, and the DNA strands are ligated together (Fig. 8–2A; Dewar and Walter, 2017).

Cells ensure that each stretch of inter-origin DNA is replicated only once by allowing each DNA replication origin to initiate or "fire" only once per cell cycle. Origins can only initiate synthesis once each cell cycle because of a temporal separation between the formation of the pre-replicative complex (pre-RC) on the origin and the initiation of replication at the origin (origin firing) (Fragkos et al, 2015). Pre-RCs are protein complexes containing DNA-binding proteins that assemble on origins at the end of the previous mitosis (see Fig. 8–2B). Once an origin is bound by a pre-RC, it is said to be "licensed" for replication, but these licensed origins remain inert throughout the G_1 phase. It is only starting in S phase that licensed replication origins "fire," when the aforementioned replication complexes containing DNA polymerases are recruited to the pre-RC and DNA synthesis begins at the origin (see Fig. 8–2C). Pre-RC complexes cannot reassemble in S phase, nor throughout the subsequent G_2 and early M phases. This strict separation between times during which pre-RCs can assemble and hence license the origins (G_1 phase) and during which the licensed origins can fire (S phase) limits each origin to a single firing event and prevents re-replication of the DNA.

8.2.1.2 The Duplicated Genome Is Segregated Into 2 Daughter Cells During Mitosis

Segregating the replicated genomes into 2 daughter cells is the cell cycle's other primary objective. Chromosome segregation is powered and organized by microtubules. Microtubules and associated proteins form the mitotic spindle, a complex cellular apparatus that pulls apart the replicated chromosomes and then drags the separated sister chromatids to opposite ends of the mother cell (Prosser and Pelletier, 2017).

Assembly of the mitotic spindle is complicated but is facilitated by organelles called centrosomes that sit at either spindle pole and generally act to organize microtubules. Centrosomes are small (1-μm) and consist of an electron-dense pericentriolar material (PCM) centered on 2 compact (200-500 nm), barrel-shaped cylinders of microtubules arranged with 9-fold symmetry called *centrioles*. Normal cells in G_1 phase contain a single, centrally located centrosome with 2 separated centrioles (see Fig. 8–1). This single centrosome must replicate itself during the cell cycle, a process deemed the centrosome cycle

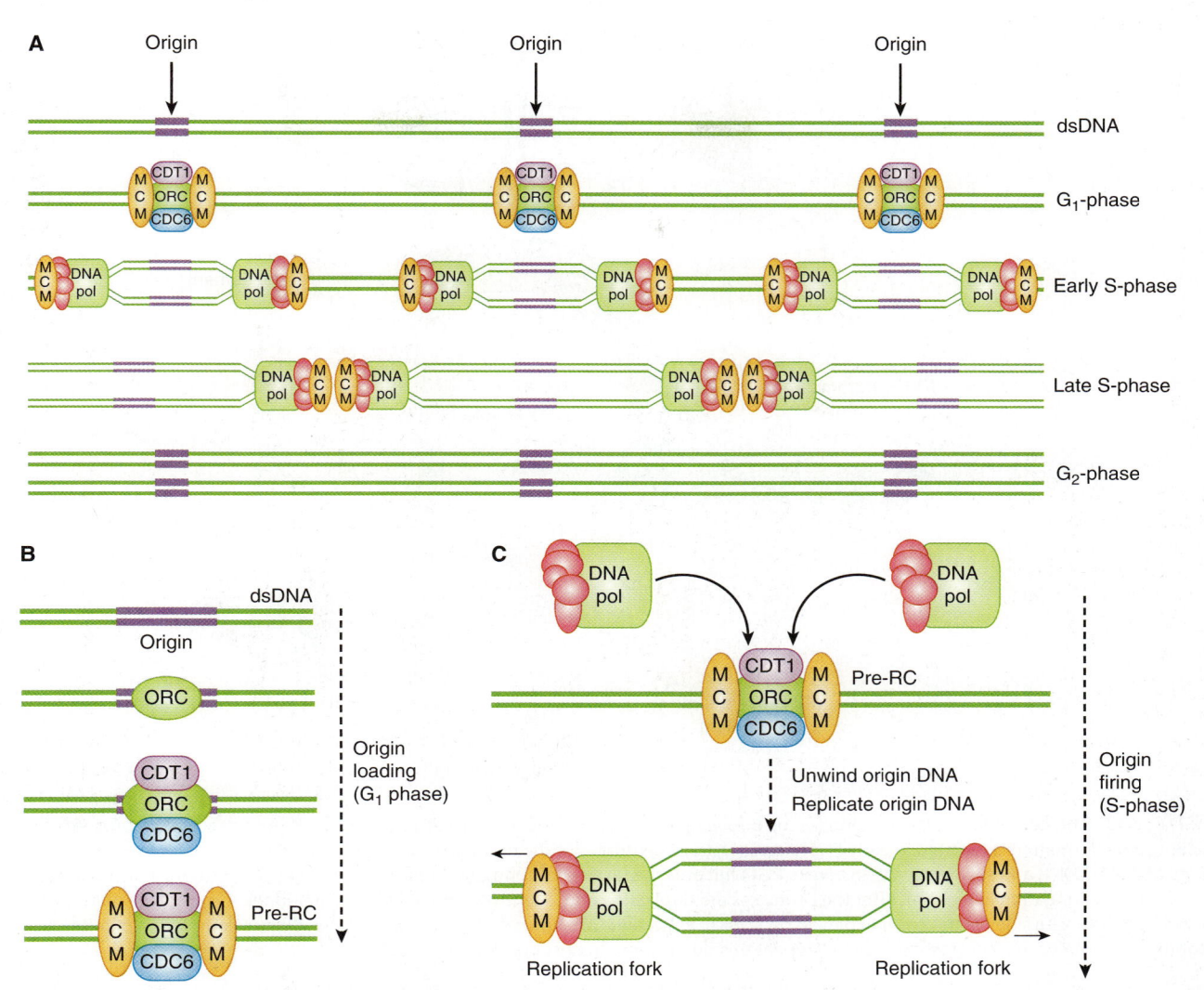

FIGURE 8–2 The loading and firing of DNA replication origins during the cell cycle. **A, B)** During G_1 phase, pre–replication complexes (pre-RCs) composed of ORC, CDT1, CDC6, and MCM proteins, termed *replication origins* (origins) assemble on stretches of double-stranded DNA (dsDNA). *ORC*, origin-recognition complex; *MCM*, minichromosome maintenance complex. **A, C)** In S phase, replication proteins, including DNA polymerase (DNA pol), are recruited by the pre-RC, leading to the unwinding of the origin DNA and the exposure of single-stranded DNA (ssDNA). The 2 exposed stands of ssDNA act as the templates for DNA replication, leading to the formation of 2 copies of dsDNA. Replication proceeds bidirectionally away from the origin, as 2 replication forks unwind DNA and then replicate the exposed ssDNA.

(Fig. 8–3; Wang et al, 2014; Nigg and Holland, 2018). First, the 2 centrioles comprising the parent centrosome disengage in G_1. Around the time of G_1/S transition, centriole duplication is initiated. Once centriole duplication is complete in late S phase, the 2 distinct centrosomes mature and separate in G_2. On entering mitosis, the 2 centrosomes separate and move to opposite sides of the cell and function as microtubule organizing centers with the bipolar spindle forming between them (Prosser and Pelletier, 2017). After mitosis, each new daughter cell contains 1 centrosome and the replication process will repeat during the next cell cycle.

At the start of mitosis, the replicated chromosomes (46 in humans) are composed of 2 sister chromatids that are coupled together along their entire length by cohesive protein complexes. Although it involves multiple parallel processes that progress in a continuous fashion, mitosis continues to be described as a series of discrete phases, defined by morphologic events observed under the microscope by early cell biologists (Fig. 8–4). Prophase begins with chromosome condensation in the nucleus. As long linear molecules of DNA, chromosomes must be compacted approximately 10,000-fold in order to be cleanly separated from one another and to be moved around the cell (Morgan, 2007). In the cytoplasm, the 2 centrosomes separate from one another and the mitotic spindle begins to form between them, moving the centrosomes to opposite sides of the cell. This process is facilitated by microtubule motor proteins, including the kinesin-5 motor (Eg5) which pushes antiparallel microtubules apart, and the minus-end directed motor dynein, which can bind and pull on microtubules anchored at the centrosome (Prosser and Pelletier, 2017).

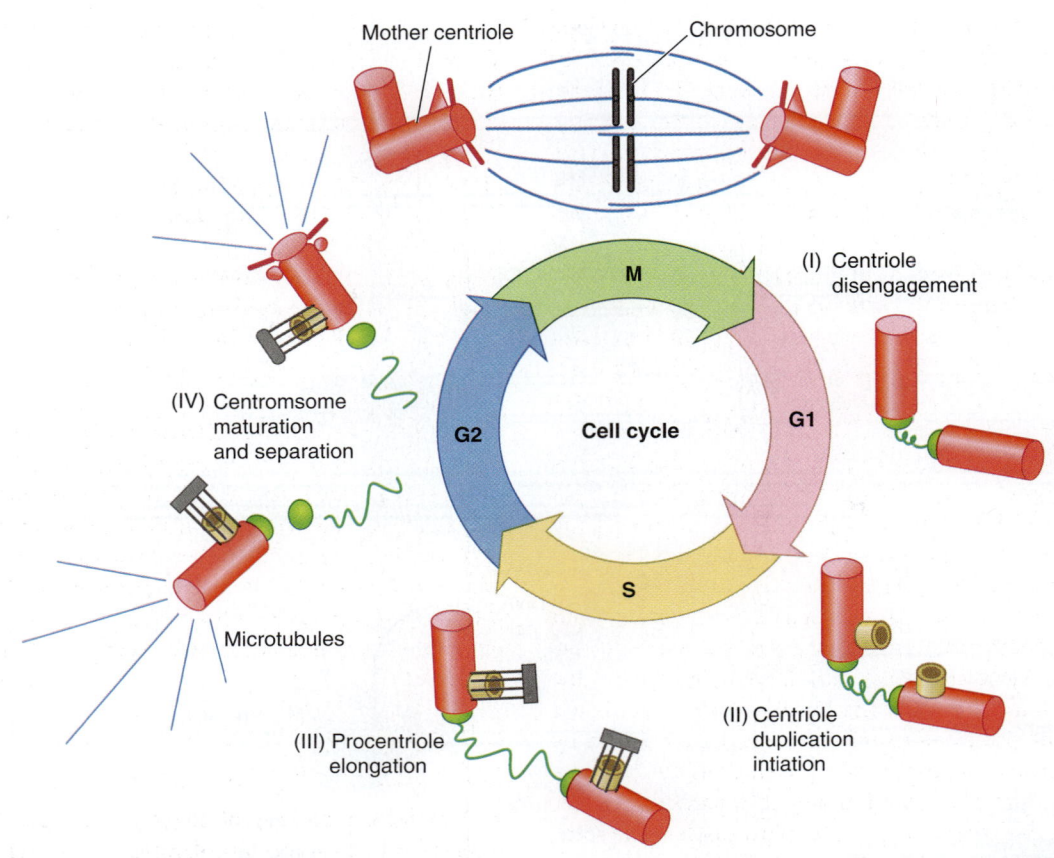

FIGURE 8-3 **The centrosome cycle.** Centrosome duplication occurs once during the cell cycle. Generation of a second centrosome for bipolar spindle formation is initiated in early G$_1$ phase. First, the 2 centrioles of the mother centrosome disengage, which is regulated by the activity of PLK1, CDK1, and separase proteins. Next, PLK4 initiates the process of centriole duplication at the G$_1$/S transition, which is followed by procentriole elongation in S phase. After the centrioles are duplicated and 2 centrosomes have been generated, centrosome maturation and separation to opposite sides of the cell is achieved by AURKA, PLK1, and CDK1 proteins in G$_2$ and M phases. On the completion of mitosis, each daughter cell contains one centrosome that will repeat this duplication process in the next cell cycle.

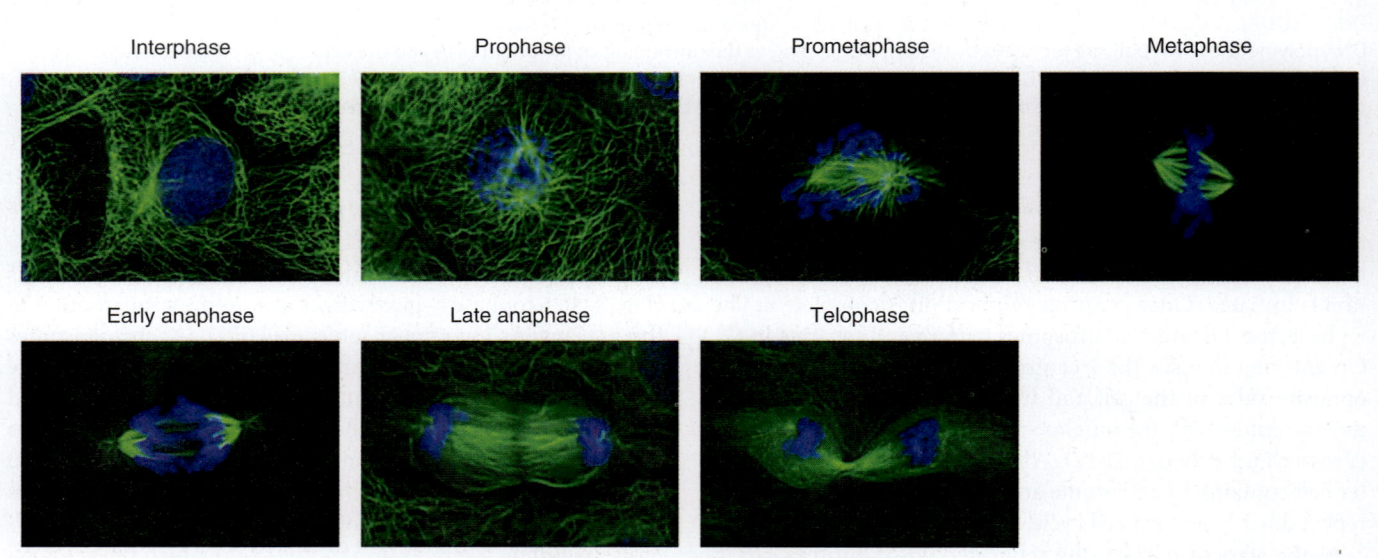

FIGURE 8-4 **The phases of mitosis.** Microtubules stained green, DNA stained blue. The events of each phase are described in the text. Note the microtubule-rich midzone between the segregated chromosomes in late anaphase. The midzone collapses into the midbody following ingression of the contractile ring during telophase. The images are of fixed and stained rat kangaroo kidney (PtK) cells, which are presented in lieu of human cells because the small numbers of chromosomes in these cells make the mitotic events clearer. (Used with permission from Jennifer Waters, Harvard Medical School.)

At the beginning of prometaphase, the nuclear envelope breaks down, allowing the microtubule spindle to physically interact with the chromosomes (Guttinger et al, 2009). At this point, the 2 sister chromatids that make up each chromosome have condensed into distinct rods. During prometaphase, the sister chromatids lose most, but not all, of their lengthwise cohesion but remain tightly juxtaposed at their centromeres (Peters et al, 2008). The centromere is a single, long (0.2-7 megabases) sequence of repetitive DNA encoded in each sister chromatid that forms a platform for the kinetochore, a large protein complex that will physically link microtubules with the sister chromatid (see Fig. 8–1). During prometaphase, each kinetochore is bound by a bundle of 20 to 25 microtubules (Walczak et al, 2010). For each sister chromatid pair, the 2 bundles emanate from opposite spindle poles. The bundles apply pulling forces on each centromere toward their respective spindle pole, but the sister chromatids remain tightly tethered at their centromeres. Under the influence of these counterbalanced pulling forces, as well as other spindle forces, each of the 46 pairs of sister chromatids becomes biorientated in the center of the spindle, aligned in a plane called the metaphase plate (Dumont and Mitchison, 2009). The cell is now in metaphase, but progresses into anaphase when an abrupt and total loss of sister chromatid cohesion occurs driven by the anaphase-promoting complex/cyclosome (APC/C), allowing the opposing microtubule bundles to separate the sister chromatids and pull them to opposite spindle poles. The spindle itself then elongates, driving the divided genomes to opposite ends of the mother cell. During the subsequent telophase, the events of early mitosis are reversed, as the chromosomes decondense, the nuclear envelopes assemble, and the spindle is taken apart (McIntosh, 2016). The process of cytokinesis, which splits the mother cell into 2 daughter cells, is initiated in late anaphase and is completed when both daughter cells are in early G_1 phase.

8.2.1.3 Gap Phases and Checkpoints Are Points of Decision Making
The G_1 and G_2 gap phases are decision-making periods, during which intracellular and extracellular signals determine whether the cell is prepared to enter the subsequent S phase and M phase (Kastan and Bartek, 2004; Malumbres and Barbacid, 2009). During G_2 phase, the key signal is intracellular, arising from the newly replicated DNA. If serious DNA damage has occurred during replication, entry into mitosis is delayed. During G_1 phase, many different kinds of extracellular and intracellular information are integrated into the decision to enter S phase. Extracellularly, the appropriate signal transduction pathways need to be activated by the binding of receptor ligands. The combination of ligands required to proliferate depends on the cell type but are generically referred to here as "growth factors" (see Chap. 6, Sec. 6.2). In some cell types, G_1 arrest can also be imposed by excessive physical contact with neighboring cells. Together, these extracellular requirements define the niches in which cells typically proliferate in vivo. Intracellularly, serious genomic damage will block cells in G_1 phase. Cells lacking nutrients, such as essential amino acids, will also arrest in G_1 phase. Supply of nutrients is unlikely to be limiting in normal animal tissues with adequate blood supply but may be limiting within solid tumors (see Chap. 12, Sec. 12.2.3). In some mammalian cell types, a minimal cell size may also be needed to enter S phase, a requirement that would help coordinate cell growth with the cell cycle (Jorgensen and Tyers, 2004).

When essential growth factors or nutrients are removed from cells, death by apoptosis or senescence may result (see Sec. 8.4). If the cells do not die or senesce, a transition in G_1 phase called the *restriction point* determines the cellular response (see Fig. 8–1; Blagosklonny and Pardee, 2002). If growth factors or nutrients are withdrawn before the restriction point, cells will enter the quiescent G_0 state. If these factors are withdrawn after the restriction point, cells will progress through a full cell cycle before transitioning into the G_0 state early in the subsequent G_1 phase. The restriction point can occur early or late in G_1 phase, depending on the cell type. In most cancers, control over the restriction point is lost. Malignant cells acquire abilities to bypass the normal cellular checkpoints that govern cell-cycle entry, enabling them to proliferate without the requirement for extracellular mitogenic signals.

8.2.2 Primary Effectors of Cell-Cycle Control

The molecular biology of the cell cycle has been explored intensively with important discoveries having been made in yeasts, frog eggs, fruit flies, cultured mammalian cells, and mice. The molecular wiring of the cell cycle has largely been conserved during eukaryotic evolution and employs the full gamut of cellular regulatory mechanisms: transcription, translation, post-translational modifications (eg, phosphorylation), protein degradation, protein localization, and microRNAs. Central to cell-cycle regulation are molecular mechanisms involving cyclins, cyclin-dependent kinases (CDKs) and E3 ubiquitin ligases.

8.2.2.1 Cyclin-Dependent Kinase Activity Is Tightly Regulated
CDKs are the central regulators of the cell cycle (Malumbres, 2014). CDK activities largely define the phases of the cell cycle, whereas changes in CDK activity drive transitions between these phases. CDKs exert these effects by phosphorylating hundreds of different proteins throughout the cell, although the abundance of CDKs is constant throughout the cell cycle. Multiple, overlapping, post-translational mechanisms ensure that the catalytic activity of different CDKs is highly regulated in space and time (Fig. 8–5A).

CDK activity is almost entirely dependent on the binding of regulatory proteins called cyclins (see Fig. 8–5A). Once bound, a CYCLIN not only greatly stimulates the enzymatic activity of the CDK, it also influences substrate selection by the CDK. Based on sequence similarity, the human genome encodes at least 20 CDKs and 29 CYCLINs, but only a subset of the CYCLIN-CDK pairs have been shown to directly regulate the cell cycle (Malumbres et al, 2009). In normal cells, CDK1 forms complexes with A- and B-type CYCLINs, CDK2

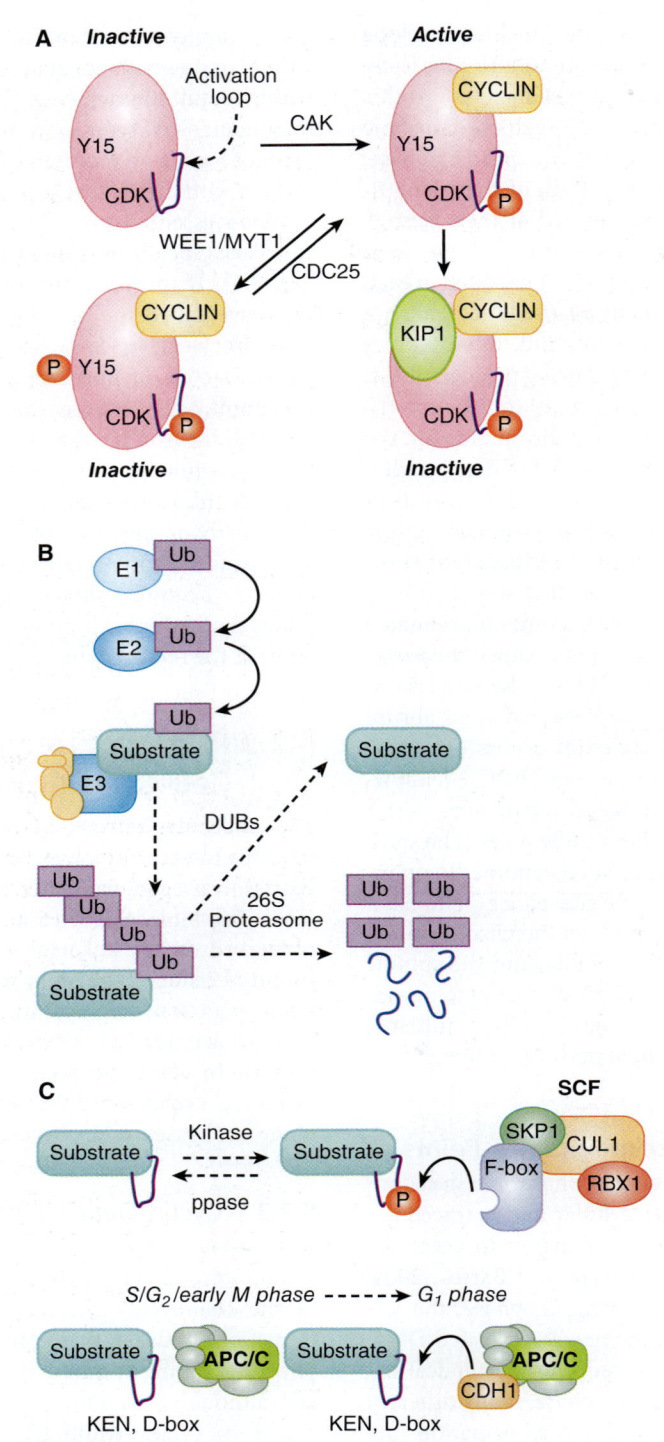

FIGURE 8–5 Molecular mechanisms central to cell-cycle control. A) CDKs are the central regulators of the cell cycle. Multiple mechanisms control CDK kinase activity. To become active kinases, CDKs must bind CYCLINs, which leads to the phosphorylation (P) of their activation loop by the CDK-activating kinase (CAK). CYCLIN-bound CDKs can, however, become inactivated by phosphorylation on a different residue (Y15) by WEE1/MYT1 kinases. This inhibitory phosphorylation is removed by CDC25 phosphatases. CDKs can also be inactivated on binding CDK inhibitors (CKIs), such as KIP1. **B)** Several important cell-cycle proteins are destroyed by ubiquitin-mediated proteolysis. Ubiquitin (Ub) is activated by the E1 ubiquitin-activating protein and the covalent bond then transferred to an E2 ubiquitin-conjugating enzyme. E3 ubiquitin ligases bind to both the E2 and to the substrate protein, catalyzing the formation of a covalent bond between the ubiquitin and the substrate. Iterative rounds of ubiquitination generate a multiubiquitinated substrate, which is recognized by the 26S proteasome and degraded into peptides. If the substrate is also recognized by deubiquitinating enzymes (DUBs), the DUBs may hydrolyze the covalent bond with ubiquitin from the substrate, preempting substrate degradation. **C)** SCF complexes often recognize substrates when the F-box protein binds to a phosphorylated peptide (degron) in the substrate protein. The rate at which these substrates are degraded is set by the activity of the kinase or the phosphatase (ppase), which is often cell-cycle regulated. In contrast, anaphase-promoting complex/cyclosome (APC/C) complexes recognize substrates that contain degrons called D-boxes or KEN-boxes. APC complexes are only active during late mitosis and G_1 phase when they have bound to an activating subunit, CDC20 or CDH1.

forms complexes with E- and A-type CYCLINs, and CDK4 and CDK6 form complexes with D-type CYCLINs. In mice and humans, CYCLINs are expressed in small families of 2 to 3 proteins each, with the expression of different isoforms often being tissue-specific. For example, CYCLIN A1 is expressed solely in the male germline in mice, while CYCLIN A2 is expressed in all other cells. CYCLINs also specify the intracellular location of CDK activity, as localized CYCLINs can focus CDK activity to the nucleus, the cytoplasm, or the Golgi apparatus. The location of some CYCLIN-CDK complexes changes dynamically during the cell cycle.

Typically, A-, B-, and E-type CYCLINs oscillate in abundance throughout the cell cycle, defining windows of potential CDK1 and CDK2 activity (see Fig. 8–6A, B). Cyclin expression levels are regulated by transcription and ubiquitin ligase complex-mediated degradation. In contrast, the abundance of D-type CYCLINs does not change appreciably during the cell cycle. When a CYCLIN binds a CDK, a threonine (eg, T160) in the activation loop of the CDK becomes accessible for phosphorylation by the CDK-activating kinase (CAK) (see Fig. 8–5A; Merrick et al, 2008). In human cells, CAK is found in a complex that is constitutively active throughout the cell cycle (Lolli and Johnson, 2005).

CDK activity is further shaped by repressive influences (see Fig. 8–5A). The MYT1 and WEE1 kinases inhibit CYCLIN B–CDK1 complexes by phosphorylating amino acids of CDK1 (Malumbres, 2014). CDC25 phosphatases remove the phosphates from these amino acids. CDK activity can also be curbed by 2 families of CDK inhibitor proteins (CKIs) (Fig. 8–1). The INK4 family of CKIs bind to CDK4 and CDK6 and prevent their binding to D-type CYCLINs. The CIP/KIP family of CKIs are more generalized inhibitors, binding and inhibiting the activity of CYCLIN E–CDK2, CYCLIN A-CDK2, and CYCLIN B–CDK1 (Malumbres et al, 2009).

8.2.2.2 Ubiquitin-Mediated Proteolysis and E3 Ligases Degrade Cell-Cycle Regulators
Critical cell-cycle events are triggered by the destruction of regulatory proteins. Protein degradation is rapid and irreversible—these properties are advantageous when regulating a dynamic and unidirectional process such as the cell cycle. The primary cellular mechanism for targeted protein degradation is ubiquitin-mediated proteolysis in which the small protein ubiquitin is covalently attached to target proteins (see Chap. 6, Sec. 6.2.8). This process requires the activity of an E1 ubiquitin-activating enzyme, an E2 ubiquitin-conjugating enzyme, and an E3 ubiquitin ligase (see Fig. 8–5B; Skaar et al, 2014). Substrate selectivity in ubiquitin-mediated proteolysis appears to be entirely conferred by the binding interaction between the substrate and the E3 ligase. The same substrate can be ubiquitinated multiple times: it is the presence of multiple ubiquitins attached to a substrate protein that result in that protein binding to and being degraded by the 26S proteasome. Deubiquitinating enzymes (DUBs) can, however, hydrolyze the covalent bond between a substrate and ubiquitin, counteracting the actions of the E3 ligase. For any given ubiquitinated protein, the rate of proteolysis by the 26S proteasome is set by the relative activity of the E3 ligase and the DUB (see Fig. 8–5B; Komander et al, 2009).

Two RING E3 ubiquitin ligase families have prominent roles in cell-cycle regulation—the Skp, Cullin, F-box-containing complex (SCF), and the anaphase promoting complex/cyclosome (APC/C) (see Figs. 8–5C and 8–6C; Senft et al, 2018). These protein complexes are evolutionarily related to one another and share similar modular structures, with a catalytic core binding to multiple substrate-binding proteins. The catalytic cores of SCF complexes bind via adaptor proteins (SKP1) to multiple substrate-binding proteins known as F-box proteins (eg, SKP2, β-TRCP) (Senft et al, 2018). As individual F-box proteins are typically able to bind many different substrates, SCF complexes catalyze the ubiquitination of a myriad of target proteins. Degradation of SCF substrates is required for cell-cycle transitions; for example, destruction of the cell cycle inhibitory proteins KIP1 and WEE1 by the SCF complex enables G_1/S and G_2/M transitions, respectively. The APC/C is a large complex composed of at least 14 different subunits and

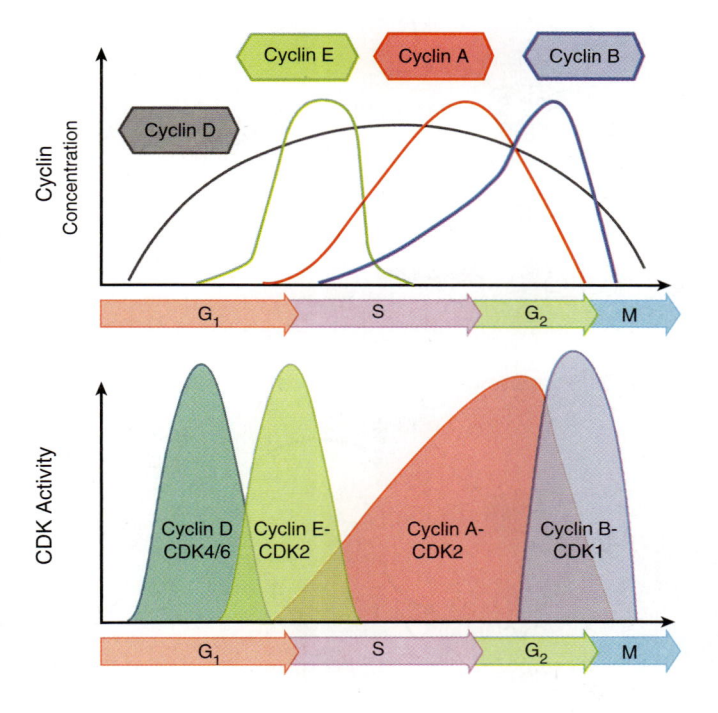

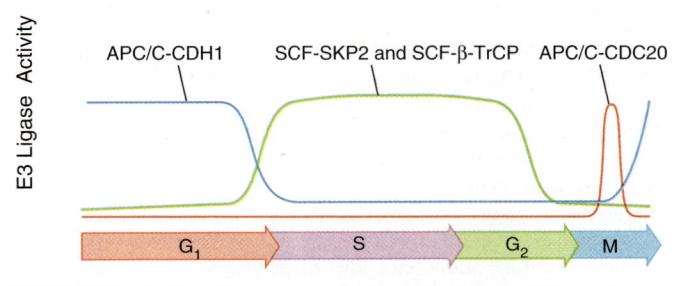

FIGURE 8–6 The abundance and activity levels of the proteins regulating the cell cycle oscillate between phases. **A)** Cyclin protein levels, and **B)** CDK-Cyclin complex activities fluctuate throughout the cell cycle to regulate specific cell-cycle phases and transitions. **C)** The activity of the APC/C and SCF ubiquitin ligase complexes also oscillates throughout the cycle to regulate cyclin and CDK activity levels.

binds to one of 2 coactivators (CDC20 or CDH1) that facilitate binding of substrate proteins in a cell cycle–dependent manner (Sivakumar and Gorbsky, 2015). When bound to CDC20 (denoted hereafter as APC/C-CDC20), as its name implies, the APC/C initiates anaphase and mitotic exit through its degradation of CYCLIN-B and the separase inhibitor, Securin, which enables chromosome separation. When the APC/C is bound to CDH1 (denoted hereafter as APC/C-CDH1), it degrades several mitotic factors including cyclins late in mitotic exit and CDC20, CDC25A, and SKP2 during the G_1 phase of the cell cycle (Sivakumar and Gorbsky, 2015). Given the importance of ubiquitination in governing the cell cycle, genes encoding E3 ligase components are often inactivated through various genetic mechanisms in cancer cells (Ge et al, 2018; Senft et al, 2018). Therapeutic targeting of E3 ubiquitin ligase complexes has been proposed as a strategy to deregulate cell-cycle control in cancer cells to induce cell death.

8.2.3 Molecular Mechanisms Regulating Progression Through the Cell Cycle

The cell cycle can be considered as an oscillation between 2 biochemical states. The first state lasts from anaphase to the end of the next G_1 phase, whereas the second state lasts from the beginning of S phase to metaphase (Fig. 8–7). In the first state, CDK1 and CDK2 activity is low, APC/C–CDH1 activity is high, and pre-RC assembly on replication origins is permitted. In the second state, CDK2 activity is high, APC/C-CDH1 activity is low, and pre-RC assembly on replication origins is not allowed. Each biochemical state is highly stable as a result of multiple positive feedback loops that continually reinforce that state. Switching between the 2 stable states requires special mechanisms that overcome the positive feedback that maintains each state. The points at which the cell switches between the 2 states, the G_1/S transition and the metaphase-anaphase transition (governed by the spindle assembly checkpoint, SAC), are key points of cell-cycle control. The G_2/M transition is a third critical control point at which the high CYCLIN B–CDK1 activity that controls early mitosis first appears (Kastan and Bartek, 2004).

8.2.3.1 G_1 Phase is a Period of Low CDK1 and CDK2 Activity and High APC/C-CDH1 Activity Replication origins become capable of initiating DNA replication during G_1 phase when pre-RCs assemble on them (see Fig. 8–2B; Fragkos et al, 2015). The origin DNA is bound directly by the origin recognition complex (ORC). ORC is then bound by CDC6 and CDT1, which, in turn, recruit minichromosome maintenance complexes (MCMs) to the origin (Fragkos et al, 2015). The absence of CDK1 and CDK2 kinase activity and the high activity of APC/C-CDH1 during G_1 phase combine to create a biochemical environment that allows pre-RC assembly (see below).

During G_1 phase, CDK1 and CDK2 are not bound to CYCLINs so their kinase activity is very low (see Fig. 8–5A). CYCLIN A2 and CYCLIN B protein levels are very low during G_1 phase because both proteins are substrates of the APC/C-CDH1 complex (see Fig. 8–6). CDH1 is itself a substrate of CYCLIN A2–CDK2 and CYCLIN B–CDK1 complexes, which generates a self-reinforcing positive feedback loop that lasts throughout G_1 phase (Fig. 8–7A, inner loop). When phosphorylated, CDH1 dissociates from the APC/C complex, abolishing APC/C activity (Sivakumar and Gorbsky, 2015). Therefore, the low activity of CDK1 and CDK2 in G_1 phase prevents CDH1 from becoming phosphorylated and the activity of the APC/C-CDH1 complex remains high, which, in turn, keeps CYCLIN A2 and CYCLIN B levels low. An additional positive feedback loop reinforces low CDK1 and CDK2 kinase activity (Fig. 8–7A, outer loop). In this loop, APC/C-CDH1 targets the F-box protein SKP2 for degradation (Wei et al, 2004). As the SKP2-bound SCF complex (denoted SCF-SKP2) targets the CKI KIP1 for degradation (Malek et al, 2001; Wei et al, 2004), high APC/C-CDH1 activity

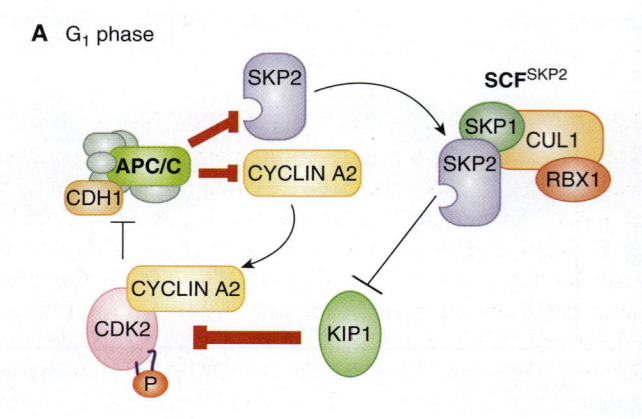

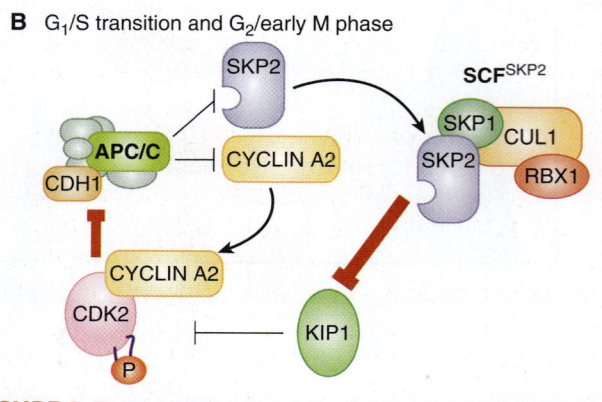

FIGURE 8–7 Positive feedback loops between APC/C-CDH1 and CYCLIN-CDK1/2 complexes create self-reinforcing states that help define the 2 primary biochemical states in the eukaryotic cell cycle. **A)** In G_1 phase, APC/C and CDH1 are associated so APC/C-CDH1 activity is high. This high APC/C-CDH1 activity results in the degradation of CYCLIN A2 and SKP2. Because of the low abundance of these 2 proteins, CYCLIN A2–CDK2 and SKP2-bound SCF complexes (SCF-SKP2) are rare. Low SCF-SKP2 activity results in relatively high KIP1 abundance. KIP1 helps suppress the activity of any CYCLIN A2–CDK2 complexes that do form. CYCLIN B–CDK1 has a role similar to CYCLIN A2–CDK2 in the positive feedback loops, but is not shown for simplicity. **B)** At the G_1/S transition and in S/G_2/early M phase, the balance of power is reversed. Now, CYCLIN A2 is abundant, so CYCLIN A2–CDK2 complexes form and suppress the activity of APC/C-CDH1. Similarly, SKP2 is abundant, so SCF-SKP2 complexes form and cause the degradation of KIP1.

during G$_1$ phase indirectly stabilizes the CKI KIP1. KIP1 can then bind to and inactivate any CYCLIN B–CDK1 or CYCLIN A2–CDK2 complexes that do form.

Quiescence or G$_0$ is not simply an indefinitely prolonged G$_1$ period. Like G$_1$ phase cells, G$_0$ phase cells have low CDK1 and CDK2 activity and high APC/C-CDH1 activity. However, in contrast to G$_1$ phase cells, G$_0$ phase cells have little to no CYCLIN D–CDK4/6 activity, as a result of sharply repressed CYCLIN D transcription (Fischer and Müller, 2017). In G$_0$ phase cells, pre-RCs are not assembled on replication origins, apparently because the abundance of some pre-RC components is very low (Williams et al, 1998). The entry of quiescent cells into G$_1$ phase is a prolonged process that includes the synthesis of D-type cyclins, decreasing levels of KIP1, the accumulation of CDC6, CDT1, MCM, and the assembly of pre-RCs. D-type cyclins are transcriptionally induced and the gene encoding KIP1 is transcriptionally repressed downstream of growth factor signaling (Sherr and Roberts, 1999; Chen et al, 2009; Fischer and Müller, 2017).

8.2.3.2 The G$_1$/S Transition Marks the Rise of CDK1/2 Activity

At the G$_1$/S transition, the positive feedback loops that suppress CDK2 activity and maintain the high activity of APC/C-CDH1 are overturned (see Fig. 8–7B). CYCLIN D–CDK4/6 complexes are thought to have 2 key roles early in this process. First, CYCLIN D–CDK4/6 functions noncatalytically to bind KIP1 protein, and prevents KIP1 from inhibiting CYCLIN E–CDK2 and CYCLIN A-CDK2 (Sherr and Roberts, 1999). Second, CYCLIN D–CDK4/6 phosphorylates 3 related "pocket proteins": the retinoblastoma (RB) protein, p107, and p130. Phosphorylation of these proteins leads to their release from the E2F family of transcription factors (Fig. 8–8; Chen et al, 2009). E2Fs complex with the dimerization partner (DP) protein and bind to sequences found in the promoters of a broad spectrum of genes, many of which encode proteins important for S phase entry or DNA synthesis. Phosphorylation of the 3 pocket proteins by CYCLIN D–CDK4/6 decreases their affinity for E2Fs, resulting in the inhibitory E2Fs (E2F4, E2F5) leaving the nucleus and the activating E2Fs (E2F1, 2, 3) inducing a broad transcriptional program in late G$_1$ phase (Fig. 8–8; Bertoli et al, 2013).

The E2F transcriptional program includes the genes encoding CYCLIN E, CYCLIN A2, and CDK2 (Bertoli et al, 2013). Once translated, these 3 proteins collectively overturn the G$_1$ state of inactive CDK1 and CDK2 and active APC/C-CDH1. Newly formed CYCLIN E–CDK2 complexes phosphorylate RB and further stimulate the expression of E2F1-3 target genes in a positive feedback loop (Fig. 8–8). CYCLIN E–CDK2 and CYCLIN A2–CDK2 also phosphorylate CDH1, causing CDH1 to dissociate from the APC/C (see Fig. 8–7A, inner loop) (Sivakumar and Gorbsky, 2015). The loss of APC/C-CDH1 activity leads to the accumulation of its substrate SKP2. Rising SCF-SKP2 activity in late G$_1$ phase targets KIP1 for degradation, contributing to the rise in CYCLIN E–CDK2 and CYCLIN A2–CDK2 activity (see Fig. 8–7A, outer loop) (Skaar et al, 2014). These interlocking feedback loops, which are initiated late in G$_1$ phase and cause the G$_1$/S transition, stabilize the

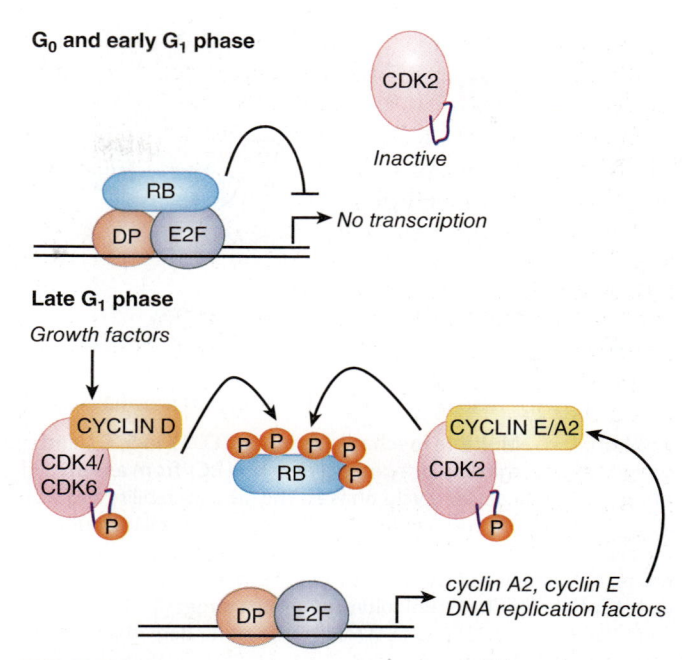

FIGURE 8–8 In late G$_1$ phase, the transcription of *cyclin E*, *cyclin A2*, and DNA replication factors is driven by the E2F1-3 transcription factors. Five types of E2F bind to DNA-binding sites in the promoters of hundreds to thousands of genes with the assistance of the DP protein. In G$_0$ and early G$_1$ phases, these genes are repressed by either E2F4-5/p130 complexes (not shown) or E2F1-3/RB complexes. Phosphorylation of the 3 pocket proteins (RB, p130, p107) by CYCLIN D–CDK4/6 causes the pocket proteins to dissociate from the E2Fs during G$_1$ phase, freeing E2F1-3 to activate transcription. The onset of E2F-dependent transcription is also likely to be the molecular basis for the restriction point.

new S/G$_2$/early M phase state of high CDK2 activity and low APC/C-CDH1 activity (see Fig. 8–6).

The switch from low to high CDK2 activity and from high to low APC/C-CDH1 activity is thought to be the molecular basis of the restriction point (Blagosklonny and Pardee, 2002; Bertoli et al, 2013). That is, at some point in G$_1$ phase, this switching process becomes irreversible and no longer requires growth-signaling pathways. As discussed above, these signaling pathways are thought to drive the G$_1$/S transition by (a) stimulating the synthesis and activity of CYCLIN D–CDK4/6 complexes, and (b) transcriptionally repressing and directly inactivating the CDK inhibitor KIP1.

8.2.3.3 The Initiation of DNA Replication and the Block to Overreplication

The rise of CYCLIN A2–CDK2 activity at the G$_1$/S transition triggers DNA replication. In at least some cell types, CYCLIN E–CDK2 also contributes to this process (Kalaszczynska et al, 2009). Initiation of DNA replication requires activity of both CDK2 and DBF4-dependent kinase (DDK) complexes at the G$_1$/S transition (Fragkos et al, 2015). CDK and DDK-mediated phosphorylation of replication factors in the pre-RC complex leads to the recruitment of replication proteins to that origin. The DNA double helix at the origin is subsequently unwound by the MCM helicase. These events attract DNA polymerase

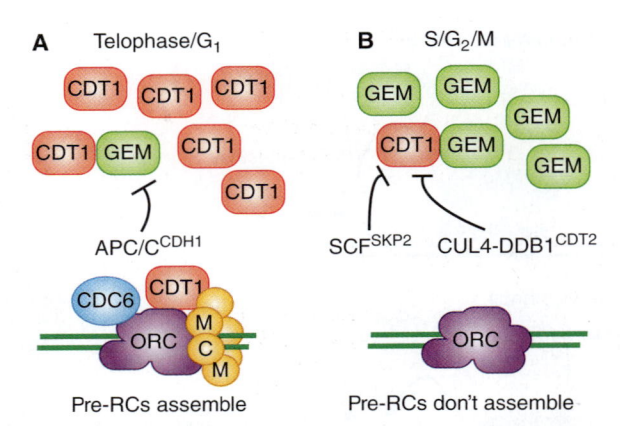

FIGURE 8–9 Multiple mechanisms inhibit CDT1 in S, G$_2$, and early M phase, thereby preventing new pre-RCs from assembling during these cell-cycle phases. The protein stability and abundance of CDT1 and Geminin (GEM) are inversely related during the cell cycle. CDT1 is stable and abundant during telophase and G$_1$ phase (A), whereas GEM is stable and abundant during S, G2, and early M phase (B). The E3 ubiquitin ligases that target CDT1 (SCF-SKP2 and CUL4-DDB1-CDT2) and GEM (APC/C-CDH1) for degradation in each phase are shown.

complexes, which bind to the unwound ssDNA at the origin and initiate DNA replication (see Fig. 8–2).

The reloading of pre-RC complexes on replication origins in S, G$_2$, and early M phase is prevented primarily by eliminating activity of the licensing factor CDT1 (Fig. 8–9A; Fragkos et al, 2015). Overlapping mechanisms are likely necessary to ensure that pre-RC complexes do not reappear on any of the tens of thousands of replication origins over the many hours it takes to complete S, G$_2$, and early M phases. CDT1 is subject to degradation by E3 ligases including SCF-SKP2 and is inactivated by Geminin (GEM) protein binding (Fig. 8–9B), which inhibits CDT1 activity and recruitment of MCM complexes to replication origins. GEM itself is an APC/C-CDH1 substrate that starts to accumulate at the G$_1$/S transition when APC/C-CDH1 is inactivated. Therefore, CDT1 and GEM are binding partners that have reciprocal patterns of degradation and abundance during the cell cycle.

During DNA replication, the 2 emerging sister chromatids become connected by a protein complex called Cohesin. By keeping the sister chromatids tightly connected, Cohesin is critical for the segregation of the 2 chromatids into separate daughter cells during mitosis. Cohesin is also important for the repair of dsDNA breaks (DSBs) by recombination between sister chromatids (Peters and Nishiyama, 2012).

8.2.3.4 G$_2$ and the Entrance to Mitosis

In late G$_2$ phase, mammalian cells experience a surge of CYCLIN B–CDK1 activity that initiates the events of early mitosis. Throughout the S and G$_2$ phase, the concentration of CYCLIN B rises, being induced by the FOXM1 transcription factor (see Fig. 8–6; Fischer and Müller, 2017). The newly translated CYCLIN B binds to unphosphorylated CDK1. The binding of CYCLIN B allows phosphorylation of CDK1 on the activation loop, generating a transiently active CYCLIN B–CDK1 kinase (see Fig. 8–5A; Deibler and Kirschner, 2010). This complex is quickly recognized in the cytoplasm by MYT1 and in the nucleus by WEE1, 2 protein kinases that phosphorylate other amino acids of CDK1 and thereby quell the kinase activity of the CYCLIN B–CDK1 complex (see Fig. 8–5A; O'Farrell, 2001; Lindqvist et al, 2009). Throughout S and G$_2$ phase, these inactive, phosphorylated CYCLIN B–CDK1 complexes accumulate in the cell.

In late G$_2$ phase, the stockpiled complexes are suddenly activated by a rapid loss of the inhibitory phosphorylations, a process that is driven by at least 2 positive feedback loops (O'Farrell, 2001; Lindqvist et al, 2009). In the first positive feedback loop, CYCLIN B–CDK1 phosphorylates and activates the CDC25 phosphatases, which remove the inhibitory phosphate groups, making these enzymes critical regulators of mitotic entry (see Fig. 8–5A). In the second positive feedback loop, CYCLIN B–CDK1 inactivates WEE1 and MYT1, thereby blocking any further inhibitory phosphorylation of CDK1. The activity of CYCLIN B–CDK1 in late G$_2$ phase is blocked by severely damaged or unreplicated DNA, a checkpoint that prevents cells from attempting to segregate damaged chromosomes (see Sec. 8.3 and Chap. 9, Sec. 9.4; Kastan and Bartek, 2004).

8.2.3.5 The Events of Early Mitosis Culminate in Sister Chromatid Separation

The early events of mitosis are orchestrated by 4 mitotic kinases: CDK1, Polo-like kinase 1 (PLK1), Aurora kinase (AUR) A, and AUR B (Nigg, 2001). Correspondingly, more than 1000 proteins become phosphorylated specifically during mitosis (Dephoure et al, 2008). All 4 mitotic kinases are activated at the G$_2$/M transition or in prophase. CYCLIN B–CDK1 activation has been discussed. Activation of PLK1, AUR A, and AUR B results from phosphorylation and from binding interactions that localize these kinases to critical locations in the mitotic cell (Fig. 8–10). At the end of mitosis, all 4 of the mitotic kinases are inactivated, in large part as a result of the resurgence of APC/C activity. CYCLIN B is targeted for degradation by APC/C-CDC20 during metaphase, whereas the degradation of PLK1, AUR A, and AUR B by APC/C-CDH1 begins in anaphase (Sivakumar and Gorbsky, 2015).

The strength and location of CYCLIN B–CDK1 activity during early mitosis helps determine the sequence of early events (see Fig. 8–10; Gavet and Pines, 2010). CYCLIN B–CDK1 activity is first apparent in the cytoplasm and on the centrosomes. In early prophase, cytoplasmic CYCLIN B–CDK1 causes adherent cells to "round up" and, in collaboration with PLK1, causes the 2 centrosomes to separate and mature (Gavet and Pines, 2010). CYCLIN B–CDK1 then moves into the nucleus and by late prophase the complex is predominantly nuclear. Nuclear CYCLIN B–CDK1 triggers chromosome condensation, as well as the breakdown of the nuclear envelope, in part by phosphorylating and disassembling the meshwork of intermediate filaments called lamins that lines the inner nuclear membrane.

On dissolution of the nuclear envelope, which marks the start of prometaphase, microtubules gain access to the

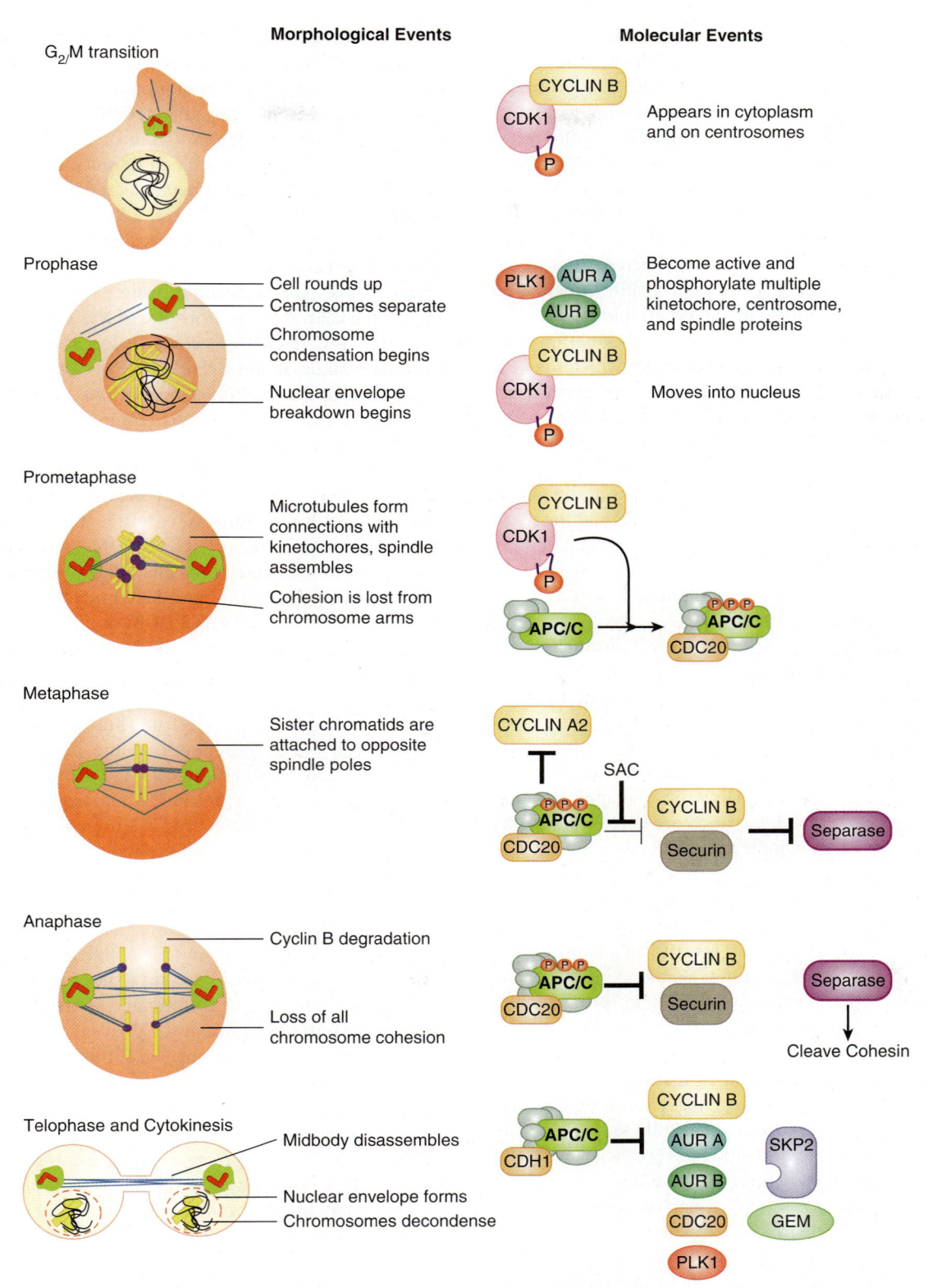

FIGURE 8-10 Major morphologic and molecular events of mitosis. Schematic (left) images of cells in the primary stages of mitosis. Uncondensed DNA is in black, condensed DNA is in yellow, and microtubules are in blue. Purple spheres on DNA represent kinetochores. Orthogonal red rectangles within green spheres represent centrosomes. The concentration of active CYCLIN B–CDK1 complexes is roughly indicated by the intensity of orange in the cytoplasm and nucleus. See text for details on the major molecular events. *P*, phosphorylation; *SAC*, spindle assembly checkpoint.

chromatin. Microtubule interaction with the condensing chromosomes leads to the self-organization of the mitotic spindle between the 2 centrosomes (see Fig. 8–10). This process is highly complex and requires numerous proteins that move and stabilize microtubules (Gatlin and Bloom, 2010; Prosser and Pelletier, 2017). During prometaphase, 20 to 25 microtubules bind the kinetochore of each sister chromatid (Walczak et al, 2010). By metaphase, each sister chromatid pair has formed a bipolar attachment to the mitotic spindle: one sister chromatid's kinetochore is connected by microtubules to one spindle pole, whereas the other sister chromatid's kinetochore is connected by microtubules to the other spindle pole (see Fig. 8–10). Each microtubule bundle exerts pulling forces on the kinetochore toward the spindle pole from which the bundle emanates. Although their kinetochores and centromeres are being pulled in opposite directions, the sister chromatids do not separate as a result of the Cohesin complexes that continue to physically connect them. The balance of these pulling and resistive forces, among other forces present in the mitotic spindle, cause each sister chromatid pair to align at the metaphase plate. By phosphorylating multiple centrosome, spindle, and kinetochore proteins, the 4 mitotic kinases play key roles in shaping the mitotic spindle and aligning sister chromatid pairs (Prosser and Pelletier, 2017).

The loss of cohesion between the sister chromatid pairs occurs in 2 steps. During prophase and prometaphase, most of the Cohesin along the chromosomal arms dissociates, allowing the chromosomal arms to partially separate by metaphase (Peters and Nishiyama, 2012). But Cohesin located at the centromeres does not dissociate until the onset of anaphase. The 2-step loss of cohesion explains the X-shaped structure of chromosomes in karyotypes, which are derived from cells arrested in metaphase by spindle poisons.

The APC/C becomes active early in mitosis when CDC20 binds to the APC/C following extensive phosphorylation of the APC/C by CYCLIN B–CDK1 (Sivakumar and Gorbsky, 2015). The bound APC/C-CDC20 is active against some substrates in prometaphase, including CYCLIN A2, but remains inactive toward other critical substrates in prometaphase because of the inhibitory effects of the spindle assembly checkpoint (SAC; see Fig. 8–10). Once all of the kinetochores have attached to microtubules and each sister chromatid pair is under tension, cells are in metaphase, the SAC is inactivated, and the APC/C-CDC20 becomes fully active. This fully active APC/C-CDC20 then ubiquitinates 3 crucial substrates: securin and the 2 B-type Cyclins (B1 and B2) (Sivakumar and Gorbsky, 2015). Securin is a binding partner and inhibitor of the protease Separase, whereas CYCLIN B–CDK1 phosphorylation of separase represses separase activity. Anaphase is initiated when the APC/C-CDC20 simultaneously removes these 2 blocks to separase protease activity. Separase then cleaves the Cohesin subunit SCC1 (kleisin), which causes the removal of centromeric Cohesin and any Cohesin remaining on the chromosome arms (Peters and Nishiyama, 2012). Once cohesin is removed, the sister chromatids are free to respond to the pulling forces exerted on their kinetochores and progress toward opposite spindle poles.

8.2.3.6 Late Mitosis Ends With 2 Genetically Identical Daughter Cells
The events of late anaphase and telophase are largely driven by the loss of protein phosphorylations that were applied earlier in mitosis by the CYCLIN B–CDK1, PLK1, and AUR B mitotic kinases (Sullivan and Morgan, 2007). Also key to late mitosis is the appearance of APC/C-CDH1 activity (see Fig. 8–10). With the degradation of CYCLIN B during metaphase and anaphase, CYCLIN B–CDK1 kinase activity is much lower by telophase, allowing CDH1 to become dephosphorylated and bind to the APC/C (see Fig. 8–10). APC/C-CDH1 has a much broader substrate range than APC/C-CDC20. As CDC20 is one of the substrates of APC/C-CDH1, APC/C-CDC20 activity is lost in late mitosis (see Fig. 8–6; Sivakumar and Gorbsky, 2015).

The loss of protein phosphorylations applied earlier in mitosis by CYCLIN B–CDK1 is required to disassemble the mitotic spindle, decondense the separated chromosomes, and form nuclear envelopes around the 2 daughter genomes. The dephosphorylation of CDK1 substrates is an active process catalyzed by phosphatases (Wurzenberger and Gerlich, 2011). The assembly of pre-RCs on DNA replication origins also occurs in telophase, with the APC/C playing an important role. The ubiquitin-dependent proteolysis of CYCLIN A2 in prometaphase and CYCLIN B1 and B2 in metaphase by APC/C-CDC20 re-establishes the low-CDK1/2 activity state required for pre-RC formation (see above). In late anaphase and telophase, APC/C-CDH1 maintains the degradation of these CYCLINs. APC/C-CDH1 also initiates the destruction of GEM (the binding inhibitor of the pre-RC component CDT1) and SKP2 (which targets CDT1 for degradation via the SCF-SKP2 complex) (Sivakumar and Gorbsky, 2015). As a result of APC/C-CDH1 activity, CDT1 can accumulate in telophase, bind to ORC at DNA replication origins, and recruit the remaining components of the pre-RC. The DNA replication origins are now prepared to initiate DNA synthesis in the next S phase (see Fig. 8–2).

Separation of the daughter cells (cytokinesis) is caused by the gradual constriction of a contractile ring attached to the inner face of the plasma membrane (Mierzwa and Gerlich, 2014). The contractile force at the cleavage furrow appears to be provided by filaments of myosin II motor protein interacting with filaments of actin, which forms an actomyosin ring around the central spindle. During anaphase, the contractile ring forms on the inner plasma membrane at the spindle midzone, equidistant from each mass of chromosomes. This division site is normally created at the cell equator so the cell divides in half, but asymmetric spindle positioning leading to asymmetric cell cleavage is common during development and in stem cell divisions. During late anaphase and telophase, the spindle's morphology changes due to cleavage furrow ingression at the midzone, before being compacted into a bundle of microtubules called the midbody. This dense body of microtubules forms an intercellular bridge with 1 to 2 μm diameter between nascent daughter cells. During the process of ingression leading up to abscission, membrane vesicles fuse with the cleavage furrow to provide the increased plasma membrane required for 2 smaller daughter cells. Membrane vesicles are then directed by the midbody to fill the remaining hole, which completes the physical separation process of abscission, resulting in the production of 2 daughter cells. Protein regulator of cytokinesis (PRC1) is a microtubule bundling protein with an important role in central spindle assembly through its organization of microtubules and recruitment of other midzone proteins. The central spindle complex and the chromosome passenger complex are additional complexes involved in cytokinesis (Mierzwa and Gerlich, 2014).

8.2.4 Cell Growth

Although the term *growth* is often used loosely to refer to proliferation, the term *cell growth* specifically refers to increases in cell size. Fundamentally, cell growth is a net increase in biomass, primarily proteins, RNA, and membrane lipids. For cells to proliferate and maintain their size, cell growth must, on average, double the size of the mother cell by the time of mitosis. So, in addition to doubling the amount of DNA and the number of centrosomes with each cell cycle, a cell must grow sufficiently to double all its other constituent parts—ribosomes, mitochondria, lysosomes, etc.

It remains unclear how intertwined cell growth and the cell cycle are in human cells. Growth of some cells can become uncoupled from the cell cycle, arguing that they are distinct processes. For example, during the formation of the oocytes, which are giant single cells, cell growth occurs in the absence of any cell division. The uncoupling of cell growth and the cell cycle can also occur in somatic cells when the cell cycle is arrested by a DNA damage checkpoint (see Sec. 8.3.1). Such cell-cycle arrest usually allows cell growth to continue, resulting in oversized cells. In general, cell growth is more limiting for cell proliferation than is the cell cycle, because in animal cells the events of the cell cycle can be accomplished in far less time than it takes to double the mass of the cell. Because different amounts of time are necessary to double cell mass and to complete the cell cycle, coordination between cell growth and the cell cycle must exist at some level or else cell size would fluctuate wildly, which is not observed (Lloyd, 2013).

For a given human cell, cell growth, like the cell cycle, requires the appropriate combination of growth factors to bind to the cell (see Chap. 6, Sec. 6.2.7). Growth factor signaling pathways that control cell growth include pathways regulated by receptor tyrosine kinases (RTKs) that transmit extracellular signals through intracellular signal transduction pathways into downstream transcriptional programs (see Fig. 8–11). The most well-described growth-promoting pathway is the IGF/PI3K/AKT/MTOR pathway which culminates in a MYC-driven transcriptional program (Laplante and Sabatini, 2012).

The mammalian target of rapamycin (mTOR) and phosphatidylinositol-3 kinase (PI3K) signaling network (see Chap. 6, Sec. 6.2.4 and Chap. 7, Sec. 7.5.4) is a central regulator of animal cell growth and proliferation. Activation of this pathway is triggered by upstream growth factor binding to RTKs. This network integrates large amounts of extracellular and intracellular information into the decision to activate the AKT kinase and the mTORC1 kinase complex (Laplante and Sabatini, 2012). These 2 kinases then activate multiple downstream processes that drive cell growth, the cell cycle, and block cell death (see Fig. 8–11). Genetic alterations that increase AKT and mTORC1 activity can be oncogenic as described below. Mutations in the gene encoding PTEN (see Chap. 7, Sec. 7.6.2), a phosphatase that counteracts PI3K, or mutations in *PIK3CA*, can constitutively activate AKT and are common in many cancers (Sanchez-Vega et al, 2018). Activating mutations or amplification of the genes encoding growth factor receptors upstream of AKT and mTORC1 (eg, ERBB2 and EGFR; see Chap. 7, Sec. 7.5.3) are also common in cancer (Liu et al, 2009). Dozens of inhibitors of AKT/mTOR signaling have entered clinical development. However, only temsirolimus and everolimus (inhibitors of mTORC1 complex) and idelalisib and copanlisib (PI3K inhibitors) have received FDA approval for the treatment of cancer patients (Janku et al, 2018).

A key downstream effector of cell growth is the gene *MYC*, which is the oncogene most frequently amplified in cancers (Dang, 2012). This proto-oncogene encodes the transcription factor MYC, which is activated downstream of growth-promoting signal transduction pathways (see Fig. 8–11). MYC binds to target genes containing E-box DNA sequences with its binding partner MAX. The widespread transcriptional program activated by MYC overexpression can stimulate cell growth, in part by inducing genes involved in metabolism and ribosome synthesis, processes intrinsically related to mass accumulation and cell growth. MYC/MAX can also stimulate the cell cycle by activating the transcription of *CYCLIN D1*, *CYCLIN D2*, and *CDK4*, whereas a MYC/MAX/MIZ1 complex represses the genes encoding the inhibitory CIP1 (e.g. p21) and INK4B (e.g. p15) proteins.

To grow, cells need to either import or synthesize large amounts of amino acids, nucleotides, and fatty acids. In addition, large amounts of adenosine triphosphate (ATP) are required to polymerize these building blocks into proteins, RNA, and membrane lipids. Consequently, growing cells have special metabolic requirements (Ward and Thompson, 2012). The anabolic state is programmed by growth factor signaling pathways and transcription factors, particularly the PI3K/mTOR network and MYC discussed above. The anabolic state is characterized by a number of features, including rapid uptake and metabolism of glucose. The rapid uptake of glucose by some cancer cells reflects their higher rate of glycolysis. Indeed, some cancer cells produce more pyruvate—the end product of glycolysis—than can be oxidized by the tricarboxylic acid (TCA) cycle in the mitochondria. The excess pyruvate is converted to lactic acid and secreted, a phenomenon commonly known as the Warburg effect (see Chap. 12, Sec. 12.3.1; Jones and Thompson, 2009; Vander Heiden et al, 2009). Although usually thought of as an energy generating pathway, glycolysis—via the interlinked pentose phosphate pathway—also has important roles in supplying cellular building blocks, including the reducing equivalent nicotinamide adenine dinucleotide phosphate (NADPH) which is used in many anabolic reactions; the nucleotide precursor ribose-5-phosphate; the phospholipid precursor glycerol-3-phosphate; and the precursors for amino acids (Jones and Thompson, 2009; Vander

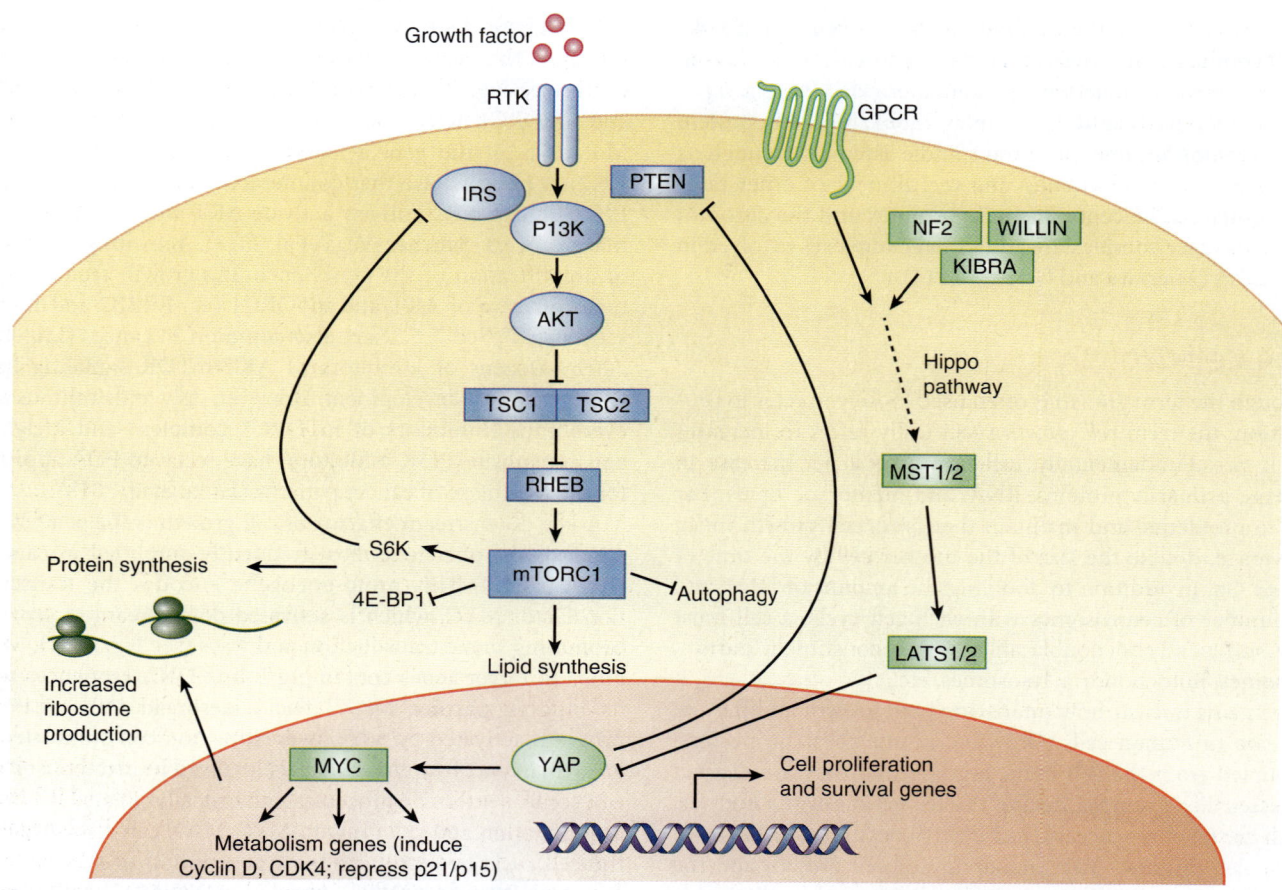

FIGURE 8–11 Simplified cell growth pathway. Extracellular growth factors stimulate receptor tyrosine kinases (RTKs) that transmit these signals through an intracellular pathway. The end result of signal transduction is the activation of transcriptional regulators such as MYC, which induces the expression of metabolism and cell-cycle genes and suppresses transcription of CDK inhibitors. The Hippo pathway is a suppressor of cell growth signaling.

Heiden et al, 2009). The need to produce building blocks like NADPH to allow for rapid cell growth may be the molecular explanation for why some cancer cells engage in such rapid glycolysis that lactic acid must be secreted from the cell.

In order to prevent aberrant growth, cells have mechanisms to negatively regulate growth. The Hippo pathway is capable of inducing cell death and differentiation, and inhibiting cell proliferation and growth (Harvey et al, 2013; see Fig. 8–11). At the core of the Hippo pathway is a highly conserved kinase cascade that controls phosphorylation of the major downstream effectors of Hippo signaling, the transcription regulators YAP and TAZ. When the Hippo cascade is activated, by cell stress for example, YAP/TAZ is phosphorylated, which results in its cytoplasmic retention and inhibition of cell growth. When dephosphorylated, YAP/TAZ facilitates gene transcription by its interaction with transcription factors such as TEAD1-4 that regulate various cellular phenotypes including growth. In addition to the core kinase cascade, YAP/TAZ may also be inhibited by upstream Hippo pathway components (KIBRA, WILLIN, and NF2) that can physically bind to YAP/TAZ at cellular junctions, thereby sequestering them from the nucleus. Not surprisingly, Hippo pathway disruption and YAP overexpression are common in cancer, and often associated with poor prognosis (Harvey et al, 2013).

8.2.5 Modifications to Control of Cell Proliferation in Cancer

The first tumor suppressor gene discovered in humans was *RB1*, whose loss was found to be the cause of familial retinoblastoma (see Chap. 7, Sec. 7.6.4). Soon after, *CYCLIN D1* was isolated as an oncogene in a subset of parathyroid adenomas. The *CDKN2A* locus, which encodes the CDK4/6 inhibitory protein P16, and the TP53 activator ARF, was then identified as a tumor suppressor in familial melanomas. These findings illustrate a recurring feature of malignancy, whereby most cancers contain genetic or epigenetic alterations that loosen control over the G_1/S transition. Large genomic profiling studies of more than 9000 clinical tumor specimens conducted by The Cancer Genome Atlas consortium have confirmed that molecular alterations, including mutations, gene dosage (ie, DNA amplifications or deletions) and epigenetic alterations (ie, DNA methylation) are highly recurrent in cancer genomes and affect key regulatory genes involved in cell cycle, proliferation, and growth-regulating pathways (Sanchez-Vega et al, 2018). Typical alterations include those that activate genes driving the G_1/S transition and cell proliferation (eg, CCND1, CCNE1, CDK2, CDK4, CDK6, E2F, MYC, PIK3CA, YAP) or those that inactivate negative regulators of cell cycle progression and cell growth (eg, p16, KIP1, RB1, PTEN, NF2). These alterations allow cancer cells to enter the cell cycle promiscuously and grow without bounds, defying the extracellular signals that limit the growth and proliferation of their normal counterparts.

8.2.6 Therapeutic Targeting of Cell Proliferation and Growth in Cancer

Chemotherapy and microtubule binding agents (MTBAs) are used routinely in the clinical management of cancer although they do not target specific molecular alterations that drive cancer biology (see Chap. 18, Sec. 18.3.4). These agents are aimed at killing actively dividing cells with little evidence of preferential activity toward cancer cells; cytotoxic effects against nonmalignant, cycling cells explains why they cause side effects (see Chap. 17, Sec. 17.5). Efforts have been made to identify tumor-specific vulnerabilities and to develop corresponding drugs to target them, with the goal of improving the therapeutic index (Dominguez-Brauer et al, 2015; Otto and Sicinski, 2017).

Preclinical development and clinical evaluation of numerous agents designed to inhibit specific cell cycle and cell growth regulators is ongoing (see Chap. 19, Sec. 19.6; Fig. 8–12). These drugs exploit features such as defective control over the G_1/S transition, loss of the TP53 response, aneuploidy, or the presence of extra centrosomes, which represent vulnerabilities of cancer cells. Further perturbation of these pathways (eg, G_1/S transition) or potentiation of these malignant features (eg, aneuploidy; see Sec. 8.3.5) may induce prolonged cell-cycle arrest or cellular phenotypes (eg, elevated genomic instability) that are not compatible with survival. Functional genomic approaches and efforts to characterize alterations in tumor genomes including mutations in oncogenes and tumor suppressors have been instrumental in identifying cell cycle– and cell growth–influencing genes, whose products can be targeted, and have spurred the development of anticancer drugs.

Early generation cell-cycle inhibitors including those targeting PLK1, Aurora kinases, and multiple CDKs (eg, pan-CDK–targeting agents such as flavopiridol and dinaciclib) have shown some clinical activity in hematologic malignancies but failed to show efficacy in clinical trials for solid tumors. Although preclinical studies validated these targets in multiple cancer types, they were essential to nonmalignant cells (Dominguez-Brauer et al, 2015; Otto and Sicinski, 2017). These drugs exert cytotoxic effects primarily through target inhibition in mitotic cells, and their limited activity in solid tumors may be due to their relatively low mitotic index compared to hematologic tumors.

Improvement in efficacy of cell cycle–targeting agents required refinement of therapeutic targets (ie, essential in tumor tissue while sparing normal cells), improved patient selection (ie, biomarkers to identify tumors sensitive to a given strategy), and improved pharmacologic selectivity to avoid off-target effects. The greatest success to date has been development of selective CDK4/6 inhibitors (eg, palbociclib, ribociclib, and abemaciclib), which all improve clinical outcomes when added to endocrine therapy for hormone receptor–positive (HR+) HER2-negative breast cancer (see Chap. 19, Sec. 19.6.1; Thu et al, 2018b). The effectiveness of CDK4/6 inhibitors is dependent on RB status, with RB-competent tumors displaying sensitivity to these drugs whereas RB-inactivated tumors are resistant: loss of RB function is rarely observed in untreated HR+/HER2-negative breast cancer, providing the appropriate molecular context for the successful application of these agents. When development of acquired resistance to CDK4/6 inhibitor therapy occurs in metastatic disease, loss of RB is a recurrent finding. Evaluation of whether additional components of the CDK4/6-RB1-CCND1 axis are clinically relevant predictors of response to CDK4/6 inhibitors is ongoing. Selective CDK4/6 inhibitors are generally well tolerated, with a much-improved therapeutic index compared to early pan-CDK inhibitors (eg, flavopiridol, seliciclib, dinaciclib). The improved toxicity profile for these compounds likely reflects their specificity in CDK inhibition, and the fact that CDK4 and CDK6 are interphase CDKs that are not essential for cycling nonmalignant cells (Malumbres and Barbacid 2009).

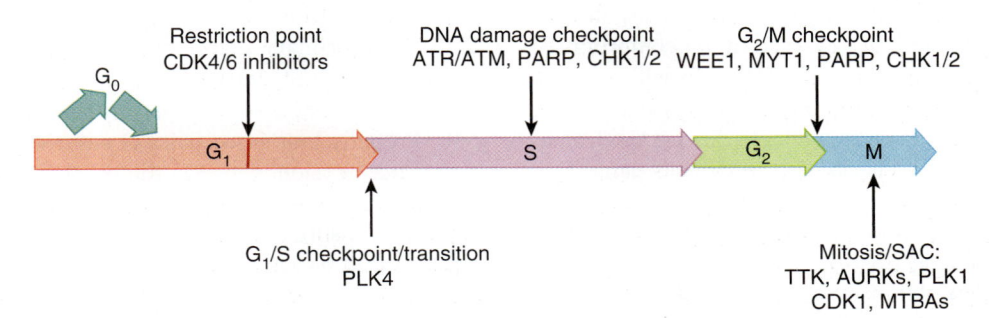

FIGURE 8–12 **Therapeutic vulnerabilities of the cell cycle in cancer.** Cancer cells can be therapeutically targeted at multiple points throughout the cell cycle, including cell-cycle transitions and checkpoints. *SAC*, spindle assembly checkpoint; *MTBAs*, microtubule binding agents.

Ongoing clinical trials include continued evaluation of PLK1 and Aurora kinase inhibitors and studies of additional cell-cycle inhibitors, as well as inhibitors of several proteins involved in regulating cell-cycle checkpoints and genomic instability (Fig. 8–12, discussed in Sec. 8.3.5) (Dominguez-Brauer et al, 2015; Otto and Sicinski, 2017).

8.3 GENOMIC INSTABILITY AND CHECKPOINT PATHWAYS

Most cancers show evidence of genomic instability, which can be defined as the propensity to continually alter the genomic state, through gain or loss of genetic material or single nucleotide changes (see Chap. 9, Sec. 9.2). Mutations that increase genomic instability are probably selected for early in the evolution of cancers because they promote genetic diversity that enables cancer cells to acquire phenotypes to support their proliferation and growth. Many familial cancer syndromes are caused by mutations in genes encoding DNA repair and checkpoint proteins that result in nucleotide and chromosomal instability (see Chap. 9, Sec. 9.5). Genomic instability can be classified as nucleotide instability, which is characterized by a high rate of acquired point mutations (eg, single nucleotide variants); microsatellite instability, defined as the expansion or reduction in number of short oligonucleotide polymorphic repeat sequences (ie, microsatellites); or as chromosomal instability, which involves amplification or deletion of genomic regions (ie, changes in gene dosage) and the fusion, loss, or gain of whole chromosomes (Pikor et al, 2013). Duplication and segregation of the genome during the cell cycle inexorably increases the risk of genomic instability. Checkpoints that arrest the cell cycle in response to DNA damage or to misalignment of chromosomes in mitosis exist to guard against such risks (Kastan and Bartek, 2004; Fig. 8–1).

8.3.1 The DNA Damage Checkpoints

The cell cycle is intimately associated with the detection and repair of DNA damage (see Chap. 9, Sec. 9.5). When the cell sustains genomic damage beyond a threshold level, the cell cycle arrests. Arresting the cell cycle gives time to repair this damage before entering either S phase or mitosis, thereby preventing the replication or segregation of compromised chromosomes (Kastan and Bartek, 2004). Cells with severely damaged DNA can undergo malignant transformation, as demonstrated by the many hereditary cancer syndromes caused by defective DNA checkpoint and repair genes (see Chap. 9, Sec. 9.5). To protect the body from this threat, a cell's response to DNA damage can often end in that cell's death (see Sec. 8.4; Ciccia and Elledge, 2010).

There is a 2-way flow of information between the DNA damage response and the cell cycle. Serious DNA damage arrests the cell cycle, but the cell cycle also regulates the response to DNA damage. Mechanisms that correct common chemical changes to DNA bases, such as base excision repair and nucleotide excision repair, operate constitutively (see Chap. 9, Sec. 9.3). In contrast, a cell's response to DSBs, likely the most dangerous type of DNA damage, can depend on its cell-cycle phase. During G_1 phase, cells primarily repair DSBs through a nonhomologous end-joining (NHEJ) process, in which broken ends are directly ligated together, often leading to the loss or insertion of base pairs (ie, indels). During S and G_2 phases, cells continue to repair DSBs by NHEJ, but also deploy homologous recombination (HR), which typically uses the replicated sister chromatid as a template for correcting damaged DNA. In contrast to NHEJ, HR is considered an error-free DSB repair pathway (see Chap. 9, Sec. 9.3.4).

The signaling pathways involved in DNA damage response (DDR) involve sensing of the damage, recruitment of DDR proteins to the genetic lesion, and execution of the signaling cascades for repair. These pathways rely on ATM and CHK2 for detecting DSBs at the G_1/S checkpoint, and ATR and CHK1 for responding to replication stress and single-strand DNA lesions at the G_2/M checkpoint (Ciccia and Elledge, 2010). However, many other proteins are critically involved in the signaling that is initiated on activation of these checkpoints, most notably, TP53 (see Chap. 7, Sec. 7.6.1). Moreover, in addition to sensing DNA damage at these checkpoints, inhibition of cell-cycle progression is important for checkpoint function.

Serious DNA damage like DSBs activate DNA damage kinases that trigger cell-cycle arrest through phosphorylation of proteins that control the G_1/S and G_2/M transitions. These phosphorylation events lead to the stabilization and activation of both the transcription factor TP53 and the CKI p21 (CIP1), whose transcription is induced by TP53. TP53 also induces a broad transcriptional program of DNA repair proteins (Zilfou and Lowe, 2009). p21 suppresses CYCLIN E–CDK2 and CYCLIN A2–CDK2 activity, preventing entry into S phase. For cells in S and G_2 phase, DNA damage kinases inactivate all 3 CDC25 phosphatases and activate WEE1 kinase (Otto and Sicinski, 2017). These actions arrest cells before the G_2/M transition point by preventing the surge of CYCLIN B–CDK1 activity that drives cells into mitosis.

8.3.2 The Spindle Assembly Checkpoint

The spindle assembly checkpoint (SAC) is essential for delaying anaphase until all replicated chromosomes are bioriented and under tension (Lara-Gonzalez et al, 2012; Musacchio, 2015). The primary defect detected by the SAC is kinetochores that are not attached to spindle microtubules. A single unattached kinetochore can prevent anaphase in mammalian cells. Properly bioriented pairs of sister chromatids will also experience tension between their tethered centromeres, as the 2 microtubule bundles pull the 2 kinetochores in opposite directions. Insufficient levels of tension between centromeres can also lead to activation of the SAC, although the mechanism is incompletely understood.

The SAC blocks anaphase by preventing the full activation of the APC/C-CDC20. The result is stabilized Securin and CYCLIN B, which can suppress Separase and maintain the metaphase state for a long, though not indefinite, period of time. TTK protein kinase (TTK) is a key protein involved in establishing the SAC. Through phosphorylation of its substrates, TTK (also known as monopolar spindle 1, MPS1) recruits various SAC proteins to the kinetochore to generate the mitotic checkpoint complex (MCC). The MCC is a multiprotein complex that functions as the SAC effector signal to inhibit APC/C-CDC20 ubiquitin ligase activity (Lara-Gonzalez et al, 2012; Musacchio, 2015).

8.3.3 Mitotic Errors and Aneuploidy

In the multi-hit genetic model of oncogenesis, it is proposed that genomic instability that arises during S phase can contribute to cancer formation. For instance, errors by DNA polymerases can introduce point mutations in genes, whereas DSBs can cause chromosomal translocations that lead to the aberrant expression of oncogenes. Cancers are marked not just by such discrete genetic changes but also by changes in the overall number of chromosomes (aneuploidy), which presumably arise from errors in mitosis. More than 90% of clinically detected solid tumors are aneuploid. Although they typically have less bizarre karyotypes than solid tumors, hematopoietic cancers also frequently show translocations or loss or gain of 1 or more chromosomes (Sansregret et al, 2018). Thus, cancer cells must maintain a fine balance between levels of genomic instability that are advantageous for tumor evolution and excessive levels that induce cellular stress and even death (Burkard and Weaver, 2017).

It is not clear whether aneuploidy is a cause or a consequence of cancer (Sansregret et al, 2018). Aneuploidy is generally detrimental to the proliferation of normal cells, presumably because it creates imbalances in the expression levels of the hundreds or thousands of genes present on a single chromosome. Dysregulation of such a large cohort of genes imposes substantial proteotoxic and energy stress on cells (Holland and Cleveland, 2012; Sansregret et al, 2018). As a general rule, molecular mechanisms proposed to cause cancer are thought to increase—not decrease—the rate of cell proliferation, raising the question as to how aneuploidy might be a cause of cancer? First, in contrast to the general presumption that drivers of cancer must increase the rate of cell proliferation, cell proliferation in solid tumors is often considerably slower than in normal renewing tissues (see Chap. 12, Sec. 12.1). Second, populations of aneuploid cells will have greater genetic variability, and the altered expression of multiple genes resulting from aberrant karyotypes may generate advantageous phenotypes. Such phenotypic diversity could allow aneuploid populations of cancer cells to evolve rapidly in response to physiological stresses, such as hypoxia or immune responses, or to medical interventions, such as chemotherapy (Sansregret et al, 2018).

The mitotic segregation errors and DDR deficiencies that occur in malignant cells can induce aneuploidy and contribute to the genomic instability of cancer cells. Mechanisms that produce aneuploidy in dividing cancer cells include but are not limited to chromosomal instability due to impaired checkpoint functions that compromise the cell's ability to correct improper kinetochore-microtubule attachments, defective chromosome segregation induced by centrosomal abnormalities, formation of tetraploid cells, and catastrophic events such as chromothripsis (Holland and Cleveland, 2012; Vitre and Cleveland, 2012; Sansregret et al, 2018).

Chromosome instability (CIN) results from the failure to properly segregate 1 copy of the sister chromatid pair to each of the 2 daughter cells, which results in 2 aneuploid daughter cells. In normal cells, missegregation of a chromosome—leading to 1 daughter cell inheriting both sister chromatids—is a rare event, occurring once every 50 to 100 cell cycles. However, in some cancer cell lines, chromosomes can be missegregated nearly every cell cycle (Thompson and Compton, 2008). One mechanism underlying missegregation is the formation of merotelic attachments between the kinetochore and microtubules of the mitotic spindle. Such attachments, in which one of the sister chromatids is attached to both spindle poles, satisfy the mitotic checkpoint but often lead to lagging chromosomes that segregate inappropriately or generate micronuclei. The chromosome passenger complex, which includes Aurora B, is the cellular machinery responsible for correcting faulty chromosome-spindle attachments (Carmena et al, 2012). Failure of the mitotic checkpoint to inhibit anaphase until all chromosomes are properly attached to the spindle is another potential mechanism for chromosome missegregation, although cancer cells often exhibit an impaired but not completely abrogated mitotic checkpoint. Chromosomes may also segregate inappropriately if the cohesion of sister chromatids happens prematurely, which may occur if cancer cells have impaired function of the cohesion complex. Lastly, replication stress prior to mitosis can promote aneuploidy through telomere fusions that generate dicentric chromosomes, which are then randomly segregated into daughter cells (Holland and Cleveland, 2012; Sansregret et al, 2018).

Extra centrosomes are a common feature of cancers that may arise through cell fusion, cytokinesis failure, or overduplication of centrioles with subsequent centrosome assembly (Vitre and Cleveland, 2012). In normal cells, centrosomes are similar to chromosomes in that they are replicated during S phase and then segregated during mitosis (see Sec. 8.2.1.2). In fact, cells appear to use a similar strategy to ensure that both chromosomes and centrosomes replicate only once per cell cycle: there are distinct windows of time for becoming competent for replication and for actually undergoing replication (Nigg and Holland, 2018). However, cell-cycle defects that weaken the blocks against centriole re-replication appear to arise during the evolution of many cancers. At the start of mitosis, the presence of extra centrosomes results in a spindle with more than 2 poles being formed (ie, multipolar spindle). If the multipolar spindle is stable, the resulting anaphase typically generates 3 or more daughter cells. In such cases, the daughter cells usually die as a consequence of profound aneuploidy. Frequently, however, multipolar spindles collapse into pseudo-bipolar spindles prior to anaphase, with the extra centrosome clustered around one of the 2 spindle poles. Such divisions generate only 2 daughter cells but often result in chromosome missegregation as a result of additional attachments being made to kinetochores by the extra centrosome (Holland and Cleveland,

2012; Sansregret et al, 2018). Therefore, cancer cells with centrosome amplification are heavily reliant on centrosome clustering mechanisms to avoid the generation of lethal multipolar spindles during mitosis. The kinesin protein, KIFC1, has been identified as a critical mediator of centrosome clustering and represents a dependency of cells with centrosome amplification (Patel et al, 2018; Sansregret et al, 2018).

Tetraploid cells can arise when anaphase or cytokinesis fails. Some tissues, such as the liver, give rise intentionally to tetraploid cells. In most cell types, however, tetraploidy results from mitotic segregation errors and can lead to death or G_1 arrest in the subsequent cell cycle. Tetraploid cancer cells formed from mitotic errors may be able to survive because of compromised Hippo signaling (Fig. 8–11), which is commonly disrupted in cancer (Harvey et al, 2013) and is consistent with the concept that the Hippo pathway governs a tetraploidy checkpoint (Ganem et al, 2014; Zhang et al, 2017). Because centrosomes are not segregated when tetraploid cells form, tetraploid cells almost always exhibit centrosome amplification, which is a trigger for Hippo signaling. The effects of supernumerary centrosomes on spindle formation may help explain the high rates of chromosomal instability in tetraploid cells.

A small fraction of tumors (2%-3%) experience chromothripsis—the acquisition of tens to hundreds of rearrangements in a localized genomic region in one catastrophic event. Chromothripsis events may be driven by DNA damage in micronuclei, which form after failed segregation of lagging chromosomes in aberrant mitoses (Crasta et al, 2012). These events can generate a massive wave of aneuploidy during a single cell division.

8.3.4 Modifications of Cell-Cycle Checkpoints in Cancer

To support sustained proliferation and avoidance of cell death in the face of abnormal signaling, mitotic defects, and aneuploid genomes, cancer cells acquire genetic alterations that enable them to satisfy or bypass the checkpoints that exist to prevent these abnormalities in normal cells. For example, inactivation of the *RB1* gene enables cancer cells to bypass the restriction point to enable G_1/S transition, as described. Thus, cancer cells often exhibit alterations to components of the DNA damage checkpoints and downstream DNA damage repair processes that are considered to be guardians of the genome. A comprehensive analysis of genetic and epigenetic disruption of genes involved in DNA damage checkpoint and response pathways in 33 cancer types and nearly 10,000 tumors indicated that *TP53* was the most frequently disrupted gene (~35%). The DNA damage checkpoint genes *ATM* and *ATR* were disrupted in ~5% and ~3.5% of tumors, respectively. Other genes related to the function of these checkpoints were altered in 1% to 5% of tumors including *BRCA1*, *BRCA2*, several mismatch repair genes, and genes in the Fanconi anemia (DNA repair) pathway (Knijnenburg et al, 2018).

The mitotic checkpoint is reported as frequently disrupted in cancer cells, but complete inactivation is thought to be lethal (Kops et al, 2005). Mutations in several SAC components including *TTK*, *BUB1*, *BUBR1*, *MAD1*, and *MAD2* have been observed in multiple cancers, although at low frequencies (1%-5% of tumors), whereas overexpression of *BUB1*, *BUBR1*, and *TTK* is much more prevalent (Knijnenburg et al, 2018). SAC deregulation may facilitate chromosomal instability levels that are beneficial for tumor development and progression, although tumor cells may be heavily dependent on retaining at least some SAC function to provide time for adequate mitotic segregation of their aneuploid genomes, which may explain the relative infrequency of mutations affecting SAC genes in tumors. The SAC may be dispensable for cell survival when the APC/C has a reduced function (Wild et al, 2016). Correspondingly, impairment of the APC/C has been shown to confer cancer resistance to inhibitors of TTK protein kinase (TTK), which is required to establish SAC activity (Sansregret et al, 2017; Thu et al, 2018a).

8.3.5 Targeting Genomic Instability and Cell-Cycle Checkpoints for Cancer Therapy

Genomic instability and deregulation of cell-cycle checkpoints are features of nearly all tumor types and represent major vulnerabilities for dividing cancer cells (Fig. 8–12). Because checkpoints exist to preserve genomic integrity by preventing cells from acquiring detrimental or lethal genomic alterations, exploiting the dependency of cancer cells on maintaining a minimum checkpoint activity sufficient for viable mitotic segregation of their aneuploid genomes is an attractive therapeutic target. This strategy holds promise because in theory, a substantial therapeutic window is achievable as normal cells have properly functioning and redundant pathways to protect them from genomic instability.

Drugs under development aimed at targeting this feature of cancer cells include those that abrogate the intra-S, G_1/S, and DNA damage checkpoints such as ATM, ATR, PARP1, CHK2, and inhibitors that target centrosome dynamics and G_2/M checkpoints including Aurora kinases, PLK4 and TTK (Fig. 8–12). These drugs aim to induce intolerable levels of genomic instability specifically in already unstable cancer cells. Cancer cells are often dependent on DNA damage response pathways for repairing damage induced by genomic instability to sustain their survival. Thus, inhibition of critical damage response effectors like ATM and ATR offers a rational strategy for inducing cancer cell death (Weber and Ryan, 2015). Aurora kinases (eg, AURKA, AURKB) are important mediators of G_1/S transition, centrosome maturation, mitotic spindle formation, chromosome passenger complex, and cytokinesis. Their recurrent upregulation and involvement in important process throughout the cell cycle makes AURKs attractive therapeutic targets; however, the high toxicity of AURK inhibitors evaluated thus far has limited their utility in the clinic. Nevertheless, a number of next-generation AURK-targeting agents are being investigated

(Otto and Sicinski, 2017). CFI-400945, an ATP-competitive inhibitor of PLK4, the governor of centriole duplication, causes centrosome abnormalities, multipolar spindles, and potentiation of aneuploidy that leads to cancer cell death in model systems (Mason et al, 2014), and has demonstrated preliminary evidence of antitumor activity in patients (Veitch et al, 2019). Others drugs aim to compromise the G_2/M checkpoint by targeting proteins such as WEE1. These inhibitors induce premature progression through targeted checkpoints and can result in death by mitotic catastrophe (see Sec. 8.4.6.2) due to lethal accumulation of DNA damage, particularly in cancers with defective G_1 checkpoints due to TP53 inactivation (Otto and Sicinski, 2017). Inhibitors of TTK (aka MPS1) are another promising class of drugs that induce cell death through abrogation of the SAC (Mason et al, 2017). Again, the therapeutic goal of these inhibitors is to increase genomic instability and cause arrest or death specifically of aneuploid cancer cells by rushing them through the mitotic checkpoint (Dominguez-Brauer et al, 2015).

8.4 CELL DEATH

The balance between cell viability and cell death is critical for all organisms and involves a network of proteins and communication among several signaling pathways. Impaired cell death is associated with various human pathologies, including immunodeficiency, autoimmunity, neurodegenerative diseases, and cancer. Similar to proliferation, cell death is essential for embryonic and postnatal development and for tissue homeostasis. During these processes, death occurs in a highly regulated way; however, cells can also undergo accidental cell death, which is an unregulated phenomenon that occurs in response to extreme and intolerable cellular aggravations such as physical, chemical, or mechanical stresses.

Different types of regulated cell death occur in mammalian cells, with the primary modes including apoptosis (or programmed cell death), necrosis, and autophagy (Fuchs and Steller, 2015). Morphologic changes within dying cells constitute important criteria for distinguishing between apoptosis, necrotic, and autophagic cell death. Changes associated with apoptosis include rounding up of the cell, plasma membrane blebbing, cytoplasm shrinkage, alteration of membrane asymmetry, and condensation and fragmentation of the nucleus (Fig. 8–13). Cells at late stages of apoptosis become fragmented into apoptotic bodies that are eliminated by phagocytic cells without triggering inflammation. Necrosis-associated cellular changes are manifested by swelling of the cell, mitochondria, and cytoplasmic organelles, followed by focal rupture of the plasma membrane. Moderate chromatin condensation is also displayed by necrotic cells. More advanced stages of necrosis are associated with disintegration of all cellular components and inflammation (see Fig. 8–13). Transcriptional changes, protein levels, and posttranslational modifications, affecting apoptotic regulators such as the BCL-2 family of proteins for example (see below), can also help differentiate among the different types of cell death (Fuchs and Steller, 2015; Galluzzi et al, 2018). Autophagy, which is a process that can lead to cell survival through breakdown and recycling of cellular macromolecules, can also be a mode of cell death (Levy et al, 2017). Autophagic cell death is achieved by degradation of cellular components through the formation of autophagosomes that morphologically appear as vacuolization of the dying cell (Fig. 8–13; see Chap. 12, Sec. 12.3.7). Mitotic catastrophe and immunogenic cell death are additional concepts that are described below since they have important consequences in the context of cancer and anti-neoplastic therapy (Fuchs and Steller, 2015; Galluzzi et al, 2018).

8.4.1 Mechanisms of Apoptosis

Apoptosis is triggered in mammalian cells in response to endogenous stimuli (eg, growth factor deprivation) or exogenous stimuli (eg, irradiation or genotoxic chemotherapeutic drugs) (Bock and Tait, 2019; Singh et al, 2019). Apoptosis is also induced in response to inadequate cell-matrix interactions—a specific type of apoptosis known as *anoikis* (Galluzzi et al, 2018).

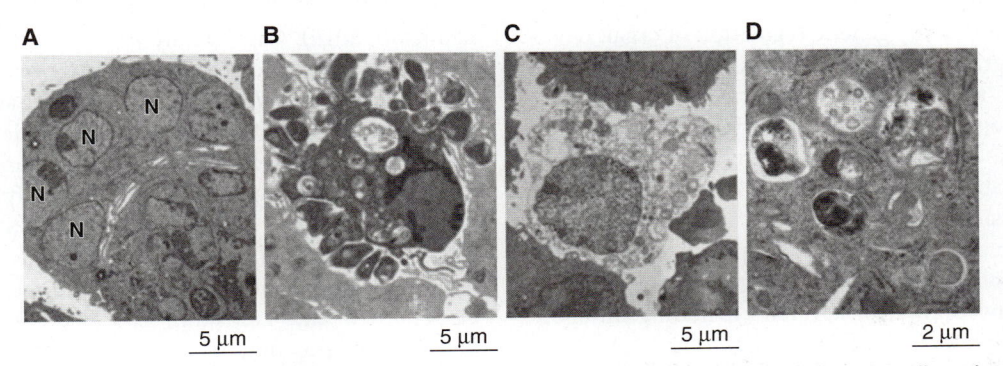

FIGURE 8–13 Morphologic changes within dying cells. Transmission electron microscopy images of cancer cells undergoing various modes of cell death. (**A**) Cell undergoing mitotic catastrophe with characteristic multi-nucleation. N=nuclei. (**B**) Apoptotic cell displaying typical features including chromatin condensation and plasma membrane blebbing. (**C**) Cell with necrotic features such as nuclear membrane dilation and cellular swelling. (**D**) Autophagic cell displaying characteristic vacuolization. (Reproduced with permission from Vitale I, Galluzzi L, Castedo M, et al, Mitotic catastrophe: a mechanism for avoiding genomic instability. *Nat Rev Mol Cell Biol* 2011;12(6):385-392.)

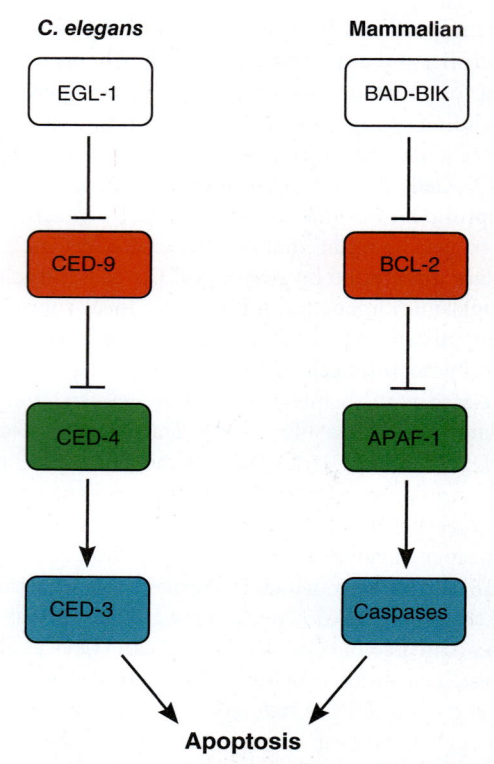

FIGURE 8–14 Major regulators of apoptosis in *Caenorhabditis elegans* and their mammalian orthologs. Schematic of the major components of the apoptotic pathway in *C elegans* (left). Mammalian cells have evolved several orthologs to the pro- and antiapoptotic proteins of *C elegans* (right; see text).

The first evidence that apoptosis is genetically regulated arose from studies of the nematode *Caenorhabditis elegans* (Kinchen and Hengartner, 2005). During the development of this invertebrate, 131 of the 1090 somatic cells died by apoptosis, and genetic screens identified several genes required for this process. Loss-of-function mutations of *C elegans egl-1*, *ced-3*, or *ced-4* or gain-of-function mutations of *ced-9* result in survival of the 131 cells programmed to die. (Fig. 8–14). Sydney Brenner, Robert Horvitz, and John Sulston were awarded the Nobel Prize in Medicine or Physiology in 2002 for their elucidation of the genetic regulation of organ development and programmed cell death in *C elegans*. Biochemical and genetic studies have demonstrated the existence of multiple analogs of the *C elegans* apoptotic proteins in mammalian cells. These studies also demonstrated the existence of 2 major apoptotic pathways: the death receptor (also known as extrinsic) apoptotic pathway and the mitochondrial (also known as intrinsic) apoptotic pathway (Fig. 8–15). Mammalian apoptotic pathways are highly controlled, and their regulation involves various proteins including antiapoptotic (eg, BCL-2 and BCL-XL) and proapoptotic (eg, BID and BAX) proteins (Fig. 8–16).

Biochemical studies have proven instrumental for the identification and characterization of the components involved in the initiation, propagation, or inhibition of the mammalian apoptotic signaling pathways. Genetic studies in mice engineered with a disruption within, or overexpression of, specific pro- or antiapoptotic genes have been critical in demonstrating the in vivo apoptotic functions of these proteins, and have helped to identify developmental defects and diseases associated with impaired apoptosis (McIlwain et al, 2013; Fuchs and Steller, 2015).

8.4.1.1 BCL-2 Family Members and Their Roles in Apoptosis
The mammalian *Bcl-2* gene, a homolog of the *C elegans Ced-9*, is a prototypical member of the BCL-2 family that includes antiapoptotic proteins, such as BCL-2, BCL-XL, BCL-W, BCL2A1, and MCL-1, and proapoptotic proteins, such as BAX, BCL-XS, BAK, BAD, BIK, BIM, BID, NOXA, and PUMA (see Fig. 8–16; Bock and Tait, 2019). These proteins share several conserved domains known as "BCL-2 homology" (BH) regions including BH1, BH2, BH3, and BH4. These domains allow the formation of homo- and heterodimers between BCL-2 family members and are integral for the function of these proteins. Proteins of the BCL-2 family are essential for the initiation and regulation of mammalian apoptosis (Bock and Tait, 2019). In response to oncogenic activation or DNA damage, the transcription factor TP53 induces transcription and expression of a number of proapoptotic BCL-2 family members (eg, BAX, NOXA and PUMA) that lead to activation of caspases resulting in apoptosis (see Fig. 8–15; Hafner et al, 2019). In addition, overexpression of BCL-2 in mammalian cells inhibits the release of cytochrome C as well as other factors important for apoptosis (eg, apoptosis-inducing factor [AIF], second mitochondria–derived activator of caspases [SMAC], and the serine protease OMI) from the mitochondrial intermembrane space into the cytosol. Overexpression of BCL-2 also prolongs the survival of cells and increases their resistance to apoptosis (Delbridge et al, 2016).

8.4.1.2 Role of Caspases in Apoptosis
Mammalian caspases, "cysteine-dependent aspartate specific proteases," are analogs of the *C elegans* protein ced3. The first caspase (CASP1 or ICE) was identified in 1993 on the basis of its similarity to ced3. More than 14 mammalian caspases have since been cloned (Fig. 8–17; McIlwain et al, 2013; Van Opdenbosch and Lamkanfi, 2019). Caspases are present in the cytosol in their inactive forms (procaspases or zymogens). To be activated, they require proteolytic cleavage at specific aspartate residues. Active caspases are heterotetrameric complexes composed of 2 large subunits (20 kDa) and 2 small subunits (10 kDa) (see Fig. 8–17). Although caspases are primarily known for their apoptotic function, caspases such as CASP1 and CASP11 (ortholog of human caspases 4 and 5) also play important roles in inflammation (Karki and Kanneganti, 2019; Van Opdenbosch and Lamkanfi, 2019). CASP8 also possesses nonapoptotic functions (see below).

Caspases possess a wide range of expression patterns throughout mammalian tissues. The finding that caspases are able to sequentially process and activate other caspases, together with the structural studies of these proteins, has allowed the classification of caspases into "initiators" (eg, CASP8, CASP9, and CASP10) or "executioners" of

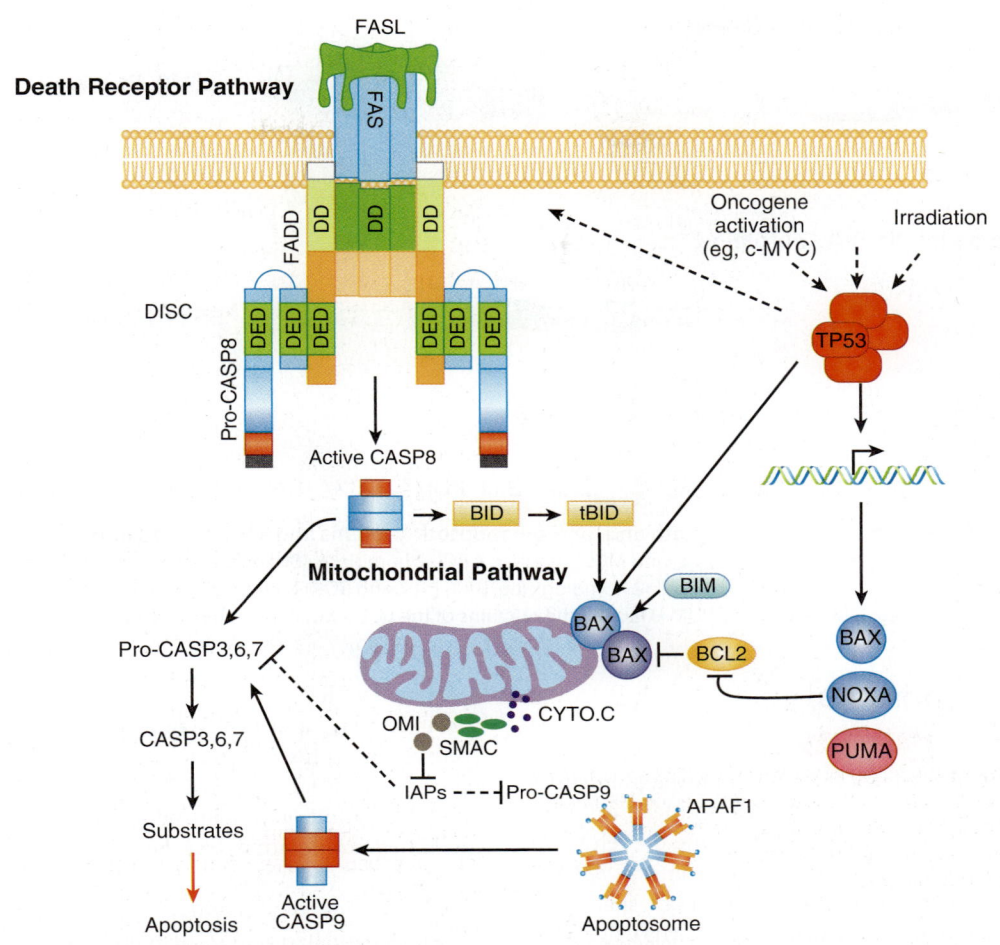

FIGURE 8-15 Schematic of the 2 major apoptotic pathways in mammalian cells. The death receptor (or extrinsic) pathway is exemplified by the events that occur following engagement of FAS (CD95) by its ligand FASL (CD95L). FAS/FASL interaction leads to the trimerization of the FAS receptor and the recruitment of the adapter protein FADD to the cytoplasmic tail of FAS. The interaction FAS/FADD is mediated by their respective death domains (DDs). This interaction allows the recruitment of CASP8 (and CASP10 in human cells) and the formation of the death-inducing signaling complex (DISC). The presence of these caspases in the DISC results in their oligomerization, autoactivation, and subsequent processing of downstream effector caspases (CASP3, -6, and -7). Once activated, effector caspases cleave various cellular proteins leading to apoptotic cell death. The mitochondrial (or intrinsic) apoptotic pathway is triggered in response to various stimuli including oncogenic activation and DNA damage. Activation of the tumor suppressor and transcription factor TP53 in response to cellular stresses leads to the transcriptional activation of several proapoptotic genes (eg, BAX, PUMA, NOXA, and FAS). Activation of BAX and BAK leads to outer membrane permeabilization and the release to the cytosol of a number of mitochondrial proteins including OMI, SMAC, and cytochrome C (CYTO.C). CYTO.C clusters with APAF-1 and the pro-CASP9, forming the apoptosome. The oligomerization of pro-CASP9 within the apoptosome leads to its activation and the subsequent processing of downstream caspases and cell death. Caspases can also be negatively regulated by inhibitors of apoptosis (IAPs) which can bind to caspases to inhibit their function. In certain cell types, the cleavage of BID by CASP8 generates tBID, a truncated form of BID that translocates to the mitochondria and cooperates with BAX-BAK in inducing the mitochondrial apoptotic pathway.

apoptosis (eg, CASP3, CASP6, and CASP7) (Van Opdenbosch and Lamkanfi, 2019). Thousands of potential caspase substrates have been identified, including cytoskeleton proteins (eg, actin and gelsolin), nuclear proteins (eg, lamin A and B), proteins involved in DNA damage repair (eg, PARP, RAD51, and DNA-PKcs), cell-cycle proteins (eg, p21, p27, CDC27, and RB), cytokines (eg, IL-1 and IL-18), antiapoptotic proteins (eg, BCL-2, BCL-XL, and the inhibitor of the caspase-activated DNase [CAD] also known as DNA fragmentation factor [DFF]), and proapoptotic proteins (eg, caspases, BID, and BAX) (Julien and Wells, 2017). CAD is inactive when associated with its inhibitor ICAD. In response to apoptotic stimuli, ICAD is cleaved by caspases, allowing the release of the active endonuclease CAD, resulting in internucleosomal DNA cleavage, a characteristic of apoptosis (Julien and Wells, 2017; Larsen and Sorensen, 2017).

Several caspases also have proinflammatory functions. These caspases include CASP1, 4, 5, 11, and 12 (Van Opdenbosch and Lamkanfi, 2019). CASP8 is important in other cellular functions, including blood vessel formation during embryogenesis, nuclear factor kappa B (NF-κB) activation and mitogen- or antigen-induced proliferation of T and B cells. The hierarchical involvement of caspases in the extrinsic and intrinsic apoptotic pathways, impaired apoptosis in their absence, as well as their nonapoptotic functions all highlight the importance of these proteins in regulating cell biology.

Anti-apoptotic BCL-2 proteins

BH4 — BH3 — BH1 — BH2 — TM   BCL-2, BCL-W
BCL-X, A1 and MCL1

Pro-apoptotic BCL-2 proteins

BH3 — BH1 — BH2 — TM   BAX, BAK and BOK

Pro-apoptotic BH3-only proteins

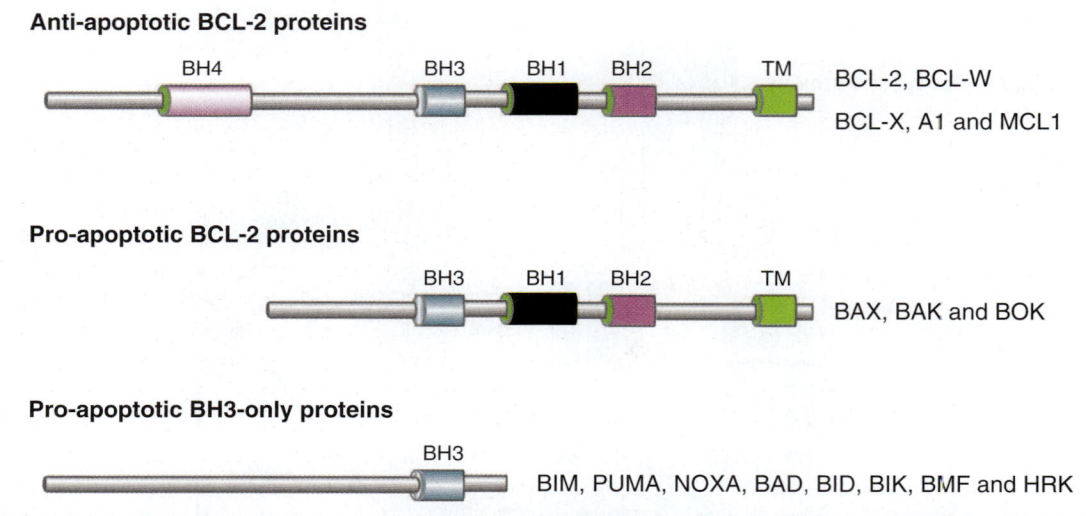

BH3   BIM, PUMA, NOXA, BAD, BID, BIK, BMF and HRK

FIGURE 8–16 BCL-2 family members include both anti- and proapoptotic proteins and are classified into different groups. The antiapoptotic group of BCL-2 homologs (eg, BCL-2, BCL-XL, and MCL1) contain 4 BCL-2 homology (BH) domains (BH1 to BH4), and a transmembrane domain (TM). Members of the proapoptotic group of BCL-2 homologs (eg, BAX, BAK, and BOK) contain TM, BH1, BH2, and BH3, but lack BH4. Finally, the BH3-only proteins (eg, BIM, NOXA, and PUMA) lack all the domains of the BCL-2 family members with the exception of BH3.

8.4.2 The Mitochondrial Apoptotic Pathway

Apoptotic stimuli, which trigger the mitochondrial or intrinsic apoptotic pathway, activate BAX and BAK and lead to mitochondrial outer membrane permeabilization and the release of proteins important for apoptosis (eg, cytochrome C, SMAC, and OMI) from the mitochondrial intermembrane space into the cytosol (see Fig. 8–15; Bock and Tait, 2019). Mitochondrial membrane permeabilization is suppressed by the antiapoptotic BCL-2 family members (eg, BCL-2 and BCL-XL), as they bind and inhibit activated BAX or BAK as well as other BH3-only proteins. Once in the cytosol, cytochrome C forms the apoptosome with APAF-1 (apoptosis activating factor-1, a mammalian analog of Ced-4) and CASP9, leading to activation of CASP9, which, in turn, processes and activates downstream effector caspases. This leads to cleavage of various cellular substrates and cell death.

Caspase activity is modulated by various members of the family of inhibitors of apoptosis (IAPs). IAPs were originally discovered in baculoviruses and shown to suppress the host cell death response to viral infection (Altieri, 2010). Identified IAPs include the X-linked IAP (XIAP), Survivin, and cellular IAP1 and 2 (c-IAP1 and c-IAP2). Several IAPs bind directly to caspases such as CASP3, 7, and 9 and inhibit their functions. This IAP-mediated inhibition of caspases can be antagonized by the proteins SMAC and OMI (see Fig. 8–15; Bock and Tait, 2019). When SMAC and OMI are released from the mitochondrial intermembrane space into the cytosol, they bind directly to XIAP and suppress its inhibition of caspases. In addition to their roles in apoptosis, IAPs are also involved in other processes including NF-κB signaling, cell division, and cellular stress responses.

The mitochondrial apoptotic pathway is essential for the response to DNA damage and oncogenic activation, and deregulation of the mitochondrial apoptotic pathway has been associated with diseases, including cancer. The tumor suppressor TP53 plays a critical role in this apoptotic pathway as it controls the transactivation of a number of essential proapoptotic BCL-2 family members including PUMA, BAX, and NOXA. In addition to controlling different cellular processes, including proliferation (see Sec. 8.4.1), the activated oncogene c-MYC (see Chap. 7, Sec. 7.5.2) also induces apoptosis in a TP53-dependent manner (see Fig. 8–15; Meyer and Penn, 2008). Deregulated c-MYC also promotes the accumulation of the tumor suppressor ARF that sequesters MDM2 in the nucleolus, thus releasing TP53 from MDM2-mediated inhibition.

Posttranslational modifications (eg, phosphorylation, ubiquitylation, and SUMOylation) play important roles in regulating the mitochondrial apoptotic pathway. For example, ubiquitination of BCL-2 family members (eg, BCL-2, BAX, BIK, NOXA, BID, BIM, and MCL-1) or caspases (eg, CASP3, CASP7, CASP8, and CASP9) leads to their proteasomal degradation, thus controlling their levels of expression (Vucic et al, 2011; Zamaraev et al, 2017).

8.4.3 The Death Receptor Apoptotic Pathway

The death receptor or extrinsic apoptotic pathway is initiated by the interaction of the death receptors, members of the tumor necrosis factor (TNF) receptor superfamily, with their ligands (Green, 2019). The death receptors share the presence of an approximately 80–amino acid motif known as the death domain (DD) in their cytoplasmic tails. Six human death receptors have been identified and include FAS (also known as CD95 or APO-1), TNFR-1, death receptor (DR) 3, DR4 (also known as TRAILR1), DR5 (also known as TRAILR2), and DR6. Several ligands for these death receptors have been identified and include TNF and LT (TNFR1), FASL (FAS), TL1A (DR3), and APO2L/TRAIL (DR4 and DR5).

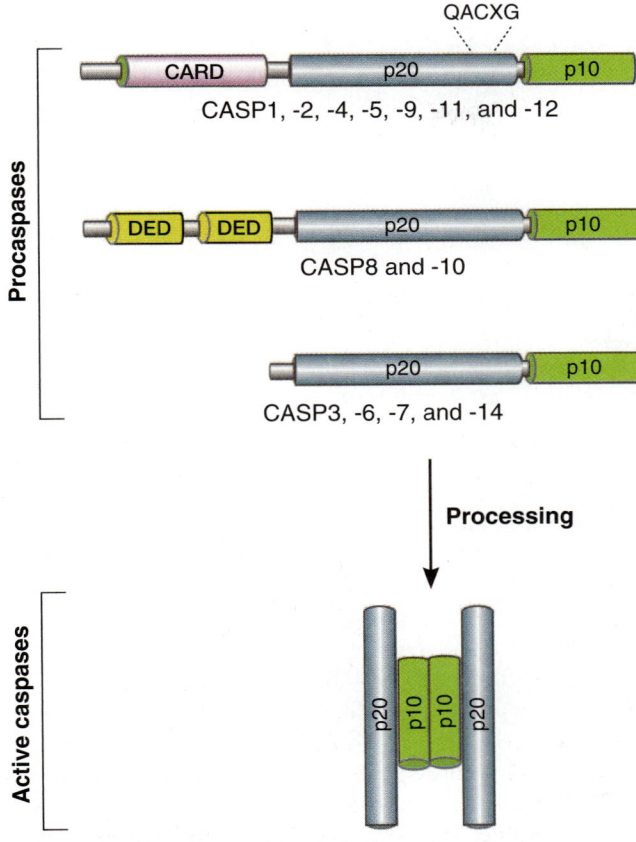

FIGURE 8–17 Mammalian caspases. Caspases exist in an inactive form (procaspases) that require autoprocessing or proteolytic cleavage by upstream caspases in order to be activated. The first group of caspases (CASP1, -2, -4, -5, -9, -11, and -12) contain caspases that contain caspase recruitment domain (CARD) and the subunits p20 and p10. The second group include CASP8 and CASP10, which possess 2 N-terminal death effector domains (DEDs) and the subunits p20 and p10. The third group contains CASP3, -6, -7, and -14. These caspases contain only the 2 subunits, p20 and p10. The processing of procaspases allows the formation of active caspases that consist of heterotetrameric complexes composed of 2 p20 and 2 p10 subunits.

The death receptor apoptotic pathway is exemplified by the FAS-induced apoptotic signaling pathway (see Fig. 8–15; Green, 2019). Following FAS/FASL interaction, the FAS receptor proteins aggregate to form a trimer and recruit the adaptor protein FADD (FAS-associated death domain) that contains 2 protein interaction domains, a death domain, and a death effector domain (DED). FAS/FADD interaction allows the recruitment of the DED-containing initiator pro-CASP8 (as well as pro-CASP10 in humans) and the formation of the death-inducing signaling complex (DISC), which functions as a platform for caspase activation to stimulate the extrinsic apoptotic pathway. Dimerization of pro-CASP8 within the DISC allows its autoprocessing, activation, and the formation and release of its active tetrameric form into the cytosol. Active CASP8 in the cytosol processes its substrates including the effector CASP3, CASP6, and CASP7 and the BH3-only protein BID. Cellular FLICE-like inhibitory protein (cFLIP), a pseudo-CASP8 protein with a nonfunctional catalytic domain, inhibits the death receptor apoptotic pathway by precluding the recruitment of CASP8 to the DISC.

TP53 also affects the death receptor apoptotic pathway as demonstrated by TP53 transactivation of FAS and DR5 in response to DNA damage (see Figs. 8–15 and 8–18). Posttranslational modifications, including ubiquitylation, phosphorylation, SUMOylation, and S-nitrosylation, also play important roles in the death receptor apoptotic pathway (Zamaraev et al, 2017). For example, in response to stimulation of DR4 or DR5, the E3 ligase CULLIN-3 polyubiquitinates CASP8 present at the DISC. This ubiquitination event recruits the ubiquitin-binding polypeptide p62 that mediates CASP8 aggregation, increasing its activation and processing (Jin et al, 2009).

Communication between the death receptor and apoptotic pathways is best demonstrated by CASP8 cleavage of BID (Green, 2019). This cleavage generates a truncated form of BID (tBID) that cooperates with BAX to form openings in the outer mitochondrial membrane, leading to release of proteins including cytochrome C from the mitochondrial intermembrane space (see Fig. 8–15). This CASP8 processing of BID amplifies the death receptor apoptotic pathway. In addition, stimulation of the mitochondrial pathway leads to the activation of the effector caspases, such as CASP3 and CASP6 that can subsequently process and activate CASP8.

Impaired apoptosis owing to alterations in components of the death receptor apoptotic pathway has been observed in human and mouse cells. For example, resistance to stimuli that activate this pathway is observed in cells deficient for CASP8, FADD, FAS, FASL, or in cells overexpressing c-FLIP (Strasser et al, 2009). Like the mitochondrial apoptotic pathway, the death receptor apoptotic pathway also plays critical roles in development and tissue homeostasis and is dysregulated in a number of diseases as well as cancer.

8.4.4 Apoptosis, Developmental Defects, and Disease

Deregulation of apoptosis is associated with human diseases, including cancer, immunodeficiency, and autoimmunity (Singh et al, 2019). Studies of genetically modified mice deficient in or overexpressing anti- or proapoptotic proteins also demonstrate an essential role of apoptosis in the prevention of embryonic and postnatal developmental defects, and in restraining the development of various diseases, including autoimmunity and tumorigenesis.

BCL-2 inhibits apoptosis in response to a wide range of stimuli that target the mitochondrial apoptotic pathway. In addition to cancer, overexpression of the prosurvival BCL-2 family members also promotes the development of other diseases, including autoimmunity (Singh et al, 2019). Transgenic mice expressing human BCL-2 in B-cell lineage and Bim-deficient mice develop an autoimmune disorder characterized by antinuclear antibodies and glomerulonephritis (Delbridge et al, 2016). Deficiency of the prosurvival BCL-2 family members (eg, BCL-2, BCL-XL, or MCL-1) results in increased cell death and promotes the development of a number of pathologies

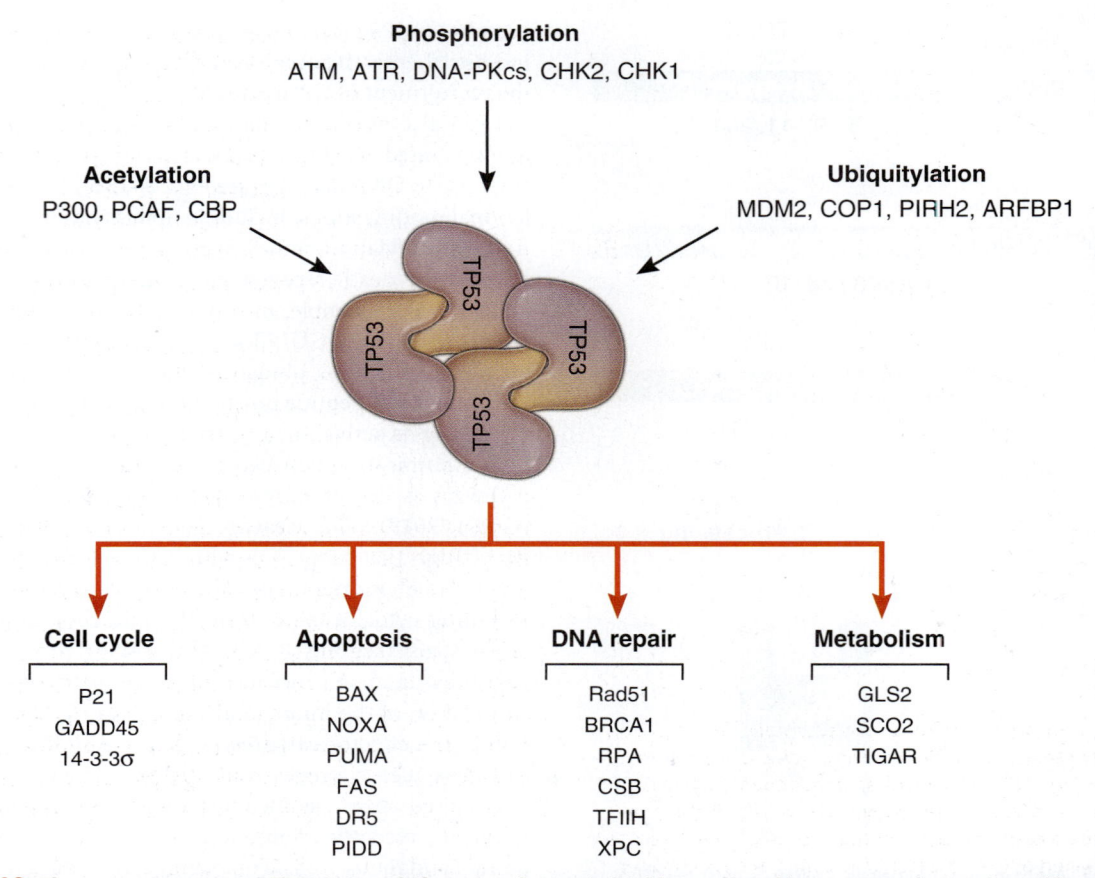

FIGURE 8–18 The tumor suppressor TP53 is a multifunctional protein highly regulated by posttranslational modifications. Examples of proteins involved in TP53 posttranslational modifications (eg, acetylation, phosphorylation, and ubiquitylation) are indicated. Activated TP53 plays major roles in a number of cellular processes including cell cycle, apoptosis, DNA repair, and metabolism. Examples of TP53 transcriptional targets involved in these cellular processes are indicated (see also Chap. 7, Sec. 7.6.1).

(Delbridge et al, 2016). For example, mice deficient for BCL-2 display polycystic kidney disease, loss of mature B and T cells as a consequence of increased apoptosis, and die by 6 weeks of age. Inactivation of Bcl-XL in mice results in embryonic lethality by day 14 of gestation, underscoring the critical role of BCL-XL in the regulation of programmed cell death. Mice deficient for Bax and Bak suffer early postnatal death; however, the few double mutants that survive develop lymphoid tumors and autoimmunity (Delbridge et al, 2016).

8.4.5 Mechanisms Leading to Necrosis

Although necrosis was thought initially to be a nonregulated process, subsequent studies demonstrated that necroptosis, a programmed type of necrosis, is regulated by a network of proteins (Fuchs and Steller, 2015). Unlike apoptosis, necrosis and necroptosis do not involve the activation of caspases. Instead, this process is mediated by RIPK1 (receptor-interacting protein kinase 1), RIPK3, and MLKL (mixed-lineage kinase domain-like pseudokinase) (Fig. 8–19). RIPK1 interacts with components of the apoptotic machinery, including CASP8, and thus is involved in the control of cell fates through both major forms of cell death. Mechanistic studies have dissected many of the complexities of these pathways, and genetic data from knockout mice lacking key apoptosis and necrosis proteins have demonstrated important interactions between the mechanisms that control apoptotic and necrotic cell death (Weinlich et al, 2017).

8.4.6 Additional Mechanisms Associated With Cell Death

Several other cellular mechanisms are involved in processes that may lead to cell death, including autophagy, mitotic catastrophe, and immunogenic cell death and these are described below.

8.4.6.1 Autophagy Autophagy is a regulated process that facilitates cell adaptation to stress, whereby damaged or excess cellular components are recycled by lysosome-mediated degradation of membrane-bound vesicles called autophagosomes (see Chap. 12, Sec. 12.3.6). Different stimuli can trigger autophagy, including redox, metabolic, proteomic, or genotoxic stress, and the macromolecules generated by this catabolic process may be broken down and recycled or used for metabolic reactions. Autophagy is considered a cell survival mechanism, as inactivation of autophagy-related (ATG) genes

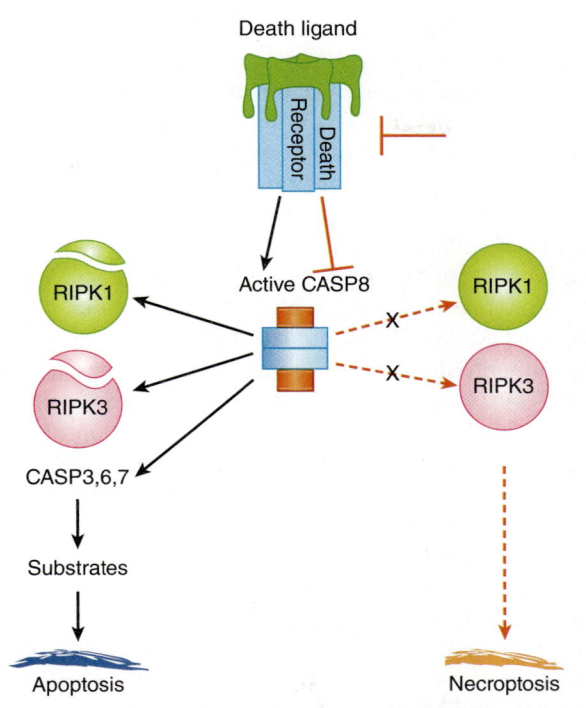

FIGURE 8–19 Representation of the crosstalk between apoptosis and necroptosis. In response to the binding of ligands to death receptors (eg, TNFR1) on the plasma membrane, active CASP8 inactivates RIPK1 and RIPK3 by proteolytic cleavage and also processes downstream caspases to promote apoptosis. If death receptor signaling is impaired or CASP8 is lost or inhibited, the executioner caspases are not activated and RIPK1 and RIPK3 are not cleaved and thus remain active. Active RIPK1 and RIPK3 trigger necroptosis, a programmed necrotic cell death.

has been shown to accelerate cell death, but autophagy can also lead to cell death (Fuchs and Steller, 2015; Levy et al, 2017).

There is overlap between the autophagy and apoptotic pathways. Beclin 1, the key protein responsible for autophagosome production, contains a BH3 domain and complexes with BCL-2 and BCL-XL. This complex resides at the endoplasmic reticulum and functions to inhibit autophagy, and its dissociation is required to drive the autophagic process (Fuchs and Steller, 2015). Furthermore, autophagic cell death has been shown to upregulate apoptosis, inhibiting autophagy has been shown to downregulate apoptosis, and CASP8 inhibition can activate autophagic cell death. The crosstalk between these 2 pathways suggests that they may engage one another to elicit their effects, and autophagy-mediated cell death may be a backup process to induce cell death in the absence of competent apoptotic signaling (Mohammad et al, 2015).

8.4.6.2 Mitotic Catastrophe

Mitotic catastrophe can occur after abnormal or failed mitosis and is proposed to be a mechanism that exists to prevent genomic instability that could promote tumor development and progression (Galluzzi et al, 2018). Death resulting from this process may exhibit features characteristic of apoptosis or necrosis (Fig. 8–13A), suggesting that mitotic catastrophe may be an event that triggers other cell death mechanisms. Cells undergoing mitotic catastrophe exhibit major nuclear aberrations as a result of chromosomal alterations and DNA breaks, leading to cells with micronuclei and multinucleation. The sequelae of mitotic catastrophe seem to rely on detection by the spindle assembly checkpoint and/or TP53, with death initiated by CASP2 and often involving an intrinsic apoptosis mechanism (Galluzzi et al, 2018).

Mitotic catastrophe may be induced by DNA-damaging compounds, radiation, or agents that disrupt the mitotic spindle apparatus (eg, microtubule-binding agents) (see Chap. 15, Sec 15.3.1). Such perturbations result in arrest of the cells experiencing mitotic errors, and prolonged arrest may result in cellular senescence or mitotic death. Additionally, such cells may undergo mitotic slippage, the escape of cells from mitotic arrest without chromosome segregation and cell division, which produces G_1 cells with aberrant tetraploid DNA content (Vitale et al, 2011). These cells that prematurely exit mitosis may experience mitotic catastrophe-mediated cell death during the following interphase. Aside from chemical stimuli, centrosome amplification can predispose cells to mitotic catastrophe through the formation of multipolar spindles if centrosome clustering is not achieved. Thus, the innate susceptibility of centrosome-amplified cancer cells to succumb to mitotic catastrophe provides a potential therapeutic window for anticancer agents that potentiate centrosome amplification and drive mitotic catastrophe. This strategy is being explored by drugs like CFI-400945, a PLK4 inhibitor (Veitch et al, 2019).

8.4.6.3 Immunogenic Cell Death

A cell whose death initiates an immune response with specificity toward antigens expressed by the dying cells is said to undergo immunogenic cell death (ICD) (Galluzzi et al, 2018). This feature of cell death can be induced by distinct stimuli including infectious pathogens (eg, viral infection), radiation therapy, hypericin-based photodynamic therapy, high hydrostatic pressure, and chemotherapeutic drugs. Death induced by these stimuli leads to the release or exposure of damage-associated molecular patterns (DAMPs) that are sensed by pattern-recognition receptors (PRRs) on innate and adaptive immune cells, which triggers an immune response capable of immunologic memory (Galluzzi et al, 2018). ICD is defined based on vaccination and rechallenge experiments. For example, cancer cells killed by the agent in question are inoculated into syngeneic, immunocompetent mice followed by rechallenge of these vaccinated mice with the living cancer cells. If the cell death–inducing agent was immunogenic and produced memory effector cells, tumors will not grow in the rechallenge experiment. Production of DAMPs can be triggered by inflammasome signaling, endoplasmic reticulum stress (eg, unfolded protein response), autophagy, membrane permeabilization, and cellular degradation during apoptotic and necrotic processes. Immunogenic DAMPs generated by dying cells include extracellular release of HMGB1, ATP secretion, calreticulin exposure at the cell surface, production of type I interferons, and release of cancer cell–derived nucleic acids (Galluzzi et al, 2018).

Immunogenic cell death is particularly relevant for cancer therapy. Numerous studies have shown that cell death induced by chemotherapeutic drugs or radiation therapy can induce an immunogenic, type I interferon response through production of DAMPs internally within the cell (eg, mitochondrial DNA, single-stranded DNA, or viral RNA) or through the release of double-stranded DNA and RNA species or other DAMPs (eg, calreticulin, ATP) from cancer cells (Galluzzi et al, 2018). The type I interferon response activates antigen-presenting cells that can then orchestrate an antitumor immune response. Type I interferons can also trigger autocrine and paracrine signaling pathways within cancer cells that can result in cell death, as well as in the expression of interferon-stimulated genes such as CXCL10, a chemo-attractant for T cells. Thus, ICD-inducing therapies can mediate tumor killing through direct cytotoxic effects and indirectly through stimulation of the immune system. This provides a rationale for combining traditional chemotherapies with new immunotherapies such as immune checkpoint blockade, to enhance therapeutic efficacy (see Chap. 21; Sec. 21.5.4). However, it has also been shown that type I and type II interferon responses can be immunosuppressive and promote resistance to cancer therapies because they induce interferon gamma in activated T cells (Minn, 2015; Benci et al, 2016). Interferon gamma stimulates expression of the inhibitory ligand, PD-L1 on antigen-presenting cells and tumor cells, which functions to dampen the antitumor cytotoxic activity of infiltrating T cells, thereby contributing to therapy resistance.

8.4.7 Modifications to Control of Cell Death in Cancer

In addition to promoting the development of neurodegenerative diseases and immune disorders, defective apoptosis also promotes cancer development. Studies of mouse models have confirmed the important role apoptosis plays in suppressing tumorigenesis (Delbridge and Strasser, 2015). Correspondingly, resisting programmed cell death has been proposed as one of 10 hallmarks of cancer (Hanahan and Weinberg, 2011), and numerous genetic and epigenetic mechanisms can enable cells to escape cell death. These mechanisms include loss of function of TP53, aberrant activation of antiapoptotic proteins, inactivation of proapoptotic proteins, and deregulation of the effectors responsible for implementing apoptotic and necroptotic signaling cascades.

Several tumor suppressors (eg, TP53) and oncogenes (eg, c-MYC, BCL-2) are involved in the regulation of apoptosis. The *P53* gene, important for promoting apoptosis and suppressing proliferation, is mutated in approximately 35% of human tumors, and mouse models for Trp53 deficiency have shown increased predisposition for various types of tumors (Lozano, 2010) (Hafner et al, 2019). TP53 is required for the apoptotic response to various stimuli, including DNA damage, oncogenic activation, hypoxia, and ribosomal stress. As a transcription factor, TP53 controls the expression of genes involved in many different cellular processes such as apoptosis, proliferation, metabolism, and DNA repair (see Fig. 8–18). Apoptotic genes that are transcriptionally activated by TP53 include *Bax*, *Noxa*, and *Puma* (Hafner et al, 2019).

The *BCL-2* gene was identified initially in studies of human follicular B-cell lymphoma carrying the translocation t(14-18). This chromosomal translocation results in the overexpression of BCL-2 and inhibition of apoptosis. The antiapoptotic protein MCL-1 is also overexpressed in human malignancies including B-cell lymphoma and myeloma (Delbridge and Strasser, 2015). Homozygous deletion of BIM has been reported in ~20% of human mantle cell lymphomas and epigenetic silencing of BIM or PUMA was found in cancers including lymphomas (Delbridge et al, 2016).

Loss of CASP8 expression driven by DNA hypermethylation of its promoter has been observed in human neuroblastomas with N-MYC amplification, small cell lung carcinoma, and in relapsed glioblastoma multiforme. Inactivation of human *CASP8* by somatic mutation is a recurrent event observed in multiple tumor types, including squamous cell carcinoma of the head and neck (8%), colorectal (4%), breast (1%), and endometrial cancer (7%) (Lawrence et al, 2014).

Cancer cells may harbor alterations that lead to overexpression of IAPs and FLIP that inhibit the intrinsic and extrinsic apoptotic pathways to avoid cell death. Genetic or epigenetic disruptions to genes encoding upstream death receptors such as TRAIL or FAS receptors have been reported in various cancer types. Autophagy has also been shown to play a role in mediating resistance to chemotherapeutic agents through its ability to maintain homeostasis in the face of cellular stress (Mohammad et al, 2015). Elucidation of mechanisms of tumor resistance to cell death has provided the molecular insights necessary to develop therapies targeting these escape mechanisms to enhance cancer therapy.

Novel compounds that modulate cell death, particularly apoptosis, have potential as therapeutic agents, because avoidance of cell death represents a major mechanism of resistance to anticancer therapies. Venetoclax (ABT-199), a BH3-mimetic that antagonizes BCL-2, is approved for the treatment of some hematologic malignancies and acts to augment cell death–regulating pathways in cancer cells (see Chap. 19, Sec. 19.7.3; Singh et al, 2019). As with other targeted approaches, the efficacy of this and related drugs is likely to depend on the state of proteins or pathways being targeted in cancer cells. Because numerous mechanisms conferring resistance to cell death have been identified, biomarkers indicative of specific cell death escape mechanisms may be required to inform the most relevant contexts for therapeutic application of these strategies.

SUMMARY

- The entry of resting cells into cycle, and the orderly progression of cells to synthesize DNA and subsequently to divide at mitosis is tightly regulated by the synthesis, activation, and subsequent degradation of proteins.
- Different CDKs are activated by phosphorylation after binding to corresponding CYCLINs, and allow progression around the cell cycle. Other families of proteins inhibit CDKs, so that both positive and

negative effectors contribute to regulation of cell-cycle progression.
- Expression of molecules that regulate the cell cycle may become disturbed in malignant cells, which results in a loss of control of cell proliferation, and this constitutes a hallmark of cancer.
- Various checkpoints arrest the cell cycle in response to DNA damage or to difficulties in segregating the chromosomes, but these may also be disrupted in the development of malignancy.
- Therapies targeting the cell cycle, including CDK4/6 inhibitors and drugs targeting proteins with key roles in mediating cell-cycle checkpoints have been approved or are being evaluated in clinical trials for the treatment of cancer.
- Different cell death mechanisms, including programmed apoptosis and necroptosis, exist in mammalian cells. Communication between these cell death mechanisms has been identified and is thought to balance prosurvival and prodeath signals.
- Resistance to cell death is achieved by multiple mechanisms and is a hallmark of human cancer.
- Specific inhibitors that promote cell death have been developed and approved. Clinical development of strategies employing these agents is ongoing.

REFERENCES

Altieri DC. Survivin and IAP proteins in cell-death mechanisms. *Biochem J* 2010;430(2):199-205.

Benci JL, Xu B, Qiu Y, et al. Tumor interferon signaling regulates a multigenic resistance program to immune checkpoint blockade. *Cell* 2016;167(6):1540-1554.e12.

Bertoli C, Skotheim JM, de Bruin RAM. Control of cell cycle transcription during G1 and S phases. *Nat Rev Mol Cell Biol* 2013;14(8):518-528.

Blagosklonny MV, Pardee AB. The restriction point of the cell cycle. *Cell Cycle* 2002;1(2):103-110.

Bock FJ, Tait SWG. Mitochondria as multifaceted regulators of cell death. *Nat Rev Mol Cell Biol* 2019;21(2):85-100.

Burgers PMJ, Kunkel TA. Eukaryotic DNA replication fork. *Annu Rev Biochem* 2017;86:417-438.

Burkard ME, Weaver BA. Tuning chromosomal instability to optimize tumor fitness. *Cancer Discov* 2017;7(2):134-136.

Carmena M, Wheelock M, Funabiki H, Earnshaw WC. The chromosomal passenger complex (CPC): from easy rider to the godfather of mitosis. *Nat Rev Mol Cell Biol* 2012;13(12):789-803.

Chen HZ, Tsai SY, Leone G. Emerging roles of E2Fs in cancer: an exit from cell cycle control. *Nat Rev Cancer* 2009;9(11):785-797.

Ciccia A, Elledge SJ. The DNA damage response: making it safe to play with knives. *Mol Cell* 2010;40(2):179-204.

Crasta K, Ganem NJ, Dagher R, et al. DNA breaks and chromosome pulverization from errors in mitosis. *Nature* 2012;482(7383):53-58.

Dang CV. MYC on the path to cancer. *Cell* 2012;149(1):22-35.

Deibler RW, Kirschner MW. Quantitative reconstitution of mitotic CDK1 activation in somatic cell extracts. *Mol Cell* 2010;37(6):753-767.

Delbridge ARD, Strasser A. The BCL-2 protein family, BH3-mimetics and cancer therapy. *Cell Death Differ* 2015;22(7):1071-1080.

Delbridge AR, Grabow S, Strasser A, et al, Thirty years of BCL-2: translating cell death discoveries into novel cancer therapies. *Nat Rev Cancer* 2016;16(2):99-109.

Dephoure N, Zhou C, Villen J, et al, A quantitative atlas of mitotic phosphorylation. *Proc Natl Acad Sci U S A* 2008;105(31):10762-10767.

Dewar JM, Walter JC. Mechanisms of DNA replication termination. *Nat Rev Mol Cell Biol* 2017;18(8):507-516.

Dominguez-Brauer C, Thu KL, Mason JM, Blaser H, Bray MR, Mak TW. Targeting mitosis in cancer: emerging strategies. *Mol Cell* 2015;60(4):524-536.

Dumont S, Mitchison TJ. Force and length in the mitotic spindle. *Curr Biol* 2009;19(17):R749-R761.

Fischer M, Müller GA. Cell cycle transcription control: DREAM/MuvB and RB-E2F complexes. *Crit Rev Biochem Mol Biol* 2017;52(6):638-662.

Fragkos M, Ganier O, Coulombe P, et al. DNA replication origin activation in space and time. *Nat Rev Mol Cell Biol* 2015;16(6):360-374.

Fuchs Y, Steller H. Live to die another way: modes of programmed cell death and the signals emanating from dying cells. *Nat Rev Mol Cell Biol* 2015;16(6):329-344.

Galluzzi L, Buqué A, Kepp O, Zitvogel L, Kroemer G. Immunogenic cell death in cancer and infectious disease. *Nat Rev Immunol* 2017;17(2):97-111.

Galluzzi L, Vitale I, Aaronson SA, et al. Molecular mechanisms of cell death: recommendations of the Nomenclature Committee on Cell Death 2018. *Cell Death Differ* 2018;25(3):486-541.

Ganem NJ, Cornils H, Chiu S-Y, et al. Cytokinesis failure triggers hippo tumor suppressor pathway activation. *Cell* 2014;158(4):833-848.

Gatlin JC, Bloom K. Microtubule motors in eukaryotic spindle assembly and maintenance. *Semin Cell Dev Biol* 2010;21(3):248-254.

Gavet O, Pines J. Progressive activation of cyclinB1-Cdk1 coordinates entry to mitosis. *Dev Cell* 2010;18(4):533-543.

Ge Z, Leighton JS, Wang Y, Peng X, Chen Z, Chen H, Sun Y, Yao F, Li J, Zhang H, Liu J, Shriver CD, Hu H, Cancer Genome Atlas Research Network, Piwnica-Worms H, Ma L, Liang H. Integrated genomic analysis of the ubiquitin pathway across cancer types. *Cell Rep* 2018;23(1):213-226.e3.

Guttinger S, Laurell E, Kutay U. Orchestrating nuclear envelope disassembly and reassembly during mitosis. *Nat Rev Mol Cell Biol* 2009;10(3):178-191.

Hafner A, Bulyk ML, Jambhekar A, et al, The multiple mechanisms that regulate p53 activity and cell fate. *Nat Rev Mol Cell Biol* 2019;xvl(4):199-210.

Hanahan D, Weinberg RA. Hallmarks of cancer: the next generation. *Cell* 2011;144(5):646-674.

Harvey KF, Zhang X, Thomas DM. The Hippo pathway and human cancer. *Nat Rev Cancer* 2013;13(4):246-257.

Holland AJ, Cleveland DW. Losing balance: the origin and impact of aneuploidy in cancer. *EMBO Rep.* 2012;13(6):501-514.

Janku F, Yap TA, Meric-Bernstam F. Targeting the PI3K pathway in cancer: are we making headway? *Nat Rev Clin Oncol* 2018;15(5):273-291.

Jin Z, Li Y, Pitti R, et al, Cullin3-based polyubiquitination and p62-dependent aggregation of caspase-8 mediate extrinsic apoptosis signaling. *Cell* 2009;137(4):721-735.

Jones RG, Thompson CB. Tumor suppressors and cell metabolism: a recipe for cancer growth. *Genes Dev* 2009;23(5):537-548.

Jorgensen P, Tyers M. How cells coordinate growth and division. *Curr Biol* 2004;14(23):R1014-R1027.

Julien O, Wells JA. Caspases and their substrates. *Cell Death Differ* 2017;24(8):1380-1389.

Kalaszczynska I, Geng Y, Iino T, et al. Cyclin A is redundant in fibroblasts but essential in hematopoietic and embryonic stem cells. *Cell* 2009;138(2):352-365.

Karki R, Kanneganti TD. Diverging inflammasome signals in tumorigenesis and potential targeting. *Nat Rev Cancer* 2019;19(4):197-214.

Kastan MB, Bartek J. Cell-cycle checkpoints and cancer. *Nature* 2004;432(7015):316-323.

Kinchen JM, Hengartner MO. Tales of cannibalism, suicide, and murder: programmed cell death in *C. elegans*. *Curr Top Dev Biol* 2005;65:1-45.

Knijnenburg TA, Wang L, Zimmermann MT, et al; Cancer Genome Atlas Research Network. Genomic and molecular landscape of DNA damage repair deficiency across the cancer genome atlas. *Cell Rep* 2018;23(1):239-254.e6.

Komander D, Clague MJ, Urbé S. Breaking the chains: structure and function of the deubiquitinases. *Nat Rev Mol Cell Biol* 2009;10(8):550-563.

Kops GJPL, Weaver BAA, Cleveland DW. On the road to cancer: aneuploidy and the mitotic checkpoint. *Nat Rev Cancer* 2005;5(10):773-785.

Laplante M, Sabatini DM. mTOR signaling in growth control and disease. *Cell* 2012;149(2):274-293.

Lara-Gonzalez P, Westhorpe FG, Taylor SS. The spindle assembly checkpoint. *Curr Biol* 2012;22(22):R966-R980.

Larsen BD, Sorensen CS. The caspase-activated DNase: apoptosis and beyond. *FEBS J* 2017;284(8):1160-1170.

Lawrence MS, Stojanov P, Mermel CH, et al. Discovery and saturation analysis of cancer genes across 21 tumour types. *Nature* 2014;505(7484):495-501.

Levy JMM, Towers CG, Thorburn A. Targeting autophagy in cancer. *Nat Rev Cancer* 2017;17(9):528-542.

Lindqvist A, Rodriguez-Bravo V, Medema RH. The decision to enter mitosis: feedback and redundancy in the mitotic entry network. *J Cell Biol* 2009;185(2):193-202.

Liu P, Cheng H, Roberts TM, Zhao JJ. Targeting the phosphoinositide 3-kinase pathway in cancer. *Nat Rev Drug Discov* 2009;8:627-644.

Lloyd AC. The regulation of cell size. *Cell* 2013;154(6):1194-1205.

Lolli G, Johnson LN. CAK-cyclin-dependent activating kinase: a key kinase in cell cycle control and a target for drugs? *Cell Cycle* 2005;4(4):572-577.

Lozano G. Mouse models of p53 functions. *Cold Spring Harb Perspect Biol* 2010;2(4):a001115.

Malek NP, Sundberg H, McGrew S, et al, A mouse knock-in model exposes sequential proteolytic pathways that regulate p27Kip1 in G1 and S phase. *Nature* 2001;413(6853):323-327.

Malumbres M, Barbacid M. Cell cycle, CDKs and cancer: a changing paradigm. *Nat Rev Cancer* 2009;9(3):153-166.

Malumbres M. Cyclin-dependent kinases. *Genome Biol* 2014;15(6):122.

Mason JM, Lin DC-C, Wei X, et al. Functional characterization of CFI-400945, a Polo-like kinase 4 inhibitor, as a potential anticancer agent. *Cancer Cell* 2014;26(2):163-176.

Mason JM, Wei X, Fletcher GC, et al, Functional characterization of CFI-402257, a potent and selective Mps1/TTK kinase inhibitor, for the treatment of cancer. *Proc Natl Acad Sci U S A* 2017;114(12):3127-3132.

McIlwain DR, Berger T, Mak TW. Caspase functions in cell death and disease. *Cold Spring Harb Perspect Biol* 2013;5(4):a008656.

McIntosh JR. Mitosis. *Cold Spring Harb Perspect Biol* 2016;8(9).

Merrick KA, Larochelle S, Zhang C, et al, Distinct activation pathways confer cyclin-binding specificity on Cdk1 and Cdk2 in human cells. *Mol Cell* 2008;32(5):662-672.

Meyer N, Penn LZ. Reflecting on 25 years with MYC. *Nat Rev Cancer* 2008;8(12):976-990.

Mierzwa B, Gerlich DW. Cytokinetic abscission: molecular mechanisms and temporal control. *Dev Cell* 2014;31(5):525-538.

Minn AJ. Interferons and the immunogenic effects of cancer therapy. *Trends Immunol* 2015;36(11):725-737.

Mohammad RM, Muqbil I, Lowe L, et al. Broad targeting of resistance to apoptosis in cancer. *Semin Cancer Biol* 2015;35(suppl):S78-S103.

Morgan DO. *The Cell Cycle: Principles of Control*. London, UK: New Science Press; 2007.

Musacchio A. The molecular biology of spindle assembly checkpoint signaling dynamics. *Curr Biol* 2015;25(20):R1002-R1018.

Nigg EA. Mitotic kinases as regulators of cell division and its checkpoints. *Nat Rev Mol Cell Biol* 2001;2(1):21-32.

Nigg EA, Holland AJ. Once and only once: mechanisms of centriole duplication and their deregulation in disease. *Nat Rev Mol Cell Biol* 2018;19(5):297-312.

O'Farrell PH. Triggering the all-or-nothing switch into mitosis. *Trends Cell Biol* 2001;11(12):512-519.

Otto T, Sicinski P. Cell cycle proteins as promising targets in cancer therapy. *Nat Rev Cancer* 2017;17(2):93-115.

Patel N, Weekes D, Drosopoulos K, et al. Integrated genomics and functional validation identifies malignant cell specific dependencies in triple negative breast cancer. *Nat Commun* 2018;9(1):1044.

Peters JM, Nishiyama T. Sister chromatid cohesion. *Cold Spring Harb Perspect Biol* 2012;4(11).

Peters JM, Tedeschi A, Schmitz J. The cohesin complex and its roles in chromosome biology. *Genes Dev* 2008;22:3089-3114.

Pikor L, Thu K, Vucic E, et al, The detection and implication of genome instability in cancer. *Cancer Metastasis Rev* 2013;32(3-4):341-352.

Prosser SL, Pelletier L. Mitotic spindle assembly in animal cells: a fine balancing act. *Nat Rev Mol Cell Biol* 2017;18(3): 187-201.

Sanchez-Vega F, Mina M, Armenia J, et al. Oncogenic signaling pathways in the cancer genome atlas. *Cell* 2018;173(2): 321-37.e10.

Santamaria D, Barriere C, Cerqueira A, et al. CDK1 is sufficient to drive the mammalian cell cycle. *Nature* 2007;448(7155): 811-815.

Sansregret L, Patterson JO, Dewhurst S, et al. APC/C dysfunction limits excessive cancer chromosomal instability. *Cancer Discov* 2017;7(2):218-233.

Sansregret L, Vanhaesebroeck B, Swanton C. Determinants and clinical implications of chromosomal instability in cancer. *Nat Rev Clin Oncol* 2018;15(3):139-150.

Senft D, Qi J, Ronai ZA. Ubiquitin ligases in oncogenic transformation and cancer therapy. *Nat Rev Cancer* 2018; 18(2):69-88.

Sherr CJ, Roberts JM. CDK inhibitors: positive and negative regulators of G1-phase progression. *Genes Dev* 1999;13(12):1501-1512.

Singh R, Letai A, Sarosiek K. Regulation of apoptosis in health and disease: the balancing act of BCL-2 family proteins. *Nat Rev Mol Cell Biol* 2019;20(3):175-193.

Sivakumar S, Gorbsky GJ. Spatiotemporal regulation of the anaphase-promoting complex in mitosis. *Nat Rev Mol Cell Biol* 2015;16(2):82-94.

Skaar JR, Pagan JK, Pagano M. SCF ubiquitin ligase-targeted therapies. *Nat Rev Drug Discov* 2014;13(12):889-903.

Strasser A, Jost PJ, Nagata S. The many roles of FAS receptor signaling in the immune system. *Immunity* 2009;30(2):180-192.

Sullivan M, Morgan DO. Finishing mitosis, one step at a time. *Nat Rev Mol Cell Biol* 2007;8(11):894-903.

Thompson SL, Compton DA. Examining the link between chromosomal instability and aneuploidy in human cells. *J Cell Biol* 2008;180(4):665-672.

Thu KL, Silvester J, Elliott MJ, et al. Disruption of the anaphase-promoting complex confers resistance to TTK inhibitors in triple-negative breast cancer. *Proc Natl Acad Sci U S A* 2018;115(7):E1570-E1577.

Thu KL, Soria-Bretones I, Mak TW, et al, Targeting the cell cycle in breast cancer: towards the next phase. *Cell Cycle* 2018;17(15):1871-1885.

Van Opdenbosch N, Lamkanfi M. Caspases in cell death, inflammation, and disease. *Immunity* 2019;50(6):1352-1364.

Vander Heiden MG, Cantley LC, Thompson CB. Understanding the Warburg effect: the metabolic requirements of cell proliferation. *Science* 2009;324(5930): 1029-1033.

Veitch ZW, Cescon DW, Denny T, et al, Safety and tolerability of CFI-400945, a first-in-class, selective PLK4 inhibitor in advanced solid tumours: a phase 1 dose-escalation trial. *Br J Cancer* 2019;121(4):318-324.

Vitale I, Galluzzi L, Castedo M, et al, Mitotic catastrophe: a mechanism for avoiding genomic instability. *Nat Rev Mol Cell Biol* 2011;12(6):385-392.

Vitre BD, Cleveland DW. Centrosomes, chromosome instability (CIN) and aneuploidy. *Curr Opin Cell Biol* 2012;24(6):809-815.

Vucic D, Dixit VM, Wertz IE. Ubiquitylation in apoptosis: a post-translational modification at the edge of life and death. *Nat Rev Mol Cell Biol* 2011;12(7):439-452.

Walczak CE, Cai S, Khodjakov A. Mechanisms of chromosome behaviour during mitosis. *Nat Rev Mol Cell Biol* 2010;11(2):91-102.

Wang G, Jiang Q, Zhang C. The role of mitotic kinases in coupling the centrosome cycle with the assembly of the mitotic spindle. *J Cell Sci* 2014;127(pt 19):4111-4122.

Ward PS, Thompson CB. Signaling in control of cell growth and metabolism. *Cold Spring Harb Perspect Biol* 2012;4(7):a006783.

Weber AM, Ryan AJ. ATM and ATR as therapeutic targets in cancer. *Pharmacol Ther* 2015;149:124-138.

Wei W, Ayad NG, Wan Y, et al. Degradation of the SCF component Skp2 in cell-cycle phase G1 by the anaphase-promoting complex. *Nature* 2004;428(6979):194-198.

Weinlich R, Oberst A, Beere HM, Green DR. Necroptosis in development, inflammation and disease. *Nat Rev Mol Cell Biol* 2017;18(2):127-36.

Wertz IE, Dixit VM. Regulation of death receptor signaling by the ubiquitin system. *Cell Death Differ* 2010;17(1):14-24.

Wild T, Larsen MSY, Narita T, Schou J, Nilsson J, Choudhary C. The spindle assembly checkpoint is not essential for viability of human cells with genetically lowered APC/C activity. *Cell Rep* 2016;14(8):1829-1840.

Williams GH, Romanowski P, Morris L, et al. Improved cervical smear assessment using antibodies against proteins that regulate DNA replication. *Proc Natl Acad Sci U S A* 1998;95(25):14932-14937.

Wurzenberger C, Gerlich DW. Phosphatases: providing safe passage through mitotic exit. *Nat Rev Mol Cell Biol* 2011;12(8):469-482.

Youle RJ, Strasser A. The BCL-2 protein family: opposing activities that mediate cell death. *Nat Rev Mol Cell Biol* 2008;9(1):47-59.

Zamaraev AV, Kopeina GS, Prokhorova EA, et al. Post-translational modification of caspases: the other side of apoptosis regulation. *Trends Cell Biol* 2017;27(5):322-339.

Zhang S, Chen Q, Liu Q, et al. Hippo signaling suppresses cell ploidy and tumorigenesis through Skp2. *Cancer Cell* 2017;31(5):669-684.e7.

Zilfou JT, Lowe SW. Tumor suppressive functions of p53. *Cold Spring Harb Perspect Biol* 2009;1(5):a001883.

Genomic Stability and DNA Repair

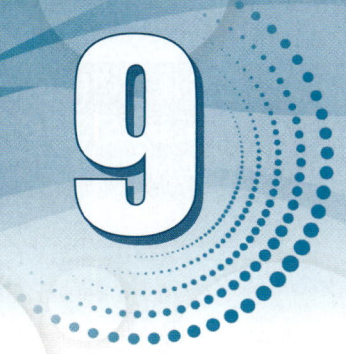

Guillaume Laflamme, Yahya Benslimane, and Damien D'Amours

Chapter Outline

9.1 Introduction
9.2 Genetic Instability as the Basis for Malignant Transformation
    9.2.1 Intrinsic Causes of Genetic Instability
    9.2.2 Extrinsic Causes of Genetic Instability
9.3 DNA Repair Pathways
    9.3.1 Mismatch Repair
    9.3.2 Base Excision Repair
    9.3.3 Nucleotide Excision Repair
    9.3.4 DNA Double-Strand Break Repair: Homologous Recombination
    9.3.5 DNA Double-Strand Break Repair: Nonhomologous End-Joining
    9.3.6 DNA Crosslink Repair: Fanconi Anemia Proteins
9.4 Cell-Cycle Checkpoints and Genome Stability
    9.4.1 DNA Damage Checkpoints
    9.4.2 Mitotic Spindle Checkpoints
    9.4.3 Checkpoint Silencing by Adaptation or Inactivation

9.5 Human DNA Repair Disorders and Familial Cancers
    9.5.1 Ataxia Telangiectasia
    9.5.2 Xeroderma Pigmentosum and Related Disorders
    9.5.3 Hereditary Nonpolyposis Colon Cancer
    9.5.4 Li-Fraumeni Syndrome
    9.5.5 Fanconi Anemia
    9.5.6 BRCA1/2
9.6 Assays of DNA Damage and Repair
9.7 Regulation of Telomere Length and Cancer
    9.7.1 Telomeres Protect Chromosomal Ends from Recognition as DNA Damage
    9.7.2 Telomere Regulation in Normal Cell Proliferation
    9.7.3 Shelterin and Telomere Integrity
    9.7.4 Telomere Maintenance and Cancer
Summary
References

9.1 INTRODUCTION

There is overwhelming evidence that mutations can cause cancer. Major evidence for the genetic origin of cancer includes (1) the observation of Ames that many carcinogens are also mutagens (Ames et al, 1981) and (2) the finding that genetically determined traits associated with a deficiency in the enzymes necessary to repair lesions in DNA are associated with an increased risk of cancer. Mutations may occur in the germline of an individual and be represented in every cell in the body, or they may occur in a single somatic cell and be identified in a tumor following clonal proliferation. As described in Chapter 7, all species have numerous genes called *cellular oncogenes* (or *proto-oncogenes*), many of which are homologous to the transforming oncogenes carried by specific RNA retroviruses. Some human tumors have mutations in these oncogenes that may have led to their activation. However, there is no evidence for germline mutations in cellular oncogenes, perhaps because such mutations in the germline are lethal even in the heterozygous state. In contrast, there is good evidence for germline mutations affecting *tumor-suppressor genes*, which can lead to familial clustering of cancer or transmission of predisposition to tumors. In such cases, the loss of function of a tumor-suppressor gene is inherited in a Mendelian manner.

The maintenance of genetic information is important for prevention of genetic instability and carcinogenesis. In this chapter, intrinsic and extrinsic causes of genomic instability are discussed and the biochemical pathways that act to repair DNA lesions and the function of cell-cycle checkpoints following DNA damage are described. The methods used to evaluate DNA damage sensing and repair are detailed and human disorders that result in defective DNA damage sensing and repair are discussed. Finally, the maintenance of chromosomal length and telomere integrity is highlighted. Throughout the chapter, examples are given of the importance of each of these factors in the genesis, diagnosis, and treatment of human cancer.

9.2 GENETIC INSTABILITY AS THE BASIS FOR MALIGNANT TRANSFORMATION

9.2.1 Intrinsic Causes of Genetic Instability

Cellular carcinogenesis is known to require sequential mutations in DNA (see Chap. 5, Sec. 5.1). Damaged DNA is produced by numerous mechanisms, including (1) spontaneous reactions of DNA with the aqueous environment, (2) influence of metabolic by-products such as reactive oxygen or nitrogen species, (3) action of environmental mutagens such as radon and chemical exposure, and (4) errors during DNA replication. These mechanisms can produce abasic sites, deamination, base alterations, and single-strand and double-strand DNA breaks, with as many as 10^5 DNA lesions per cell per day (Hoeijmakers, 2009; Ciccia and Elledge, 2010). Unless the cell can protect and maintain the integrity of the genome, these genetic alterations may cause cancer by activating proto-oncogenes and/or inactivating tumor-suppressor genes. Natural mutation rates appear sufficient to drive the selection required for formation of many tumors (Bodmer et al, 2008). Some inactivating mutations occur in genes responsible for maintaining genomic integrity or DNA repair, which facilitate the development of a *mutator* cellular phenotype (Fig. 9–1; Loeb, 1991). Regardless of the nature of the genotoxic insult, genomic instability is believed to be the main "enabler" of malignant transformation.

There are mechanisms other than mutation that lead to genetic instability, including *gene amplification*, whole chromosome gain/loss, and the epigenetic modification of chromatin-associated transcriptional states through *gene methylation* and *gene acetylation* (see also Chap. 3, Sec. 3.1). In cells that display *gene amplification*, gene expression is

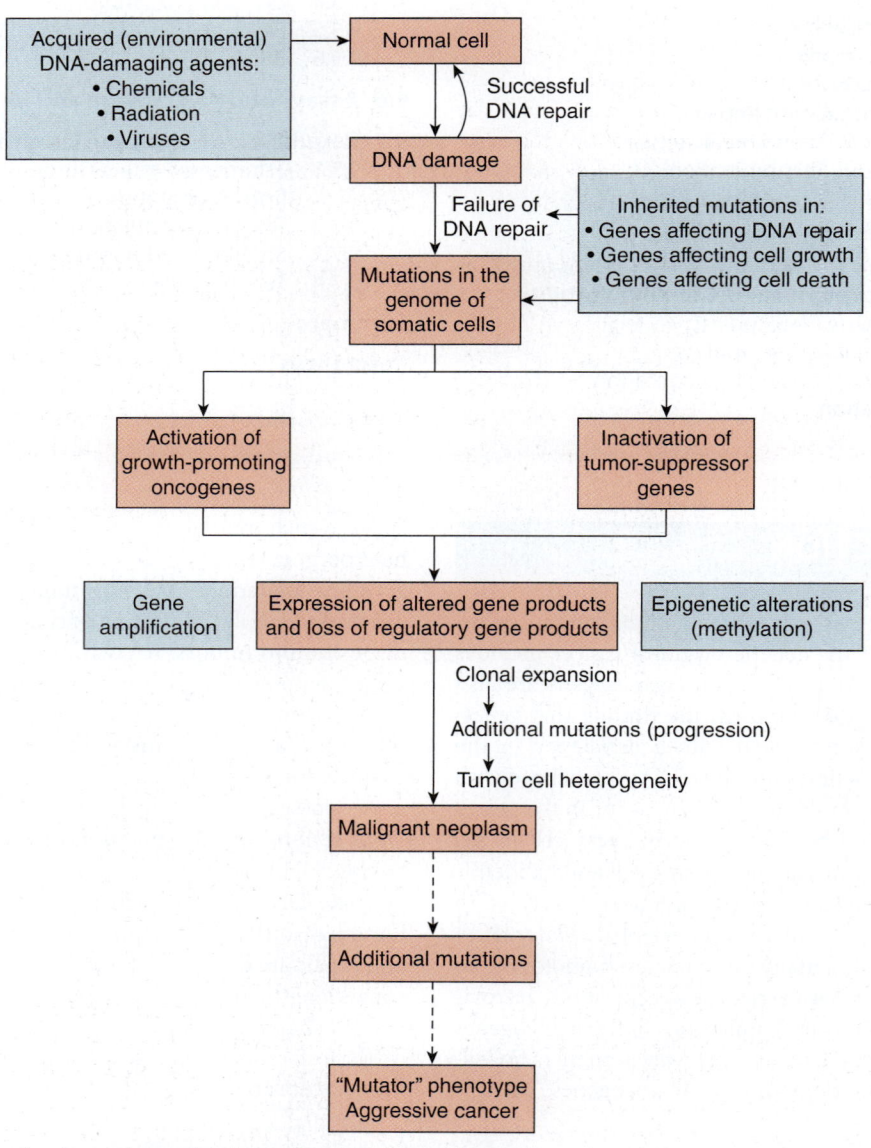

FIGURE 9–1 Genetic and epigenetic mechanisms of genetic instability.

aberrantly and constitutively enhanced above normal levels required for tissue homeostasis. Gene-amplified cells can display discrete cytogenetic changes, such as *double-minute (DM) chromosomes* or *homogeneously staining regions (HSRs)*. Cells may also acquire drug-resistance via mutation, gene amplification, or epigenetic changes (see Chap. 18). Consequently, the prevalence of drug-resistant variants in a cell population is an indirect measure of genetic instability. For instance, monitoring of specific markers of drug resistance in tissue culture has revealed that gene amplification can occur at a high frequency in transformed cells (10^{-7} to 10^{-3} events per cell per generation), yet it is almost undetectable in normal diploid fibroblasts (a frequency of less than 10^{-8} events per cell per generation; Tlsty, 1990).

If the amplified gene is a positive regulator of DNA replication or cell-cycle progression, gene overexpression may result in increased cellular proliferation, leading to clonal selection and malignant transformation. Some amplified oncogenes, such as human epidermal growth receptor 2 (*HER2*) in breast cancer and the *N-MYC* gene in neuroblastoma, are predictors of poor prognosis in those patients who harbor tumors containing them (see Chap. 7, Sec. 7.4-7.5, and Chap. 20, Sec. 20.3).

The structure and activity of chromatin can be altered by post-translational modifications such as acetylation, phosphorylation, methylation, and ubiquitylation. *Methylation* of DNA plays an important role in control of gene expression and normal cellular differentiation (see also Chap. 3) and is observed commonly in tumor-suppressor genes that cause familial cancers. In these tumors, there is methylation of normally unmethylated cytosine phosphate guanine (CpG) islands within the DNA. Methylation-induced transcriptional silencing can affect many genes that are important in tumor progression: they include genes involved in cell-cycle control (eg, p16^{INK4a}; see Chap. 8, Sec. 8.2), transcription, hormone biology (ie, estrogen and progesterone receptor genes; see Chap. 20, Sec. 20.2), intracellular signal transduction (see Chap. 6), apoptosis (see Chap. 8, Sec. 8.4), DNA repair, and tumor-suppressor genes (eg, retinoblastoma [Rb]; see Chap. 7, Sec. 7.6). Given that methylation is potentially reversible, it creates a target for novel therapeutic strategies involving gene reactivation. For example, both retinoic acid and 5′-*aza*-deoxycytidine can reverse DNA methylation and reactivate gene expression of normal regulatory genes (eg, cyclin-dependent kinases), thereby leading to regression of some human leukemias.

Histones are the core protein components of chromatin, and their acetylation status regulates, in part, gene expression. Two groups of enzymes, the histone deacetylases (HDACs) and the histone acetyl transferases (HATs), regulate the level of histone acetylation. Deacetylated histones are generally tightly coiled with the DNA and are associated with silencing of gene expression; in contrast, the acetylation of histones leads to the uncoiling of chromatin and is associated with gene expression. Inhibition of HDACs in cancer cells can lead to transcriptional activation of approximately 2% of human genes, including tumor-suppressor genes. Treating cells with HDAC inhibitors increases cell-cycle arrest, induction of apoptosis, and cancer cell differentiation, in vitro and in vivo, by promoting p21^{WAF} CDK-mediated cell-cycle inhibition and downregulation of pro-proliferative Raf/Mek/Erk cell signaling (see Chap. 6, Sec. 6.2). Several HDAC inhibitors have shown antitumor activity and have been approved for treatment of hematologic malignancies, but they have limited activity against solid tumors (Falkenberg and Johnstone, 2014; see Chap. 20, Sec. 20.4).

Normal tissues may have different inherent abilities to maintain their genetic integrity when faced with similar exogenous or endogenous damaging stimuli. Comparison of primary stromal versus primary epithelial cell cultures suggests that normal epithelial cells may be predisposed to genetic instability. Stromal cells (eg, fibroblasts) eventually lose the ability to proliferate in culture (termed *cellular senescence*) as a result of loss of chromosomal telomere DNA (see Sec. 9.6). Other cell types, such as human mammary epithelial cultures (HMECs), exhibit genetic alterations caused by loss of DNA repair and checkpoint control during cell proliferation that enable increased population doublings; rare cells can then escape cellular senescence and become immortalized (Lecot et al, 2016; Fig. 9–2). There are also differences between stromal and epithelial cultures in their ability to initiate cell-cycle checkpoints following DNA damage. These factors may contribute to the higher incidence of epithelial-based compared to stromal-based tumors in humans. There is also evidence that genetic stability is maintained in stem cells when compared to somatic cells, in part due to altered regulation of DNA repair (Woodward and Bristow, 2009).

The identification of specific biomarkers of genetic instability in premalignant human tissues is an important objective of a large number of studies (see also Chap. 2). This information can be used to ascertain whether an individual requires screening for early detection of cancer, lifestyle change, or treatment with a chemopreventive agent (if available) based on the biomarker panel, familial susceptibility, and carcinogenic insult. Tissue biomarkers can be related to mechanisms of DNA repair, cell-cycle checkpoint control, altered oncogenes or tumor-suppressor genes, or chromosomal aberrations. Biopsies have been obtained from high-risk patients (eg, bronchial biopsies from chronic smokers, oral or laryngeal biopsies from individuals with premalignancy) and examined for chromosome instability using in situ hybridization (Hittelman, 2001). Biopsies often show evidence of chromosome instability throughout the exposed tissue, with multifocal clonal outgrowths that can persist for many years, and that may account for continued risk of lung cancer following smoking cessation. Consistent with this view, recent studies indicate that chromosome instability promotes metastasis in models of triple-negative breast cancer and lung adenocarcinoma (Bakhoum et al, 2018). Future investigation may lead to the discovery of new compounds that can limit genetic instability or its effects in a given tissue, thereby preventing cancer. Recent advances indicate this might be achieved by manipulation of effectors of checkpoint responses, such as BubR1, or by senolysis (ie, the selective elimination of senescent cells; Childs et al, 2017). However, these approaches are not without risk since modulation of senescence may result in detrimental effects on cells homeostasis and patients (Sieben et al, 2018).

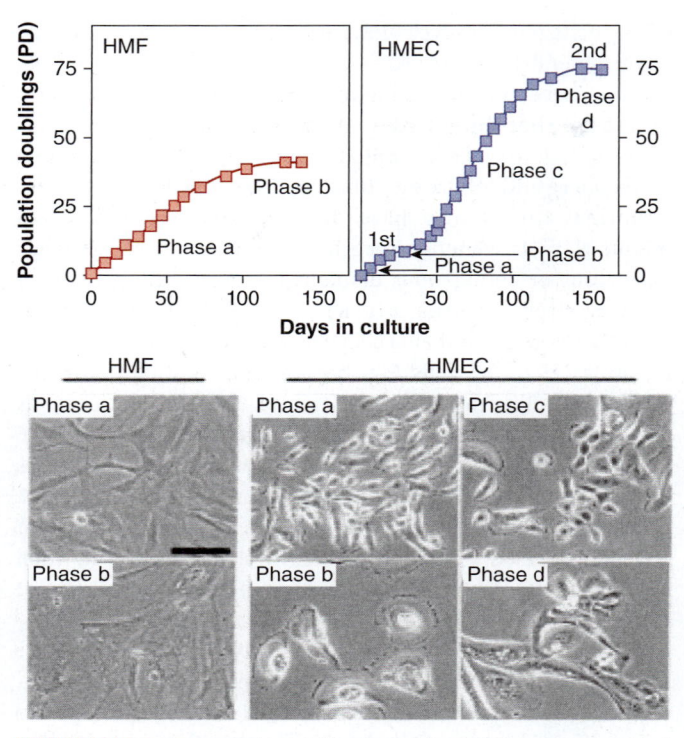

FIGURE 9–2 Genetic instability in epithelial tissues compared to stromal tissues. Data showing that human mammary fibroblasts (HMFs; left upper panel) undergo a limited number of cell divisions (phase a) before undergoing irreversible arrest, called *senescence* (phase b). In contrast, human mammary epithelial cultures (HMECs; upper right panel) exhibit an initial growth phase (phase a) that is followed by a transient growth plateau (termed *selection* or phase b), from which proliferative cells emerge to undergo further population doublings (phase c; approximately 20-70 doublings) before entering a second growth plateau (phase d). Seen in the panels below are representative cell images from each phase for each cell type. HMECs emerge from senescence, exhibit eroding telomeric sequences (see Sec. 9.7) and, ultimately, enter telomere-based crisis to generate the types of chromosomal abnormalities seen in the earliest lesions of breast cancer and point to differences between epithelial cells and fibroblasts during neoplastic transformation. (Reproduced with permission from Romanov SR, Kozakiewicz BK, Holst CR, et al: Normal human mammary epithelial cells spontaneously escape senescence and acquire genomic changes. *Nature* 2001 Feb 1;409(6820):633-637.)

9.2.2 Extrinsic Causes of Genetic Instability

Many extracellular factors also place pressure on the genome. Extrinsic sources of genetic instability include ultraviolet light (UV), ionizing radiation (IR), and chemical carcinogens (see Chap. 6).

9.2.2.1 Ultraviolet Radiation There is a correlation between latitude (average sun exposure) and the incidence of malignant tumors of the skin, with the tumors tending to occur on sun-exposed areas, such as the face. Genetic background is also a determining factor, especially low skin pigmentation, as this allows a high UV dose to be delivered to the cells at risk in the basal layer of the epidermis. Chronic exposure to sunlight is required for carcinogenesis, suggesting the need for multiple interactions of UV radiation with the target cells.

UV-induced tumors in mice demonstrate point mutations in the *Tp53* tumor-suppressor gene (see Chap. 7, Sec. 7.6), and these mutations are primarily C-to-T transitions (Kress et al, 1992). More than 50% of skin cancers in humans (both squamous and basal cell carcinomas) also have characteristic p53 mutations (Ziegler et al, 1993). Many of these mutations are CC-to-TT transitions and are characteristic of misrepair or lack of repair of pyrimidine dimers in the DNA induced by the exposure to the UV radiation (Daya-Grosjean et al, 1995). Such dimers may be repaired by numerous processes, including nucleotide excision repair (see Sec. 9.3.3). There is an increased risk of skin cancer in patients with xeroderma pigmentosum (XP), an inherited disease in which there is a deficiency in nucleotide excision repair (de Gruijl et al, 2001). The high incidence of p53 mutations found in preneoplastic lesions may cause genomic instability, which is consistent with the frequent loss of heterozygosity (LOH; see Chap. 7, Sec. 7.2) seen in basal cell carcinoma (BCC; 9q) and squamous cell carcinoma (SCC; 3p, 9q, 13p, 17p, 17q), although LOH has also been observed in the absence of p53 mutations. The LOH at 9q is associated with deletion or mutation of the patched (PTCH) gene (see Chap. 6, Sec. 6.4), and 70% to 90% of BCC in XP patients have PTCH mutations (Daya-Grosjean and Sarasin, 2000). The PTCH gene is part of the Hedgehog (Hh) signaling pathway that can cause activation of the Gli transcription factors in human cells. One of the downstream targets of Gli is the *BCL2* gene, which acts to inhibit apoptosis (see Chap. 6, Sec. 6.4). Activation of this pathway may also override the G_1-arrest associated with the p21 (*WAF1*) gene (see Chap. 8, Sec. 8.3).

In familial cutaneous melanoma, there are markers on 9p21 that map to the *INK4a,b* locus, which codes for the cyclin-dependent kinase inhibitors p16 and p15 (see Chap. 8, Sec. 8.2). Alternate splicing of this locus encodes another protein, p14^{ARF}, which can stabilize p53 by binding to the product of *HDM2* gene (the human ortholog of MDM2) to interfere with degradation of p53 (see Chap. 7, Sec. 7.6). Loss of INK4a (p16) appears to be the most important defect in familial cutaneous melanoma, whereas, in sporadic disease, point mutations typical of UV irradiation can be observed in this gene. Mutations affecting telomere length regulators (see Sec. 9.7) are also significant drivers of melanoma and other cancers (Heidenreich and Kumar, 2017). Finally, up to 70% of melanomas exhibit BRAF mutations that are associated with UV-induced lesions (Besaratinia and Pfeifer, 2008). Thus, skin cancers are clearly associated with UV damage to DNA.

9.2.2.2 Ionizing Radiation The carcinogenic risks of radiation exposure have been derived from many sources, including occupational exposures (eg, early radiologists and uranium miners), therapeutic exposures (eg, unavoidable treatment of normal tissues in cancer therapy, or treatment of ankylosing spondylitis), and accidental exposures (see Chap. 15 and 16). Most information comes from studies of A-bomb survivors in Hiroshima and Nagasaki, from studies of civilian populations exposed to radioactive materials released during the Chernobyl accident, and from studies of exposures during medical radiographic examinations, particularly of pregnant women, which resulted in fetal exposure to irradiation. These people were exposed to acute doses of radiation (eg, Bazyka et al, 2018), and extrapolation of the risks associated with lower levels of continuous exposure has relied on more limited information from occupational exposures and on experimental studies and modeling. Studies of radiation transformation in cultured cells point toward a high-frequency initial step followed by a rare second step (Little, 2000). The important initial effect of radiation appears to be the induction of genetic instability (Syljuasen et al, 2001; Morgan et al, 2002), which then allows for a higher probability of "rare" mutations that lead to malignant transformation. These observations, that radiation tends to increase the incidence of the types of tumors that arise naturally in the population, and that exposure at earlier ages leads to increased relative risk, are consistent with the concept that radiation acts to induce genetic instability.

The mechanism(s) by which genetic instability is induced by radiation and maintained in the population are uncertain, but probably include (1) mutations in genes involved in control of DNA synthesis or DNA repair, such as the mismatch repair system (see Sec. 9.3.1); (2) the induction of chromosome instability; and (3) persistent aberrant production of oxygen radicals that can damage DNA (Little, 2000; Morgan et al, 2002). Irradiated cells acquire further mutations and chromosome instability for many generations after exposure both in vitro and in vivo (Morgan et al, 2002).

Hanahan and Weinberg (2010) reviewed the evidence for a model whereby the induction of genetic instability is a key driver of subsequent mutagenic events that induce malignant transformation. Ionizing radiation induces deletions, translocations, or inversion of DNA sequences that may induce genetic instability secondary to DNA repair and cell-cycle checkpoint defects (Cox, 1994). Alternatively, chromosome breakage followed by faulty repair and translocation or amplification of DNA segments are also possible mechanisms for activation of genetic instability.

9.3 DNA REPAIR PATHWAYS

About 10^5 DNA lesions are produced every day in a typical cell (Sec. 9.2.1). To prevent fixation and propagation of these genetic lesions in progenitor cells, organisms in all domains of life have evolved multiple mechanisms to detect and remove these lesions. An improved understanding of the mechanisms of DNA repair in mammals came from the isolation of repair-deficient rodent cells (eg, Chinese hamster ovary [CHO] mutants) with unusual sensitivity to different classes of DNA-damaging agents (Thompson et al, 1982). Some mutants exhibited extreme sensitivity to UV light and crosslinking agents, such as mitomycin C, but little or no sensitivity to x-rays. Other cells exhibited sensitivity to x-rays and chemical agents known to cause DNA breakage, but little or no sensitivity to UV light or crosslinking agents. These various phenotypes, which mimicked those characterized previously in bacteria and yeast, indicated the involvement of several DNA repair pathways. Some of these repair pathways are so highly conserved that yeast proteins can substitute for their human counterparts and vice versa in complementation assays. This high degree of conservation has been instrumental in the cloning and functional characterization of the human homologs of yeast DNA repair genes.

Some frequent lesions, such as those formed by oxidation or DNA-reactive carcinogens, induce structurally distinct mutagenic and cytotoxic damage to the DNA (see Chap. 5, Sec. 5.2). Some of these adducts are recognized and repaired directly by a class of enzymes that are used only once (Yi and He, 2013). For example, induction of $O(6)$-methylguanine (O^6-meG) by oxidation or N-nitroso compounds is recognized by $O(6)$-alkylguanine DNA *alkyltransferase,* which reverts the O^6-meG to guanine in a single-step irreversible reaction that inactivates the enzyme and prevents mutagenic G:C→A:T transitions.

An important property in DNA repair is the fidelity of the repair pathway, leading to the concepts of error-prone and error-resistant (or error-free) DNA repair. Many DNA lesions can block transcription of RNA, and persistent blockage of RNA synthesis can lead to cell death. These lesions are often repaired through the *transcription-coupled repair* pathway (see Sec. 9.3.3); this pathway is designed to displace the stalled RNA polymerase and drive a high-priority repair mechanism. For lesions that block progression of the replication fork during DNA replication, several error-prone DNA polymerases have been described that have increased flexibility and low fidelity to allow for replicative bypass (ie, translesion DNA synthesis) of the base damage contained within DNA (Lange et al, 2011). These polymerases can be used temporarily by the cell during acute DNA replication damage and, subsequently, substituted by more accurate DNA polymerases. Use of these lower-fidelity bypass DNA polymerases can contribute to high error rates during DNA replication and may lead to malignant transformation. This process is diagrammed in Figure 9–3 and is known as *translesion DNA synthesis.*

Discrete biochemical pathways of DNA repair are described in the following sections. These pathways can be divided into different classes depending on the specific DNA lesion they are designed to repair, and include (1) mismatch repair, (2) base excision repair, (3) nucleotide excision repair, (4) single-strand break repair, and (5) homologous and nonhomologous repair of DNA double-strand breaks (DSBs).

9.3.1 Mismatch Repair

The mismatch repair (MMR) pathway is enacted when the proofreading activity of DNA-polymerases fails, resulting in the incorporation of incorrect bases during the process of DNA replication. The MMR pathway is also required when the polymerase creates helical distortions by inserting or deleting bases in short oligonucleotide repeats (microsatellites) during replication. These helical distortions are termed *insertion-deletion loops* (Li, 2008; Kunkel and Erie, 2015). The process of MMR consists of 3 steps: (1) recognition of the mismatched DNA

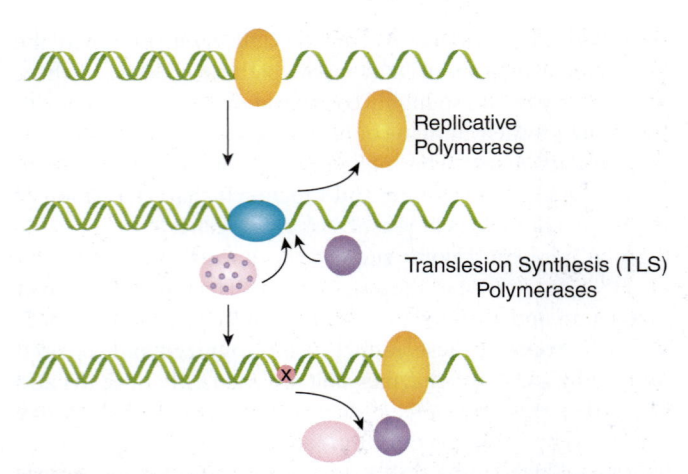

FIGURE 9–3 Translesion DNA synthesis. The "DNA polymerase switch model" for translesion synthesis and mutagenesis. This cartoon shows the replicative DNA polymerase (yellow sphere) blocked at a template lesion site. Cells contain several different DNA polymerases (other indicated spheres) that transiently replace the replicative DNA polymerase. After a short patch of synthesis in the vicinity of the lesion, the replicative DNA polymerase resumes high fidelity and processive synthesis.

bases, (2) excision of the error-containing bases, and (3) DNA synthesis by polymerases and ligation (Fig. 9–4). The protein products of MMR genes form heterodimer complexes, and different protein pairs recognize specific mismatched nucleotides or insertion-deletion loops in DNA. For example, the MSH2 protein forms a heterodimer with an additional MMR protein, MSH6 or MSH3, and the resulting complexes are called MutS-α or MutS-β, respectively. MUTS-α is required for the recognition of DNA base-base mismatches, whereas MutS-α and MutS-β have partially redundant functions for the recognition of DNA insertion-deletion loops. A second heterodimer forms between the MMR gene product MLH1 and PMS2 or MLH3 to form MutLα and MutLβ, respectively. The MutL complexes coordinate the interplay between the initial mismatch recognition complex and subsequent protein interactions required to complete MMR. The latter proteins include proliferating cell nuclear antigen (PCNA), DNA polymerases δ and ε, and possibly DNA helicases that unwind the DNA helix to facilitate DNA synthesis (Hoeijmakers, 2001).

9.3.2 Base Excision Repair

Spontaneous oxidative damage is known to occur in cells producing 10^4 to 10^5 oxidative residues, such as 8-*oxo*-deoxyguanosine (8-oxoG), per cell per day among the approximately 3×10^9 bases in the human genome. DNA base damage,

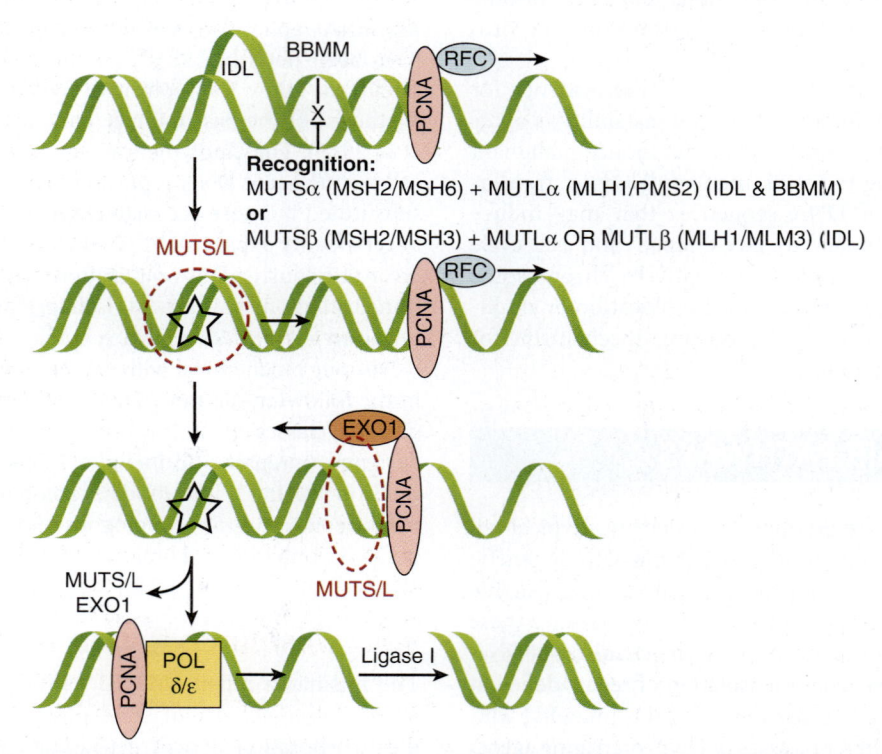

FIGURE 9–4 Mismatch repair (MMR). The mismatch repair pathway is initiated either when a base is misincorporated to create a base–base mismatch (BBMM) or when insertion-deletion loops (IDLs) are created during replication in microsatellite regions. These lesions are recognized by different complexes: MSH2/MSH6 (MutSα) + MLH1/PMS2 (MutLα) recognize BBMMs and IDLs, whereas MSH2/MSH3 (MutSβ) + MutLα or MLH1/MLH3 (MutLβ) can also recognize IDLs. Whichever MutS/L complex is used, it translocates along DNA until it reaches the proliferating cell nuclear antigen (PCNA) associated with the replication factor complex (RFC) at the site of the replication fork. Next, the nuclease EXO1 is loaded and activated, which resects the fork backward past the lesion, at which point MutS/L and EXO1 are unloaded. The DNA polymerase δ and ε (POL δ/ε) fills the gap and Ligase I seals the nick if necessary.

occurring via endogenous oxidative processes or exogenous DNA damage (eg, from ionizing radiation) is repaired by the *base excision repair (BER)* pathway (David et al, 2007). BER involves the enzymatic removal of the damaged DNA base by DNA glycosylases, which cleave glycosidic bonds and are specific to particular DNA base lesions. Two classes of DNA glycosylases differ in their reaction mechanism: monofunctional enzymes leave the DNA strand intact and bifunctional DNA glycosylases cleave the DNA backbone (Fig. 9–5). For example, the OGG1 protein is a bifunctional 8-oxoguanine DNA glycosylase that removes spontaneous or ionizing radiation–induced lesions to prevent cellular mutations. During BER, the initial base removal step leaves an apurinic or apyrimidinic site that resembles a single-strand DNA break. Such single-strand breaks can be induced by free radicals or by ionizing radiation without the action of DNA glycosylases, and repair of these 2 types of lesions (base damage and single-strand breaks) converge into this common pathway, as shown in Figure 9–5. The major pathway is *short-*patch base excision repair and involves the replacement of a single nucleotide following DNA backbone cleavage at the base excision site. A minor pathway is the *long-patch* base excision-repair pathway, which enables the repair of 2 to 13 damaged nucleotides.

Knockout mice engineered to lack core proteins in the BER pathway die as embryos, attesting to its important role in development. Genetic mouse knockout models that are disrupted in various glycosylase genes have shown only mild increases in genetic mutations. Nevertheless, this limited increase in mutagenesis incidence is likely to be relevant for human health, as patients carrying germline mutations in MUTYH, a glycosylase responsible for 8-oxoG removal by BER, suffer from a hereditary syndrome associated with enhanced colorectal carcinogenesis (see Table 9–1). The limited impact of glycosylase inactivation on rates of mutagenesis may reflect partial redundancy in the substrate repertoire of glycosylases and/or overlap with transcription-coupled repair processes described below. Base excision repair may be defective in cells that have mutations in p53 as the p53 protein can stimulate BER by direct interactions with APE1 and DNA-Polβ (Offer et al, 2001). Indeed, the gene locus encoding the glycosylase 8-oxoguanine glycosylase (OGG1) on chromosome 3p25-26 is frequently lost in lung cancers, consistent with a purported role in preventing carcinogenesis. The effect associated with loss/reduction of glycosylase activity is not limited to cancer as mice carrying mutations in glycosylase-encoding genes are severely affected in multiple aspects of their physiology (reviewed in Sampath, 2014).

Inhibitors of poly(ADP-ribose) polymerase (PARP) have been approved for cancer treatment (see Chap. 19, Sec. 19.6). As shown in Figure 9–5, PARP activity is required at an intermediate step preceding DNA synthesis during BER or when single-stranded DNA regions are recognized. When PARP is inhibited, accumulation of single-stranded gaps leads to collapse of DNA replication forks during S phase. Homologous recombination (see below) can rescue these collapsed forks and prevent DSB formation. However, when homologous recombination is defective, such as in *BRCA2*-deficient breast cancers, treatment with PARP inhibitors can lead to accumulation of DSBs and cell death (Helleday, 2010; Lord and Ashworth, 2017). In this instance, PARP inhibitors are not lethal to normal cells that do not harbor the *BRCA2* deficiency. This general concept of lethality specific to inhibition in 2 cellular processes (ie, functional pathways or networks) is termed *synthetic lethality*. The synthetic lethality can arise—as in this case—when lethality ensues due to a defective gene and a chemical that inhibits another gene-encoded function

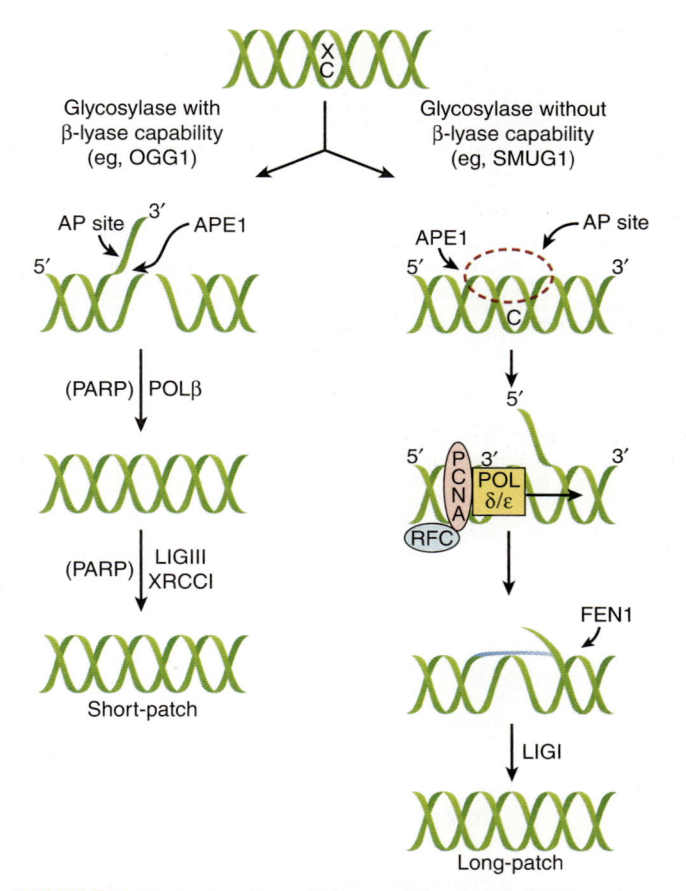

FIGURE 9–5 **Mechanism of base excision repair (BER) and single-strand break repair (SSBR).** Damaged bases are removed by the BER pathway and single-strand breaks are repaired by components of the same pathway. There are 2 subpathways, known as *short-* and *long-patch BER*, and pathway choice depends on the initial glycosylase enzyme that is required to recognize and remove the particular base lesion. When the enzyme includes β-lyase activity, the base is removed, leaving an apyrimidinic (AP)-site with a nick in the DNA backbone and a flap 3′ to the removed base. The APE1 endonuclease removes this flap and the POLβ enzyme fills in the gap. Simultaneously the single-stranded DNA recruits the poly(ADP-ribose) polymerase (PARP) enzyme that facilitates recruitment of ligase III and XRCC1 that seal the nick. Because only a single nucleotide is replaced, this is called *short-patch* BER. In the complementary long-patch BER pathway, the recognition glycosylase does not contain β-lyase activity and leaves an AP site with an intact DNA backbone. The APE1 endonuclease catalyzes the formation of a flap 5′ to the removed base, and PCNA, POLδ/ε, and replication factor C (RFC) initiate synthesis and create a longer flap of 2 to 10 nucleotides. The FEN1 nuclease cleaves the overhang and the nick is sealed by ligase I.

TABLE 9–1 Cancer prone human syndromes with defective DNA repair.

Syndrome	Affected Repair Pathway	Defective Protein	Main Type of Genomic Defect	Major Cancer Predisposition
Xeroderma pigmentosum (XP)	Nucleotide excision repair	XP CS	Point mutations	UV-induced skin cancer
Cerebro-oculo-facio-skeletal syndrome (COFS)	Nucleotide excision repair	ERCC1	Not reported, but likely point mutations	Unknown
Ataxia telangiectasia (AT)	DNA DSB response	ATM	Chromosome aberrations	Lymphomas, leukemia, breast
AT-like disorder (ATLD)	DNA DSB response	MRE11	Chromosome aberrations	Lymphomas (and likely breast)
Nijmegen breakage syndrome (NBS)	DNA DSB response	NBS1	Chromosome aberrations	Lymphomas
Nijmegen breakage syndrome–like disorder (NBSLD)	DNA DSB response	RAD50	Chromosome aberrations	Unknown
BRCA1/BRCA2	Homologous recombination	BRCA1, BRCA2	Chromosome aberrations	Breast and ovarian cancers
Werner syndrome	Homologous recombination	WRN helicase	Chromosome aberrations	Multiple sites
Bloom syndrome	Homologous recombination	BLM helicase	Chromosome aberrations—sister-chromatid exchange	Multiple sites
Cohesinopathies (Cornelia de Lange syndrome [CdLS], Roberts syndrome [RS], Warsaw breakage syndrome [WBS])	Homologous recombination and other defects	SMC1A, SMC3, SCC2/NIPBL, ECO1/ESCO2	Chromosome aberrations (reported in several but not all cases of cohesinopathies)	Unknown
Hereditary nonpolyposis colorectal cancer (Lynch syndrome, constitutional mismatch repair deficiency [CMMRD] syndrome)	Mismatch repair	MLH1, MSH2, MSH6, PMS2, PMS1	Microsatellite instability	Colorectal cancer
Polyposis-associated colorectal cancer syndromes (NTHL1-associated polyposis [NAP], MUTYH-associated polyposis [MAP], and polymerase proofreading-associated polyposis [PPAP]).	Base excision repair and/or replication proofreading	NTHL1, MUTYH, POLE, POLD1	Point mutations	Colorectal tumors, endometrial cancer and others
Fanconi anemia	DNA crosslink repair	FANC-D2	Chromosome aberrations	Multiple sites
Li-Fraumeni	DNA DSB Response	p53 (in ~75% of Li-Fraumeni cases)	Cell-cycle checkpoints	Multiple sites (with early onset)
Riddle	DNA DSB Response	RNF168	Cell-cycle checkpoints, DSB repair	Unknown
Seckel	Repair of replication damage	ATR	Cell-cycle checkpoints	Unknown

(a so-called chemo-genetic interaction) or when 2 unlinked mutations, neither of which is lethal on its own, are combined (a so-called genetic interaction). Synthetic lethality is a common concept in yeast and fly genetics, and it has become an exciting area of research for novel cancer therapies (see Chap. 19, Sec. 19.6).

9.3.3 Nucleotide Excision Repair

In aqueous solution, DNA is susceptible to absorption of photons in the range of 200 to 300 nm, which increases reactivity of pyrimidine bases to produce 6-4 photoproducts (6-4PPs) and interstrand crosslinks in the form of cyclobutane pyrimidine dimers (CPDs; eg, thymine-thymine linkages). These lesions, and other bulky chemical adducts, thermodynamically destabilize duplex DNA and are removed by nucleotide excision repair (NER), which is a complex DNA repair pathway involving more than 30 genes (Schärer, 2013; Marteijn et al, 2014). Many of the NER genes were originally cloned using complementation analyses of cells derived from patients with xeroderma pigmentosum (XP) or Cockayne syndrome (CS), and are referred to as XPA-XPG or CSA-CSB in protein nomenclature. Patients with these syndromes have severe sensitivity to UV light and a high incidence of skin cancer (Fig. 9–6).

The process of NER consists of 4 steps: (1) recognition of the damaged DNA; (2) dual incision of the damaged DNA strand on each side of the lesion leading to the excision of an oligonucleotide of 24 to 32 residues; (3) filling in of the

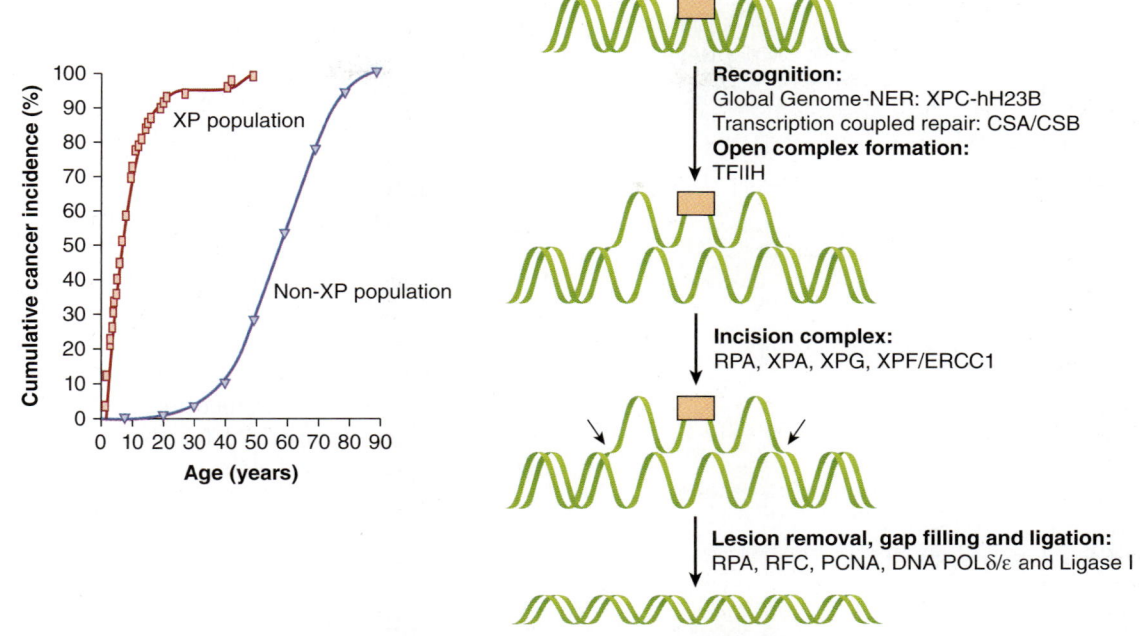

FIGURE 9-6 Nucleotide excision repair (NER) and xeroderma pigmentosum (XP). *Left:* Incidence of skin cancer in people with XP compared to the normal population with similar exposure to the sun. The 1000-fold excess risk of UV-induced skin cancer is secondary to defective repair of UV-induced DNA lesions in XP patients. *Right:* NER proceeds by initial recognition of the lesion by 1 of 2 different complexes, depending on whether "global genome"-nucleotide excision repair (GG-NER) or "transcription-coupled" repair (TCR) is used. In GG-NER helical distortions stimulate recognition by the XP complementation group C (XPC)-hHR23B complex. Subsequently, XPA is recruited and transcription factor IIH (TFIIH) causes formation of an "open complex." The single-stranded regions of DNA are recognized by RPA. Two endonucleases, XPG and XPF/ERCC1, cut 3' and 5' to the lesion, respectively. The approximately 30-nucleotide gap is filled by POLδ/ε and the nick is sealed by ligase I. In TCR, the RNA polymerase II transcription machinery is thought to facilitate recognition of the lesion that, along with the CS proteins A and B (CSA/B), contribute to recognition of the lesion and induction of NER in a similar mechanism to GG-NER. The entire process of NER takes several minutes to complete.

resulting gap by DNA polymerase; and (4) ligation of the nick (Spivak, 2015). In human cells, NER requires at least 6 core protein complexes for recognition of damage and dual incision including XPA, XPC-hHR23B (human homolog of RAD23B), RPA (replication protein A), TFIIH (transcription factor IIH), XPG, and ERCC1-XPF (excision repair cross complementation 1). Other factors are required for DNA synthesis and ligation to complete repair: PCNA, RFC (replication factor C), DNA polymerase δ or α, and DNA ligase I (de Laat et al, 1999). The process of NER is diagrammed in Figure 9–6.

NER consists of 2 subpathways that differ in their mode of recognition of the helical distortions that DNA lesions produce. *Global genome repair* (GG-NER) is transcription-independent and surveys the entire genome for DNA lesions. The 6-4 photoproducts, which distort the DNA more than the 4 cyclobutane pyrimidine dimes (CPDs), are removed rapidly, through recognition by the XPC-HH23B protein complex in GG-NER. In contrast, CPDs are repaired very slowly by GG-NER and are removed more efficiently from the transcribed strand of expressed genes by *transcription-coupled repair* (TCR). During TCR, the stalled RNA polymerase induces the recognition of the DNA lesions on the transcribed strand, and this process is facilitated by CSA and CSB proteins (Friedberg, 2001). The TCR and GG-NER pathways converge after this recognition step to form the open complex and removal of the damage as shown in Figure 9–6.

Access of NER components to the DNA lesions may be impaired by chromatin. The concept of "access-repair-restore" has been proposed for the process of NER (Smerdon and Lieberman, 1978). Different chromatin remodeling factors, including members of the SWI/SNF family, were shown to be recruited to the site of NER in an XPC-dependent fashion (Lans et al, 2012): they promote the decompaction of chromatin and thereby facilitate NER.

9.3.4 DNA Double-Strand Break Repair: Homologous Recombination

DNA DSBs are among the most toxic DNA lesions: they can arise from ionizing radiation and certain chemotherapeutic drugs, endogenously generated reactive oxygen species, as well as excessive mechanical stress applied on chromosomes (Zhou et al, 1998; Mehta and Haber, 2014). They can also be produced when DNA replication forks encounter DNA single-strand breaks, following defective replication of chromosome ends (ie, at telomeres; see Sec. 9.7) or when topoisomerase enzymes are inhibited (eg, by etoposide) preventing the ability of these enzymes to rejoin DSBs. In addition, DNA DSBs are generated to initiate recombination between homologous chromosomes during meiosis and occur as intermediates during developmentally regulated rearrangements, such

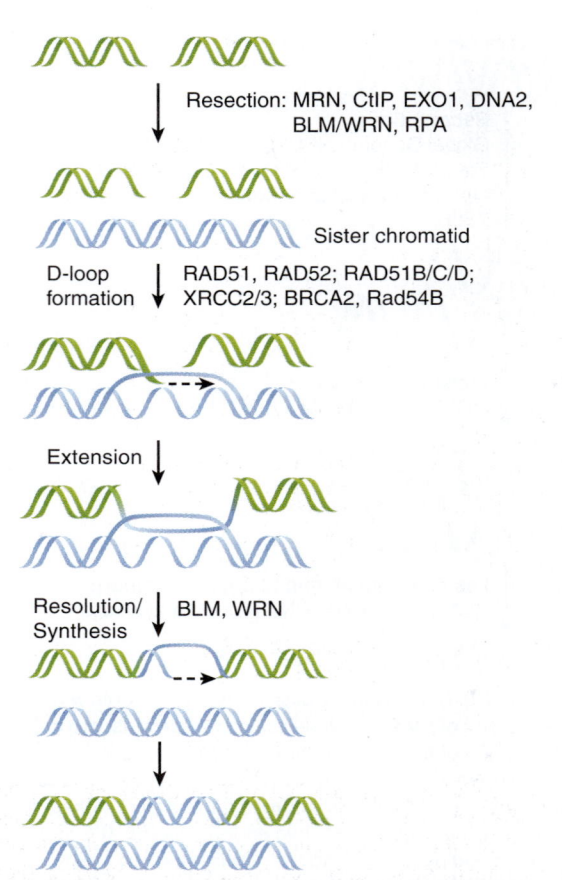

FIGURE 9–7 Homologous recombination (HR) of DNA double-strand breaks (DSBs). HR is a major pathway for DSB repair and requires the presence of a sister chromatid. Here, single-stranded DNA overhangs are created and stabilized by nucleases (MRN [MRE11-RAD50-NBS1] complex, CtIP, EXO1, DNA2), helicases (BLM, WRN), and the single-strand DNA-binding protein RPA. These RPA-coated overhangs are then exchanged to create RAD51-coated overhangs, a process facilitated by the RAD52 group of proteins (RAD52, RAD51B/C/D; XRCC2/3), BRCA2, and RAD54B, that also contributes to scanning for homologous DNA regions. This RAD51-filament can then invade the complementary DNA-duplex to form a D-loop. DNA polymerases then extend this invading strand and the corresponding strand on the opposite side of the DSB.

as V(D)J recombination during the generation of immunoglobulins (see Chap. 22, Sec. 22.3).

In human cells, repair of DNA DSBs occurs either by *homologous recombination* (HR; Fig. 9–7) or *nonhomologous end-joining* (NHEJ; Fig. 9–8). The preferred pathway depends on the tissue type, the extent of DNA damage, the cell-cycle phase in which the cell is damaged, and the relative need for repair fidelity. There may also be cooperation between the 2 pathways (Richardson and Jasin, 2000). Repair by HR requires homology between the broken DNA strand and the template strand used in repair. Typically, this homology is provided by a newly replicated sister chromatid and, as a result, HR is restricted to the S and G_2 phases of the cell cycle (see Fig. 9–7). The HR pathway results in error-free repair of DNA DSBs because the intact undamaged template is used to pair new DNA bases between the damaged and undamaged strands during DNA synthesis.

The HR pathway is highly conserved, likely owing to its role in the maintenance of genome integrity. Figure 9–7 depicts a general schematic of HR processes where a DSB is initially recognized by the MRN complex (MRE11-RAD50-NBS1). MRE11 possesses both single-stranded DNA (ssDNA) endonuclease and 3′ to 5′ exonuclease activities, which are enhanced by the CtIP protein. Together with the 5′ to 3′ exonuclease EXO1 and endonuclease DNA2, these proteins collaborate with DNA helicases (ie, BLM and WRN) to form resected ssDNA at the DSB site, which is rapidly coated with replication protein A (RPA). Exchange of RPA for the RAD51 protein is facilitated by *RAD52 epistasis group* proteins, XRCC2/3, BRCA1/2, and RAD54B, which also contribute to strand invasion of the sister chromatid forming a displacement loop, or D-loop (Heyer et al, 2010; Svendsen and Harper, 2010). DNA synthesis extends the invading strand, and the D-loop is resolved or dissolved under the actions of structure-specific endonucleases and helicases, respectively. There are several subpathways of HR that vary in their ability to prevent crossover of genetic information from the strand acting as the template for DNA synthesis during the formation of the so-called Holliday junctions (see Fig. 9–7; Helleday et al, 2007; Heyer et al, 2010).

Biochemical and genetic studies in yeast have allowed the cloning of human homologs of proteins involved in HR. In the budding yeast *Saccharomyces cerevisiae*, the *RAD52* group of genes encode key effectors of HR such as RAD50, RAD51, RAD52, RAD54, RAD55, RAD57, RAD59, MRE11, and XRS2 (the latter known as p95 or NBS1-Nibrin in mammalian cells). $Rad51^{-/-}$ mice are embryonic lethal, attesting to the importance of this critical HR protein in meiosis and development. Study of the initial stages of embryogenesis in $Rad51^{-/-}$ mice show that lethality is preceded by chromosomal rearrangements and deletions: DNA replication errors and replication-associated DNA strand breaks are converted into DNA DSBs in HR-defective cells (Lim and Hasty, 1996). In cells derived from $Rad54^{-/-}$ mice (which are developmentally normal), there is also decreased HR and hypersensitivity to DNA crosslinking agents such as mitomycin C (Essers et al, 1997). The *RAD52* gene is essential for DNA DSB repair in *S cerevisiae*, but $Rad52^{-/-}$ mice are viable and fertile and do not show a DNA DSB repair deficiency. Instead, the central role of *S cerevisiae* Rad52 appears to be performed by the mammalian orthologs of BRCA2 (Holloman, 2011).

The BRCA1/2 breast cancer–susceptibility proteins (see also Chap. 7, Sec. 7.6) play a central role in HR. Both BRCA1 and BRCA2 proteins form discrete nuclear foci during S phase following exposure to DNA-damaging agents. Although RAD51 colocalizes at subnuclear sites with BRCA1, their interaction is thought to be indirect, with only 1% to 5% of BRCA1 in somatic cells associating with RAD51 (Marmorstein et al, 1998). In contrast, the BRCA2 protein contains 8 BRC repeats, each encompassing 30 to 40 residues, which are major sites for binding to RAD51 by a substantial fraction of the total intracellular pool of BRCA2 (Davies et al, 2001). BRCA2-deficient cells have 10-fold lower levels of HR when compared to BRCA2-proficient cells (Moynahan et al, 2001). Mechanistically, BRCA2 acts as the main mediator of Rad51 filament

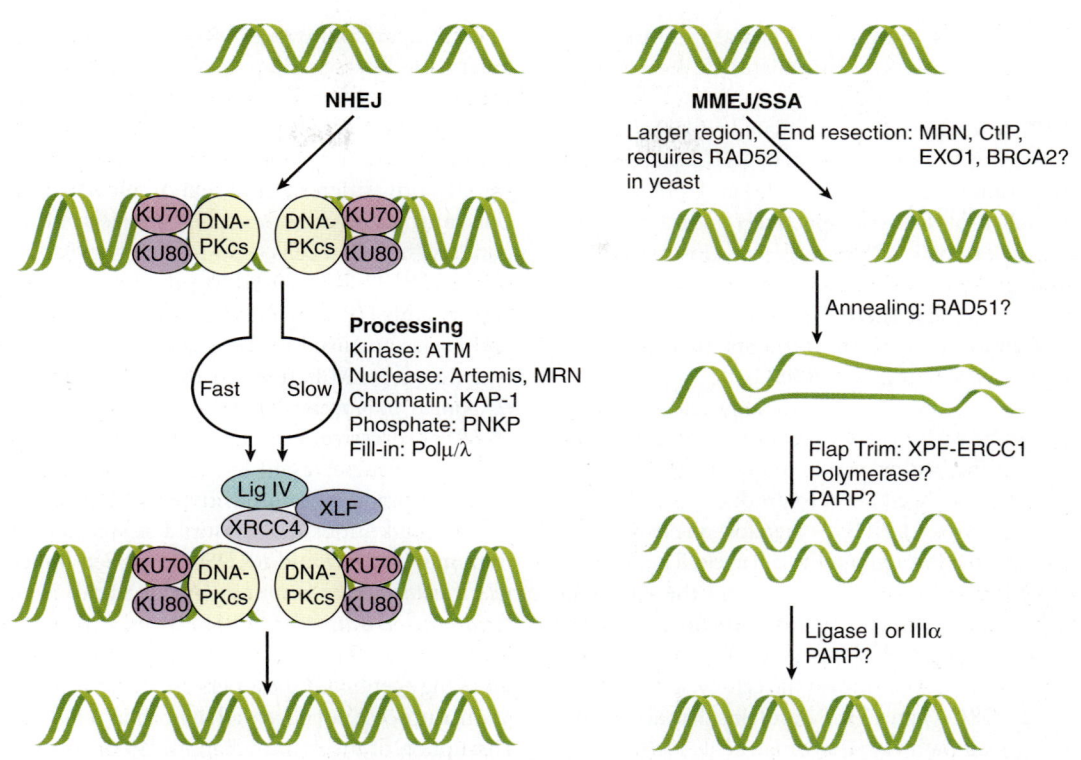

FIGURE 9–8 **NHEJ of DNA DSBs.** NHEJ is composed of subpathways that repair the DNA lesion. In the "fast" NHEJ pathway, the KU70/80 heterodimer recognizes the DNA ends and recruits the DNA-dependent protein-kinase catalytic subunit (DNA-PKcs), which autophosphorylates and forms the active DNA-PK complex. Downstream the ligase IV/XRCC4 dimer associates with the XLF/Cernunnos proteins and joins the DNA ends together. In some cases, the DSB ends at the break are unligatable and require processing in the so-called slow NHEJ pathway. Repair of these ends depends at least in part on the ATM kinase and is processed by nucleases such as MRE11 or Artemis, kinases or phosphatases like PNKP, or filled in by Polμ/λ. Once competent for ligation, these ends follow the same XRCC4/ligase IV pathway above. Some lesions may require chromatin modification by KAP-1 for repair. A less well understood parallel pathway is microhomology-mediated end joining (MMEJ)/single-strand annealing (SSA), which can be thought of as a hybrid pathway for DSB repair. The distinguishing features of MMEJ and SSA are poorly defined, but are differentiated primarily by the extent of the homologous regions involved and the requirement of RAD52 for SSA in yeast. The initial step includes end resection to expose homologous regions by nucleases, including MRE11, CtIP, EXO1, and BRCA2. The annealing of the homologous single-strand overhangs is facilitated by the RAD51 protein, and the remaining flaps are trimmed by XPF-ERCC1. The nicks are sealed with ligase I or IIIα. Despite the disadvantage of its low fidelity, this pathway can act quickly, as required of an emergency mechanism, and, unlike HR, it does not depend on sister DNA molecules, which exist in the cells only after DNA replication.

formation on single-stranded DNA, an essential early step in the process of DNA repair by homologous recombination. Mutational inactivation of this step can lead to gross chromosomal rearrangements, LOH at tumor-suppressor gene loci, and carcinogenesis. When a single-stranded gap is met by the DNA replication machinery, a single DSB may be produced, which utilizes HR as a mechanism to restart replication forks if the delay is not prolonged.

Several human cancers, including ovarian, breast, prostate, and pancreatic, have mutations or altered expression and function of the *MRE11*, *RAD51/RAD52/RAD54*, and *BRCA1/2* genes. This observation suggests that tumorigenesis is associated with altered HR in sporadic tumors. Increased levels of RAD51 in certain cancer cell lines is associated with altered phosphorylation, ubiquitination of RAD51, as well as altered *RAD51* transcription, in part due to abnormal c-ABL- and STAT5-mediated tyrosine kinase signaling pathways (see Chap. 6, Sec. 6.3). This upregulation can lead to acquired radioresistance and chemoresistance (Daboussi et al, 2002).

9.3.5 DNA Double-Strand Break Repair: Nonhomologous End Joining

DNA DSBs can also be repaired by the NHEJ pathway (outlined in Fig. 9–8). In NHEJ, DNA ends at the DSBs are first recognized by high-affinity binding of the KU70/80 heterodimer, which causes a conformational change that recruits the DNA-dependent protein-kinase catalytic subunit (DNA-PKcs). Autophosphorylation of DNA-PKcs at multiple sites is essential for NHEJ to occur and appears to mediate DNA-PKcs dissociation from the break site (Dobbs et al, 2010). Most DNA DSBs have chemically altered ends that need to be processed to allow ligation; for example, when 5′-phosphates are not present and/or 3′-phosphate groups need to be removed to create blunt ends. These structures are repaired by "end processors" that are partially dependent on the activity of the kinase mutated in ataxia telangiectasia (ATM [ataxia-telangiectasia, mutated]) and include the Artemis protein, CtIP and MRN complexes, which are nucleases; PNKP, which is both a 5′ kinase and

3′-phosphatase and DNA Polμ/λ. Once ends are restored, the XRCC4-ligase IV complex, which is stimulated by the XRCC4-like factor (XLF), then rejoins the ends to complete the repair (Chang et al, 2017). Microhomology-mediated end joining and single-strand annealing, are subpathways of NHEJ that require extensive end resection to reveal short (5-25) and longer (>30) homologous stretches of DNA, respectively (see Fig. 9–8). Because of the more extensive DNA ends resection associated with microhomology-mediated end joining and single-strand annealing, it is believed that these 2 pathways contribute to deletions and chromosomal rearrangements that result in genomic instability (McVey and Lee, 2008).

Unlike HR, NHEJ does not require homology, and the NHEJ proteins simply link the ends of DNA breaks together; this process usually results in the loss or gain of a few nucleotides during modification of the damaged DNA to produce ligatable ends (5′-phosphate and 3′-hydroxyl). NHEJ is therefore an error-prone pathway but is operational throughout the cell cycle. There is evidence that RAD52 (an HR-related protein), and the KU70/80 heterodimer, a DNA end-binding protein that functions in NHEJ, compete for binding to DSBs and channel the repair of DSBs into HR or NHEJ respectively, depending on the cell-cycle stage (van Gent et al, 2001). The BRCA1 and 53BP1 proteins may also direct the choice of DNA repair pathway (Bouwman et al, 2010).

The major protein complexes implicated in the NHEJ pathway are the DNA-dependent protein kinase (DNA-PK) complex and the XRCC4/ligase IV complex. Human DNA-PK consists of an approximately 460-kDa DNA-PK catalytic subunit (DNA-PKcs), and a DNA end-binding KU heterodimer (consisting of 70-kDa and 80-kDa protein subunits). The catalytic subunit exhibits homology to the phosphatidylinositol-3 kinase (PI3K) superfamily at its C-terminus, which contains the protein kinase domain required for the phosphorylation of DNA-PK–associated proteins during repair. Mutations in the genes encoding DNA-PKcs (*PRKDC*), Ku70 (*XRCC6*), or Ku80 (in humans, Ku86, encoded by *XRCC5*) result in sensitivity to ionizing radiation and reduced ability to repair radiation-induced DNA DSBs. XRCC4 forms a stable complex with DNA ligase IV and XLF, and probably links detection of the initial lesion by DNA-PK to the actual ligation reaction carried out by ligase IV (Pang et al, 1997; see Fig. 9–8).

Key insights into the cellular activity of the DNA-PK complex was obtained from studies on the severe combined immunodeficiency (SCID) model mouse, which lacks mature T and B cells and is radiosensitive. The DNA-PKcs protein in the SCID mouse is mutated and unstable because of a loss of the last 83 amino acid residues at the C-terminus of the protein. Consequently, DNA-PK activity is severely reduced in tissues derived from this animal. Immunodeficiency is secondary to an inability to process and rejoin the broken DNA molecules produced endogenously during rearrangement of immunoglobulins and T-cell receptor loci (see Chap. 22, Sec. 22.3). These animals also show chromosomal instability in their normal cells and are susceptible to lymphoma, suggesting a tumor-suppressive role of DNA-PK (Khanna and Jackson, 2001). Consistent with phenotypes observed in the animals, fibroblasts derived from *Prkdc-*, *Xrcc5-*, or *Xrcc6*-deficient mice present delayed kinetics of DSB repair and overall lower DSB rejoining following ionizing radiation (see Chap. 15 and 16). Human cells defective in components of NHEJ are also severely impaired in DSB repair, although their preference for repair by specific subpathways of NHEJ (ie, classic or microhomology-mediated end joining) is significantly different from that of mice, likely because human cells normally express much higher levels of Ku/DNA-PK compared with rodent cells (~50-fold higher; Fattah et al, 2010).

The MRE11-RAD50-NBS1 protein complex (termed MRN) acts in both HR and NHEJ pathways (see Figs. 9–7 and 9–8) and is also involved in the maintenance of telomere integrity (see Sec. 9.6). Mutations in the *NBS1* gene (also called p95 or Nibrin in humans) result in *Nijmegen breakage syndrome* (NBS), a recessive disorder with some phenotypic similarities to ataxia telangiectasia (AT) (see Sec. 9.5), including chromosomal instability, radiosensitivity, and an increased incidence of lymphoid tumors (D'Amours and Jackson, 2002). Mutations in human *MRE11* and *RAD50* have been linked to the *ataxia-telangiectasia–like disorder* (ATLD) and *Nijmegen breakage syndrome–like disorder* (NBSLD), respectively. Cells from NBS, AT, NBSLD, and ATLD patients are hypersensitive to DSB-inducing agents and show persistent DNA synthesis after irradiation, a process not observed in normal cells (Girard et al, 2000). Disruption of the mammalian *Rad50* or *Mre11* genes results in nonviable mice attesting to their importance in development. Biochemical studies of the yeast and human protein complexes reveal that MRE11 has a 3′ to 5′ Mn^{2+}-dependent exonuclease activity on DNA substrates with blunt or 5′ protruding ends and endonuclease activity on hairpin and single-stranded DNA substrates. This substrate preference suggests that MRE11 may expose single-stranded regions on DNA DSB. Such ssDNA exposure may promote the use of HR or may activate separate pathways related to NHEJ, called microhomology-mediated end joining and single-strand annealing (see Fig. 9–8).

DNA DSB repair defects and increased radiosensitivity have been reported for a DNA-PKcs–deficient human glioblastoma tumor cell line. Moreover, 6 individuals carrying mutations in the gene encoding DNA-PKcs have been described in the literature and presented diverse clinical phenotypes often associated with recurrent infections (Esenboga et al, 2018). The diversity in the phenotypic profiles observed upon loss of DNA-PK/KU activity may reflect differences in the relative levels of DNA-PKcs protein in rodent and human tissues, as well as varying levels of DNA-PKcs and KU80 protein expression among different tissue types. Evidence suggests there is no simple relationship between tumor cell radiosensitivity and the absolute level of ATM or DNA-PK protein expression (Chan et al, 1998).

9.3.6 DNA Crosslink Repair: Fanconi Anemia Proteins

The Fanconi anemia pathway is a specialized pathway for the repair of interstrand crosslinks (ICLs). ICLs are highly toxic lesions that prevent DNA strand separation, interfering with the processes of transcription and replication. People with deficiencies in any of 19 Fanconi anemia complementation (FANC) proteins have a predisposition to cancer. In this

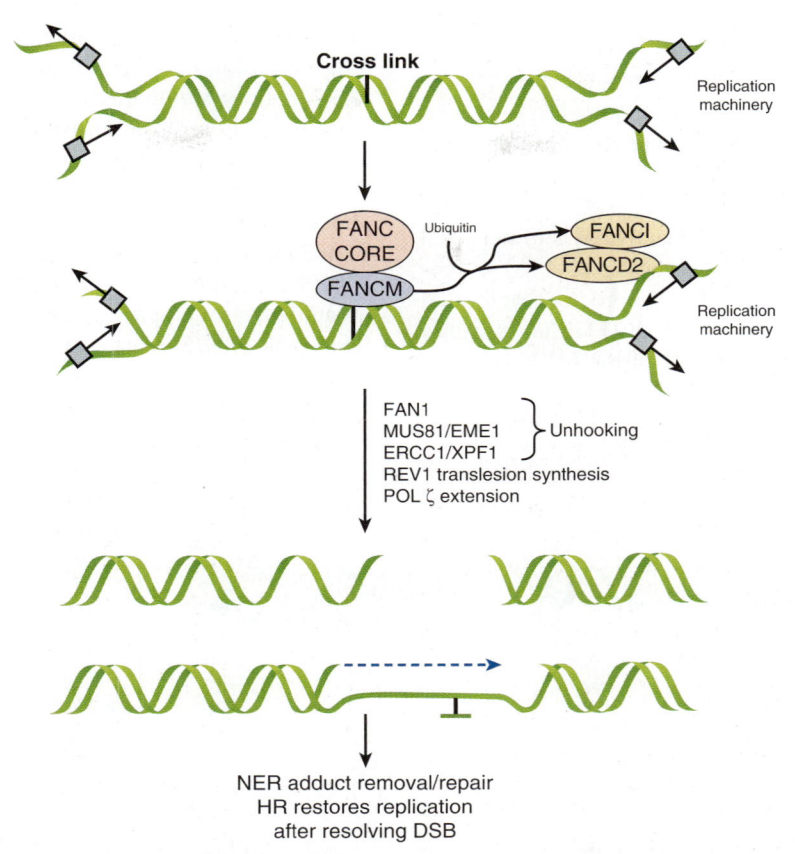

FIGURE 9–9 Fanconi anemia pathway for repairing interstrand crosslinks. Large protein complexes mediate recognition and repair of interstrand crosslinks by the Fanconi anemia pathway. Initially, when replicating DNA meets an interstrand crosslink, the FANCM protein complex recognizes the lesion and recruits the "FA core complex" consisting of FANCs A, B, C, L, E, F, and G. This induces ubiquitylation of FANCD2 and FANCI, facilitating the downstream processes. The crosslink is then unhooked by FAN1, Mus81/Eme1, and ERCC1/XPF1. Although the exact mechanism is poorly understood, Rev1 and Polζ replicate across the lesion. The NER pathway removes the "flipped out" base and repairs the lesion while HR pathway components restore the replication fork after the DSB is resolved.

pathway, unique FANC proteins coordinate a repair mechanism including components of translesion synthesis, HR and NER (Fig. 9–9). When a replication fork approaches an interstrand crosslink, the DNA is not able to form an open configuration for the passage of the polymerase. The FANCM protein initially recognizes the lesion, which recruits an FA-core complex and creates a large E3 ubiquitin ligase that promotes the ubiquitylation of FANCD2 and FANCI proteins that subsequently localize to the damage site and coordinate downstream functions of nucleases (eg, FAN1), DNA polymerases, NER components, and BRCA1/2-mediated HR (Kee and D'Andrea, 2010). Together these mechanisms lead to the restart of the replication fork, thereby preventing cell death or genomic rearrangements (Moldovan and D'Andrea, 2009).

9.4 CELL-CYCLE CHECKPOINTS AND GENOME STABILITY

The cellular response to DNA damage is a multifaceted program whereby mammalian cells activate multiple distinct pathways in an integrated manner after exposure to genotoxic stress. Damaged cells induce feedback control mechanisms known as *checkpoints* that arrest cell-cycle progression and, when necessary, induce cell death. Checkpoint pathways can halt cell-cycle progression at multiple stages of the cell cycle to ensure that cells do not replicate or divide with damaged DNA (see Chap. 8, Sec. 8.3). These checkpoints are initiated by protein kinases (Blackford and Jackson, 2017) and are followed by a cascade of molecular events that include posttranslational modification (ie, phosphorylation, poly(ADP-ribosyl)ation, sumoylation, and ubiquitylation) of proteins surrounding the break (Dantuma and van Attikum, 2016). Three related kinases, ATM, ATR (ATM- and Rad3-related), and DNA-PKcs, act upstream of several signaling cascades that sense damaged chromosomes and block cell-cycle progression (Blackford and Jackson, 2017). There are 2 general types of cell-cycle checkpoints: (1) mitotic spindle checkpoints are responsible for ensuring that microtubules are assembled into a functional mitotic spindle that connects sister kinetochores to opposite centrosomes prior to division, whereas (2) DNA integrity checkpoints delay progression through the cell cycle in response to DNA damage or replication defects (ie, G_1 to S, intra-S and G_2 to M; see also Chap. 8, Sec. 8.3) (London and Biggins, 2014).

9.4.1 DNA Damage Checkpoints

A concerted response to DNA DSBs includes the localization of several regulatory proteins to break sites, a process that stimulates phosphorylation of substrates near genomic lesions. Figure 9–10 outlines the DNA DSB-sensing pathways that lead to phosphorylation of downstream effector proteins. The ATM protein is normally held inactive as a dimer until DNA damage induces autophosphorylation of ATM monomers leading to enhanced kinase activity, a process that is often stimulated by the MRN complex (Paull, 2015). The activation of ATM can also occur independently of the MRN complex via oxidation of disulfide bonds between different kinase molecules, forming a covalent dimer (Paull, 2015). This activation of ATM (and simultaneous activity of DNA-PKcs) induces phosphorylation of the histone protein H2AX on serine-139 forming γ-H2AX (see Sec. 9.6), which serves as a platform for the assembly of other components, including MDC1. ATM phosphorylation of MDC1 triggers recruitment of the RNF8 E3-ubiquitin ligase, which cooperates with UBC13 to ubiquitylate H2AX and H2A histones. In turn, the RNF168-UBC13 ubiquitin ligase complex is recruited to extend ubiquitin chains (Doil et al, 2009; Stewart et al, 2009). These events are thought

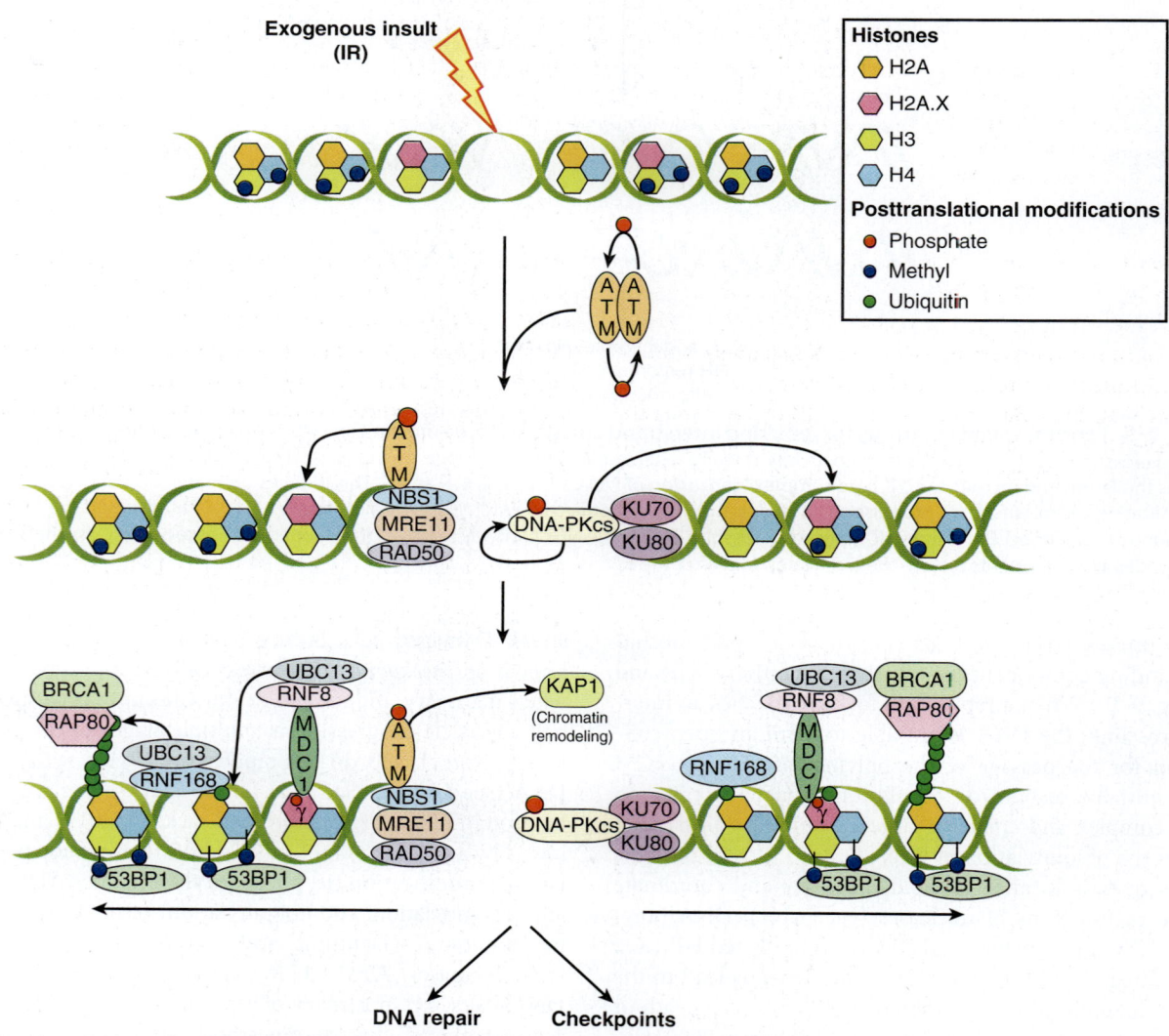

FIGURE 9–10 Signaling pathways in response to DNA DSBs induced by ionizing radiation. Signaling pathways that recognize DNA DSBs are multifaceted and likely include overlapping functions that serve to ensure checkpoints are activated even when some components do not respond properly. In addition to their role in checkpoints, these cascades also contribute to repair. When ionizing radiation (IR) creates DSBs, it leads to activation of the ATM kinase by autophosphorylation and dissociation into monomers from the inactive dimer; this process is facilitated by the MRN complex. Simultaneously, the DNA-PK complex (DNA-PKcs/KU70/KU80) (see Sec. 9.3.5) is activated, and together with ATM, phosphorylates the histone H2AX at serine-139 (forming γ-H2AX) in megabase domains spanning the break. This serves as a platform for the assembly of mediator of DNA damage checkpoint 1 (MDC1) which is also phosphorylated by ATM. This then recruits the E3 ubiquitin ligase RNF8, which, along with the E2-ubiquitin ligase, UBC13, ubiquitylates H2A and H2AX. This further recruits the RNF168 E3-ubiquitin ligase that, through poorly understood mechanisms, leads to the recruitment of RAP80/BRCA1 and the p53-binding protein 1 (53BP1). Multiple protein-protein interactions, facilitated by "mediator" proteins (ie, MDC1, RNF8/168, 53BP1) surrounding the DSB are thought to concentrate the "effector" proteins (ie, p53, etc) in the vicinity of "sensor" proteins (ie, ATM, MRN) to facilitate the enactment of downstream processes, including DNA repair and checkpoints.

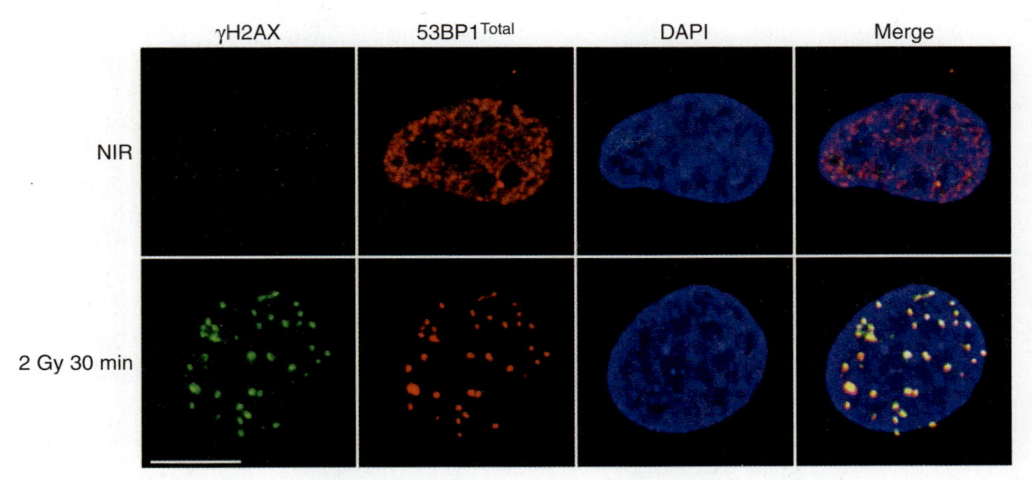

FIGURE 9–11 DNA damage-induced foci and the H2AX response. Confocal immunofluorescent images of normal human fibroblasts (GM05757) either untreated (nonirradiated [NIR]) or irradiated with 2 Gy and fixed at 30 minutes post-IR. Cells were stained for phosphorylated H2AX (γ-H2AX) and total 53BP1. IR induces γ-H2AX intranuclear foci whereas 53BP1 redistributes from a pan-nuclear nonnucleolar pattern into discrete foci that colocalize with γ-H2AX in the DAPI-stained nucleus (shown in blue) as shown by yellow coloration. Scale bar is 10 μm. Many DSB-responsive proteins form foci in this manner (eg, MRE11, ATM, MDC1).

to modify chromatin in such a way that proteins, including 53BP1 and the RAP80-BRCA1 complex can associate along the break site. Phosphorylation of SMC1 and SMC3—2 core subunits of the cohesin complex—by ATM also contributes to the establishment of a robust checkpoint response in S phase (Kitagawa et al, 2004; Bauerschmidt et al, 2011). Following the initial wave of kinase activation and substrate phosphorylation, downstream effectors of ATM, including p53 and CHK2, are actively recruited to sites of DNA damage (Al-Hakim et al, 2010; Panier and Durocher, 2009). This model implies that the local concentration of kinase activity and downstream effector proteins contributes to the initiation of cell-cycle checkpoints, and that it also facilitates repair mechanisms such as those discussed above. Many of these proteins have been found to colocalize in a spatiotemporal manner at IR-induced nuclear foci as shown in Figure 9–11 for γ-H2AX and 53BP1.

As discussed above, a number of lesions in DNA can stall replication forks during S phase, which exposes single-stranded (ss) tracts in the genome. To protect these tracts from degradation, replication protein A (RPA) rapidly coats ssDNA and creates a structure that recruits ATR interacting protein (ATRIP) and ATR to stalled replication forks. ATR and ATM kinases cooperate to activate/phosphorylate many of the same checkpoint effectors, leading to cell-cycle arrest (Fig. 9–12) (Blackford and Jackson, 2017). Shortly after the formation of DNA DSBs/ssDNA tracks, the activation of signaling cascades by ATM or ATR results in the enrichment of numerous downstream effectors to damaged sites (Bensimon et al, 2011). Recent experiments have shown that ATM and ATR kinases share upward of 700 protein targets, revealing functional overlap and redundancies built in checkpoint signaling cascades (eg, Bensimon et al, 2010). These overlapping pathways increase the likelihood that a strong checkpoint response will be established.

The colocalization of ATM with its effectors initiates a G_1-to-S checkpoint response that depends on the post-translational stabilization of the p53 protein via direct phosphorylation on serine 15 (Canman et al, 1998). ATM also phosphorylates threonine residue 68 on the Chk2 protein, which can, in turn, phosphorylate p53. These phosphorylation events lead to nuclear accumulation of p53 by interfering with a nuclear export site contained within the amino terminus of the p53 protein and by preventing degradation of p53 by MDM2 (see Chap. 7, Sec. 7.X; Liang and Clarke, 2001). Because p53 acts primarily as a transcription factor, its stabilization following DNA damage is a probable mechanism to activate the cyclin D/E-kinase complex inhibitor, $p21^{WAF}$, which leads to hypophosphorylation of the Rb protein to effect G_1 cell-cycle arrest (see Chap 8, Sec. 8.2). A second G_1 checkpoint pathway is also activated that targets the CDC25A phosphatase that is essential for G_1/S transition (Falck et al, 2001).

Further important targets of ATM-mediated phosphorylation are the BRCA1, NBS1, and FANCD2 proteins, which initiate both DNA repair and an S phase DNA damage checkpoint (eg, Lim et al, 2000). The ATM-mediated phosphorylation of NBS1 seems to be required for proper execution of an S phase checkpoint as removal of the ATM-induced phosphosites (ie, Ser278, 343, or 397) in mutant NBS1 leads to radioresistant DNA synthesis, a phenotype associated with AT cells.

Following their activation by ATM and ATR, CHK1 and CHK2 phosphorylate a conserved site (Ser216) on protein phosphatase CDC25C, which results in its inactivation and recognition by the 14-3-3σ protein. The inactive CDC25C is then incapable of removing an inhibitory phosphate group on Tyr-15 of CDK1 (CDC2), which then prevents entry into mitosis. In addition, p53-dependent transcriptional repression of the *CDC2* and *CCNB1* (which encodes cyclin B) promoters may contribute to the maintenance of the G_2/M checkpoint in mammalian cells, which in turn may allow for repair of chromosomal or chromatid damage prior to cellular division. The elegant crosstalk between ATM and ATR and factors involved in DNA repair, DNA damage signaling, and cell-cycle control

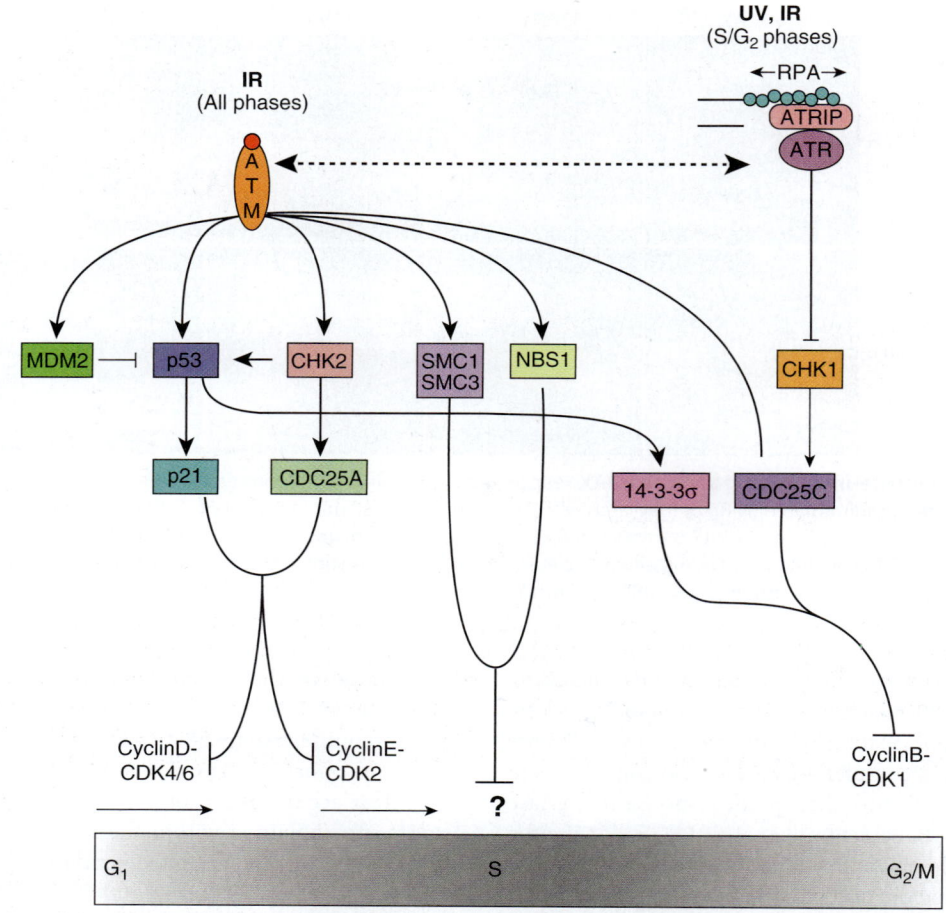

FIGURE 9–12 Cell-cycle checkpoint activation downstream of ATM (ataxia-telangiectasia, mutated) and ATR (ATM- and Rad3-related). Induction of DSBs by IR activates ATM, which phosphorylates MDM2 preventing p53 proteasomal degradation. ATM also activates, via phosphorylation, CHK2, which, in turn, phosphorylates CDC25A to inactivate its phosphatase activity and block Cyclin E-CDK2-Rb–mediated S phase entry. The stabilization of p53 is accompanied by ATM- and CHK2-phosphorylation which activate transcription of p53 target genes, such as p21. As a CDK inhibitor p21 blocks Cyclin D-CDK4/5 and Cyclin E-CDK2 and, therefore, S phase entry. Activated ATM also phosphorylates the cohesin subunits SMC1 and SMC3, as well as NBS1 protein that slow progression through S phase by poorly defined mechanisms. DNA damage incurred during S phase (by IR or UV) may create ssDNA. This ssDNA is coated by RPA recruiting ATR via its coactivator, ATRIP. Active ATR phosphorylates CHK1, which inactivates CDC25C. ATM activity and p53-induction of 14-3-3σ also inactivate CDC25C. Inactive CDC25C cannot remove inhibitory phosphate groups on CDK1 and therefore blocks Cyclin B-mediated transition to mitosis. Crosstalk between ATM and ATR leads to simultaneous activation of many of these pathways, as described in the text.

act to maintain genomic stability and inhibit carcinogenesis (see Fig. 9–12).

9.4.2 Mitotic Spindle Checkpoints

The accurate segregation of chromosomes is a crucial event for the maintenance of genome integrity. This process is tightly controlled by the ubiquitin-dependent destruction of securin, the inhibitor of separase, a site-specific protease that cleaves and inactivates a subunit of the cohesin complex. On cleavage of cohesin at the metaphase-anaphase transition, sister chromatids are released from the topological entrapment of cohesin rings, thereby allowing segregation to occur via the forces applied on chromosomes by the mitotic spindle (Uhlmann, 2016). Shortly thereafter, ubiquitination and proteolytic degradation of cyclin B by the anaphase promoting complex (APC) inactivates CDK1 kinase and allows mitotic exit to occur (Gavet and Pines, 2010). The timing of late mitotic events such as chromosome segregation and mitotic exit are regulated by at least 2 distinct checkpoint mechanisms. The *spindle assembly checkpoint (SAC)* monitors the interaction between chromosomes and microtubules at highly specialized chromosomal regions called *kinetochores* (London and Biggins, 2014). This checkpoint prevents chromosome segregation by blocking the ubiquitin-dependent degradation of securin until all kinetochores are attached to microtubules of the mitotic spindle. If attachment defects persist, cells may undergo mitotic slippage and/or cell death (Brito and Rieder, 2006; Haschka et al, 2018). The kinetochore-associated MAD2, BUBR1, BUB1, and BUB3 proteins are critical constituents of the SAC pathway: MAD2 and BUBR1 regulate mitotic progression by direct interaction and inhibition of the APC machinery, and BUB1 and BUB3

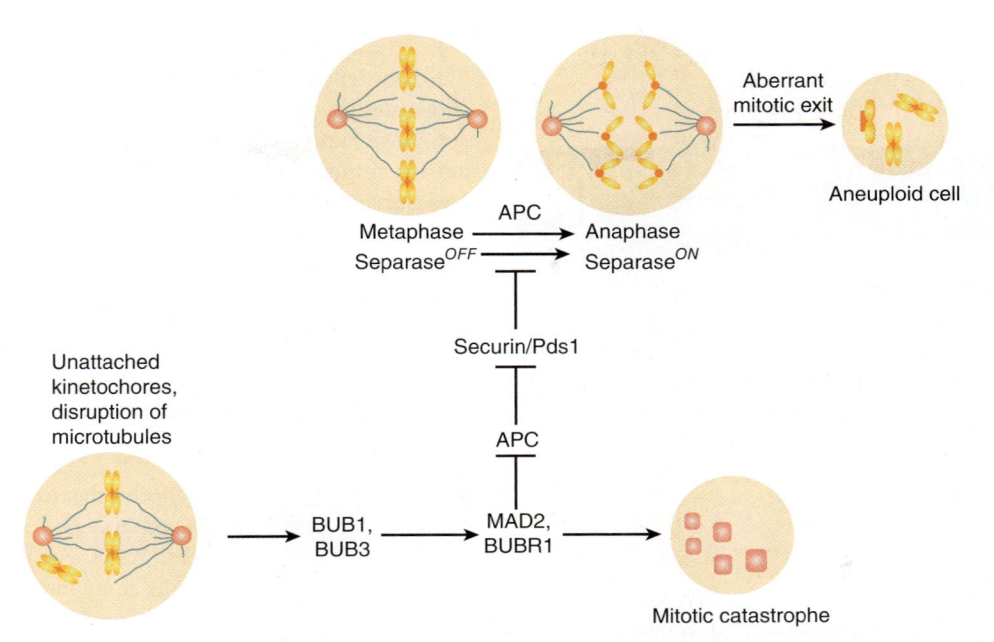

FIGURE 9–13 Improper chromosome alignment on the mitotic spindle can activate the spindle checkpoint mediated by the BUB1, BUB3, BUBR1, and MAD2 proteins that localize to kinetochores. An intact spindle checkpoint induces metaphase arrest through inhibition of the APC and stabilization of the Separase inhibitor, Securin/Pds1. Defective spindle checkpoint function results from either loss of BUB1- and BUB3-dependent signaling or abrogation of MAD2, BUBR1-mediated inhibition of the APC. Under conditions where sister chromatids have not achieved biorientation on the mitotic spindle, misregulation of spindle checkpoint activity will lead to premature degradation of Securin/Pds1, early activation of Separase, and errors in chromosome segregation, thus generating aneuploid cells.

also mediate mitotic arrest after disruption of microtubules (Haschka et al, 2018), as shown in Figure 9–13. Cells that lack either BUB1 or BUB3 do not undergo mitotic arrest when treated with spindle-disrupting agents, such as the chemotherapy drugs docetaxel or vinblastine. A second spindle feedback mechanism, the *tension checkpoint*, operates in mitotic cells to ensure that chromosome segregation is not initiated until all sister kinetochores on replicated chromatids are attached to microtubules originating from different centrosomes (London and Biggins, 2014). This state is known as biorientation, and it is monitored by the tension generated at sister kinetochores when they are pulled in opposite directions by microtubules originating from 2 different centrosomes. The chromosomal passenger complex (CPC) is the central regulator of the tension checkpoint, and it is composed of the aurora B kinase in complex with INCENP, survivin, and borealin. If activated by a lack of tension at kinetochores, aurora B phosphorylation of several kinetochore proteins, notably the NDC80 complex, will result in the removal of improper attachments and activation of the SAC (Haase et al, 2017; Yoo et al, 2018). Securin degradation and chromosome segregation can only occur when the SAC and tension checkpoints are fully satisfied, and thus silenced.

9.4.3 Checkpoint Silencing by Adaptation or Inactivation

Although most healthy cells will induce a robust cell-cycle arrest on checkpoint activation, checkpoint mechanisms are not absolute and cells can eventually evade checkpoint arrest using a number of normal or pathologic mechanisms. Notably, cells can adapt to bypass checkpoint arrest induced by low levels of persistent DNA damage or spindle dysfunction (Rieder and Maiato, 2004; Serrano and D'Amours, 2014). This adaptation behavior is a normal response incorporated in many checkpoint mechanisms and depends on a conserved family of protein kinases, the Polo-like kinase (PLK) (Toczyski et al, 1997; Syljuasen et al, 2006; Rossio et al, 2010; Ratsima et al, 2016). At clinically relevant doses of DNA/microtubule-targeted chemotherapy, adaptation to checkpoint arrest appears to occur frequently, thus highlighting its relevance to treatment (Kubara et al, 2012).

Mutational inactivation of checkpoint effectors can also lead to pathologic/premature release from checkpoint-induced cell-cycle arrest, with dire consequences on genomic stability. Genetic defects in the spindle checkpoint, for example, can lead to whole chromosome loss during mitosis and meiosis with links to the pathogenesis of several human tumors. In human colon and breast carcinoma cells, BUB1 mutations have been identified that facilitate the transformation of cells that lack BRCA2. In other studies, Mad2 haploinsufficiency elevated the rate of lung tumor development in $Mad2^{+/-}$ mice compared with age-matched controls (Stewart et al, 2003). There is also therapeutic potential from abrogation of cell-cycle checkpoints using agents targeted at particular kinases (eg, UCN-01 for CHK1) in cells that already lack other checkpoints (ie, p53-mediated). This checkpoint inactivation results in catastrophic mitotic death as a result of cell-cycle progression into mitosis with unrepaired DNA DSBs (Lapenna and Giordano, 2009; Haschka et al, 2018).

9.5 HUMAN DNA REPAIR DISORDERS AND FAMILIAL CANCERS

Several human disease syndromes are associated with pronounced cellular sensitivity to DNA-damaging agents because of hereditary deficiencies in DNA repair or in signaling pathways that are activated by DNA damage (Table 9–1). People suffering from several of these syndromes show marked chromosomal instability and predisposition to malignancy, as discussed below.

9.5.1 Ataxia Telangiectasia

The AT syndrome is an autosomal recessive disease characterized by cerebellar degeneration, immunodeficiency, chromosomal instability, cancer predisposition, radiation sensitivity (see Chap. 16, Sec. 16.3), and cell-cycle abnormalities (Rotman and Shiloh, 1998; Weissberg et al, 1998). A mutation in a single gene coding for ATM is responsible for this syndrome. The *ATM* gene encodes a large protein that possesses a highly conserved C-terminal kinase domain related to PI3K (see Durocher and Jackson, 2001). Most mutations in ATM result in truncation and destabilization of the protein, but certain missense and splicing errors produce a less severe phenotype. Cells derived from AT patients and $Atm^{-/-}$ mice display hypersensitivity to ionizing but not UV radiation; they also exhibit chromosomal instability and a mild DNA DSB rejoining defect. ATM-deficient cells also have radioresistant DNA synthesis and further defects in the G_1/S, S, and G_2/M phase DNA damage checkpoints. At the clinical level, the pleiotropic symptoms associated with AT may be explained partly by modification of cellular metabolism. For example, the loss of ATM function is associated with increased oxidative damage, particularly in cerebellar Purkinje cells, implicating a role for ATM in the response to reactive oxygen species and possibly explaining the cerebellar degeneration observed in AT-affected individuals (Rotman and Shiloh, 1998).

People with AT have a high incidence of lymphoid malignancy, and ATM-deficient mice also develop lymphomas, implying that inactivation of the ATM gene is important in the pathogenesis of lymphoid malignancy. LOH at 11q22-23 (ie, the location of the ATM gene) is a common event in lymphoid malignancy. Frequent inactivating mutations of the ATM gene have been reported in patients with Hodgkin and non-Hodgkin lymphoma, rare sporadic T-cell prolymphocytic leukemia (T-PLL), B-cell chronic lymphocytic leukemia (B-CLL), and, most recently, mantle cell lymphoma (MCL). Furthermore, AT heterozygotes may have a slightly increased risk of breast cancer when compared to the normal population. These data suggest that ATM functions as a tumor-suppressor gene (Rotman and Shiloh, 1998).

Interestingly, other diseases such as Ataxia-telangiectasia–like disorder (ATLD) and Nijmegen breakage syndrome (NBS) show similar phenotypes to AT, illustrating the functional complexity and cooperative nature of ATM-dependent mechanisms responsible for the suppression of genetic instability (see Sec. 9.4). The mechanism for the developmental defects in these patients is not well understood, but these syndromes have been instrumental in the understanding of the molecular pathways that control the responses to DNA damage, particularly DNA DSBs.

9.5.2 Xeroderma Pigmentosum and Related Disorders

The human XP, CS, and trichothiodystrophy disorders exhibit cellular UV sensitivity as a consequence of deficiency in NER (see Sec. 9.3.3; Hoeijmakers, 2001). For reasons that are not understood, only XP patients are cancer-prone with a dramatic 1000-fold increase in the incidence of UV-induced skin cancer. This predisposition is caused by mutations in 1 of 7 XP genes (XPA-XPG) in their cells. CS is characterized by a transcription-coupled repair (TCR) defect secondary to mutations in CSB and CSA genes. CS patients exhibit neurodegeneration and premature aging related to inappropriate apoptosis. Trichothiodystrophy patients share many features of CS patients but also have brittle hair, nails, and scaly skin, secondary to reduced expression of epidermal matrix proteins.

9.5.3 Hereditary Nonpolyposis Colon Cancer

Hereditary nonpolyposis colon cancer (HNPCC) is the most common form of hereditary colon cancer, accounting for 5% to 8% of all colon cancers. People with HNPCC also have an excess of endometrial, small bowel, and renal cancers. This familial cancer syndrome occurs secondarily to genetic instability acquired through deficient MMR by virtue of mutations in 6 different mismatch repair (MMR) loci (see Sec. 9.3.1) (Harfe and Jinks-Robertson, 2000). Replication of repetitive DNA sequences, termed *microsatellites*, can result in gains or losses of these repeated units giving rise to *microsatellite instability* (MSI). The MMR system suppresses MSI. Cells from HNPCC patients (and patients with sporadic colorectal tumors) can acquire runs of approximately 4 to 40 repeated mononucleotides or dinucleotides, such as TTTT or CACACA, at multiple sites within the genome as a consequence of MSI.

More than 300 different predisposing MMR genetic mutations have been documented in human cancers, mainly affecting *MLH1* (approximately 50%), *MSH2* (approximately 40%), and *MSH6* (approximately 10%) (Friedberg, 2001). Genetically predisposed individuals with HNPCC carry a defective copy of an MMR gene in every cell, and mutation rates in tumor cells with MMR deficiency are 100- to 1000-fold higher than in normal cells. Somatic inactivation of the remaining wild-type copy in a target tissue, typically colon, gives rise to a profound

DNA repair defect and increased rates of mutation in cells (ie, a "mutator" phenotype) with progressive accumulation of mutations in *APC*, *TP53*, or other genes that contribute to colon cancer development (Li and Martin, 2016).

9.5.4 Li-Fraumeni Syndrome

One of the most frequently mutated genes in human tumors is *TP53*, which encodes the p53 protein. The pivotal roles of p53 in response to DNA damage and genetic instability include, but are not limited to, cell-cycle checkpoints, apoptosis, and modulation of DNA repair (see Chap. 7, Sec 7.5). The Li-Fraumeni syndrome occurs in people with germline mutations of *TP53*. Originally characterized in 1969 in early-onset cancers in relatives of children with rhabdomyosarcoma, p53 is mutated in diverse tumor types and in various families with inherited cancers (Palmero et al, 2010). In people with the Li-Fraumeni syndrome, 50% develop cancer before age 40 years, and 90% develop cancer before age 60 years. Patients present tumors of various histopathologies, which include sarcomas and brain and breast cancers. Although mutations in other genes (eg, *CHK2*) have been suggested as alternative predisposing factors for Li-Fraumeni syndrome, the evidence for such involvement is controversial (Palmero et al, 2010). Finally, new recommendations for enhanced surveillance procedures have been presented recently to ensure early tumor detection and treatment in Li-Fraumeni patients (Kratz et al, 2017).

9.5.5 Fanconi Anemia

Fanconi anemia (FA) is a very rare autosomal recessive disorder with 1 in 300 people carrying mutations in 1 FANC gene; 1 to 5 in 1 million people are affected by this disorder (D'Andrea, 2010). Although rare, this syndrome has led to the identification of 19 "complementation group" proteins that are mutated or lost in FA patients and that comprise a distinct pathway in mammalian cells (see Sec. 9.3.6). The definitive test for FA is to treat lymphocytes from patients with diepoxybutane, a DNA-crosslinking agent, and assess chromosome breakage. In FA patients, this treatment leads to accumulation of breaks owing to an inability to repair interstrand crosslinks in DNA. Tumors (eg, leukemia, head and neck) develop in at least 20% of FA patients, and this number would likely be much higher if bone marrow failure and other manifestations of the syndrome did not lead to early death of afflicted individuals.

9.5.6 BRCA1/2

Germline mutations in a single copy of the BRCA1 or BRCA2 tumor-suppressor gene occur in approximately 1 in 250 women and lead to early-onset breast and ovarian cancer (Narod and Foulkes, 2004). Most tumors from carriers display LOH such that both copies of the gene become mutated, rendering the cell BRCA1 or BRCA2 null. Mechanistic roles for BRCA1/2 have been observed in various DNA repair pathways, including the FA (see Sec. 9.3.6) and HR (see Sec. 9.3.4) pathways, as well as in cell-cycle checkpoints and maintenance of ploidy (O'Donovan and Livingston, 2010). The potential of PARP inhibitors to generate synthetic lethality when combined with the HR defect of BRCA1/2-defective tumors is being tested in clinical trials (Oza et al, 2017; Somlo et al, 2017).

9.6 ASSAYS OF DNA DAMAGE AND REPAIR

The ability to precisely measure the nature and extent of DNA damage in tissues, as well as the capacity of cells to repair this damage, is highly relevant for therapy and research. Table 9–2 outlines techniques that have been used to measure different types of DNA strand breaks; modifications of some of these assays also allow quantification of base damage and photoproducts. Techniques such as velocity sedimentation, filter elution, assays for chromosomal damage, and DNA electrophoresis have been used to study specific DNA lesions caused by radiation (Whitaker et al, 1991; Fairbairn et al, 1995). Two techniques, fluorescence in situ hybridization (FISH; see Chap. 2, Sec 2.2) and premature chromosome condensation (PCC), allow the quantification of single- or double-strand breaks following doses of ionizing radiation as low as 1 Gy (Sasai et al, 1994). Other techniques, such as pulsed-field gel electrophoresis (PFGE) or the comet assay (Fairbairn et al, 1995), can facilitate the separation and quantification of large DNA fragments secondary to single- or double-strand DNA breaks following radiation, but, with the exception of the comet assay, require much higher (>10 to 20 Gy) doses because of their lower sensitivity. DNA DSBs are of particular importance as they are the most lethal form of DNA damage (see Chap. 15, Sec. 15.4). Next-generation sequencing has greatly increased the sensitivity of detection of different types of DNA damage as well as the mapping of their genomic location with nucleotide resolution (reviewed in Bouwman and Crosetto, 2018).

Ionizing radiation leads to rapid phosphorylation of nucleosomal histone protein, H2AX. γ-H2AX is the phosphorylated form that can be quantified using a specific antibody as an intracellular marker of DNA DSBs (see Figs. 9–10 and 9–11). This early event precedes the actions of enzymes involved in HR and NHEJ repair of these breaks. Interestingly, genome-wide localization of γ-H2AX by immunopurification (CHIP-chip) has revealed different fragile sites in the genome that are prone to double-stranded breaks (Szilard et al, 2010). Microscopically visible nuclear foci, each containing thousands of γ-H2AX molecules covering about 2 Mb of DNA surrounding the break, can be detected using antibody staining and fluorescence microscopy. The number of γ-H2AX foci has been directly correlated to the number of DNA DSBs in [125]IUdR-treated cells as each ^{125}I decay yields a DNA DSB and each DNA DSB yielded a visible γ-H2AX focus (Sedelnikova et al, 2002). These foci resolve such that approximately 50% of breaks remain after 2 hours and almost all breaks are rejoined by 24 hours following the radiation exposure. It is probable

TABLE 9–2 Assays for the detection of DNA damage following ionizing radiation.

Assay	Dose Range	Technique	Limitations
1. Sucrose Velocity Sedimentation	SSB > 5 Gy DSB > 15 Gy	Larger DNA fragments sediment to a greater extent.	Insensitive to clinically relevant low radiation doses
2. Filter elution	SSB > 1 Gy (alkaline elution) DSB > 5 Gy (neutral elution)	Smaller DNA fragments elute more quickly through a filter of defined pore size.	Uncertain effects of DNA conformation, cell cycle, cell number, and lysis
3. Nucleoid sedimentation	SSB 1 to 20 Gy	Irradiated cells show altered DNA supercoiling within nucleus.	Uncertain which DNA lesion(s) are being detected
4. Pulse-field gel electrophoresis (PFGE)	DSB > 2 Gy	Allows for resolution of DNA DSB, which can be quantified by relative migration within the gel.	Uncertain effects of DNA conformation; high number of cells in S phase may bias results of assay
5. Comet assay	SSB > 1 Gy (alkaline lysis) DSB > 2 Gy (neutral lysis)	Following lysis, individual nuclei are subjected to agarose gel electrophoresis. The DNA that moves out of the nucleus (head) to form the "tail" of the comet is quantitated to provide a measure of DNA damage.	Requires image analysis system to quantify DNA damage; increased numbers of cells in S phase may bias assay
6. Fluorescence in situ hybridization (FISH)	Doses > 1 Gy	Chromosome-specific probes, which can be detected with a fluorescent ligand, are used to identify radiation-induced translocations.	May be difficult to interpret in tumor cells that contain translocations prior to irradiation
7. Premature chromosome condensation (PCC)	Doses > 1 Gy	An irradiated interphase cell is fused to a mitotic cell. The chromosomes in the interphase cell undergo premature condensation, allowing radiation-induced chromosome damage to be scored.	May be difficult to interpret in tumor cells that contain chromosome aberrations prior to irradiation
8. γ-H2AX intranuclear foci	Doses > 0.05 Gy	Immunofluorescence microscopy or flow cytometry using an antibody to γ-H2AX phosphoprotein.	Requires image analysis system. No standard for size of foci to count

DSB, double-strand breaks; *SSB*, single-stranded breaks.
Reproduced with permission from Whitaker SJ, Powell SN, McMillan TJ. Molecular assays of radiation-induced DNA damage. *Eur J Cancer* 1991;27(7):922-928.

that residual nuclear foci (≥24 hours post-IR) represent non-rejoined DNA DSBs and lead to subsequent cell lethality (MacPhail et al, 2003). There are other mechanisms that activate γ-H2AX, such as apoptosis and oncogene signaling (Lobrich et al, 2010). This method has also been adapted to detect other types of lesions, such as 6-4PPs, to which antibodies have been generated (Vermeulen, 2011).

Recent advances in imaging and fluorescence technologies allow the visualization and generation of discrete DNA DSBs in tissues and cells. For example, use of high-fluence, targeted laser microirradiation induces DNA DSBs in a spatially restricted manner within the nucleus: these techniques can monitor the recruitment of repair proteins to DNA damage, and when used with advanced techniques such as fluorescence recovery after photobleaching (FRAP) can determine the residence of repair proteins at the DNA damage site in live cells. Conclusions drawn from such assays are augmented usually by more traditional techniques outlined in Table 9–2.

The development of the CRISPR technology (see Chap. 2, Sec. 2.3) has allowed researchers to control the generation of localized DNA DSBs. This system combines a nuclease (Cas9) in complex with an RNA scaffold (sgRNA) that also contains a 20-bp protospacer sequence complementary to the target region in the genome (reviewed in Sander and Joung 2014). The generation of these precise DSBs can be combined with the use of Sanger sequencing or next-generation sequencing of the target site to study the repair fate of the DSBs as well as the mutagenicity of each break site (Bothmer et al, 2017; Brinkman et al, 2018). By designing different protospacer sequences, it is possible to target the Cas9 nuclease to induce a break in different DNA sequences or chromatin environments and probe the DNA repair machinery for different repair outcomes (van Overbeek et al, 2016).

9.7 REGULATION OF TELOMERE LENGTH AND CANCER

Human cells have evolved a complex network of proteins that bind to chromosome ends, called *telomeres*, to protect them from being inappropriately recognized as DNA damage. Disruption of this nucleoprotein complex, either through loss of telomere DNA or disruption of protein function at the telomere, induces a DNA damage response leading to cell death or cessation of cell division (reviewed in Doksani and de Lange, 2014). Cells that retain the capacity to proliferate, such as stem cells and cancer cells, must thus find a mechanism to maintain telomere integrity. Most often, cancer cells achieve this protection through the activation of an enzyme that adds new telomere DNA onto chromosome ends, called *telomerase*. More rarely, maintenance of telomeres is achieved through recombination, exchange, or copying of existing telomere DNA tracts through mechanisms collectively referred to as "alternative lengthening of telomeres" (ALT) (Apte and Cooper, 2017). Interestingly, tumors that possess aberrantly long telomeres but show no detectable telomere maintenance mechanism have been reported (Dagg et al, 2017; Viceconte et al, 2017). These cancer cells lose telomeric DNA with every cell division and yet retain the ability to proliferate, suggesting that telomere maintenance mechanisms are only necessary when telomere integrity is compromised after extensive shortening (Taboski et al, 2012). Together, telomerase and the nucleoprotein complex that protects telomeres ensure the maintenance of telomere integrity in dividing mammalian cells.

Experiments in the fruit fly *Drosophila melanogaster* and in maize established the importance of telomeres in genome stability (reviewed in Greider, 1996). These initial experiments determined that DNA damage could result in the loss of the terminal "knob" of linear chromosomes. Loss of telomeres in maize led to fusion or loss of chromosomes and an ensuing cycle of chromosome breakage, chromosome fusion, and anaphase bridges during cell division that is referred to as the *breakage-fusion-bridge* cycle. Telomere integrity is now known to be critical to the viability of normal and malignant cells in many organisms, and loss of telomere DNA is an important contributor to genomic instability.

9.7.1 Telomeres Protect Chromosomal Ends From Recognition as DNA Damage

Most linear chromosomes terminate in a long, noncoding repetitive tract of G-rich, telomeric-DNA that varies in its sequence and average length between organisms. In humans, telomeres are composed of 4 to 15 kilobase pairs (kbp) of the hexanucleotide sequence 5′-TTAGGG-3′ followed by 100 to 150 nucleotides of a single-stranded TTAGGG-3′ overhang. The 3′ single-stranded overhang is looped back on itself in a structure termed the *t-loop* (reviewed in de Lange, 2004). Internal to the telomeric tract, there are several kilobases of degenerate telomeric sequence, called *subtelomeric DNA*. The subtelomeric and telomeric regions exist in a nucleoprotein complex containing several telomere-binding proteins and chromatin-associated proteins. This nucleoprotein complex possesses a distinct nucleosomal structure that is thought to protect the chromosome ends from being perceived as damaged DNA, although in response to uncapping of telomere DNA, overt chromatin remodeling is not observed nor is it required for the DNA damage response (Wu and de Lange, 2008; Timashev et al, 2017; Vancevska et al, 2017; Fig. 9–14). Telomere dysfunction, either by erosion of telomere DNA or through loss of telomere end protection, can trigger the recruitment of several DSB response factors, including γ-H2AX, 53BP1, the MRN complex, and phosphorylated ATM. These resultant telomere-dysfunction–induced foci (TIF) coincide with the activation of the checkpoint kinases ATR and/or ATM, which, in turn, phosphorylate CHK1 and CHK2 and lead to p53- and p21-dependent cell apoptosis or cycle arrest. In some instances, such TIFs can persist long after the original insult (Rossiello et al, 2014). These TIFs are further modulated by Telomere-repeat containing RNAs (TERRA), which are transcribed from subtelomeres and contain G-rich telomeric repeats. This modulation of TIFs occurs through the association of TERRA transcripts with telomeres and recruitment of DNA repair and chromatin remodeling factors (reviewed in Cusanelli and Chartrand, 2015). Thus, many factors that play a role in the DNA damage response elsewhere in the genome also play important roles at the telomere.

To prevent the gradual erosion of linear DNA that arises as a result of the inability of DNA polymerases to completely replicate the 5′ ends of linear DNA, termed the *end replication problem*, a special cellular mechanism must compensate for telomere loss. This mechanism entails the addition of new G-rich, single-stranded telomere DNA to chromosome ends by telomerase, which carries its own telomere-complementary RNA template (see Fig. 9–14). At its core, this enzyme employs a reverse transcriptase (*telomerase reverse transcriptase [TERT]*) and the RNA template (*telomerase RNA-TR*) to direct new telomere DNA synthesis, 1 nucleotide at a time, onto chromosome ends (reviewed in Greider and Blackburn, 1996).

Telomeric sequences added by telomerase compensate for the gradual erosion of chromosome ends to enable cells undergoing multiple divisions during cell proliferation such as stem cells and cancer cells to maintain telomere length and chromosome stability. New telomere DNA synthesis is coordinated with replication of the telomeric DNA tract by conventional DNA polymerases, and telomerase interacts with subunits of the DNA replication machinery (reviewed in Price et al, 2010). Concomitant with or following replication, the 5′ and 3′ ends of telomeric DNA are processed to regenerate the overhangs and/or t-loops, and involve the highly regulated recruitment of nuclease complexes that include MRE11, CtIP, EXO1, and others (reviewed in Muraki and Murnane, 2018). During de novo telomere DNA synthesis by TERT, the telomerase RNA template is reverse transcribed into telomeric DNA (see Fig. 9–14). The assembly of active telomerase in vivo requires other components. For example, dyskerin and its protein partners NHP2, NOP10, and GAR1 bind to the 3′ terminal H/ACA box on telomerase RNA to modulate telomerase assembly and stability (Egan and Collins, 2010). TCAB1 (telomerase Cajal body protein 1) interacts with dyskerin and recognizes the CAB box in the telomerase RNA. It also facilitates telomerase assembly, catalysis, recruitment to telomeres, and trafficking to Cajal bodies (Stern et al, 2012; Chen et al, 2018; reviewed in Venteicher and Artandi, 2009). A recently published cryo-electron microscopy structure of the human telomerase RNP showcases the architecture of the different subunits that make up the active telomerase enzyme (Nguyen et al, 2018).

9.7.2 Telomere Regulation in Normal Cell Proliferation

In humans, normal cells often express low or undetectable levels of telomerase activity because of transcriptional repression of the *TERT* gene, and therefore undergo telomere shortening with each subsequent cell division. Normal cells do not replicate indefinitely in culture. The eventual loss of replicative potential is termed *cellular senescence* or the *Hayflick limit*. The time to the cessation of cell division correlates closely with critically eroded telomeres (called telomere signal-free ends [TSFEs]) (Allsopp et al, 1992; Allsopp and Harley, 1995).

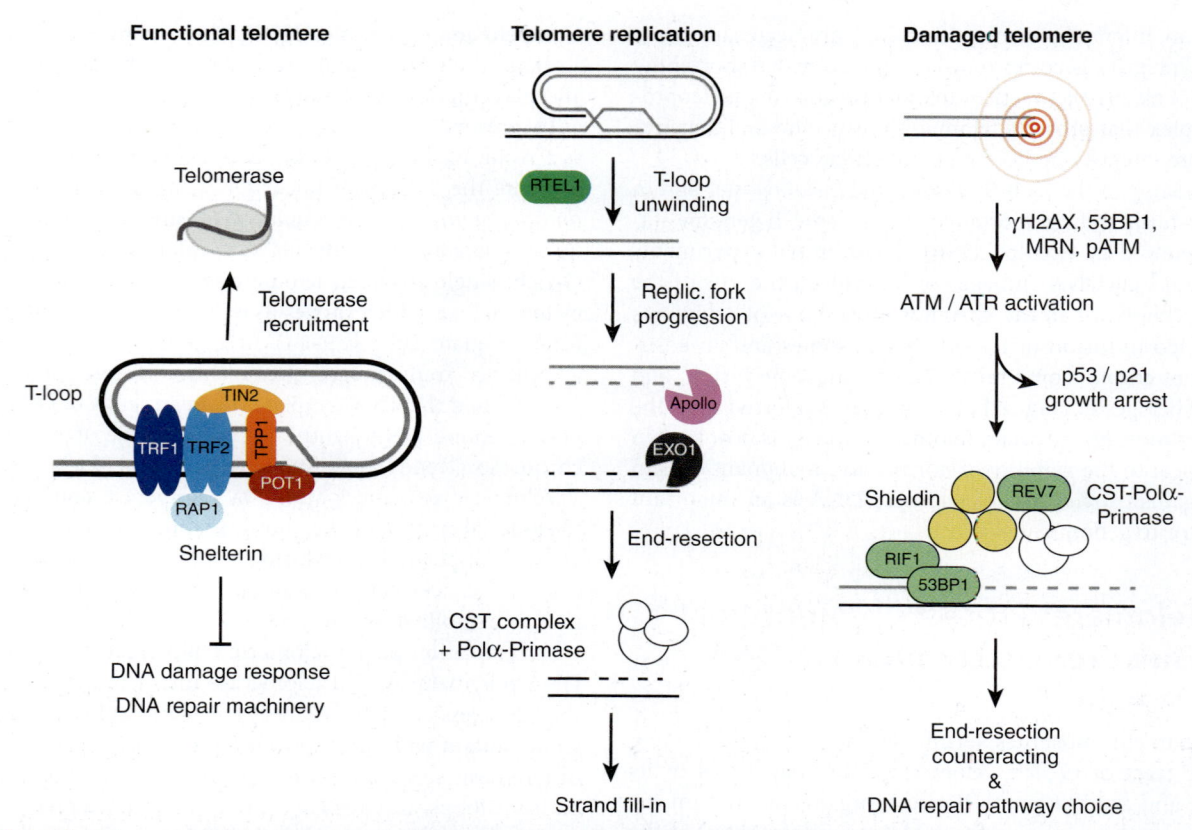

FIGURE 9–14 Telomere maintenance by telomerase and shelterin and the consequences of telomere dysfunction. Telomeres are bound by a complex called Shelterin (TIN2, TRF1, TRF2, POT1, RAP1, TPP1) and form a loop (t-loop) as a protection from DNA damage and degradation. The access of telomerase is limited by telomere-bound POT1 and TRF1 and the activity of ATM and ATR is limited by TRF2 and POT1 (left). During DNA replication, the activity of RTEL1 is needed to unwind the t-loop to allow the progression of the replication fork. End resection (by the Apollo and EXO1 nucleases) and strand fill-in (by the CST complex with Polα-Primase) are both required to regenerate a 3' overhang that will form the t-loop and protect chromosome ends (middle). Dysfunctional telomeres that arise via loss of telomere DNA repeats or loss of protection of shelterin induce DNA damage foci formation in telomeres (TIF) and activate ATM or ATR kinases leading to p53/p21-dependent cell apoptosis, cell-cycle arrest, and cellular senescence. In the case of a deprotected telomere, the DNA repair machinery acts through the coordinated activities of 53BP1-RIF1-REV7, Shieldin and the CST-Polα-Primase complex (right).

In the absence of the tumor-suppressor genes, p53 or pRb, cells can undergo additional population doublings before eventually reaching a proliferative block, called *crisis*. TSFEs are also a feature of cellular crisis in normal cells and many cancer cell types (reviewed in Cleal et al, 2018). At crisis, telomere fusion leads to mitotic arrest that is dependent on the spindle assembly checkpoint. This prolonged mitosis triggers more telomere deprotection that eventually leads to apoptosis (Hayashi et al, 2015). Only a small fraction of cells (approximately 1 in 10^7) survive by either activating expression of the endogenous *hTERT* gene or other telomerase-independent mechanisms, such as ALT (see below). Stem cells from various human tissues express telomerase during proliferative bursts, although usually at levels sufficient only to maintain telomere integrity and insufficient to elicit overall telomere lengthening (reviewed in Blasco, 2007). Aberrant telomere lengthening is also deleterious and can be counteracted by rapid telomere loss called telomere trimming, a process that serves to keep telomere length in equilibrium (reviewed in Li and Denchi, 2018).

The hypothesis that cellular senescence is causally linked to "critically short" telomeres is supported by a tight correlation between them, and the finding that reintroduction of TERT into human primary cells renders them capable of indefinite proliferation. Indeed, reintroduction of this single gene indefinitely prolongs the life span of human cells in culture (Bodnar et al, 1998; Vaziri and Benchimol, 1998). Despite being "immortal" in a culture dish, TERT-reconstituted human cells appear to preserve their normal morphology, response to external stress, and karyotype (Morales et al, 1999; Vaziri et al, 1999). Thus, TERT does not possess the classical characteristics that define an oncogene (Greider, 1998a), although in combination with other oncogenes TERT promotes the malignant transformation of normal cells (reviewed in Hahn, 2002). It is important to appreciate that senescence is a multifaceted phenotype that can be induced by myriad triggers other than critically short telomeres (He and Sharpless, 2017).

In mice, disruption of the genes encoding the telomerase RNA (*Terc*) or *Tert* leads to telomere shortening in all tissues and proliferative defects in multiple tissues and eventual germline sterility (reviewed in Liu and Harrington, 2012). Crossing telomerase-deficient mice with p53-deficient mice can extend the number of fertile generations (Chin et al, 1999), but eventually the germline cells from telomerase/p53-deficient mice also undergo apoptosis; thus p53-independent mechanisms are involved in monitoring telomere integrity and genome instability in dividing cells. Tissue defects are related not to overall short telomere lengths per se but to the inability to repair critically eroded telomeric tracts.

Telomere shortening has been linked to human syndromes with early mortality. For example, mutations in the telomerase components, TERT, TERC, DKC, NHP2, and NOP10 (as well as in RTEL1 and in a shelterin component, TIN2—see below) are associated with rare human genetic disorders, including dyskeratosis congenita, Hoyeraal-Hreidarsson syndrome, aplastic anemia, and idiopathic pulmonary fibrosis (reviewed in Bertuch, 2016). Most of these diseases are haploinsufficiency disorders, and a single inactive allele is sufficient to confer disease. Partial loss of function of telomerase activity also leads to various forms of hematopoietic cancer. Similar disease phenotypes are recapitulated in murine models in which one or both copies of telomerase subunits or telomere-associated proteins have been deleted or mutated, alone or in combination with factors that promote genome instability (reviewed in Liu and Harrington, 2012).

These findings suggest a potential paradox for diseases in which telomerase activation could potentially ameliorate disease. On the one hand, overexpression of telomerase leads to telomere extension and can extend the life span of cells derived from people with dyskeratosis congenita harboring mutations in the telomerase RNA (Agarwal et al, 2011) and telomerase activation ameliorates lung fibrosis in mice with limiting telomerase function (Le Saux et al, 2013; Povedano et al, 2018). On the other hand, a burgeoning number of genetic and epigenetic alterations have been identified in the *TERT* promoter in many cancer types, leading to an increase in telomerase expression and/or longer telomeres (Stern et al, 2015; Leao et al, 2018).

9.7.3 Shelterin and Telomere Integrity

In mammals, telomeres are bound by a 6-subunit complex called shelterin, which contains the telomere-binding proteins TRF1, TRF2, and POT1, and their associated proteins RAP1, TPP1, and TIN2 (de Lange, 2018; see Fig. 9–14). TRF1 and TRF2 bind to duplex telomeric DNA and anchor shelterin along the telomere repeats; POT1 binds to the single-stranded G-rich DNA overhang at telomeres; TIN2 is a protein scaffold for TRF1 and TRF2 and recruits POT1 to the complex via TPP1; and RAP1 associates with shelterin via binding to TRF2. Shelterin can form stable subcomplexes with different subunit stoichiometries in vitro, which could bind to different regions of the telomere in cells (Lim et al, 2017). This might explain how shelterin is able to serve several regulatory roles at the telomere, including telomerase access to the telomere, telomere replication and integrity, t-loop assembly and stability, and the ability to attenuate ATM- and ATR-dependent DNA damage responses (reviewed in de Lange, 2018). Shelterin function is conserved across a wide number of species, even in *Drosophila* where telomeres are maintained via a telomerase-independent mechanism of retrotransposition (Cenci et al, 2005; Longhese, 2008). Other conserved complexes that protect telomere integrity include the RPA-like protein complex CST (named after Cdc13/CTC1, STN1, TEN1) that regulates telomerase-mediated telomere extension and C-strand fill-in at telomeres and at other nontelomeric sites (Price et al, 2010; Lue, 2018). CST interacts with Shieldin, another multi-subunit complex that counteracts DNA resection at DSBs and telomeres (reviewed in Setiaputra and Durocher, 2019). These protective functions have clear clinical relevance, because loss-of-function mutations in Shieldin promote the resistance of *BRCA1*-deficient and *BRCA2*-deficient tumor cells to PARP inhibitors (Noordermeer et al, 2018; Tomida et al, 2018).

9.7.4 Telomere Maintenance and Cancer

To support long-term proliferative potential, an overwhelming majority of cancer cells express telomerase activity or, more rarely, maintain telomeres via telomerase-independent mechanisms (as described below). Evidence that telomerase inhibition kills cancer cells selectively was provided by studies showing that overexpression of dominant interfering variants of hTERT elicits telomere erosion and apoptosis in several cancer cell lines (Hahn et al, 1999; Herbert et al, 1999; Zhang et al, 1999). Several other lines of evidence now indicate that tumor cells must maintain minimally functional telomere reserves in order to retain proliferative potential. Below a critical threshold length (the so-called fusogenic range), the resultant telomere-telomere fusions that arise in cancers, such as chronic lymphocytic leukemia, are associated with coding sequence and copy number alterations, and are thus believed to be a significant factor in the evolution of the cancer genome architecture (Escudero et al, 2019; Norris et al, 2019).

In approximately 15% of cancers (across a wide variety of cancer types), cells maintain telomeres via HR and other telomere recombination events using an ALT mechanism (reviewed in Sobinoff and Pickett, 2017). ALT cells possess promyelocytic leukemia-like nuclear bodies called APBs (ALT-associated PML bodies) that contain telomeric DNA, telomere DNA binding proteins, and DNA repair proteins and may represent sites permissive for telomere recombination. ALT cells also possess long and heterogeneous telomere lengths, and carry extrachromosomal telomere DNA called t-circles (Sobinoff and Pickett, 2017). The chromatin state of telomeres seems to be critical for the activation of ALT in telomerase-negative cells, as suggested by the crisis bypass when chromatin remodeling factors such as ASF1 or ATRX are inactivated (O'Sullivan et al, 2014; Clynes et al, 2015; Napier et al, 2015). The activation of ALT is facilitated by multiple mechanisms that include dysregulation of chromatin, and other genetic events that favor break-induced telomere synthesis; for example, stalled replication fork recovery, alternative nonhomologous end joining, and repair of telomere DSBs serve important roles in repressing ALT activity (Sobinoff and Pickett, 2017). Some of these alterations are found to be drivers in the development of glioma and have suggested that ALT, and the epigenetic alterations that permit it, might serve to be an important therapeutic target in certain cancers (Haase et al, 2018).

Given the importance of telomere maintenance for long-term cellular proliferation, several telomerase targeting chemotherapeutic and immunotherapeutic strategies have been proposed but have shown limited anticancer efficiency (Harley, 2008). This apparent paradox stresses the importance of fully understanding telomere biology in order to leverage that knowledge into anticancer therapies. Optimization of these telomerase targeting clinical trials for earlier disease stages and patient stratification might be the key to higher success of these trials (Zanetti, 2017).

SUMMARY

- Genetic stability is crucial to the prevention of carcinogenesis. Many proteins involved in cell-cycle checkpoint control, chromosomal stability, DNA repair, and telomerase activity act in concert with one another during cell proliferation to maintain the integrity of the genome.
- Determining the tissue specificity of the proteins involved in these responses will be important to understand the relative susceptibility of different tissues to endogenous and exogenous carcinogens.
- Different types of lesions occur in DNA and are repaired by dedicated pathways: DNA-base mismatches (mismatch repair), damaged bases of the DNA (base excision repair), UV lesions or bulky DNA adducts (nucleotide excision repair), double-strand breaks (homologous recombination and nonhomologous end joining), and DNA interstrand crosslinks (Fanconi Anemia pathway).
- DNA double-strand breaks are the most toxic type of DNA damage. Checkpoint signaling cascades respond to these lesions in situ to enact DNA repair mechanisms and cell-cycle arrest to suppress mutagenesis and cell death.
- Human DNA repair- and checkpoint-deficient syndromes as well as murine "gene knockout" models provide important cellular and biochemical clues as to the temporal activity of many proteins within DNA damage signaling cascades.
- To support long-term proliferative potential, cancer cells often express telomerase activity or, more rarely, maintain telomeres via ALT. Because telomeres in actively dividing tumor cells are often short, telomerase is an attractive target for therapeutic intervention in cancer. Abnormal telomere regulation can lead to genetic instability.
- Our understanding of these pathways has led to the development of molecular cancer diagnostics and therapies specific to certain proteins which normally act as gatekeepers of genomic stability.

ACKNOWLEDGEMENT

We are grateful to the members of the D'Amours laboratory for their comments on the manuscript. We also wish to thank previous authors of this chapter, namely Shane M. Harding, Robert G. Bristow, and Lea Harrington, for their substantial contribution to the text. Work in D.D.'s laboratory is supported by a Foundation Grant from CIHR (FDN–167265) and a Canada Research Chair in Chromatin Dynamics & Genome Architecture (Tier 1). G.L. is supported by a merit studentship from the Fonds de Recherche du Québec-Santé (FRQ-S).

REFERENCES

Agarwal S, Loh YH, McLoughlin EM, et al. Telomere elongation in induced pluripotent stem cells from dyskeratosis congenita patients. *Nature* 2011;464:292-296.

Allsopp RC, Harley CB. Evidence for a critical telomere length in senescent human fibroblasts. *Exp Cell Res* 1995;219:130-136.

Allsopp RC, Vaziri H, Patterson C, et al. Telomere length predicts replicative capacity of human fibroblasts. *Proc Natl Acad Sci U S A* 1992;89:10114-10118.

Al-Hakim A, Escribano-Diaz C, Landry M-C, et al. The ubiquitous role of ubiquitin in the DNA damage response. *DNA Repair (Amst)* 2010;9:1229-1240.

Ames BN, Cathcart R, Schwiers E, Hochstein P. Uric acid provides an antioxidant defense in humans against oxidant- and radical-caused aging and cancer: a hypothesis. *Proc Natl Acad Sci U S A* 1981;78:6858-6862.

Apte MS, Cooper JP. Life and cancer without telomerase: ALT and other strategies for making sure ends (don't) meet. *Crit Rev Biochem Mol Biol* 2017;52:57-73.

Bakhoum SF, Ngo B, Laughney AM, et al. Chromosomal instability drives metastasis through a cytosolic DNA response. *Nature* 2018;553:467-472.

Bauerschmidt C, Woodcock M, Stevens D, et al. Cohesin phosphorylation and mobility of SMC1 at ionizing radiation-induced DNA double-strand breaks in human cells. *Exp Cell Res* 2011;317:330-337.

Bazyka D, Prysyazhnyuk A, Gudzenko N, et al. Epidemiology of late health effects in Ukrainian Chernobyl Cleanup Workers. *Health Phys* 2018;115:161-169.

Bensimon A, Aebersold R, Shiloh Y. Beyond ATM: the protein kinase landscape of the DNA damage response. *FEBS Lett* 2011;585:1625-1639.

Bensimon A, Schmidt A, Ziv Y, et al. ATM-dependent and -independent dynamics of the nuclear phosphoproteome after DNA damage. *Sci Signal* 2010;3:rs3.

Bertuch AA. The molecular genetics of the telomere biology disorders. *RNA Biol* 2016;13:696-706.

Besaratinia A, Pfeifer GP. Sunlight ultraviolet irradiation and BRAF V600 mutagenesis in human melanoma. *Hum Mutat* 2008;29:983-991.

Blackford AN, Jackson SP. ATM, ATR, and DNA-PK: the trinity at the heart of the DNA damage response. *Mol Cell* 2017;66:801-817.

Blasco MA. Telomere length, stem cells and aging. *Nat Chem Biol* 2007;3:640-649.

Bodmer W, Bielas JH, Beckman RA. Genetic instability is not a requirement for tumor development. *Cancer Res* 2008;68:3558-3560; discussion 3560-3561.

Bodnar AG, Ouellette M, Frolkis M, et al. Extension of lifespan by introduction of telomerase into normal human cells. *Science* 1998;279:349-352.

Bothmer A, Phadke T, Barrera LA, et al. Characterization of the interplay between DNA repair and CRISPR/Cas9-induced DNA lesions at an endogenous locus. *Nat Commun* 2017;8:13905.

Bouwman BAM, Crosetto N. Endogenous DNA double-strand breaks during DNA transactions: emerging insights and methods for genome-wide profiling. *Genes (Basel)* 2018;9.

Bouwman P, Aly A, Escandell JM, et al. 53BP1 loss rescues BRCA1 deficiency and is associated with triple-negative and BRCA-mutated breast cancers. *Nat Struct Mol Biol* 2010;17:688-695.

Brinkman EK, Chen T, de Haas M, et al. Kinetics and fidelity of the repair of Cas9-Induced double-strand DNA breaks. *Mol Cell* 2018;70:801-813.e806.

Brito DA, Rieder CL. Mitotic checkpoint slippage in humans occurs via cyclin B destruction in the presence of an active checkpoint. *Curr Biol* 2006;16:1194-1200.

Canman CE, Lim DS, Cimprich KA, et al. Activation of the ATM kinase by ionizing radiation and phosphorylation of p53. *Science* 1998;281:1677-1679.

Cenci G, Ciapponi L, Gatti M. The mechanism of telomere protection: a comparison between Drosophila and humans. *Chromosoma* 2005;114:135-145.

Chan DW, Gately DP, Urban S, et al. Lack of correlation between ATM protein expression and tumour cell radiosensitivity. *Int J Radiat Biol* 1998;74:217-224.

Chang HHY, Pannunzio NR, Adachi N, Lieber MR. Non-homologous DNA end joining and alternative pathways to double-strand break repair. *Nat Rev Mol Cell Biol* 2017;18:495-506.

Chen L, Roake CM, Freund A, et al. An activity switch in human telomerase based on RNA conformation and shaped by TCAB1. *Cell* 2018;174:218-230.e213.

Childs BG, Gluscevic M, Baker DJ, et al. Senescent cells: an emerging target for diseases of ageing. *Nat Rev Drug Discov* 2017;16:718-735.

Chin L, Artandi SE, Shen Q, et al. p53 deficiency rescues the adverse effects of telomere loss and cooperates with telomere dysfunction to accelerate carcinogenesis. *Cell* 1999;97:527-538.

Ciccia A, Elledge SJ. The DNA damage response: making it safe to play with knives. *Mol Cell* 2010;40:179-204.

Cleal K, Norris K, Baird D. Telomere length dynamics and the evolution of cancer genome architecture. *Int J Mol Sci* 2018;19.

Clynes D, Jelinska C, Xella B, et al. Suppression of the alternative lengthening of telomere pathway by the chromatin remodelling factor ATRX. *Nat Commun* 2015;6:7538.

Cordonnier AM, Fuchs RP. Replication of damaged DNA: molecular defect in xeroderma pigmentosum variant cells. *Mutat Res* 1999;435:111-119.

Cox R. Molecular mechanisms of radiation oncogenesis. *Int J Radiat Biol* 1994;65:57-64.

Cusanelli E, Chartrand P. Telomeric repeat-containing RNA TERRA: a noncoding RNA connecting telomere biology to genome integrity. *Front Genet* 2015;6:143.

D'Andrea AD. Susceptibility pathways in Fanconi's anemia and breast cancer. *N Engl J Med* 2010;362:1909-1919.

Daboussi F, Dumay A, Delacote F, Lopez BS. DNA double-strand break repair signalling: the case of RAD51 post-translational regulation. *Cell Signal* 2002;14:969-975.

Dagg RA, Pickett HA, Neumann AA, et al. Extensive proliferation of human cancer cells with ever-shorter telomeres. *Cell Rep* 2017;19:2544-2556.

D'Amours D, Jackson SP. The Mre11 complex: at the crossroads of DNA repair and checkpoint signalling. *Nat Rev Mol Cell Biol* 2002;3:317-327.

Dantuma NP, van Attikum H. Spatiotemporal regulation of posttranslational modifications in the DNA damage response. *EMBO J* 2016;35:6-23.

David SS, O'Shea VL, Kundu S. Base-excision repair of oxidative DNA damage. *Nature* 2007;447:941-950.

Davies AA, Masson JY, McIlwraith MJ, et al. Role of BRCA2 in control of the RAD51 recombination and DNA repair protein. *Mol Cell* 2001;7:273-282.

Daya-Grosjean L, Dumaz N, Sarasin A. The specificity of p53 mutation spectra in sunlight induced human cancers. *J Photochem Photobiol B* 1995;28:115-124.

Daya-Grosjean L, Sarasin A. UV-specific mutations of the human patched gene in basal cell carcinomas from normal individuals and xeroderma pigmentosum patients. *Mutat Res* 2000;450:193-199.

de Gruijl FR, Van Kranen HJ, Mullenders LH. UV-induced DNA damage, repair, mutations and oncogenic pathways in skin cancer. *J Photochem Photobiol B* 2001;63:19-27.

de Laat WL, Jaspers NG, Hoeijmakers JH. Molecular mechanism of nucleotide excision repair. *Genes Dev* 1999;13:768-785.

de Lange T. Shelterin-mediated telomere protection. *Annu Rev Genet* 2018;52:223-247.

de Lange T. T-loops and the origin of telomeres. *Nat Rev Mol Cell Biol* 2004;5:323-329.

Dobbs TA, Tainer JA, Lees-Miller SP. A structural model for regulation of NHEJ by DNA-PKcs autophosphorylation. *DNA Repair (Amst)* 2010;9:1307-1314.

Doil C, Mailand N, Bekker-Jensen S, et al. RNF168 binds and amplifies ubiquitin conjugates on damaged chromosomes to allow accumulation of repair proteins. *Cell* 2009;136:435-446.

Doksani Y, de Lange T. The role of double-strand break repair pathways at functional and dysfunctional telomeres. *Cold Spring Harb Perspect Biol* 2014;6:a016576.

Durocher D, Jackson SP. DNA-PK, ATM and ATR as sensors of DNA damage: variations on a theme? *Curr Opin Cell Biol* 2001;13:225-231.

Egan ED, Collins K. Specificity and stoichiometry of subunit interactions in the human telomerase holoenzyme assembled in vivo. *Mol Cell Biol* 2010;30:2775-2786.

Escudero L, Cleal K, Ashelford K, et al. Telomere fusions associate with coding sequence and copy number alterations in CLL. *Leukemia* 2019.

Esenboga S, Akal C, Karaatmaca B, et al. Two siblings with PRKDC defect who presented with cutaneous granulomas and review of the literature. *Clin Immunol* 2018;197:1-5.

Essers J, Hendriks RW, Swagemakers SM, et al. Disruption of mouse RAD54 reduces ionizing radiation resistance and homologous recombination. *Cell* 1997;89:195-204.

Fairbairn DW, Olive PL, O'Neill KL. The comet assay: a comprehensive review. *Mutat Res* 1995;339:37-59.

Falck J, Lukas C, Protopopova M, Lukas J, Selivanova G, Bartek J. Functional impact of concomitant versus alternative defects in the Chk2-p53 tumour suppressor pathway. *Oncogene* 2001;20:5503-5510.

Falkenberg KJ, Johnstone RW. Histone deacetylases and their inhibitors in cancer, neurological diseases and immune disorders. *Nat Rev Drug Discov* 2014;13:673-691.

Fattah F, Lee EH, Weisensel N, Wang Y, Lichter N, Hendrickson EA. Ku regulates the non-homologous end joining pathway choice of DNA double-strand break repair in human somatic cells. *PLoS Genet* 2010;6:e1000855.

Friedberg EC. How nucleotide excision repair protects against cancer. *Nat Rev Cancer* 2001;1:22-33.

Gavet O, Pines J. Progressive activation of CyclinB1-Cdk1 coordinates entry to mitosis. *Dev Cell* 2010;18:533-543.

Girard PM, Foray N, Stumm M, et al. Radiosensitivity in Nijmegen breakage syndrome cells is attributable to a repair defect and not cell cycle checkpoint defects. *Cancer Res* 2000;60:4881-4888.

Greider CW. Telomerase activity, cell proliferation, and cancer. *Proc Natl Acad Sci U S A* 1998a;95:90-92.

Greider CW. Telomere length regulation. *Annu Rev Biochem* 1996;65:337-365.

Greider CW, Blackburn EH. Telomeres, telomerase and cancer. *Sci Am* 1996;274:92-97.

Haase J, Bonner MK, Halas H, et al. Distinct roles of the chromosomal passenger complex in the detection of and response to errors in Kinetochore-Microtubule attachment. *Dev Cell* 2017;42:640-654.e645.

Haase S, Garcia-Fabiani MB, Carney S, et al. Mutant ATRX: uncovering a new therapeutic target for glioma. *Expert Opin Ther Targets* 2018;22:599-613.

Hahn WC. Immortalization and transformation of human cells. *Mol Cells* 2002;13:351-361.

Hahn WC, Stewart SA, Brooks MW, et al. Inhibition of telomerase limits the growth of human cancer cells. *Nat Med* 1999;5:1164-1170.

Hanahan D, Weinberg RA. Hallmarks of cancer: the next generation. *Cell* 2010;144:646-674.

Harfe BD, Jinks-Robertson S. DNA mismatch repair and genetic instability. *Annu Rev Genet* 2000;34:359-399.

Harley CB. Telomerase and cancer therapeutics. *Nat Rev Cancer* 2008;8:167-179.

Haschka M, Karbon G, Fava LL, et al. Perturbing mitosis for anti-cancer therapy: is cell death the only answer? *EMBO Rep* 2018;19.

Hayashi MT, Cesare AJ, Rivera T, et al. Cell death during crisis is mediated by mitotic telomere deprotection. *Nature* 2015;522:492-496.

He S, Sharpless NE. Senescence in health and disease. *Cell* 2017;169(6):1000-1011.

Heidenreich B, Kumar R. Altered TERT promoter and other genomic regulatory elements: occurrence and impact. *Int J Cancer* 2017;141:867-876.

Helleday T. Homologous recombination in cancer development, treatment and development of drug resistance. *Carcinogenesis* 2010;31:955-960.

Helleday T, Lo J, Van Gent DC, Engelward BP. DNA double-strand break repair: from mechanistic understanding to cancer treatment. *DNA Repair (Amst)* 2007;6:923-935.

Herbert B, Pitts AE, Baker SI, et al. Inhibition of human telomerase in immortal human cells leads to progressive telomere shortening and cell death. *Proc Natl Acad Sci U S A* 1999;96:14276-14281.

Heyer W-D, Ehmsen KT, Liu J. Regulation of homologous recombination in eukaryotes. *Annu Rev Genet* 2010;44:113-139.

Hittelman WN. Genetic instability in epithelial tissues at risk for cancer. *Ann N Y Acad Sci* 2001;952:1-12.

Hoeijmakers JH. DNA damage, aging, and cancer. *N Engl J Med* 2009;361:1475-1485.

Hoeijmakers JH. Genome maintenance mechanisms for preventing cancer. *Nature* 2001;411:366-374.

Holloman WK. Unraveling the mechanism of BRCA2 in homologous recombination. *Nat Struct Mol Biol*. 2011;18:748-754.

Jiricny J. The multifaceted mismatch-repair system. *Nat Rev Mol Cell Biol* 2006;7:335-346.

Kee Y, D'Andrea AD. Expanded roles of the Fanconi anemia pathway in preserving genomic stability. *Genes Dev* 2010;24:1680-1694.

Khanna KK, Jackson SP. DNA double-strand breaks: signaling, repair and the cancer connection. *Nat Genet* 2001;27:247-254.

Kitagawa R, Bakkenist CJ, McKinnon PJ, et al. Phosphorylation of SMC1 is a critical downstream event in the ATM-NBS1-BRCA1 pathway. *Genes Dev* 2004;18:1423-1438.

Kratz CP, Achatz MI, Brugieres L, et al. Cancer screening recommendations for individuals with Li-Fraumeni syndrome. *Clin Cancer Res* 2017;23:e38-e45.

Kress S, Sutter C, Strickland PT, Mukhtar H, Schweizer J, Schwarz M. Carcinogen-specific mutational pattern in the p53 gene in ultraviolet B radiation-induced squamous cell carcinomas of mouse skin. *Cancer Res* 1992;52:6400-6403.

Kubara PM, Kerneis-Golsteyn S, Studeny A, et al. Human cells enter mitosis with damaged DNA after treatment with pharmacological concentrations of genotoxic agents. *Biochem J* 2012;446:373-381.

Kunkel TA, Erie DA. Eukaryotic mismatch repair in relation to DNA replication. *Annu Rev Genet* 2015;49:291-313.

Lange SS, Takata K, Wood RD. DNA polymerases and cancer. *Nat Rev Cancer* 2011;11:96-110.

Lans H, Marteijn JA, Vermeulen W. ATP-dependent chromatin remodeling in the DNA-damage response. *Epigenetics Chromatin* 2012;5:4.

Lapenna S, Giordano A. Cell cycle kinases as therapeutic targets for cancer. *Nat Rev Drug Discov* 2009;8:547-566.

Le Saux CJ, Davy P, Brampton C, et al. A novel telomerase activator suppresses lung damage in a murine model of idiopathic pulmonary fibrosis. *PLoS One* 2013;8:e58423.

Leao R, Apolonio JD, Lee D, Figueiredo A, Tabori U, Castelo-Branco P. Mechanisms of human telomerase reverse transcriptase (hTERT) regulation: clinical impacts in cancer. *J Biomed Sci* 2018;25:22.

Lecot P, Alimirah F, Desprez PY, Campisi J, Wiley C. Context-dependent effects of cellular senescence in cancer development. *Br J Cancer* 2016;114:1180-1184.

Liang SH, Clarke MF. Regulation of p53 localization. *Eur J Biochem* 2001;268:2779-2783.

Li GM. Mechanisms and functions of DNA mismatch repair. *Cell Res* 2008;18:85-98.

Li JSZ, Denchi EL. How stem cells keep telomeres in check. *Differentiation* 2018;100:21-25.

Li SKH, Martin A. Mismatch repair and colon cancer: mechanisms and therapies explored. *Trends Mol Med* 2016;22:274-289.

Lim CJ, Zaug AJ, Kim HJ, Cech TR. Reconstitution of human shelterin complexes reveals unexpected stoichiometry and dual pathways to enhance telomerase processivity. *Nat Commun* 2017;8:1075.

Lim DS, Hasty P. A mutation in mouse rad51 results in an early embryonic lethal that is suppressed by a mutation in p53. *Mol Cell Biol* 1996;16:7133-7143.

Lim DS, Kim ST, Xu B, et al. ATM phosphorylates p95/nbs1 in an S-phase checkpoint pathway. *Nature* 2000;404:613-617.

Little JB. Failla Memorial Lecture. Changing views of cellular radiosensitivity. *Radiat Res* 1994;140:299-311.

Little JB. Radiation carcinogenesis. *Carcinogenesis* 2000;21:397-404.

Liu Y, Harrington L. Murine models of dysfunctional telomeres and telomerase. In: Autexier C, Lue NF, eds. *Telomerases: Chemistry, Biology, and Clinical Applications*. 1st ed. New York, NY: John Wiley; 2012:213-242.

Lobrich M, Shibata A, Beucher A, et al. gammaH2AX foci analysis for monitoring DNA double-strand break repair: strengths, limitations and optimization. *Cell Cycle* 2010;9:662-669.

Loeb LA. Mutator phenotype may be required for multistage carcinogenesis. *Cancer Res* 1991;51:3075-3079.

London N, Biggins S. Signalling dynamics in the spindle checkpoint response. *Nat Rev Mol Cell Biol* 2014;15:736-747.

Longhese MP. DNA damage response at functional and dysfunctional telomeres. *Genes Dev* 2008;22:125-140.

Lord CJ, Ashworth A. PARP inhibitors: synthetic lethality in the clinic. *Science* 2017;355:1152-1158.

Lue NF. Evolving linear chromosomes and telomeres: a C-strand-centric view. *Trends Biochem Sci* 2018;43:314-326.

MacPhail SH, Banath JP, Yu TY, Chu EH, Lambur H, Olive PL. Expression of phosphorylated histone H2AX in cultured cell lines following exposure to x-rays. *Int J Radiat Biol* 2003;79:351-358.

Marmorstein LY, Ouchi T, Aaronson SA. The BRCA2 gene product functionally interacts with p53 and RAD51. *Proc Natl Acad Sci U S A* 1998;95:13869-13874.

Marteijn JA, Lans H, Vermeulen W, et al. Understanding nucleotide excision repair and its roles in cancer and ageing. *Nat Rev Mol Cell Biol* 2014;15:465-481.

McVey M, Lee SE. MMEJ repair of double-strand breaks (directors cut): deleted sequences and alternative endings. *Trends Genet* 2008;24:529-538.

Mehta A, Haber JE. Sources of DNA double-strand breaks and models of recombinational DNA repair. *Cold Spring Harb Perspect Biol* 2014;6:a016428.

Moldovan GL, D'Andrea AD. How the Fanconi anemia pathway guards the genome. *Annu Rev Genet* 2009;43:223-249.

Morales CP, Holt SE, Ouellette M, et al. Absence of cancer-associated changes in human fibroblasts immortalized with telomerase. *Nat Genet* 1999;21:115-118.

Morgan WF, Hartmann A, Limoli CL, Nagar S, Ponnaiya B. Bystander effects in radiation-induced genomic instability. *Mutat Res* 2002;504:91-100.

Moynahan ME, Pierce AJ, Jasin M. BRCA2 is required for homology-directed repair of chromosomal breaks. *Mol Cell* 2001;7:263-272.

Muraki K, Murnane JP. The DNA damage response at dysfunctional telomeres, and at interstitial and subtelomeric DNA double-strand breaks. *Genes Genet Syst* 2018;92:135-152.

Napier CE, Huschtscha LI, Harvey A, et al. ATRX represses alternative lengthening of telomeres. *Oncotarget* 2015;6:16543-16558.

Narod SA, Foulkes WD. BRCA1 and BRCA2: 1994 and beyond. *Nat Rev Cancer* 2004;4:665-676.

Nguyen THD, Tam J, Wu RA, et al. Cryo-EM structure of substrate-bound human telomerase holoenzyme. *Nature* 2018;557:190-195.

Noordermeer SM, Adam S, Setiaputra D, et al. The shieldin complex mediates 53BP1-dependent DNA repair. *Nature* 2018;560:117-121.

Norris K, Hillmen P, Rawstron A, et al. Telomere length predicts for outcome to FCR chemotherapy in CLL. *Leukemia* 2019;33:1953-1963.

O'Donovan PJ, Livingston DM. BRCA1 and BRCA2: breast/ovarian cancer susceptibility gene products and participants in DNA double-strand break repair. *Carcinogenesis* 2010;31:961-967.

Offer H, Milyavsky M, Erez N, et al. Structural and functional involvement of p53 in BER in vitro and in vivo. *Oncogene* 2001;20:581-589.

O'Sullivan RJ, Arnoult N, Lackner DH, et al. Rapid induction of alternative lengthening of telomeres by depletion of the histone chaperone ASF1. *Nat Struct Mol Biol* 2014;21:167-174.

Oza AM, Tinker AV, Oaknin A, et al. Antitumor activity and safety of the PARP inhibitor rucaparib in patients with high-grade ovarian carcinoma and a germline or somatic BRCA1 or BRCA2 mutation: integrated analysis of data from Study 10 and ARIEL2. *Gynecol Oncol* 2017;147:267-275.

Palmero EI, Achatz MI, Ashton-Prolla P, Olivier M, Hainaut P. Tumor protein 53 mutations and inherited cancer: beyond Li-Fraumeni syndrome. *Curr Opin Oncol* 2010;22:64-69.

Pang D, Yoo S, Dynan WS, Jung M, Dritschilo A. Ku proteins join DNA fragments as shown by atomic force microscopy. *Cancer Res* 1997;57:1412-1415.

Panier S, Durocher D. Regulatory ubiquitylation in response to DNA double-strand breaks. *DNA Repair (Amst)* 2009;8:436-443.

Paull TT. Mechanisms of ATM activation. *Annu Rev Biochem* 2015;84:711-738.

Povedano JM, Martinez P, Serrano R, et al. Therapeutic effects of telomerase in mice with pulmonary fibrosis induced by damage to the lungs and short telomeres. *Elife* 2018;7.

Price CM, Boltz KA, Chaiken MF, Stewart JA, Beilstein MA, Shippen DE. Evolution of CST function in telomere maintenance. *Cell Cycle* 2010;9:3157-3165.

Ratsima H, Serrano D, Pascariu M, et al. Centrosome-dependent bypass of the DNA damage checkpoint by the polo kinase Cdc5. *Cell Rep* 2016;14:1422-1434.

Richardson C, Jasin M. Coupled homologous and nonhomologous repair of a double-strand break preserves genomic integrity in mammalian cells. *Mol Cell Biol* 2000;20:9068-9075.

Rieder CL, Maiato H. Stuck in division or passing through: what happens when cells cannot satisfy the spindle assembly checkpoint. *Dev Cell* 2004;7:637-651.

Romanov SR, Kozakiewicz BK, Holst CR, Stampfer MR, Haupt LM, Tlsty TD. Normal human mammary epithelial cells spontaneously escape senescence and acquire genomic changes. *Nature* 2001;409:633-637.

Rossiello F, Herbig U, Longhese MP, Fumagalli M, d'Adda di Fagagna F. Irreparable telomeric DNA damage and persistent DDR signalling as a shared causative mechanism of cellular senescence and ageing. *Curr Opin Genet Dev* 2014;26:89-95.

Rossio V, Galati E, Ferrari M, et al. The RSC chromatin-remodeling complex influences mitotic exit and adaptation to the spindle assembly checkpoint by controlling the Cdc14 phosphatase. *J Cell Biol* 2010;191:981-997.

Rotman G, Shiloh Y. ATM: from gene to function. *Hum Mol Genet* 1998;7:1555-1563.

Sampath H. Oxidative DNA damage in disease—insights gained from base excision repair glycosylase-deficient mouse models. *Environ Mol Mutagen* 2014;55:689-703.

Sancar A, Lindsey-Boltz LA, Unsal-Kacmaz K, Linn S. Molecular mechanisms of mammalian DNA repair and the DNA damage checkpoints. *Annu Rev Biochem* 2004;73:39-85.

Sander JD, Joung JK. CRISPR-Cas systems for editing, regulating and targeting genomes. *Nat Biotechnol* 2014;32:347-355.

Sasai K, Evans JW, Kovacs MS, Brown JM. Prediction of human cell radiosensitivity: comparison of clonogenic assay with chromosome aberrations scored using premature chromosome condensation with fluorescence in situ hybridization. *Int J Radiat Oncol Biol Phys* 1994;30:1127-1132.

Schärer OD. Nucleotide excision repair in eukaryotes. *Cold Spring Harb Perspect Biol* 2013;5:a012609.

Sedelnikova OA, Rogakou EP, Panyutin IG, Bonner WM. Quantitative detection of (125)IdU-induced DNA double-strand breaks with gamma-H2AX antibody. *Radiat Res* 2002;158:486-492.

Serrano D, D'Amours D. When genome integrity and cell cycle decisions collide: roles of polo kinases in cellular adaptation to DNA damage. *Syst Synth Biol* 2014;8:195-203.

Setiaputra D, Durocher D. Shieldin—the protector of DNA ends. *EMBO Rep.* 2019;20.

Sieben CJ, Sturmlechner I, van de Sluis B, van Deursen JM. Two-step senescence-focused cancer therapies. *Trends Cell Biol* 2018;28:723-737.

Smerdon MJ, Lieberman MW. Nucleosome rearrangement in human chromatin during UV-induced DNA-repair synthesis. *Proc Natl Acad Sci U S A* 1978;75:4238-4241.

Sobinoff AP, Pickett HA. Alternative lengthening of telomeres: DNA repair pathways converge. *Trends Genet* 2017;33:921-932.

Somlo G, Frankel PH, Arun BK, et al. Efficacy of the PARP inhibitor veliparib with carboplatin or as a single agent in patients with germline BRCA1- or BRCA2-associated metastatic breast cancer: California Cancer Consortium Trial NCT01149083. *Clin Cancer Res* 2017;23:4066-4076.

Spivak G. Nucleotide excision repair in humans. *DNA Repair (Amst)* 2015;36:13-18.

Stern JL, Theodorescu D, Vogelstein B, Papadopoulos N, Cech TR. Mutation of the TERT promoter, switch to active chromatin, and monoallelic TERT expression in multiple cancers. *Genes Dev* 2015;29:2219-2224.

Stern JL, Zyner KG, Pickett HA, Cohen SB, Bryan TM. Telomerase recruitment requires both TCAB1 and Cajal bodies independently. *Mol Cell Biol* 2012;32(13):2384-2395.

Stewart GS, Panier S, Townsend K, et al. The RIDDLE syndrome protein mediates a ubiquitin-dependent signaling cascade at sites of DNA damage. *Cell* 2009;136:420-434.

Stewart ZA, Westfall MD, Pietenpol JA. Cell-cycle dysregulation and anticancer therapy. *Trends Pharmacol Sci* 2003;24:139-145.

Svendsen JM, Harper JW. GEN1/Yen1 and the SLX4 complex: solutions to the problem of Holliday junction resolution. *Genes Dev* 2010;24:521-536.

Syljuasen RG, Jensen S, Bartek J, et al. Adaptation to the ionizing radiation-induced G2 checkpoint occurs in human cells and depends on checkpoint kinase 1 and Polo-like kinase 1 kinases. *Cancer Res* 2006;66:10253-10257.

Syljuasen RG, Krolewski B, Little JB. Molecular events in radiation transformation. *Radiat Res* 2001;155:215-221.

Szilard RK, Jacques PE, Laramee L, et al. Systematic identification of fragile sites via genome-wide location analysis of gamma-H2AX. *Nat Struct Mol Biol* 2010;17:299-305.

Taboski MA, Sealey DC, Dorrens J, et al. Long telomeres bypass the requirement for telomere maintenance in human tumorigenesis. *Cell Rep* 2012;1:91-98.

Thompson LH, Brookman KW, Dillehay LE, et al. Hypersensitivity to mutation and sister-chromatid-exchange induction in CHO cell mutants defective in incising DNA containing UV lesions. *Somatic Cell Genet* 1982;8:759-773.

Timashev LA, Babcock H, Zhuang X, de Lange T. The DDR at telomeres lacking intact shelterin does not require substantial chromatin decompaction. *Genes Dev* 2017;31:578-589.

Tlsty TD. Normal diploid human and rodent cells lack a detectable frequency of gene amplification. *Proc Natl Acad Sci U S A* 1990;87:3132-3136.

Toczyski DP, Galgoczy DJ, Hartwell LH. CDC5 and CKII control adaptation to the yeast DNA damage checkpoint. *Cell* 1997;90:1097-1106.

Tomida J, Takata KI, Bhetawal S, et al. FAM35A associates with REV7 and modulates DNA damage responses of normal and BRCA1-defective cells. *EMBO J* 2018;37.

Uhlmann F. SMC complexes: from DNA to chromosomes. *Nat Rev Mol Cell Biol* 2016;17:399-412.

van Gent DC, Hoeijmakers JH, Kanaar R. Chromosomal stability and the DNA double-strand break connection. *Nat Rev Genet* 2001;2:196-206.

van Overbeek M, Capurso D, Carter MM, et al. DNA repair profiling reveals nonrandom outcomes at Cas9-mediated breaks. *Mol Cell* 2016;63:633-646.

Vancevska A, Douglass KM, Pfeiffer V, et al. The telomeric DNA damage response occurs in the absence of chromatin decompaction. *Genes Dev* 2017;31:567-577.

Vaziri H, Benchimol S. Reconstitution of telomerase activity in normal human cells leads to elongation of telomeres and extended replicative life span. *Curr Biol* 1998;8:279-282.

Vaziri H, Squire JA, Pandita TK, et al. Analysis of genomic integrity and p53-dependent G1 checkpoint in telomerase-induced extended-life-span human fibroblasts. *Mol Cell Biol* 1999;19:2373-2379.

Venteicher AS, Artandi SE. TCAB1: driving telomerase to Cajal bodies. *Cell Cycle* 2009;8:1329-1331.

Vermeulen W. Dynamics of mammalian NER proteins. *DNA Repair (Amst)* 2011;10:760-771.

Viceconte N, Dheur MS, Majerova E, et al. Highly aggressive metastatic melanoma cells unable to maintain telomere length. *Cell Rep* 2017;19:2529-2543.

Weissberg JB, Huang DD, Swift M. Radiosensitivity of normal tissues in ataxia-telangiectasia heterozygotes. *Int J Radiat Oncol Biol Phys* 1998;42:1133-1136.

Whitaker SJ, Powell SN, Mcmillan TJ. Molecular assays of radiation-induced DNA damage. *Eur J Cancer* 1991;27:922-928.

Woodward WA, Bristow RG. Radiosensitivity of cancer-initiating cells and normal stem cells (or what the Heisenberg uncertainly principle has to do with biology). *Semin Radiat Oncol* 2009;19:87-95.

Wu P, de Lange T. No overt nucleosome eviction at deprotected telomeres. *Mol Cell Biol* 2008;28:5724-5735.

Yi C, He C. DNA repair by reversal of DNA damage. *Cold Spring Harb Perspect Biol* 2013;5:a012575.

Yoo TY, Choi JM, Conway W, et al. Measuring NDC80 binding reveals the molecular basis of tension-dependent kinetochore-microtubule attachments. *Elife* 2018;7.

Zanetti M. A second chance for telomerase reverse transcriptase in anticancer immunotherapy. *Nat Rev Clin Oncol* 2017;14:115-128.

Zhang X, Mar V, Zhou W, Harrington L, Robinson MO. Telomere shortening and apoptosis in telomerase-inhibited human tumor cells. *Genes Dev* 1999;13:2388-2399.

Zhou PK, Sproston AR, Marples B, West CM, Margison GP, Hendry JH. The radiosensitivity of human fibroblast cell lines correlates with residual levels of DNA double-strand breaks. *Radiother Oncol* 1998;47:271-276.

Ziegler A, Leffell DJ, Kunala S, et al. Mutation hotspots due to sunlight in the p53 gene of nonmelanoma skin cancers. *Proc Natl Acad Sci U S A* 1993;90:4216-4220.

Tumor Progression and Metastasis

Virginie Defamie and Rama Khokha

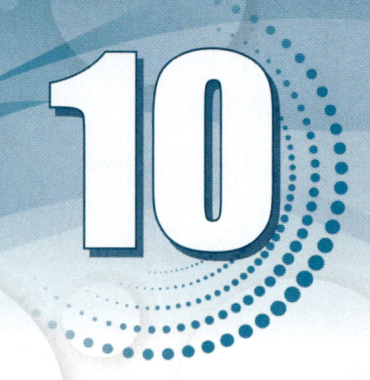

Chapter Outline

10.1 Tumor Progression
  10.1.1 Cellular Aspects of Tumor Progression
  10.1.2 Molecular Genetics of Tumor Progression

10.2 Tumor Microenvironment
  10.2.1 Extracellular Matrix
  10.2.2 Cellular Proteinases and Their Inhibitors
  10.2.3 Cell Adhesion Molecules
  10.2.4 The Pathophysiological Microenvironment

10.3 Metastasis
  10.3.1 The Spread of Cancer
  10.3.2 Detachment from the Primary Tumor, Local Invasion, and Intravasation
  10.3.3 Survival in the Bloodstream
  10.3.4 Circulating Tumor Cells
  10.3.5 Extravasation
  10.3.6 Initiation of a New Growth (Colonization)

10.4 Dynamics of Metastasis
  10.4.1 Metastatic Organotropism
  10.4.2 Metastatic Inefficiency
  10.4.3 Metastatic Dormancy and Relapse
  10.4.4 Cancer Stem Cells in Recurrence and Metastasis

10.5 Molecular Mechanisms of Metastasis
  10.5.1 Protease Activity at the Invasive Front
  10.5.2 Protease Activity in the Tumor Microenvironment
  10.5.3 Cancer-Associated Fibroblasts
  10.5.4 Tumor-Associated Macrophages
  10.5.5 Epithelial-to-Mesenchymal Transition
  10.5.6 Pre-metastatic Niches and Exosomes

10.6 Genetic Evolution of Metastasis

10.7 Treatment to Prevent Metastasis

Summary

References

10.1 TUMOR PROGRESSION

10.1.1 Cellular Aspects of Tumor Progression

Cancer is not a static disease. In many tumors, there appears to be an orderly progression from benign tissue to premalignant lesion to frank malignancy. In other tumors, premalignant lesions may not have been identified, but it is likely the tumor has passed through less-malignant stages before detection. The pathologic and clinical criteria for tumor progression are often specific to a given type of tumor, but include local spread along tissue planes and into various tissue spaces and cavities. Tumors also have the capacity to invade and spread from their origins to other organs in the body; this process is referred to as *metastasis*. Increasing numbers and types of genetic abnormalities accompany tumor progression and metastasis.

More than 60 years ago, Foulds defined tumor progression as "the acquisition of permanent, irreversible qualitative changes in one or more characteristics of a neoplasm" that cause the tumor to become more autonomous and malignant (Foulds, 1954). In 1986, Nowell proposed that such changes arise because cancer cells tend to be genetically unstable and described a conceptual model to explain the process of tumor progression (Fig. 10–1) (Nowell, 1986).

The key features of this model are the generation of mutant cells within a tumor and the selection and outgrowth of more autonomous cells to become dominant subclones in the population, leading to progression of the tumor and increasing malignancy. Many studies have confirmed the genetic instability of malignant cells (see Chap. 7, Sec. 7.2 and Chap. 9, Sec. 9.2) and have identified both genetic and epigenetic alterations using genome-wide analyses (see Chap. 2, Sec. 2.2). Consistent with this model, multiple studies have identified different clonal populations within tumors (see Chap. 13, Sec. 13.2), raising the possibility for a minor (resistant) subpopulation to cause tumor recurrence following therapy (McGranahan and Swanton, 2017). The growth and development of various cells within a tumor are subject to constraints associated

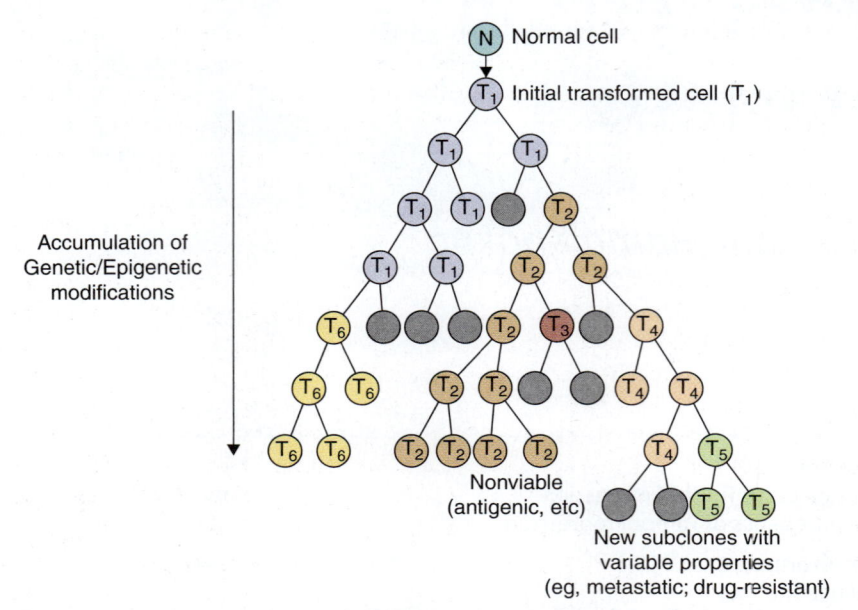

FIGURE 10–1 Schematic showing the clonal evolution of tumors. New subclones arise by mutation and/or epigenetic modifications. Many of these may become extinct (indicated by dark shading) but others may have a growth advantage and become dominant. All of the subclones (indicated by T_2 to T_6) may share common clonal markers, but many of them have new properties leading to heterogeneity. (Nowell, 1986).

with interactions among the tumor cells, the stromal cells, and the extracellular environment. Thus, the normal homeostatic mechanisms that control cell proliferation in the body (see Chap. 6 and Chap. 8, Sec. 8.2) are not lost completely in tumor cells, but rather the cells may become less responsive to them. In addition, tumor cells acquire autonomous means to grow, becoming less dependent on extraneous growth factors (Kopfstein and Christofori, 2006). The main characteristics acquired by cancer cells are depicted in Figure 10–2. These findings are consistent with the original concepts of Foulds that there are many different paths to malignancy: tumors are evolving cell communities with properties that continue to change as they grow (Foulds, 1954). The role of the stromal cell populations and the extracellular microenvironment are recognized as critical elements in tumor development and progression (Hanahan and Weinberg, 2011).

10.1.2 Molecular Genetics of Tumor Progression

Genetic instability of tumor cells may arise as a result of genetic and/or epigenetic changes. Epigenetic changes such as methylation of cytosine bases in DNA or modifications to chromatin structure (eg, by methylation, acetylation), and post-translational modification of histones can modify the expression of genes and are important mechanisms for "silencing" genes during normal differentiation (see Chap. 3). Genetic changes may occur by point mutation, deletion, gene amplification, chromosomal translocation, or other mechanisms (see Chap. 9, Sec. 9.2). For instance, consistent copy number gains on chromosome 8q22 and high metadherin expression is strongly associated with high risk of tumor metastasis and worse prognosis in breast cancer (Vogelstein et al, 2013). A cell is continually exposed to both external and internal stresses, such as reactive oxygen species, which may cause DNA damage. Moreover, there are inherent errors made by DNA polymerases whenever DNA is being replicated. Normally such damage is either repaired by the various DNA repair mechanisms in the cell (see Chap. 9, Sec. 9.3), or damaged cells undergo apoptosis (see Chap. 8, Sec. 8.4). However, cancer cells

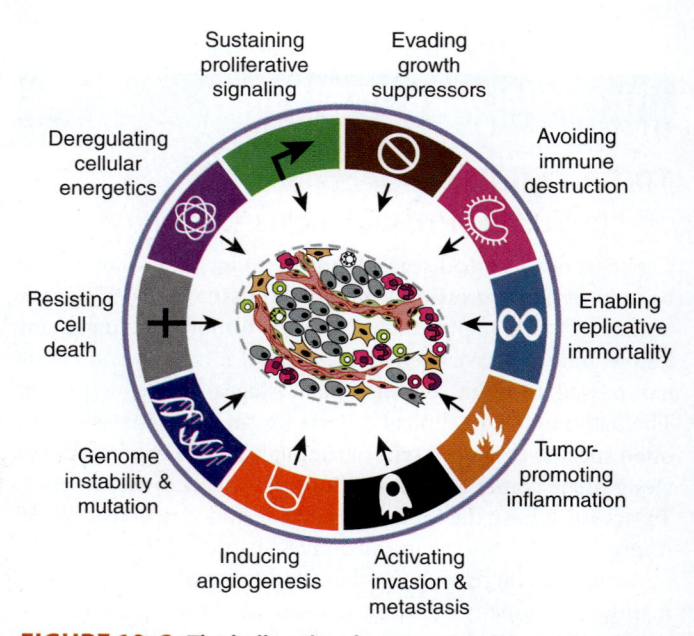

FIGURE 10–2 The hallmarks of cancer. The biology of cancer can be divided into 10 categories representing distinctive and complementary capabilities that enable tumor growth and metastatic dissemination.

have an increased frequency of mutation because of deficiencies in their ability to repair lesions in DNA and/or decreased activation of apoptosis, so that mutated cells may survive and proliferate. For example, the breast cancer–related genes, BRCA1/2, are linked with DNA double-strand break repair (see Chap. 9, Sec. 9.5). Oxidative lesions and deficiencies of mismatch repair have been demonstrated in tumor cells, particularly those from patients with certain types of colon cancer. A deficiency in mismatch repair can result in up to a 1000-fold increase in the mutation frequency. Failures in DNA damage repair may result in mutations or alterations in the expression of the many oncogenes and tumor-suppressor genes that are associated with different human cancers (see Chap. 7). Mutations in these genes are not necessarily more frequent than in other genes; rather these "driver mutations" are selected during the process of cancer development, and thus are the ones that are most frequently detected. Cancer cells may also carry many "passenger" mutations, so-called because they play little or no known role in their cancer phenotype.

The multiple changes that must occur in cells during tumor development and progression are illustrated by the model established by Vogelstein and colleagues describing the progression of colon cancer (Fearon and Vogelstein, 1990; Fig. 10–3). This model provides a paradigm for multistep carcinogenesis that has been applied to many other cancers (eg, breast, pancreatic, bladder, and lung), although the steps do not always occur in a specific order. These concepts have been reinforced by evidence that sequential modifications involving activation of oncogenes or inactivation of tumor suppressors can result in the transformation of normal human cells. Thus, a molecular description of tumor progression envisages that cancers progress as a result of a series of (selected) genetic and epigenetic changes. Some of these changes are shared between different cancers, but changes unique to specific types of cancer also occur and the sequence of the multisteps may not follow the same timeline in individual cancers of the same type. For example, large-scale chromosomal alterations that disrupt hundreds of genes have been observed in pancreatic cancers and represent macro-evolutionary events contributing to tumor progression (Notta et al, 2016).

As a result of genetic and epigenetic changes, cells within animal and human tumors demonstrate considerable heterogeneity in their phenotypes (Mazor et al, 2016). This heterogeneity includes karyotype, surface markers, biochemical pathway activity, cell proliferation, metastatic ability, and response to therapy. Next-generation sequencing has shown that the degree of intratumor heterogeneity can be highly variable, with up to 8000 coding mutations found within primary tumors or between primary and metastatic or recurrent lesions (Johnson et al, 2014). The ability of tumor cells to disseminate and form metastases represents the most malignant characteristic of a cancer. As described in Section 10.3, metastases probably arise from a small subset of cells within a primary tumor that has undergone genetic or epigenetic changes

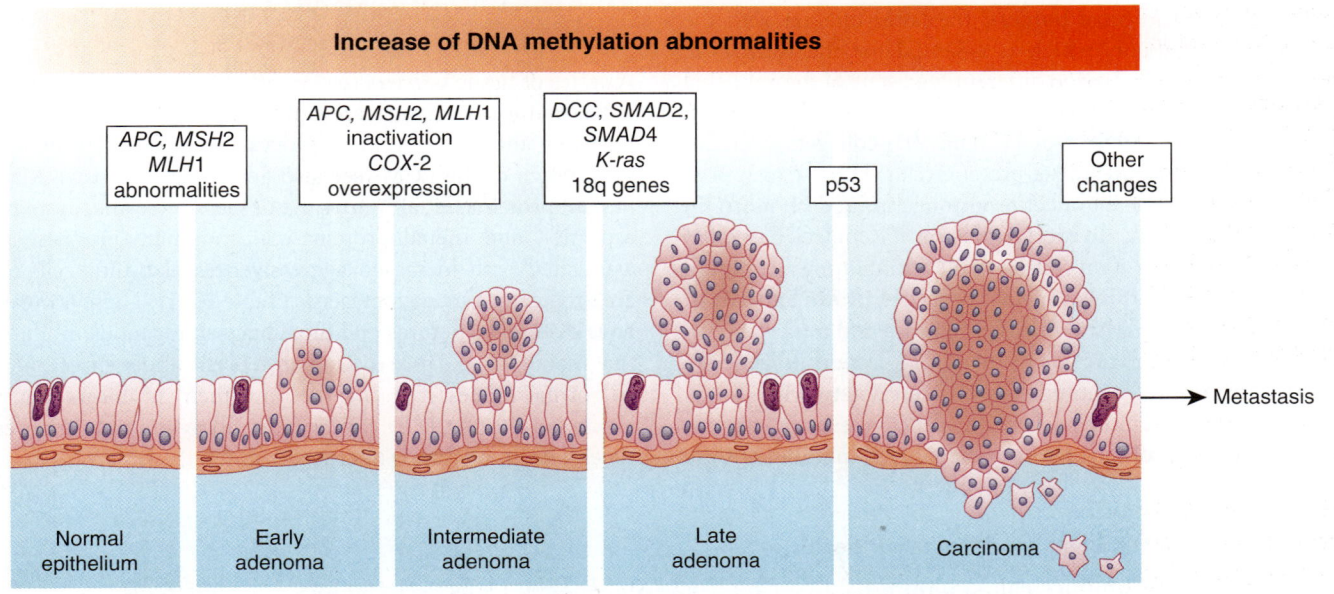

FIGURE 10–3 **Genetic and epigenetic changes associated with colorectal tumorigenesis.** Adenoma polyposis coli (APC) mutations initiate the neoplastic process, and tumor progression results from mutations in the other genes indicated. Patients with familial adenomatous polyposis (FAP) inherit APC mutations and develop numerous dysplastic aberrant crypt foci (ACF), some of which progress as they acquire the other mutations indicated in the figure. DNA methylation is one of the most important epigenetic events, which is thought to occur during the early stages of oncogenic transformation. The tumors from patients with hereditary nonpolyposis colorectal carcinoma (HNPCC) go through a similar although not identical series of mutations; DNA repair deficiency speeds up this process. K-ras is an oncogene that requires only 1 genetic event for its activation. The other specific genes indicated are tumor-suppressor genes that require 2 genetic events (1 in each allele) for their inactivation. Chromosome 18q21 may contain several different tumor-suppressor genes involved in colorectal neoplasia, with DCC (deleted in colon cancer), SMAD2 and SMAD4 genes proposed as candidates. A variety of other genetic alterations have each been described in a small fraction of advanced colorectal cancers. These may be responsible for the heterogeneity of biological and clinical properties observed among different cases.

enhancing their ability to metastasize. Metastases at different sites have been found to derive either from a single subclone in the primary tumor, showing low inter-metastatic heterogeneity (Schwarz et al, 2015) or originate from distinct subclones of the primary tumor (Turajlic and Swanton, 2016) (see Sec. 10.6). Moreover, tracking of pancreatic tumor progression using multicolor lineage tracing in the Kras/p53 mouse model has shown evidence of polyclonal seeding of metastasis in the lung, liver, and peritoneum, suggesting cooperation between cancer subclones facilitating their metastatic colonization (Maddipati and Stanger, 2015). Similarly, collective migration and invasion of polyclonal clusters of cells within the circulation and at metastatic sites were shown in a model of breast cancer (Cheung et al, 2016). Finally, the tumor stroma can also contribute to tumor heterogeneity. In pancreatic cancers, the dense desmoplastic stroma, often representing 60% to 90% of the tumor volume, shows substantial differences in its cellular and structural content and is thought to associate with patient outcome (Laklai et al, 2016).

10.2 TUMOR MICROENVIRONMENT

10.2.1 Extracellular Matrix

Most mammalian cells are in contact with an extracellular matrix (ECM; see also Chap. 12, Sec. 12.2). The composition and structure of the ECM are specific to location and developmental stage. For example, epithelial cells have specialized lateral, apical, and basal borders: the latter interact with the basement membrane, which is essential for the formation, maintenance, and polarized differentiated state of the epithelial cell sheet. The basement membrane, a specialized form of ECM, is composed of laminin, type IV (and VII) collagen, entactin/nidogen, and heparan sulfate proteoglycan (HSPG), as well as smaller amounts of fibronectin, vitronectin, and chondroitin sulfate proteoglycans. To exert tissue-specific control, basement membranes vary in composition while maintaining a common set of structural and mechanical properties (Rowe and Weiss, 2009). There are at least 7 forms of laminin and 6 type IV collagen chains that interact with other ECM proteins to generate a 3-dimensional (3D) interlocking structural network.

In contrast to epithelial cells, mesenchymal cells are not attached to each other or to a basement membrane, but are surrounded by an ECM that contains the interstitial collagen types I to III, elastin, proteoglycans, fibronectin, and vitronectin. Other specialized tissue-specific ECM molecules include tenascin, thrombospondin, and osteopontin. The highly organized 3D matrix provides an adhesive environment for cells and other molecules, such as growth factors. The ECM binds to cell surface molecules (cell adhesion molecules [CAMs]; see Sec. 10.2.3), which interact with specific signal transduction pathways in the cell. Regulated proteolysis is essential for normal cell-ECM communication. Proteinases act on an array of substrates, including the ECM, CAMs, growth factors, and cytokines, as well as their receptors and binding proteins. Growth factors can be embedded within the matrix or anchored to the cell surface in close proximity to their cell surface receptors (see Chap. 6) and become bioavailable only on proteinase mediated cleavage.

The interaction of cells with the ECM is essential for growth and survival, and the ECM can also regulate the differentiation of a variety of cell types. Depriving normal cells of such interactions results in the induction of apoptosis (anoikis) in epithelial and endothelial cells, or cell-cycle arrest in fibroblasts (Buchheit et al, 2014). Transformed cells are often defective in secreting fibronectin and in laying down an organized matrix, and a common property of malignant cells is their ability to survive and proliferate with a lower dependence on interactions with an ECM than normal cells.

10.2.2 Cellular Proteinases and Their Inhibitors

A series of tissue barriers (eg, basement membrane and interstitial connective tissue) are traversed by tumor cells during invasion and metastasis by processes involving proteolytic breakdown of the ECM (see also Secs. 10.3 and 10.5). Mammalian proteinases fall into 4 major classes (serine, cysteine-, aspartic-, and metalloproteinases), and many of these are associated with increased aggressiveness of tumor cells and are implicated during metastasis (Table 10–1). These proteases have distinct structures and most have endogenous inhibitors that maintain a balance to keep proteolysis under strict control in normal tissues. The enzymes and their inhibitors may be expressed aberrantly by cancer cells and by multiple other cell types within the tumor microenvironment.

TABLE 10–1 Proteinases in specific catalytic classes.

Catalytic Type	Numbers (Human/Mouse)	Associated with Malignancy	Specific Inhibitors	Substrates
Cysteine	143/153	Cathepsins B, L, H	Kinogens, cystatins, stefins	ECM
	15/14	Calpains 1, 2, 3, 4, 6, 9, 10	Calpastatin	Focal adhesion proteins, Cell signaling proteins
Aspartic	21/27	Cathepsin D	Not known	ECM
Metallo	186/197	MMPs 2, 3, 7, 9, 11, 13, 14	TIMPs	ECM, GFs/cytokines
Serine	176/227	uPA, tPA	PAIs	Plasminogen, latent MMPs

ECM, extracellular matrix; GF, growth factor; MMP, matrix metalloproteinase; PAI, plasminogen activator inhibitor; TIMP, tissue inhibitor of metalloproteinase; tPA, tissue plasminogen activator; uPA, urokinase plasminogen activator.
Data from Puente XS, Sánchez LM, Overall CM, et al: Human and mouse proteases: a comparative genomic approach. Nat Rev Genet 2003 Jul;4(7):544-558.

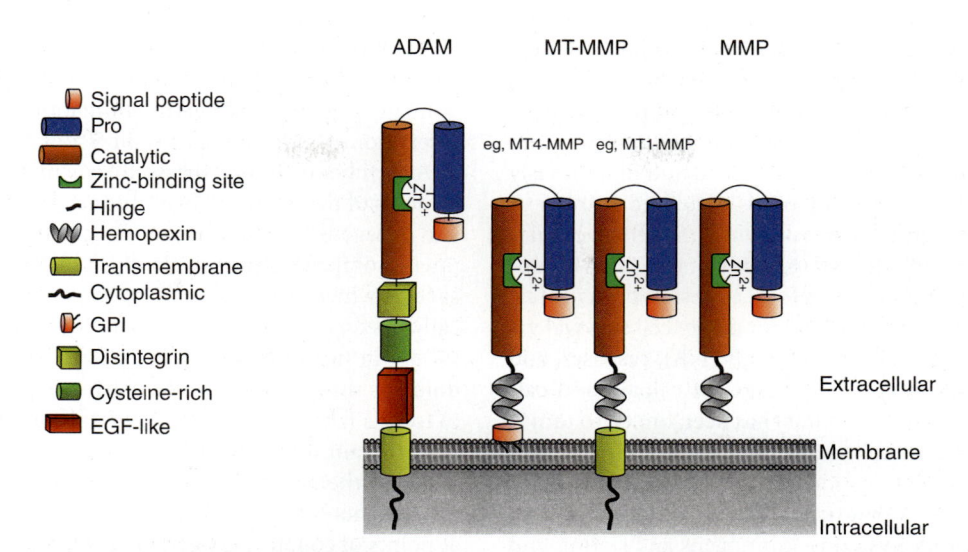

FIGURE 10-4 Modular structure of MMPs, MT-MMPs, and ADAMs. Matrix metalloproteinases (MMPs) are secreted as soluble enzymes but 6 of them are membrane-type MMPs (MT-MMPs) that are associated with the cell membrane by either a transmembrane domain (MT1-, MT2-, MT3-, MT5-MMP) or a glycosylphosphatidyl-inositol (GPI) anchor (MT4- and MT6-MMP). The pro-domain blocks their protease activity. The ADAMs (A Disintegrin And Metalloproteinase) are membrane-anchored proteinases and they share the catalytic domain with the MMPs. However, they lack the hemopexin-like domain (responsible for substrate binding) and they harbor 3 additional domains: cysteine-rich domain, epidermal growth factor (EGF)-like domain, and the disintegrin domain. The disintegrin domain can mediate cell–cell and cell–matrix interaction by binding integrins while the cysteine-rich domain allows the binding of several extracellular matrix (ECM) constituents. (Modified with permission from Noël A, Gutiérrez-Fernández A, Sounni NE, et al. New and paradoxical roles of matrix metalloproteinases in the tumor microenvironment. *Front Pharmacol* 2012 Jul 17;3:140.)

Metalloproteinases comprise the biggest family of proteases in the human genome with 186 members: subfamilies such as MMPs (matrix metalloproteinases) and ADAMs (A Disintegrin And Metalloproteinase), including membrane type (MT)-MMPs, are the major enzymes responsible for degradation of ECM proteins (Fig. 10–4). Extracellular MMPs are often secreted in a latent form (pro-MMP), and activated subsequently. The MMPs chelate 2 zinc ions: one is present in the active site and the other associates with the pro-MMP to stabilize the inactive state (Egeblad and Werb, 2002). These enzymes can be auto-catalyzed, activated by other MMPs, or activated by a serine proteinase. Cell surface–anchored proteases, such as MT-MMPs, are activated by proprotein convertases, some of which are also critical for the localization and cell-surface activation of soluble pro-MMPs. For example, MT1-MMP is essential for the activation of pro-MMP-2 at the cell surface. Interactions among different classes of proteases also generate complex proteolytic cascades, which can amplify their activity. Within the metalloproteinase family, the ADAMs are unique in that they possess both adhesion and proteolytic domains (Reiss and Saftig, 2009). These transmembrane proteases act as "sheddases" to release cell surface anchored growth factors and cytokines in a process called *ectodomain shedding*; in addition, they are critical for the activation of receptor-mediated pathways such as NOTCH and epidermal growth factor receptor (EGFR) (Murphy, 2009; see Chap. 6). ADAM8, 10, 17, and 28 have been implicated in cancer formation and progression, with the strongest evidence for ADAM17. Also known as tumor necrosis factor α (TNF-α) converting enzyme or TACE, ADAM17 downstream signaling culminates in increased cell proliferation, migration, invasion, and metastasis. In mouse models, deficiency of *ADAM17* results in decreased growth of cancer cell lines and of xenografted tumors, whereas high levels of ADAM17 are associated with poor prognosis of diverse types of primary cancers (Mullooly et al, 2016).

Plasminogen activators (urokinase type [uPA] and tissue type [tPA]) are serine proteinases that act on circulating plasminogen to release plasmin and have long been associated with malignant cells. The activity of plasminogen and plasmin is localized to the cell surface by the uPA receptor (uPAR), which also associates with integrins and can bind to vitronectin in the ECM (Laufs et al, 2006). Increased expression of uPA has been correlated with metastasis in a number of cancers including human epidermal growth receptor 2 (HER2)-positive breast cancer (see Chap. 19, Sec. 19.4). The level of expression of plasminogen activator inhibitor (PAI)-1 also provides an independent unfavorable prognostic factor for the development of metastases in women with hormone receptor- and lymph node-positive breast cancer (Schmitt et al, 2011). Among serine proteases, kallikreins are coded by a contiguous cluster of protease genes and have been studied extensively for their utility as serum cancer biomarkers. For example, prostate-specific antigen (PSA) is a kallikrein used routinely for evaluation of prostate cancer progression.

Cathepsins are cysteine proteases on intracellular membranes localized to endosomal or lysosomal vesicles. Cathepsins can also be found outside the cell during pathologic conditions and their presence in body fluids is a prognostic indicator for several cancers (Olson and Joyce, 2015). Slight structural differences between the 11 cathepsins are responsible for differences in substrate specificity and inhibition by their endogenous inhibitors. Cathepsins B, H, and L are associated particularly with tumor progression. An imbalance between the cathepsins and their inhibitors can occur during tumor progression and may be responsible for direct digestion of the ECM or activation of other proteolytic enzymes, such as uPA.

Calpains are intracellular cysteine proteases directly activated by calcium. Among the calpain family, μ-calpain and m-calpain are the most commonly described and ubiquitously expressed. They catalyze the proteolysis of a large number of specific substrates resulting in cytoskeletal remodeling, cellular signaling, apoptosis, and cell survival. For instance, they induce cell migration through cleavage of focal adhesion proteins (eg, focal adhesion kinase and talin) and modulate cell survival via cleavage of inhibitor of nuclear factor-κB (IκB), caspases, and BCL-2 proapoptotic proteins. Expression of calpain and calpastatin (their endogenous inhibitor) has been linked to tumor progression and response to therapy (Storr et al, 2011).

Proteinase inhibitors are produced by both malignant and normal cells. Examples of these inhibitors are PAI-1 and PAI-2, the cathepsin inhibitors, cystatins, kininogens and stefins, and tissue inhibitors of metalloproteinases (TIMPs). Under physiological conditions, a balance between activated proteinases and their inhibitors keeps proteolysis under strict control, but when this balance is disrupted, (malignant) cells can invade tissues. Downregulation of TIMP-1 activity in immortalized murine fibroblasts, using transfected antisense RNA (see Chap. 2, Sec 2.3.3), confers invasive capacity and ability to form metastatic tumors in nude mice. Increased levels of TIMP-1, TIMP-2, or TIMP-3 reduce the invasive and metastatic ability of malignant cells. Gain- and loss-of-function studies have addressed the causal role of specific TIMPs and cystatins with various processes underlying tumorigenesis (Jackson et al, 2017). However, the relationship between advanced malignancy and increased proteolytic activity (such as that arising from increased MMP or decreased TIMP expression) is not simple. For example, increased MMP activity during cancer progression can be associated with a favorable prognosis, as for MMP-12 in colon cancer, and increased TIMP expression is a poor prognostic indicator in many studies (Egeblad and Werb, 2002). The recognition that proteolysis influences basic cellular processes, including cell division, differentiation, dissociation, and death highlights the complexity of the proteolytic balance and the difficulty of predicting how changes in this balance may affect cancer progression.

10.2.3 Cell Adhesion Molecules

Cell-cell and cell-ECM interactions during invasion and metastasis depend on molecules expressed on the cell surface, including integrins and cadherins, as well as the ligands that bind to these molecules. Cell adhesion molecules (CAMs) are transmembrane proteins with extracellular and intracellular domains; the intracellular domains are usually connected to the cytoskeleton or to signaling molecules (Fig. 10–5). Although originally named for cell adhesion, CAMs have multiple functions, including a major role in signaling from outside to inside a cell and vice versa. The formation and breaking of adhesive bonds between tumor cells and their environment provide information to the cell and may lead to changes in the expression of genes that determine cell proliferation, invasion, or other processes.

Integrins are expressed in all cell types and are involved in the regulation of cellular functions during embryonic development, wound healing, inflammation, homeostasis, bone resorption, apoptosis, cell proliferation, and metastasis. They are a family of widely expressed transmembrane receptors for proteins of the ECM, such as fibronectin, laminin, vitronectin, and collagens. These adhesion molecules are obligate heterodimers, comprising noncovalently associated α and β subunits, each of which spans the plasma membrane and possess, typically, a short cytoplasmic domain. Receptor diversity and versatility in ligand binding are determined by the extracellular domains through the specific pairing of 18 α and 8 β subunits, to form a family of 24 recognized heterodimers. The cytoplasmic domain of the β subunit interacts directly with components of the actin cytoskeleton, such as α-actinin and talin, allowing its localization to focal adhesion plaques that form at points of contact between integrins and the ECM. The focal adhesion plaques represent the submembranous termini of actin stress fibers thus providing a structural bridge between the ECM and the actin cytoskeleton (Fig. 10–5), and also contain a number of protein tyrosine kinases, such as focal adhesion kinase, p125, and integrin-linked kinase. Integrins are unique in their capacity to signal bidirectionally, acting as part of signal-transduction complexes that allow cells to "sense" (and respond to) their extracellular environment (Hamidi and Ivaska, 2018). Integrin activation may act to prolong and intensify signaling from growth factor receptors and can be a positive mediator of angiogenesis (see Chap. 11, Sec. 11.4.7). It has been reported that so-called cancer stem cells (CSCs) (see Chap. 13, Sec, 13.2) are dependent on integrin signaling triggered by ECM proteins such as periostin and tenascin C, which are enriched in the stem cell niche. Several integrin subunits (α6, β1, and β3) are thought to be important for the self-renewal and maintenance of the CSC phenotype at the primary tumor and to serve as CSC markers (Seguin et al, 2015). Alpha6 is the most widely observed in breast, prostate, squamous cell carcinoma, and colorectal cancers. How or whether these proteins play a role in the reported plasticity of this phenotype in cancer cells is currently unclear.

Cadherins are intercellular adhesion receptors that play important roles in assembling adherens junctions and desmosomes. Distinct members of the cadherin family are principal constituents of each type of junction, mediating calcium-dependent adhesion between similar cells. There are more than 20 recognized cadherins and protocadherins. E-cadherin (*CDH1*), the major epithelial cadherin, contains 4 conserved extracellular domains, a fifth extracellular domain possessing conserved cysteine residues, a transmembrane domain, and a cytoplasmic domain. Calcium-binding sites lie between adjacent extracellular domains. The cytoplasmic domain associates with cellular proteins such as catenins, which link cadherins to the actin cytoskeleton and to signal-transduction components (Cavallaro et al, 2002). An important connection between cadherins, catenins, and tumor progression was made with the observation that the APC (adenoma polyposis coli) tumor-suppressor protein (see Fig. 10–3) and β-catenin form physiological complexes

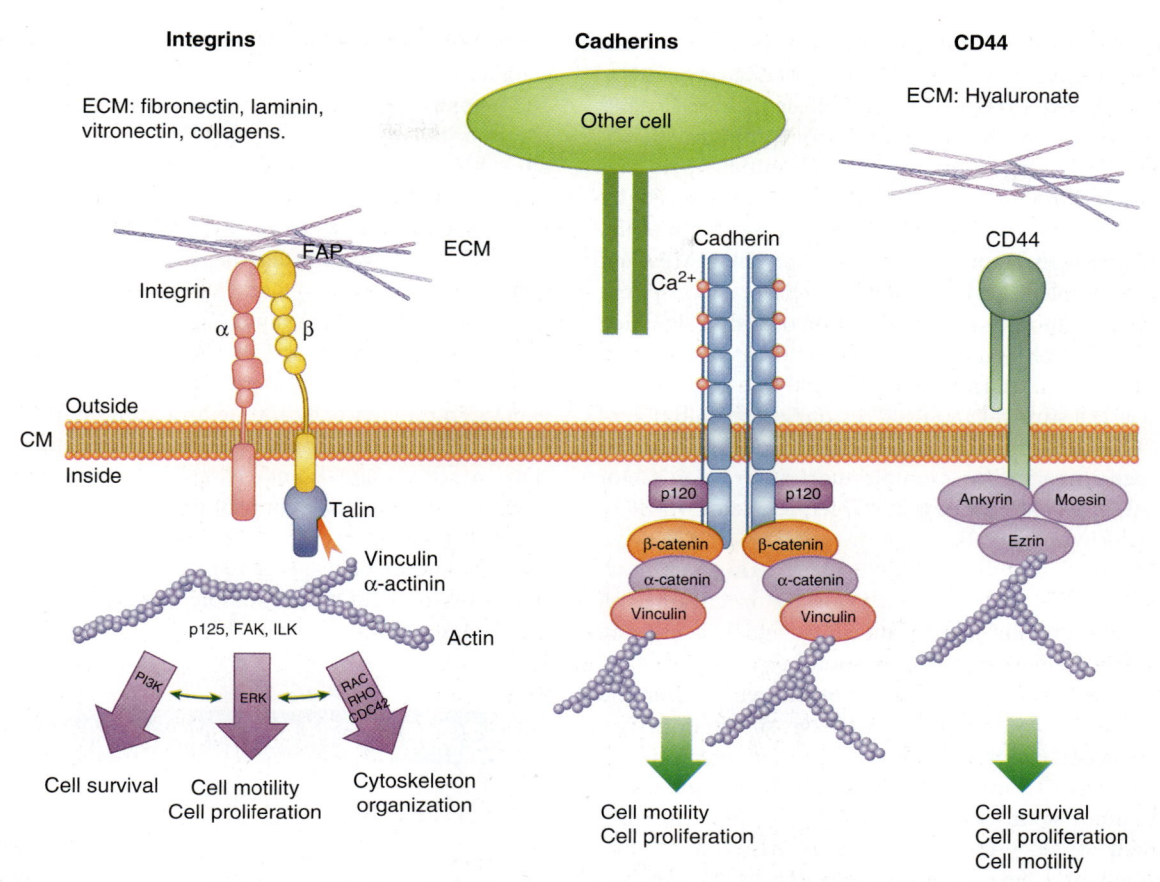

FIGURE 10–5 Schematic of integrin, cadherin, and CD44 receptors with linkage to their major downstream signal transduction pathways. An integrin receptor contains 2 subunits (α and β); different combinations of α and β subunits lead to the structural and functional variety of the integrin receptors. Integrin receptors are important players in the "outside-in" signaling system; they can sense the changes in the environment and transduce the signals into the cell through the signal transduction pathways shown. Cadherins are defined by their signature calcium-binding domains. Different cadherins can have various numbers of repeats of calcium-binding domains. Cadherins can also activate important signaling pathways, such as WNT signaling, through their intracellular association with (p120, α, and β) catenins. CD44 has many isoforms; the standard isoform is designated CD44s, whereas the splice variants are designated CD44v. The extracellular domain binds extracellular matrix (ECM) components whereas its intracellular domain can associate with ezrin, which is also an important player in metastasis. The function of CD44 is largely controlled by its post-translational modifications.

with axin and glycogen synthase kinase (GSK)-3β, in which β-catenin can be phosphorylated by GSK-3β and targeted for ubiquitin-mediated degradation (for review, Hankey et al, 2018). This complex thereby acts to control the level of β-catenin in the cell. Besides binding APC and cadherins, β-catenin can enter the nucleus and associate with LEF/TCP transcription factors, upregulating genes involved with cell proliferation such as c-Myc and cyclin D1 (see Chap. 8, Sec. 8.2.2.1 and Chap. 7, Figure 7-10). Mutations in APC, which are associated with the formation of adenomas in the colon, cluster within the β-catenin–binding region, yielding truncated APC peptides that are unable to bind to β-catenin. This reduces its degradation and increases its availability to diffuse to the nucleus and activate cell proliferation. Degradation of β-catenin is also disrupted if the activity of GSK-3β is blocked by activation of the WNT-signaling pathway (see Chap. 6, Sec. 6.4.1). Loss of E-cadherin and increased levels of N-cadherin (CDH2) are correlated with cellular invasiveness and, as discussed in Section 10.5.5, are associated with epithelial-to-mesenchymal transition (EMT). Disruption of cadherin-catenin complexes leads to disruption of the cytoskeleton, which, in turn, may affect signal transduction, as there is evidence that cytoskeletal proteins can act as a scaffold for the components of signal transduction pathways.

CD44 is a cell-surface glycoprotein and a receptor for hyaluronate, a component of the ECM expressed by stromal and cancer cells. CD44 is expressed widely and exists in multiple forms with variable glycosylation. All CD44 isoforms contain a cytoplasmic domain, which may link CD44 to actin filaments through interactions with ankyrin, ezrin, and moesin. Alternative splicing of the messenger RNA (mRNA) to produce these variable isoforms (CD44v) is regulated in a tissue-specific manner or by antigen activation in lymphocytes. These isoforms possess overlapping and distinct cellular functions. For example, CD44v isoforms act as co-receptors by sequestering growth factors on the cell surface and presenting these to cognate receptors (Orian-Rousseau, 2002). Cancer cells that undergo EMT and/or acquire stem cell–like properties have increased CD44 expression (Mani et al, 2008; see also Chap. 13, Sec. 13.3.2). In pancreatic cancer cells, an EMT phenotype depended on upregulation of CD44 expression, with CD44s being the most prevalent isoform (Zhao et al, 2016). CD44v isoforms are expressed in metastasis of several types of solid tumors and associated with poorer prognosis (Chen et al, 2018). CD44 expression in tumor cells initiates cytoskeletal changes and modulates the activities of multiple cellular signaling pathways including MAPK, Hippo, β-catenin, AKT, transforming growth factor beta (TGF)-β, Emprin, MMPs, and STAT3. For example, CD44 attenuates the tumor cell response to stress-induced apoptosis via modulation of Hippo signaling and induces cell proliferation by regulating β-catenin activity. CD44 expression in cancer-associated fibroblasts promotes breast cancer cell survival and drug resistance by inhibition of apoptosis. CD44 also modulates the activities of MMPs linked to tumor cell invasion, for example the transcription factor Snai1 (Snail), a CD44 downstream target, regulates MMP-14 expression during pancreatic cancer invasion.

The ERM proteins (containing ezrin, radixin, and moesin motifs) link the actin network cytoskeleton and the cell membrane and provide a mechanism by which a cell can sense environmental changes and respond to growth factors. ERM proteins normally form aggregates with each other and assume an inactive conformation. After tyrosine and threonine phosphorylation, ezrin becomes activated, which allows for its translocation from the cytoplasm to the plasma membrane, bringing F-actin to the cell surface. The ERM proteins are abundant at cell protrusions such as membrane ruffles and microvilli, and have been implicated in tumor progression. ERM proteins take part in a number of signaling pathways (RhoGTPases, PI3K/AKT, WNT/β-catenin, CD44, RTKs) known to be crucial for cancer progression (Clucas and Valderrama, 2015). Ezrin has been proposed to regulate assembly of E-cadherin–dependent adherence junctions through Rac1 activation and the trafficking of E-cadherin to the plasma membrane. It has also been identified as a metastasis-associated gene in breast, lung, prostate, pancreatic, and oral squamous cell carcinomas, osteosarcoma, and rhabdomyosarcoma. High moesin expression has been correlated to high-grade glioblastoma tumors. Indeed, moesin affects actin cytoskeleton reorganization as well as CD44 localization to cell protrusions favoring an invasive phenotype.

10.2.4 The Pathophysiological Microenvironment

As a solid tumor grows, the rate of cancer cell proliferation surpasses the ability of the vasculature to supply growth factors, nutrients, and oxygen, and to remove the catabolites produced by the cells. The tumor neo-vasculature is often primitive and chaotic compared to the normal tissue vessels and suffers from functional abnormalities (see also Chap. 11, Sec. 11.5). As a result, there is an imbalance between supply and demand, leading to a microenvironment containing regions of hypoxia, low glucose levels, low pH, and elevated interstitial fluid pressure (IFP) (see Chap. 12, Sec. 12.4). On hypoxic stress, ATP is transported out of cancer cells and converted into adenosine by hypoxia-inducible factor (HIF)–sensitive, membrane-bound ectoenzymes. Adenosine binds surface receptors on tumor and immune cells leading to modulation of innate and adaptive immunity (Antonioli et al, 2013). Mechanisms that facilitate tumor escape from immune surveillance include impaired activity of CD4[+] T and CD8[+] T, NK cells, and dendritic cells. In parallel, activation of Treg cells, protumor M2-macrophages, expansion of myeloid-derived suppressor cells (MDSCs), increased activity of major immune-suppressive cytokines, expression of PD-L1 ligands, and stimulation of PD-1 on the lymphocytes resulting in tumor cell tolerance (see also Chap. 21, Sec. 21.5.4). There is considerable spatial heterogeneity in the microenvironment of an individual tumor (see Chaps. 12, and 13). This heterogeneity leads to a diversity of nutrients, local signals and cell-cell interactions, and unequal drug distribution, all contributing to emergence of resistant cell populations and cells harboring metastatic capacity (Junttila and de Sauvage, 2013). Overall, this complex tumor microenvironment plays multiple roles in tumor progression and metastasis and determines the tumor response to therapy.

10.3 METASTASIS

10.3.1 The Spread of Cancer

The 2 major routes of metastatic spread are via lymphatic vessels and/or blood vessels. Metastases are subdivided into 2 groups: those in regional lymph nodes having disseminated via the lymphatic circulation, and those that arise in distant organs, which are spread mostly via the blood circulation. Most deaths caused by cancer are due to metastases. The T (= tumor) N (= nodes) M (= metastasis) system of cancer staging is used widely in clinical management: cancers are divided into stages based on tumor size, extent of involved lymph nodes, and presence or absence of distant metastases. Prognosis is correlated with the stage of the disease at diagnosis, and treatment decisions depend on it. Local treatment is of limited effectiveness in the presence of metastatic disease and systemic therapies are used to a greater extent.

The kinetics of tumor spread varies between individuals, and it does not always correlate with the size of the primary tumor. The ability to establish metastases is not present in all primary tumor cells. Cells that leave primary tumors and establish metastases must avoid cell-cycle arrest and apoptosis but require additional abilities. Tumor cells are generally very inefficient at forming metastases (see Sec. 10.4.2) and often are detected in the blood circulation of patients without evidence of metastatic disease. Oncogene-driven tumors in mouse models do not necessarily develop distant metastases. Tumor cells often gain metastatic abilities by turning on endogenous gene programs involved in normal tissue development and homeostasis to gain motility and survival advantages for metastasis (see Sec. 10.5.5). For instance, the invasive and migratory functions that are responsible for normal epithelial cell branching (eg, in the mammary gland) can be hijacked by tumor cells to

A. Reduced cell adhesion
TWIST, Snail
Slug, TGF-β
ADAM10

B. Invasion
MMPs-cathepsins
Chemokines
Cytoskeletal remodelling (RhoC)

C. Intravasation
VEGF
FGF
ROS

D. Immune escape and survival
Coagulation factors
Platelet released EGF, VEGF, HGF, TGF-β

E. Extravasation and vasculature remodeling
MMPs, COX-2, EREG, ANGPT4

F. Metastatic colonization, growth, and angiogenesis
MMPs
Growth factors
Proinflammatory cytokines

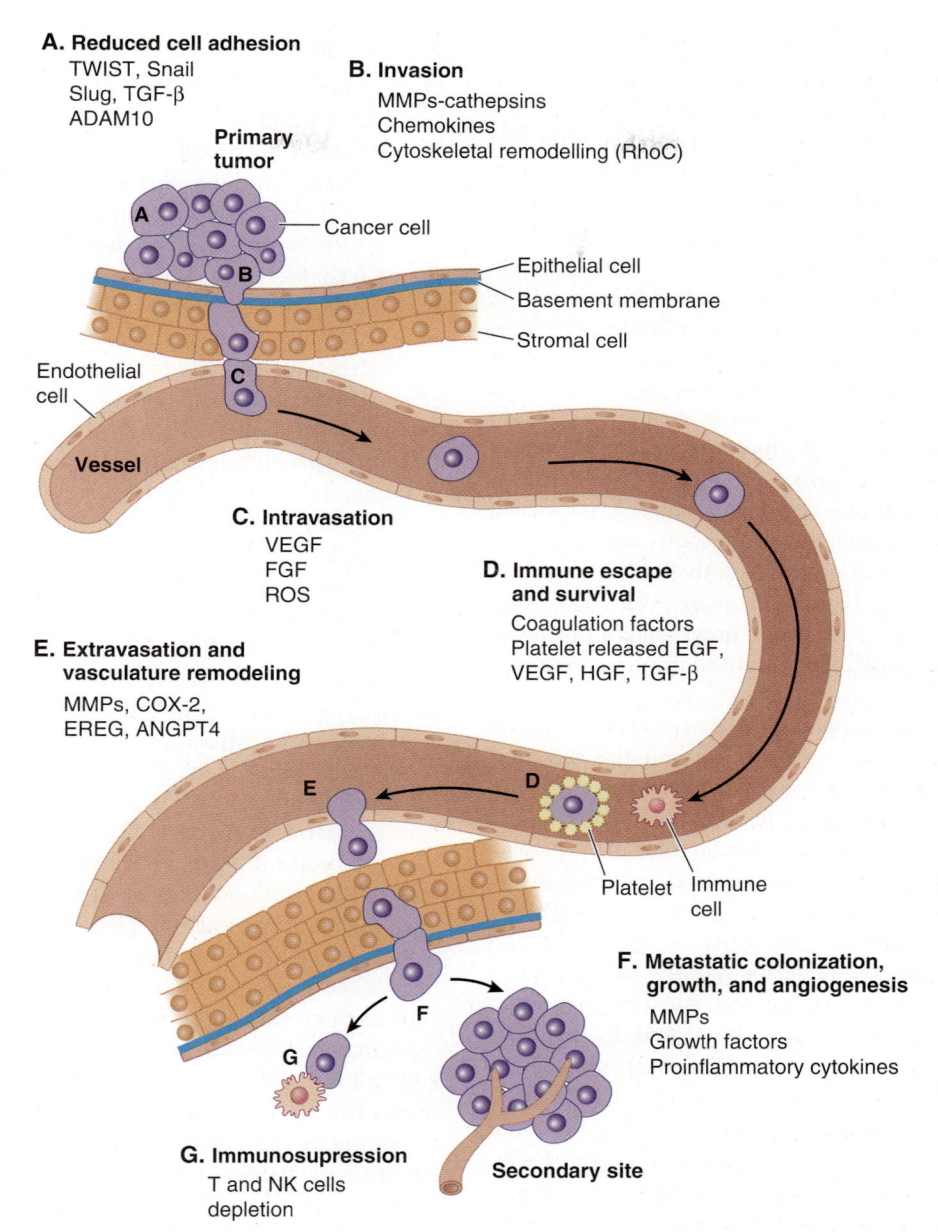

G. Immunosupression
T and NK cells depletion

FIGURE 10–6 Schematic of the sequential steps in the metastatic process. First, metastatic cells must break free from the primary tumor by (A) reducing their adhesion to neighboring cells and (B) clearing a path for migration into the stroma. During intravasation (C) cancer cells can cause endothelial cell retraction by releasing compounds such as vascular endothelial growth factor (VEGF) or endothelial cell death by releasing reactive oxygen species (ROS). In the bloodstream, cancer cells can bind to platelets (D) and gain protection from the immune system. After reaching the secondary site, cancer cells can exit the bloodstream (E) by inducing endothelial cell retraction or death. The colonization step (F) requires survival and proliferation signals. Cancer cells co-opt the local environment by releasing proinflammatory cytokines and matrix metalloproteinases (MMPs), inducing their neighbors to release growth factors. Angiogenesis (F) and immunosuppression (G) will allow the micrometastases to grow.

expand into surrounding tissue (Ewald et al, 2008). Metastasis is often divided into a few defined steps: invasion, intravasation and survival in the circulation, extravasation, and finally, establishment of a new growth (Fig. 10–6). These steps provide a simplified view of the complex set of biological events involved in the process. In each step, the factors influencing the survival and tumor-initiating activity of the cells are important determinants of metastasis.

10.3.2 Detachment from the Primary Tumor, Local Invasion, and Intravasation

Cancer cells can migrate as single cells through the ECM or migrate collectively at the tumor invasion front. Detachment or shedding of cells into blood or lymphatic vessels (intravasation) may occur as a result of prior invasion of the tumor mass into vessels or because the abnormal vasculature of tumors permits passage of cells into the circulation. Angiogenic factors such as vascular endothelial growth factors (VEGFs) and fibroblast growth factors (FGFs) can induce vascular remodeling (see Chap. 11) and thereby facilitate intravasation. Tumor blood vessels are less well organized and leaky in comparison to their normal counterparts, providing additional opportunities for cell penetration. The poor alignment of endothelial cells in tumor vessels has been reported to allow circulating tumor cells (CTCs) to home back to the original tumor, as has been observed in a mouse model of breast cancer (Kim et al, 2009). This phenomenon of cross-seeding is enhanced by tumor-derived chemoattractive cytokines such as interleukin (IL)-6 and IL-8. Tumor cells can fine-tune surface molecules to interact with endothelial cells so as to increase their survival. For example, tumor cells can downregulate KAI1/CD82, a surface molecule that interacts with the Duffy antigen receptor for chemokine (DARC) on the endothelial cell to induce senescence of tumor cells (Bandyopadhyay et al, 2006). Loss of CD82 is correlated with metastatic progression in patients, and the knockout of DARC abrogates the tumor-suppressive effect of CD82.

Cytoskeletal rearrangements within cancer cells combined with adhesive interactions between cells and the secretion of MMPs and cathepsins drive their invasion and migration through the stroma (Quail and Joyce, 2013). Detachment of cancer cells from the primary tumor mass may involve decreased expression of adhesion molecules involved in the "homotypic" adhesion of cells to one another or may depend on the expression of motility factors (eg, hepatocyte growth factor [HGF], autotaxin, or autocrine motility factor), which are glycoproteins found to promote cell movement through interaction with cell-surface molecules linked to the Rho/Rac/Cdc42 guanosine triphosphatase (GTPase) intracellular signaling system. The EMT process, in which a polarized epithelial cell assumes a mesenchymal-like cell phenotype, could facilitate cancer cell migration (see Sec. 10.5.5). Several MMPs, as well as ADAM10, can cleave cell adhesion proteins such as cadherins and integrins (Radisky and Radisky, 2010). Transcription factors such as Snail and Twist1 create a shift in cadherin expression (E-cadherin loss or N-cadherin gain), which facilitates cell depolarization and motility.

Tumor cells may gain motility by overexpressing RhoC, a small calcium-dependent GTPase that is responsible for sensing extracellular signals and controlling cytoskeletal actin organization. RhoC-deficient mice have normal primary tumor formation but reduced cancer cell motility and drastically reduced metastases (Hakem, 2005). Local invasion and intravasation also involve breakdown of the ECM and basement membrane. Various proteases, including MMPs, play a major role in this process: overexpression of each TIMP in cancer cell lines of diverse origins inhibits their migration, invasion, metastasis, and subsequent growth (Cruz-Munoz and Khokha, 2008), and adenoviral delivery of TIMP-2 to pre-established MDA-MB-231 breast epithelial tumor xenografts delays their invasion and metastasis [(Li et al, 2001); see Secs. 10.2.2 and 10.5.1].

10.3.3 Survival in the Bloodstream

Once tumor cells break free of constraints at the primary site, they can gain access to the blood (or lymphatic) vessels. While in the blood, tumor cells may travel with platelets to evade immune surveillance and lysis by NK cells, ensuring their survival (Lambert et al, 2017). Platelets are small, terminally differentiated anuclear cells shed from megakaryocytes that are essential for blood clotting, and this is exploited by tumor cells. With the help of coagulation factors, activated platelets can form tumor cell–platelet aggregates and, in combination with the adhesive properties of platelets, this leads to arrest of tumor cells in the capillaries of target organs. Many platelet-surface molecules and platelet-derived factors enhance metastasis. For example, mice deficient in the platelet-specific receptor glycoprotein Ib-alpha (GPIb-α) have a 15-fold reduction of lung metastatic foci in an experimental metastasis model. In addition, α-granules released by platelets contain many growth-promoting factors, such as EGF, VEGF, HGF, and TGF-β (Gay and Felding-Habermann, 2011).

Most tumor cells that reach the circulation are arrested in the first capillary bed that they encounter (first-pass capillary bed). Early experimental studies in which radiolabeled tumor cells were injected into the systemic or portal veins indicated that most cells are arrested initially in the lung or liver capillaries, respectively. Cell encoding markers, such as green fluorescent protein (GFP) or luciferase, have provided direct visualization of tumor cell arrest following intravenous injection (Hoffman, 2002). Combined with such labels, the technique of intravital videomicroscopy (IVVM) has confirmed the early arrest of tumor cells in "first-pass" capillary beds and permitted dynamic study of events in the process of experimental metastasis as discussed below (MacDonald et al, 2002). It is this effect that probably accounts for the high level of metastases in lung and liver, but some tumor cells succeed in passing through the first-pass organ to become CTCs or to establish metastases in other (preferred) sites.

10.3.4 Circulating Tumor Cells

Distant metastases arise usually through the distribution of tumor cells into the circulating blood. Tumor cell dissemination can be an early event and may persist throughout the growth of the primary tumor, although the survival time of such cells in the circulation is quite short (half-life of 1 to 2.4 hours). Small numbers of CTCs can be detected in the blood of patients, and CTC counts are prognostic for outcome of a wide range of cancers (Joosse et al, 2015). However, the isolation and characterization of CTCs remain challenging partly because of their low frequency, which is estimated to be 1 in 1-10 million normal peripheral blood cells (Alix-Panabières, 2012).

Methodologies to enrich for CTC are based on their physical properties, including size/deformability-based filtration, density-gradient centrifugation, and electrical property–based di-electrophoresis separation. Those based on their biological properties include either positive selection procedures targeting surface markers exclusively found on CTCs or negative selection methods involving depletion of blood cells. The most common surface protein used in CTC detection is epithelial cell adhesion molecule (EpCAM), because many tumors are of epithelial cell origin. Among the numerous EpCAM-based CTC detection technologies, the US Food and Drug Administration (FDA)-approved CellSearch® system is used in monitoring patients with metastatic breast, colorectal, or prostate cancer. It classifies a CTC as a positive event if the cell size is ≥4 μm, DAPI⁺ (4,6-diamino-2-phenylindole), pan-keratin⁺, and CD45⁻. An additional fluorescence channel can be used for detection of therapy relevant markers such as the androgen receptor (AR), the prostate-specific antigen (PSA), the human epidermal growth factor receptor 2 (ERBB2), and the epidermal growth factor receptor (EGFR) (Riethdorf et al, 2007). However, because metastasis formation might involve downregulation of EpCAM (eg, during the EMT process), other CTC phenotypes should be included in future studies of CTCs. Whole-genome copy number analysis and gene expression profiling have been used to characterize CTCs. In breast cancer, HER2 expression on CTCs is associated with poor prognosis, and in gastric cancer, uPAR expression on CTCs is associated with metastatic relapse (Tachtsidis et al, 2016). CTCs that express angiogenesis and hypoxia-associated markers such as VEGF, VEGFR-2, FAK, and HIF-1 are also thought to be associated with aggressive disease and poor prognosis (Bednarz-Knoll et al, 2011). Analysis of CTCs in cancer patients has the potential to improve our understanding of the biology of tumor cell dissemination and to refine the management of metastatic disease.

10.3.5 Extravasation

After tumor cells arrive at the distant organ, they may extravasate into the new tissue. As discussed in Sections 10.2.2 and 10.5.1, this process involves the activity of proteases, of which MMPs play a major role. Several groups have reported studies of extravasation using intravital video microscopy (IVVM). Chambers and colleagues observed that the majority of arrested cells were able to extravasate, even cells with reduced proteolytic capability or nonmalignant fibroblasts, suggesting that this process may not be a major barrier to the metastatic process (MacDonald et al, 2002). In contrast, other IVVM studies found that extravasation was a formidable barrier to metastasis, and tumor cells were observed to proliferate intravascularly. Yet others observed that tumor cell extravasation was dependent on CAMs and could occur in precapillary vessels following stimulation of the endothelial cells by inflammatory growth factors. Because the structural organization of capillary walls varies in different organs, tumor cells may need specific capabilities for infiltration at different sites. Studies of gene expression in patients with advanced metastatic disease have indicated that tumor cells trapped in the lung capillaries produce factors such as epiregulin (EREG), cyclooxygenase-2 (COX-2), MMP-1, and cytokine angiopoietin-like 4 (ANGPTL4) to remodel the pulmonary vasculature (Minn et al, 2005). These factors modify the integrity of lung endothelia and provide entry points into the lung parenchyma. Genetic and pharmaceutical inhibition of these factors reduced metastatic extravasation. Some of the involved genes seem to encode general metastasis-promoting factors; for example, COX-2 is a potent mediator of metastasis to the brain, and RNA interference-mediated knockdown of COX-2 expression decreases the ability of certain breast cancer cell lines to metastasize to brain (Bos et al, 2009). Genes such as $α_{2,6}$-sialyltransferase can facilitate passage through the blood-brain barrier by enhancing adhesion to brain endothelial cells and can act as a specific promoter of brain metastasis. Other cell-surface molecules, such as chemokine receptors (eg, CXCR4) and growth factor receptors (eg, c-MET), have also been reported to augment metastasis. Conceivably, they accomplish this by recruiting tumor cells to target organs and enhancing their survival and proliferation.

10.3.6 Initiation of a New Growth (Colonization)

Following infiltration, most tumor cells die as a result of selective pressure from the foreign environment, but a few tumor cells may initiate growth inside the target organ. This escape from death may be accomplished by their incorporation into specific sites (niches) that are receptive to tumor growth (see Sec. 10.5.6). There is also evidence that tumor cells initiating metastatic growth can modify the environment of the target organ to support their outgrowth. For example, metastatic cells can disrupt normal bone homeostasis through the secretion of parathyroid hormone-related peptide (PTHrP), IL-6, and TNF-α and thus stimulate the release of receptor activator of nuclear factor-κB ligand (RANKL) by osteoblasts (Fig. 10–7). RANKL, in turn, activates myeloid progenitor cells to differentiate into osteoclasts that can digest bone structures creating space for establishment of metastasis. The lytic activity also releases TGF-β, insulin-like growth factor I (IGF-I), and bone morphogenetic proteins (BMPs), which enhance tumor cell survival. The efficiency of this vicious cycle can be potentiated when tumor cells suppress the production of the RANKL antagonist osteoprotegerin (OPG) (Jones et al, 2006). Denosumab, a monoclonal antibody targeting RANKL, has been approved for treating patients with bone metastasis. Metastatic outgrowths rely on successful recruitment of endothelial cells, myeloid cells, and stromal fibroblasts. Production of VEGF enables Lewis lung carcinoma micrometastatic cells to recruit Id1⁺ bone marrow–derived endothelial cell progenitors that trigger angiogenesis and proliferation of metastatic cells (Gao et al, 2008). In addition, several microRNAs (miRNAs; see Chap. 2, Sec 2.3.3) can promote metastatic colonization in breast cancer and melanoma by inducing recruitment of endothelial cells and angiogenesis (Chou et al, 2013).

Host immunity is a major defense against metastatic growth. Depletion of cytotoxic T cells or NK cells has been shown to

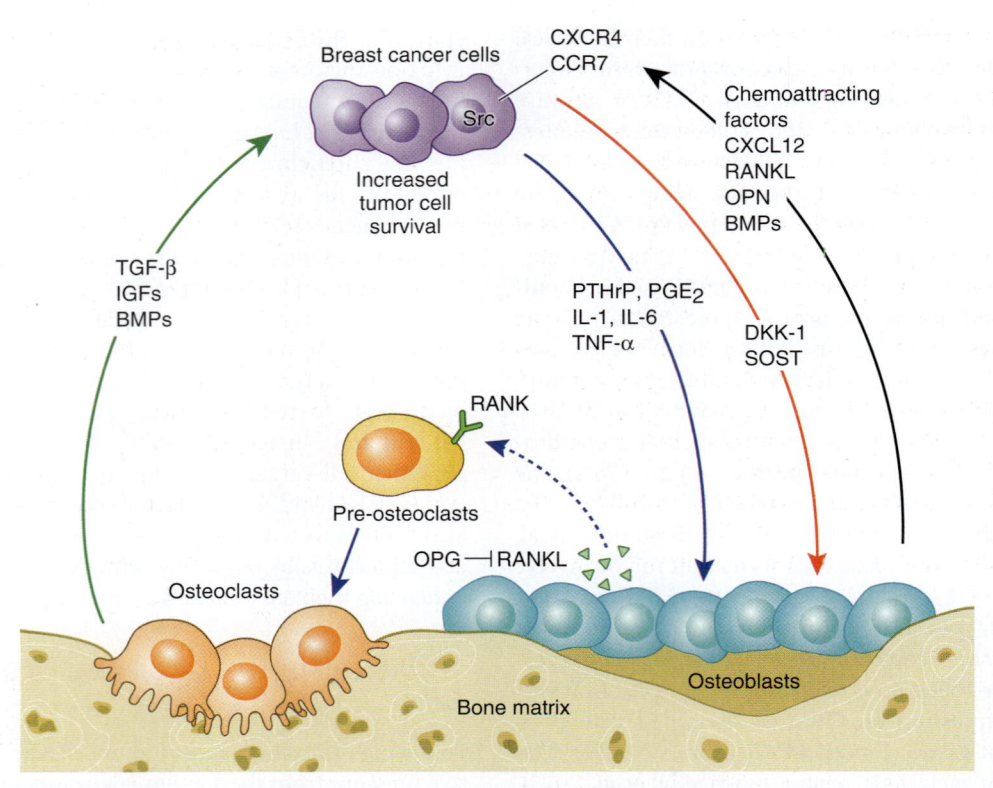

FIGURE 10-7 Breast cancer bone metastasis formation. Osteoblasts secrete chemoattracting factors to recruit breast cancer cells (black arrow). Breast tumor cells release factors that stimulate osteoblasts to enhance osteoclast differentiation and activity (blue arrows). As a result, bone-resorbing activity of mature osteoclasts increases, and bone-embedded growth factors are released from the bone matrix–promoting tumor growth (green arrow). The efficiency of this vicious cycle is potentiated when tumor cells suppress the production of the RANKL antagonist OPG. In addition, tumor cells secrete factors (DKK-1, SOST) that inhibit osteoblast differentiation and activity, thereby contributing to cancer-induced bone destruction (red arrow). (Adapted with permission from Le Pape F, Vargas G, Clézardin P. The role of osteoclasts in breast cancer bone metastasis. *J Bone Oncol* 2016 Apr 8;5(3):93-95.)

increase metastasis (Bidwell et al, 2012) and inhibition of the tyrosine kinase Mer, a negative regulator of NK cells, suppresses metastasis (Paolino et al, 2014). Moreover, each organ possesses specific endogenous immune cell composition and thus can exhibit different susceptibility to metastasis. The liver, for example, is rich in NK cells, and neutralization of proapoptotic NK cell–derived ligand TRAIL or the genetic depletion of NK cells can increase hepatic metastasis in mice (Takeda et al, 2001).

10.4 DYNAMICS OF METASTASIS

10.4.1 Metastatic Organotropism

Some cancer types predominantly spread preferentially to one organ (eg, prostate cancer to bone, pancreatic cancer to liver) or show sequential organ-specific colonization (eg, colorectal cancer frequently metastasizes first to the liver and later to lungs and brain). Other cancer types, such as breast cancer, lung cancer, or melanoma, are able to colonize different organ sites, either sequentially or synchronously. All of the subtypes of breast cancer are prone to bone metastases, whereas some of them also target additional organs including brain and liver

(Table 10-2). Paget's soil-and-seed hypothesis postulated that tumor cell–host organ interactions can favor or hinder metastatic development (Paget, 1889). The structure and organization of capillaries and adjacent parenchyma and tissue function vary widely in different organs; therefore, organ-specific adhesive interactions between endothelial cells and tumor cells or between tumor cells and growth factors in the organ can influence the establishment of metastatic growth. Liver and bone marrow possess fenestrated endothelia facilitating

TABLE 10-2 Typical sites of metastasis of the common tumors.

Tumor Type	Principal Sites of Metastasis
Lung	Brain, bone, adrenal gland, and liver
Breast	Bone, lung, liver, and brain
Prostate	Bone
Colon	Liver, lung, and brain
Pancreas	Liver and lung
Skin	Lung, brain, skin, and liver
Sarcoma	Lung
Uveal	Liver

extravasation of circulating tumor cells compared to capillaries in other organs. Factors such as the dynamics of blood flow also contribute to organ preference; thus, although kidneys, liver, and brain equally receive 10% to 20% of blood volume, each shows a very different pattern of metastasis. Beyond vasculature, the organ preference to seed metastasis depends on multiple factors including cancer cell features, host immune microenvironment, and cancer cell cross-talk with local cells. Bone cells like osteoblasts secrete a variety of chemo-attracting factors (eg, CXCL12, RANKL, OPN, or BMPs) that recruit breast cancer cells expressing the corresponding chemokine receptors (eg, CXCR4 and CCR7). Elevated Src signaling in cancer cells expressing CXCR4 also gives a survival advantage and increases the probability of establishing metastasis over time. High expression of CXCR4 and the Src signature in tumor cells is associated with relapse of breast cancer in bone (Zhang et al, 2009). Further, once established in the bone, cancer cells actively modify the microenvironment and co-opt osteoblast and osteoclast functions to form different types of metastases, that is, osteoblastic lesions by prostate and osteolytic lesions by breast or lung cancers (see Fig. 10–7) (Weilbaecher et al, 2011). Recently, tumor-derived exosomes have been shown to influence organotropic behavior; thus, expression of the integrin α6β4 heterodimer on the surface of tumor-derived exosomes promotes their homing to the lung, whereas αvβ5 targets them to the liver. The binding of exosomes to ECM molecules at distant sites helps to prepare the targeted organ for the arrival of CTCs by participating in pre-metastatic niche formation (Hoshino et al, 2015) (see Sec. 10.5.6).

Animal models have been developed to study the organ specificity of metastasis. The classic example of serial selection is the isolation of the B16F10 cell population from B16 mouse melanoma cells (Fidler, 1973). The procedure involved intravenous injection of cancer cells, isolation of cells that had formed lung metastases, and their expansion *in vitro* before reinjection into isogenic animals (Fig. 10–8). After 10 such passages, a population of cells was obtained (termed B16F10 cells) that was approximately 5 times as efficient at forming experimental lung metastases after intravenous injection as the starting B16F1 cell population. These cells were not more capable of forming spontaneous lung metastasis when implanted at a local site, suggesting that selecting for increased ability to grow in lung does not affect the invasive properties necessary for initial escape from the primary tumor. This process has been successfully replicated for murine mammary, osteosarcoma, rhabdomyosarcoma, lung and colon tumors.

10.4.2 Metastatic Inefficiency

The number of CTCs far exceeds the number of overt metastatic lesions observed in patients, suggesting the inefficiency of the metastatic colonization process. In mouse models, intravenously injected cancer cells that reach the lungs die in large numbers within 2 days, and similar observations have been made for micrometastases in liver following tumor cell injection into the portal vein. Even injection of cancer stem cells has shown rapid clearance of the cells and lack of metastatic

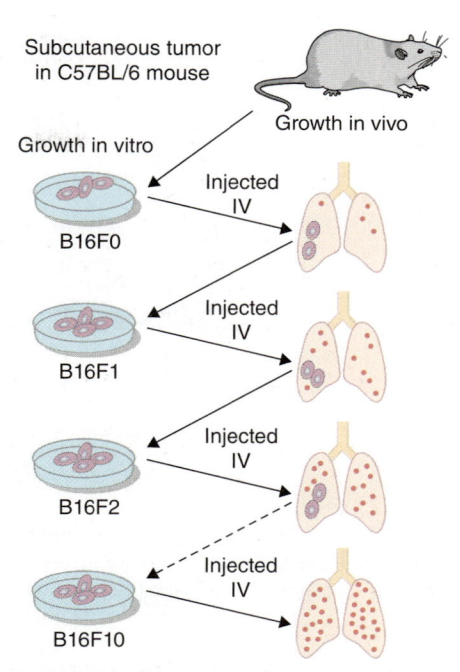

FIGURE 10–8 Procedure used for selecting highly metastatic cell populations from B16 melanoma cells. The B16F10 cells were selected after 10 successive intravenous (IV) injections of cancer cells isolated from lung metastases and expanded *in vitro*.

colonization (Massagué and Obenauf, 2016). The inefficiency of the metastatic process leads to the question as to whether metastasis is a random or a specific process. A small subpopulation of the cells in a tumor might express properties that confer a high probability of being able to form metastases, but it is also possible that all tumor cells might have an equal (low) probability of forming metastases, but only a few manage to survive through the various stages of the process (see Sec. 10.3). Support for the specific nature of metastasis derives from experimental studies, including those described in Section 10.3.2 and Figure 10–8. Also, when clones of B16 melanoma cells were isolated, expanded in culture, and the cells tested for their ability to form experimental metastases, the variability in metastases for cells from a single clone was found to be much less than that observed when different clones were compared (Fidler and Kripke, 1977). These results, which were replicated in a number of cell lines, indicated a wide heterogeneity in metastatic ability between different clones and are consistent with the presence of preexisting metastatic variants within a cell population (Fig. 10–9). The clonal heterogeneity model of metastasis formation (Hill et al, 1984) proposes that although some of the multiple properties necessary for a cell to metastasize may be relatively stable, others are expressed transiently, giving rise to unstable clonal heterogeneity. Metastasis is often divided into a few sequenced steps: invasion, intravasation and survival in the circulation, extravasation, and finally, establishment of a new growth (Fig. 10–6). These steps provide a simplified view of the complex set of biological events involved in the process. In each step, the factors influencing the survival and tumor-initiating activity of the cells are important determinants of metastasis (see Sec. 10.3).

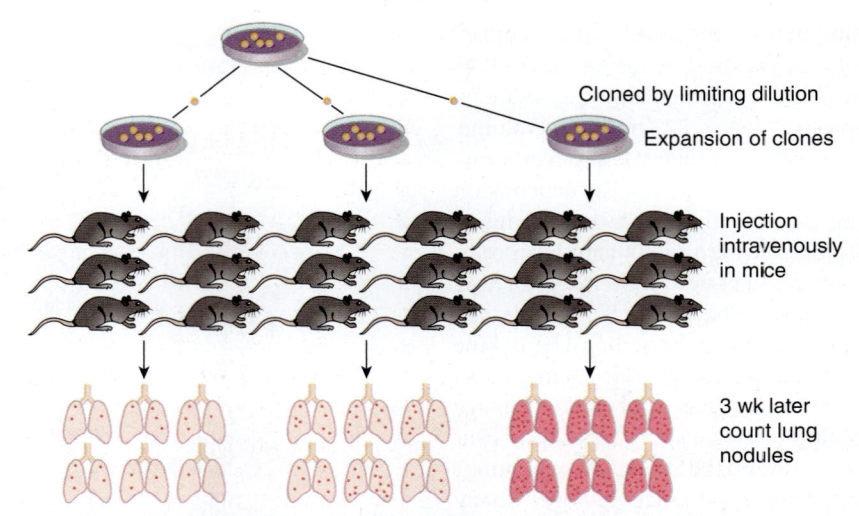

FIGURE 10–9 Experimental testing of clonal heterogeneity. After establishment of a series of clones from a tumor cell population and their expansion *in vitro*, the clones are tested for metastatic ability *in vivo*. Although there is some variability in the number of nodules observed in different animals injected with cells from the same clone, there is much greater variability between the clones.

10.4.3 Metastatic Dormancy and Relapse

Patients, particularly those with breast, prostate, or kidney carcinomas or melanoma may experience metastatic relapse several years after initial diagnosis and local treatment. For example, most breast cancer metastases are detected within 10 years of surgery but metastatic outgrowth can occasionally occur after 20 years or later. Late relapse in breast cancer correlates with molecular subtypes: most patients with HER2+ or triple-negative breast cancers relapse early (<5 years from surgery), developing lung, brain, or liver metastases. In contrast, ER+ cancers have a relatively constant rate of relapse over several years and tend to develop predominantly bone metastases. Currently, relatively little is known about the mechanisms by which single cancer cells or micrometastases enter a dormant state and remain in target organs for years before resuming metastatic growth. Stromal signals that impose tumor dormancy have been identified in mouse xenograft models. TGF-β and BMPs, members of the TGF-β family, promote quiescence, and inhibit self-renewal in disseminated tumor cells (Bragado et al, 2013). The perivascular niche has also been implicated in the regulation of cancer-cell dormancy: although normal vasculature provides a dormant niche, a sprouting neovasculature induces micrometastatic outgrowth (Ghajar et al, 2013). Studies of melanoma, lymphoma, and prostate adenocarcinoma models suggest that immunosurveillance mechanisms can contribute to halting the expansion of micrometastases (Eyles et al, 2010). The extracellular matrix plays a role in dormant cell reactivation: environments that are rich in type I collagen or fibronectin inhibit dormancy (Barkan et al, 2010), whereas extensively crosslinked collagen fibers, such as those created by HIF1-induced lysyl oxidase, induce reactivation by enhancing integrin-mediated conversion of mechanical forces into biochemical signals (Cox et al, 2013). Because dormant tumor cells are not actively dividing, they are hard to treat, as most drug treatments target dividing cells.

10.4.4 Cancer Stem Cells in Recurrence and Metastasis

One proposed model of cancer dissemination is that only a subpopulation of tumor cells exhibiting cancer stem cell features (see Chap. 13, Sec 13.3.2) can initiate the formation of metastasis. For example, in human colorectal cancers, the abundance of CD26+ tumor-initiating cells correlates with the development of liver metastases. Injection of these cells in the cecal wall of mice gives rise to liver metastases, whereas the remaining tumor cells lack this capacity (Pang et al, 2010). In human primary pancreatic carcinomas, the ability to form metastases is reported to be restricted to the CD133+CXCR4+ tumor-initiating cell subpopulation found at the invasive edges of the tumor (Hermann et al, 2007). Gene expression analysis of single breast cancer cells showed that early metastatic cells possess a stem cell–like signature, suggesting that metastases are initiated and maintained by cells exhibiting cancer stem cell properties (Lawson et al, 2015). Moreover, circulating human breast cancer cells expressing stem cell markers, generate bone, liver, and lung metastases when inoculated into immunodeficient mice (Baccelli et al, 2013). Other studies suggest that metastasis-initiating cells enter into dormancy and undergo reactivation in response to niche signals similar to those regulating normal adult stem cells. For example, the extracellular matrix protein tenascin C induces the reactivation and outgrowth of breast cancer micrometastases by increasing both NOTCH and WNT signaling (Oskarsson et al, 2011). Finally, studies of several human cancer types demonstrate that primary tumors harboring cells with stem cell signatures and displaying long-term self-renewal capacity are associated with poor prognosis and metastatic relapse (Oskarsson et al, 2014). However, the low efficiency of metastasis formation makes it uncertain whether such signatures relate to features specific to the metastatic process or more generally to features associated with tumor cell growth.

10.5 MOLECULAR MECHANISMS OF METASTASIS

10.5.1 Protease Activity at the Invasive Front

Proteolysis must function at the tumor cell surface to facilitate invasion and degradation of the basement membrane. Extracellular proteinases, transmembrane proteinases, cell-surface molecules, and intracellular factors all contribute to generating pericellular zones of proteolysis. Mechanisms known to underlie the proteolytic activation at the cell membrane include the activation of plasmin by uPA and its receptor uPAR, and the activation of pro-MMP-2 within a trimolecular complex generated by MT1-MMP, MMP-2, and TIMP-2 (Hernandez-Barrantes et al, 2000). MT1-MMP activity associated with tumor progression has been observed at the leading edge of migrating cells. For the cell surface activation of pro-MMP-2 in the trimolecular complex, MT1-MMP must itself be activated by a proprotein convertase called furin. Mature furin can cycle between the Golgi and the cell surface, and activate MT1-MMP at both locations. The association of pro-MMP-2 with $\alpha_2\beta_1$ integrin-bound collagen provides a reserve of the enzyme for subsequent activation of the trimolecular complex. By comparing multiple MMPs in experimental systems that use 3D matrix composites, it was found that MT1-, MT2-, or MT3-MMPs constitute the minimal requirement for migration across a basement membrane, and that MT1-MMP is the dominant protease mobilized for cancer cell trafficking through ECM barriers (Rowe and Weiss, 2009). Several secreted MMPs, especially MMP-2 and MMP-9, have also been shown to facilitate tumor cell invasion and motility, although their primary function *in vivo* may be to facilitate bulk ECM turnover during tissue remodeling (Kessenbrock et al, 2010).

The integrin $\alpha_v\beta_3$ can localize active MMP-2 to the cell surface. Their co-localization was observed on newly developing blood vessels and on the tumor invasive front. The inhibition of their binding reduced tumor growth and angiogenesis (Silletti, 2001). MT1-MMP catalyzes shedding of the α_3 integrin ectodomain in ovarian carcinoma cells, and this associates with formation of multicellular aggregates, an important step in ovarian cancer metastasis (Moss et al, 2009). Shedding of MMP-9–dependent E-cadherin may also play a role in the dissemination of ovarian cancer cells. CD44 provides a means of anchoring active MMP-9 to the cell surface of invadopodia in breast cancer and melanoma cells and was found to be critical for MMP-9–mediated cell migration (Dufour et al, 2010). The association of CD44 with hyaluronic acid has been shown to increase MMP-2 secretion, and CD44 has been found to recruit MMP-7 and direct localization of MT1-MMP to the cell membrane. These findings highlight the complex spatial coordination between adhesion molecules and enzymatic activity, which bring about controlled activation of metalloproteinases and, ultimately, the digestion of ECM at the leading edge of invasive tumor cells.

10.5.2 Protease Activity in the Tumor Microenvironment

Studies using transgenic and knockout mouse models of MMPs and TIMPs have documented that proteolysis affects the early, as well as the late, stages of cancer progression (see Sec. 10.2.2). Protease activity impacts directly on cell proliferation, cell survival, angiogenesis, and inflammation (Table 10–3). Metalloproteinases and TIMPs alter the release of potent growth factors such as VEGF, TGF-β, and IGF-II, which are either sequestered in the ECM or exist in complexes with their binding proteins. Proteolytic cleavage of already synthesized factors results in altered bioavailability of growth signals to cancer cells and impacts on cell proliferation. Activation of EGFR (see Chap. 6, Sec. 6.2.1), which is overexpressed in many human cancers, follows ADAM-mediated release of members of the EGF family of growth factors, including amphiregulin, TGF-α, and heparin binding (HB)-EGF. Similarly, activation of NOTCH receptor (see Chap. 6, Sec. 6.4.2), which requires

TABLE 10–3 MMPs and cancer progression.

Biological Effect	Activity
Cell Invasion	
MT1-MMP, MMP-2, MMP-9, ADAMs	Proteolytic, degradation of ECM
Cell adhesion and EMT	
MT-MMPs, ADAM10	Integrins
ADAM10	Notch cleavage and subsequent activation
MMP-1, -7 ADAM10	Shedding of E-cadherin
MMP-28	Proteolytic activation of TGF-β
Cell proliferation	
MMP-1, -2, -3, -7, -9, -11, -19, ADAM12	Release of sequestered IGF proteins by proteolysis of IGF-binding proteins
MMP-3, -7, ADAM17, ADAM10	Shedding of membrane-anchored ligands of EGFR (HB-EGF, TGF-α, and amphiregulin)
Cell apoptosis	
MMP-7, ADAM10	Cleavage of Fas ligand
Tumor angiogenesis	
MMP-2, -9	Degradation of COL-IV, perlecan
MMP-3, -10, -11	Release of VEGF and bFGF
Immune surveillance and inflammation	
MMP-9, -2, -14	Release of active TGF-β (Suppress T-lymphocyte reaction against cancer cells)
ADAM17	Release of TNF-α (proinflammation)
MMPs (e.g. MMP-9)	Chemokine processing and activation (CXCL8/IL-8)
MMPs (MMP-1, -3)	Chemokine processing and inactivation (CCL8/MCP-2)

ADAM, A Disintegrin And Metalloproteinase; *ECM*, extracellular matrix; *EGFR*, epidermal growth factor receptor; *FGF*, fibroblast growth factor; *HB*, heparin binding; *IGF*, insulin-like growth factor; *MT1*, membrane type 1; *MMP*, matrix metalloproteinase; *TGF-β*, transforming growth factor β; *TNF-α*, tumor necrosis factor α; *VEGF*, vascular endothelial growth factor.
Data from Gialeli C, Theocharis AD, Karamanos NK. Roles of matrix metalloproteinases in cancer progression and their pharmacological targeting. *FEBS J* 2011 Jan;278(1):16-27.

3-step proteolytic cleavages with ADAMs performing the second cleavage, participates in the EMT process during tumor progression and metastasis (Yuan et al, 2015). Additionally, ADAM10, expressed by stromal fibroblast–derived exosomes, can induce Notch signaling to promote growth of tumor xenografts and their metastatic dissemination (Shimoda and Khokha, 2017). MMPs and TIMPs also influence apoptotic signals, such as those feeding into Fas-mediated death receptor signaling (see Chap. 8, Sec. 8.4.3). Proteolytic activity also regulates capillary ingrowth, vascular stability, and access of tumor cells to vascular and lymphatic networks. Overall, manipulation of the expression of TIMPs reveals that they inhibit angiogenesis, invasion, and metastasis, but their effects on cell proliferation and apoptosis are both tissue-specific and context-dependent (Jackson et al, 2017).

Several non-neoplastic host cells, including fibroblasts, endothelial cells, leukocytes, and bone marrow–derived cell populations, are recruited during tumor development, and the composite of these stromal and cancer cells creates a complex microenvironment. Metalloproteinase activity contributes to generating this microenvironment and can further facilitate tumor progression. The TIMP-metalloproteinase balance regulates a repertoire of substrates and signal transduction pathways that are central to inflammation and immune cell activity. For example, metalloproteinase activity, as regulated by the TIMP3-ADAM17 interaction, is important for the systemic release of proinflammatory cell surface–bound TNF-α. Chemokines that influence immune cell motility are similarly processed by proteases. MMP cleavage of members of the monocyte chemoattractant protein (MCP) family of chemokines renders them receptor antagonists with inflammation-dampening effects (Hromas, 2002). MMP-1 and MMP-3 process CCL8/MCP-2, which has antitumor activity in a melanoma model.

Tumor-associated neutrophils control and facilitate aspects of the metastatic process, and high neutrophil burden is a poor prognostic indicator. Neutrophils exhibit plasticity and can be polarized to an N1 antitumoral or N2 protumoral phenotype in response to the microenvironment. Neutrophil recruitment to the tumor and polarization to the protumorigenic N2 phenotype is dependent on cytokines that are processed by MMPs. For example, MMP-9 cleaves the first five amino acids of tumor-produced CXC-chemokine ligand 8 (CXCL8; also known as IL-8), which increases its activity (Powell and Huttenlocher, 2016). Other chemokines, including CXCL1/KC (neutrophil-attracting) and CXCL11 (Th1-lymphocyte-attracting), are also substrates of MMPs and, thus, proteolysis can affect neutrophil content and T-cell response (see Chap. 21).

10.5.3 Cancer-Associated Fibroblasts

Cancer-associated fibroblasts (CAFs) coevolve with cancer cells during tumor progression and participate in paracrine communication (Fig. 10–10). Pericytes (contractile cells wrapping around endothelial cells) are another population that co-evolves with tumor progression. CAFs were thought initially to arise from local fibroblasts by acquiring a modified "activated" phenotype, but later studies linked their origin to bone marrow–derived cells or transdifferentiation from epithelial or even endothelial cells. TGF-β is a critical activating factor for CAFs, which are identified through the expression of markers (ie, α-smooth muscle actin [α-SMA]; fibroblast specific protein-1 [FSP-1]/S100A4; FAP; neuron-glial antigen-2 [NG-2]; platelet-derived growth factor-β receptor [PDGFR-β]), whereas pericytes are defined more loosely but depend on PDGF and TGF-β signaling. CAFs contribute to cancer promotion by the delivery of key growth (HGF, FGF) and survival signals (insulin-like growth factors [IGFs]) that counter death signals and activate downstream oncogenic signaling. They provide ECM components for interaction with integrins resulting in the activation of specific signal transduction pathways. CAFs also overexpress multiple MMP and ADAM proteinases involved in enhancing cytokine and growth factor bioactivity. Experimentally, fibroblasts that lack TIMPs acquire a CAF phenotype, expressing multiple growth factors/cytokines and can accelerate tumor growth and metastasis. CAFs express chemokines (SDF-1 or CXCL12, IL-6, CXCL8) and angiogenic factors (VEGFs, FGFs) that lead to the generation of a proangiogenic and proinflammatory microenvironment. When co-injected with tumor cells, CAFs promote xenograft growth and are observed at sites of metastases, where they induce angiogenesis by SDF-1–mediated recruitment of endothelial progenitors and activation of pericytes to alter vessel permeability. The gene expression profiles of CAFs demonstrate heterogeneity in individual tumors and allow identification of CAF subsets, which may have prognostic value. The importance of these cells is emphasized by the observation that mice deficient in specific CAF markers show decreased metastasis, and that CAFs may alter the drug-sensitivity of cancer cells (Östman and Augsten, 2009).

10.5.4 Tumor-Associated Macrophages

Macrophages are very plastic cells, constantly adapting in response to environmental stimuli such as cytokines and other signaling mediators. They can undergo a cell "polarization" process wherein they express different surface markers and functional programs. Classically activated macrophages (M1) produce proinflammatory cytokines and reactive oxygen/nitrogen species crucial for host defense and tumor cell killing. The alternatively activated macrophages (M2) produce anti-inflammatory cytokines and are involved in the resolution of inflammation. Tumor-associated macrophages (TAMs) tend to display an M2-like phenotype that promotes cancer progression (Fig. 10–10), and high TAM content in a tumor correlates with poor prognosis in patients (Qian and Pollard, 2010). TAMs, located in the perivascular areas or at the invasive edge of the tumors, are recruited by tumor-derived chemoattractants. On arrival, TAMs supply promigratory factors such as EGF, promote proteolytic remodeling of the extracellular matrix, induce migration and invasion of tumor cells, and support immunoevasion (Aras and Zaidi, 2017).

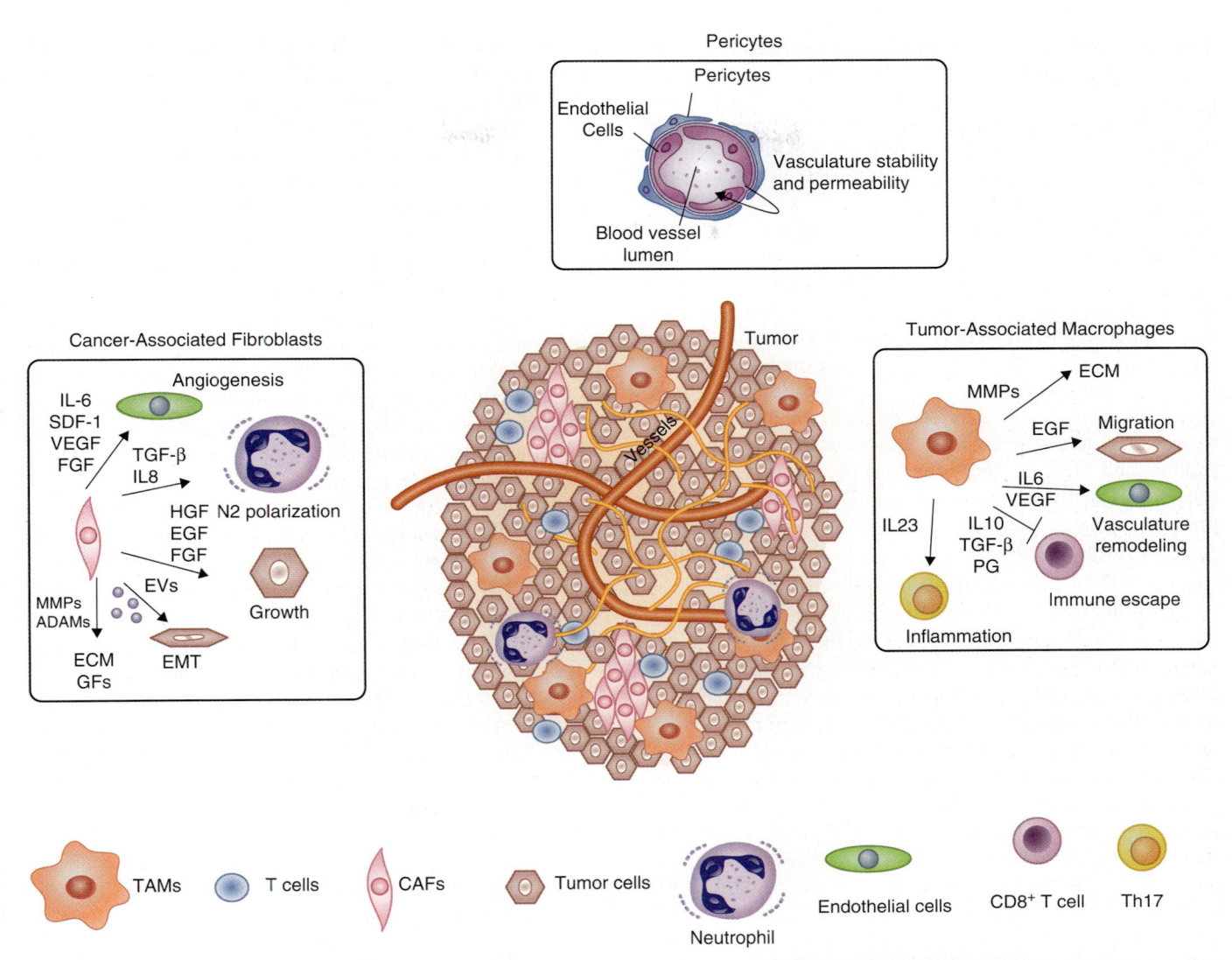

FIGURE 10–10 Mutual interactions between tumor cells and the microenvironment promote progression to metastasis. Tumor cells can influence their microenvironment and induce the production of tumor-promoting factors from neighboring or incorporated nonmalignant cells such as cancer-associated fibroblasts and tumor-associated macrophages. By releasing growth factors, exosomes, cytokines, and matrix metalloproteinases (MMPs), these stromal cells induce cancer cell proliferation and motility, angiogenesis, and extracellular matrix (ECM) remodeling, and influence the immune defense toward tumor cells. Pericytes participate in the tumor vasculature remodeling, where they either stabilize the blood vessels favoring tumor growth or compromise vessel structure integrity, facilitating tumor cell invasion/extravasation. PG, prostaglandin

The inflammatory state of TAMs is controlled by the transcription factor NF-κB, which is activated through toll-like receptors (TLRs; see Chap. 21). Specific inhibition of NF-κB activity in myeloid cells through ablation of IkB kinase (IKK)-α results in a reduction of inflammation and inhibition of tumor progression. The secretion of cytokine IL-6 by TAMs causes the endothelial lining of tumor vessels to become leaky, resulting in the recruitment of more inflammatory cells and providing escape routes into the bloodstream for tumor cells. An anatomical structure consisting of macrophages, endothelial cells, and tumor cells named the tumor microenvironment for metastasis (TMEM) is recognizable in histologic sections and is predictive of metastatic potential in primary human breast cancers (Rohan et al, 2014).

TAMs are also involved in immunosuppression either by directly inhibiting the CD8+ T-cell response through direct cell-cell interaction with T cells or by secreting immunosuppressive cytokines and proteases such as IL-10, TGF-β, arginase-1, and prostaglandins, which inhibit T-cell activation and proliferation. TNF-α produced by TAMs can activate the NF-κB and AP-1 family of transcription factors in the tumor cells, stimulating their cell proliferation and survival. Moreover, inactivation of STAT3 (a transcription factor that functions to suppress inflammation; see Chap. 6, Sec. 6.3.1) in myeloid cells is associated with abundant expression of inflammatory cytokines such as TNF-α and IL-6 that promote chronic colitis and invasive colorectal cancer in animal models (Grivennikov et al, 2009). Another crucial cytokine produced by TAMs is IL-23, which enhances the activity of Th17 cells while inhibiting T-regulatory cells. The Th17 cells belong to the T-helper cell subclass with strong inflammatory effects and are generally associated with tumor progression.

10.5.5 Epithelial-to-Mesenchymal Transition

The epithelium is a highly polarized structure composed of polygonal-shaped cells with abundant cell-cell tight junctions. It lines the outer surface, as well as the surface of inner organs, of the body. Epithelial cells make contact with a basal membrane, and both cell-cell and cell-matrix adhesions are necessary for their survival. Different epithelial cell populations are heterogeneous, depending on the tissue/organ involved. In contrast, mesenchymal cells are spindle-shaped and migratory; they support tissue/organ development. EMT (Fig. 10–11; see also Chap. 13, Sec. 13.3.1) is a process during which an epithelial cell loses its apical-basal polarity and becomes a mesenchymal-like cell with increased migratory ability, resistance to apoptosis, and increased production of ECM components (Kalluri and Neilson, 2003). During this process, epithelial cells often lose the expression of cell-surface and cytoskeletal proteins mediating adhesion, such as E-cadherin, cytokeratin, zona occludens 1 (ZO-1), and laminin. Instead, they gain proteins associated with mesenchymal cell phenotypes such as N-cadherin, vimentin, fibronectin, and α-SMA. The resulting mesenchymal-like cell can detach from the basal membrane and migrate away from the epithelial layer. This process occurs in the embryo at different stages of maturation and development of organs, and in wound healing. It is hypothesized that in tumors this embryonic program may be reactivated to drive an initial step in metastasis, but may then be reversed by mesenchymal-to-epithelial transition (MET) when the cell establishes a new growth (Ye and Weinberg, 2015).

Cancer cell lines with loss of E-cadherin expression show higher tumorigenicity as xenografts in nude mice, and in some cancers, E-cadherin levels relate inversely to prognosis. Mutations in the E-cadherin gene (*CDH1*) causing either loss or truncation of the protein have been identified in human breast and gastric cancers, possibly rendering these tumors more prone to EMT and metastasis. Similarly, epigenetic mechanisms such as transcriptional repression and promoter silencing by hypermethylation (see Chap. 3, Sec 3.1) also contribute to E-cadherin downregulation in various carcinomas. Transcription factors that play roles in EMT such as Twist1, Snai1 (Snail), and Snai2 (Slug) also repress E-cadherin expression (Medici et al, 2008).

In various *in vitro* studies, TGF-β has been shown to induce EMT-like changes in epithelial cell lines. Two pathways downstream of TGF-β are at least partially responsible for its transforming effect, SMAD and p38/RhoA (see Chap. 6, Sec. 6.4.4). Other signals that induce EMT include HGF, which activates the receptor tyrosine kinase C-MET, as well as EGF and PDGF, activating their respective receptors. Multiple studies have linked noncoding miRNAs (see Chap. 2, Sec 2.3.3) as regulators of EMT, both positively and negatively. miRNA family

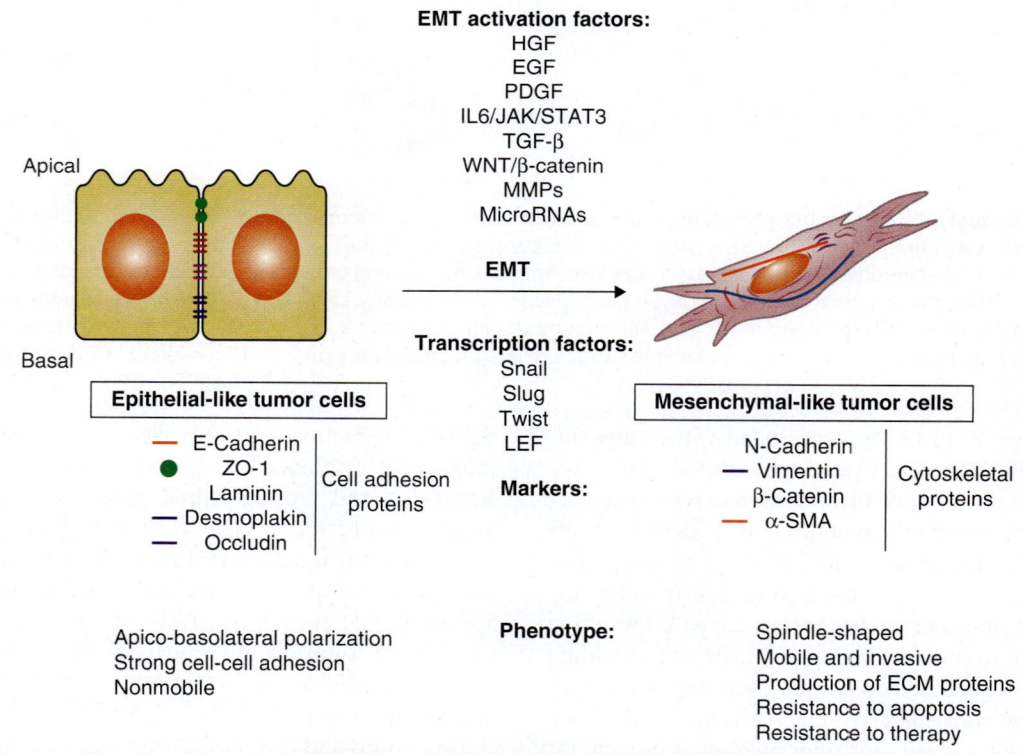

FIGURE 10–11 Epithelial tumor cells often undergo epithelial-to-mesenchymal transition (EMT) to gain anchorage-independent survival and motility during tumor progression. Epithelial cells usually express markers such as E-cadherin, ZO-1, laminin, and desmoplakin. Through the aberrant expression of transcription factors such as Snai-1 (Snail) and Snai-2 (Slug), these epithelial cells lose their epithelial markers and start to express mesenchymal markers, such as N-cadherin, vimentin, β-catenin, and α-SMA. Many of these markers are also functionally associated with the epithelial or mesenchymal characteristics. For example, E-cadherin and N-cadherin activate different intracellular programs that give rise to the epithelial-like or mesenchymal-like properties.

members, miR-200 and miR-205, prevent EMT by inhibiting Zeb-1 and Zeb-2, known repressors of E-cadherin expression. In contrast, miR-21 expression is elevated in many carcinomas and supports TGF-β–dependent EMT (Shi et al, 2010).

Although this phenotype switch has been extensively studied, strong evidence from human tumor specimens is still lacking and an EMT requirement for metastasis is debatable. Indeed, in the majority of carcinomas, metastatic cells show aberrant expression of a few mesenchymal markers and retain epithelial characteristics such as apical-basal polarity, cohesive migration, and keratin expression. Furthermore, the transcription factors Snai1, Snai2, and Twist1 that serve as EMT markers can also mediate dedifferentiation and maintenance of the stem cell state, features predictive of early metastatic spread and poor prognosis (Chui, 2013). Thus, expression of mesenchymal markers may be reflective of the reversion to a more primitive dedifferentiated state rather than the initiation of a directed metastatic program. Recent studies in mouse models have also questioned the importance of EMT in the induction of metastatic spread by using conditional deletions of EMT-related genes and signaling pathways. They demonstrated that EMT is dispensable for metastatic dissemination of breast and pancreatic cancer cells but rather contributes to chemoresistance (Fischer et al, 2015; Zheng et al, 2015).

10.5.6 Pre-metastatic Niches and Exosomes

An important concept in the metastatic process is that a "pre-metastatic niche" can be created in distant organs to which CTCs can "home" (Peinado et al, 2017). The pre-metastatic niche represents an abnormal, tumor growth–favoring microenvironment; its formation involves the induction of vascular leakiness and is followed by ECM remodeling, activation of resident stromal cells, and immune cell infiltration (Fig. 10–12). Different classes of systemic mediators, such as primary tumor-derived inflammatory cytokines, exosomes (extracellular vesicles, EVs), and extracellular matrix remodeling enzymes, have been shown to recruit bone marrow–derived cells to support metastatic colonization in the lung, liver, or bone marrow. Pre-metastatic niches were identified in lymph nodes in mouse and in cancer patients. For example, the provasculogenic VEGF receptor 1 (VEGFR1$^+$) myeloid progenitor cells can colonize lymph nodes primed by factors released by the primary tumor before the arrival of CTCs (Karaca et al, 2011) and lymphangiogenesis precedes CTC arrival at future sites of lymph node metastasis (Hirakawa et al, 2005). Other factors such as clot formation by platelets in pre-metastatic organs reduce shear stress and interstitial flow,

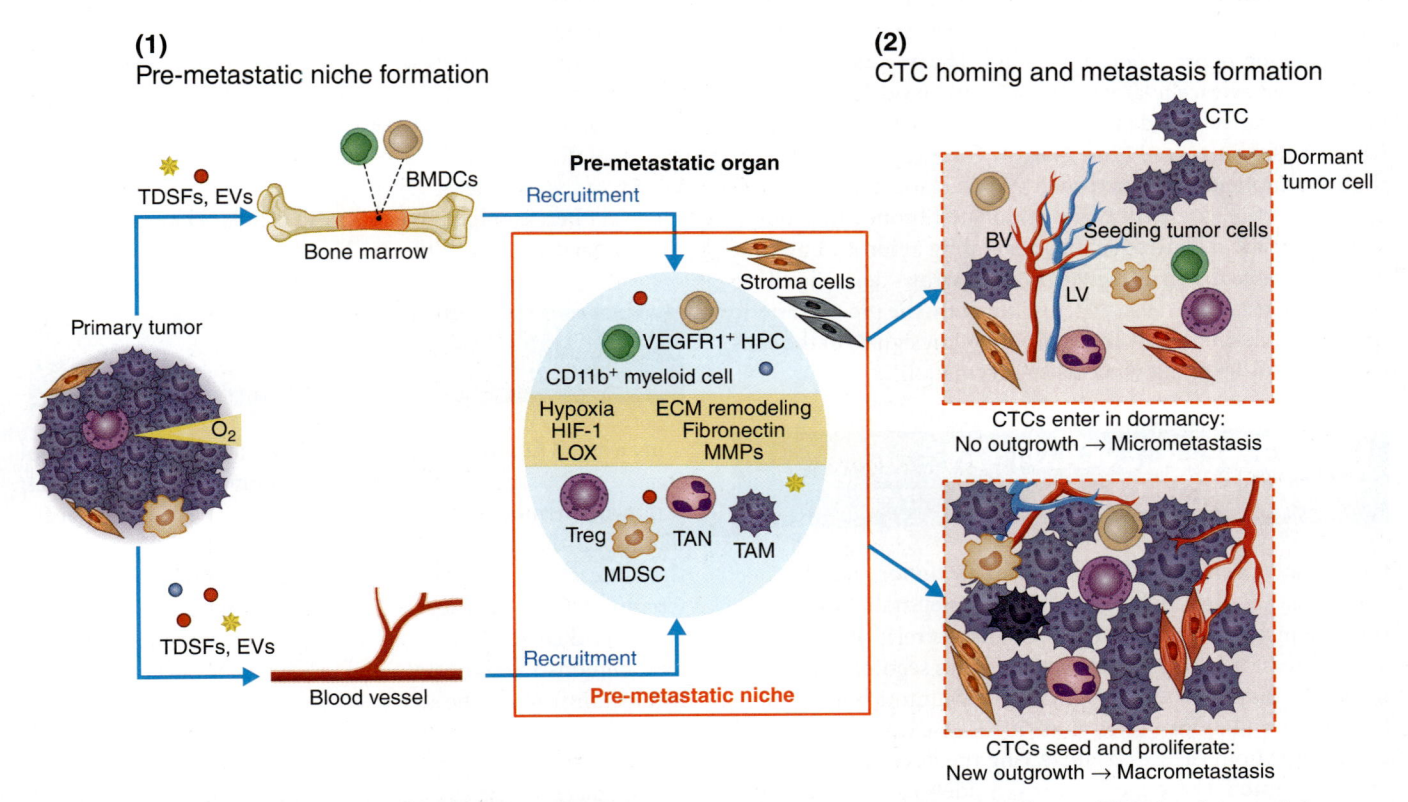

FIGURE 10–12 Formation of the pre-metastatic niche and metastasis. (1) Tumor-derived secreted factors (TDSFs) and extracellular vesicles (EVs) induce the recruitment of bone marrow–derived cells (BMDCs) such as VEGFR1$^+$ hematopoietic progenitor cells (HPCs) and CD11b$^+$ myeloid cells to secondary organ sites. TDSFs and EVs also promote immune cells recruitment (myeloid-derived suppressor cells [MDSCs], Treg cells, tumor-associated macrophages [TAMs], and tumor-associated neutrophils [TANs]). The recruited cells, the local stromal cells, hypoxia, and extracellular matrix (ECM) remodeling create a microenvironment favoring metastatic tumor cell survival and colonization. (2) Circulating tumor cells (CTCs) that home to the pre-metastatic niche can enter dormancy or proliferate and form metastases. BV, blood vessels; LV, lymphatic vessels. (Adapted with permission from Liu Y, Cao X. Characteristics and Significance of the Pre-metastatic Niche. *Cancer Cell* 2016 Nov 14;30(5):668-681.)

thereby providing docking sites for the arrest of CTCs (Gay and Felding-Habermann, 2011; Labelle et al, 2014). The MMP inhibitor TIMP-1 can generate an hepatic pre-metastatic niche through stromal CXCL12-CXCR4-dependent recruitment of neutrophils (Seubert et al, 2015). Furthermore, targeting STAT3 in the primary tumor and in myeloid cells impairs the recruitment and accumulation of myeloid bone marrow–derived cells into the pre-metastatic niche and inhibits tumor metastasis (Deng et al, 2012). In preclinical models of breast cancer, activation of hypoxia-inducible factor 1 (HIF1, see Chap. 12, Sec. 12.4.2) is involved in pre-metastatic niche formation, and tumor release of hypoxia-induced lysyl oxidase (LOX) was associated with the formation of osteolytic lesions in bone (Cox et al, 2015).

Exosomes are derived from the multivesicular endosome pathway and enriched in endosome-derived components. They are extracellular vesicles characterized by a size of 30-100 nm in diameter. They are released from cells on activation, malignant transformation, stress, or death, and are found in biological fluids, including blood and urine. These structures contain proteins (receptors, antigens), lipids, and nucleic acids (DNA, mRNA, miRNA), and can be endocytosed by other cells or interact with their cell surface receptors through fusion. This process occurs frequently in platelets and tumor cells, providing a means for transfer of bioactive molecules to stimulate tumor progression, immune response, invasion, angiogenesis, and metastasis (Lobb et al, 2017). Exosomes are important for the formation of pre-metastatic niches. The injection of tumor cell–derived extracellular vesicles in mouse models of skin and pancreatic cancers leads to pre-metastatic niche formation in lymph nodes, lung, and bone marrow (Peinado et al, 2011). In the liver, Kupffer cells are activated by pancreatic tumor–derived exosomes to release TGF-β and stimulate fibronectin production by hepatic stellate cells, thus generating a fibrotic environment favorable to recruitment of bone marrow–derived cells to the liver (Costa-Silva et al, 2015). Ultimately, the pre-metastatic niche must deliver survival and proliferation signals to the cancer cells in order to allow metastasis formation.

10.6 GENETIC EVOLUTION OF METASTASIS

Comparative genomic studies of primary tumor and matched metastasis are used to define patterns of metastatic dissemination. For instance, analysis of primary, locally relapsed, and metastatic breast tumors has shown that clones seeding metastasis or relapse disseminate late from primary tumors but continue to acquire mutations (Yates et al, 2017). Metastatic subclones can emerge both early and late during the development of the primary tumor. There are 2 general models of metastatic dissemination: the linear and the parallel progression models. In both, the primary tumor and its metastases are clonally related. In the linear model, the metastasis-competent clone arises late in tumorigenesis and, thus, the degree of primary-metastasis genetic divergence is small because the metastasis is seeded by the most advanced primary clone. In the parallel progression model, the metastatic clone disseminates from the primary tumor early, and both the primary tumor and the metastasis evolve in parallel, resulting in genetic divergence between the primary and metastatic lesions. Moreover, the same subclone in the primary tumor can seed multiple metastases in different organs (metastases monophyletic) or multiple metastatic subclones in the primary tumor disseminate independently of each other, in different target organs, in parallel and at different times (metastases polyphyletic). Furthermore, polyclonal seeding, in which multiple clones from the primary tumor seed the same metastasis, can occur in parallel or at different times. The colonization by the initial clone has provided a metastatic niche favoring homing of other clones.

Self-seeding, a process by which metastatic cells can reinfiltrate their tumor of origin can falsely make the primary and metastatic tumors appear to be closely related. In human prostate cancer, a recurrence at the site of the resected primary tumor was found to be divergent from the original primary tumor and was in fact seeded by a clone derived from a bone metastasis (Hong et al, 2015). Another source of error in primary-metastasis divergence is the limited sampling of the primary tumor and metastasis (eg, by a single biopsy) where the representation of clonal heterogeneity is incomplete; thus, sampling of multiple locations within a tumor and its metastasis is needed in order to establish the clonal evolution of metastatic processes. A recent development in clinical practice is to collect postmortem samples from cancer patients allowing exhaustive sampling of metastatic sites. This sampling procedure has the potential to provide information on the patterns of metastatic dissemination within and across tumor types. All of the above modes of dissemination have been observed across cancers and within individual cases. Overall, no clear correlation has been made yet between the molecular and cellular characteristics of the primary tumor and the mode of metastatic progression.

10.7 TREATMENT TO PREVENT METASTASIS

Only a small number of patients with metastatic cancer can be treated successfully by conventional therapies such as surgical removal, chemotherapy, and radiotherapy. Drugs have been developed that target specifically the metastatic process, but the success and clinical use of these drugs is limited (Perret and Crépin, 2008). As described above, metastatic dissemination can be broken down into various stages and preclinical models have demonstrated the potential to block metastasis formation by blocking each of the stages. For example, avoiding the arrest of CTCs via the use of anticoagulant drugs has been achieved in animals by treatment with heparin, warfarin, and inhibitors of platelet aggregation (prostacyclin and dipyridamole), but these agents have not shown activity in treating human cancer. Similarly, the use of peptides that block the integrin motif RGD, which is involved in binding of cells to fibronectin, was also largely ineffective in clinical studies, although they showed considerable promise in preclinical studies. A major problem is that microscopic metastases are often seeded before the primary tumor is diagnosed, so that drugs targeting the metastatic process are then given too late to be effective.

Adjuvant systemic therapy, given after local treatment of the primary tumor, is aiming at preventing outgrowth of metastasis. Adjuvant therapy has improved the survival of people with many types of cancer, and adjuvant hormonal therapy and chemotherapy are standard treatment for many women with breast cancer (see Chaps. 17-20). These agents are most likely eradicating small metastases rather than attacking the metastatic process. Recently, a meta-analysis has suggested that adjuvant therapy with osteoclast-inhibitory bisphosphonates could suppress bone metastasis and increase survival in postmenopausal women with breast cancer (Early Breast Cancer Trialists Collaborative Group, 2015); the mechanisms underlying this effect remain unknown.

Recent advances in sequencing and microarray technologies (see Chap. 2) have enabled genome-wide analyses of primary tumors and -omic approaches (eg, genome, transcriptome, proteome, or methylome). A group of 70 genes (known as the Amsterdam signature) expressed in primary breast tumors allows survival prediction and the likelihood of metastasis development (van de Vijver et al, 2002). A 21-gene signature including several genes associated with cell proliferation, known as Oncotype DX® Breast Recurrence Score, is used to determine which women (hormone receptor [HR]–positive, HER2-negative, axillary node–negative) with early-stage breast cancer will benefit from adjuvant chemotherapy to decrease the probability of subsequent metastasis. By identifying and treating only the responsive patients, it is anticipated that the test will spare about 70% of women the side effects of chemotherapy (Siow et al, 2018).

SUMMARY

- Metastasis is the major cause of death in cancer patients.
- Cancer is a multistep process that progresses through benign and premalignant changes to frank malignancy. It involves a number of genetic or epigenetic changes that may be very extensive in late-stage cancer.
- Clonal heterogeneity within the primary tumor is a source for the selection of metastatic cancer cells.
- Several major steps are involved in the process of metastasis, including the ability to invade into and out of blood vessels, to survive in the circulation, and to arrest and grow at a new site.
- A range of properties, particularly those relating to cell adhesion, secretion of proteolytic enzymes, and initiation of a new growth, are involved in this process.
- Metastasis is an inefficient process and may depend partially on random survival factors but also on specific attributes that dictate organ-site specificity in the development of metastases.
- A single cancer cell or micrometastases can enter a dormant state and remain in target organs for years before resuming metastatic growth, contributing to late recurrence in patient.
- A pre-metastatic niche is an abnormal, tumor growth–favoring microenvironment in distant organs, created by tumor-derived factors, stromal and immune cells, to facilitate the homing of circulating tumor cells.
- Cellular interactions with the ECM play an important role in the development of metastasis. The formation and breakdown of adhesive bonds, mediated through CAMs, such as integrins and cadherins, provides signals leading to changes in gene expression, cell proliferation, invasion, and other processes.
- Proteolytic enzymes, such as the families of serine proteases and metalloproteinases, play important functions in the breakdown of extracellular matrix components to enhance the invasive properties of tumor cells and to release and/or activate growth factors that assist the growth of tumor cells at a new metastatic site.
- Infiltrating stromal cells, particularly cancer-associated fibroblasts and tumor-associated macrophages, play an important role in tumor growth and metastasis.
- Specific changes in cellular phenotype from epithelial to mesenchymal-like as well as stem cell–like properties (cancer stem cells) may play a role in the ability of cancer cells to metastasize.

REFERENCES

Alix-Panabières C. EPISPOT assay: detection of viable DTCs/CTCs in solid tumor patients. *Recent Results Cancer Res* 2012;195:69-76.

Antonioli L, Blandizzi C, Pacher P, Haskó G. Immunity, inflammation and cancer: a leading role for adenosine. *Nat Rev Cancer* 2013;13(12):842-857.

Aras S, Zaidi MR. TAMeless traitors: macrophages in cancer progression and metastasis. *Br J Cancer* 2017;117(11):1583-1591.

Baccelli I, Schneeweiss A, Riethdorf S, et al. Identification of a population of blood circulating tumor cells from breast cancer patients that initiates metastasis in a xenograft assay. *Nat Biotechnol* 2013;31(6):539-544.

Bandyopadhyay S, Zhan R, Chaudhuri A, et al. Interaction of KAI1 on tumor cells with DARC on vascular endothelium leads to metastasis suppression. *Nat Med* 2006;12(8):933-938.

Barkan D, El Touny LH, Michalowski AM, et al. Metastatic growth from dormant cells induced by a Col-i-enriched fibrotic environment. *Cancer Res* 2010;70(14):5706-5716.

Bednarz-Knoll N, Alix-Panabières C, Pantel K. Clinical relevance and biology of circulating tumor cells. *Breast Cancer Res* 2011;13(6):228.

Bidwell BN, Slaney CY, Withana NP, et al. Silencing of Irf7 pathways in breast cancer cells promotes bone metastasis through immune escape. *Nat Med* 2012;18(8):1224-1231.

Bos PD, Zhang XHF, Nadal C, et al. Genes that mediate breast cancer metastasis to the brain. *Nature* 2009;459(7249):1005-1009.

Bragado P, Estrada Y, Parikh F, et al. TGF-β2 dictates disseminated tumour cell fate in target organs through TGF-β-RIII and p38α/β signalling. *Nat Cell Biol* 2013;15(11):1351-1361.

Buchheit CL, Weigel KJ, Schafer ZT. Cancer cell survival during detachment from the ECM: multiple barriers to tumour progression. *Nat Rev Cancer* 2014;14(9):632-641.

Cavallaro U, Schaffhauser B, Christofori G. Cadherins and the tumour progression: is it all in a switch? *Cancer Lett* 2002;176(2):123-128.

Chen C, Zhao S, Karnad A, Freeman JW. The biology and role of CD44 in cancer progression: therapeutic implications. *J Hematol Oncol* 2018;11(1):1-23.

Cheung KJ, Padmanaban V, Silvestri V, et al. Polyclonal breast cancer metastases arise from collective dissemination of keratin 14-expressing tumor cell clusters. *Proc Natl Acad Sci* 2016;113(7):E854-E863.

Chou J, Lin JH, Brenot A, Kim J, Provot S, Werb Z. GATA3 suppresses metastasis and modulates the tumour microenvironment by regulating microRNA-29b expression. *Nat Cell Biol* 2013;15(2):201-213.

Chui MH. Insights into cancer metastasis from a clinicopathologic perspective: epithelial-mesenchymal transition is not a necessary step. *Int J Cancer* 2013;132(7):1487-1495.

Clucas J, Valderrama F. ERM proteins in cancer progression. *J Cell Sci* 2015;128(6):1253-1253.

Costa-Silva B, Aiello NM, Ocean AJ, et al. Pancreatic cancer exosomes initiate pre-metastatic niche formation in the liver. *Nat Cell Biol* 2015;17(6):816-826.

Cox TR, Bird D, Baker AM, et al. LOX-mediated collagen crosslinking is responsible for fibrosis-enhanced metastasis. *Cancer Res* 2013;73(6):1721-1732.

Cox TR, Rumney RMH, Schoof EM, et al. The hypoxic cancer secretome induces pre-metastatic bone lesions through lysyl oxidase. *Nature* 2015;522(7554):106-110.

Cruz-Munoz W, Khokha R. The role of tissue inhibitors of metalloproteinases in tumorigenesis and metastasis. *Crit Rev Clin Lab Sci* 2008;45(3):291-338.

Deng J, Liu Y, Lee H, et al. S1PR1-STAT3 signaling is crucial for myeloid cell colonization at future metastatic sites. *Cancer Cell* 2012;21(5):642-654.

Dufour A, Zucker S, Sampson NS, Kuscu C, Cao J. Role of matrix metalloproteinase-9 dimers in cell migration. *J Biol Chem* 2010;285(46):35944-35956.

Early Breast Cancer Trialists Collaborative Group. Adjuvant bisphosphonate treatment in early breast cancer: meta-analyses of individual patient data from randomised trials. *Lancet* 2015;386(10001):1353-1361.

Egeblad M, Werb Z. New functions for the matrix metalloproteinases in cancer progression. *Nat Rev Cancer* 2002;2(3):161-174.

Ewald AJ, Brenot A, Duong M, Chan BS, Werb Z. Collective epithelial migration and cell rearrangements drive mammary branching morphogenesis. *Dev Cell* 2008;14(4):570-581.

Eyles J, Puaux AL, Wang X, et al. Tumor cells disseminate early, but immunosurveillance limits metastatic outgrowth, in a mouse model of melanoma. *J Clin Invest* 2010;120(6):2030-2039.

Fearon ER, Vogelstein B. A genetic model for colorectal tumorigenesis. *Cell* 1990;61(5):759-767.

Fidler I, Kripke M. Metastasis results from preexisting variant cells within a malignant tumor. *Science* 1977;197(4306):893-895.

Fidler IJ. Selection of successive tumour lines for metastasis. *Nat New Biol* 1973;242(118):148-149.

Fischer KR, Durrans A, Lee S, et al. Epithelial-to-mesenchymal transition is not required for lung metastasis but contributes to chemoresistance. *Nature* 2015;527(7579):472-476.

Foulds L. The experimental study of tumor progression; a review. *Cancer Res* 1954;14(5):327-339.

Gao D, Nolan DJ, Mellick AS, Bambino K, McDonnell K, Mittal V. Endothelial progenitor cells control the angiogenic switch in mouse lung metastasis. *Science* 2008;319(5980):195-198.

Gay LJ, Felding-Habermann B. Contribution of platelets to tumour metastasis. *Nat Rev Cancer* 2011;11(2):123-134.

Ghajar CM, Peinado H, Mori H, et al. The perivascular niche regulates breast tumour dormancy. *Nat Cell Biol* 2013;15(7):807-817.

Gialeli C, Theocharis AD, Karamanos NK. Roles of matrix metalloproteinases in cancer progression and their pharmacological targeting. *FEBS J* 2011;278(1):16-27.

Grivennikov S, Karin E, Terzic J, et al. IL-6 and Stat3 are required for survival of intestinal epithelial cells and development of colitis-associated cancer. *Cancer Cell* 2009;15(2):103-113.

Hakem A. RhoC is dispensable for embryogenesis and tumor initiation but essential for metastasis. *Genes Dev* 2005;19(17):1974-1979.

Hamidi H, Ivaska J. Every step of the way: integrins in cancer progression and metastasis. *Nat Rev Cancer* 2018;18(9):533-548.

Hanahan D, Weinberg RA. Hallmarks of cancer: the next generation. *Cell* 2011;144(5):646-674.

Hankey W, Frankel WL, Groden J. Functions of the APC tumor suppressor protein dependent and independent of canonical WNT signaling: implications for therapeutic targeting. *Cancer Metastasis Rev* 2018;37(1):159-172.

Hermann PC, Huber SL, Herrler T, et al. Distinct populations of cancer stem cells determine tumor growth and metastatic activity in human pancreatic cancer. *Cell Stem Cell* 2007;1(3):313-323.

Hernandez-Barrantes S, Toth M, Bernardo MM, et al. Binding of active (57 kDa) membrane type 1-matrix metalloproteinase (MT1-MMP) to tissue inhibitor of metalloproteinase (TIMP)-2 regulates MT1-MMP processing and Pro-MMP-2 activation. *J Biol Chem* 2000;275(16):12080-12089.

Hill R, Chambers A, Ling V, Harris J. Dynamic heterogeneity: rapid generation of metastatic variants in mouse B16 melanoma cells. *Science* 1984;224(4652):998-1001.

Hirakawa S, Kodama S, Kunstfeld R, Kajiya K, Brown LF, Detmar M. VEGF-A induces tumor and sentinel lymph node lymphangiogenesis and promotes lymphatic metastasis. *J Exp Med* 2005;201(7):1089-1099.

Hoffman RM. Green fluorescent protein imaging of tumor cells in mice. *Lab Anim (NY)* 2002;31(4):34-41.

Hong MK, Macintyre G, Wedge DC, et al. Tracking the origins and drivers of subclonal metastatic expansion in prostate cancer. *Nat Commun* 2015;6:6605.

Hoshino A, Costa-Silva B, Shen TL, et al. Tumour exosome integrins determine organotropic metastasis. *Nature* 2015;527(7578):329-335.

Hromas R. Cutting the head off chemokines. *Blood* 2002;100(4):1110-1110.

Jackson HW, Defamie V, Waterhouse P, Khokha R. TIMPs: versatile extracellular regulators in cancer. *Nat Rev Cancer* 2017;17(1):38-53.

Johnson BE, Mazor T, Hong C, et al. Mutational analysis reveals the origin and therapy-driven evolution of recurrent glioma. *Science* 2014;343(6167):189-193.

Jones DH, Nakashima T, Sanchez OH, et al. Regulation of cancer cell migration and bone metastasis by RANKL. *Nature* 2006;440(7084):692-696.

Joosse SA, Gorges TM, Pantel K. Biology, detection, and clinical implications of circulating tumor cells. *EMBO Mol Med* 2015;7(1):1-11.

Junttila MR, de Sauvage FJ. Influence of tumour microenvironment heterogeneity on therapeutic response. *Nature* 2013;501(7467):346-354.

Kalluri R, Neilson EG. Epithelial-mesenchymal transition and its implications for fibrosis. *J Clin Invest* 2003;112(12):1776-1784.

Karaca Z, Tanriverdi F, Unluhizarci K, et al. VEGFR1 expression is related to lymph node metastasis and serum VEGF may be a marker of progression in the follow-up of patients with differentiated thyroid carcinoma. *Eur J Endocrinol* 2011;164(2):277-284.

Kessenbrock K, Plaks V, Werb Z. Matrix metalloproteinases: regulators of the tumor microenvironment. *Cell* 2010;141(1):52-67.

Kim M-Y, Oskarsson T, Acharyya S, et al. Tumor self-seeding by circulating cancer cells. *Cell* 2009;139(7):1315-1326.

Kopfstein L, Christofori G. Metastasis: cell-autonomous mechanisms versus contributions by the tumor microenvironment. *Cell Mol Life Sci* 2006;63(4):449-468.

Labelle M, Begum S, Hynes RO. Platelets guide the formation of early metastatic niches. *Proc Natl Acad Sci* 2014;111(30):E3053-E3061.

Laklai H, Miroshnikova YA, Pickup MW, et al. Genotype tunes pancreatic ductal adenocarcinoma tissue tension to induce matricellular fibrosis and tumor progression. *Nat Med* 2016;22(5):497-505.

Lambert AW, Pattabiraman DR, Weinberg RA. Emerging biological principles of metastasis. *Cell* 2017;168(4):670-691.

Laufs S, Schumacher J, Allgayer H. Urokinase-receptor (u-PAR)—an essential player in multiple games of cancer: a review on its role in tumor progression, invasion, metastasis, proliferation/dormancy, clinical outcome and minimal residual disease. *Cell Cycle* 2006;5(16):1760-1771.

Lawson DA, Bhakta NR, Kessenbrock K, et al. Single-cell analysis reveals a stem-cell program in human metastatic breast cancer cells. *Nature* 2015;526(7571):131-135.

Le Pape F, Vargas G, Clézardin P. The role of osteoclasts in breast cancer bone metastasis. *J Bone Oncol* 2016;5(3):93-95.

Li H, Lindenmeyer F, Grenet C, et al. AdTIMP-2 inhibits tumor growth, angiogenesis, and metastasis, and prolongs survival in mice. *Hum Gene Ther* 2001;12(5):515-526.

Liu Y, Cao X. Characteristics and significance of the pre-metastatic niche. *Cancer Cell* 2016;30(5):668-681.

Lobb RJ, Lima LG, Möller A. Exosomes: key mediators of metastasis and pre-metastatic niche formation. *Semin Cell Dev Biol* 2017;67:3-10.

MacDonald IC, Groom AC, Chambers AF. Cancer spread and micrometastasis development: quantitative approaches for in vivo models. *BioEssays* 2002;24(10):885-893.

Maddipati R, Stanger BZ. Pancreatic cancer metastases harbor evidence of polyclonality. *Cancer Discov* 2015;5(10):1086-1097.

Mani SA, Guo W, Liao M-J, et al. The epithelial-mesenchymal transition generates cells with properties of stem cells. *Cell* 2008;133(4):704-715.

Massagué J, Obenauf AC. Metastatic colonization by circulating tumour cells. *Nature* 2016;529(7586):298-306.

Mazor T, Pankov A, Song JS, Costello JF. Intratumoral heterogeneity of the epigenome. *Cancer Cell* 2016;29(4):440-451.

McGranahan N, Swanton C. Clonal heterogeneity and tumor evolution: past, present, and the future. *Cell* 2017;168(4):613-628.

Medici D, Hay ED, Olsen BR. Snail and slug promote epithelial-mesenchymal transition through β-catenin–T-cell factor-4-dependent expression of transforming growth factor-β3. *Mol Biol Cell* 2008;19(11):4875-4887.

Minn AJ, Gupta GP, Siegel PM, et al. Genes that mediate breast cancer metastasis to lung. *Nature* 2005;436(7050):518-524.

Moss NM, Liu Y, Johnson JJ, et al. Epidermal growth factor receptor-mediated membrane type 1 matrix metalloproteinase endocytosis regulates the transition between invasive versus expansive growth of ovarian carcinoma cells in three-dimensional collagen. *Mol Cancer Res* 2009;7(6):809-820.

Mullooly M, McGowan PM, Crown J, Duffy MJ. The ADAMs family of proteases as targets for the treatment of cancer. *Cancer Biol Ther* 2016;17(8):870-880.

Murphy G. Regulation of the proteolytic disintegrin metalloproteinases, the "Sheddases." *Semin Cell Dev Biol* 2009;20(2):138-145.

Noël A, Gutiérrez-Fernández A, Sounni NE, et al. New and paradoxical roles of matrix metalloproteinases in the tumor microenvironment. *Front Pharmacol* 2012;3:140.

Notta F, Chan-Seng-Yue M, Lemire M, et al. A renewed model of pancreatic cancer evolution based on genomic rearrangement patterns. *Nature* 2016;538(7625):378-382.

Nowell PC. Mechanisms of tumor progression. *Cancer Res* 1986;46(5):2203-2207.

Olson OC, Joyce JA. Cysteine cathepsin proteases: regulators of cancer progression and therapeutic response. *Nat Rev Cancer* 2015;15(12):712-729.

Orian-Rousseau V. CD44 is required for two consecutive steps in HGF/c-Met signaling. *Genes Dev* 2002;16(23):3074-3086.

Oskarsson T, Acharyya S, Zhang XH-F, et al. Breast cancer cells produce tenascin C as a metastatic niche component to colonize the lungs. *Nat Med* 2011;17(7):867-874.

Oskarsson T, Batlle E, Massagué J. Metastatic stem cells: sources, niches, and vital pathways. *Cell Stem Cell* 2014;14(3):306-321.

Östman A, Augsten M. Cancer-associated fibroblasts and tumor growth—bystanders turning into key players. *Curr Opin Genet Dev* 2009;19(1):67-73.

Paget S. The distribution of secondary growths in cancer of the breast. *Lancet* 1889;133:571-573.

Pang R, Law WL, Chu ACY, et al. A subpopulation of CD26+ cancer stem cells with metastatic capacity in human colorectal cancer. *Cell Stem Cell* 2010;6(6):603-615.

Paolino M, Choidas A, Wallner S, et al. The E3 ligase Cbl-b and TAM receptors regulate cancer metastasis via natural killer cells. *Nature* 2014;507(7493):508-512.

Peinado H, Lavotshkin S, Lyden, D. The secreted factors responsible for pre-metastatic niche formation: old sayings and new thoughts. *Semin Cancer Biol* 2011;21(2):139-146.

Peinado H, Zhang H, Matei IR, et al. Pre-metastatic niches: organ-specific homes for metastases. *Nat Rev Cancer* 2017;17(5):302-317.

Perret GY, Crépin M. New pharmacological strategies against metastatic spread. *Fundam Clin Pharmacol* 2008;22(5):465-492.

Powell DR, Huttenlocher A. Neutrophils in the tumor microenvironment. *Trends Immunol* 2016;37(1):41-52.

Puente XE, Sánchez LM, Christopher M, Overall CM, López-Otín C. Human and mouse proteases: a comparative genomic approach. *Nat Rev Genet* 2003;4:544-558.

Qian B-Z, Pollard JW. Macrophage diversity enhances tumor progression and metastasis. *Cell* 2010;141(1):39-51.

Quail DF, Joyce JA. Microenvironmental regulation of tumor progression and metastasis. *Nat Med* 2013;19(11):1423-1437.

Radisky ES, Radisky DC. Matrix metalloproteinase-induced epithelial-mesenchymal transition in breast cancer. *J Mammary Gland Biol Neoplasia* 2010;15(2):201-212.

Reiss K, Saftig P. The "A Disintegrin And Metalloprotease" (ADAM) family of sheddases: physiological and cellular functions. *Semin Cell Dev Biol* 2009;20(2):126-137.

Riethdorf S, Fritsche H, Muller V, et al. Detection of circulating tumor cells in peripheral blood of patients with metastatic breast cancer: a validation study of the CellSearch system. *Clin Cancer Res* 2007;13(3):920-928.

Rohan TE, Xue X, Lin H-M, et al. Tumor microenvironment of metastasis and risk of distant metastasis of breast cancer. *J Natl Cancer Inst* 2014;106 (8).

Rowe RG, Weiss SJ. Navigating ECM barriers at the invasive front: the cancer cell–stroma interface. *Annu Rev Cell Dev Biol* 2009;25:567-595.

Schmitt M, Harbeck N, Brünner N, et al. Cancer therapy trials employing level-of-evidence-1 disease forecast cancer biomarkers uPA and its inhibitor PAI-1. *Expert Rev Mol Diagn* 2011;11:617-634.

Schroeder A, Heller DA, Winslow MM, et al. Treating metastatic cancer with nanotechnology. *Nature Reviews Cancer* 2011;12:39.

Schwarz RF, Ng CKY, Cooke SL, et al. Spatial and temporal heterogeneity in high-grade serous ovarian cancer: a phylogenetic analysis. *PLoS Med* 2015;12(2):e1001789.

Seguin L, Desgrosellier JS, Weis SM, Cheresh, DA. Integrins and cancer: regulators of cancer stemness, metastasis, and drug resistance. *Trends Cell Biol* 2015;25(4):234-240.

Seubert B, Grünwald B, Kobuch J, et al. Tissue inhibitor of metalloproteinases (TIMP)-1 creates a premetastatic niche in the liver through SDF-1/CXCR4-dependent neutrophil recruitment in mice. *Hepatology* 2015;61(1):238-248.

Shi M, Liu D, Duan H, Shen B, Guo N. Metastasis-related miRNAs, active players in breast cancer invasion, and metastasis. *Cancer Metastasis Rev* 2010;29(4):785-799.

Shimoda M, Khokha R. Metalloproteinases in extracellular vesicles. *Biochim Biophys Acta Mol Cell Res* 2017;1864(11, pt A):1989-2000.

Silletti S. Disruption of matrix metalloproteinase 2 binding to integrin alpha vbeta 3 by an organic molecule inhibits angiogenesis and tumor growth in vivo. *Proc Natl Acad Sci* 2001;98(1):119-124.

Siow ZR, De Boer R, Lindeman G, Mann GB. Spotlight on the utility of the Oncotype DX® breast cancer assay. *Int J Womens Health* 2018;10:89-100.

Storr SJ, Carragher NO, Frame MC, Parr T, Martin SG. The calpain system and cancer. *Nat Rev Cancer* 2011;11(5): 364-374.

Tachtsidis A, McInnes LM, Jacobsen N, Thompson EW, Saunders CM. Minimal residual disease in breast cancer: an overview of circulating and disseminated tumour cells. *Clin Exp Metastasis* 2016;33(6):521-550.

Takeda K, Hayakawa Y, Smyth MJ, et al. Involvement of tumor necrosis factor-related apoptosis-inducing ligand in surveillance of tumor metastasis by liver natural killer cells. *Nat Med* 2001;7(1):94-100.

Turajlic S, Swanton C. Metastasis as an evolutionary process. *Science* 2016;352(6282):169-175.

van de Vijver MJ, He YD, van 't Veer LJ, et al. A gene-expression signature as a predictor of survival in breast cancer. *N Engl J Med* 2002;347(25):1999-2009.

Vogelstein B, Papadopoulos N, Velculescu VE, Zhou S, Diaz LA, Kinzler KW. Cancer genome landscapes. *Science* 2013;339(6127):1546-1558.

Weilbaecher KN, Guise TA, McCauley LK. Cancer to bone: a fatal attraction. *Nat Rev Cancer* 2011;11(6):411-425.

Yates LR, Knappskog S, Wedge D, et al. Genomic evolution of breast cancer metastasis and relapse. *Cancer Cell* 2017;32(2):169-184.

Ye X, Weinberg RA. Epithelial-mesenchymal plasticity: a central regulator of cancer progression. *Trends Cell Biol* 2015;25(11):675-686.

Yuan X, Wu H, Xu H, et al. Notch signaling: an emerging therapeutic target for cancer treatment. *Cancer Lett* 2015; 369(1):20-27.

Zhang XHF, Wang Q, Gerald W, et al. Latent bone metastasis in breast cancer tied to src-dependent survival signals. *Cancer Cell* 2009;16(1):67-78.

Zhao S, Chen C, Chang K, et al. CD44 expression level and isoform contributes to pancreatic cancer cell plasticity, invasiveness, and response to therapy. *Clin Cancer Res* 2016;22(22):5592-5604.

Zheng X, Carstens JL, Kim J, et al. Epithelial-to-mesenchymal transition is dispensable for metastasis but induces chemoresistance in pancreatic cancer. *Nature* 2015;527(7579):525-530.

Angiogenesis

Janusz Rak and Urban Emmenegger

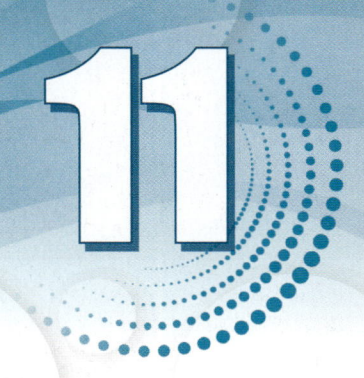

Chapter Outline

- 11.1 Introduction: The Tumor-Vascular Interface
- 11.2 Constituents of the Vascular System
- 11.3 Processes Leading to Vessel Formation
  - 11.3.1 Developmental Vasculogenesis, Angiogenesis, and Vascular Remodeling
  - 11.3.2 Arteriogenesis and Vascular Repair
  - 11.3.3 Mechanisms of Angiogenesis
  - 11.3.4 Vascular Maturation
  - 11.3.5 Lymphangiogenesis
  - 11.3.6 Vasculogenic Mimicry
  - 11.3.7 Vascular Co-option
- 11.4 Molecular Regulators of Vascular Growth
  - 11.4.1 Vascular Endothelial Growth Factor Family
  - 11.4.2 Platelet-Derived Growth Factor Family
  - 11.4.3 Prokineticins
  - 11.4.4 Angiopoietins and TIE Receptors
  - 11.4.5 NOTCH Pathway
  - 11.4.6 Ephrins and EPH Receptors
  - 11.4.7 Vascular Integrins, Cadherins, and Adhesion Molecules
  - 11.4.8 Angiogenesis-Regulating Proteases
  - 11.4.9 Angiogenesis Stimulators and Inhibitors
  - 11.4.10 Coagulation System and Platelets as Regulators of Tumor Angiogenesis
  - 11.4.11 Extracellular Vesicles in Tumor Neovascularization
- 11.5 Tumor Angiogenesis
  - 11.5.1 Constituent Processes of Tumor Neovascularization
  - 11.5.2 Onset and Progression of Angiogenesis in Cancer
  - 11.5.3 Mechanisms Triggering Tumor Neovascularization
  - 11.5.4 Hypoxia as a Trigger of Tumor Angiogenesis
  - 11.5.5 Tumor Vasculogenesis
  - 11.5.6 Proangiogenic Effects of Oncogenic Pathways
  - 11.5.7 Inflammation
  - 11.5.8 Angiogenic Activation of Tumor Stroma
- 11.6 Unique Characteristics and Modifiers of Tumor Angiogenesis
  - 11.6.1 Impact of Genetic Background on Tumor Angiogenesis
  - 11.6.2 Modulation of Tumor Angiogenesis by Vascular Ageing and Comorbidities
  - 11.6.3 Properties of the Tumor Microcirculation
  - 11.6.4 Tumor Lymphangiogenesis
  - 11.6.5 Tumor-Initiating Cells and Blood Vessels
- 11.7 Blood Vessel–Directed Anticancer Therapies
  - 11.7.1 Antiangiogenic Therapies
  - 11.7.2 Vascular Disrupting Agents
  - 11.7.3 Antiangiogenic Effects of Agents Targeting Oncogenic Pathways
  - 11.7.4 Antiangiogenic Effects of Other Therapeutics
  - 11.7.5 Challenges and Opportunities Associated With Targeting Tumor Blood Vessels
- Summary
- References

11.1 INTRODUCTION: THE TUMOR-VASCULAR INTERFACE

An important feature of malignancies is the emergence of new and abnormal contact points between cancer cells and the host vascular system (Folkman, 2007). Prior to transformation, many epithelial tissues (eg, in the gut, skin, and exocrine glands) are anatomically separated from the vasculature by basement membranes and/or connective tissue layers. These barriers are compromised during the malignant process, resulting in abnormal interactions between vascular components (endothelial cells, blood cells, plasma, or lymph) and cancer cells at this new *tumor-vascular interface* (Rak, 2009).

Tumor-vascular interactions are important for disease progression, because of several "outside-in" effects, such as supply of oxygen, nutrients, growth factors, metabolites,

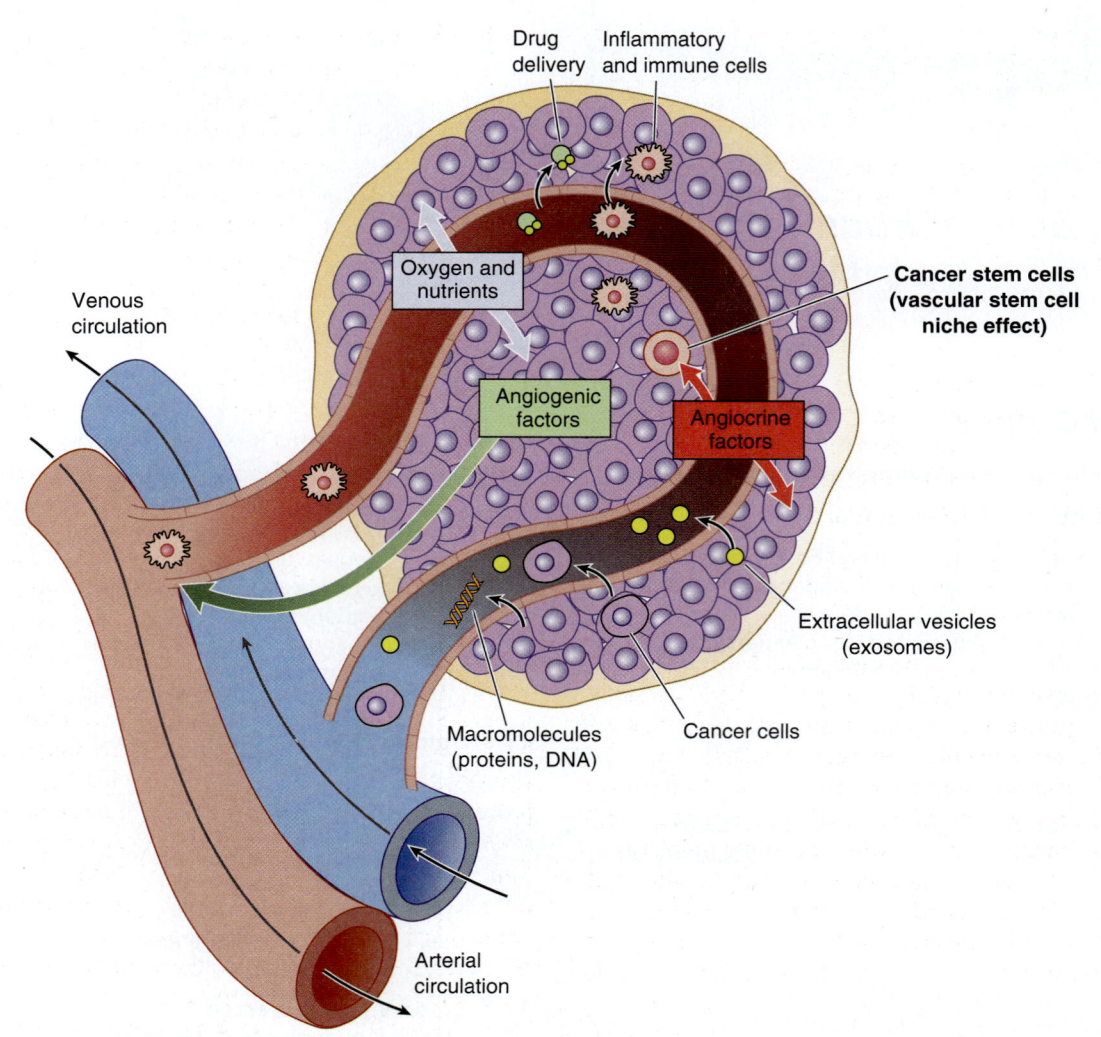

FIGURE 11–1 Tumor-vascular interface. Reciprocal interactions, adjacencies, and interdependencies between cancer cell populations and their supplying vascular cells and structures. Tumor and host cells deploy angiogenic factors that recruit new blood vessels and regulate the state of those proximal to the tumor mass. Conversely, vascular endothelial cells release angiocrine growth factors that influence growth, survival, and motility of cancer cells and supply cancer stem cells with a vascular niche. Blood inflow (perfusion) delivers oxygen, nutrients, endocrine regulators, bone marrow–derived cells (BMDCs), immune cells, and drugs to the tumor mass. Blood outflow from the tumor carries metabolic waste products, systemically acting cytokines, as well as metastatic cancer cells, tumor-related macromolecules, such as DNA, or proteins and extracellular vesicles (exosomes) that mediate long-range intercellular communication including preparation of pre-metastatic niche effects (see text).

and paracrine (angiocrine) effects of endothelial cells (Rafii et al, 2016). This progression also includes adhesive tumor-vascular interactions, formation of a vascular stem cell niche (Gilbertson and Rich, 2007), recruitment/retention of host immune, inflammatory, and bone marrow–derived progenitor cells, as well as delivery of drugs, hormones, and regulatory molecules (Fig. 11–1). The vascular interface also mediates important "inside-out" processes, notably, through intravasation of metastatic cancer cells, release into the circulation of angiogenesis-regulating, proinflammatory, procoagulant, hormonal, immunomodulatory and metabolic (eg, cachexia-inducing) signals, as well as shedding of tumor-related extracellular vesicles (exosomes) containing biologically active molecules (Rak, 2009). The dynamic nature of the tumor-vascular interface is influenced by a succession of genetic and epigenetic alterations in cancer cells, microenvironmental influences (hypoxia, inflammation), as well as the host's genetic background, accompanying diseases (comorbidities), aging, and other processes (Folkman, 2007).

The term *angiogenesis* was first used by John Hunter in 1787, and reintroduced in 1935 by Artur Tremain Hertig, to describe non-cancer-related blood vessel growth processes. Investigations led gradually to a description of vascular expansion associated with a developing cancer, along with pioneering experimental methods (Roy-Chowdhury and Brown, 2007). In the early 1970s, the concept of targeting angiogenesis for therapeutic purposes (antiangiogenesis) was proposed by Judah Folkman (Folkman, 1971). This form of therapy is now a part of the clinical management of several malignancies. Further development of these approaches depends on our understanding of responses of the vascular system to an emerging malignancy at both local and systemic levels.

11.2 CONSTITUENTS OF THE VASCULAR SYSTEM

Blood circulation ensures the delivery of oxygen, nutrients, macromolecules, hormones, and cells (eg, immune, inflammatory, or reparative stem cells) to the vicinity of every living cell, while removing catabolites and waste products. To remain viable, each mammalian cell must be located no further than 100 to 180 μm from the nearest functional (perfused) capillary blood vessel. Directionality, efficiency, and organ-specificity of the blood flow are developmentally preprogrammed by the geometry, physical properties, and hierarchical architecture (arborization) of the vascular system. Thus, cardiac output is directed through the tree of arteries of decreasing caliber and changing wall structure, including elastic, muscular-type, and contractile arteries, as well as smaller and precapillary arterioles, which eventually branch into capillary blood vessels. Capillaries converge to form the postcapillary venules, followed by small, midsize, and large veins that differ from their corresponding arteries by lower pressure, bloodstream velocity, and content of blood (low oxygen levels), as well as by thinner wall structure and (in some segments) the presence of intraluminal valves to maintain flow directionality.

Each blood vessel is composed of a crucial inner lining made of endothelial cells, which are surrounded by 1 or more supportive layers containing mural cells with contractile characteristics of smooth muscle cells or pericytes, sheaths (laminae) of extracellular matrix (ECM), and other components (eg, innervation). Collectively, these structures (Fig. 11-2) support a luminal surface not susceptible to blood coagulation with mechanical resistance, contractility, spatial architecture, and a web of homeostatic intercellular interactions (Carmeliet and Jain, 2011a).

Capillaries are thin-walled tubes of endothelial cells (ECs), with lumens of 8 to 20 μm in diameter; their exterior is wrapped in a basement membrane (BM) rich in type IV collagen, which also envelopes discontinuous layers of smooth muscle-like cells (SMCs), here known as pericytes. Although capillaries in most of the vascular beds are permeable to fluids and certain micromolecules (oxygen, ions) they are highly restrictive to macromolecules. In the brain, such molecular passage is controlled tightly by the blood-brain barrier, while being less restrictive in endocrine organs (Carmeliet and Jain, 2011). Structurally, the blood-brain barrier is composed of endothelial cells (with associated adherens as well as tight junctions), pericytes, and astrocytes. Blood-brain barrier endothelial cells selectively regulate the influx and efflux of molecules via ABC transporter pumps (see Chap. 18, Sec 18.4.3) and solute carriers as well as receptor-mediated transporters.

Fluid released (extravasated) through the capillary walls into the intercellular tissue space (interstitium) is collected by lymphatic capillaries (lymphatics), which are open ended and thin walled, have a discontinuous or absent basement membrane, and lack pericytes (see Fig. 11-2). Lymphatics drain their content (lymph) to regional lymph nodes, whereas the larger lymphatic channels converge and drain to the thoracic duct, which carries the lymph to the left subclavian vein. In humans, up to 2 liters of interstitial fluid carrying macromolecules and cells enter the lymphatic system daily (Tammela and Alitalo, 2010).

Each of the cellular constituents of the vascular system exhibits unique molecular and phenotypic properties (Fig. 11-3):

Endothelial cells line the entire inner surface of the circulatory system. Normally quiescent (99.9%), with a slow turnover time ranging between 6 weeks and many years, these cells may proliferate rapidly during wound healing and, in female reproductive organs, at the time of cyclical hormonal changes. Endothelial cells exhibit a characteristic flat morphology, anticoagulant luminal surfaces, and express several relatively lineage-specific molecules (pan-endothelial markers), including CD31 (PECAM), CD144 (VE-cadherin), von Willebrand factor (vWF), CD202b (tunica interna endothelial cell kinase-2, TIE2; encoded by the *tek* gene), CD34 (sialomucin), CD146 (P1H12 antigen/MUC18), and CD105 (endoglin). These cells may display regional differences dependent on vessel type, caliber, and organ site (Chang et al, 2017).

Mural cells (smooth muscle cells and pericytes) are heterogeneous with different surface marker configurations (eg, Nestin$^+$/NG2$^+$ [nerve/glial antigen 2] and Nestin$^-$/NG2$^+$). They maintain the integrity of the endothelial tube and provide blood vessels with mechanical resistance, functional stability, and vasoconstrictive properties. In capillaries, pericytes form processes that extend along the vessel axis making contact with several endothelial cells to which they deliver survival signals. Mural cell-specific antigens (markers) include α smooth muscle actin (αSMA), desmin, CD13, 3G5 ganglioside, CD248 (endosialin), NG2, RGS5, and platelet-derived growth factor receptor beta (PDGFRβ) (Carmeliet and Jain, 2011).

Bone marrow–derived regulatory and progenitor cells (BMDCs) maintain vascular homeostasis at the systemic level (see Fig. 11-3). Local cytokine release leads to the recruitment and retention of various populations of BMDCs. These populations include endothelial progenitor cells (EPCs; also known as circulating endothelial progenitor-like or colony forming cells or endothelial colony forming cells) that are implicated in formation of new blood vessels, vascular regrowth, and metastasis, but their origin and ability to differentiate into mature ECs and contribute to the vessel wall still remains controversial. These cells must be distinguished from myeloid pro-angiogenic cells with similar phenotype. While bone marrow is the major source of EPCs, other tissues (eg, adipose tissue, local endothelia) may also contribute to the pool of circulating EPCs. Tumor-associated endothelial cells have been reported to contain a subset of cells with multipotential (stemlike) properties and the capability to differentiate into chondrocytes and bone cells, and to trigger calcification (Dudley et al, 2008).

Among BMDCs, myeloid cells play regulatory roles during remodeling and maintenance of the vasculature, including changes occurring in the course of cancer. The best-described subpopulations of these cells in murine and human tissues encompass (1) tumor-associated M2-type macrophages (F4/80$^+$/CD11b$^+$); (2) monocytes expressing TIE2 receptor (TIE2$^+$/CD11b$^+$); (3) myeloid bone marrow–derived regulatory cells (VEGFR1$^+$/CXCR4$^+$/CD11b$^+$);

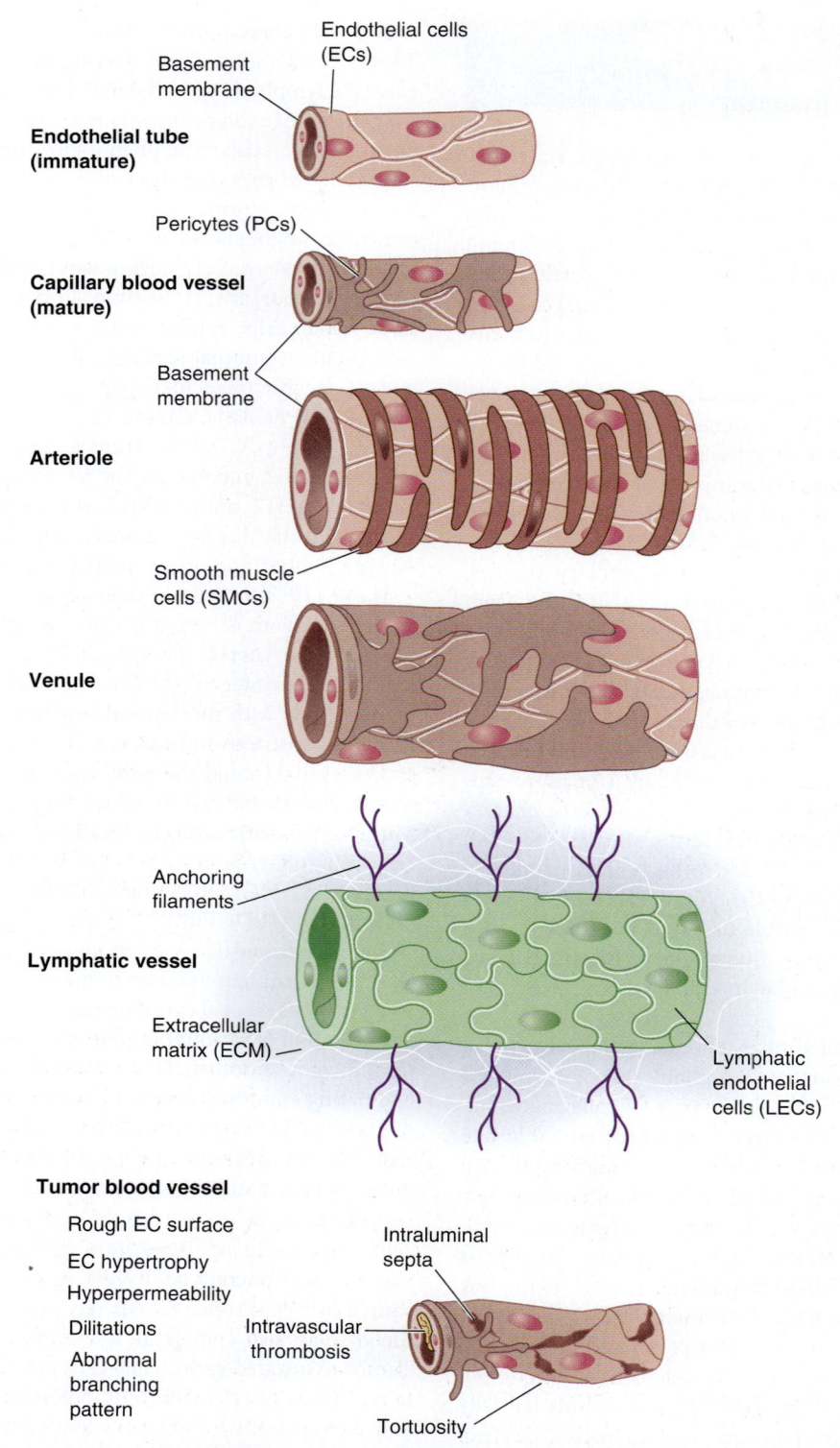

FIGURE 11–2 Structural constituents of the microvasculature. The cellular architecture of blood vessels reflects their functions, including newly formed endothelial tube (top), capillary blood vessels, precapillary arteriole, postcapillary venule, and lymphatic capillary. Blood vessel endothelial cells (ECs), pericytes / smooth muscle cells (PCs/SMCs), and lymphatic endothelial cells (LECs) are the key constituents of the microvasculature, including in cancer. Tumor blood vessels exhibit multiple structural and functional abnormalities, and features consistent with lack of maturation/normalization, hence referred to as vessel abnormalization (see text for details).

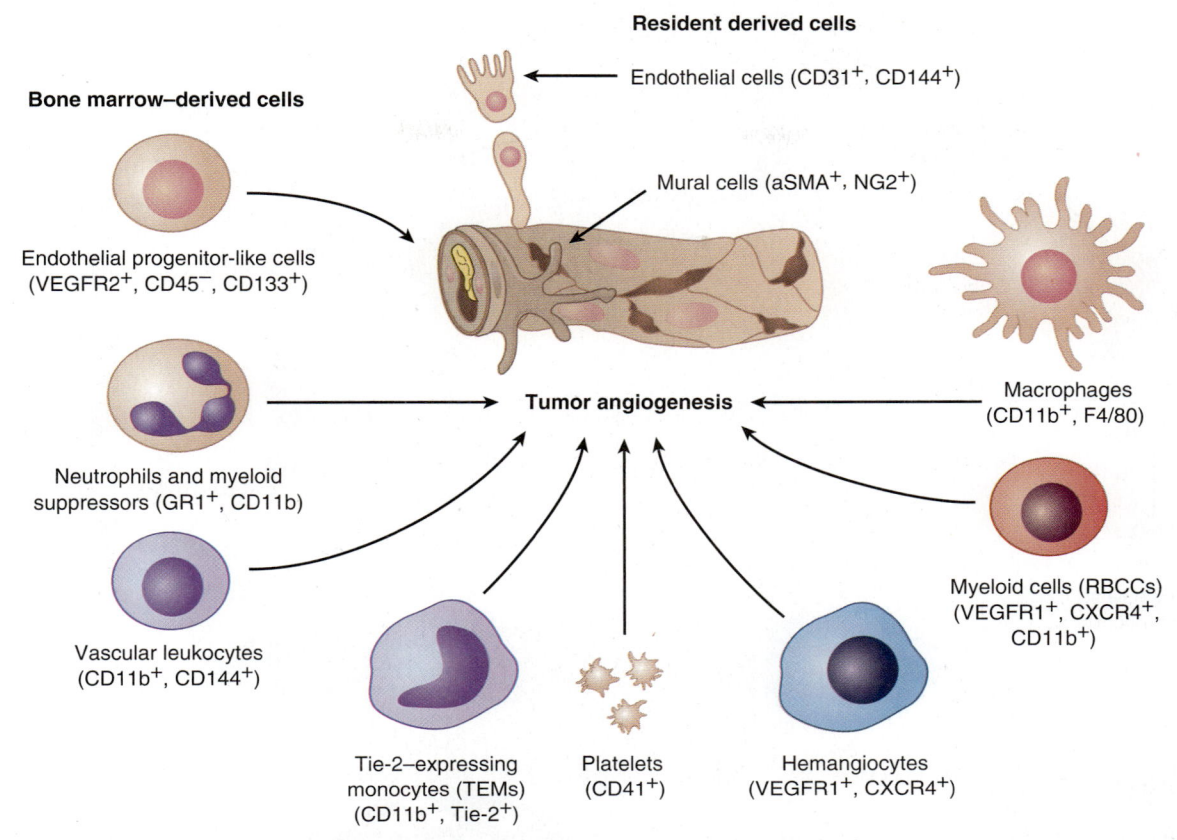

FIGURE 11–3 Cell populations involved in tumor angiogenesis. Vascular growth is coordinated by structural resident cells in the preexisting blood vessels, and by several populations of regulatory and circulating bone marrow-derived cells (EPCs and BMDCs). Although the structural contribution of endothelial progenitor-like cells (EPCs) to tumor neovascularization remains controversial, the regulatory function of these cells and that of several other types of bone marrow–derived cells (BMDCs) is increasingly well established, for example, as sources of vascular endothelial growth factor (VEGF), alternative angiogenic factors, guidance signals, proteolytic activity, and other effects. Angiogenic fibroblasts, cancer cells, and immune effectors are not included in this diagram for simplicity (see text for details).

(4) hemangiocytes (VEGFR1$^+$/CXCR4$^+$); (5) vascular leukocytes (CD11b$^+$/CD144$^+$); and (6) angiogenic neutrophils (GR1$^+$/CD11b$^+$). Subsets of these cells are also referred to as marrow-derived suppressor cells (MDSCs) because of their immunoregulatory properties. Proangiogenic properties have also been ascribed to other myeloid cells, such as mast cells (MCs), dendritic cells (DCs), and hematopoietic stem cells. Several of these cell types not only produce angiogenic factors, for example, vascular endothelial growth factors (VEGFs), but also express overlapping markers with endothelial cells (De Palma et al, 2017).

11.3 PROCESSES LEADING TO VESSEL FORMATION

11.3.1 Developmental Vasculogenesis, Angiogenesis, and Vascular Remodeling

Vasculature is the first organ system to develop during embryogenesis, around midgestation in mice (Ema and Rossant, 2003). The process (Fig. 11–4) consists of at least 4 distinct phases (Carmeliet and Jain, 2011), including (1) the emergence of endothelial progenitors (angioblasts); (2) coalescence and differentiation of angioblasts to form the primitive network of endothelial tubes (*vasculogenesis*), a structure known as the *primary capillary plexus*; (3) branching of new vascular projections (sprouts) from the preformed endothelial tubes (*angiogenesis*); and (4) remodeling, expansion, and diversification of the vascular network to form the arterial and the venous sides of the circulation, a process that defines the directionality of the blood flow.

As the vascular system matures, the ingress of mural cells (*vascular maturation*) stabilizes the endothelial channels. Some of these channels may be superfluous, or nonfunctional, which leads to their regulated regression (*pruning*) (Potente and Makinen, 2017).

11.3.2 Arteriogenesis and Vascular Repair

As branching and angiogenesis lead to the establishment of vascular hierarchy some vessels become supply lines for smaller capillaries. To meet the related volumetric and mechanical requirements, these supplying macrovessels undergo

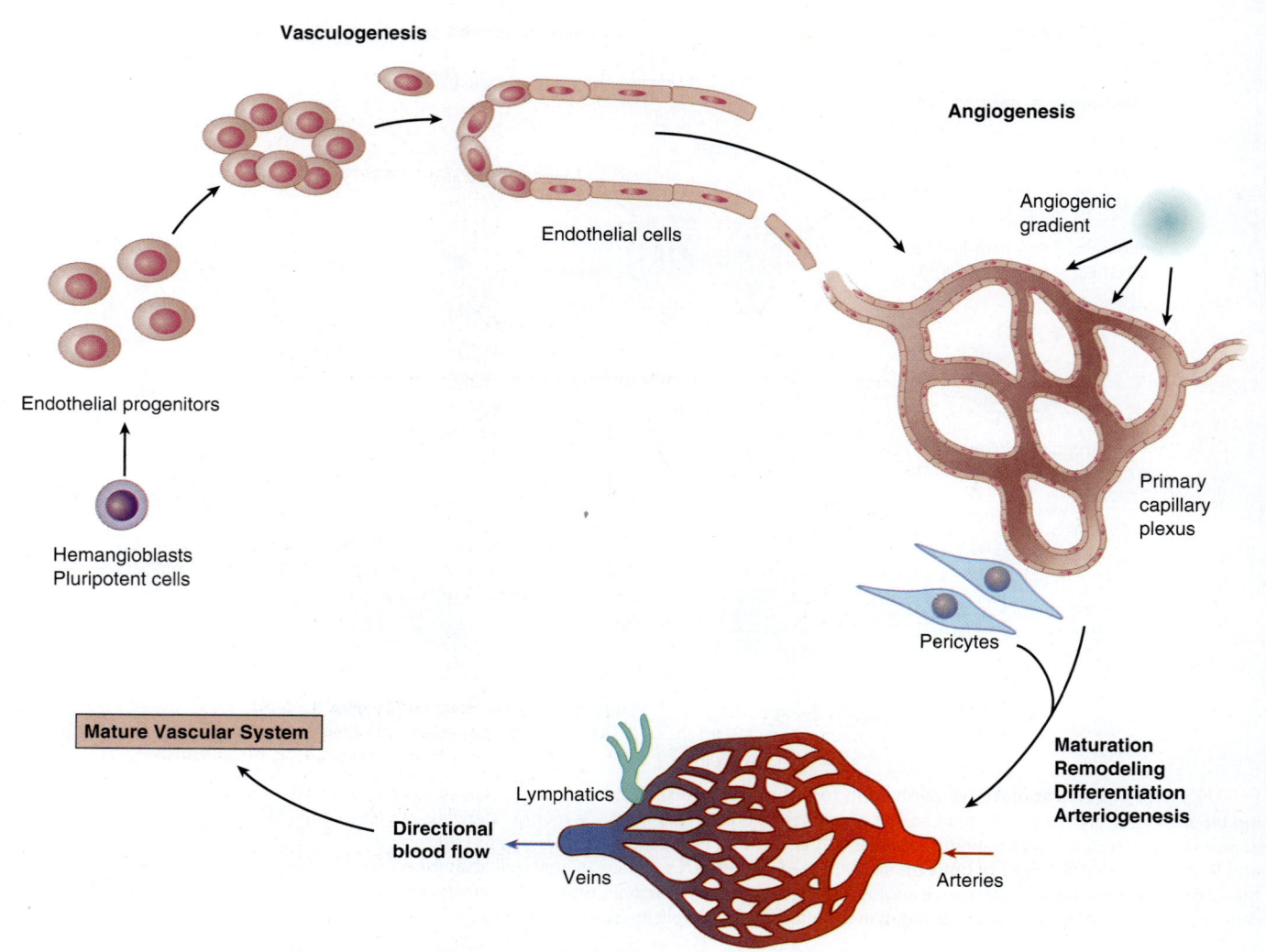

FIGURE 11–4 Development of the vascular system. A spectrum of blood vessel–forming processes is activated during development, and partially reactivated during postnatal vascular growth (wound healing, pregnancy, vascular diseases, and cancer). Endothelial cells, the key organizing elements of the vascular system, emerge from their precursors, which are a product of the lineage commitment of earlier precursors (hemangioblasts) in the embryonic mesenchyme, or may arise through transdifferentiation of other cells. *Vasculogenesis* entails coalescence of endothelial progenitors, their differentiation to endothelial cells, and formation of primitive vascular tubes, which organize themselves into a homogenous, directionless, and largely nonperfused network (primary capillary plexus). *Angiogenesis* is a process of outgrowth of vascular structures from the preexisting primary plexus, or mature vasculature. During development, angiogenesis is accompanied by the antithetical process leading to removal of superfluous vessels (*pruning*), both of which are essential for the establishment of the proper hierarchy (*arborization*) of the vascular network and for directional blood flow from arterial to the venous side of the circulation. The integrity of the emerging capillary blood vessels is ensured by arrival of pericytes (PCs; *vessel maturation*). The arterial vessels that supply blood to the expanding microcirculation undergo a remodeling and circumferential growth process, often referred to as *arteriogenesis*; see the text and references for further details.

circumferential expansion and wall remodeling (*arteriogenesis*), a process dependent on BMDCs. Bone marrow is also the principal source of EPCs that are recruited to sites of pathologic losses in endothelial lining (denudation), usually in arterial vessels or vascular grafts, and are responsible for their repair (Xu, 2006). These cells may also home to intravascular clots and facilitate formation of inner vascular channels within them (recanalization), among other functions (Carmeliet and Jain, 2011).

11.3.3 Mechanisms of Angiogenesis

Angiogenesis is a process whereby new vascular structures emerge from ones that have already been established in tissues or tumor masses (see Figs. 11–5 and 11–9). In cancer, this process is viewed as the key source of new vascular growth associated with tumor formation and metastasis, and one that occurs via at last 3 different mechanisms: (1) intussusception; (2) vascular splitting; and (3) sprouting angiogenesis. Intussusceptive angiogenesis is a form of new blood vessel formation through the division of a larger or dilated capillary vessel into smaller channels, as a result of external pressure exerted by extravascular tissue. Similar branching may be achieved through formation of intraluminal septa (splitting). In this manner, additional capillary loops make contacts with a greater volume of the adjacent tissue, but their most extensive increase occurs through processes of capillary sprouting (Carmeliet and Jain, 2011).

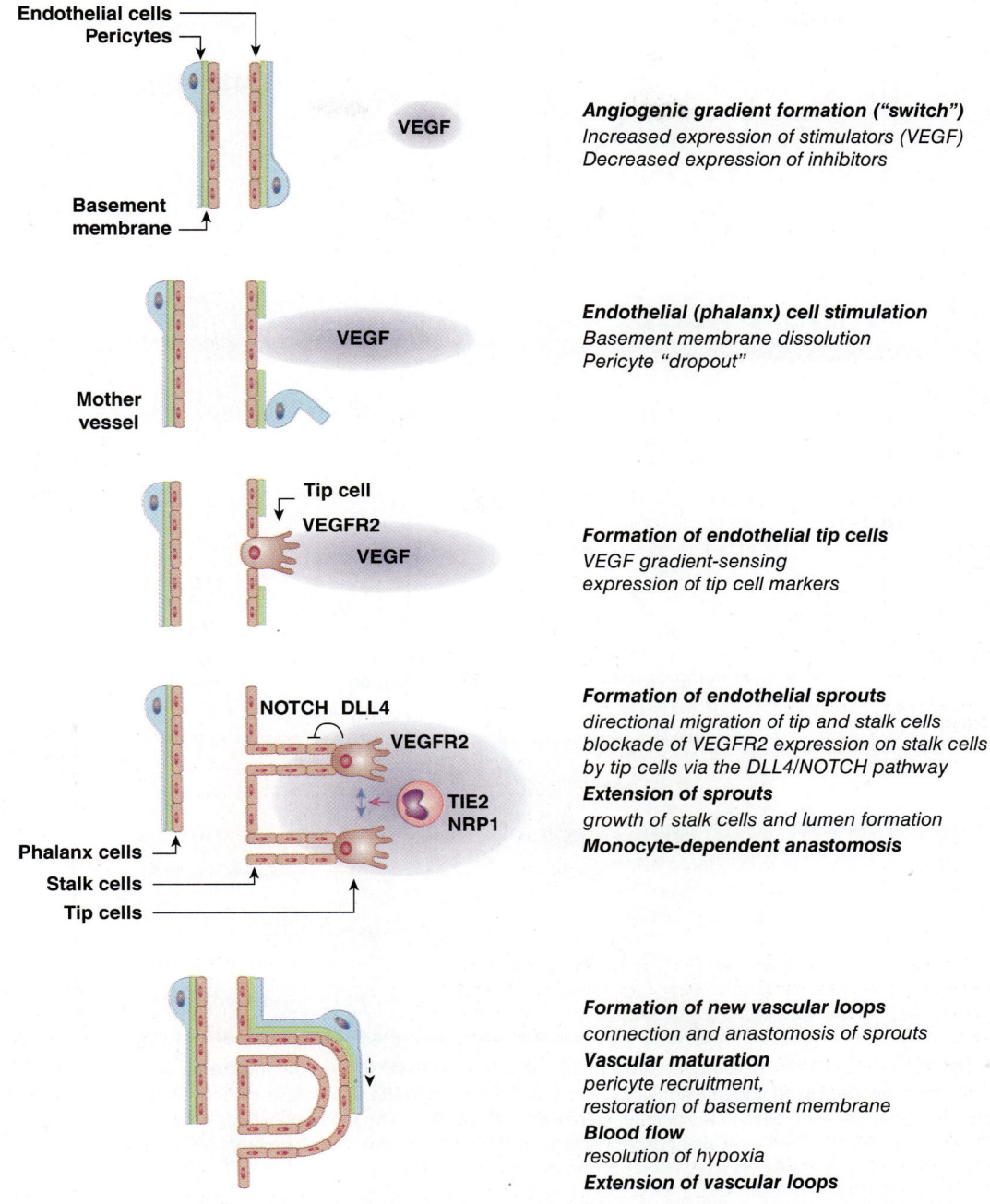

FIGURE 11-5 Sprouting angiogenesis. The change in balance between angiogenesis stimulators and inhibitors (angiogenic "switch") and especially local upregulation of vascular endothelial growth factor (VEGF) and formation of the VEGF gradient leads to stimulation of vascular responses known as sprouting angiogenesis. Stimulated blood vessels undergo a series of structural changes that consist of localized dissociation of pericytes ("dropout") from the endothelial tube, dissolution of the basement membrane, and recruitment of the angiogenesis-directing cells (tip cells) from the endothelial monolayer (phalanx cells). Capillaries enlarge (to form "mother vessels") and deploy cohorts of endothelial cells (stalk cells) led by VEGF gradient-seeking tip cells that express high levels of VEGFR2 and DLL4. Interaction of tip cell–related DLL4 with NOTCH on following stalk cells suppresses their VEGFR2 expression and ensures that they do not become superfluous tip cells. Vascular sprouts extend and undergo lumen formation (hollowing). TIE-2/NRP1–expressing monocytes orchestrate the encounter and connection (anastomosis) of nearby sprouts (or their link to preexisting vessels) to complete the formation of a functional vascular loop. Capillary loops can extend further to promote increased tissue perfusion, a process known as looping angiogenesis, and operative during formation of granulation tissue.

Sprouting angiogenesis constitutes the main vascular program leading to the expansion of capillary networks both in health and disease (see Fig. 11-5). The exposure of a precapillary vessel to a gradient of proangiogenic activity (eg, VEGF expression induced by hypoxia; see Sec. 11.5.3 and Chap. 12, Sec. 12.4.2) leads to several orchestrated responses, that begin with vessel dilatation giving rise to a thin-walled, regionally distended structure known as a "mother vessel" (Dvorak, 2015b). This transition reflects the activation state of the still intact monolayers of endothelial cells, here referred to as

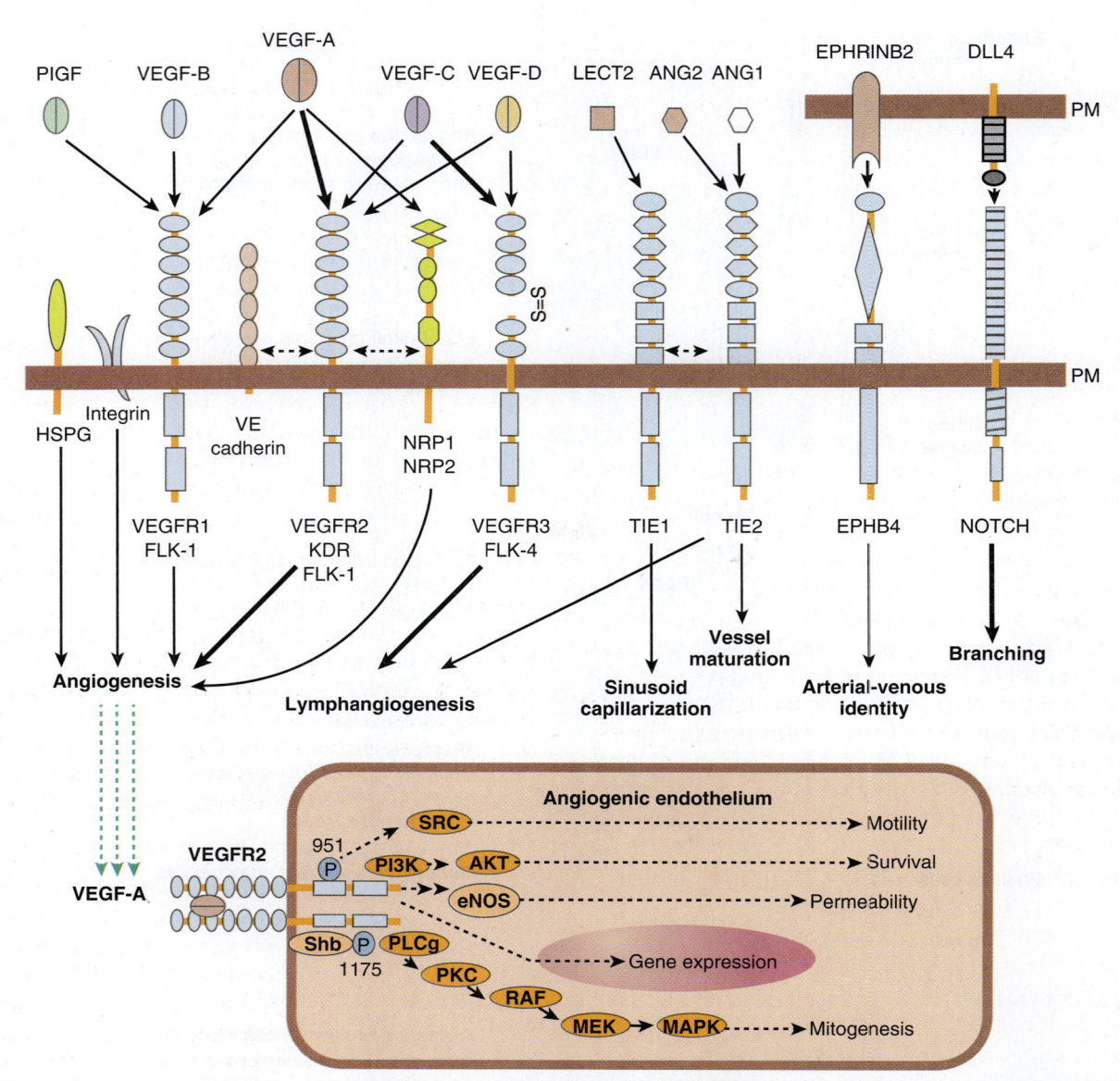

FIGURE 11-6 Key elements of the signaling circuitry involved in blood vessel formation and tumor angiogenesis. Top panel: Ligands, receptors, and coreceptors involved in angiogenic signaling. Note that EphrinB2 and DLL4 are transmembrane ligands. Domain structure, signaling properties, targets, and crosstalk are detailed in the related references. Bottom panel: Outline of signaling pathways and their effector mechanisms downstream of VEGF-A/VEGFR2. Numbers indicate phosphorylated tyrosines. *PM*, cellular plasma membrane; *HSPG*, heparan sulfate proteoglycan.

phalanx cells. Formation of mother vessels is often followed by focal detachment of pericytes from the endothelial tube, which thereby becomes liberated from structural constraints, more exposed to extravascular stimuli, and capable of deployment of endothelial cells. The centerpiece of these complex endothelial-pericyte interactions is the upregulation of angiopoietin 2 (ANG2) in the endothelium, following exposure to high levels of VEGF. ANG2 acts as an autocrine antagonist of the TIE2 receptor tyrosine kinase expressed on the surface of endothelial cells (compare Figs. 11–5 and 11–6). ANG2 binding relieves phosphorylation of TIE2, as a result of displacement of its natural pericyte-derived agonist, angiopoietin 1 (ANG1), which disrupts ANG1-induced vessel-stabilizing endothelial-pericyte interactions (Augustin et al, 2009). As a consequence, endothelial cells may now form new outgrowths following focal dissolution of the capillary basement membrane by release of matrix metalloproteinases (MMPs; see Chap. 10, Sec. 10.2.2). MMPs also liberate additional angiogenic factors from the extracellular matrix (Carmeliet and Jain, 2011).

The continued exposure of liberated endothelial phalanx cells to extravascular angiogenic gradients triggers the process of coordinated formation, movement, and extension of multicellular structures known as *angiogenic sprouts* (see Fig. 11–5). Each sprout is composed of a single specialized endothelial *tip cell* equipped with hairlike, ligand-sensing projections (filopodia), containing high concentrations of VEGF receptors (especially VEGFR2) (Carmeliet and Jain, 2011). Tip cells also express other molecules such as platelet-derived growth factor B (PDGF-B), and the transmembrane protein known as Delta-like ligand 4 (DLL4). The latter acts as the key ligand for

NOTCH receptors present on adjacent endothelial *stalk cells* trailing each migrating tip cell (see Chap. 6, Sec. 6.4.2). This interaction activates the NOTCH pathway, which suppresses VEGFR2 expression in stalk cells to prevent their conversion into ectopic tip cells. Indeed, when the DLL4/NOTCH interaction is inhibited, excessive numbers of tip cells and sprouts emerge, leading to hyperdense, nonperfused, and dysfunctional capillary networks, a phenomenon known as *nonproductive angiogenesis* (Noguera-Troise et al, 2006). This regulation is fine-tuned through regulation of Jagged 1, which competes with DLL4 for binding to NOTCH. The NOTCH pathway also integrates angiogenesis and arteriogenesis (Potente and Makinen, 2017).

Tip cells serve as guidance devices for endothelial sprouts, the numbers and directions of which they control, as they move along the path of angiogenic (VEGF) gradients (Gerhardt et al, 2003). Cohorts of stalk cells follow each tip cell and contribute to the sprout extension by directional collective migration and division of cells at the sprout base. Eventually neighboring sprouts connect or fuse to preexisting loops (anastomose), which is regulated by a subset of tissue macrophages expressing TIE2 and Neuropilin 1 (NRP1) receptors (Potente and Makinen, 2017). Formation of functional capillary loops requires generation of the vascular lumen through intra- or interendothelial processes of space formation (hollowing), likely dependent on activation of cellular vesicle transport and chloride channels of the chloride intracellular ion channel family (CLIC) proteins (Tung et al, 2012). At this point, blood may begin to flow through the newly formed capillary tubes as they undergo further maturation (see Fig. 11–5).

11.3.4 Vascular Maturation

Maturation of microvessels involves the assembly of a mural cell layer around the newly formed endothelial tube (Carmeliet and Jain, 2011). Angiogenic endothelial cells, including tip cells, secrete PDGF-B, which is deposited onto heparin sulfate proteoglycan chains and serves as a chemoattractant for regional pericytes expressing PDGFRβ. Pericytes also secrete ANG1, which orchestrates their interactions with endothelial cells and acts as an endothelial survival factor by activating the TIE2 receptor. Vascular maturation is also critically dependent on sphingosine 1 phosphate (S1P), which regulates N-cadherin, an adhesion molecule that links endothelial cells and pericytes. Upon their attachment to the endothelial tube (see Fig. 11–2), pericytes differentiate to a more mature phenotype, a process thought to be regulated by transforming growth factor beta 1 (TGFβ1) (Gaengel et al, 2009). Pericyte coverage of endothelial structures and the vascular maturation (stabilization) processes are profoundly affected by the endothelial oxygen sensor prolyl hydroxylase 2 (PHD2), and by other mechanisms responsible for cellular integrity, response to hypoxia, and survival (see Chap. 12, Sec. 12.4.2). Vascular maturation provides newly formed capillaries with structural support and mechanical resistance, and reduces endothelial cell demand for soluble survival factors, such as VEGF (Carmeliet and Jain, 2011).

11.3.5 Lymphangiogenesis

Formation of new lymphatics from preexisting lymphatic vessels is called *lymphangiogenesis*. Studies of lymphatic endothelial cells (LECs) and lymphangiogenesis have markedly accelerated after description of their distinct markers, such as the prospero homeobox transcription factor (PROX-1), podoplanin (PDPN), and lymphatic vessel hyaluronan receptor-1 (LYVE-1). Formation of lymphatics also depends on the activity of the forkhead transcription factor FOX2c, as well as two VEGF-related growth factors, VEGF-C and VEGF-D, and their unique receptor (VEGFR-3/FLT-4) that is expressed preferentially by LECs (see Fig. 11–6). Another pathway involved in lymphatic vessel formation is EPHRIN-B2, that is co-expressed on the vessel surface with its receptor EPHB4, and which together control lymphatic sprouting and remodeling. Moreover, in LECs (unlike in vascular endothelium), both ANG2 and ANG1 activate the TIE2 receptor and promote lymphangiogenesis. Indeed, a germline *Ang2* deletion in mice leads to lymphatic defects, which can be rescued by the expression of Ang1 (Augustin et al, 2009).

Lymphangiogenesis and angiogenesis are intricately linked to ensure the balance between blood supply and recovery of interstitial lymph. For example, while proteolytically unprocessed VEGF-C/D selectively stimulates VEGFR-3 on LECs, the proteolytic processing of these factors allows them to bind to VEGFR2 on angiogenic endothelial cells. Such cells may also express VEGFR3 and respond to both VEGF-A and VEGF-C/D ligands.

Lymphangiogenesis is fine-tuned by additional signaling cues that include interactions between VEGF-C and Neuropilin-2 (NRP2), a coreceptor for VEGFR3. This process is modulated by β_1 and α_9 integrins, hepatocyte growth factor (HGF), insulin-like growth factors 1 and 2 (IGF-1 and IGF-2), PDGF-B, fibroblast growth factors (FGFs), and other inputs collectively leading to formation of the lymphatic microcirculation. Lymphatics must be separated anatomically from blood vessels to prevent mixing of blood and lymph. This separation is induced by thrombosis of connecting channels due to interactions between podoplanin and c-type lectin-like receptor 2 (CLEC2) receptors on platelets (Tammela and Alitalo, 2010).

11.3.6 Vasculogenic Mimicry

In some contexts, nonendothelial cells may adopt endothelial-like phenotypes and line vascular channels (Hendrix et al, 2003). This process occurs in the normal placenta, where trophoblast epithelium enters the myometrium at sites of spiral arteries. Such entry causes epithelial-to-endothelial transformation of trophoblastic cells, including the expression of several markers normally associated with vascular endothelium (CD31, CD144, integrin $\alpha_v\beta_3$). Aberrant differentiation also occurs after subcutaneous injection of pluripotent embryonic stem cells into mice and results in formation of aggressive teratomas, which contain blood vessels partially derived from these stem cells. Such endothelial transdifferentiation events were described in patients with chronic myelogenous leukemia, lymphoma, and uveal melanoma. Regulators implicated in these events include tissue factor (TF), TF pathway inhibitor 2 (TFPI-2), phosphatidylinositol 3 kinase (PI3K), focal adhesion kinase (FAK), MMPs, ephrins, and laminin chains (Welti et al, 2013).

11.3.7 Vascular Co-option

Cancer cells can exploit preexisting tissue vasculature by growing around, and enveloping, the vessels. This nonangiogenic process has been observed in highly vascular organs, such as lung and brain, as well as in melanoma and in liver metastases of colorectal cancer. Vascular cooption is increasingly considered to be as one of predominant mechanisms of neovascularization of different cancer types and a source of resistance to angiogenesis inhibitors (Kuczynski et al 2019). Although cancer cells can grow and migrate along blood vessels, this interaction may also trigger blood vessel thrombosis, occlusion, and regression (Carmeliet and Jain, 2011).

11.4 MOLECULAR REGULATORS OF VASCULAR GROWTH

Formation of new vascular networks, whether in health or disease, is based on the ability of the constituent cells to coordinate their responses through intercellular communication. The mediators of these interactions can be divided into several categories, including (1) specialized ("professional") signaling effectors required for vascular homeostasis; (2) pleiotropic effectors endowed with angiogenesis-regulating activities (stimulators and inhibitors), along with other functions; and (3) other regulators that link angiogenesis to processes such as hemostasis, bone marrow stimulation, neuronal growth, or immunity (Carmeliet and Jain, 2011). Although this molecular network contains redundancies, feedbacks, and complex response patterns, there are individual key molecules that can serve as potential targets for blood vessel directed therapies (Table 11–1 and Figs. 11–5 to 11–10). Key elements of this molecular circuitry are shown in Figure 11–6 and are discussed below.

11.4.1 Vascular Endothelial Growth Factor Family

VEGF-A, also known as VEGF or vascular permeability factor (VPF), is the key member of a larger family of related polypeptides, which also includes VEGF-B, VEGF-C, VEGF-D, VEGF-E, VEGF-F, and placenta growth factor (PlGF), all also related to platelet-derived growth factor (PDGF) (Ferrara and Adamis, 2016). These ligands form functional homo- and heterodimers and interact with at least 3 different receptor tyrosine kinases (VEGFR1/FLT-1, VEGFR2/KDR/FLK-1, and VEGFR3/FLT-4), and with 2 neuropilin coreceptors (NRP1 and NRP2). The relatively selective (albeit nonexclusive) expression of VEGFRs by endothelial cells (of blood vessels, lymphatics, and in tumors) allows VEGFs to control vascular processes in a potent and combinatorial manner (see Fig. 11–6). Thus, VEGFR1 binds VEGF-A, VEGF-B, and PlGF, whereas VEGFR2 interacts mainly with VEGF-A (and VEGF-E), and VEGFR3 interacts preferentially with intact VEGF-C and VEGF-D. NRP1, also involved in neuronal guidance by binding class 3 semaphorin SEMA3A, is expressed by endothelial cells, where it acts as a VEGF-A coreceptor in concert with VEGFR2. NRP1 binds only certain VEGF-A splice isoforms (eg, VEGF165), contributing to their distinct activities (Carmeliet and Jain, 2011).

Germline deletion of each VEGF receptor in mice leads to early embryonic lethality amid vascular defects suggesting their essential roles in vascular development and angiogenesis. VEGFR2 is responsible for VEGF-A-dependent angiogenic signaling, a process that involves receptor phosphorylation and recruitment of intracellular proteins (see Fig. 11–6). Although VEGFR1 also binds VEGF-A with high affinity (10-fold greater than VEGFR2), the phosphorylation of this receptor in endothelial cells is weak, and deletion of its kinase domain is relatively inconsequential for vascular development. Indeed, VEGFR1 is often expressed as a soluble splice variant (sFLT-1), which acts as a natural VEGF antagonist (VEGF "sink"). However, VEGFR1 does possess an important regulatory function for macrophages, and certain cancer cells, in which it mediates migratory responses to VEGF (Carmeliet and Jain, 2011).

The crucial role of VEGF-A is underscored by embryonic lethality and profound vascular defects in mouse embryos lacking even a single *vegf* allele (haplo-insufficiency). Indeed, VEGF-A acts as a potent mitogen, as well as a motility and survival factor for endothelial cells, and a chemo-attractant for their progenitors. These powerful influences are finely regulated by the organ- and context-specific alternative splicing of the VEGF-A transcript, resulting in several protein isoforms. The main species generated during this process are designated according to the number of their constituent amino acids and include VEGF121 (121 amino acids), VEGF145, VEGF165, VEGF189, and VEGF206. VEGF splicing removes various sequences from within the region encoded by exons 6 and 7, while leaving the sequences corresponding to exons 1 to 5 and 8 largely intact (Ferrara and Adamis, 2016). Consequently, VEGF-A splice isoforms differ in their binding to NRP1, heparin, cellular membranes, and the extracellular matrix, and in their ability to diffuse through tissues. For example, the shortest VEGF121 isoform is highly diffusible, VEGF189 is mostly cell bound, whereas VEGF165 expresses intermediate properties and possesses the greatest angiogenic activity. The latter is a function of reduced diffusion rates and thereby a more stable angiogenic gradient that allows VEGF165 (Vegfa164 in the mouse) to accumulate within the interstitial space in tissues. This gradient favors directional responses of tip cells and robust sprouting. In addition, unlike VEGF121, VEGF165 interacts with both VEGFR2 and NRP1, which is thought to contribute to more pronounced endothelial responses. The VEGF-A splicing process also results in the expression of alternative ligands endowed with antagonistic (antiangiogenic) activities: for example, one variant, VEGF165b (which comprises exon 8b in C-terminal position instead of exon 8a found in VEGF165), exerts a modulating influence on responses of blood vessels

TABLE 11–1 Key molecular regulators of tumor angiogenesis.

Examples of angiogenic effectors required for endothelial and mural cell function		
Regulator	**Main Receptor(s)**	**Biological Activity**
VEGF-A/VEGF	VEGFR2 (VEGFR3, VEGF1), NRP1	Stimulator of angiogenic functions, migration and survival of ECs, including formation of tip cells
VEGF-C	VEGFR3 (VEGFR2)	Stimulator of lymphangiogenesis (LECs), and of angiogenesis (ECs)
ANG1	TIE2	Positive regulator of endothelial-mural interactions, EC survival and vessel maturation
ANG2	TIE2	Negative regulator of endothelial-mural interactions, stimulator of lymphangiogenesis
DLL4	NOTCH	Inhibitor of tip cell formation
JAG1	NOTCH	Stimulator of tip cell formation
EphrinB2	EPHB4	VEGFR internalization/signaling, arterial identity, tube formation
PDGF-B	PDGFRβ	Recruitment of mural cells, vessel maturation
TGFβ1	TGFβRII	Differentiation of mural cells, ECM formation
Integrins ($α_v$, $β_1$, $β_5$)	ECM proteins	EC survival, migration, morphogenesis
Examples of stimulators involved in pathologic angiogenesis		
PlGF	VEGFR1	Stimulates angiogenesis by interaction with ECs and BMDCs
acidic FGF (FGF-1)	FGFRs 1-4	Stimulator of EC mitogenesis, survival, and angiogenesis
basic FGF (FGF-2)	FGFRs 1-4	Stimulator of EC mitogenesis, survival, and angiogenesis
FGF-3	FGFRs 1-4	Stimulator of EC mitogenesis, survival, and angiogenesis
FGF-4	FGFRs 1-4	EC mitogen, survival, and angiogenesis factor
IL-8	CXCR1	Stimulator of ECs and inflammatory cells
IL-6	IL-6R	Stimulator of inflammatory angiogenesis
TNFα	TNFR1 (p55)	EC stimulator and VEGF inducer
Bv8	GPCR	Stimulator of endocrine and tumor ECs
PD-ECGF/TP	GPCR	Stimulator of angiogenesis
Angiogenin	170 kD receptor	Stimulator of angiogenesis and RNAse
MMP9	ECM proteins	Matrix metalloproteinase that breaks down ECM and releases angiogenic growth factors
Examples of endogenous angiogenesis inhibitors		
Inhibitor	**Biological Activity**	
TSP-1	Interacts with CD36 receptor, integrins, and other proteins causing growth inhibition and apoptosis of angiogenic ECs	
Endostatin	Proteolytic fragment of collagen XVIII with antiangiogenic activity	
Angiostatin	Proteolytic fragment of plasminogen with antiangiogenic activity	
Tumstatin	Proteolytic fragment of collagen IV alpha 3 chain with antiangiogenic activity	
sFlt-1/sVEGFR1	Soluble splice variant of VEGFR1 neutralizing VEGF and blocking VEGFR2 signaling	
VEGF165b	Splice variant of VEGF with antiangiogenic activity	
PEX	210–amino acid fragment of MMP2 inhibiting EC invasion and MMP activity	
INF α (β)	Inhibits release of angiogenic growth factors	

Abbreviations: *Ang (1, 2)*, angiopoietin; *BMDC*, bone marrow–derived cells; *Bv8*, *Bombina variegata*-secreted protein 8; *DLL4*, delta-like ligand 4; *EC*, endothelial cell; *FGF*, fibroblast growth factor; *GPCR*, G protein–coupled receptor; *IFN*, interferon; *IL-8*, interleukin 8; *IL-6*, interleukin 6; *JAG1*, Jagged 1; *LEC*, lymphatic endothelial cell; *MMP*, matrix metalloproteinase; *PDGF*, platelet-derived growth factor; *PD-ECGF/TP*, platelet-derived endothelial cell growth factor/thymidine phosphorylase; *PlGF*, placenta growth factor; *TNFα*, tumor necrosis factor alpha; *TSP-1*, thrombospondin 1; *VEGF*, vascular endothelial growth factor.
See text for more details (Folkman, 1971, 2007; Kerbel, 2008; Carmeliet and Jain, 2011).

to angiogenic growth factors during tissue remodeling and inflammation (Harper and Bates, 2008).

The remaining members of the VEGF family play more restricted roles in vascular processes, and germline deletions of the respective genes do not lead to a haplo-insufficient phenotype in mice. VEGF-C and VEGF-D control lymphangiogenesis, whereas VEGF-B provides additional survival protection to endothelial cells. The effects of these factors can become prominent under pathologic conditions such as tumor angiogenesis (eg, in the case of PlGF; Carmeliet and Jain, 2011). Finally, although VEGF-related factors were originally viewed as having mainly paracrine effects, VEGF-A is expressed at low, but functionally meaningful, levels by endothelial cells, so that autocrine effects contribute to vascular homeostasis and arteriogenesis (Pitulescu et al, 2017).

11.4.2 Platelet-Derived Growth Factor Family

This family of VEGF-related growth factors consists of 4 members: PDGF-A, PDGF-B, PDGF-C, and PDGF-D, the homo- or heterodimers of which interact preferentially with one of 2 main cellular receptor tyrosine kinases (RTKs), namely, PDGFRα and PDGFRβ. Although PDGFs play multiple roles in development, disease, and cancer, they are also central to vascular growth, especially blood vessel maturation. Thus, PDGF-BB homodimers are produced at high levels in endothelial tip cells and in phalanx cells of arteriogenic vessels, where they attract mural cells harboring PDGFRβ (Andrae et al, 2008). Other members of this family may also contribute to various angiogenic events indirectly, for example, by influencing the expression of angiogenesis-related genes (eg, VEGF) in cancer cells and fibroblasts (Carmeliet and Jain, 2011).

11.4.3 Prokineticins

This family of VEGF-unrelated growth factors was found to induce VEGF-like effects, especially in endothelial cells of endocrine glands and other organs. This stimulation includes growth, migration, permeability, fenestration (formation of trans-endothelial openings), and angiogenesis. Members of this family consist of the endocrine gland VEGF/prokineticin 1 (EG-VEGF/PK1) and *Bombina variegata*–secreted protein 8/prokineticin 2 (Bv8/PK2), which both interact with their respective G-protein-coupled receptors (PK-R1 and PK-R2). Prokineticins are found in cancer, where they may be produced by myeloid cells and contribute to VEGF-independent angiogenesis (Monnier and Samson, 2010).

11.4.4 Angiopoietins and Tie Receptors

At least 3 related ligands known as angiopoietins (ANG1, 2, and 4) play diverse roles in endothelial cell survival, vascular development and maturation, as well as angiogenesis and lymphangiogenesis in humans (Ang3 is a mouse ortholog of ANG4). Angiopoietins interact with the TIE2/TEK receptor tyrosine kinase (RTK) that is expressed preferentially (but not exclusively) on ECs. ECs also harbor a related receptor known as TIE1, which binds LEC2 and regulates TIE1 activity during pathological remodelling (capillarization) of liver sinusoids. Both TIE1 and TIE2 receptors are essential for vascular development. Their activity is controlled by the vascular endothelial receptor tyrosine phosphatase (VE-PTP). The best-understood function of the angiopoietin/TIE2 circuitry is in the regulation of endothelial cell survival, vascular permeability, and recruitment of mural cells. ANG1 is expressed by perivascular tissues and acts as a TIE2 agonist. In contrast, ANG2 is produced largely by endothelial cells exposed to VEGF, and it blocks ANG1/TIE2 interaction, thereby destabilizing endothelial-pericyte contacts (see Fig. 11–6). Thus, in the presence of VEGF, exposure to ANG2 promotes vascular sprouting, but when VEGF levels are low, ANG2 promotes vascular regression (see Augustin et al, 2009, for review).

11.4.5 Notch Pathway

Cell-cell contact-dependent regulatory interactions often involve NOTCH receptors (NOTCH 1 to 4) and their 5 cell-associated (juxtacrine) ligands, including Jagged 1 and 2 (JAG 1 and 2), as well as Delta-like ligand 1, 3, and 4 (DLL1, DLL3, and DLL4) along with several alternative (non-canonical) ligands (see also Chap. 6, Sec 6.4.2). NOTCH 1 and 4 are expressed by endothelial cells (NOTCH 4 preferentially) and, along with DLL4, are required for proper vascular development. DLL4 is expressed in angiogenic tip cells and plays a pivotal role in maintaining their identity, whereas JAG1 may be involved in modulating these effects and in recruitment of additional tip cells. JAG1 may also mediate direct interactions between endothelial and mural cells, or between tumor cells and the vasculature. Another NOTCH ligand, DLL1, is involved in vascular remodeling and arteriogenesis. Interactions with these ligands trigger proteolytic release of the intracellular domain of NOTCH (ICN/NICD), which is responsible for modulation of gene expression and cellular effects (Tung et al, 2012).

11.4.6 Ephrins and EPH Receptors

The definition of arterial and venous identity in the developing vascular system is largely attributed to the unique bidirectional signaling mechanism mediated by transmembrane ligands of the ephrin family, notably Ephrin B2 (on arterial endothelial cells) and their EPHB4 receptors (on endothelial cells of adjacent veins; see Fig. 11–6). These molecules define the arterial and venous identity of endothelial cells and interact on parallel blood vessels. The expression of other Ephrins (eg, A1, A2, B1, and B3) and additional EPH receptors (EPHB2, EPHB3) is also observed in endothelial cells, including those in tumors. Ephrins are implicated in various angiogenesis-related processes, such as endothelial–pericyte interactions, interactions of blood vessels with tumor cells, and cooperation with other angiogenic factors. The latter is exemplified by Ephrin B2-dependent regulation of VEGFR2 endocytosis and signaling (Wang et al, 2010).

11.4.7 Vascular Integrins, Cadherins, and Adhesion Molecules

Adhesion molecules connect endothelial cells with their extraluminal, intercellular, and intraluminal surroundings (see Fig. 11–7). Thus, direct interaction between the abluminal surfaces of endothelial cells and the extracellular matrix (basement membrane) is essential for survival, homeostasis, and angiogenic activity of these cells. Quiescent endothelial cells are anchored to the permanent basement membrane, which is composed of laminin and collagen type IV. In contrast, angiogenic endothelial cells are surrounded by provisional extracellular matrix (ECM) containing fibrin, vitronectin, fibronectin, and partially proteolyzed collagens. These various interactions are mediated by a family of heterodimeric, transmembrane receptors, known as *integrins* (each composed

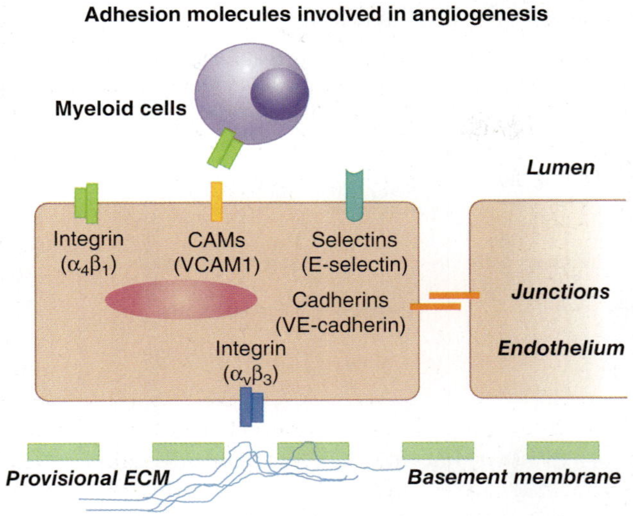

Adhesion molecules involved in angiogenesis

FIGURE 11–7 Adhesive mechanisms involved in angiogenesis and endothelial cell function. Endothelial cells interact homotypically through gap and tight junctional mechanisms, the latter involving endothelial cell lineage–specific VE-cadherin (CD144). Interactions with provisional ECM composed of proteolyzed collagen, fibrin, and vitronectin are mediated by $\alpha_v\beta_3/\beta_5$ integrins. Cell adhesion molecules (CAMs), selectins, and integrins mediate interactions with circulating cells and platelets, playing a role in mechanosensing, inflammation, and permeability; see text for details.

of α and β subunits), which recognize specific motifs within their target ECM proteins (eg, RGD peptides; see also Chap 10, Sec 10.2.3).

Integrins function as hubs that localize and regulate the activities of other angiogenic effectors, including VEGFR2, other receptors, MMPs, angiopoietins, and intracellular signal-transducing kinases (PKB/AKT, FAK, ILK, SRC). Growth factors upregulate the expression of integrins on the surface of endothelial cells in both blood vessels ($\alpha_v\beta_3$, $\alpha_v\beta_5$, $\alpha_1\beta_1$, $\alpha_2\beta_1$, $\alpha_4\beta_1$, $\alpha_5\beta_1$) and lymphatics ($\alpha_1\beta_1$, $\alpha_2\beta_1$, $\alpha_4\beta_1$, $\alpha_9\beta_1$) (Avraamides et al, 2008). Pharmacologic disruption of the adhesive function of certain integrins ($\alpha_v\beta_3$) can result in antiangiogenic effects, but gene-targeting studies suggested a more complex involvement, and enhanced tumor angiogenesis is observed in β_3/β_5-deficient mice (Avraamides et al, 2008). Mutations of vascular integrins may either reduce (β_3 mutant, $\alpha_1\beta_1$) or increase ($\alpha_2\beta_1$) adult angiogenesis (Avraamides et al, 2008).

In contrast to the outward-oriented adhesion that is mediated by endothelial integrins, vascular endothelial cadherin (VE-cadherin/CD144) mediates formation of intercellular adherens junctions between endothelial cells within the vascular tube. These junctions contribute to the unique properties of the endothelial lining that include barrier function, restricted permeability, and homotypic adhesion. VE-cadherin is expressed selectively by cells of endothelial lineage and serves as their genetic marker. Gene targeting studies reveal that VE-cadherin is essential for vascular development, and for the function of some of its key regulators, such as VEGFR2. N-cadherin is also expressed by endothelial cells, albeit not as selectively, and is required for vascular integrity and developmental angiogenesis. Cadherin-mediated adherens junctions

along with tight junctions (involving claudins) influence the functional integration of the endothelial lining (Giannotta et al, 2013).

Interactions between the intraluminal parts of endothelial cells and circulating immune, myeloid, inflammatory, progenitor cells and platelets are mediated by diverse adhesion molecules, including selectins (eg, E-selectin), integrins ($\alpha_4\beta_1$/VLA4), and members of the immunoglobulin family of cell adhesion molecules (CAMs, eg, ICAM-1/2 and VCAM1), all of which play important roles in angiogenesis and inflammation (Francavilla et al, 2009).

11.4.8 Angiogenesis-Regulating Proteases

During blood vessel formation, the dissolution of the endothelial basement membrane, liberation of progenitor cells from the bone marrow, release of VEGF and other growth factors from their ECM stores, and the activation/modulation of the coagulation system, all involve various classes of proteases and their endogenous inhibitors (van Hinsbergh et al, 2006). MMPs and their tissue inhibitors (TIMPs 1 to 4), expressed in the tumor microenvironment (see Fig. 11–8 and Chap. 10, Sec. 10.2.2), participate in ECM breakdown, generation of angiogenesis-regulating protein fragments, control of tumor and endothelial cell invasion, and may also act as ligands of cellular receptors. The main MMPs involved in tumor angiogenesis are MMP-1, MMP-2, MMP-9, and MMP-14. Their role is illustrated by the impairment of tumor neovascularization in mice with disrupted *Mmp9* gene expression (Kessenbrock et al, 2010). Other proteases involved in angiogenesis include cathepsins, coagulation factor VIIa, thrombin (IIa), urokinase-type plasminogen activator (uPA), as well as members of the disintegrin and metalloproteinase domain (ADAM) and thrombospondin motif-containing (ADAMTS) families of proteases. In addition, cellular surfaces carry enzymatic activities displayed as either receptor-bound, glycosylphosphatidyl-inositol (GPI)-linked, or transmembrane proteins. Examples of such outwardly oriented cell-associated catalytic proteins include membrane-type MMPs (MT-MMPs), aminopeptidases (APN/CD13), dipeptidyl peptidases (DPPIV/CD26), and other enzymes that are able to stimulate angiogenesis by pericellular proteolysis, release of active peptides from the extracellular matrix, or by protein-protein interactions (van Hinsbergh et al, 2006).

11.4.9 Angiogenesis Stimulators and Inhibitors

The mechanisms described above are required for the execution of one or more neovascularization programs (Fig. 11–9), but they are not necessarily the only or initial triggers of tumor angiogenesis. In cancer and other angiogenesis-dependent diseases, vascular growth may be initiated by a global shift in expression of several molecules, and the related cumulative change in the regulatory environment, the constituents of which are broadly classified as angiogenesis stimulators

Proteases involved in angiogenesis

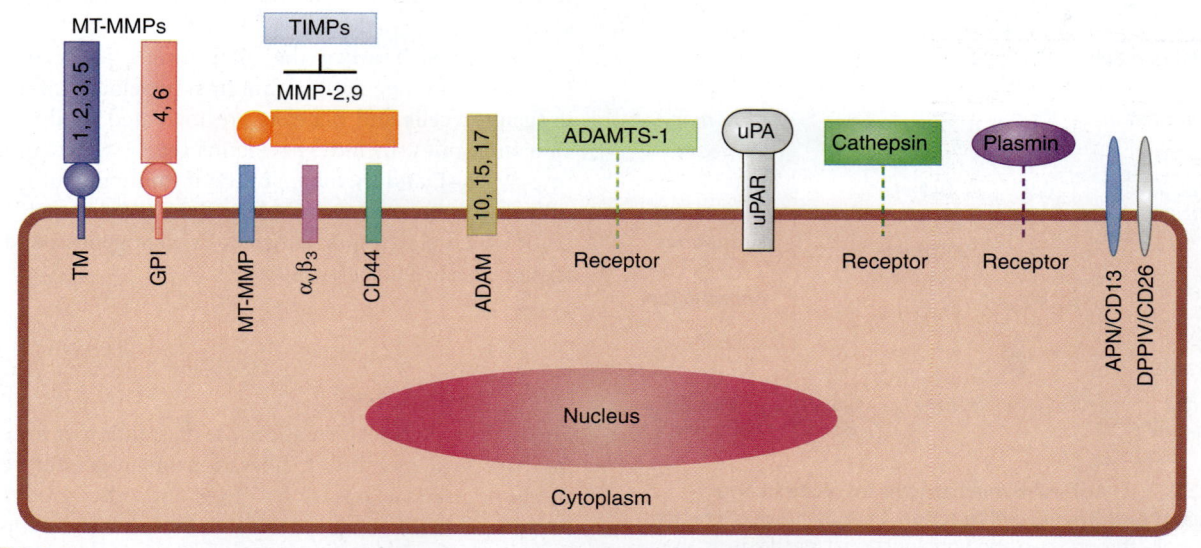

FIGURE 11–8 Proteolytic mechanisms involved in angiogenesis and endothelial cell function. Families of cellular and pericellular proteases involved in angiogenesis: *ADAM*, a disintegrin and metalloproteinase domain–containing protein; *ADAMTS*, a disintegrin and metalloproteinase domain–containing protein with thrombospondin motif; *APN*, aminopeptidase; *DPPIV*, diaminopeptidase; *GPI*, glycosyl-phosphatidylinositol anchor; *MT-MMP*, membrane-type matrix metalloproteinase; *TIMPs*, tissue inhibitors of metalloproteinases; *TM*, transmembrane region; *uPA*, urokinase plasminogen activator; *uPAR*, uPA receptor.

and inhibitors (see Table 11–1). The onset of angiogenesis ("angiogenic switch"; see Fig. 11–10) is triggered when the balance between these opposing influences is tilted beyond a certain discrete threshold, and in favor of stimulators (Folkman, 2007). Although this transition may appear as a binary event, the biologic mechanisms involved can be complex, discontinuous, incremental, or oscillatory. The angiogenic threshold and the magnitude of EC responses may also differ depending on the genetic background and several other factors. Furthermore, the composition of angiogenic factors may change over time during tumor progression (see Fig. 11–10), leading to a series of transitions rather than a single switch (Folkman, 2007).

Stimulators of angiogenesis include factors acting directly on endothelial cells, such as VEGF, PlGF, FGF1/2, HGF, or interleukin 8 (IL-8). Their angiogenic effects can also result from indirect actions of their potent inducers, for example, transforming growth factors alpha or beta (TGFα, TGFβ) and several other cytokines and chemokines (eg, pleiotrophin). Some of these factors may act by recruitment of inflammatory cells (eg, IL-6) or bone marrow progenitors (eg, VEGF or stromal-derived factor 1 [SDF1]), or through concomitant stimulation of both endothelial and inflammatory cell populations (eg, IL-8; Kerbel, 2008).

The endogenous angiogenesis inhibitors are thought to maintain blood vessels in their quiescent state, or limit the magnitude of angiogenic responses, both locally and systemically (Folkman, 2007). These inhibitors belong to different classes of molecules, including certain ECM proteins, such as thrombospondins 1 and 2 (TSP1 and TSP2), proteolytic fragments of ECM components (endostatin, tumstatin, arresten), fragments of enzymes and zymogens (angiostatin, PEX domain), fragments of coagulation-related chemokines (platelet factor 4 [PF4]), and of hormones (prolactin 16-kDa fragment), along with cytokines (interferons α, β, and γ), and other factors detailed elsewhere (Folkman, 2007; see Table 11–1 and Sec. 11.7).

11.4.10 Coagulation System and Platelets as Regulators of Tumor Angiogenesis

The discovery of VEGF in 1983 (Senger et al, 1983), and its role as a vascular permeability factor (VPF), linked angiogenesis to the coagulation system, especially through the observation of the associated extravascular leakage of plasma and formation of a proangiogenic fibrin matrix (Dvorak, 2015b). Although tumor angiogenesis was found to occur in the absence of fibrinogen and fibrin, proangiogenic activities can be ascribed to several effectors of the coagulation system, such as tissue factor (thromboplastin), and thrombin/thrombin receptors (Mackman and Davis, 2011). These factors may act directly on endothelial cells, or stimulate the expression of VEGF, IL-8, and other angiogenic proteins by their cancer or stromal counterparts. Circulating platelets may serve as reservoirs and carriers of angiogenic factors (eg, VEGF) and inhibitors (PF4, TSP-1): platelets take up, accumulate, and segregate such factors in their granules and may selectively release them at sites of angiogenesis (Klement et al, 2009).

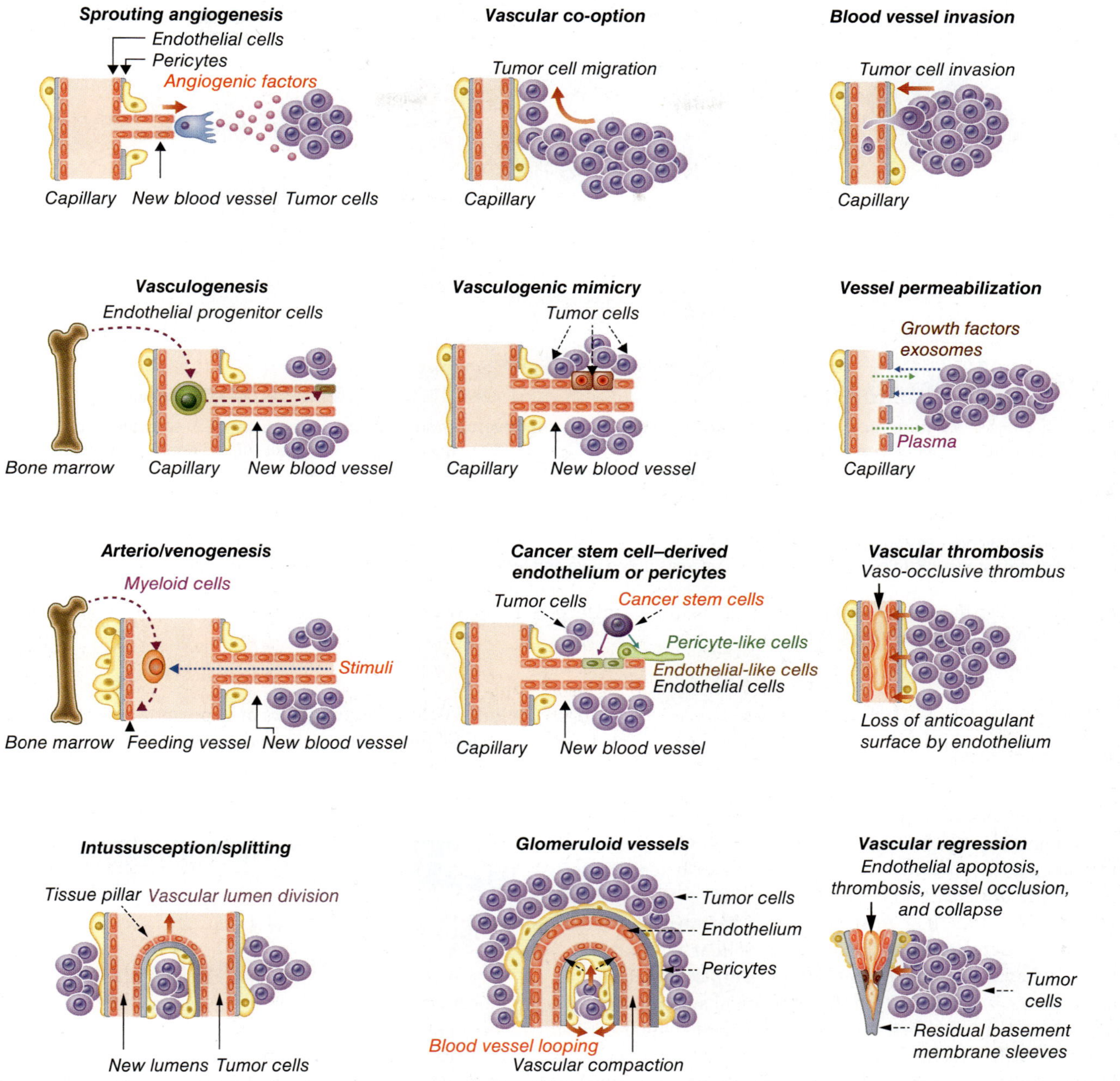

FIGURE 11–9 Processes contributing to tumor neovascularization. While sprouting *angiogenesis* is among the most studied vascular mechanisms in cancer, several other processes may contribute to tumor neovascularization. First row (top): *Vascular co-option* involves cancer cells seeking, growing and migrating around preexisting blood vessels; *blood vessel invasion* represents a destructive form of blood vessel seeking behavior of cancer cells, which results in breaching the vascular wall and cancer cell intravasation. Second row: *Vasculogenesis* is a process of recruitment of endothelial cell progenitors (mostly from the bone marrow) to lodge and contribute to the endothelial lining of growing blood vessels; *vasculogenic mimicry* consists in positioning of cancer cells within the functional blood vessel lining during which cancer cells may adopt some of the phenotypic features of endothelial cells; *vessel permeabilization* results from interactions between blood vessels and adjacent tumor masses, which may produce vascular endothelial growth factors (VEGF) or other mediators of vascular permeability (e.g. exosomes). Formation of intercellular gaps, transcellular vacuoles, fenestrae, and wall porosities allows bidirectional leakage of macromolecules or even cells between plasma and perivascular space, including formation of extravascular blood lakes and fibrin clots. Third row: *Arterio/venogenesis* involves circumferential extension of feeding vessels that supply the tumor capillary bed. This process may occur within or outside of the tumor mass and is regulated by circulating myeloid cells; *cancer stem cell (CSC)–derived endothelium and pericytes* occur in certain tumors via differentiation of CSCs to endothelial cells or pericytes with respective contributions to the tumor microvasculature; *vascular thrombosis* occurs when tumor cells induce clotting of blood in adjacent capillaries or larger vessels resulting in loss of patency and perfusion, followed by tissue necrosis. Fourth row (bottom): *Intussusception or splitting* is a process where external tissue pillars, for example, a pushing cancer cell mass, or intravascular septa divide a larger vessel into smaller capillary loops, thereby increasing vascular access; *glomeruloid vessels* form through pulling forces of pericytes whereby capillary looping occurs, resulting in a "bundle" of vascular channels; *vascular regression (pruning)* may result from detrimental interactions between perivascular cancer cells and the vessel wall, or following anti-VEGF therapy; endothelial apoptosis, and detachment leads to thrombosis, occlusion, and collapse of the vessel, often leaving behind a sleeve of the vascular basement membrane; see text for details.

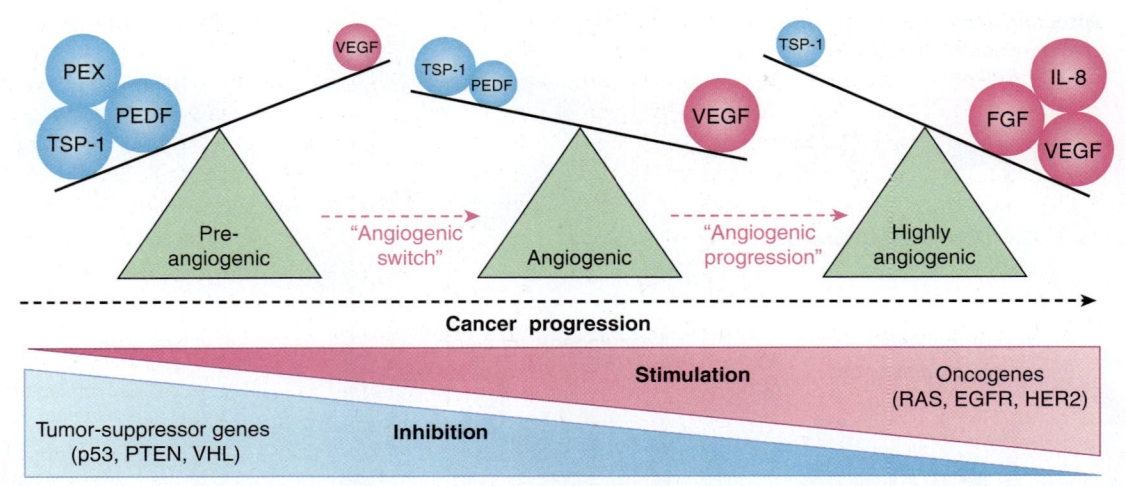

FIGURE 11–10 Angiogenic switch and progression during tumor development. The preangiogenic state in early tumor development is marked by the preponderance of angiogenesis inhibitors (eg, TSP-1, PEDF, PEX), which override the effects of angiogenic stimulators (VEGFs) expressed at low levels. Aggressive tumor growth is triggered by the change in balance between these factors, leading to the increase in the net stimulatory activity and the onset of angiogenesis ("angiogenic switch"). The underlying qualitative and quantitative changes in levels of angiogenesis stimulators and inhibitors are driven by the tumor microenvironment (hypoxia, inflammation) and by genetic progression of cancer cells (mutations in oncogenes and tumor suppressors). Continued escalation of these molecular changes with progressive disease may result in an exuberant proangiogenic microenvironment with increasingly active and redundant stimulatory networks (angiogenesis progression). However, excessive amounts of VEGF activity may be incompatible with robust angiogenesis. Abbreviations: *FGF*, fibroblast growth factor; *IL-8*, interleukin 8; *PEDF*, pigment epithelium derived factor; *PEX*, noncatalytic fragment of matrix metalloproteinase; *TSP-1*, thrombospondin 1; *VEGF*, vascular endothelial growth factor/VEGF-A; see text for details.

11.4.11 Extracellular Vesicles in Tumor Neovascularization

In addition to purely molecular signals (eg, soluble VEGF), endothelial cells and other elements of the tumor microenvironment may receive and secrete more complex (multimolecular) messages, which are encapsulated in heterogeneous membrane structures known as extracellular vesicles (EVs). Larger EVs (100-1000 nm), known as *microvesicles* (ectosomes or microparticles), form at the cellular plasma membrane, whereas smaller vesicles (30-150 nm), often referred to as *exosomes*, originate within the endosomal system of parental cells and are enriched for tetraspanins and cellular export proteins. Other distinct categories of EVs include apoptotic bodies, large oncosomes, exosome-like membrane vesicles, and several other subtypes generated through processes of cell budding, migration, or fragmentation. EVs carry diverse repertoires of bioactive and diagnostically important cargo, including lipids, metabolites, proteins, nucleic acids (RNA, DNA), or even organelles, such as mitochondria. EVs possess a unique ability to protect and selectively transfer their cargo between cellular populations, including cancer cells and the vascular compartment. Indeed, cancer-related EVs carry angiogenic growth factors (VEGF, FGF), inflammatory cytokines (IL-1), enzymes (eg, MMPs), enzyme inducers such as extracellular MMP inducer (EMMPRIN), and other mediators, including bioactive messenger RNA (mRNA), microRNA, and DNA. A unique property of cancer-derived EVs is their content of active oncoproteins and oncogenic nucleic acids that may enter and reprogram endothelial cells, stimulate their growth, trigger vascular permeability, and modulate angiogenesis (Rak, 2013). Moreover, EVs are known to influence (educate) myeloid and stromal cells and impact the coagulation system, thereby exerting multifaceted and often disease-specific effects on the tumor-vascular interfaces (Rak, 2013).

11.5 TUMOR ANGIOGENESIS

11.5.1 Constituent Processes of Tumor Neovascularization

Cancer cells are dependent on their proximity to vascular networks for their growth, survival, and metastatic dissemination (Folkman, 2007). These requirements are satisfied through tumor neovascularization, which may be regarded as a caricature of normal blood vessel development (Fig. 11–9) described in prior sections. Tumor angiogenesis, arterio-/venogenesis and vasculogenesis collectively lead to cancer-driven growth, remodeling and expansion of abnormal vascular structures with contributions of host endothelial, mural, and bone marrow–derived cell populations. Conversely, cancer cells may seek out, grow, and migrate around pre-existing blood vessels in a process called co-option, exhibit patterns of intravascular or perivascular invasion, or physically contribute to the vascular wall by adopting features of endothelial cells (vasculogenic mimicry). Moreover, cancer stem cells (eg, in glioma) may differentiate to become endothelial- or pericyte-like cells and occupy the respective compartments within the vascular network (see Chap. 13, Sec. 13.3.2). Tumor cells may also trigger changes in microvascular patterning, structure, and patency, through processes of intussusception, glomeruloid body formation, increased vascular permeability, occlusive thrombosis or vascular regression/pruning (Fig. 11–9).

Because of the frequent upregulation of VEGF in human cancers and the central role of this factor in developmental and reparative angiogenesis, the VEGF pathway is often viewed as dominant in tumor neovascularization. Historically, the indispensability of sprouting angiogenesis and VEGF signals for tumor growth and metastatic progression underwent considerable (excessive) generalization resulting in the majority of clinically used antiangiogenic drugs being directed against VEGF or VEGFRs (Table 11–2). Increasingly a broader view of tumor angiogenesis (neovascularization) inspires new biologic and therapeutic studies. For simplicity, in subsequent sections the term "angiogenesis" will be used more broadly to describe bona fide angiogenic and other less understood neovascularization processes in cancer.

11.5.2 Onset and Progression of Angiogenesis in Cancer

In cancer, processes of angiogenesis, vascular maturation, and patterning are disorganized, resulting in aberrant vessel structures, including excessive proliferation and incomplete and heterogeneous coverage with pericytes. These defects and their biologic mechanisms provide targets for blood vessel–directed therapies in cancer. For example, immature tumor blood vessels are vulnerable to VEGF-directed therapies, as endothelial cells devoid of pericyte contacts are more dependent on VEGF for their survival (Ferrara and Adamis, 2016). Limited effects of such therapy may coincide in certain settings with preponderance of more mature and better-perfused tumor blood vessels resistant to VEGF deprivation. Moreover, a shift to more functional vessels following therapeutic inhibition of angiogenesis was suggested as a means to improve tumor blood flow (normalization) and thereby the intratumoral delivery of anticancer agents (Jain, 2001). Alternatively, pericytes might serve as therapeutic targets in cancer, especially where they support a substantial proportion of tumor blood vessels (Carmeliet and Jain, 2011). Finally, angiogenic pathways such as VEGF possess a potent immunoregulatory component and their purposeful modulation may enhance the activity of immunotherapy agents (Rivera and Bergers, 2015). For blood vessel targeting to succeed as an anticancer strategy, it is imperative to understand the context, triggers, and modulators of tumor neovascularization.

11.5.3 Mechanisms Triggering Tumor Neovascularization

The onset of tumor neovascularization (including angiogenesis) is often viewed as an early event in disease progression, and one that permits the emerging tumor mass to expand beyond the size of 1 to 2 mm in diameter. The "preangiogenic" phase of tumor growth is defined by the limits of oxygen and macromolecule diffusion from the preexisting host vasculature (see Chap. 12, Sec. 12.2.3). Other factors that influence and limit preangiogenic tumor growth include the ability of cancer cells to tolerate hypoxia and metabolic deprivation (see Chap. 12, Sec. 12.4.2), as well as the degree to which such cells can use vascular co-option and other alternative, nonangiogenic mechanisms to gain access to vascular networks. Beyond the boundaries of perivascular diffusion, cancer cells either undergo growth arrest, or there may be a balance between cell migration, growth, and cell death, without a net increase in tumor mass. Intrinsic factors (transformation) combined with the exposure to a hypoxic and a nutrient-deprived environment may drive the onset of angiogenesis due to changes in the cellular phenotype (Folkman, 2007). The resulting "angiogenic switch" (see Fig. 11–10) is often attributed to the net increase in the activity of angiogenesis-stimulating influences over those of inhibitors (Folkman, 2007).

Cancer cells play a central role in these events, and their influence may be either direct (as producers of angiogenic factors) or indirect, for example, related to hypoxia in the tissue microenvironment, recruitment/activation of proangiogenic stromal cells, induction of inflammatory responses and/or "education" of host cells by cancer-related exosomes (Rak, 2009). Within the same lesion, cancer cells may differ in their proangiogenic activity, and this heterogeneity can also change over time. In some settings, such as brain tumors, such proangiogenic capacity may be more pronounced for tumor-initiating or cancer stem cells (Gilbertson and Rich, 2007). The major underlying trigger of a cancer cell–related angiogenic phenotype lies with the interplay between intracellular oncogenic pathways and responses to the extracellular tumor microenvironment, especially hypoxia and inflammation (see Chap. 12, Sec. 12.4.2).

11.5.4 Hypoxia as a Trigger of Tumor Angiogenesis

Hypoxia acts as a primary trigger of blood vessel formation during development, ischemia, and wound healing. Hypoxia is usually defined as drop in tissue oxygen below the normoxic level of 10 to 15 mm Hg (see Chap. 12, Sec. 12.4) and may originate from changes such as increased oxygen consumption, low capillary density, poor blood perfusion, and the presence of vascular occlusion. Hypoxic regions (and areas of necrosis) are common in advanced solid tumors, and their presence is usually associated with poor prognosis. Poor oxygenation evokes cellular responses involving the expression of genes that control intrinsic coping mechanisms, such as glycolytic metabolism, cellular quiescence, cell survival, and DNA repair, as well as those responsible for extracellular effects such as erythropoiesis and angiogenesis (Bristow and Hill, 2008).

The best described among the hypoxia response pathways is the activation of hypoxia-inducible transcription factors 1 and 2 (HIF1/2; see Chap. 12, Sec. 12.4.2). Several angiogenesis-related genes are targets of the HIF pathway, including VEGF, SDF1, ANG2, PlGF, PDGF-B, stem cell factor (SCF), and endothelial VEGFR1. Hypoxia also leads to downregulation of some angiogenesis inhibitors, notably thrombospondin 1 (TSP1). In addition, HIF-mediated transcription is involved in angiogenic responses of endothelial cells, and contributes to vascular permeability and structural aberrations

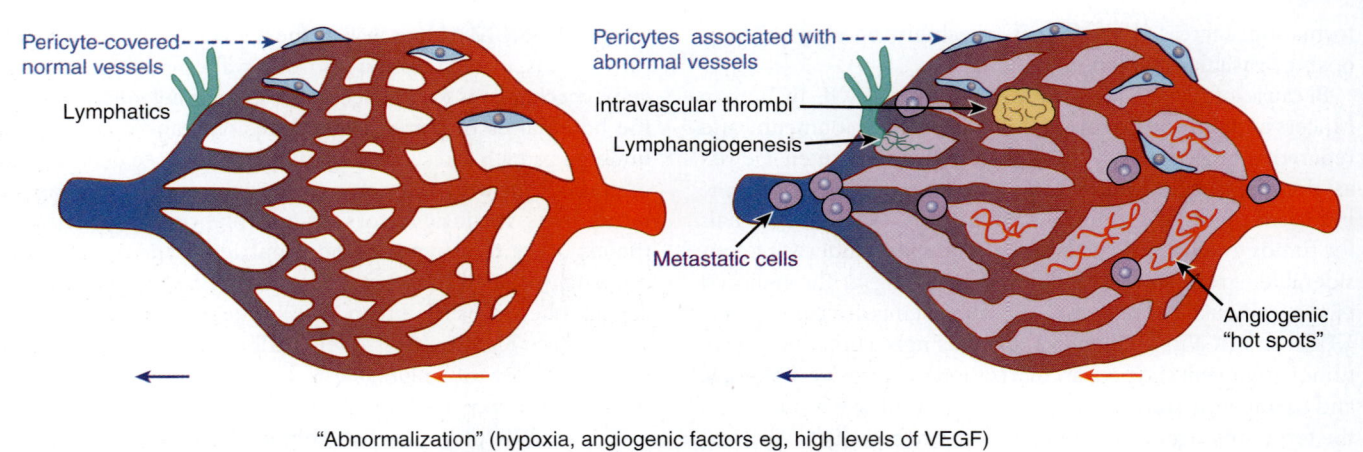

Normal microcirculation

(i) Structural characteristics

- Continuous endothelium
- Intact basement membrane
- Complete and close pericyte coverage
- Innervation
- Proper arborization and quasifractal branching
- Gradual changes in lumen diameter
- No shunts or corkscrew structures
- No blunt ends or tortuosities
- Organ-specific architecture

(ii) Functional characteristics

- Quiescent endothelial cells
- Intact junctional structures
- Patent and perfused vascular branches
- Proper tissue oxygenation and viability
- Nonleaky nonhemorrhagic capillaries
- Intact barrier function
- Properly organized fenestrations and transport
- Intact anticoagulant luminal surfaces
- Proper lymphatic drainage (normal interstitial pressure)

(iii) Molecular characteristics

- Expression of pan-endothelial markers
- Low VEGF/VEGFR pathway activity
- High ANG1/TIE2 pathway activity
- Absence of tumor endothelial markers (eg, TEM8)

Tumor (abnormal) microcirculation

(i) Structural characteristics

- Discontinuous endothelium
- Incomplete basement membrane
- Loose and incomplete pericyte coverage
- No innervation
- Abnormal and chaotic branching
- Paradoxical changes in lumen diameter
- Shunts and corkscrew structures
- Blunt ends and tortuosities
- Heterogenous vascular density ("hot spots")

(ii) Functional characteristics

- Proliferating, activated endothelial cells
- Abnormal/absent junctional structures
- Sluggish flow, poorly perfused vascular branches
- Tissue hypoxia and necrosis
- Leaky and hemorrhagic capillaries (blood lakes)
- Penetrable for metastatic cells
- Abnormal fenestrations and transport
- Intravascular thrombi
- Poor lymphatic drainage (high interstitial pressure)

(iii) Molecular characteristics

- Expression of pan-endothelial markers
- High VEGF/VEGFR pathway activity
- High ANG2/TIE2 pathway activity
- Expression of tumor endothelial markers (eg, TEM8)

FIGURE 11-11 Tumor-related changes in vascular characteristics. Disorganized regulatory network in the tumor microenvironment leads to formation of blood vessels that are structurally, functionally, and molecularly abnormal (vessel "abnormalization"). Some of these abnormalities provide targets for antiangiogenic therapy that can selectively obliterate tumor blood vessels. Blood vessel–directed agents may either destroy blood vessels or restore, at least partially, some of their normal characteristics (vessel normalization); see text for details.

("abnormalization"; Fig. 11–11) that enable the shedding of metastatic cancer cells into the bloodstream (Carmeliet and Jain, 2011). Finally, hypoxia provokes tumor cell invasiveness (Rey and Semenza, 2010) and HIF may help to maintain the cancer stem cell phenotype (Hill et al, 2009). Several other transcription factors may contribute to proangiogenic responses under hypoxia, including nuclear factor kappa B (NF-κB), NF-IL6, MTF-1, and EGR-1.

Hypoxia triggers both angiogenesis (locally) and arteriogenesis (remotely), but the nature of these 2 events is fundamentally different (Carmeliet and Jain, 2011). Hypoxia serves as a potent inducer of local VEGF production (along with other factors), which in normal tissues acts as a self-limiting growth stimulus for capillaries. The increase in blood vessel numbers and volume improves perfusion and leads to tissue reoxygenation, which normally (but not in cancer) causes cessation of the hypoxic stimulus. Arteriogenic enlargement of feeding vessels is required to supply blood to the increased volume of angiogenic capillaries. This process occurs upstream of the hypoxic (tumor) tissue and leads to remodeling of the feeding vessel walls through the effects of shear forces, nitric oxide (NO), and recruitment of regulatory monocytes (Dvorak, 2015b).

11.5.5 Tumor Vasculogenesis

Vasculogenesis involves incorporation of circulating endothelial precursor-like cells (frequently referred to as EPCs) into the capillary wall of the emerging vasculature. Although the nature and extent of this process is controversial, the presence of circulating cells with EPC-like characteristics in tumor-bearing animals and in cancer patients is well established. The ability of such cells to populate certain vascular structures varies from as little as 0.01% to 5% of tumor blood vessels in mice and humans with incorporated EPCs, to rarely higher rates of up to 50%, mostly in mice (Ahn and Brown, 2009). The incorporation of EPC-like cells into tumor blood vessels may, however, be stimulated by the microenvironmental stress (eg, hypoxia), or antiangiogenic, antivascular, and anticancer therapy because of the release of bone marrow–activating cytokines (Kerbel, 2008). It is presently thought that the role of EPC-like cells is mostly regulatory and their structural contribution to new blood vessels is minimal.

11.5.6 Proangiogenic Effects of Oncogenic Pathways

Cancer cells often feature strongly proangiogenic properties (eg, overproduction of VEGF), even without exposure to hypoxia (Rak, 2009). This intrinsic and constitutive proangiogenic phenotype is triggered by the expression of several dominant oncogenes, examples of which include *HRAS, KRAS, SRC, MYC, EGFR,* and *HER2*. In addition, the loss of function of tumor-suppressor genes, such as *TP53, PTEN, CDKN2A,* and *VHL*, is also associated with potent angiogenic effects, often acting in a cumulative manner (see Chap. 7, Secs. 7.5 and 7.6). These changes exert their pleiotropic influence on the cellular angiogenic transcriptome and proteome (angiome), via activation of kinase cascades, transcription factors, and microRNA networks (see Chap. 7, Sec. 7.4.3), the latter exemplified by the miR-17-92 cluster (Landskroner-Eiger et al, 2013).

The most studied proangiogenic effects of oncogenic mutations include upregulation of the key vascular stimulators such as VEGF, FGF, IL-6, IL-8, or angiopoietins coupled with downregulation of angiogenesis inhibitors, especially TSP-1, endostatin, tumstatin, and pigment epithelium-derived factor (PEDF; Rak, 2009). However, oncogene-regulated mediators of angiogenesis also include phospholipids, proteolytic enzymes, and extracellular vesicles (eg, exosomes) containing multiple angiogenic proteins, lipids, and nucleic acids (Rak, 2013).

Activated oncogenic pathways often mimic or exacerbate cellular responses to hypoxia. For example, the extremely high levels of VEGF, florid angiogenesis, and hypervascularity observed in clear cell renal carcinoma are largely attributed to the high frequency (>70%) of the loss-of-function mutations affecting the *VHL* gene. The resulting activation of HIF-dependent responses (see Chap. 12, Sec. 12.3.2 and 12.4.2) drives transcription of VEGF and other vascular changes, even in the absence of overt oxygen deprivation. Hypoxia-dependent upregulation of VEGF is also dramatically exacerbated by oncogenic RAS (Rak, 2009). Less is known about the impact of oncogenic driver mutations on nonangiogenic processes of tumor neovascularization (eg, vessel co-option), but this area is under investigation (Frentzas et al, 2016).

11.5.7 Inflammation

Inflammatory cells and their soluble mediators profoundly affect tumor neovascularization. The sources of inflammatory reactions in cancer can be either extrinsic (infection), intrinsic (oncogenic mutations), immunologic, or microenvironmental (De Palma et al, 2017). These processes trigger recruitment of multiple inflammatory cell types, especially M2-polarized (tumor-promoting) macrophages and other bone marrow–derived myeloid regulatory cells (BMDCs; see Fig. 11–3). A growing interest surrounds TIE2-expressing macrophages, mast cells, and granulocytes, many of which produce proteolytic enzymes, proangiogenic growth factors, cytokines, and chemokines (VEGF-A, Bv8, IL-8) at the tumor site. VEGF-A exerts promigratory effects on macrophages but inhibits antitumor immune responses, thereby tilting the regulatory balance toward tumor-promoting processes (Rivera and Bergers, 2015). Both tumor cells and stroma may contribute to these events through the activation of cellular "defense" mechanisms orchestrated by transcription factors (eg, NF-κB, HIF, and STAT [signal transducer and activators of transcription]; see also Chap. 6, Sec 6.2.6), in response to changes in the microenvironment (De Palma et al, 2017).

11.5.8 Angiogenic Activation of Tumor Stroma

The presence of diverse host cell types (stroma) within the tumor mass is central to the onset of angiogenesis. Stromal cells likely contribute to endothelial cell quiescence in normal tissues by producing architectural constraints and angiogenesis inhibitors. In cancer, stromal cells may undergo functional changes often described as "activation," or may sustain genetic mutations. Cancer-associated fibroblasts (CAFs) represent a prominent component of tumor stroma (see Chap. 12, Sec. 12.2.1), derived from phenotypic reprogramming of resident connective tissue cells, changes in endothelial cells (endothelial-to-mesenchymal transition), or analogous processes involving cancer cells (ie, epithelial-to-mesenchymal transition; Kalluri, 2016). CAFs produce VEGF-A, and may also elaborate other angiogenic factors. For example, secretion of PDGF-C by these cells was found to contribute to the resistance of tumors to therapies directed at VEGF-A (Kalluri, 2016). Proangiogenic properties are also attributed to adipocytes, which may contribute to the link between cancer and obesity. Hypoxia, paracrine interactions, activation of the coagulation system, inflammation, and oncogenic lesions may all contribute to the recruitment and stimulation of the angiogenic tumor stroma in a process that resembles a perpetual "wound healing" response (Dvorak, 2015b).

11.6 UNIQUE CHARACTERISTICS AND MODIFIERS OF TUMOR ANGIOGENESIS

Although tumors invariably express various elements of the proangiogenic phenotype, the dynamics of the related vascular responses is often context-dependent. Such host-dependent influences may be a function of individual characteristics of cancer patients, for example, their genetic background, age, comorbidities such as metabolic conditions (eg, obesity, diabetes), atherosclerosis, and thrombosis, postsurgical tissue responses, and variable constitutive levels of circulating growth factors and hormones among others. Several examples (below) illustrate how host-related factors may impact various aspects of tumor angiogenesis, including microvessel density, endothelial cell proliferation, vascular branching, and recruitment of BMDCs.

11.6.1 Impact of Genetic Background on Tumor Angiogenesis

A similar angiogenic stimulus may evoke angiogenic responses of differential nature and magnitude because of relatively subtle changes in the host genetic background. For example, different strains of mice exhibit inherently different angiogenic reactions in response to stimulation with the same recombinant angiogenic growth factor (Folkman, 2007). Tumor angiogenesis is constitutively altered in mice deficient for the ID1 transcriptional repressor, β_1 and β_3/β_5 integrins, and other factors (Carmeliet and Jain, 2011). In mice with subtle variation in *vegf-a* gene expression levels, alterations are observed in angiogenesis and tumor neovascularization, whereas *VEGF* gene polymorphisms in humans may impact responses to antiangiogenic therapy (see Sec. 11.7.1.3; Sung et al, 2010). An additional chromosome 21, associated with Down syndrome, impedes VEGF production and angiogenesis through the action of DSCR1 and DYRK1a genes (Reynolds et al, 2010). Moreover, otherwise phenotypically silent heterozygosity of host cells for certain tumor-suppressor genes, such as *NF1*, may influence regulation of angiogenesis, inflammation, and tumor progression (Yang et al, 2008).

11.6.2 Modulation of Tumor Angiogenesis by Vascular Ageing and Comorbidities

Cancers are more prevalent in adults and elderly than in children, and the age of cancer onset can influence tumor angiogenesis. This form of host influence is exemplified by differences in vascular phenotypes of malignancies affecting children, adolescents, and young adults (although multiple factors may be involved) and by the age-related differences in common cancers. For example, the age at diagnosis of kidney cancer may vary by up to 5 decades. During this time, the vascular system undergoes profound changes, including alterations in the state of endothelial, bone marrow, inflammatory, and other cellular compartments. Aging impacts responses to hypoxia, impedes production of angiogenic growth factors and efficiency of vascular repair, increases procoagulant tendencies, and leads to cardiovascular decline (Lahteenvuo and Rosenzweig, 2012). For example, age-related alterations in the vasculature may increase tumor responses to antiangiogenic effects of VEGF inhibitors in mice (Meehan et al, 2014). It is noteworthy that aging processes at the cellular level may lead to the phenomenon known as senescence-associated secretory phenotype (SASP), which includes upregulation of several cytokines, angiogenic factors, proteolytic enzymes and release of exosomes, collectively resulting in perturbations of vascular physiology. SASP occurring at the level of tumor microenvironment, endothelium, progenitor cell populations, parenchyma, or stroma is likely to impact angiogenesis, but its exact role is still poorly understood (Oubaha 2016). While extensive studies are lacking it is likely that in the clinic the effects and side effects of antiangiogenic therapies could also be further compounded by complex age-related comorbidities affecting the macro- and microvasculature, for example, in atherosclerosis (Rak, 2009).

11.6.3 Properties of the Tumor Microcirculation

Tumor blood vessels exhibit high levels of architectural, cellular, and molecular heterogeneity, in comparison to normal tissues and between tumor types and tumor microregions (Carmeliet and Jain, 2011). These anomalies include loss of proper arborization (hierarchy), unusual patterns of branching (eg, trifurcation), paradoxical lumen dilatations, formation of corkscrew and blind-ended structures, and abnormal vascular connections (shunts). Tumor blood vessels may contain capillaries with either incomplete or hypertrophic endothelial cell lining (eg, in brain tumors), which may fold into intraluminal projections and septa, and interact poorly with the surrounding pericytes (see Fig. 11–11). Perivascular microhemorrhages and spaces filled with blood (blood lakes) are common in certain tumors along with vascular occlusion and regression. Regional abnormalities of the vessel wall often result in the leakage of plasma, macromolecules, and clotting factors into the extravascular space (see Fig. 11–9). Tumor angiogenesis exhibits organ-specific differences because of site-specific features of the vascular system. For example, in glioblastoma, the microvasculature exhibits hyperproliferative and hypertrophic characteristics, frequent and diagnostically relevant microthrombosis, glomeruloid blood vessels, areas of vascular collapse, elevated permeability, edema, and compromised blood-brain barrier (Gilbertson and Rich, 2007). Extravascular and intravascular activation of the coagulation system and deposition of crosslinked fibrin, as well as formation of occlusive thrombi and systemic risk of thrombosis are observed frequently in cancer patients (Dvorak, 2015b). A combined effect of vascular changes results in sluggish, intermittent, often bidirectional and inefficient blood flow, poor tissue perfusion, hypoxia, hemorrhage, and necrosis (Folkman, 2007).

Structural abnormalities of tumor blood vessels are associated with a shift in the endothelial cell phenotype. Thus, tumor-associated endothelial cells may proliferate, have altered metabolism, and exhibit changes in shape, as well as unusual and heterogeneous expression of molecular markers (Carmeliet and Jain, 2011). For example, tumor endothelial cells may express phosphatidylserine on their surface and overexpress proangiogenic receptors (eg, VEGFR2 or TIE2) and molecules normally absent in the vasculature; these are often referred to as tumor endothelial markers (TEMs; Seaman et al, 2007).

Tumor endothelial cells may also exhibit regional differences in phenotype or genetic abnormalities, such as aneuploidy (Hida et al, 2004), marker chromosomes, or expression of mutant oncogenes. This suggests that some tumor cells may directly contribute to endothelial or pericyte layers of the microvasculature (Krishna Priya et al, 2016) or that they may have a destabilizing effect on endothelial genome. Some of the unique features of tumor-associated endothelial cells enable their therapeutic targeting (Seaman et al, 2007).

11.6.4 Tumor Lymphangiogenesis

Solid tumors often exhibit high interstitial fluid pressure indicative of poor lymphatic drainage (see also Chap. 12, Sec. 12.2.3). Although functional lymphatics may be compromised in cancer, the disease progression is commonly associated with lymphangiogenesis, expression of lymphangiogenic growth factors (VEGF-C/D) and their receptors (VEGFR3). The expression of VEGF-C/D in cancer cells increases their capacity to disseminate to regional lymph nodes where lymphangiogenesis and pre-metastatic niche formation may facilitate tumor cell colonization. Agents that block lymphangiogenesis are being developed to exert anticancer and antimetastatic activity (Tammela and Alitalo, 2010).

11.6.5 Tumor-Initiating Cells and Blood Vessels

The ability to initiate clonal neoplastic growth, disease recurrence, and metastasis is often attributed to a subset of cancer (stem) cells or tumor-initiating cells (see Chap. 13, Sec 13.3.2). Because the expression of stem cell properties, regulators, and markers (eg, Oct4) can be induced by hypoxia, some stem cells may reside in tumor regions distant from the vasculature (Hill et al, 2009). In contrast, normal neuroectodermal stem cells and their malignant counterparts appear to be located in areas adjacent to blood vessels, and in regions referred to as *perivascular niches* (Gilbertson and Rich, 2007). In glioblastoma, tumor-initiating cells expressing CD133 were found to exhibit elevated production of VEGF and increased proangiogenic activity, largely due to the constitutive activation of the hypoxia response pathway mediated by HIF2. Tumor-initiating cells may also exhibit altered coagulant properties, and their abundance may be altered following antiangiogenic therapy. Although the links between angiogenesis and cancer stem cells are rather complex, their tumor-initiating activity implicitly involves the vasculature (eg, during metastasis). Cancer stem cells have also been proposed to differentiate to endothelial cells or pericytes, but these processes remain controversial (Krishna Priya et al, 2016). Stemness may represent a part of the phenotypic spectrum of cancer cells and be influenced by the vasculature (Lu et al, 2013).

11.7 BLOOD VESSEL–DIRECTED ANTICANCER THERAPIES

The concept of targeting blood vessels to achieve anticancer effects was developed initially by Folkman (Folkman, 1971). After nearly 5 decades of experimental and clinical exploration, this treatment modality is now a part of clinical management for several human cancers (see Table 11–2), with numerous agents approved by the Food and Drug Administration (FDA) in the United States and in other constituencies. Targeting tumor blood vessels in cancer is based on functional and molecular differences that separate properties of the tumor microcirculation from the corresponding normal vasculature. Agents and techniques that target tumor blood vessels may act on endothelial cells, or on mural cells directly (direct inhibitors). Alternatively, therapeutic agents may interfere with events and cells stimulating or supporting the tumor vasculature (indirect inhibitors; Fig. 11–12; Jayson et al, 2016). Although the biology of all cancers is intimately and universally linked with the vascular system, their growth and progression may not be equally (or at all) dependent on a particular mediator or vascular process, such as angiogenesis; hence the activities of various agents vary between different disease contexts.

11.7.1 Antiangiogenic Therapies

Antiangiogenic agents are designed to block the formation of new tumor blood vessels through approaches ranging from targeting the specific signaling circuitry of endothelial cells (eg, by blocking VEGF or VEGFR2), to exploiting naturally occurring angiogenesis inhibitory pathways (see Table 11–2). Whether a particular agent possesses antiangiogenic activity can be determined using several functional assays conducted either on cultured endothelial cells or in animals (Folkman, 2007). Those tests usually analyze survival, proliferation, migration, and formation of tube-like structures by cultured endothelial cells, ingrowth of capillaries into the chick chorioallantoic membrane (CAM), sprouting at avascular anatomical sites in animals (eg, corneal micropocket assays), or in pellets of ECM (Matrigel™) implanted subcutaneously into mice. In animal models and in the clinic, antiangiogenic activity may also be deduced from tumor responses as measured by functional imaging (see Chap. 14, Sec. 14.5.3), which allows the assessment of tissue metabolism, oxygenation, vascular permeability, or blood flow (Jain et al, 2009). Despite a lack of clinically validated markers of antiangiogenic activity, numerous antiangiogenic agents have been evaluated, and they can be broadly assigned into several main (historical) categories as summarized in Table 11–2 and Figure 11–12.

TABLE 11–2 Examples of blood vessel–targeting agents developed to treat cancer.

Drug	Type	Target	Stage of Development
Antiangiogenic agents (AAs)			
1. Molecularly targeted agents designed to obliterate key angiogenic pathways			
Bevacizumab	Neutralizing huMoAb	VEGF	Approved for human use
Ramucirumab	Neutralizing huMoAB	VEGFR2	Approved for human use
Sunitinib, sorafenib, pazopanib, vandetanib, axitinib, regorafenib, nintedanib, lenvatinib, cabozantinib	TKI	VEGFR1-3 > other (proangiogenic) RTKs	Approved for human use
Aflibercept (VEGF-trap)	Soluble decoy "receptor-body"	VEGF-A, VEGF-B, PlGF	Approved for human use
Cilengitide	Cyclic pentapeptide	$\alpha v\beta 3/\beta 5$ integrin	In ongoing clinical development
2. Indirectly acting agents with antiangiogenic activity designed to block oncogenic pathways			
Trastuzumab	Neutralizing huMoAb	HER-2	Approved for human use
Cetuximab	Neutralizing huMoAb	EGFR	Approved for human use
Gefitinib, erlotinib	TKI	EGFR	Approved for human use
Lapatinib	TKI	EGFR, HER-2	Approved for human use
Imatinib	TKI	ABL, PDGFRβ, KIT	Approved for human use
3. Agents with antiangiogenic activity originally developed for non-antiangiogenic indications			
Chemotherapy (metronomic)	Various agents	Pleiotropic antiangiogenic and immunomodulatory effects	Under clinical exploration
Thalidomide and analogues (Lenalidomide)	Small molecule	Inflammatory pathways	Approved in multiple myeloma
4. Antivascular agents / vascular disrupting agents (VDAs)			
Vadimezan (ASA 404)	Flavonoid	EC survival	Clinical development halted after failed phase III trials
Combretastatin A 4-phosphate (CA4P, fosbretabulin), plinabulin	Tubulin binding	Tubulin assembly	Clinical development halted (fosbretabulin) or ongoing (plinabulin)

Abbreviations: *ABL*, Abelson murine leukemia viral oncogene homolog 1 kinase; *EGFR*, epidermal growth factor receptor; *HER-2*, epidermal growth factor receptor 2; *huMoAb*, humanized monoclonal antibody; *KIT*, mast/stem cell growth factor receptor; *PDGFRβ*, platelet-derived growth factor receptor β; *PlGF*, placenta growth factor; *RTK*, receptor tyrosine kinase; *TKI*, tyrosine kinase inhibitor; *VEGFR*, vascular endothelial growth factor receptor.
See text for more details (Ferrara and Adamis, 2016; Folkman, 1971, 2007; McKeage and Baguley, 2010).

11.7.1.1 First-Generation, Exogenous Antiangiogenic Agents

In early studies, several natural compounds or their derivatives were found empirically to possess activities inhibiting endothelial cells. Examples include the fungal product fumagillin (and its derivative TNP470), penicillamine (a copper chelator), carboxyaminotriazole, suramin, and 2-methoxyestradiol (2ME2) (Folkman, 2007). The mechanisms of action of many of these agents remain unclear, and there are no approved clinical indications for their use as anticancer agents. In contrast, the pleiotropic antiangiogenic and immunomodulating effects of thalidomide, and those of related agents such as lenalidomide, are the basis of their use in the treatment of multiple myeloma (Cook and Figg, 2010). Thalidomide's antiangiogenic activity is at least partially linked to the teratogenic effects of this drug and its grim earlier legacy.

11.7.1.2 Agents Based on the Activity of Endogenous Angiogenesis Inhibitors

The ability of tissues to elaborate endogenous angiogenesis inhibitors inspired drug development aimed at therapeutic antiangiogenesis (Folkman, 2007). Several agents have been evaluated, including antiangiogenic cytokines such as interferon-α (IFNα), antiangiogenic fragments of ECM proteins (endostatin), fragments of plasminogen (angiostatin, K5), and peptides related to TSP1 (ABT-510). Typically, the mechanisms of antiangiogenic activity of these agents are either complex, or have not been fully elucidated. Although the clinical efficacy of most endogenous angiogenesis inhibitors in cancer has been modest at best, IFNα was used for the treatment of renal cell cancer, but recently has been largely replaced by VEGFR-targeted tyrosine kinase inhibitors (TKIs) and other agents.

11.7.1.3 Molecularly Targeted Antiangiogenic Agents

Our improved understanding of molecular pathways involved in angiogenesis led to the development of several targeted antiangiogenic agents. These can be broadly divided into 3 categories: (1) neutralizing (monoclonal) antibodies against angiogenic ligands, or their receptors (eg, bevacizumab, ramucirumab); (2) decoy molecules designed to neutralize angiogenic factors by virtue of binding them to high-affinity

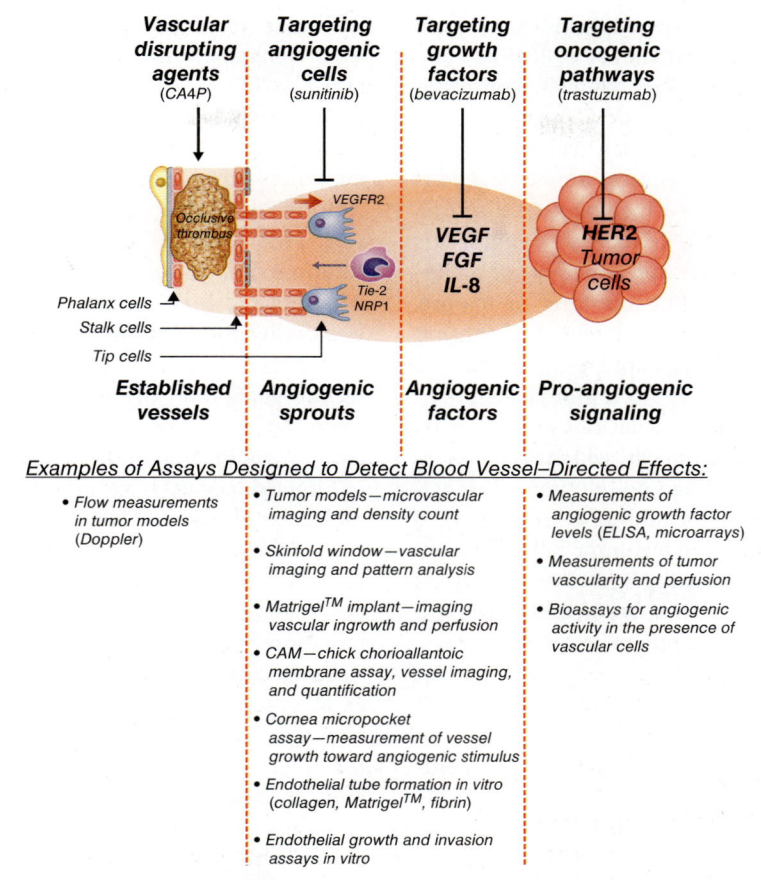

FIGURE 11–12 Some of the main strategies to target tumor vasculature. Development of the tumor microcirculation can be therapeutically opposed in several ways, including by blocking mechanisms of the "angiogenic switch" through the use of antagonists of oncogenic and signaling pathways, such as for example trastuzumab, a neutralizing antibody that binds to HER-2 oncoprotein. Targeting other driver mutations or hypoxic mediators (HIF) may have similar effects. Angiogenic factors, such as vascular endothelial growth factors (VEGFs), can also be obliterated using neutralizing antibodies (eg, bevacizumab). Cells involved in angiogenic responses, namely, endothelial cells, pericytes, and myeloid cells, can be prevented from responding to angiogenic growth factors by agents blocking their receptors (eg, sunitinib or pazopanib). These cells can also be targeted using direct angiogenesis inhibitors such as thrombospondins, tumstatin, integrin inhibitors, metronomic chemotherapy, and other agents. While these strategies generally prevent formation of new blood vessels, vascular disrupting agents (VDAs) obliterate the already established tumor vasculature by causing endothelial damage and thrombosis. Several assays have been developed to detect and measure the responses of the microcirculation to these respective insults (bottom panel); see text for details.

soluble ectodomains of the corresponding cellular receptors inserted into the inhibitor (eg, VEGF-trap/aflibercept); and (3) small-molecule TKIs of angiogenic signaling receptors such as VEGFR2 (eg, sunitinib).

Targeted antiangiogenic therapeutics in clinical use are directed primarily against the VEGF signaling pathway. In 2004, a humanized monoclonal antibody directed against VEGF-A (bevacizumab) became the first targeted antiangiogenic agent to be approved for the treatment of cancer, that is, metastatic colorectal carcinoma (Ferrara and Adamis, 2016). Subsequently, several VEGFR-targeted TKIs have entered medical practice in oncology (Table 11–2). Most of these agents are multikinase inhibitors where VEGFR is believed to be the main target (Jayson et al, 2016).

Patterns are emerging regarding the clinical use of VEGF pathway inhibitors. First, renal cell, ovarian, cervical, hepatocellular, thyroid, and neuroendocrine carcinomas are among relatively sensitive tumor types; colorectal, gastroesophageal, pulmonary, and breast malignancies are considered moderately or less sensitive; and prostate, as well as exocrine pancreatic tumors are deemed resistant (Jayson et al, 2016). Second, notwithstanding life prolongation achieved with VEGFR targeted TKI monotherapy (eg, in the management of renal cell cancer), VEGF pathway inhibitors used alone typically do not result in clinically meaningful survival benefit for most tumor types. Thus, the development of antiangiogenic agents has mostly focused on combinations, generally with chemotherapy, for common solid tumors. There are also studies to determine the role of antiangiogenesis in conjunction with radiation therapy, and a rapidly growing interest in the concurrent use of antiangiogenic agents with immunotherapeutics such as checkpoint inhibitors (Senan and Smit, 2007; Ramjiawan et al, 2017). The latter is driven both by a strong preclinical rationale for synergistic effects of such an approach, and by encouraging clinical results. Third, the successful use of VEGF pathway inhibitors has been limited to the treatment of advanced (ie, metastatic) disease. Adjuvant trials for renal cell, colorectal, breast, esophageal and ovarian cancers, as well as for melanoma have not shown a significant overall survival benefit (Jayson et al, 2016; Massari et al, 2017).

Preclinical observations that await clinical confirmation may account for the generally modest clinical benefit attributable to antiangiogenic therapeutics. Foremost, similar to other cancer treatment modalities, antiangiogenesis is not devoid of inherent or acquired therapeutic resistance. Such resistance may be due to (1) redundancy of angiogenic growth factors or HIF1α-mediated overexpression of angiogenic factors; (2) vascular remodeling resulting in mature, treatment-resistant blood vessels, or preferential expansion of VEGF-independent blood vessel subtypes; (3) reduced vascular dependence of hypoxia-resistant tumor cell subpopulations; (4) the acquisition of endothelial cell properties by otherwise VEGF-independent tumor cells, which is suggested to render them capable of integrating into the tumor vasculature in a process termed vasculogenic mimicry (see Sec. 11.3.6 for more details); (5) vessel co-option by tumor cells proficient in exploiting the presence of pre-existing host vessels in organs with abundant vasculature such as liver, brain, and lungs; and finally (6) a range of proangiogenic effects of bone marrow–derived, tumor-infiltrating leukocytes as well as of resident stromal cells (Bergers and Hanahan, 2008; Bottsford-Miller et al, 2012; Dvorak, 2015a; Frentzas et al, 2016).

Aside from mediating therapeutic resistance, treatment-induced vascular remodeling may also have undesirable consequences. Downregulation or blockade of VEGF exposes endothelial cells to the residual excess of ANG2. In the absence of VEGF-dependent survival/stimulating signals, ANG2 blocks the remaining TIE2 survival pathway and leads to endothelial cell apoptosis, resulting in vessel thrombosis, collapse, and regression (see Fig. 11–9). However, it is suggested that regression of capillaries does not obliterate the tissue "memory" of the prior capillary network. Instead, on the disappearance of endothelial cells, the tissue still contains the networks of their related basement membranes (capillary "sleeves"), which may serve as a scaffold for rapid endothelial regrowth on restoration of VEGF supply, once the antiangiogenic therapy has been discontinued (Carmeliet and Jain, 2011).

Because of frequent resistance to VEGF pathway inhibitors, there is continuing interest to develop agents targeting other antiangiogenic pathways, including ANG/TIE2 signaling (Saharinen et al, 2017). Trebananib/AMG386 (a TIE2-binding peptide fused to an Fc domain, ie, a peptibody) was the first-in-class anti-ANG-TIE2 drug tested in a phase III trial. Trebananib impairs the binding of both ANG1 and ANG2 to the TIE2 receptor, resulting in lower extremity edema (typically mild) as a class side effect. Although trebananib combined with weekly paclitaxel improved the progression-free survival in women with recurrent ovarian cancer, there was no overall survival benefit (Monk et al, 2016). The multitargeted TKI regorafenib is approved for the management of pretreated colorectal, gastrointestinal (stromal cell), and hepatocellular malignancies (Bruix et al, 2017; Saharinen et al, 2017). Although regorafenib blocks TIE2 among other proangiogenic receptor TKIs, including VEGFRs, further studies are needed to clarify the importance of TIE2 versus VEGFR inhibition for regorafenib's anticancer effects. Novel ANG/TIE2 signaling inhibitors in early clinical development either target ANG2 only, or block simultaneously ANG2 and VEGF in the case of bispecific antibodies (Saharinen et al, 2017).

Aside from VEGF/VEGFR and ANG/TIE2 inhibition, numerous other angiogenic pathways are under investigation for possible development of anticancer therapies. As examples, TKIs approved for renal cell carcinoma therapy such as sunitinib and cabozantinib target not only VEGFRs but also PDGFRs and MET kinase, and the FGFR inhibitor dovitinib was studied for third-line renal cell carcinoma therapy (Motzer et al, 2014; Choueiri et al, 2016). Ultimately, pathway-specific second-generation drugs will be essential to determine the importance of the aforementioned alternative angiogenic pathways compared to the VEGF circuitry.

Targeted agents have also been developed against other molecular effectors of angiogenesis, with more complex roles, such as the $\alpha_v\beta_3/\alpha_v\beta_5$ integrin inhibitor cilengitide. Yet cilengitide failed to improve the outcome of patients with newly diagnosed glioblastoma when combined with temozolomide and radiation therapy (Stupp et al, 2014). Other targets at various stages of clinical investigation include the endothelial-binding ECM protein EGFRL7, EPHRINB2/EPH4, and DLL4/NOTCH. The efficacy of these targeted agents as stand-alone therapies, or in combination with other therapies, remains an ongoing area of investigation.

There is a considerable interest in combinations of antiangiogenic therapies, notably VEGF/VEGFR targeted agents, with cancer immunotherapy (Khan and Kerbel, 2018). As an example, the VEGFR targeted TKI axitinib improves the overall survival of patients with previously untreated advanced renal cell carcinoma when combined with the checkpoint inhibitor pembrolizumab, compared to sunitinib monotherapy (Rini et al, 2019). A similar treatment strategy was also successful in treatment-naive, unresectable hepatocellular carcinoma by improving survival compared to sorafenib alone (Finn RS et al, 2020). These clinically active combinations further illustrate an actionable biological link between vascular and immune factors in pathogenesis of specific cancers, with a prospect of further therapeutic gains.

11.7.2 Vascular Disrupting Agents

Although antiangiogenic therapy mainly blocks new vascular growth, the preformed tumor blood vessels remain and are targets of another class of drugs, referred to as vascular disrupting agents (VDAs) (McKeage and Baguley, 2010). The goal of this therapy is to provoke a selective vascular shutdown, or "infarction," within the tumor vasculature, mainly by compromising the viability, continuity, and antithrombotic properties of the endothelial lining. Unlike antiangiogenesis, the effects of VDAs are rapid (begin within less than an hour), and result in acute intravascular thrombosis, vascular shutdown, ischemia, and tumor necrosis. Although these effects are dramatic in the center of the tumor mass, they dissipate in the periphery, leaving a viable rim of cancer cells supplied by the intact vasculature in the surrounding tissue.

The residual disease and local vascular regrowth involving mobilization of cells from the bone marrow may lead to rapid tumor relapse post-VDA treatment; this adverse effect could be mitigated by combining VDAs with other agents, including angiogenesis inhibitors, a strategy under clinical development (Siemann et al, 2017).

Two distinct classes of VDAs have entered clinical studies (see Table 11–2): (1) synthetic flavonoids such as ASA404/vadimezan, which act mainly by releasing vasoactive cytokines, and (2) tubulin-binding agents such as combretastatin A4 phosphate/fosbretabulin and plinabulin (Siemann et al, 2017). Although phase III trials with tubulin-binding agents are ongoing, ASA404 coadministered with first- or second-line platinum-based chemotherapy did not improve the survival of patients with non–small cell lung cancer in phase III trials (Lara et al, 2011; Lorusso et al, 2011). While the development of ASA 404 and fosbretabulin has been halted, plinabulin is undergoing further clinical study.

11.7.3 Antiangiogenic Effects of Agents Targeting Oncogenic Pathways

The oncogene-driven angiogenic switch in cancer cells represents another attractive therapeutic target (Rak, 2009; Fig. 11–10). Studies have demonstrated antiangiogenic effects of several oncogene-directed agents, including trastuzumab (HER2) and EGFR inhibitors such as cetuximab, gefitinib, and erlotinib, which may exert their effects by blocking signaling pathways in both cancer cells and endothelium (Samant and Shevde, 2011). In addition, multitargeted TKIs may be specifically designed to exhibit a combined inhibitory effect against endothelial VEGFRs and parenchymal EGFR (vandetanib). Indeed, combinatorial action of multikinase inhibitors (eg, sunitinib or sorafenib) may explain some aspects of their clinical activity (Cook and Figg, 2010). Other molecular targets that are being studied in this context include mammalian target of rapamycin (inhibited by temsirolimus and everolimus), proteasome complexes (inhibited by bortezomib), coagulation factors (heparin), and steroid receptors. Mechanisms of resistance to agents targeting oncogenic drivers may contribute to their transient anticancer and antiangiogenic activity observed in multiple cancers.

11.7.4 Antiangiogenic Effects of Other Therapeutics

The increased mitogenic activity of tumor-associated endothelial cells may make them susceptible to traditional cytotoxic anticancer agents and radiation, but these effects rapidly dissipate after treatment because of vascular regrowth and mobilization of bone marrow–derived cells (Kerbel, 2008). This regrowth occurs during "drug holidays" taken to allow for hematopoietic recovery. However, when chemotherapy drugs are given continuously at lower doses, drug holidays are no longer needed, and antiangiogenic, immunomodulating, and other stromal effects may be amplified, even in the presence of tumor cell resistance to the toxicity of the same agent. This approach is known as metronomic chemotherapy (Kerbel, 2008). In reported phase III trials comparing metronomic versus conventional chemotherapy strategies, the outcome is often similar, especially when metronomic chemotherapy is used as maintenance or adjuvant therapy (Lien et al 2013). The response rates to metronomic chemotherapy are generally moderate, and acquired resistance typically ensues within months (Riesco-Martinez et al, 2017).

11.7.5 Challenges and Opportunities Associated With Targeting Tumor Blood Vessels

11.7.5.1 Tumor-Specificity of Antiangiogenic Agents
The distinct nature of tumor blood vessels, the quiescence of normal endothelial cells, and the presumed absence of genetic instability of endothelial cells suggested that, unlike conventional anticancer agents, therapies directed against blood vessels should be selective, nontoxic, universally applicable, and devoid of the risk of drug resistance (Folkman, 2007). However, clinical experience has not validated these predictions. For example, inhibitors of the VEGF pathway have shown efficacy in a narrow spectrum of malignancies in which a period of therapeutic response is often followed by progression because of drug resistance (Jayson et al, 2016).

11.7.5.2 Side Effects of Blood Vessel–Directed Agents
Antiangiogenic agents may block physiological functions of angiogenic factors, or cause off-target effects that lead to toxicity (Jayson et al, 2016). Common side effects related to VEGF pathway inhibitors include arterial hypertension, proteinuria, risk of bleeding or thrombosis, impairment of wound healing, fistula formation, and intestinal perforation, due to their impact on vascular homeostasis, vascular tone, kidney or other organ functions. Most VEGFR TKIs also inhibit off-target kinases, which may result in additional side effects such as fatigue, hypothyroidism, hand-foot syndrome, diarrhea, hair changes, and other poorly understood dose-limiting toxicities (Verheul et al 2007).

11.7.5.3 Biomarkers of Therapeutic Response to Antiangiogenic Agents
The protracted nature of therapy with antiangiogenic agents and their biological complexity make the effective monitoring of their specific antivascular activities challenging. Efforts have been made to study tumor-based markers (eg, microvessel density), imaging parameters (eg, tumor perfusion assessment by dynamic contrast-enhanced MRI), single or multiple angiogenic growth factors measured in blood or urine (eg, VEGF), levels of circulating blood cells (eg, EPCs), and polymorphisms of genes involved in angiogenesis (eg, VEGFR) (Jain et al, 2009; Cidon et al, 2016). However, none of these biomarkers has been clinically validated.

11.7.5.4 Alternative Blood Vessel–Directed Therapies in Cancer
Although overwhelming evidence supports the

dependence of tumor formation and progression on blood vessels, targetable vascular mechanisms are not restricted to VEGF-dependent angiogenesis. Apart from broadening the molecular spectrum of targetable angiogenesis regulators, alternatives to the paradigm of antiangiogenesis have also emerged. Several strategies are under consideration: (1) therapeutic deregulation of vascular patterning to achieve superfluous and nonproductive angiogenesis, for example, by interference with the DLL4-NOTCH pathway (Takebe et al, 2014); (2) targeting nonangiogenic forms of tumor neovascularization, such as vascular co-option (Frentzas et al, 2016); (3) vascular normalization aiming at producing a mitigated antiangiogenic effect with the preservation of more mature tumor blood vessels and their role in prevention of acute hypoxia and maintenance of drug delivery (Cantelmo et al, 2017); and (4) angiogenesis enhancement therapy, in which a controlled increase in blood vessel growth and dilatation in the tumor is intended to maximize the effects of concomitant chemotherapy (Wong et al, 2015). The integrative role of the vascular system in both physiology and cancer continues to inspire new questions, studies, and therapeutic efforts.

SUMMARY

Neovascularization is among the most critical host tissue responses to an emerging malignancy. It creates a tumor-vascular interface, which signifies the transition from a local cellular defect to the systemic disease that most cancers eventually become. Because of these considerations, angiogenesis has become a validated therapeutic target in cancer.

The key features of tumor angiogenesis covered in this chapter are:

- Tumor growth and metastasis are dependent on the interaction (interface) between cancer cells and the vascular system.
- Several angiogenic and nonangiogenic processes contribute to tumor neovascularization
- Endothelial cells (ECs) are the central drivers of blood vessel formation.
- In growing vessels, ECs form specialized structures (sprouts), and in so doing differentiate into distinct subsets of tip, stalk, and phalanx cells.
- Endothelial homeostasis is regulated by their surrounding mural cells, as well as systemically acting bone marrow–derived cells (BMDCs) and their products (growth factors, enzymes, and extracellular matrix [ECM]).
- Vascular growth is triggered by the excess of angiogenesis-stimulating factors relative to inhibitors.
- Vascular endothelial growth factor (VEGF) and its receptors are key molecular regulators of vascular development, homeostasis, and growth, but in cancer, this pathway may become dispensable.
- Tumor blood vessels exhibit several structural, cellular, and molecular anomalies, which can be exploited as therapeutic targets.
- Numerous agents targeting tumor blood vessels have entered preclinical and clinical development, of which several have been approved to treat cancer.
- Agents targeting blood vessels are broadly divided into drugs blocking blood vessel growth (antiangiogenics) and drugs able to selectively destroy established tumor vessels (VDAs).
- Although effective in some settings (eg, renal cell cancer with very high angiogenic activity), inherent or acquired resistance to antiangiogenic agents is relatively common.

REFERENCES

Ahn GO, Brown JM. Role of endothelial progenitors and other bone marrow-derived cells in the development of the tumor vasculature. *Angiogenesis* 2009;12(2):159-164.

Andrae J, Gallini R, Betsholtz C. Role of platelet-derived growth factors in physiology and medicine. *Genes Dev* 2008; 22(10):1276-1312.

Augustin HG, Koh GY, Thurston G, Alitalo K. Control of vascular morphogenesis and homeostasis through the angiopoietin-TIE system. *Nat Rev Mol Cell Biol* 2009;10(3): 165-177.

Avraamides CJ, Garmy-Susini B, Varner JA. Integrins in angiogenesis and lymphangiogenesis. *Nat Rev Cancer* 2008; 8(8):604-617.

Bergers G, Hanahan D. Modes of resistance to anti-angiogenic therapy. *Nat Rev Cancer* 2008;8(8):592-603.

Bottsford-Miller JN, Coleman RL, Sood AK. Resistance and escape from antiangiogenesis therapy: clinical implications and future strategies. *J Clin Oncol* 2012;30:4026-4034.

Bristow RG, Hill RP. Hypoxia and metabolism. Hypoxia, DNA repair and genetic instability. *Nat Rev Cancer* 2008; 8(3):180-192.

Bruix J, Qin S, Merle P, et al. Regorafenib for patients with hepatocellular carcinoma who progressed on sorafenib treatment (RESORCE): a randomised, double-blind, placebo-controlled, phase 3 trial. *Lancet* 2017;389(10064):56-66.

Cantelmo AR, Pircher A, Kalucka J, Carmeliet P. Vessel pruning or healing: endothelial metabolism as a novel target? *Expert Opin Ther Target* 2017;21(3):239-247.

Carmeliet P, Jain RK Molecular mechanisms and clinical applications of angiogenesis. *Nature* 2011;473(7347):298-307.

Chang J, Mancuso MR, Maier C, et al. Gpr124 is essential for blood-brain barrier integrity in central nervous system disease. *Nat Med* 2017;23(4):450-460.

Chen HX, Cleck JN. Adverse effects of anticancer agents that target the VEGF pathway. *Nat Rev Clin Oncol* 2009;6(8):465-477.

Choueiri TK, Escudier B, Powles T, et al. Cabozantinib versus everolimus in advanced renal cell carcinoma (METEOR): final results from a randomised, open-label, phase 3 trial. *Lancet Oncol* 2016;17(7):917-927.

Cidon EU, Alonso P, Masters B. Markers of response to antiangiogenic therapies in colorectal cancer: where are we now and what should be next? *Clin Med Insights Oncol* 2016;10(Suppl 1):41-55.

Cook KM, Figg WD. Angiogenesis inhibitors: current strategies and future prospects. *CA Cancer J Clin* 2010;60(4):222-243.

De Palma M, Biziato D, Petrova TV. Microenvironmental regulation of tumour angiogenesis. *Nat Rev Cancer* 2017;17(8):457-474.

Dudley AC, Khan ZA, Shih SC, et al. Calcification of multipotent prostate tumor endothelium. *Cancer Cell* 2008;14(3):201-211.

Dvorak HF. Tumor stroma, tumor blood vessels, and antiangiogenesis therapy. *Cancer J* 2015a;21(4):237-243.

Dvorak HF. Tumors: wounds that do not heal-redux. *Cancer Immunol Res* 2015b;3:1-11.

Ema M, Rossant J. Cell fate decisions in early blood vessel formation. *Trends Cardiovasc Med* 2003;13(6):254-259.

Ferrara N, Adamis AP. Ten years of anti-vascular endothelial growth factor therapy. *Nat Rev Drug Discov* 2016;15(6):385-403.

Finn RS, Qin S, Ikeda M, et al. Atezolizumab plus Bevacizumab in Unresectable Hepatocellular Carcinoma. *N Engl J Med*. 2020;382:1894-1905.

Folkman J. Tumor angiogenesis: therapeutic implications. *N Engl J Med* 1971;285(21):1182-1186.

Folkman J. 2007. Angiogenesis: an organizing principle for drug discovery? *Nat Rev Drug Discov* 2007;6(4):273-286.

Francavilla C, Maddaluno L, Cavallaro U. The functional role of cell adhesion molecules in tumor angiogenesis. *Semin Cancer Biol* 2009;19(5):298-309.

Frentzas S, Simoneau E, Bridgeman VL, et al. Vessel co-option mediates resistance to anti-angiogenic therapy in liver metastases. *Nat Med* 2016;22(11):1294-1302.

Gaengel K, Genove G, Armulik A, Betsholtz C. Endothelial-mural cell signaling in vascular development and angiogenesis. *Arterioscler Thromb Vasc Biol* 2009;29(5):630-638.

Gerhardt H, Golding M, Fruttiger M, et al. VEGF guides angiogenic sprouting utilizing endothelial tip cell filopodia. *J Cell Biol* 2003;161(6):1163-1177.

Giannotta M, Trani M, Dejana E. VE-cadherin and endothelial adherens junctions: active guardians of vascular integrity. *Dev Cell* 2013;26(5):441-454.

Gilbertson RJ, Rich JN. Making a tumour's bed: glioblastoma stem cells and the vascular niche. *Nat Rev Cancer* 2007;7(10):733-736.

Gougis P, Wassermann J, Spano JP, Keynan N, Funck-Brentano C, Salem JE. Clinical pharmacology of anti-angiogenic drugs in oncology. *Crit Rev Oncol Hematol* 2017;119:75-93.

Harper SJ, Bates DO. VEGF-A splicing: the key to anti-angiogenic therapeutics? *Nat Rev Cancer* 2008;8(11):880-887.

Hendrix MJ, Seftor EA, Hess AR, Seftor RE. Vasculogenic mimicry and tumour-cell plasticity: lessons from melanoma. *Nat Rev Cancer* 2003;3(6):411-421.

Hida K, Hida Y, Amin DN, et al. Tumor-associated endothelial cells with cytogenetic abnormalities. *Cancer Res* 2004;64(22):8249-8255.

Hill RP, Marie-Egyptienne DT, Hedley DW. Cancer stem cells, hypoxia and metastasis. *Semin Radiat Oncol* 2009;19(2):106-111.

Jain RK. Normalizing tumor vaculature with anti-angiogenic therapy: a new paradigm for combination therapy. *Nat Med* 2001;7(9):987-989.

Jain RK, Duda DG, Willett CG, et al. Biomarkers of response and resistance to antiangiogenic therapy. *Nat Rev Clin Oncol* 2009;6(6):327-338.

Jayson GC, Kerbel R, Ellis LM, Harris AL. Antiangiogenic therapy in oncology: current status and future directions. *Lancet (London, England)* 2016;388(10043):518-529.

Kalluri R. The biology and function of fibroblasts in cancer. *Nat Rev Cancer* 2016;16(9):582-598.

Kerbel RS. Tumor angiogenesis. *N Engl J Med* 2008;358(19):2039-2049.

Kessenbrock K, Plaks V, Werb Z. Matrix metalloproteinases: regulators of the tumor microenvironment. *Cell* 2010;141(1):52-67.

Khan K, Kerbel RS. Improving immunotherapy outcomes with anti-angiogenic treatments and vice versa. *Nat Rev Clin Oncol* 2018;15:310-324.

Klement GL, Yip TT, Cassiola F, et al. Platelets actively sequester angiogenesis regulators. *Blood* 2009;113(12):2835-2842.

Krishna Priya S, Nagare RP, Sneha VS, et al. Tumour angiogenesis—origin of blood vessels. *Int J Cancer* 2016;139(4):729-735.

Kuczynski E, Vermeulen PB, Pezzella F, Kerbel RS, Reynolds AR. Vessel co-option in cancer. *Nature Rev. Clin. Oncol* 2019;16:469-493.

Lahteenvuo J, Rosenzweig A. Effects of aging on angiogenesis. *Circ Res* 2012;110(9):1252-1264.

Landskroner-Eiger S, Moneke I, Sessa WC. miRNAs as modulators of angiogenesis. *Cold Spring Harb Perspect Med* 2013;3(2):a006643.

Lara PN Jr, Douillard JY, Nakagawa K, et al. Randomized phase III placebo-controlled trial of carboplatin and paclitaxel with or without the vascular disrupting agent vadimezan (ASA404) in advanced non-small-cell lung cancer. *J Clin Oncol* 2011;29(22):2965-2971.

Lien K, Georgsdottir S, Sivanathan L, Chan K, Emmenegger U. Low-dose metronomic chemotherapy: a systematic literature analysis. *Eur J Cancer* 2013;49(16):3387-3395.

Lorusso PM, Boerner SA, Hunsberger S. Clinical development of vascular disrupting agents: what lessons can we learn from ASA404? *J Clin Oncol* 2011;29(22):2952-2955.

Lu J, Ye X, Fan F, et al. Endothelial cells promote the colorectal cancer stem cell phenotype through a soluble form of Jagged-1. *Cancer Cell* 2013;23:171-185.

Mackman N, Davis GE. Blood coagulation and blood vessel development: is tissue factor the missing link? *Arterioscler Thromb Vasc Biol* 2011;31(11):2364-2366.

Massari F, Di Nunno V, Ciccarese C, et al. Adjuvant therapy in renal cell carcinoma. *Cancer Treat Rev* 2017;60:152-157.

McKeage MJ, Baguley BC. Disrupting established tumor blood vessels: an emerging therapeutic strategy for cancer. *Cancer* 2010;116(8):1859-1871.

Meehan B, Garnier D, Dombrovsky A, et al. Ageing-related responses to antiangiogenic effects of sunitinib in atherosclerosis-prone mice. *Mech Ageing and Dev* 2014;140:13-22.

Monk BJ, Poveda A, Vergote I, et al. Final results of a phase 3 study of trebananib plus weekly paclitaxel in recurrent ovarian cancer (TRINOVA-1): Long-term survival, impact of ascites, and progression-free survival-2. *Gynecol Oncol* 2016;143(1):27-34.

Monnier J, Samson M. Prokineticins in angiogenesis and cancer. *Cancer Lett* 2010;296(2):144-149.

Motzer RJ, Porta C, Vogelzang NJ, et al. Dovitinib versus sorafenib for third-line targeted treatment of patients with metastatic renal cell carcinoma: an open-label, randomised phase 3 trial. *Lancet Oncol* 2014;15(3):286-296.

Noguera-Troise I, Daly C, Papadopoulos NJ, et al. Blockade of Dll4 inhibits tumour growth by promoting non-productive angiogenesis. *Nature* 2006;444(7122):1032-1037.

Oubaha M, Miloudi K, Deja A, et al. Senescence-associated secretory phenotype contributes to pathological angiogenesis in retinopathy. *Science Trans Med* 2016:362ra144.

Pitulescu ME, Schmidt I, Giaimo BD, et al. Dll4 and Notch signalling couples sprouting angiogenesis and artery formation. *Nat Cell Biol* 2017;19(8):915-927.

Potente M, Makinen T. Vascular heterogeneity and specialization in development and disease. *Nat Rev Mol Cell Biol* 2017;18(8):477-494.

Rafii S, Butler JM, Ding BS. Angiocrine functions of organ-specific endothelial cells. *Nature* 2016;529(7586):316-325.

Rak J. Ras oncogenes and tumour vascular interface. In: Thomas-Tikhonenko A, ed. *Cancer Genome and Tumor Microenvironment*, New York, NY: Springer; 2009:133-165.

Rak J. Extracellular vesicles—biomarkers and effectors of the cellular interactome in cancer. *Front Pharmacol* 2013;4:21.

Ramjiawan RR, Griffioen AW, Duda DG. Anti-angiogenesis for cancer revisited: Is there a role for combinations with immunotherapy? *Angiogenesis* 2017;20(2):185-204.

Rey S, Semenza GL. Hypoxia-inducible factor-1-dependent mechanisms of vascularization and vascular remodelling. *Cardiovasc Res* 2010;86:236-242.

Reynolds LE, Watson AR, Baker M, et al. Tumour angiogenesis is reduced in the Tc1 mouse model of Down's syndrome. *Nature* 2010;465(7299):813-817.

Riesco-Martinez M, Parra K, Saluja R, Francia G, Emmenegger U. Resistance to metronomic chemotherapy and ways to overcome it. *Cancer Lett* 2017;400:311-318.

Rini BI, Plimack ER, Stus V, et al. Pembrolizumab plus Axitinib versus Sunitinib for Advanced Renal-Cell Carcinoma. *N Engl J Med* 2019;380:1116-1127.

Rivera LB, Bergers G. Intertwined regulation of angiogenesis and immunity by myeloid cells. *Trends Immunol* 2015;36(4):240-249.

Roy-Chowdhury S, Brown CK. Cytokines and tumor angiogenesis. In: Caligiuri MA, Lotze MT, eds. *Cancer Drug Discovery and Development*. Totowa, NJ: Humana Press Inc; 2007:245-266.

Saharinen P, Eklund L, Alitalo K. Therapeutic targeting of the angiopoietin-TIE pathway. *Nat Rev Drug Discov* 2017;16(9):635-661.

Samant RS, Shevde LA. Recent advances in anti-angiogenic therapy of cancer. *Oncotarget* 2011;2(3):122-134.

Seaman S, Stevens J, Yang MY, Logsdon D, Graff-Cherry C, St CB. Genes that distinguish physiological and pathological angiogenesis. *Cancer Cell* 2007;11(6):539-554.

Senan S, Smit EF. Design of clinical trials of radiation combined with antiangiogenic therapy. *Oncologist* 2007;12(4):465-477.

Senger DR, Galli SJ, Dvorak AM, Perruzzi CA, Harvey VS, Dvorak HF. Tumor cells secrete a vascular permeability factor that promotes accumulation of ascites fluid. *Science (New York, NY)* 1983;219(4587):983-985.

Siemann DW, Chaplin DJ, Horsman MR. Realizing the potential of vascular targeted therapy: the rationale for combining vascular disrupting agents and anti-angiogenic agents to treat cancer. *Cancer Invest* 2017;35(8):519-534.

Stupp R, Hegi ME, Gorlia T, et al. Cilengitide combined with standard treatment for patients with newly diagnosed glioblastoma with methylated MGMT promoter (CENTRIC EORTC 26071-22072 study): a multicentre, randomised, open-label, phase 3 trial. *Lancet Oncol* 2014;15(10):1100-1108.

Sung HK, Michael IP, Nagy A. Multifaceted role of vascular endothelial growth factor signaling in adult tissue physiology: an emerging concept with clinical implications. *Curr Opin Hematol* 2010;17(3):206-212.

Takebe N, Nguyen D, Yang SX Targeting notch signaling pathway in cancer: clinical development advances and challenges. *Pharmacol Ther* 2014;141(2):140-149.

Tammela T, Alitalo K. Lymphangiogenesis: Molecular mechanisms and future promise. *Cell* 2010;140(4):460-476.

Tung JJ, Tattersall IW, Kitajewski J. Tips, stalks, tubes: notch-mediated cell fate determination and mechanisms of tubulogenesis during angiogenesis. *Cold Spring Harb Perspect Med* 2012;2(2):a006601.

van Hinsbergh V, Engelse MA, Quax PH. Pericellular proteases in angiogenesis and vasculogenesis. *Arterioscler Thromb Vasc Biol* 2006;26(4):716-728.

Verheul HM, Pinedo HM. Possible molecular mechanisms involved in the toxicity of angiogenesis inhibition. *Nat Rev Cancer* 2007;7(6):475-485.

Wang Y, Nakayama M, Pitulescu ME, et al. Ephrin-B2 controls VEGF-induced angiogenesis and lymphangiogenesis. *Nature* 2010;465(7297):483-486.

Welti J, Loges S, Dimmeler S, Carmeliet P. Recent molecular discoveries in angiogenesis and antiangiogenic therapies in cancer. *J Clin Invest* 2013;123(8):3190-3200.

Wong PP, Demircioglu F, Ghazaly E, et al. Dual-action combination therapy enhances angiogenesis while reducing tumor growth and spread. *Cancer Cell* 2015;27(1):123-137.

Xu Q. The impact of progenitor cells in atherosclerosis. *Nat Clin Pract Cardiovasc Med* 2006;3(2):94-101.

Yang FC, Ingram DA, Chen S, et al. Nf1-dependent tumors require a microenvironment containing Nf1$^{+/-}$ and c-kit-dependent bone marrow. *Cell* 2008;135(3):437-448.

Tumor Growth, Microenvironment, Metabolism, and Hypoxia

Neesha Dhani, Richard P. Hill, and Ian F. Tannock

Chapter Outline

12.1 Tumor Growth and Cell Kinetics
  12.1.1 Growth of Human Tumors
  12.1.2 Cell-Cycle Analysis
  12.1.3 Cell Proliferation in Normal Tissues
  12.1.4 Cell Proliferation in Tumors
  12.1.5 Cell Proliferation and Prognosis

12.2 The Tumor Microenvironment
  12.2.1 Cellular Populations in Tumors
  12.2.2 Extracellular Matrix
  12.2.3 Nutrient Concentration and pH

12.3 Tumor Metabolism
  12.3.1 Aerobic Glycolysis (The Warburg Effect)
  12.3.2 Regulation of Tumor Metabolism
  12.3.3 Glutamine Metabolism
  12.3.4 Redox Status
  12.3.5 Metabolic Oncogenes and Tumor Suppressors
  12.3.6 Autophagy

12.4 Tumor Hypoxia
  12.4.1 Measuring Hypoxia
  12.4.2 The Hypoxic Response
  12.4.3 Hypoxia and Outcomes of Cancer Treatment
  12.4.4 Targeting Hypoxia to Improve Treatment

Summary

References

12.1 TUMOR GROWTH AND CELL KINETICS

Tumors grow because the homeostatic mechanisms that maintain the appropriate number of cells in normal tissues are defective, leading to an imbalance between cell proliferation and cell death and to expansion of the cell population. Methods based on autoradiography with tritiated thymidine in the 1950s and 1960s, and the subsequent application of flow cytometry, have allowed a detailed analysis of tumor growth in terms of the kinetics of proliferation of the constituent cells. The proliferative rate of tumor cells varies widely between tumors; slowly proliferating or nonproliferating cells are common, and there is often a high rate of cell death.

12.1.1 Growth of Human Tumors

Because tumors are generally treated rather than observed, most of the data on growth rates of untreated human cancers are from studies undertaken before the development of effective therapies. Accurate measurements could be made only on tumors from selected sites, and most studies have examined either superficial tumors (eg, those in the skin or breast) or lung metastases using serial chest radiographs. Because there is a limited observation period between the time of tumor detection and either death of the host or initiation of therapy, such measurements represent only a small fraction of the history of the tumor's growth (see Fig. 12–1).

Despite these limitations, Steel (1977) was able to review measurements of the rate of growth of more than 600 human tumors, with the following general conclusions:

1. There is wide variation in growth rate, even among tumors of the same histologic type and site of origin.
2. Childhood tumors and adult tumors that are known to be responsive to chemotherapy (eg, lymphoma, cancer of the testis) tend to grow more rapidly than less-responsive tumors.
3. Over a limited period of observation, the time for the tumor volume to double was often constant, implying exponential growth. Doubling times for lung metastases of common tumors in humans were in the range of 2 to 3 months.

Exponential growth of tumors will occur if the rates of cell production and of cell loss or death are proportional to the number of cells present in the population. Exponential growth often leads to the false impression that tumor growth is accelerating with time (see Fig. 12–1). Increase in the diameter of a human tumor from 0.5 to 1.0 cm may escape detection, whereas an increase from 5 to 10 cm is dramatic and is likely to cause new clinical symptoms. Both require 3 volume

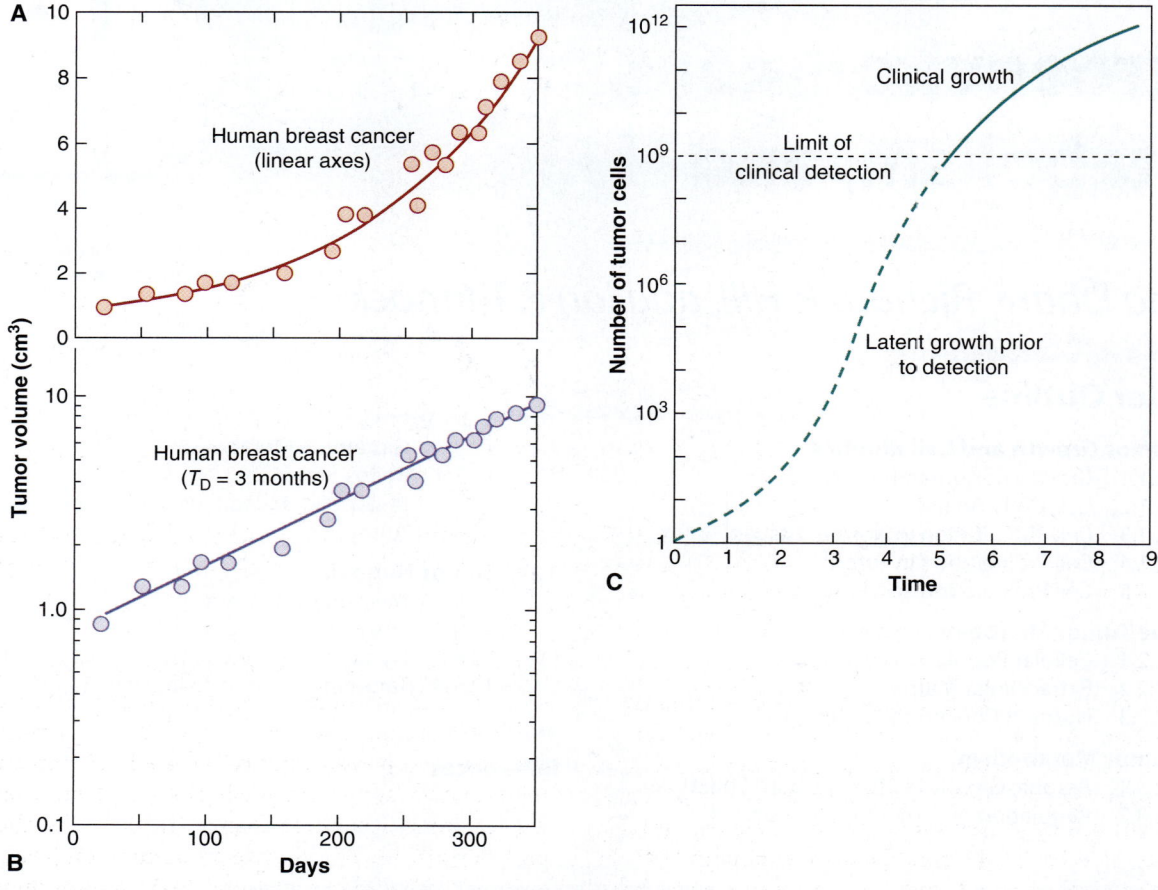

FIGURE 12–1 **A)** Growth rate of a human breast cancer using linear axes. **B)** Growth of the same tumor using a logarithmic scale for tumor volume. **C)** Hypothetical growth curve indicating initial latency and later slowing of tumor growth.

doublings, and during exponential growth, they will occur over the same period of time.

Many internal tumors are unlikely to be detected until they grow to approximately 0.5 to 1.0 g (~10-13 mm in diameter), and tumors of this size will contain approximately $5-10 \times 10^8$ cells. Cells in some tumors contain a clonal marker, suggesting that tumors arise from a single cell, and a tumor containing approximately 10^9 cells will have undergone approximately 30 doublings in volume prior to clinical detection (because of cell loss, this will involve more than 30 consecutive divisions of the initial cell). After 10 further doublings in volume, the tumor would weigh approximately 1 kg (~10^{12} cells), a size that may be lethal to the host. Thus, the range of size over which a tumor is detectable clinically represents a rather short and late part of its total growth history (Fig. 12–2). There is evidence (eg, for breast cancer) that the probability of seeding of metastases increases with the size of the primary tumor, but the long preclinical history of the tumor may allow cells to metastasize prior to detection. Thus "early" clinical detection may be expected to reduce, but not prevent, the subsequent appearance of metastases.

The growth rate of a human tumor in its preclinical phase can only be estimated indirectly or inferred from observations of spontaneous or induced tumors in animals. Tumor growth may be slow at very early stages of development when tumor cells may have to overcome immunologic and other host defense mechanisms, and induce proliferation of blood vessels to support them (see Chap. 11, Sec. 11.5, and Chap. 21, Sec. 21.4). Deceleration of growth of large tumors is also observed, probably as a result of increasing cell death and decreasing cell proliferation as tumor nutrition deteriorates (see Sec. 12.2.3). Also, tumors often contain a high proportion of nonmalignant cells, such as macrophages, lymphocytes, granulocytes, and fibroblasts (see Sec. 12.2.1, and the proliferation and migration of these cells will influence changes in tumor volume.

12.1.2 Cell-Cycle Analysis

As discussed in Chapter 8, Section 8.2.1, the cell cycle is divided into a short mitotic (M) phase that can be recognized morphologically, a subsequent variable G_1 phase (G=gap; referred to as G_0 in cells of slowly proliferating tissues if there is no evidence of cell cycle progression), a discrete period of DNA synthesis (or S-phase), and a G_2 phase that precedes mitosis. Initially, autoradiography was used to detect the selective uptake of radioactive (^{3}H or ^{14}C) thymidine during the S-phase of the cell cycle, and assessing the passage of these radiolabeled cells into mitosis provided information about the duration of phases of the cell cycle in tumors and normal tissues. These methods have now been supplanted by automated techniques

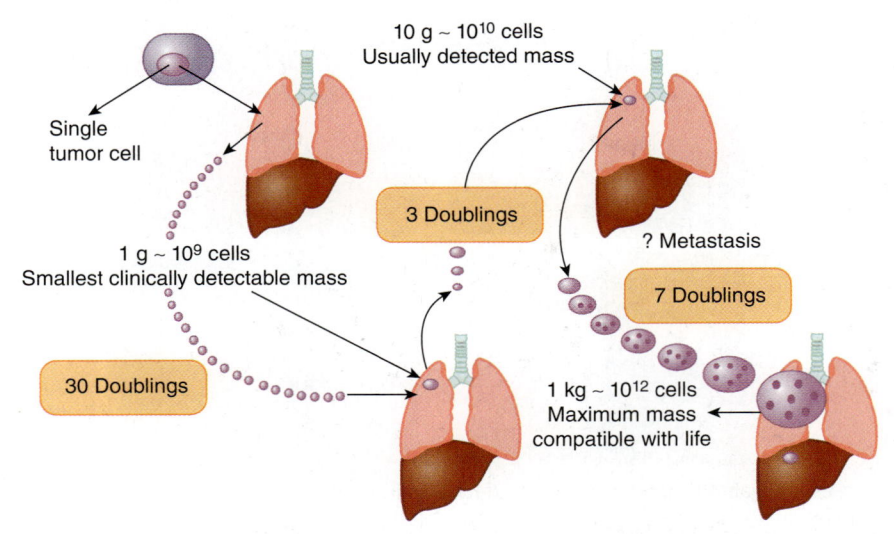

FIGURE 12–2 A human solid tumor must undergo approximately 30 to 33 doublings in volume from a single cell before it achieves a detectable size at a weight of 1 to 10 g. Metastases may have been established prior to detection of the primary tumor. Only a few further doublings of volume lead to a tumor whose size is incompatible with life.

based on flow cytometry that separates and sorts cells based on cellular fluorescence. Cells can be tagged with fluorescent markers (eg, monoclonal antibodies) to a wide range of molecules, including cell-surface receptors, molecules involved in signaling pathways, and proteins that are expressed in different phases of the cell cycle. Several fluorescent dyes (eg, propidium iodide, Hoechst 33342, acridine orange) bind to DNA in proportion to DNA content, and the fluorescence emission is displayed as a DNA distribution (Fig. 12–3A); cells can also be sorted on the basis of their fluorescence intensity. Minimally toxic agents, such as 5-bromodeoxyuridine (BrdU), can be incorporated into newly synthesized DNA (like tritiated thymidine) and recognized by fluorescence-tagged antibodies.

Analysis of the distribution of uptake of these precursors in relation to DNA content (Fig. 12–3B) can then provide estimates of the proportion of cells with 2N DNA content (ie, G_1 and most nonproliferating cells), 4N DNA content (G_2 and mitotic cells), and intermediate DNA content (S-phase cells), whereas time-dependent changes in these distributions can provide estimates of cell-cycle phase duration (Darzynkiewicz et al, 2011; Kim and Sederstrom, 2015). Many tumors are aneuploid (ie, the content of DNA in G_1-phase tumor cells differs from that of normal cells) allowing separation of tumor cells and normal cells within the tumor. Some proteins (eg, the nuclear protein Ki67) appear to be expressed uniquely in cycling cells and can be recognized by fluorescence-labeled

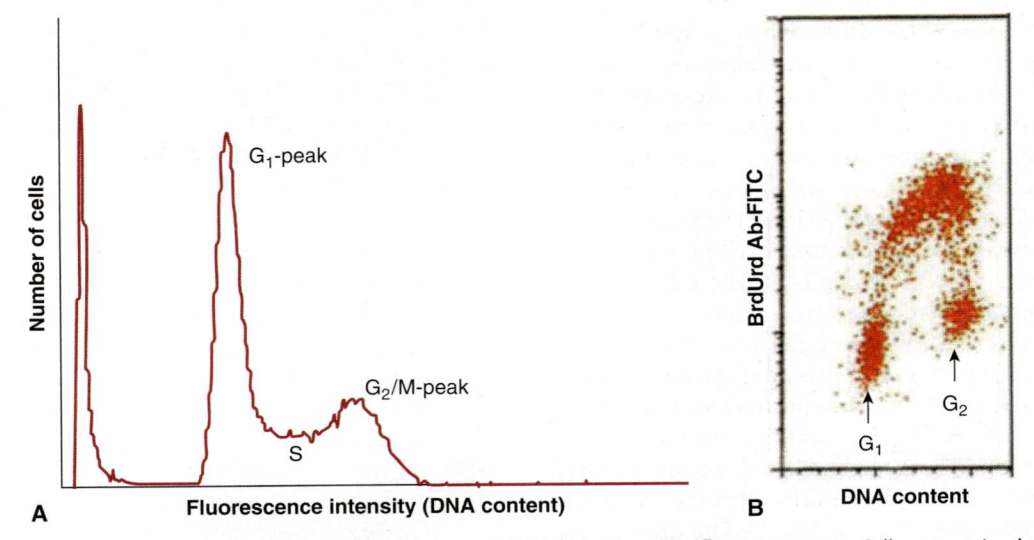

FIGURE 12–3 A) DNA distribution for a human bladder cancer cell line produced by flow cytometry. Cells were stained with a fluorescent dye whose uptake is proportional to DNA content (acridine orange). The peak at the origin represents cellular debris. B) Use of flow cytometry to sort HL-60 cells on the basis of their uptake of bromodeoxyuridine (BrdUrd) (recognized by an antibody tagged to fluorescein isothiocyanate [FITC]) in relation to DNA content; cells in different cell-cycle phases are indicated. (B) Reproduced with permission from Darzynkiewicz Z, Traganos F, Zhao H, et al: Cytometry of DNA replication and RNA synthesis: Historical perspective and recent advances based on "click chemistry". *Cytometry A* 2011 May;79(5):328-337.)

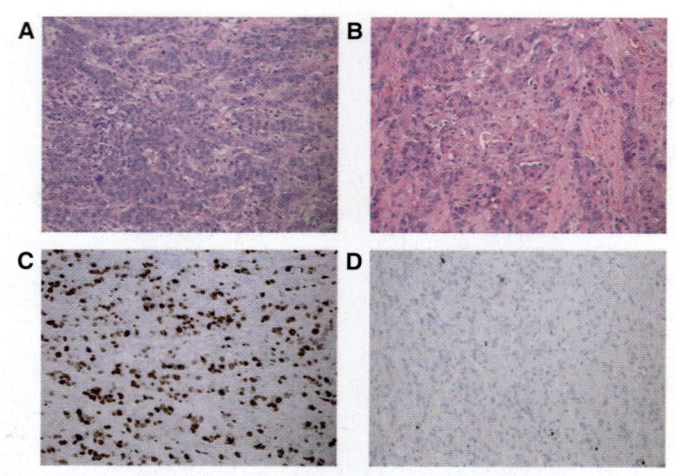

FIGURE 12–4 Hematoxylin-eosin–stained sections (upper) and Ki67-stained sections (lower) of human breast cancers with high (**A, C**) and low (**B, D**) proliferative rates. (Used with permission from Dr. Hal Berman, Princess Margaret Cancer Centre.)

antibodies; the proportion of cells expressing Ki67 is used commonly as a marker of cell proliferation (Fig. 12–4; Kim and Sederstrom, 2015). Ki67 as a marker of proliferation is also applied to tissue sections.

Tumors grow because of proliferation of their constituent cells but most tumors also contain slowly proliferating or nonproliferating cells, and the term *growth fraction* describes the proportion of cells in the tumor population that is proliferating. Most anticancer drugs (including many targeted agents) are more toxic to proliferating cells, and the growth fraction (Ki67–positive cancer cells) therefore indicates the proportion of tumor cells that might be sensitive to cycle-dependent chemotherapy.

12.1.3 Cell Proliferation in Normal Tissues

In most normal tissues of the adult, only a small proportion of cells are proliferating. The remaining cells have either lost their capacity for proliferation through differentiation, or are G_0 cells that can proliferate in response to an appropriate stimulus. Examples of the latter include stem cells in the bone marrow (see below) and cells in skin that participate in wound healing. Thymidine labeling and flow cytometry have been used to compare the overall rate of cell proliferation in a variety of normal tissues (Table 12–1). The side effects of chemotherapy that are common to many drugs (eg, myelosuppression, mucositis, hair loss, and sterility) are observed in tissues that undergo renewal because of the presence of rapidly proliferating cells within them, reflecting the greater activity of most anticancer drugs against proliferating cells (see Chap. 17, Sec. 17.5.2). Acute effects of radiation injury are also observed in these tissues, because irradiated cells often die when they attempt mitosis (see Chap. 15, Sec. 15.3.1). The proliferation and differentiation of hemopoietic cells in the bone marrow and epithelial cells in the intestine are described below as examples of renewal tissues in which the pattern of cell proliferation is an important determinant of anticancer therapy.

12.1.3.1 Bone Marrow Morphologically recognizable cells in bone marrow and blood have an orderly progression of differentiation from myeloblasts to polymorphonuclear granulocytes, from pronormoblasts to red blood cells, and from megakaryocytes to platelets (see Chap. 17, Fig. 17–10). The earlier bone marrow precursor cells cannot be recognized morphologically, but can be enriched by flow cytometry using fluorescent markers to antigens that are expressed selectively on their surface, such as CD34 (Doulatov et al, 2010). The hematopoietic stem cell may undergo self-renewal or may produce progeny that are early precursor cells, which proliferate and differentiate to produce cells of the granulocyte (G), erythroid (E), megakaryocyte (Meg), monocyte (M), and lymphoid (L) lineages. Recognizable precursors of granulocytes and red cells have a very short cell-cycle time (median ~12 hours), but more mature cells in each series undergo differentiation without proliferation. Stem cells and other early precursor cells proliferate rarely under resting conditions, but may proliferate to restore the bone marrow population following depletion of more mature functional cells (eg, by cancer chemotherapy) or after bone marrow ablation and transplantation.

TABLE 12–1 Proliferative rates of selected normal tissues in adults.

Rapid	Slow	None
Bone marrow	Lung	Muscle
GI mucosa	Liver	Bone
Ovary	Kidney	Cartilage
Testis	Endocrine glands	Nerve
Hair follicles	Vascular endothelium	

Note: Acute side effects of chemotherapy occur commonly in rapidly proliferating tissue. Rapidly proliferating tissues undergo renewal in the adult within weeks, with replacement of mature functional cells by rapidly proliferating precursors. Slowly proliferating tissues have minimal mitotic activity unless they are damaged, when proliferation can lead to replacement of lost tissue
Abbreviations: *GI*, gastrointestinal.

The pattern of proliferation and differentiation in the bone marrow provides an explanation for the decrease in mature granulocytes at 10 to 14 days after cycle-active chemotherapy and their recovery by 21 to 28 days (see Chap. 17, Fig. 17–10). The rapidly proliferating intermediate precursor cells are most likely to be killed by chemotherapy. Effects on granulocytes and other normal cells in the peripheral blood are not seen immediately because the later-maturing cells are nonproliferating. Recovery of the bone marrow occurs when earlier precursors are stimulated to proliferate by release of growth factors, following death of the mature functional cells.

The growth factors that stimulate hematopoietic precursor cells to proliferate and differentiate into lineage-specific cells have been characterized, and several analogs are now produced by recombinant techniques for clinical use. Granulocyte colony-stimulating factor (G-CSF) stimulates early cells in the granulocyte series and is used to decrease the duration and extent of myelosuppression after chemotherapy, which lowers the incidence of infection and hospitalization (Choi et al, 2014). Erythropoietin is produced by the kidney to stimulate erythroid cell precursors; recombinant erythropoietin and molecules derived from it (erythroid-stimulating factors) are used to treat anemia and accompanying fatigue, and to decrease the need for blood transfusion, but can be associated with increased blood clotting (Hadland and Longmore, 2009). Thrombopoietin stimulates the maturation of megakaryocytes and production of platelets to guard against bleeding, but various factors limit the clinical utility of thrombopoietin analogs (Hitchcock and Kaushansky, 2014).

12.1.3.2 Intestine
The functional part of the small intestine consists of numerous villi that project into the lumen and provide a large absorptive surface (Fig. 12–5). The villi are lined by a single layer of differentiated epithelial cells that do not proliferate, with apoptotic cell death (see Chap. 8, Sec. 8.4) and shedding of cells into the lumen occur at the top of the villi. These cells are replaced by upward migration of cells lining crypts, which lie between and at the base of the villi. There is a high rate of cell proliferation in the crypts of the intestine, but proliferation of cells at the base of the crypts occurs more slowly (Fig. 12–5) and some of these cells act as progenitors or intestinal stem cells for the entire crypt and surrounding villi. Proliferation and differentiation of cells in the crypts is controlled by a variety of factors including Wnt and Notch signaling, and epigenetic regulation such as histone methylation and acetylation (see Chap. 6, Sec. 6.4; Fre et al, 2009; Roostaee et al, 2016). Some cycle-dependent drugs and radiation may cause severe mucosal damage to the intestine, resulting in diarrhea and/or intestinal bleeding, although this toxicity is less often dose-limiting for anticancer drugs than toxicity to the bone marrow (see Chap. 17; Sec. 17.5.3).

12.1.4 Cell Proliferation in Tumors

Typical values for the percent of proliferating cells expressing Ki67 (ie, the "growth fraction") are in the range of 10% to 40% for many types of human solid tumors; higher values are

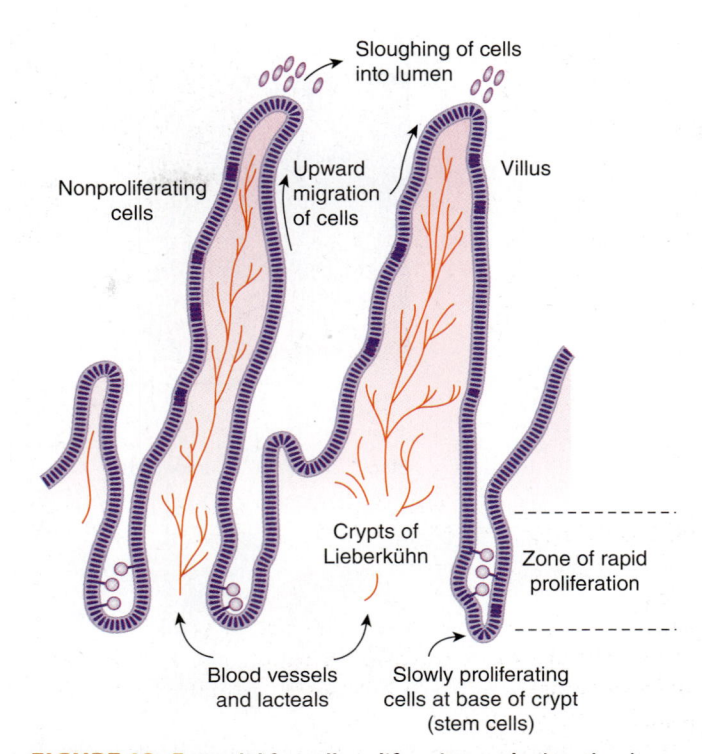

FIGURE 12–5 Model for cell proliferation and migration in the small intestine. Slowly proliferating cells near the base of the crypts act as stem cells for the entire cell population. Other cells in the lower two-thirds of the crypts proliferate rapidly, with nuclei of mitotic cells visible in the lumens of the crypts. Cells migrate up the villi to replace those sloughed into the lumen. The crypt cells are under control of various genetic and epigenetic signals, leading to plasticity in their properties.

evident in faster-growing malignancies, including acute leukemia and some lymphomas. The rate of cell proliferation is usually less than that of some cells in normal renewing tissues such as the intestine or bone marrow. Thus, growth of tumors is not simply the result of an increased rate of cell proliferation as compared to the normal tissue of origin. Rather, there is defective maturation, and the population of malignant cells increases because the rate of cell production exceeds the rate of cell death or removal from the population. The rate of cell production in most human tumors is much higher than the rate of tumor growth, implying a high rate of loss or death of tumor cells; this is typically in the range of 75% to 90% of the rate of cell production (compared with 100% in normal renewing tissues of adults).

Studies of human and animal tumors demonstrate considerable heterogeneity in markers of proliferation within different parts of the same tumor or its metastases. Factors that may contribute to this heterogeneity include differentiation, as there is often an inverse relationship between differentiation and proliferative rate, the presence of genetically distinct clones of cells that arise because of ongoing mutations as a tumor progresses (see Chap. 13; Sec. 13.2.3), and variability in nutrient availability within the tumor microenvironment (see Sec. 12.2.3). Necrosis occurs commonly in solid tumors, and orderly structures ("tumor cords") can sometimes be observed

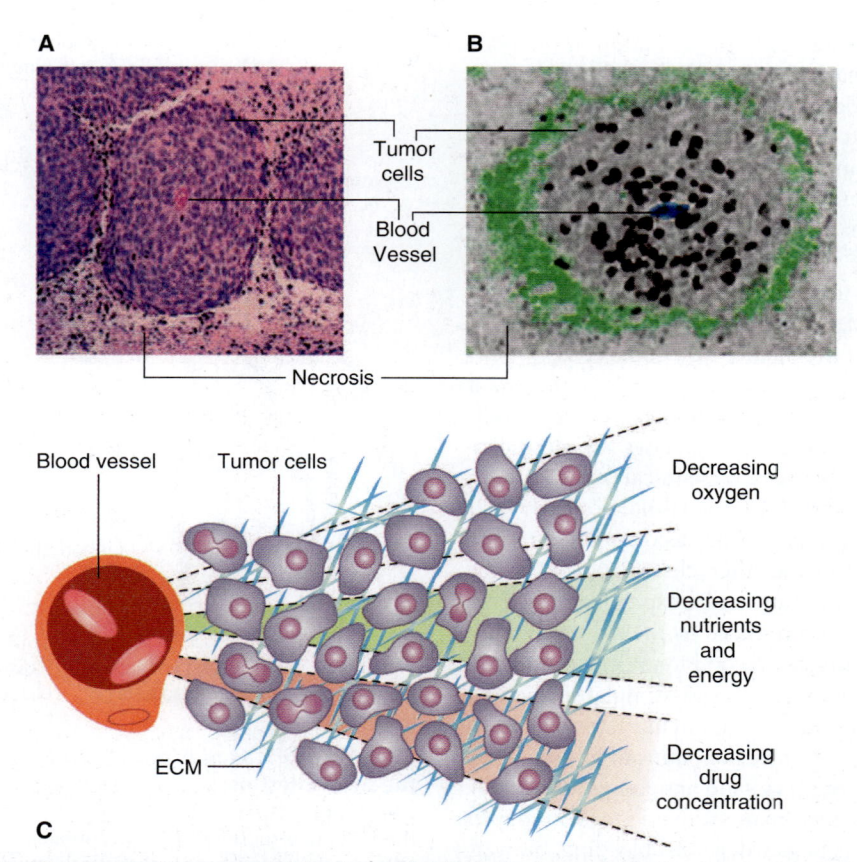

FIGURE 12–6 A) Viable cells surrounding a tumor blood vessel. B) Relation between the frequency of Ki67–positive (black) proliferating cells and distance from tumor blood vessels recognized by an antibody to CD31 in an experimental tumor. C) Diffusion gradients of oxygen and other metabolites in solid tumors. (Reproduced with permission from Minchinton AI, Tannock IF. Drug penetration in solid tumours. *Nat Rev Cancer* 2006 Aug;6(8):583-592.)

in which a tumor blood vessel and tumor necrosis are separated by a distance that in humans is commonly about 150 to 200 μm. This is the approximate distance oxygen can diffuse in tissue before being completely metabolized by the cells in the tissue (Fig. 12–6; Thomlinson and Gray, 1955; see also Sec. 12.4). The presence of such structures facilitated studies of cell proliferation in relation to the blood supply. Not surprisingly, well-nourished tumor cells close to blood vessels have more proliferating cells than poorly nourished cells close to a region of necrosis (see Fig. 12–6; Minchinton and Tannock, 2006). The presence of slowly or nonproliferating cells at a distance from functional blood vessels has implications for tumor therapy: such cells may be resistant to radiation because of hypoxia (see Sec. 12.4.4 and Chap. 16, Sec. 16.4.1), and to anticancer drugs because of their low proliferative rate and limited drug access (see Chap. 18, Sec. 18.4.7).

12.1.5 Cell Proliferation and Prognosis

The relationship between proliferative parameters and response to treatment with chemotherapy is complex. There may be a higher chance of response to chemotherapy in malignancies with a high proportion of proliferating cells, although intrinsic drug sensitivity of the cells is likely to be the major determinant of response. In contrast, malignancies with a high proportion of proliferating cells grow more rapidly both in the absence of effective treatment and during regrowth after partially effective therapy. A further confounding factor arises because analysis of DNA distributions does not provide information about the proliferative status of the cells that are able to regenerate the tumor, the putative tumor stem cells.

A technique for dissolving paraffin, followed by dispersion and staining of the cells, has allowed flow cytometry to be applied to the study of fixed tissue that is stored in paraffin blocks. This technique can provide a useful retrospective analysis of the relationship between kinetic parameters of human tumors and the subsequent response to treatment (Hedley et al, 1993).

Multiple studies of the relationship between cell-cycle parameters and outcome for several types of tumor have been reported. In many studies, an index of proliferation (eg, % Ki67+ cells) gives prognostic information that is additional to the traditional prognostic factors of tumor stage and grade. In general, aneuploid tumors have a poorer prognosis than diploid tumors, and tumors with a higher proportion of proliferating cells have a poorer prognosis than tumors with a lower proportion of proliferating cells (eg, Hedley et al, 1993). The expression within tumors of cyclins, cyclin-dependent kinases (CDKs), and their inhibitors (see Chap. 8, Sec. 8.2) has also been reported to influence outcome, with the general, but not universal, finding that upregulation of positive regulators of the cell cycle (ie, cyclins and CDKs) are associated with poorer outcome, whereas upregulation of inhibitors is associated with better outcome (eg, Keyomarsi et al, 2002; Williams and Stoeber, 2012).

12.2 THE TUMOR MICROENVIRONMENT

Tumors are complex, heterogeneous structures (see Chap. 13). Molecular changes in cells occurring during malignant transformation incite stromal reactions, which attract a diversity of fibroblasts, endothelial cells, and other vascular components and immune infiltrates. These cellular components are embedded in a complex matrix of structural proteins and glycoproteins, which themselves may promote or restrain tumor cell proliferation through tumor-stromal interactions. The unique growth and metabolic properties of malignant cells, distinct from those of normal tissues, lead to further modulation of environmental factors in tumors such as oxygen levels, nutrient availability, pH, and interstitial fluid pressure. The cellular and acellular components, and their pathophysiological context, are referred to as the *tumor microenvironment* (Fig. 12–7).

As a growing tumor adapts to meet the increasing demands of a metabolically active cellular mass, its composition changes because of the requirements of its cellular constituents as well as the stresses imposed by the external environment. This evolution results in spatial and temporal heterogeneity in the microenvironment both between and within tumors.

Given the relevance of the tumor microenvironment in tumor growth and in resistance and response to treatment, studying the microenvironmental characteristics of tumors is essential for understanding basic mechanisms of tumor biology as well as for more effective drug development.

12.2.1 Cellular Populations in Tumors

Several types of cells populate the stromal tumor compartment. Whereas some of these reside in host tissue prior to tumor development, others are recruited to the tumor microenvironment in response to signals mediated by secreted growth factors and chemokines. These cell populations have important functions in maintaining and promoting tumor growth.

12.2.1.1 Cancer-Associated Fibroblasts Cancer-associated fibroblasts (CAFs) are usually the most prominent component of the cellular microenvironment in tumors. Also referred to as tumor-associated fibroblasts (TAFs), they form a morphologically diverse population of mesenchymal cells present in tumors at all stages, from early carcinoma-in-situ to metastatic disease (Kalluri, 2016). CAFs are morphologically and functionally distinct from their nonpathologic counterparts, which are quiescent and metabolically indolent. In normal tissues, fibroblasts are activated in response to stimuli generated by tissue injury, adopting a stellate morphology as they become "normal activated fibroblasts" (NAFs). NAFs function to maintain the integrity of the extracellular matrix, promote wound healing, and regulate inflammation. Once the

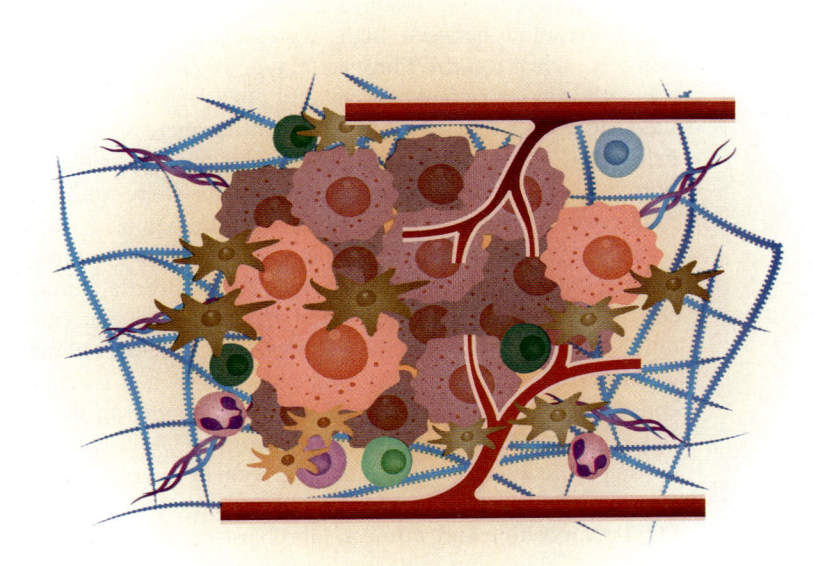

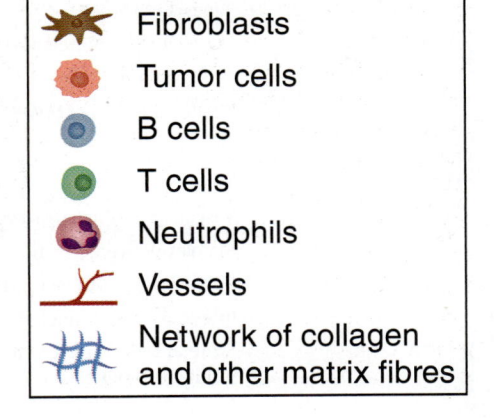

FIGURE 12–7 Components of the tumor microenvironment (TME). A malignant tumor mass includes malignant epithelial cells supported by a variety of stromal cells including cancer-associated fibroblasts and immune cells all embedded in a complex extracellular matrix. The growing tumor attempts to meet its metabolic demands by recruiting endothelial cells to develop a new tumor vascular and lymphatic network, which are often dysfunctional. Mismatch in metabolic supply and demand leads to the development of gradients of oxygen and pH with some cells residing in chronically acidic, hypoxic regions. Acute disruption of blood flow through tumor vasculature also promotes pockets of hypoxia.

initial tissue insult has been controlled, fibroblast activation is dampened, and NAFs return to a dormant state.

In contrast, fibrotic and malignant diseases are characterized by chronic tissue injury—essentially a "nonhealing wound." This pathophysiology maintains fibroblasts in a constant state of activation as either fibrosis-associated fibroblasts (FAFs) or CAFs/TAFS, with primarily epigenetic mechanisms mediating an ongoing activation to produce hyperactivated fibroblasts with a contractile, myofibroblastic appearance (CAFs are also referred to as myofibroblasts: Kang et al, 2015; Kalluri, 2016). The consequent tumor "fibrosis," also referred to as tumor desmoplasia or "tumor scar," is a prominent feature of some human cancers like pancreatic cancer where it may compromise 80% to 90% of a tumor mass.

In addition to their activated morphology and molecular programs, pertinent characteristics of CAFs include their enhanced migratory capacity and increased proliferation, which are driven partly by autocrine growth factor–induced signaling and partly by metabolic adaptations that support increased biosynthetic activity. Their diverse secretome includes angiogenic factors, other growth factors and cytokines, and matrix proteinases (Table 12–2) all of which serve to support CAFs in promoting tumor angiogenesis, immune cell recruitment, and promotion of epithelial tumor cell migration/invasion (Kalluri, 2016; see Chap. 10, Sec. 10.2, for details of extracellular matrix [ECM] components). ECM remodeling mediated by CAFs may also contribute to maintenance of a cancer stem cell niche, with the WNT, Hedgehog, and Notch pathways implicated in this context (see Chap. 6; Sec. 6.4).

The dominant subpopulation of CAFs within a tumor likely arises from activation and expansion of quiescent fibroblasts within the tissue of origin, whereas others are recruited from distant sites (eg, from the bone marrow) or evolve through transdifferentiation of endothelial or epithelial cells through *endothelial-mesenchymal* (EndoMT; Huang et al, 2016) or *epithelial-mesenchymal transition* (EMT; see also Chap. 10, Sec. 10.5.5, and Chap. 13, Sec. 13.3.1). Evidence for EMT comes from studies demonstrating similar genomic aberrations in epithelial and stromal tumor compartments (Baulida, 2017), but this accounts probably for a small proportion of stromal cells.

An early event in fibroblast activation is upregulation of α-smooth muscle actin (α-SMA), which helps to facilitate cell migration into areas of tissue damage. α-SMA is often considered to be a marker of activated fibroblasts and of CAFs in tumors. Several other markers have been explored for their ability to identify activated CAFs, some of which are listed in Table 12–2, but none is a highly sensitive or specific marker for CAFs. These markers have 2 primary limitations: (1) Lack of specificity because several of them may also be expressed by other cells within tumors; for example, focal adhesion proteins (FAPs) are also expressed by CD45+ immune cells, desmin by pericytes, and growth factor receptors such as platelet-derived growth factor receptor (PDGFR) and EGFR by epithelial tumor cells, and (2) Heterogeneity of expression. Many markers are dynamic, with changing expression over time, reflecting temporal evolution of CAF function. An evaluation of multiple markers at different points in the cancer trajectory will be required to improve understanding of their utility in informing CAF biology (Kalluri, 2016).

A correlation between high expression of CAF/stromal markers such as α-SMA, fibronectin, type IV collagen or laminin with inferior patient survival and poor response to treatment supports a role for CAFs in promoting aggressive tumor behavior (Paulsson and Micke, 2014). This hypothesis is supported by co-culture and animal experiments where epithelial tumor cells exhibit more aggressive malignant behavior when combined with stromal cell populations. In addition to direct cell-cell interactions in driving this effect, epithelial tumor cells behave more aggressively when exposed to cell-free conditioned media from stromal cultures. The CAF secretome, which includes growth factors and cytokines such as vascular endothelial growth factor (VEGF), hepatocyte growth factor (HGF), fibroblast growth factor (FGF), and CXCL12, promotes proliferation, survival, and migration of tumor cells but also remodeling of tumor neovasculature and modulation of ECM composition and stiffness. Fibroblast-derived exosomes also allow CAFs to promote local invasion and metastatic progression (Kalluri, 2016; see also Chap. 10, Sec. 10.5.6).

Further to their multiple roles in primary tumors, fibroblasts are also involved in establishing secondary sites of disease by facilitating the formation of "pre-metastatic niches"—distant sites that malignant cells in the circulation can home to and colonize, based on the conditioning provided by fibronectin

TABLE 12–2 Molecular markers used to identify cancer-associated fibroblasts.

Marker Type	Examples
ECM Components	Collagen I and II
	Fibronectin
	Tenascin
	Matrix metalloproteinases (MMPs)
	Lysyl oxidase
	Tissue inhibitors of MMPs (TIMPs)
	Desmin
Growth factors & cytokines	Transforming growth factor–β (TGF-β)
	Vascular endothelial growth factor–A (VEGFA)
	Platelet-derived growth factor (PDGF)
	Epidermal growth factor (EGF)
	Interleukins (IL-6 and IL-8)
	Stromal cell–derived factor (SDF1) or CXC motif chemokine ligand
	Hepatocyte growth factor (HGF)
Membrane-bound proteins/receptors	Intercellular adhesion molecule 1 (ICAM1)
	Vascular cell adhesion molecule 1 (VCAM1)
Cytoplasmic proteins including cytoskeletal components	Vimentin
	Focal adhesion protein (FAP)
	α-Smooth muscle actin

ECM, extracellular matrix.
For review, see Kalluri, 2016.

secreted by fibroblasts, and other factors that bind to it (Aguado et al, 2017).

Although substantial evidence supports a role of CAFs in tumor progression, other studies report that inhibition of specific stromal elements (including α-SMA⁺ CAFs or the stromal ligand sonic hedgehog [Shh]) result in more aggressive tumor biology (Von Ahrens et al, 2017). Our understanding of tumor-stromal interactions is evolving, but studies such as these provide insights into the disappointing results of stroma-targeting therapy like that of the novel hedgehog pathway inhibitor Saridegib in advanced pancreatic cancer; despite being supported by encouraging preclinical data, the study was terminated early because of futility. These results illustrate the complexity of tumor-stromal biology and its relationship to tumor progression.

The interface between CAFs and tumor immunity is also relevant to tumor promotion. Although CAFs are thought to promote an immunosuppressive microenvironment based primarily on in vitro studies, their relationships in vivo are more complex and context-dependent. A discussion of these factors is presented in Harper and Sainson, 2014.

12.2.1.2 Immune Cells
Immune infiltrates in tumors are diverse and dynamic and include monocytes or macrophages, neutrophils, and lymphocytes (see also Chap. 21, Sec. 21.4.4), some of which are residents of the host tissue while many others are recruited into tumors in response to secreted chemokines. Three main monocyte/macrophage populations have been described: (1) tissue-resident; (2) monocyte-derived or so-called *tumor-associated macrophages* (TAMs); and (3) undifferentiated monocytic-like cells or *myeloid-derived suppressor cells* (MDSCs). The functions of these different populations vary widely based on responses to signals received from the tumor microenvironment (TME). The TAMs have been studied most intensively: they use either classical or alternate pathways of activation to yield M1 or M2 TAMs. Although M1 TAMs participate in anti-tumor immune responses, M2 TAMs activated by pro-inflammatory cytokines (including interleukin [IL]-1, IL-6, IL-8, GM-CSF, tumor growth factor beta [TGF-β]) can have immunoinhibitory, pro-tumorigenic roles. There is plasticity in the response of TAMs, with phenotypic switching from immunostimulatory to immunoinhibitory transcriptional macrophage programming. TAMs appear to be preferentially attracted/retained in areas of hypoxia and/or necrosis within tumors, where they upregulate a variety of hypoxia-activated transcriptional programs promoting the production of additional pro-inflammatory cytokines (see Sec. 12.4.3), leading to further modification of the TME (Allavena and Mantovani, 2012).

Different cellular populations (including epithelial tumor cells themselves) produce and release a variety of chemo/cytokines, which modulate the TME. For example, tumor cell production of G-CSF and GM-CSF can induce expansion of bone marrow myeloid progenitors, thereby influencing levels of circulating and tumor-infiltrating myeloid cells (see also Chap. 17, Sec. 17.5.2), whereas neutrophils, mast cells, and eosinophils may all stimulate angiogenesis through the release of VEGF, HGF, matrix metalloproteinase 2 (MMP2), and IL-8, and other angiogenic factors (see also Chap. 11, Sec. 11.4). The crosstalk between tumor, immune, and other stromal cells, mediated by both direct cell-cell contact and autocrine/paracrine chemo/cytokine signaling, creates a microenvironment of chronic inflammation and immune-tolerance, facilitating tumor growth (Binnewies et al, 2018).

Classification schemes have been developed to describe the tumor immune microenvironment (TIME) with a focus on addressing how immunologic composition might affect response to treatment (and specifically to treatment with immune checkpoint inhibitors; see Chap. 21, Sec. 21.5.4). One classification considers tumors as either *infiltrated-excluded (I-E)* or *infiltrated-inflamed (I-I)* (Gajewski et al, 2013). I-E tumors may contain immune cells but demonstrate a relative absence of cytotoxic T-lymphocytes (CTLs) at the tumor core, which instead tend to localize at the invasive tumor edge. In I-E tumors, CTLs that do infiltrate into the tumor core demonstrate low levels of activation markers like granzyme B and interferon gamma. These tumors are hypothesized to be immunogenically "cold" and stand in direct contrast with the "hot" I-I tumors, which are characterized by high levels of PD-1–expressing CTL infiltrate, with PD-L1 expression on both tumor cells and leukocytes. A subset of I-I tumors also demonstrates evidence of tertiary lymphoid structures (TLS), which may correlate with better prognosis (Pagès et al, 2010).

Novel molecular techniques, including high-resolution single-cell RNA sequencing, flow cytometry, and multiparametric image analysis, are able to provide detailed characterization of the TIME focused specifically on the composition of immune infiltrates and quality and character of the inflammatory response.

12.2.1.3 Endothelial Cells and the Vascular Network
The formation of new blood vessel networks within tumors is essential to allow an expanding tumor mass to meet its increasing metabolic demands. This process of angiogenesis is described in Chap. 11, with its various cellular components including endothelial cells and pericytes. As described in Chap. 11, the blood supply in tumors is rather dysfunctional; regional variations in perfusion lead to variations in nutrient supply (see Sec. 12.2.3) and development of hypoxia (see Sec. 12.4).

In addition to the high permeability of dysfunctional vessels in newly formed networks, there is a lack of functional lymphatics within tumors, resulting in a substantial flow of bulk fluid through the interstitial spaces (Fukumura et al, 2010). This fluid accumulation is compounded by tumor desmoplasia and fibrosis, and results in high intratumoral fluid pressure (IFP). Although IFP in normal tissue is generally at atmospheric levels, in some tumors pressures of up to 60 mm Hg can be detected (Heldin et al, 2004; Lunt et al, 2008). High IFP has been correlated with inferior patient outcome, perhaps related in part to a more aggressive tumor biology driven by increased secretion of cytokines and growth factors (VEGF, platelet-derived growth factor [PDGF], TGF-β) and in part because of high tumor pressures impairing delivery of anticancer drugs. A few strategies have been demonstrated to reduce tumor IFP including antiangiogenic therapies and stromal targeting agents like hyaluronidase. These reductions in IFP levels tend to be transient at best, and the benefit of lowering IFP in the absence of concurrent delivery of an effective systemic therapy remains unclear (Heldin et al, 2004).

12.2.2 Extracellular Matrix

Mammalian cells are in contact with a complex extracellular matrix (ECM). The ECM provides structural support and interacts with cell adhesion molecules (CAMs) expressed on the cell surface, including integrins, cadherins, and CD44. These CAMs also interact with signal transduction pathways within the cell. The ECM contains a variety of other molecules including proteinases and their inhibitors. The ECM influences many properties of cells and is often modified in tumors; it has a profound influence on tumor progression and metastasis and has been described in detail in Chap. 10, Sec. 10.2.

12.2.3 Nutrient Concentration and pH

As discussed in Sec. 12.1, tumors grow because of proliferation of their constituent cells, which evade normal homeostatic controls. To support this proliferation, cancer cells tend to have higher rates than normal tissues of consumption of nutrients including glucose, amino acids, and lipids. Consumption of nutrients by proximal cells close to blood vessels establishes gradients of decreasing nutrient levels with increasing distances from functional blood supply, with distal cells residing in relatively nutrient poor microenvironments (Fig. 12–6). Moreover, acute disruption of blood flow through a dysfunctional tumor vascular network (as discussed in Chap. 11, Sec. 11.6.3) can result in abrupt interruptions of nutrient delivery with profound effects on tumor cell proliferation and metabolism, as discussed in Sec. 12.3.

Malignant cells accommodate to this nutrient-poor microenvironment by upregulating several cell surface nutrient transporters, thereby increasing cellular uptake. Increased uptake in the face of a diminished supply leads to further depletion of amino acids and glucose in cancer tissue in comparison with adjacent normal tissue. A further evolution enabling survival in these hostile microenvironments allows tumor cells to scavenge macromolecules from the TME. Malignant tumor cells can break down macromolecules synthesized by other cells in the TME into individual components that can be used for generation of adenosine triphosphate (ATP) and for anabolic pathways. This is separate from the process of *autophagy* through which cells reallocate their own resources (see Sec. 12.3.6). *Scavenging* allows cells to use integrin-mediated processes and macropinocytosis to internalize ECM proteins (such as collagen, laminin, fibronectin) and albumin as sources of nutrients (Finicle et al, 2018).

The dysfunctional tumor vascular network also compromises the elimination of cellular by-products of metabolism, which then accumulate in the TME of cells distal from blood vessels. These are tumor regions that are also more likely to be necrotic (see Fig. 12–6). Regions of necrosis may occur at distances of about 100 μm from the nearest blood vessel in rodent tumors, and about 150-200 μm in human tumors. The accumulation of cathepsins and other enzymes that break down macromolecules is likely to be toxic to living cells and to contribute to the formation of necrosis.

Cells remote from tumor blood vessels often reside in hypoxic regions at the distal edge of decreasing gradients in oxygen concentration. These gradients develop primarily because of limits of tissue oxygen diffusion due to oxygen consumption by cells more proximal to blood vessels. The resulting hypoxia promotes metabolic reprogramming to facilitate cell survival and growth, as described in Section 12.4.

Reprogramming under hypoxic conditions also leads to increases in intracellular pH of tumor cells (pH >7.4 vs. the approximate pH of 7.2 in normal cells) to promote cell proliferation and evasion of apoptosis (Sharma et al, 2015). Metabolic adaptations such as aerobic glycolysis (Sec. 12.3.1) with the accumulation of lactate, hydrolysis of ATP, glutaminolysis, and carbon dioxide production and bicarbonate depletion all contribute to acidosis of the extracellular tumor environment, which may be as low as 6.5, with gradients of pH leading to greater acidity in regions distant from functional blood vessels. Studies have linked tumor acidosis with local tumor invasion and metastatic dissemination and have implicated several mechanisms (Gatenby and Gillies, 2004). Although extracellular acidification leads to protease activation and consequent remodeling of cell-matrix and cell-cell interactions, the simultaneous mild alkalization of tumor intracellular pH supports cell migration through the ECM. Acidic extracellular pH also inhibits a tumor immune response, because accumulation of H^+ and lactate interfere with T-cell activation and release of cytokines. Acidity within tumors may also contribute to resistance to drug treatment by reducing the cellular uptake of chemotherapeutic agents, most of which are mildly basic. A variety of strategies targeting tumor pH and acidity has been investigated for therapeutic potential including targeting several of the pH-regulating transporters by pharmacologic inhibitors, administration of systemic buffers, and use of pH-sensitive drug-delivery systems. Unfortunately, these concepts have not yet met with clinical success (Corbet and Feron, 2017).

12.3 TUMOR METABOLISM

The tumor microenvironment and the metabolic phenotype of tumor cells are mutually interdependent. Because metabolite concentrations are governed both by supply via the vasculature and demand by the tissue changes in metabolism of both the tumor, stromal, and immune infiltrating cells have a profound effect on local microenvironmental conditions. Likewise, the metabolic phenotype of tumor cells changes to adapt to the dynamic changes in prevailing local conditions.

Characteristics of tumor cells are modified by a series of mutational and epigenetic events that alter multiple cellular signaling pathways affecting proliferation and survival.

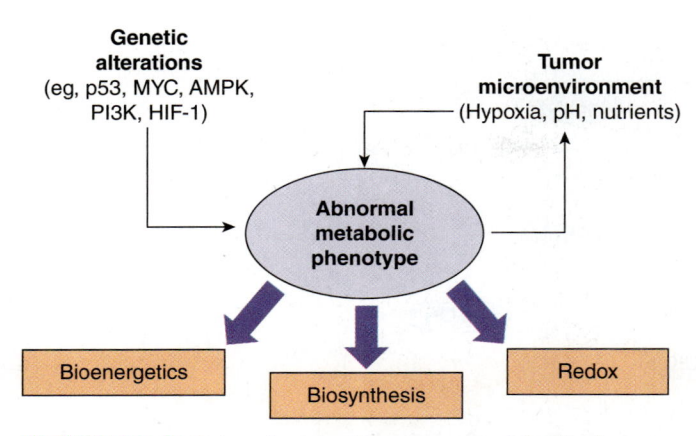

FIGURE 12–8 Determinants of the tumor metabolic phenotype. The metabolic phenotype of tumor cells is controlled by intrinsic genetic mutations and external responses to the tumor microenvironment. Oncogenic signaling pathways controlling growth and survival are often activated by loss of tumor suppressors (such as p53) or activation of oncogenes (such as PI3K, MYC and AMPK). The resulting altered signaling modifies cellular metabolism to match the requirements of cell division. Abnormal microenvironmental conditions such as hypoxia, low pH, and/or nutrient deprivation elicit responses from tumor cells that further affect metabolic activity. These adaptations serve to optimize tumor cell metabolism for proliferation by providing appropriate levels of energy in the form of adenosine triphosphate (ATP), biosynthetic capacity, and maintenance of balanced reduction-oxidation (redox) status. (HIF-1 = Hypoxia Inducible Factor-1, see Sec 12.3.2.2)

Numerous point mutations, translocations, amplifications, and deletions have been detected in cancer cells and the mutational spectrum can differ even among seemingly identical tumors. Cancer-related driver mutations can affect core signaling pathways and processes responsible for tumor formation, many of which are described in Chapter 6 and other chapters. Genetic alterations to oncogenes and tumor-suppressor genes (see Chap. 7) and the cellular response to extracellular microenvironmental conditions both contribute to the development of an abnormal metabolic phenotype. These metabolic alterations provide support for 3 of the basic needs of dividing cells (Miranda-Gonçalves et al, 2018; Fig. 12–8):

- Rapid generation of energy in the form of ATP;
- Biosynthesis of the macromolecular building blocks required to generate daughter cells;
- Maintenance of appropriate cellular reduction-oxidation (redox) status required to prevent excessive oxidative damage and to provide reducing power for anabolic enzymatic reactions.

To meet these needs, cancer cells may acquire alterations to the metabolism of all four major classes of macromolecules: carbohydrates, proteins, lipids, and nucleic acids. Many similar metabolic alterations are also observed in rapidly proliferating normal cells, where they represent appropriate responses to physiological growth signals (Newsholme et al, 1985; Van der Heiden et al, 2009). However, for cancer cells, these adaptations represent responses to the inappropriate growth and survival signals generated by acquired genetic mutations.

Furthermore, these metabolic alterations must be implemented in a stressful and dynamic tumor microenvironment, where concentrations of critical nutrients and waste products, such as glucose, glutamine, oxygen, CO_2, and lactate (which can be both a breakdown product of metabolism and be taken up by cells as a source of energy), are spatially and temporally heterogeneous (see Sec. 12.2.3).

Much of the work on cancer metabolism has focused on rapidly proliferating tumor models and cells grown in vitro. Because the rate of cell division can alter the metabolism of normal cells and tissues, some of the metabolic properties associated with malignancy may simply relate to rapid cell proliferation. These properties may differ in low-grade slow-growing tumors.

12.3.1 Aerobic Glycolysis (the Warburg Effect)

In addition to the ATP required to maintain normal cellular homeostasis, proliferating tumor cells must generate the energy required to support cell division. Furthermore, tumor cells must evade the checkpoint controls that would normally block proliferation under the stressful metabolic conditions characteristic of the abnormal tumor microenvironment. These selective pressures result in a reprogramming of core metabolic pathways. The most consistent metabolic phenotype observed in tumor cells is an increase in glycolysis, even in the presence of oxygen, whereby glucose is converted to lactate and secreted from the cell, rather than being completely oxidized to CO_2 via oxidative phosphorylation in the mitochondria (see Fig. 12–9). This phenotype is referred to as the Warburg effect, after Otto Warburg, who first described the phenomena (Warburg, 1956). This mode of glucose utilization and ATP production represents a departure from the Pasteur effect, which describes the normal suppression of glycolysis by mitochondrial respiration and the shift toward glycolytic ATP production that occurs only during periods of oxygen limitation. As a result, unlike most normal cells, many transformed cells derive a substantial amount of their energy from aerobic glycolysis, converting the majority of incoming glucose into lactate rather than metabolizing it in the mitochondria via oxidative phosphorylation. Although ATP production by glycolysis can be more rapid than by oxidative phosphorylation, it is far less efficient in terms of ATP generated per molecule of glucose consumed. This shift therefore demands that tumor cells increase their rate of glucose uptake so as to meet their energy requirements.

There is uncertainty about the selective advantage that glycolytic metabolism provides to proliferating tumor cells. Initial work by Warburg and others focused on the concept that tumor cells develop defects in mitochondrial function, and that aerobic glycolysis was a necessary adaptation to maintain ATP generation. However, functional mitochondrial defects in tumors are rare (Frezza and Gottlieb, 2009), and most tumor cells retain the capacity for oxidative phosphorylation and can use this as their source of energy if glycolysis is inhibited (Fantin et al, 2006). In fact, mitochondrial function is critical

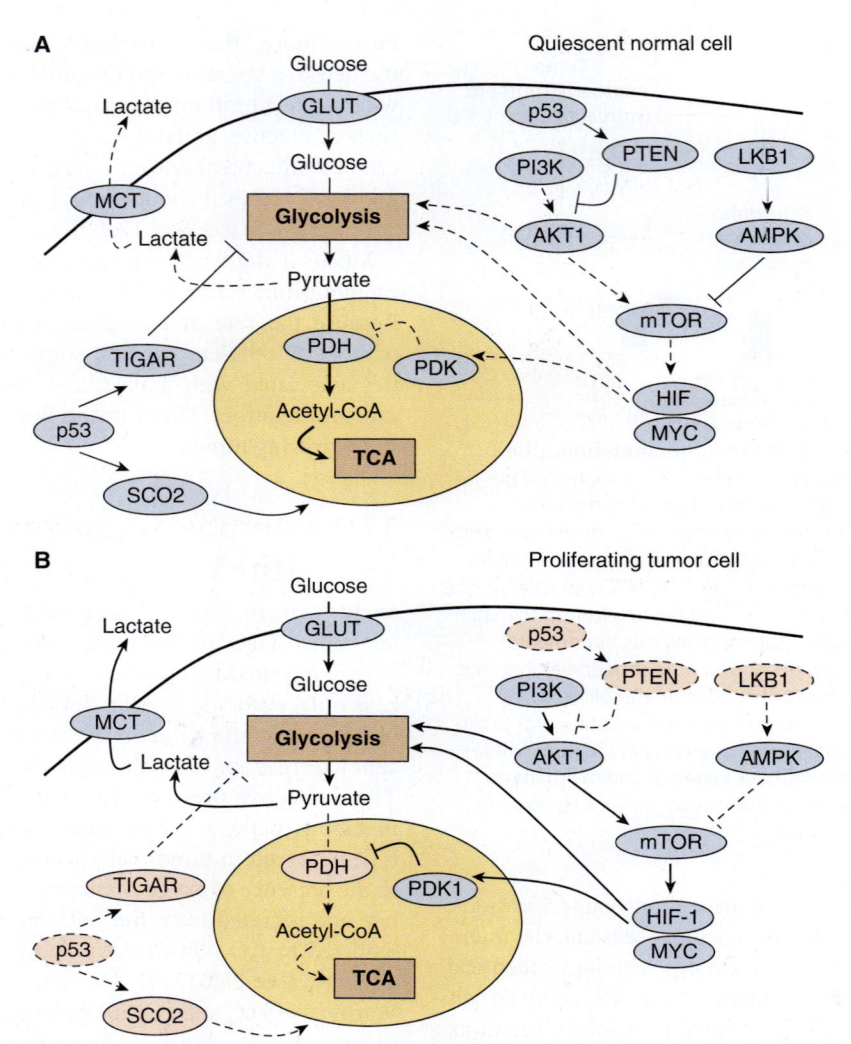

FIGURE 12–9 Molecular regulation of aerobic glycolysis. The shift to aerobic glycolysis in tumor cells (**B**) relative to normal cells (**A**) is driven by multiple oncogenic signaling pathways. Phosphatidylinositol-3 kinase (PI3K) activates the oncogenic kinase AKT1, which stimulates glycolysis by directly regulating glycolytic enzymes and by activating the mammalian target of rapamycin (mTOR) kinase. The liver kinase B1 (LKB1) tumor suppressor, through adenosine monophosphate–activated protein kinase (AMPK) activation, opposes the glycolytic phenotype by inhibiting mTOR. mTOR alters metabolism in a variety of ways, but it impacts the glycolytic phenotype by enhancing HIF1 activity, which engages a hypoxia adaptive transcriptional program. HIF-1 increases the expression of glucose transporters, glycolytic enzymes, and pyruvate dehydrogenase kinase, isozyme 1 (PDK1), which blocks entry of pyruvate into the tricarboxylic acid (TCA) cycle. MYC cooperates with HIF in activating several glycolytic genes, but also increases mitochondrial metabolism. The tumor-suppressor p53 opposes the glycolytic phenotype by suppressing glycolysis via TP53-induced glycolysis and apoptosis regulator (TIGAR), increasing mitochondrial metabolism via cytochrome C oxidase assembly protein 2 (SCO2) and supporting expression of the phosphatase and tensin homolog (PTEN) tumor suppressor. Solid lines represent more-active pathways; dashed lines represent less-active pathways. Pink protein labels indicate proteins whose function is commonly impaired in tumor cells.

for transformation in some model tumor systems (Funes et al, 2007). Other explanations include the concept that glycolysis has the capacity to generate ATP at a higher rate compared to oxidative phosphorylation, so it could be advantageous as long as glucose supplies are not limited. Also, glycolytic metabolism might arise as an adaptation to the hypoxic conditions that develop during the early avascular phase of tumor growth, thereby maintaining ATP production in the absence of oxygen. Adaptation to the resulting acidic microenvironment caused by excess lactate and carbonic acid production may further drive the evolution of the glycolytic phenotype (Gillies et al, 2008).

Another explanation for increased aerobic glycolysis in tumors is that this pathway combines the need of proliferating cells for energy with the equally important need for macromolecular building blocks and maintenance of redox homeostasis (see Sec. 12.3.4). Several biosynthetic metabolic pathways rely on glycolytic intermediates, including the hexosamine pathway, uridine diphosphate (UDP)-glucose synthesis, glycerol synthesis, and the pentose phosphate pathway (Fig. 12–10). The pentose phosphate pathway is necessary to produce nicotinamide adenine dinucleotide phosphate (NADPH), which provides reducing power for many biosynthetic reactions and maintenance of antioxidant systems. Also, by removing the

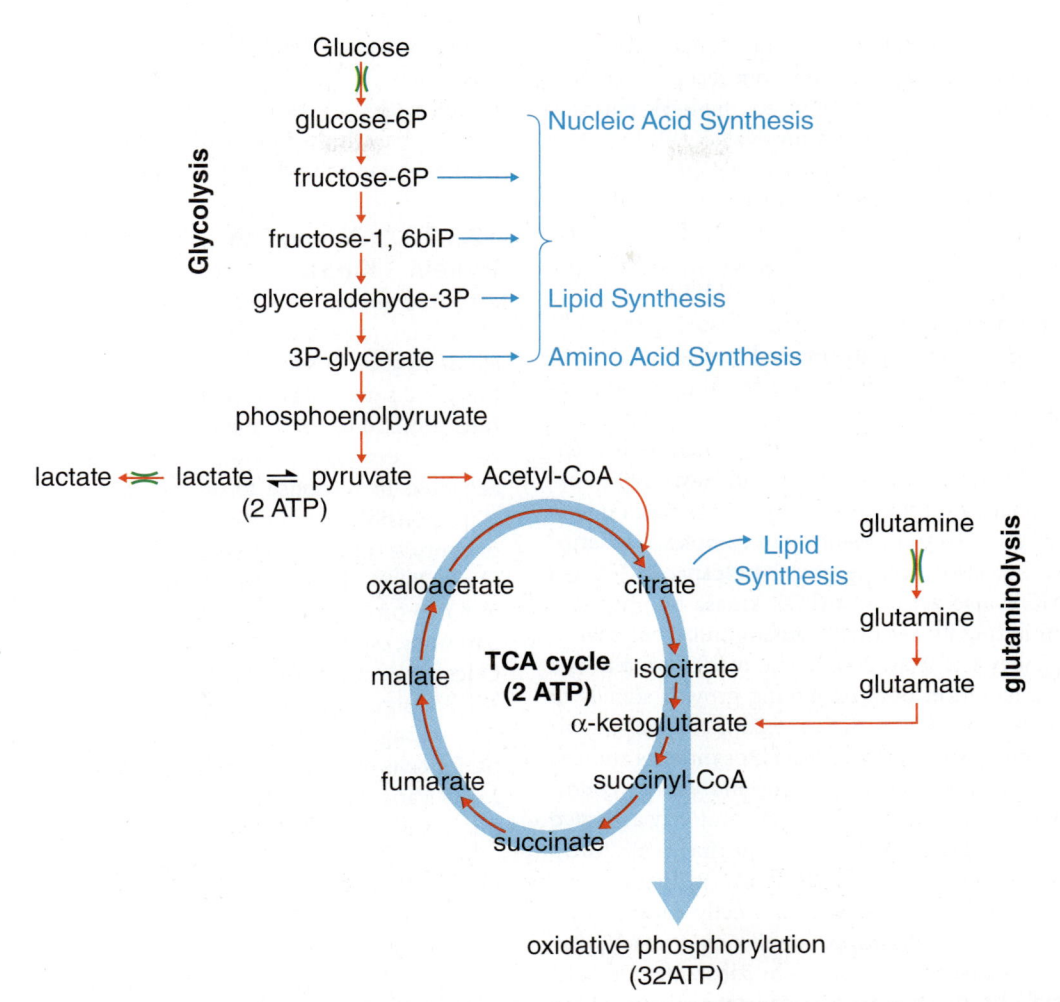

FIGURE 12–10 Relation of glycolysis to various biosynthetic pathways. Glucose is taken up into cells and converted in several steps to pyruvate. Pyruvate can enter the tricarboxylic acid (TCA) cycle (a.k.a. the Krebs cycle) leading to oxidative phosphorylation and efficient production of 36 adenosine triphosphate (ATP) molecules under aerobic conditions, or can be converted to lactate with production of 2 ATP molecules without requirement for oxygen. Intermediates of the glycolytic pathway provide building blocks for nucleic acid, lipid, and amino acid synthesis as shown. Glutamine can be a source of energy by conversion to α-ketoglutarate as shown.

burden of energy production from the mitochondria, aerobic glycolysis allows the tricarboxylic acid (TCA) cycle to act as a hub for biosynthesis of fatty acids and amino acids rather than as a site of energy generation.

The reliance of cancer cells on increased glucose uptake is useful for tumor detection and monitoring. The glycolytic phenotype of tumor cells is the basis for clinical [^{18}F] fluorodeoxyglucose positron emission tomography (FDG-PET) imaging (see Chap. 14, Sec. 14.3.3). FDG-PET employs a radioactive glucose analog that is taken up by cells along with glucose, but cannot be metabolized and is trapped intracellularly. Imaging of fluorodeoxyglucose (FDG) detects regions of high glucose uptake and allows identification and monitoring of many tumor types (Jadvar et al, 2009).

There have been attempts in experimental systems to block or modify aerobic glycolysis as part of cancer therapy, using glucose analogs such as 2-deoxyglucose, by the inhibition of lactate dehydrogenase, and by the inactivation of the monocarboxylate transporters (MCTs) responsible for conveying lactate across the plasma membrane (see Fig. 12–10), and by mitochondrial inhibitors, but these have not been sufficiently active for clinical application.

Aerobic glycolysis is not a universal feature of human cancers (Moreno-Sánchez et al, 2007), and even in relatively glycolytic tumors, oxidative phosphorylation is not shut down completely. Clinical FDG-PET data, as well as in vitro and in vivo experimental studies, show that tumor cells can use alternative fuel sources, and up to 30% of human tumors are FDG-PET–negative (Jadvar et al, 2009). Cancers, particularly in their later stages, show increased metabolic flexibility, and amino acids such as glutamine, fatty acids, and lactate can act as fuels for tumor cells under some conditions (Park et al, 2016; Elia et al, 2018).

12.3.2 Regulation of Tumor Metabolism

12.3.2.1 The PI3K Pathway The PI3K (phosphatidylinositol-3 kinase) signaling pathway is altered frequently in human cancers (see Chap. 6, Sec. 6.2.5). This pathway is activated by mutations in tumor-suppressor genes such as *PTEN* (see Chap. 7, Sec. 7.6.2), mutations in components of the PI3K complex itself, or by aberrant signaling from receptor tyrosine kinases (Wong et al, 2010). Once activated, the PI3K pathway not only provides strong growth and survival signals to tumor cells but also has profound effects on their metabolism.

The best-studied effector molecule downstream of PI3K is AKT1, also known as protein kinase B (PKB). Upon activation, AKT1 phosphorylates key signaling substrates involved in proliferation, survival, and metabolism. AKT1 stimulates ATP generation via multiple mechanisms, ensuring that cells have the bioenergetic capacity to respond to parallel growth signals. AKT1 stimulates glycolysis by increasing the expression and membrane translocation of glucose transporters, and by phosphorylating key glycolytic enzymes such as hexokinase and phosphofructokinase-2 (Robey and Hay, 2009). Prolonged AKT1 signaling inhibits the forkhead box subfamily O (FOXO) transcription factors, resulting in complex transcriptional changes that also increase glycolytic capacity (Khatri et al, 2010). AKT1 also activates mTOR kinase by phosphorylating and inhibiting its negative regulator, tuberous sclerosis 2 (TSC2) (Robey and Hay, 2009). The mTOR protein is a key metabolic integration point, coupling growth signals to nutrient availability (see Chap. 6, Sec. 6.2.5). Normally, activated mTOR stimulates protein and lipid biosynthesis and cell growth in response to sufficient nutrient and energy conditions and growth signals, but it is often constitutively activated in tumors (Guertin and Sabatini, 2007; Morita et al, 2015). mTOR directly stimulates messenger RNA (mRNA) translation and ribosome biogenesis, and indirectly causes other metabolic changes by activating or stabilizing transcription factors such as HIF-1 (see Sec. 12.4.2). The subsequent HIF-1–dependent metabolic changes are a major determinant of the glycolytic phenotype (see Fig. 12–9).

12.3.2.2 HIF-1 and MYC The HIF-1 and HIF-2 complexes are the major transcription factors responsible for changes in gene expression during the cellular response to hypoxia (see Sec. 12.4.2). The effects on metabolism have been better characterized for HIF-1. In addition to its stabilization under hypoxic conditions, HIF-1 can be activated under normoxic conditions by oncogenic signaling pathways, including PI3K, and by mutations in tumor-suppressor proteins such as von Hippel-Lindau (VHL) (Kaelin, 2008), succinate dehydrogenase (SDH), and fumarate hydratase (FH) (King et al, 2006), which cause defects in its normal degradation. HIF-1 amplifies the transcription of genes encoding glucose transporters and most of the glycolytic enzymes, increasing the capacity of the cell to perform glycolysis (Semenza, 2010). In addition, HIF-1 activates the pyruvate dehydrogenase kinases (PDKs), which phosphorylate and inactivate the mitochondrial pyruvate dehydrogenase complex, thereby reducing the flow of glucose-derived pyruvate into the TCA cycle (Papandreau et al, 2006; see Fig. 12–10) and thus reducing the rate of oxidative phosphorylation and oxygen consumption.

The oncogenic transcription factor MYC also influences cell metabolism (see Chap. 7, Sec. 7.5.2). MYC can collaborate with HIF-1 in the activation of glucose transporters, glycolytic enzymes, lactate dehydrogenase A, and pyruvate dehydrogenase kinase 1 (PDK1) (Fig. 12–9; Dang et al, 2008). However, unlike HIF-1, MYC also activates the transcription of targets that increase mitochondrial function, especially the metabolism of glutamine, which is discussed below.

12.3.2.3 Adenosine Monophosphate–Activated Protein Kinase Adenosine monophosphate (AMP)-activated protein kinase (AMPK) plays an important role in cellular responses to metabolic stress by coupling energy status to growth signals. AMPK inhibits mTOR and opposes the effects of AKT1 (see Fig. 12–9). The AMPK complex thus functions as a metabolic checkpoint, regulating the cellular response to available metabolic energy. AMPK is activated in response to an increased AMP-ATP ratio, and is responsible for shifting cells to an oxidative metabolic phenotype and inhibiting cell proliferation (Shackelford and Shaw, 2009). Tumor cells must overcome this checkpoint in order to proliferate in response to activated growth signaling pathways, especially in a nutrient-deficient microenvironment. Oncogenic mutations in signaling pathways can suppress AMPK signaling (Shackelford and Shaw, 2009), effectively uncoupling fuel signals from growth signals, and allowing tumor cells to proliferate under abnormal nutrient conditions. Many cancer cells lose appropriate AMPK signaling, which may also contribute to their glycolytic phenotype.

The gene that encodes liver kinase B1 (LKB1), the upstream kinase necessary for AMPK activation, has been identified as a tumor-suppressor gene (see Fig. 12–9). Inherited mutations in *LKB1* are responsible for Peutz-Jeghers syndrome (Jenne et al, 1998), which is characterized by the development of benign gastrointestinal and oral lesions, and an increased risk of developing a broad spectrum of malignancies. *LKB1* is also mutated in some sporadic cases of non–small cell lung cancer and cervical carcinoma. There is evidence suggesting that *LKB1* mutations are tumorigenic as a consequence of the resulting decrease in AMPK signaling and loss of mTOR inhibition (Shackelford and Shaw, 2009). Loss of AMPK signaling permits activation of mTOR and HIF-1, and may therefore support the shift toward glycolytic metabolism. Clinically, there is interest in evaluating whether AMPK agonists could be used to recouple fuel and growth signals in tumor cells and shut down cell growth. One such agonist is the commonly used antidiabetic drug metformin.

12.3.2.4 p53 As well as its function in the DNA damage response (DDR) and apoptosis pathways (see Chap. 7, Sec. 7.6.1, and Chap. 9, Sec. 9.4), the transcription factor and tumor-suppressor p53 is also an important regulator of metabolism (Vousden and Ryan, 2009). p53 induces the expression of hexokinase II, which converts glucose to glucose-6-phosphate (G6P). G6P then either enters the glycolytic pathway to produce ATP or enters the pentose phosphate pathway (PPP), which supports macromolecular biosynthesis by producing reducing potential in the form of reduced NADPH and/or ribose building blocks for nucleotide synthesis. p53 inhibits the glycolytic pathway by upregulating the expression of p53-induced glycolysis and apoptosis regulator (TIGAR), an enzyme that decreases levels of the glycolytic activator fructose-2,6-bisphosphate (see Fig. 12–9) (Vousden and Ryan, 2009). Wild-type p53 also acts to support the expression of PTEN, which inhibits the PI3K pathway, thereby suppressing glycolysis (Stambolic et al, 2001; see also Chap. 7, Sec. 7.6.2). Furthermore, p53 promotes oxidative phosphorylation by activating the expression of SCO2, which is required for assembly of the cytochrome c oxidase complex of the electron transport chain (Matoba et al, 2006). Thus, the loss of p53 may also be a major force behind the acquisition of the glycolytic phenotype.

12.3.2.5 Pyruvate Kinase

Pyruvate kinase (PK) catalyzes the final, and ATP-generating, step of glycolysis, in which phosphoenolpyruvate (PEP) is converted to pyruvate (Fig. 12–10). Multiple isoenzymes of PK exist in mammals: type L, found in the liver and kidneys; type R, expressed in erythrocytes; type M1, found in muscle and brain; and type M2, present in self-renewing cells such as embryonic and adult stem cells (Mazurek et al, 2005). Many tumor cells overexpress PKM2 and its expression by lung cancer cells confers a tumorigenic advantage over cells expressing the PKM1 isoform (Christofk et al, 2008). Although PKM1 is highly active, and would be expected to promote glycolysis and rapid energy generation, the tumor-associated PKM2 is characteristically found in a less active state (Mazurek et al, 2005; Christofk et al, 2008). Although the switch to PKM2 slows generation of ATP, it can provide an advantage to tumor cells, because it allows glucose-derived carbohydrate metabolites to be diverted to other metabolic pathways. The oncoprotein MYC promotes the expression of PKM2 over PKM1 by modulating exon splicing (David et al, 2010). MYC upregulates expression of heterogeneous nuclear ribonucleoproteins (hnRNPs), which bind to PK mRNA and lead to preferential production of PKM2.

12.3.2.6 PGC-1α

Peroxisome proliferator-activated receptor gamma co-activator 1α (PGC-1α) stimulates mitochondrial function and energy production and plays an important role in regulating metabolism (Bost and Kaminski, 2019). PGC-1α has been shown to stimulate cell migration and metastasis and to inhibit the effects of metformin, which is being evaluated for therapeutic efficacy in multiple clinical trials (Andrzejewski et al, 2017).

12.3.3 Glutamine Metabolism

Although glutamine is not an essential amino acid, oncogenic transformation can stimulate glutamine uptake and catabolism (glutaminolysis) and many tumor cells are dependent on this amino acid (Wise et al, 2008). After glutamine enters the cell via specific plasma membrane transporters, glutaminase enzymes remove an ammonium ion, converting it to glutamate, which has several fates (Fig. 12–11). Glutamate can be converted directly into glutathione (GSH) by the enzyme glutathione cysteine ligase (GCL). Reduced GSH is an abundant antioxidant in mammalian cells, and is vital to controlling the redox state of subcellular compartments. Glutamate can also be converted to α-ketoglutarate (α-KG) and enter the TCA cycle. This process supplies an alternative carbon input for the TCA cycle to act as a biosynthetic hub and permits the production of other amino acids and fatty acids. Some glutamine-derived carbon can exit the TCA cycle as malate and serve as a substrate for malic enzyme 1 (ME1), which produces NADPH (DeBerardinis et al, 2007).

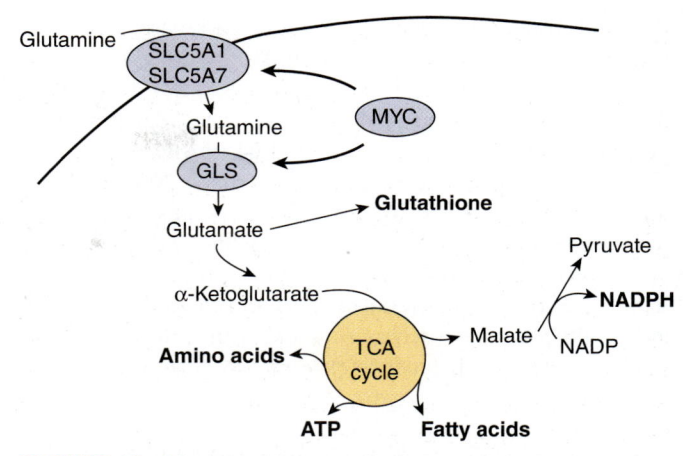

FIGURE 12–11 Glutamine metabolism. Glutamine enters cells via specific transporters (SLC5A1 and SLC5A7) and is converted to glutamate by the enzyme glutaminase (GLS). Glutamate can be converted to glutathione so as to combat oxidative stress or enter the TCA cycle as α-ketoglutarate so as to provide ATP and macromolecular building blocks for cell growth and division. Key products of glutamine metabolism are shown in bold. Oncogenic proteins, including MYC, can enhance this process at several levels and render tumor cells highly dependent on exogenous glutamine.

The oncogene MYC plays a major role in regulating glutaminolysis (Fig. 12–11; see also Chap. 7, Sec. 7.5.2) and thereby promotes both proliferation and the production of the macromolecules and reducing power. MYC increases glutamine uptake by directly increasing the expression of the glutamine transporters SLC5A1 and SLC7A1 (Gao et al, 2009). MYC also increases indirectly the level of glutaminase 1 (GLS1), the key first enzyme of glutaminolysis, by repressing the expression of microRNAs-23a/b, which function to inhibit GLS1 (see Chap. 2, Sec. 2.3.3; Gao et al, 2009). MYC supports antioxidant capacity by driving the production of NADPH via the pentose phosphate pathway, by promoting the PKM2 isoform as described above, and also by increasing the synthesis of GSH through glutaminolysis.

12.3.4 Redox Status

Redox status refers to the balance of the reduced versus the oxidized state of a biochemical system. This balance is influenced by the level of reactive oxygen species (ROS) relative to the capacity of antioxidant systems to eliminate ROS, as well as the relative concentrations of key substrates involved in oxidation-reduction reactions. ROS are a diverse class of molecules produced in all cells as a normal by-product of metabolic processes. ROS are heterogeneous: at low levels, ROS can act as signaling molecules to increase cell proliferation and survival through post-translational modification of kinases and phosphatases (Lee and Esselman, 2002). At moderate levels, ROS induce the expression of stress-responsive genes downstream of transcription factors such as HIF-1α and NRF2, which trigger the expression of proteins providing survival signals and antioxidant defense mechanisms (Gao et al, 2007). At high levels, ROS can overwhelm antioxidant systems, and damage macromolecules, including DNA, proteins, and lipids. Cells counter the detrimental effects of ROS by producing antioxidant molecules such as reduced GSH and thioredoxin (TRX), along with enzymes such as superoxide dismutase and catalase. These molecules reduce excessive ROS so as to prevent irreversible cellular damage. Several of these antioxidant systems, including GSH and TRX, rely on the reducing power of NADPH to maintain their activities. In highly proliferative tumor cells, ROS regulation is critical because of the presence of oncogenic mutations that promote aberrant metabolism and protein translation, resulting in elevated rates of ROS production. Transformed cells counteract the accumulation of ROS by upregulating antioxidant systems, creating a dynamic equilibrium between high levels of ROS production and high levels of antioxidant molecules (Trachootham et al, 2009; Fig. 12–12).

During the process of tumor formation, cells may become overloaded with the products of aberrant metabolism and lose control of redox balance. Several mechanisms downstream of commonly mutated tumor-suppressor proteins may contribute to increased oxidative stress (Fig. 12–13). For example, when the tumor-suppressor *TSC* is deleted, mTOR becomes hyperactive and leads to upregulation of protein translation and increased ROS production (Ozcan et al, 2008). In experimental systems, cells that lack retinoblastoma (RB) tumor-suppressor function, which normally participates in the

FIGURE 12–13 Tumor suppressors influence oxidative stress. Loss of the tumor suppressors tuberous sclerosis 1 (TSC), phosphatase and tensin homolog (PTEN), p53, and retinoblastoma 1 (RB), shaded in gray, leads to increased oxidative stress by increasing reactive oxygen species (ROS) production or by preventing the induction and maintenance of appropriate antioxidant defense mechanisms. TSC inhibits the mammalian target of rapamycin (mTOR), reducing the oxidative stress resulting from metabolism associated with protein translation. PTEN inhibits the ability of AKT1 to inhibit the FOXO transcription factor, which also increases oxidative stress. p53 can bolster antioxidant defenses by increasing the activity of the NRF2 antioxidant transcription factor via the p21 protein, and by stimulating glutathione production by upregulating glutaminase 2 (GLS2). The oncogenic DJ1 protein can contribute to both of these pathways by inhibiting PTEN, and by helping to stabilize NRF2. The RB tumor suppressor enhances antioxidant defenses via a number of downstream mechanisms.

antioxidant response, are more sensitive to apoptosis as a consequence of this cellular stress (Li et al, 2010). Similar results have been seen with loss of PTEN, where increased activation of AKT1 leads to inactivation of the FOXO transcription factor and increased oxidative stress because of a reduction in the antioxidant defense molecules normally maintained by FOXO (Nogueira et al, 2008).

The tumor-suppressor p53 may promote oxidative stress during the induction of apoptosis (see Chap. 8, Sec. 8.4), yet it also plays a significant role in reducing oxidative stress. Glutaminase 2 (GLS2) is upregulated by p53 and drives de novo GSH synthesis (Suzuki et al, 2010). Via the p53 target gene CDK inhibitor 1A (*CDKN1A*), which encodes p21, p53 promotes the stabilization of the NRF2 transcription factor (see Fig. 12–13) (Chen et al, 2009). NRF2 increases the expression of several antioxidant and detoxifying molecules. Loss of p53 in a cancer cell inactivates this redox maintenance mechanism. The BRCA1 tumor-suppressor protein also interacts with NRF2 to promote its stability and activation and thereby contributes to regulation of oxidative stress (Gorrini et al, 2013).

Similar mechanisms maintain appropriate redox status in both neurons and cancer cells, and understanding of ROS and oxidative stress has been enhanced by study of neurodegenerative disease. One protein involved in preventing neurodegeneration that is relevant to cancer is DJ1 (also known as PARK7). Similar to p21, DJ1 acts to stabilize NRF2 and thereby promotes antioxidant responses (Clements et al, 2006). DJ1 is mutated and inactive in several neurodegenerative disorders, most notably Parkinson disease (Gasser et al, 1997) leading to

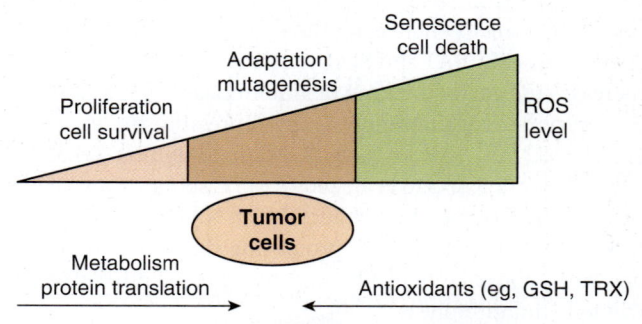

FIGURE 12–12 Relationship between reactive oxygen species (ROS) level and cancer. The impact of ROS on cell fate depends on ROS levels. Low levels of ROS provide a beneficial effect, supporting cell proliferation and survival pathways. However, once ROS levels become excessively high, they cause detrimental oxidative stress that can lead to cell death. To counter such oxidative stress, cells employ antioxidant systems such as reduced glutathione (GSH) and thioredoxin (TRX) that prevent ROS from accumulating to high levels. In cancer cells, aberrant metabolism, protein translation, and microenvironmental conditions generate abnormally high ROS levels. Through additional mutations and adaptations, cancer cells exert tight regulation of ROS and antioxidants in such a way that the cells survive and ROS are reduced to moderate levels.

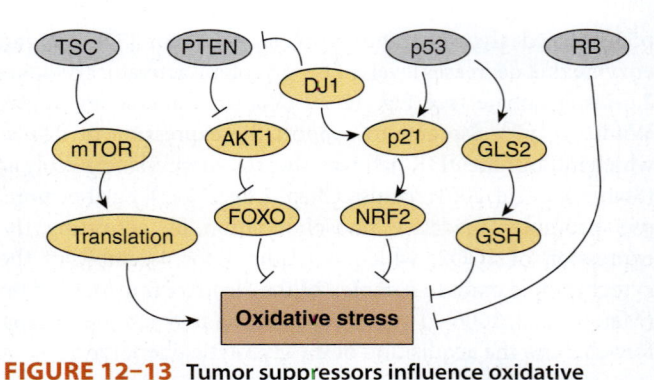

increased oxidative stress in the brain, and neuronal cell death (see Fig. 12-13). *DJ1* is also an oncogene, and in patients with lung, ovarian, and esophageal cancers, high DJ1 expression in the tumor predicts for poor outcomes (Kim et al, 2005). DJ1 stimulates AKT activity by regulating the function of the tumor-suppressor PTEN (see Fig. 12-13) (Kim et al, 2005). High DJ1 expression may also promote tumor progression by reducing the oxidative stress caused by aberrant cell proliferation and thereby preventing ROS-induced cell death.

A recent meta-analysis of people with Parkinson disease determined that they have an approximately 30% lower risk of developing cancers compared with controls (Bajaj et al, 2010). The lower risk was associated with several different cancer types, including lung, prostate, and colorectal cancers. This inverse correlation between cancer risk and Parkinson disease supports the hypothesis that loss of DJ1 prevents pro-tumorigenic redox control.

12.3.5 Metabolic Oncogenes and Tumor Suppressors

Many signaling pathways in tumors have profound effects on cellular metabolism, but few metabolic enzymes are mutated consistently. However, several metabolic enzymes have been shown to be important oncogenes and tumor suppressors.

The TCA cycle enzymes, fumarate hydratase (FH) and succinate dehydrogenase (SDH), have been identified as tumor suppressors. Loss-of-function mutations in these enzymes cause disruption of the TCA cycle and lead to hereditary cancer syndromes, predisposing patients to paraganglioma and pheochromocytoma in the case of SDH, and to leiomyoma and renal cell carcinoma in the case of FH (Selak et al, 2005). The biochemical mechanisms appear to involve the induction of a pseudo-hypoxic phenotype, caused by inhibition of enzymes responsible for the degradation of HIF-1 (Selak et al, 2005; See also Sec. 12.4.2), but other mechanisms, including an increase in ROS production, may be involved. The restricted tumor spectrum observed in these syndromes indicates that the capacity of these mutations to cause cancer depends on cellular context.

Isocitrate dehydrogenase 1 and 2 (*IDH1/2*) are genes that are mutated in several tumors, most commonly in glioma and acute myeloid leukemia (AML) (Waitkus et al, 2018; see Chap. 7, Sec. 7.5.6). These genes function normally to regulate cellular redox status by producing NADPH during the conversion of isocitrate to α-ketoglutarate in the cytoplasm and mitochondria, respectively. IDH1 and IDH2 are homologs, and structurally and functionally distinct from the nicotinamide adenine dinucleotide (NAD)–dependent enzyme IDH3, which functions in the TCA cycle to produce the reduced form of nicotinamide adenine dinucleotide (NADH) required for oxidative phosphorylation. The *IDH1* and *IDH2* mutations associated with the development of glioma and AML are restricted to critical arginine residues required for isocitrate binding in the active site of the protein (R132 in IDH1 and R172 or R140 in IDH2) (Waitkus et al, 2018). Affected patients are heterozygous for these mutations, suggesting that these alterations cause an oncogenic gain of function. The spectrum of mutation differs in the 2 diseases, with the *IDH1 R132H* mutation predominating in gliomas, whereas a more diverse collection of mutations in both *IDH1* and *IDH2* are found in AML. The specific mutations cause the IDH1 and IDH2 proteins to acquire novel enzymatic activity that converts α-ketoglutarate to 2-hydroxyglutarate (2-HG) in an NADPH-dependent manner (Dang et al, 2009; Gross et al, 2010). This change causes the mutated IDH1 and IDH2 enzymes to switch from NADPH production to NADPH consumption, with consequences for cellular redox balance. In patients bearing somatic *IDH1* or *IDH2* mutations, 2-HG builds up to high levels in glioma tissues, and in the leukemic cells and sera of AML patients and may be directly oncogenic (Dang et al, 2009; Gross et al, 2010). Thus, IDH1 and IDH2 may represent a new paradigm in oncogenesis: a driver mutation that confers metabolic enzymatic activity that produces a potential oncometabolite. Although *IDH1* and *IDH2* mutations are powerful drivers of glioma and AML, they appear to be rare or absent in other tumor types, illustrating the importance of cellular context in understanding metabolic perturbations in cancer cells (Waitkus et al, 2018).

12.3.6 Autophagy

Autophagy provides a link between cellular metabolism and hypoxia in the microenvironment of solid tumors. Autophagy means "self-eating" and is a process that is responsible for the degradation of cellular macromolecules (Fig. 12-14). It occurs through generation of a double-membrane vesicle referred to as an *autophagosome* that captures cytoplasmic contents destined for degradation. The outer membrane of the autophagosome fuses with an acidic lysosome to form an autophagolysosome, resulting in the degradation of the inner membrane and its contents by cathepsins and other enzymes present within the lysosome. The degradation products (amino acids, lipids) are delivered back to the cytoplasm and can be recycled for use in metabolic processes. Autophagy is under the control of a number of genes (designated *ATG*), and these are rarely mutated in cancer (Amaravadi et al, 2016). Autophagy occurs at a low basal rate in all cells but can be strongly induced by forms of cell stress, including those present in the microenvironment of tumors.

Autophagy serves at least 2 critical cellular functions in cancer. First, it is a mechanism for the removal and degradation of damaged organelles and misfolded protein aggregates (Koritzinsky and Wouters, 2013). This includes removal of damaged mitochondria that would otherwise "leak" electrons and produce ROS through a selective form of autophagy referred to as mitophagy. The ability to remove and degrade otherwise toxic cellular components is thought to provide a tumor-suppressor function during early tumorigenesis, and mutations in genes, such as *BECLIN-1* (or *ATG6*), that regulate the initiation of autophagy have been observed in some types of cancer (White et al, 2015). Autophagy also plays an essential metabolic function to maintain cell survival during conditions of extreme metabolic stress. Autophagy is activated

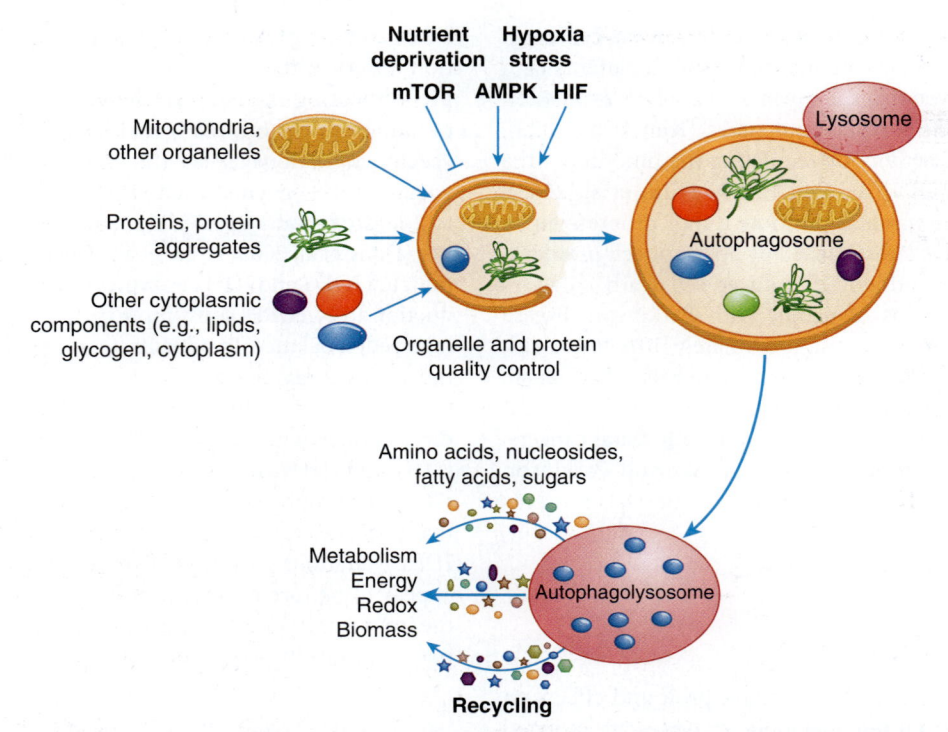

FIGURE 12-14 Process of autophagy. Under various types of stress including nutrient deprivation, hypoxia, and cancer treatment, breakdown products of metabolism are sequestered in an autophagosome. This can fuse with lysosomes where at low pH cathepsins lead to further breakdown of macromolecules. These breakdown products are released into the cytoplasm and can be recycled to provide macromolecular synthesis and metabolic energy, and to maintain REDOX status. mTOR, Mammalian target of rapamycin, AMPK, Adenosine monophosphate-activated protein kinase, HIF, Hypoxia inducible factor. (Reproduced with permission from White E, Mehnert JM, Chan CS. Autophagy, Metabolism, and Cancer. *Clin Cancer Res* 2015 Nov 15;21(22):5037-5046.)

as part of a "starvation" response when cells are unable to import oxygen and other nutrients to sustain essential metabolic pathways (Koritzinsky and Wouters, 2013). Autophagy then functions to degrade cytoplasmic components to provide essential products for sustaining cellular metabolism and energy homeostasis. This function is particularly important within hypoxic regions of solid tumors, and each of the HIF, UPR, and mTOR pathways are capable of stimulating rates of autophagy during hypoxia. In some tumors, activation of growth-promoting oncogenes including *K-RAS* is sufficient to render cells constitutively dependent on autophagy for their continued survival. Thus, in most advanced cancers, autophagy rates are markedly induced and function to promote cell survival. Consequently, autophagy and the genes/pathways that regulate it have emerged as possible therapeutic targets (see Chap. 18, Sec. 18.4.6). Strategies for inhibiting autophagy include use of agents such as hydroxychloroquine and proton pump inhibitors that disrupt lysosomal pH regulation and thus prevent autolysosome formation and degradation of captured cytoplasmic content (Levy et al, 2017).

12.4 TUMOR HYPOXIA

Under normal physiologic conditions, mammalian cells have a requirement for oxygen to function as a terminal electron acceptor in mitochondrial respiration to generate the requisite ATP to drive intracellular biochemical reactions. High consumption within solid tumors, combined with a compromised delivery system, leads to a mismatch of oxygen supply and demand and the development of regions of *hypoxia*. The existence of hypoxia within human tumors was first inferred by Thomlinson and Gray (1955), who observed regions of necrosis approximately 180 μm from tumor blood vessels; this distance is similar to the estimated diffusion distance of oxygen of ~150-200 μm based on rates of oxygen consumption by tumor tissue, and suggested that limited oxygen diffusion was the primary mechanism promoting tumor hypoxia, and that lack of oxygen led to tumor necrosis. *Chronic* or *diffusion-limited* hypoxia is characterized by gradients of decreasing oxygen tension with increasing distance from perfused vessels. It implies that within a given tumor there will exist malignant cells at different oxygen concentrations ranging from physiologically normal close to patent blood vessels to moderate hypoxia to total anoxia.

Acute or *perfusion-related* hypoxia was described later, and results from dysfunctional malignant neovascular networks, which are often immature and leaky, with structural abnormalities including blind ends and arterial-venous shunts (see Chap. 11, Sec. 11.5). Transient interruptions in blood flow occur due to microthrombi or vasospasm, or hypoxia may result from flow of plasma devoid of oxygen-transporting red corpuscles. *Perfusion related*-hypoxia is characterized by rapidly changing oxygen tensions so that malignant tumor cells are exposed to repeated cycles of hypoxia and reoxygenation. The generation of ROS may promote genomic instability and activate cell survival pathways, and acute hypoxia within tumors may have greater significance for tumor behavior than chronic hypoxia (Bayer et al, 2011).

12.4.1 Measuring Hypoxia

Although the partial pressure of oxygen (pO$_2$) in air is 150 mm Hg or 21%, physiological levels of oxygen in normal tissue range from 20 to 80 mm Hg. The average pO$_2$ in muscle is ~30 mm Hg (4%), but much higher in kidneys at ~72 mm Hg (10%). The oxygen tension within human tumors is variable, but regions of hypoxia are common as cancer cells acquire a variety of adaptive mechanisms allowing them to survive and thrive in these hostile conditions. Because pO$_2$ levels below 1% (7–8 mm Hg) lead to changes in gene expression and multiple other biological properties, this level is considered a general threshold for hypoxia. However, many other essential cellular properties may be compromised under conditions of more moderate hypoxia.

Polarographic oxygen electrodes (eg, the Eppendorf oxygen electrode) and exogenously administered hypoxia tracers (eg, EF5 and pimonidazole) have been used to provide measures of tissue oxygen status. Electrode probes provide direct measurements of pO$_2$, but the technique is disruptive of tissue and only applicable to accessible tumors; measurements have often been made in superficial, metastatic lymph nodes rather than less-accessible primary tumors. A further limitation is that electrode measurements reflect an integration of oxygen levels over a volume of tumor tissue (estimated to be equivalent to ~500 cells) and provide poor resolution of microregional differences. Also, they are unable to differentiate between viable and necrotic tumor regions, or between epithelial and stromal tumor compartments (Dhani, Fyles et al, 2015).

Exogenous hypoxia markers that can be injected into animals or patients include the nitroimidazoles, EF5, and pimonidazole. These small, diffusible molecules undergo bioactive reduction in regions of severe hypoxia (less than 1-5 mm Hg) to form covalent adducts with intracellular macromolecules that can be detected by immunohistochemical (IHC) or immunofluorescence (IF) analysis of tumor sections, or by flow cytometry of disaggregated tumor samples. Because active nitroreductases are required for enzymatic activation, bioreduction and binding does not occur in nonviable (ie, necrotic) cells, and there is no sequestration of nonreduced imidazole in oxygenated tumor regions. Analysis of whole tumor sections allows for an appreciation of microregional variability of hypoxia, and studies in both animals and people have provided evidence for substantial heterogeneity in hypoxia both within and between tumors (Fig. 12–15). Given this heterogeneity, these analyses are prone to sampling error, particularly when staining is undertaken in a limited number of sections of core biopsies acquired in patients with multiple tumor deposits. Robust assessments of hypoxia require thorough studies to characterize this heterogeneity in multiple tumor samples (Dhani, Serra et al, 2015).

The primary limitation of exogenous hypoxia markers is the requirement for prospectively designed studies where the drug

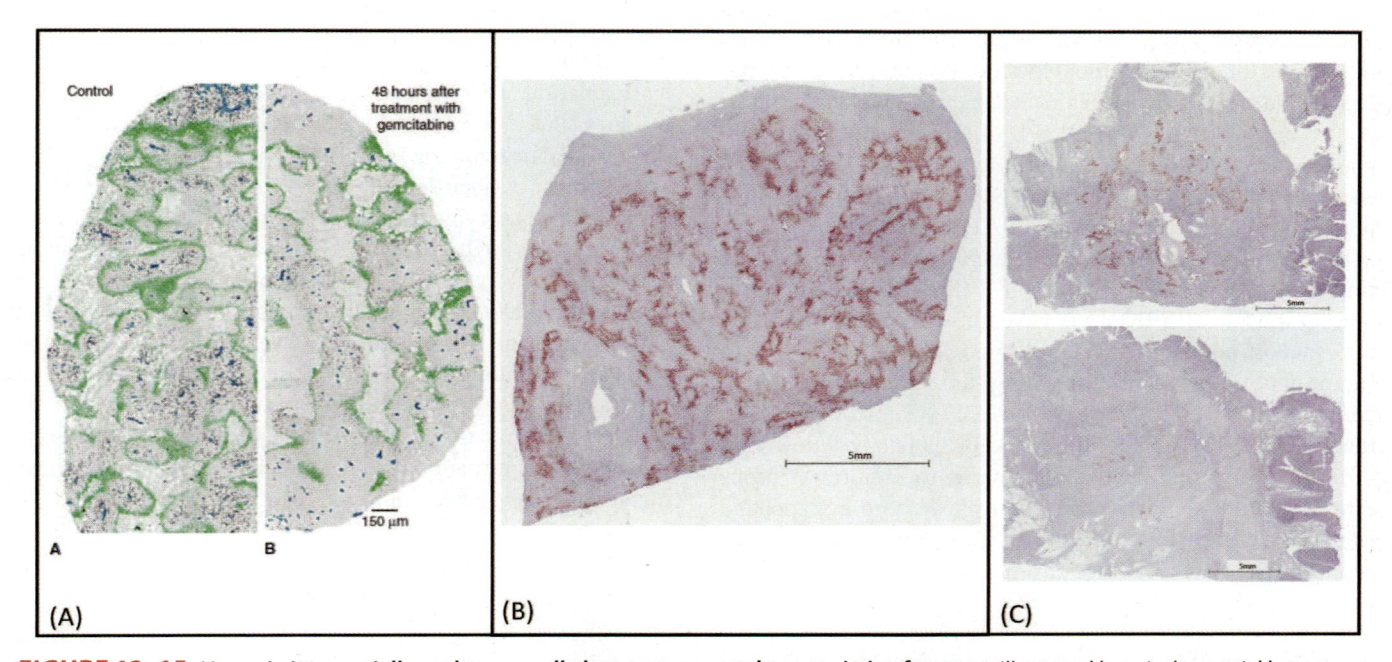

FIGURE 12–15 Hypoxia is a spatially and temporally heterogeneous characteristic of tumors. Illustrated here is the spatial heterogeneity of pimonidazole-detectable hypoxia using immunohistochemistry (IHC) in (A) murine xenografts and (B, C) tumor sections from resected pancreatic cancers (from patients with localized disease). Panels B and C demonstrates the heterogeneity of pimonidazole staining across different patients with pancreatic cancer—tumor in B has high levels of pimonidazole staining and greater extent of severe hypoxia compared with the tumor represented in C. Panel C illustrates the variability of hypoxia that can exist within the same tumor -- while the top panel has high moderately high levels of pimonidazole staining, the bottom panel from the same patient tumor demonstrates very minimal pimonidazole staining. (Panel A: Reproduced with permission from Minchinton AI, Tannock IF. Drug penetration in solid tumours. *Nat Rev Cancer* 2006 Aug;6(8):583-592.)

can be administered prior to tumor sampling. Most available tracers required intravenous administration, but the more recent development of an oral formation of pimonidazole, with its good tolerability, easy administration, and patient acceptability, has facilitated completion of clinical trials characterizing hypoxia.

Endogenous proteins that are upregulated under hypoxia can function as intrinsic markers of hypoxia. These include hypoxia-inducible factor-1α (HIF1α), glucose transporter-1 (GLUT-1), carbonic anhydrase-9 (CA-9), and osteopontin (OPN). Most of these biomarkers belong to the HIF1α-signaling network and therefore have an inverse relationship with oxygenation status, as detailed in Section 12.4.2. Endogenous markers can be assayed at either the transcriptome or proteome level in previously stored tumor samples, giving them an advantage over exogenous markers requiring prospective administration. Although transcriptome analyses of cell lysates can provide global measures of (gene) expression, antibody-based immunohistochemistry (IHC) applied to histologic sections allows evaluation of microregional variability, similar to the analysis of exogenous markers. A limitation of endogenous markers is that their interpretation may be confounded, either because of protein upregulation related to procedure-related hypoxia that leads to overestimates of the extent of hypoxia or because of degradation of labile markers (such as HIF-1) during tumor sampling/processing that leads to an underestimation of tumor hypoxia. Also, oxygen-independent, oncogene-mediated mechanisms of activation of HIF1α and related pathways can lead to imperfect correlation of these markers with hypoxia (Vaupel and Mayer, 2016).

Several gene expression signatures have been developed from analyses of both tumor samples and lysates of cancer cells exposed to hypoxia; different signatures share many similarities, including a correlation with patient outcome, but different signatures may be required for different tumor types. Some of the common genes included in hypoxia signatures include metabolic enzymes (phosphoglycerate kinase I [PGK1], PDK1, aldolase C [ALDOC]), markers of angiogenesis (angiopoietin-like 4 [ANGPTL4], chemo/cytokines [lysyl oxidase], TNF), and membrane transporters (solute carrier family 2 [SLC2A1] (Harris et al, 2015).

Functional imaging techniques such as PET (with hypoxia tracers like [^{18}F]-misonidazole or [^{18}F]-fluoroazomycinarabinofuranoside ([^{18}F]FAZA)) have the potential to provide information noninvasively about hypoxia in multiple human tumor deposits while circumventing sampling error related to core biopsies (see Chap. 14, Sec. 14.3.3). Unfortunately, PET imaging of hypoxia has been limited by its relatively low level of resolution, which is related primarily to radiotracer properties. Methods to analyze PET scans have been extrapolated from those used with other tracers with very different uptake properties and are likely not optimal for radiolabeled hypoxia tracers. As an illustration, although one study of 10 pancreatic cancer patients concluded that there was minimal uptake of the hypoxia tracer FMISO (based on analysis by SUV_{max}) (Segard et al, 2013), alternative thresholding techniques applied to analyze FAZA scans in a similar patient population demonstrated a wide range of hypoxic fraction (0% to 60%) in tumors that aligned with preliminary results from pimonidazole analysis by IHC (Metran-Nascente et al, 2016).

12.4.2 The Hypoxic Response

The cellular response to hypoxia is mediated primarily by a family of transcription factors aptly named the *hypoxia-inducible factors* (HIFs). These transcription factors are obligate heterodimer complexes, consisting of O_2-labile α-subunits and stable β-subunits. Three unique HIFα isoforms have been identified in mammalian cells including HIF1α, HIF2α, and HIF3α, with HIF1α being considered the "master regulator" of oxygen homeostasis. Although HIF1α and HIF2α (also referred to as endothelial PAS protein 1 or EPAS1) share similarities in structure and some functions, HIF3α (or IPAS), which exists as many splice variants, appears to function as a dominant-negative HIF subunit, attenuating HIF1α and HIF2α activity. Although HIF1α is expressed by all cell types, both HIF2α and HIF3α have more selective distribution limited to vascular endothelial cells, cells of myeloid lineage, type II pneumocytes, and renal interstitial cells among others (Pugh, 2016).

There is less sequence homology between the HIF1α and HIF2α transactivating domains than the DNA-binding and heterodimerization domains, which suggests that the 2 isoforms have distinct target genes; many HIF2-binding sites appear to be outside of promoter regions. HIF1 appears to mediate the acute response to hypoxia, whereas HIF2 stabilizes over longer time frames and also remains active under aerobic conditions (Löfstedt et al, 2007).

12.4.2.1 Oxygen-Dependent Mechanisms The principal mechanism by which oxygen regulates HIF activity is through proline and asparagine hydroxylation. Oxygen-dependent regulation of HIFα subunits is mediated by N-terminal transactivation domains, referred to as the *oxygen-dependent degradation domains* (ODD). At normal oxygen tension, hydroxylation at 2 distinct and highly conserved proline residues (Pro^{402} and Pro^{564} in HIF1α) target the molecules for proteasomal degradation by an E3 ubiquitin ligase (Fig. 12–16).

Additional oxygen-dependent regulation is related to activity of another enzyme, factor inhibiting HIF (FIH) (Masoud and Li, 2015; Pugh, 2016). Hydroxylation of an asparagine residue (Asn^{803} in HIF1α) by FIH blocks recruitment of the coactivator p300/CBP. This hydroxylation reaction requires both oxygen and α-ketoglutarate as substrates, and their non-availability inhibits activity of FIH, serving to stabilize HIF1α and increase its transcriptional activity (Masoud and Li, 2015). Therefore, even in the presence of adequate tissue oxygen, certain oncogenic mutations can result in an imbalance of cellular metabolites and stabilization of HIF1α.

12.4.2.2 Hypoxic Mechanisms The limitation of oxygen availability in normal cells causes reduced protein synthesis and cellular proliferation and leads ultimately to cell death via apoptosis or necrosis. However, tumor cell populations are able to initiate or upregulate adaptive responses to hypoxia, leading to modifications in metabolic, bioenergetic, and redox demands to align with oxygen supply. Such cells develop the capacity to survive and thrive under hypoxia, thereby promoting tumor progression in the face of hostile environmental conditions.

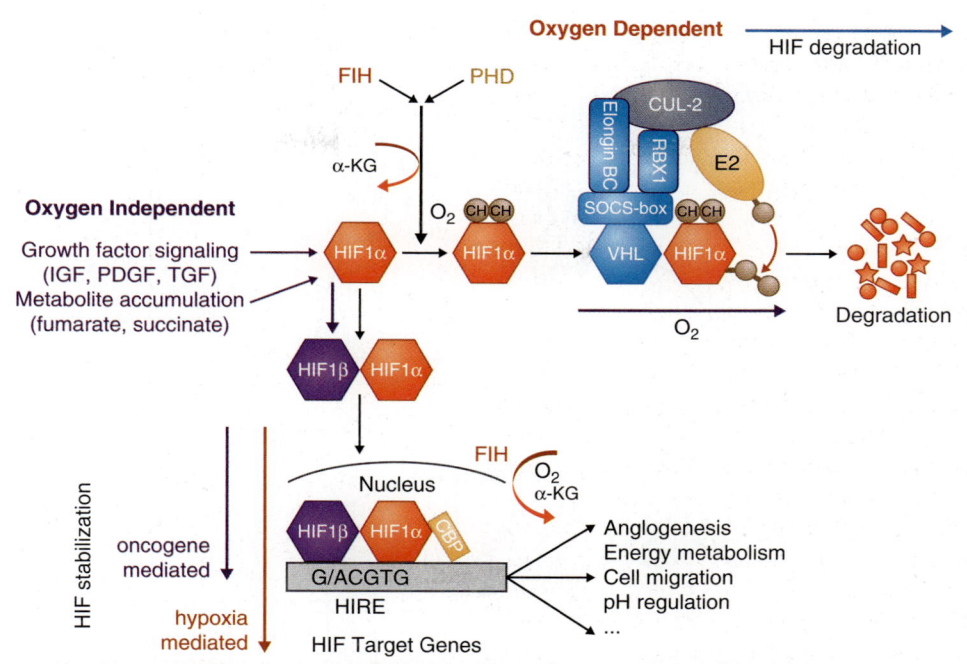

FIGURE 12–16 **HIF activity is regulated by both oxygen dependent and independent mechanisms.** Under aerobic conditions, HIF1α is hydroxylated on 2 proline residues in an oxygen-dependent reaction by one of the 3 HIF prolyl hydroxylases (HIF-PH enzymes). Hydroxylation leads to its recognition by the von Hippel-Lindau (VHL) protein, which subsequently mediates its ubiquitination by the Elongin B/C-CUL2-RBX1 complex and an E2 ubiquitin ligase. Ubiquitinated HIF1α is then degraded in the proteasome. Independent of oxygen tension, aberrant VHL activity, growth factor signaling, or the accumulation of cellular metabolites may also lead to increased levels of HIF1α. Accumulated HIF1α forms a heterodimer with HIF1β, which then translocates into the nucleus to activate HIF target genes (together with CBP) that contain a HIF consensus-binding sequence in their promoter (the hypoxia responses element). Another aspect of oxygen-dependent HIF regulation involves the activity of FIH (factor inhibiting HIF) which prevents recruitment of CBP and the activity of which is dependent on both oxygen and α-ketoglutarate (α-KG). HIF target genes encode miRNAs (eg, miR-210) and other transcription factors (eg, Twist) that themselves mediate other changes in gene expression. Affected genes promote numerous biologic changes that promote change in metabolism and angiogenesis.

Hypoxic conditions lead to increased levels of HIF1α. HIF1α molecules can then heterodimerize with constitutively active HIF1β (also referred to as aryl hydrocarbon receptor nuclear translocator [ARNT]), and the dimer then recognizes and binds hypoxia response elements (HREs) containing the consensus sequence 5'-G/ACGTG-3' (Fig. 12–16). This element is present across a wide range of genes – the number of direct HIF target genes is greater than 800 (ie, at least 1 of every 30 human genes). There is variability in HRE occupancy and hypoxic gene induction from high for HIF1α-upregulated genes to low for HIF2α-induced and HIF-repressed genes, where additional regulatory elements add specificity to target gene regulation. HIFs also modulate gene expression indirectly through transactivation of genes encoding microRNAs and chromatin-modifying enzymes (Crosby et al, 2009).

In some contexts, the "hypoxia-response" program can be activated irrespective of cellular oxygen tension. An example is the presence of VHL devoid of ubiquitin ligase activity or complete absence of the protein, both of which are associated with nuclear accumulation of HIF-1α and transcriptional activation similar to the hypoxia response (Maxwell et al, 1999). Signaling through receptors of growth factors such as insulin growth factor (IGF), PDGF, epidermal growth factor (EGF) and transforming growth factors (TGF-α and TGF-β) can act to increase expression of HIF1α through activation of phosphatidylinositol 3-kinase (PI3K) and mitogen-activated protein kinase (MAPK) pathways (see Chap. 6; Sec. 6.2), leading to increased HIF1α mRNA synthesis that exceeds the inhibitory activity of the hydroxylases (Agani and Jiang, 2013). Oncogenic activating mutations in the PI3K pathway through KRAS, HER2, EGFR, etc. as well as inactivating mutations in negative regulators of these pathways, such as PTEN, may lead to HIF1α accumulation. In addition, mTOR and the unfolded protein response (UPR) have critical roles in adaptation to hypoxia through modulation of protein translation and cellular metabolism that are HIF independent (Fig. 12–17; Wouters and Koritzinsky, 2008).

HIF activity can also be influenced by the levels of cellular metabolites. Increased cellular levels of fumarate and succinate inhibit activity of the oxygen-sensing prolyl-4-hydroxylases (PHDs), leading to modulation of HIF1α expression. Also, some cancers with a mutation in IDH1, have elevated levels of HIF1α (see Sec. 12.3.5). A possible mechanism is decreased levels of α-ketoglutarate, a direct substrate of PHDs, with IDH1 mutations thereby leading to indirect stabilization of HIF1α, but studies have been inconsistent with observation of similar levels of α-ketoglutarate in IDH1-mutant and wild-type cancers. There are, however, elevated levels of 2-hydroxyglutarate (2-HG) in IDH1 mutant cancers, but whether there is a link between 2-HG and HIF activity in these cancers remains unknown (Majmundar et al, 2010).

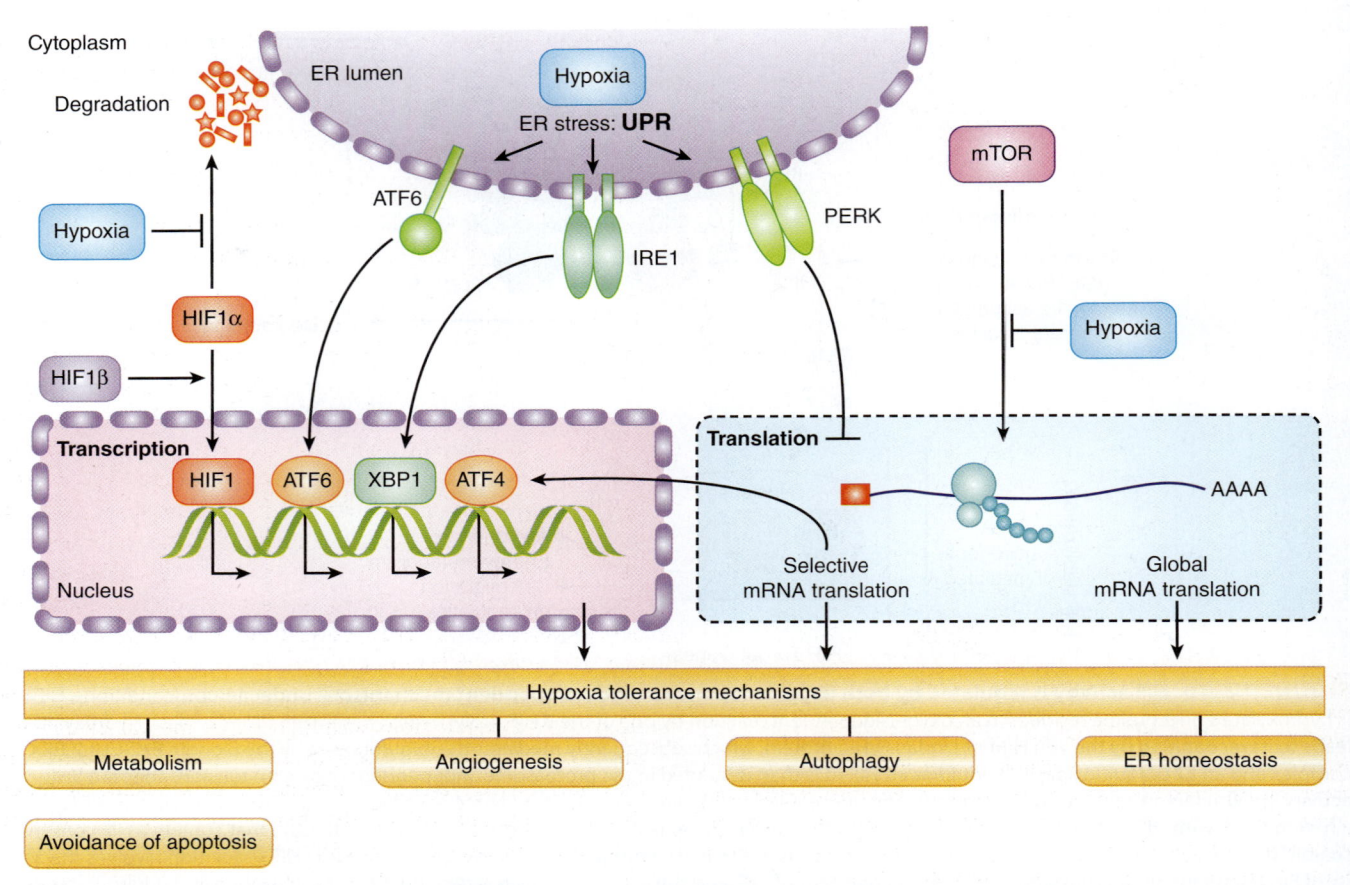

FIGURE 12–17 Cell signaling response to hypoxia. Hypoxia results in the activation of HIF and the unfolded protein response (UPR), as well as inhibition of mammalian target of rapamycin (mTOR). These distinct oxygen-sensitive signaling pathways promote adaption to hypoxic stress through a multitude of downstream effectors that influence cellular metabolism, autophagy, endoplasmic reticulum (ER) stress, and angiogenesis. The UPR consists of 3 signaling arms initiated by PERK, IRE1, and ATF6. Each of these arms results in the activation of a different transcription factor (ATF4, XBP1, and ATF6), which collectively function to prevent and mitigate the consequences of ER stress. These 3 pathways can also influence cellular phenotypes in ways that promote malignancy through increased invasion and metastasis

Most of the responses to hypoxia occur through HIF-dependent molecular mechanisms, and they impact on nearly all hallmarks of tumor progression, including cell proliferation and cell death, metabolic reprogramming, angiogenesis, invasion and metastasis, immune evasion, and treatment resistance (Fig. 12–17; LaGory and Giaccia, 2016).

12.4.2.3 Cell Proliferation and Survival

Chronic hypoxia is associated with restricted cellular differentiation, decreased proliferation, and increased apoptosis (Fig. 12–18). These effects of hypoxia on cell proliferation and apoptosis (and survival) are mediated primarily by TP53 and BCL-2. Consequently, malignant cells with reduced apoptotic capacity related to aberrant TP53 function may have a survival/growth advantage under hypoxic conditions. Mechanistic studies have demonstrated physical interactions between HIF1α and p53 leading to stabilization of p53 and increased apoptosis. This interaction is partly mediated by MDM2. Although HIF1α can increase p53 levels (through MDM2-mediated degradation), HIF2α has been demonstrated to have opposing effects, leading to reduced p53 levels (Amelio and Melino, 2015).

HIFs may also influence cellular proliferation through effects on c-MYC. Although HIF1α has been demonstrated to inhibit c-MYC transcription and promote degradation (thereby leading to decreased cellular proliferation), HIF2α may have opposite effects, leading to enhanced c-MYC activity. The decreased proliferative rate of malignant cells in hypoxic niches is well described and represents a potential cause of treatment failure because of their resistance to standard cytotoxic treatments, while hypoxia per se leads to resistance to radiation (see Sec. 12.4.3, Chap. 16, Sec. 16.4, and Chap. 18, Sec. 18.4.7.2).

Cellular stresses such as hypoxia and/or nutrient deprivation lead to an increased reliance on autophagy. This not only serves a protective function by preventing the accumulation of malfunctioning organelles (such as mitochondria) but also supplies metabolites to allow ongoing cell growth (see Sec. 12.3.6). HIF1 is directly involved in regulation of autophagy through BNIP3, BNIP3I, and Beclin-1 (Rouschop and Wouters, 2009).

12.4.2.4 Metabolic Reprogramming

Hypoxia promotes a shift in glucose metabolism from mitochondrial oxidative

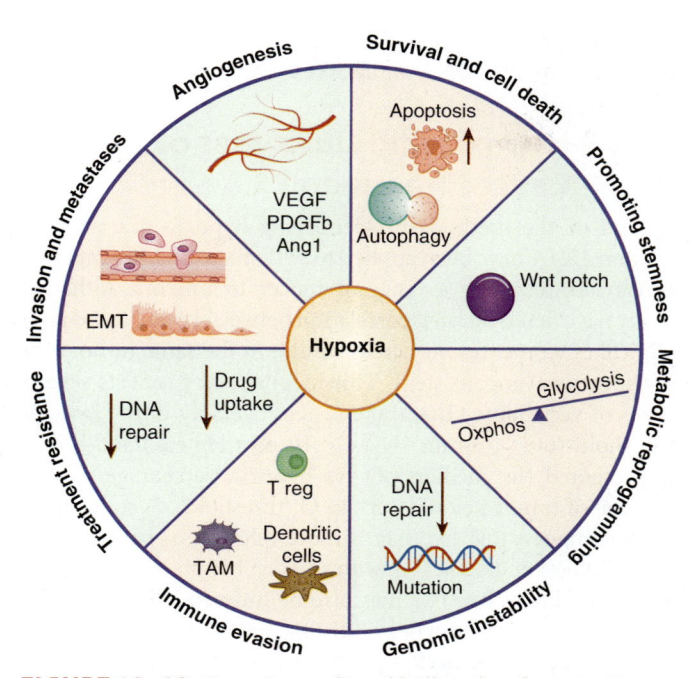

FIGURE 12–18 Hypoxia-mediated hallmarks of cancer. The hallmarks of cancer define a number of biological processes that are critical to the malignant phenotype. The cellular response to hypoxia is recognized to be mediated through many of these same mechanisms. This schematic summarizes the influence of hypoxia on some of these processes, which ultimately serves to promote a more aggressive malignant behavior. *Ang 1*, Angiopoietin 1; *EMT*, epithelial-mesenchymal transition; *oxphos*, oxidative phosphorylation; *PDGF*, platelet-derived growth factor; *TAM*, tumor-associated macrophages; *VEGF*, vascular endothelial growth factor.

phosphorylation to cytoplasmic glycolysis (Fig. 12–18). This increased glycolytic activity is a consequence of HIF1α-mediated upregulation of glucose transporters (GLUT1, GLUT3) promoting cellular uptake of glucose, and glycolytic enzymes (hexokinase, aldolase, enolase, lactic dehydrogenase, etc) to facilitate the conversion of glucose into lactic acid. Simultaneously, HIF1 suppresses mitochondrial oxidative metabolism through increased expression of pyruvate dehydrogenase kinase 1 (PDK1), inactivating pyruvate dehydrogenase (PHD) to decrease levels of acetyl-Co-A available for entry into the TCA cycle. The correlation of glycolytic activity with hypoxia is imperfect, because glycolysis also takes place in the aerobic regions of tumors (Sec. 12.3.1) (Schito and Rey, 2018).

12.4.2.5 Angiogenesis
The development of hypoxia within an early tumor mass is often the precipitating trigger of the so-called angiogenic switch (see Chap. 11, Sec. 11.5.4). Several angiogenic factors including VEGF, basic fibroblast growth factor (bFGF), and PDGF are regulated by hypoxia, and their upregulation increases access of the tumor to oxygen and nutrients by promoting angiogenesis (Fig. 12–18).

12.4.2.6 Invasion and Metastasis
Both hypoxia and HIF signaling influence several steps of the metastatic cascade, and acute hypoxia can stimulate metastasis (Cairns and Hill, 2004). A number of transcription factors involving epithelial-mesenchymal transition and increased cellular motility (including ZEB1, and SNA1) have hypoxia response elements (HREs) in their respective promoters, and are hypoxia-regulated. HIF signaling in the primary tumor also functions to condition pre-metastatic niches, thereby facilitating "metastatic homing" of malignant cells (Rankin and Giaccia, 2016).

12.4.2.7 Cancer Stem Cells
Evidence for (and against) the presence of cancer stem cells has been presented in Chap. 13, Sec. 13.3.2. The cancer stem cell hypothesis argues that a subpopulation of malignant cells within a tumor is capable of self-renewal and that these cells are responsible for tumor regrowth after treatment. These cells are hypothesized to be an important source of treatment failure since they tend to be slowly proliferative and may be relatively insensitive to the cytotoxic effects of radiotherapy and chemotherapy. The observation that normal stem cells (and in particular hematopoietic stem cells) reside in bone marrow, a relatively hypoxic microenvironment, has led to the hypothesis that hypoxic regions within tumors might serve as niches for cancer stem cell subpopulations although experimental evidence is limited. The process of EMT, itself under hypoxic regulation, may also be relevant in maintenance of so-called stemness through upregulation of the hypoxia-dependent pathways (Marie-Egyptienne et al, 2013).

12.4.2.8 The Immune Response
Intratumor hypoxia modulates the tumor immune response in a variety of ways, overall promoting an immunosuppressive and immune-tolerant environment (Fig. 12–18; Krzywinska and Stockmann, 2018; Li et al, 2018). Hypoxic regions within tumors are often found to be disproportionately infiltrated by immunosuppressive cells including tumor-associated macrophages (TAMs), myeloid-derived suppressor cells (MDSCs), and T-regulatory cells (T-regs). There is crosstalk among these immune-derived cells as well as with tumor cells and other supportive cells within the stroma, and these dynamic relationships lead to modulation of the tumor-immune response.

TAMs, recruited initially into hypoxic tumor regions in response to CSF1 and VEGF, may undergo conversion into highly immunosuppressive, M2 macrophages based on the activity of cytokines like IL-4 and IL-10 (see Sec. 12.2.1.2). TAMs in hypoxic tumor regions also upregulate expression of matrix metalloproteinase 7 (MMP7), rendering tumor cells less responsive to lysis by natural killer (NK) and T cells.

MDSCs, which accumulate in tumors as a consequence of tumor-derived secreted factors like GM-CSF, VEGF, and prostaglandins, induce T-cell anergy through restraining the effector phase of CD8+ T cells and promoting T-reg proliferation (see also Chap. 21, Sec. 21.3). HIF1α-related production of arginase and nitric oxide by MDSCs leads to further increases in immunosuppressive effects, and hypoxia itself increases expression of PD-L1 on MDSCs, thereby increasing T-cell tolerance (Noman et al, 2015).

Hypoxia acts also to divert dendritic cells, the dominant antigen-presenting cell responsible for activation of resting T cells (see Chap. 21, Sec. 21.2), away from their primary function through inhibition of differentiation and increased expression of PD-L1. These effects are modulated in part by hypoxia-induced factors such as VEGF and IL-10. The impact of hypoxia on the activity of CD8+ cytotoxic T cells (CTLs) is unclear because although hypoxic stress appears to delay development of CD8+ cells, other studies demonstrate that hypoxia may increase the cytolytic capacity of already developed CTLs. The effect of hypoxia on CD4+ cells is better described—as hypoxia-induced TGF-β production appears to cause CD4+ cells to upregulate FOXP3 expression, thereby inducing T-reg formation (Noman et al, 2015).

12.4.2.9 Genomic Instability Changes in oxygen tension in tumors can promote dynamic changes in gene expression, leading to transient alterations in cellular behavior, whereas severe hypoxia can cause more persistent genomic instability. Decreased oxygen levels reduce transcription of several genes, including some encoding proteins involved in DNA repair, including RAD51/52 and BRCA1/2 (involved in homologous recombination [HR]), KU70 and DNA-PKcs (important in nonhomologous end joining [NHEJ]) and mismatch repair (MMR) proteins MLH1, MSH6, MSH2, and PMS2 (see Chap. 9, Sec. 9.3). Several miRNAs (including miR-210 and miR-373) are upregulated by hypoxia, in turn leading to downregulation of various DNA repair pathway mediators. Defective activity of DNA repair proteins increases the frequency of persistent DNA breaks and replication errors, leading to increased genomic variants, which further accelerates genetic instability. Further, transient interruptions in blood flow lead to regions of acute hypoxia that then become reoxygenated when blood flow resumes. This leads to sudden influxes of free radicals promoting further DNA damage (Luoto et al, 2013).

12.4.3 Hypoxia and Outcomes of Cancer Treatment

Several of the methods of identifying hypoxia described in Section 12.4.1 have been applied to patients with different types of cancers receiving a range of cancer treatments. Although many have demonstrated correlation between hypoxia and poor clinical outcome, results across studies in the same tumor type are somewhat inconsistent. This inconsistency reflects several types of variability. First, there is heterogeneity in the hypoxia threshold (pO_2 < 5 mm Hg vs. < 10 mm Hg etc.) and how it is presented (ie, median pO_2 vs hypoxic percentage vs percentage of tumor below a certain O_2 threshold). Second, some studies suggest that hypoxia is more relevant in patients with earlier stages of disease (eg, with smaller, lymph node–negative tumors). Finally, hypoxia may also be differentially relevant to certain molecular subtypes of disease (eg, depending on HPV status in head and neck squamous cell cancers). Table 12–3 summarizes a few of the studies that have tried to characterize the clinical relevance of hypoxia in select tumor types. Comprehensive reviews are available which describe a wider range of studies (Table 12–3, Tharmalingham and Hoskin, 2018)).

Multiple molecular mechanisms have been implicated in hypoxia-mediated resistance to treatment (Dhani, Fyles et al, 2015). Initial observations supported the hypothesis that hypoxia caused radio-resistance based on recognition that the cytotoxicity of radiotherapy is reliant on oxygen. Cells irradiated in the presence of oxygen are about 3 times more sensitive than cells irradiated under conditions of severe hypoxia (see Chap. 16, Sec. 16.4.1, and Fig. 16–10). The primary mechanism

TABLE 12–3 Presence and relevance of tumor hypoxia in selected human cancers.

Tumor Type	Hypoxia Evaluation	Outcome (With Greater Hypoxia)	Reference
Head and neck	Eppendorf probe	Higher levels of severe hypoxia (pO_2 ≤2.5 mm Hg) associated with poor survival after primary therapy	Nordsmark et al, 2005
	PET hypoxia imaging	Higher hypoxic volume (FAZA-PET) correlated with inferior disease-free survival	Mortensen et al, 2012
		Persistent hypoxia in tumors during radiotherapy predicted for local failure (FMISO-PET)	Zips et al, 2012
	Gene expression signature	Hypoxia predictive for treatment failure in HPV-negative tumors	Linge et al, 2016
Cervix	Eppendorf probe	High levels of hypoxia (defined as % of tumor with pO_2 < 5 mm Hg) correlated with poor PFS in patients with node-negative tumors treated with radiotherapy	Fyles et al, 2002
	HIF1α (tumor) Eppendorf probe and pimonidazole	Weak correlation between HIF1α and median (Eppendorf) pO_2 and pimonidazole. HIF1α not prognostic for outcome after radiotherapy. May be an interaction with tumor size (relevant in smaller tumors)	Hutchison et al, 2004
	Eppendorf probe and pimonidazole	No correlation of hypoxia with loco-regional control or overall survival in patients receiving variety of treatments (surgery, [chemo]-radiotherapy)	Nordsmark et al, 2006
Bladder	Gene expression signature	Hypoxia predicted for worse outcome after surgery. Also predictive of response from hypoxia-directed therapy (carbogen/nicotinamide)	Yang et al, 2017
Prostate		Hypoxia correlated with higher rates of recurrence and metastasis after surgery/radiotherapy	Yang et al, 2018

FAZA, fluoroazomycin arabinoside; *FETNIM*, fluoroerythronitroimidazole; *PET*, positron emission tomography; *PFS*, progression-free survival.

(called the *oxygen fixation hypothesis*) is that oxygen interacts with (secondary) radicals on cellular molecules such as DNA, formed by their interaction with the (primary) hydroxyl radicals produced by radiation effects on water in the cell. As described in Chapter 16, this process can have a profound effect on the outcome of clinical treatment with radiotherapy; such effects provide indirect evidence that hypoxic cells in human tumors are viable and capable of regenerating a tumor. These same mechanisms are also important in the resistance of hypoxic cells to some types of chemotherapy. However, the presence of substantial hypoxia in tumors also predicts poor outcome after surgery, indicating that hypoxia is a general marker of aggressive disease (Dhani, Serra et al, 2015).

Chronically hypoxic cells within a tumor are situated far from patent blood vessels and are slowly-proliferating; these properties can lead to the resistance of these cells to drug treatment and especially to chemotherapy (see Chap. 18, Sec. 18.4.7). Malignant cells in hypoxic regions distant from functional blood vessels have a low level of exposure to most drugs, which diffuse from blood vessels and may be consumed or bound by intervening cells. Anthracyclines and taxanes are particularly compromised by this mechanism because of high rates of binding to cells closer to blood vessels, and slowly-proliferating cells are less responsive to these drugs. The low proliferation rates of hypoxic cells also affect the efficacy of some targeted agents, since the activity of many of them is also cell cycle dependent.

Cellular drug uptake may also be affected by the relatively low pH of the extracellular environment of hypoxic regions. Although basic drugs like doxorubicin have lower levels of uptake by cells in hypoxic regions, the uptake of acidic drugs like chlorambucil might be higher.

Functional defects in DNA repair induced by hypoxia might also affect the cytotoxic effects of some agents. Although hypoxia-induced downregulation of MMR (mismatch repair) genes might increase resistance to DNA-methylating agents, downregulation of NER-mediated DNA repair might increase sensitivity to platinum drugs (Shannon et al, 2003).

12.4.4 Targeting Hypoxia to Improve Treatment

The evidence that hypoxia is associated with adverse clinical outcome, and recognition that hypoxic cells are resistant to ionizing radiation and various drug treatments, provides justification for current attempts to target hypoxia as a component of anticancer treatment. Strategies that target hypoxia can be considered in four broad categories: (1) the improvement of tumor oxygenation (primarily through increasing oxygen delivery); (2) the enhancement of radiation effects through the use of hypoxic cell sensitizers; (3) hypoxia-activated prodrugs; and (4) approaches that target hypoxia-mediated molecular processes (Wilson and Hay, 2011).

12.4.4.1 Increasing Oxygen Delivery As described in Chapter 16, Section 16.4.4, there is evidence that factors that contribute to impaired delivery of oxygen to tumors, such as anemia or smoking, are associated with poor outcomes after radiotherapy. These observations led to studies to improve tumor oxygen delivery through blood transfusions, exposure to hyperbaric oxygen, or the administration of exogenous erythropoietin; some strategies have provided clinical benefit but their results have been inconsistent and they have not been widely adopted. An alternative strategy to increase tumor oxygen levels has been to decrease oxygen consumption using drugs such as metformin, but this agent has multiple effects and there are no rigorous demonstrations of benefit.

12.4.4.2 Hypoxic Cell Radiosensitizers The development and clinical use of drugs that mimic the radiosensitizing properties of oxygen are described in Chapter 16, Section 16.4.4.2. Most of these drugs are nitroimidazoles, such as misonidazole, which bind to DNA under hypoxic conditions. Results of clinical trials using misonidazole were disappointing but clinical trials using the less-toxic drug, nimorazole, have shown improved tumor control in head and neck cancer (Overgaard, 2011). Also, a meta-analysis of results for patients with head and neck cancer treated in randomized trials, using radiotherapy with hyperbaric oxygen or hypoxic cell sensitizers, indicated a small but significant improvement in local control and survival, especially if there had been selection of patients with high levels of hypoxia in their tumors (Lin and Maity, 2015).

12.4.4.3 Hypoxia-Activated Prodrugs These drugs (HAPs) are inactive under aerobic conditions, but undergo hypoxia-mediated reduction into an active metabolite with cytotoxic properties (see also Chap. 18, Sec. 18.4.7). Five discrete chemical groups (nitro groups, quinones, aromatic N-oxides, aliphatic N-oxides, and transition metals) can undergo enzymatic reduction under hypoxia—thereby providing the potential for selective cytotoxicity for hypoxic cells. The nitroaromatics, quinones, and benzotriane dioxides undergo a one-electron reduction step to yield a prodrug radical that undergoes reoxidation in a futile redox cycle. Under hypoxia, the prodrug radical either undergoes fragmentation or a second reduction step to produce the active drug. The aliphatic N-oxides such as N-oxide banoxantrone (AQ4N) are activated by 2-electron reduction catalyzed primarily by CYP isozymes. The oxygen sensitivity is conferred by the competitive oxygenation of reducing centers in the CYP catalytic cycle. These activated effector moieties may diffuse out of hypoxic zones to adjacent moderately or well-oxygenated tumor regions and induce cytotoxicity; this non–cell autonomous effect of killing surrounding cells is termed the *bystander effect*.

The 2 HAPs that have progressed furthest in development thus far are tirapazamine and evofosfamide (also known as TH-302). Unfortunately, in spite of positive preclinical data and promising efficacy in small, early-phase trials, robust clinical activity has not been confirmed in larger controlled studies. One criticism of these studies has been the lack of enrichment or stratification for tumor hypoxia, supported by observations from subgroup analyses of larger studies demonstrating clinical benefit of tirapazamine in head and neck patients with detectable hypoxia in their tumors. The negative clinical experience has decreased enthusiasm for clinical development of HAPS, although the concept continues to have therapeutic potential. It is important that patients should be selected for inclusion in future trials based on having hypoxic tumors (Hunter et al, 2016).

12.4.4.4 Targeting the Hypoxic Molecular Response

The characterization of molecular mechanisms mediating cellular response to hypoxia has led to interest in developing compounds that inhibit these pathways. A primary focus has been compounds that inhibit HIF signaling. The recognition of oncogene-mediated, hypoxia-independent mechanisms of HIF activation suggests that HIF inhibitors might be relevant to broad subgroups of patients. Several cytotoxics and molecular targeted agents already in clinical use may owe some of their anticancer activity to hypoxia targeting; the topoisomerase I inhibitors irinotecan and topotecan, and various PI3K/AKT/mTOR inhibitors all inhibit HIF1α translation. Further, several "old" drugs have been repurposed as HIF "inhibitors"—drugs like geldanamycin and some proteasome inhibitors have been demonstrated to increase HIF degradation. Direct inhibitors of HIF are also in development (Fallah and Rini, 2019).

SUMMARY

- The growth of tumors is dependent on the rate of proliferation and of death of the cells within them. In many human tumors, the rate of cell production is only slightly higher than the rate of cell death, and many cells may not be actively cycling, so that the median doubling time of tumors (typically about 2 months for common human solid tumors) is much longer than the cell-cycle time of the proliferating tumor cells (typically about 2-3 days).
- Factors that influence the rates of proliferation and cell death in tumors include nutrient molecules in the microenvironment, which, in turn, depend on angiogenesis and the expansion of the vascular network of the tumor, and the molecular signals that are influenced by endogenous and exogenous factors.
- Tumor cells grow within a unique microenvironment characterized by deficiencies in vasculature and nutrient supply. These properties result in heterogeneous regions where tumor cells are exposed to variable levels of nutrients and waste products of metabolism, with high interstitial fluid pressure and regions of low pH and hypoxia. Each of these features can influence tumor biology and tumor response to treatment in adverse ways.
- The tumor microenvironment (TME) includes supportive cells (such as fibroblasts, endothelial cells, and immune-derived cells) matrix components and environmental features (including pH, fluid pressure, and oxygenation status) of a tumor.
- Metabolic alterations in tumors help to balance 3 critical requirements of proliferating cells: supply of energy in the form of ATP; supply of macromolecular building blocks for cell growth and division; and maintenance of redox homeostasis. Tumors use commonly glycolysis for producing energy in the form of ATP; although less efficient than oxidative phosphorylation, glycolysis can utilize glucose more rapidly, and metabolic intermediates feed various biosynthetic pathways.
- Autophagy is a mechanism that facilitates cell survival in the adverse microenvironment of solid tumors. Autophagy functions to degrade cytoplasmic components to provide essential products for sustaining cellular metabolism and energy homeostasis. This function is particularly important within hypoxic regions of solid tumors where maintaining energy homeostasis becomes critical for cell survival.
- Hypoxia is a near universal and heterogeneous feature of human tumors, although its extent varies widely. Tumor hypoxia leads to a series of biological changes that can promote enhanced malignancy primarily through the action of HIF transcription factors driving several oxygen-sensitive signaling pathways.
- The cellular response to hypoxia promotes metabolic reprogramming, genomic instability, avoidance of cell death and increased survival, enhanced motility, invasion and angiogenesis, and immune evasion.
- Although high levels of hypoxia are correlated with inferior patient outcomes, a robust clinical impact from targeting hypoxia has not been realized.

ACKNOWLEDGMENT

The authors thank Dr. Julie St-Pierre, Department of Biochemistry, Microbiology and Immunology, University of Ottawa, for her constructive comments on an earlier version of this chapter.

REFERENCES

Agani F, Jiang BH. Oxygen-independent regulation of HIF-1: novel involvement of PI3K/AKT/mTOR pathway in cancer. *Curr Canc Drug Targets* 2013;13(3):245-251.

Aguado BA, Bushnell GG, Rao SS, Jeruss JS, Shea LD. Engineering the pre-metastatic niche. *Nat Biomed Eng* 2017; 1(pii):0077.

Allavena P, Mantovani A. Immunology in the clinic review series; focus on cancer: tumour-associated macrophages: undisputed stars of the inflammatory tumour microenvironment. *Clin Exp Immunol* 2012;167(2):195-205.

Amaravadi R, Kimmelman AC, White E. Recent insights into the function of autophagy in cancer. *Genes Dev* 2016;30(17):1913-1930.

Amelio I, Melino G. The p53 family and the hypoxia-inducible factors (HIFs): determinants of cancer progression. *Trends Biochem Sci* 2015;40(8):425-434.

Andrzejewski S, Klimcakova E, Johnson RM, et al. PGC-1α promotes breast cancer metastasis and confers bioenergetic flexibility against metabolic drugs. *Cell Metab* 2017;26(5):778-787.

Bajaj A, Driver JA, Schernhammer ES. Parkinson's disease and cancer risk: a systematic review and meta-analysis. *Cancer Causes Control* 2010;21(5):697-707.

Baulida J. Epithelial-to-mesenchymal transition transcription factors in cancer-associated fibroblasts. *Mol Oncol* 2017;11(7):847-859.

Bayer C, Shi K, Astner ST, Maftei CA, Vaupel P. Acute versus chronic hypoxia: why a simplified classification is simply not enough. *Int J Radiat Oncol Biol Phys* 2011;80(4):965-968.

Binnewies M, Roberts EW, Kersten K et al. Understanding the tumour immune micro-environment (TIME) for effective therapy. *Nat Med* 2018;24(5):541-550.

Bost F, Kaminski L. The metabolic modulator PGC-1α in cancer. *Am J Cancer Res* 2019;9(2):198-211.

Cairns RA, Hill RP. Acute hypoxia enhances spontaneous lymph node metastasis in an orthotopic murine model of human cervical carcinoma. *Cancer Res* 2004;64(6):2054-2061.

Chen W, Sun Z, Wang XJ, et al. Direct interaction between Nrf2 and p21(Cip1/WAF1) upregulates the Nrf2-mediated antioxidant response. *Mol Cell* 2009;34:663-673.

Choi MR, Solid CA, Chia VM, et al. Granulocyte colony-stimulating factor (G-CSF) patterns of use in cancer patients receiving myelosuppressive chemotherapy. *Support Care Cancer* 2014;22(6):1619-1628.

Christofk HR, Vander Heiden MG, Harris MH, et al. The M2 splice isoform of pyruvate kinase is important for cancer metabolism and tumour growth. *Nature* 2008;452(7184):230-233.

Clements CM, McNally RS, Conti BJ, et al. DJ-1, a cancer- and Parkinson's disease-associated protein, stabilizes the antioxidant transcriptional master regulator Nrf2. *Proc Natl Acad Sci U S A* 2006;103(41):15091-15096.

Corbet C, Feron O. Tumour acidosis: from the passenger to the driver's seat. *Nat Rev Cancer* 2017;17(10):577-593.

Crosby ME, Devlin CM, Glazer PM, Calin GA, Ivan M. Emerging roles of microRNAs in the molecular responses to hypoxia. *Curr Pharm Des* 2009;15(33):3861-3866.

Dang CV, Kim JW, Gao P, et al. The interplay between MYC and in cancer HIF. *Nat Rev Cancer* 2008;8(1):51-56.

Dang L, White DW, Gross S, et al. Cancer-associated IDH1 mutations produce 2-hydroxyglutarate. *Nature* 2009;462(7274):739-744.

Darzynkiewicz Z, Traganos F, Zhao H, Halicka HD, Li J. Cytometry of DNA replication and RNA synthesis: historical perspective and recent advances based on "click chemistry." *Cytometry A* 2011;79(5):328-337.

David CJ, Chen M, Assanah M, et al. HnRNP proteins controlled by c-Myc deregulate pyruvate kinase mRNA splicing in cancer. *Nature* 2010;463(7279):364-368.

DeBerardinis RJ, Mancuso A, Daikhin E, et al. Beyond aerobic glycolysis: transformed cells can engage in glutamine metabolism that exceeds the requirement for protein and nucleotide synthesis. *Proc Natl Acad Sci U S A* 2007;104(49):19345-19350.

Dhani N, Fyles A, Hedley D, Milosevic M. The clinical significance of hypoxia in human cancers. *Semin Nucl Med* 2015;45(2):110-121.

Dhani NC, Serra S, Pintilie M, et al. Analysis of the intra- and intertumoral heterogeneity of hypoxia in pancreatic cancer patients receiving the nitroimidazole tracer pimonidazole. *Br J Cancer* 2015;113(6):864-871.

Doulatov S, Notta F, Eppert K, Nguyen LT, Ohashi PS, Dick JE. Revised map of the human progenitor hierarchy shows the origin of macrophages and dendritic cells in early lymphoid development. *Nat Immunol* 2010;11(7):585-593.

Elia I, Doglioni G, Fendt SM. Metabolic hallmarks of metastasis formation. *Trends Cell Biol* 2018;28(8):673-684.

Falllah J, Rini BI. HIF inhibitors: Status of current clinical development. *Curr Oncol Rep* 2019;21(1):6.

Fantin VR, St-Pierre J, Leder P. Attenuation of LDH-A expression uncovers a link between glycolysis, mitochondrial physiology, and tumor maintenance. *Cancer Cell* 2006;9(6):425-434.

Finicle BT, Jayashankar V, Edinger AL. Nutrient scavenging in cancer. *Nat Rev Cancer* 2018;18(10):619-633.

Fre S, Pallavi SK, Huyghe M, et al. Notch and Wnt signals cooperatively control cell proliferation and tumorigenesis in the intestine. *Proc Natl Acad Sci USA* 2009;106(15):6309-6314.

Frezza C, Gottlieb E. Mitochondria in cancer: not just innocent bystanders. *Semin Cancer Biol* 2009;19(1):4-11.

Fukumura D, Duda DG, Munn LL, Jain RK. Tumor microvasculature and microenvironment: novel insights through intravital imaging in pre-clinical models. *Microcirculation* 2010;17(3):206-225.

Funes JM, Quintero M, Henderson S, et al. Transformation of human mesenchymal stem cells increases their dependency on oxidative phosphorylation for energy production. *Proc Natl Acad Sci U S A* 2007;104(15):6223-6228.

Fyles A, Milosevic M, Hedley D, et al. Tumor hypoxia has independent predictor impact only in patients with node-negative cervix cancer. *J Clin Oncol* 2002;20(3):680-687.

Gajewski TF, Schreiber H, Fu YX. Innate and adaptive immune cells in the tumor microenvironment. *Nat Immunol* 2013;14(10):1014-1022.

Gao P, Tchernyshyov I, Chang TC, et al. c-Myc suppression of miR-23a/b enhances mitochondrial glutaminase expression and glutamine metabolism. *Nature* 2009;458(7239):762-765.

Gao P, Zhang H, Dinavahi R, et al. HIF-dependent antitumorigenic effect of antioxidants in vivo. *Cancer Cell* 2007;12(3):230-238.

Gasser T, Müller-Myhsok B, Wszolek ZK, et al. Genetic complexity and Parkinson's disease. *Science* 1997;277(5324):388-389.

Gatenby RA, Gillies RJ. Why do cancers have high aerobic glycolysis? *Nat Rev Cancer* 2004;4(11):891-899.

Gillies RJ, Robey I, Gatenby RA. Causes and consequences of increased glucose metabolism of cancers. *J Nucl Med* 2008;49(suppl 2):24S-42S

Gorrini C, Baniasadi PS, Harris IS, et al. BRCA1 interacts with Nrf2 to regulate antioxidant signaling and cell survival. *J Exp Med* 2013;210(8):1529-1544.

Gross S, Cairns RA, Minden MD, et al. Cancer-associated metabolite 2-hydroxyglutarate accumulates in acute myelogenous leukemia with isocitrate dehydrogenase 1 and 2 mutations. *J Exp Med* 2010;207(2):339-344.

Guertin DA, Sabatini DM. Defining the role of mTOR in cancer. *Cancer Cell* 2007;12(1):9-22.

Hadland BK, Longmore GD. Erythroid-stimulating agents in cancer therapy: potential dangers and biologic mechanisms. *J Clin Oncol* 2009;27(25):4217-4226.

Harper J, Sainson RC. Regulation of the anti-tumour immune response by cancer-associated fibroblasts. *Semin Cancer Biol* 2014;25:69-77.

Harris BHL, Barberis A, West CM et al. Gene expression signatures as biomarkers of tumour hypoxia. *Clin Oncol* 2015;27(10):547-560.

Hedley DW, Shankey VT, Wheeless LL. DNA cytometry consensus conference. *Cytometry* 1993;14(5):471-500.

Heldin C-H, Rubin K, Pietras K, Ostman A. High Interstitial Fluid Pressure—an obstacle to cancer therapy. *Nat Rev Cancer* 2004;4(10):806-813.

Hitchcock IS, Kaushansky K. Thrombopoietin from beginning to end. *Br J Haematol* 2014;165(2):259-268.

Huang M, Liu T, Ma P, et al. c-Met-mediated endothelial plasticity drives aberrant vascularization and chemoresistance in glioblastoma. *J Clin Invest* 2016;126(5):1801-1814.

Hunter FW, Wouters BG, Wilson WR. Hypoxia-activated prodrugs: paths forwarded in the era of personalized medicine. *Br J Cancer* 2016;114(10):1071-1077.

Hutchison GJ, Valentine HR, Loncaster JA, et al. Hypoxia-inducible factor 1alpha expression as an intrinsic marker of hypoxia: correlation with tumor oxygen, pimonidazole measurements, and outcome in locally advanced carcinoma of the cervix. *Clin Cancer Res* 2004;10(24):8405-8412.

Jadvar H, Alavi A, Gambhir SS. ^{18}F-FDG uptake in lung, breast, and colon cancers: molecular biology correlates and disease characterization. *J Nucl Med* 2009;50(11):1820-1827.

Jenne DE, Reimann H, Nezu J, et al. Peutz-Jeghers syndrome is caused by mutations in a novel serine threonine kinase. *Nat Genet* 1998;18(1):38-43.

Kaelin WG Jr. The von Hippel-Lindau tumour suppressor protein: O_2 sensing and cancer. *Nat Rev Cancer* 2008;8(11):865-873.

Kalluri R. The biology and function of fibroblasts in cancer. *Nat Rev Cancer* 2016;16(9):582-598.

Kang N, Shah VH, Urrutia R. Membrane-to-nucleus signals and epigenetic mechanisms for myofibroblastic activation and desmoplastic stroma: potential therapeutic targets for liver metastasis? *Mol Cancer Res* 2015;13(4):604-612.

Keyomarsi K, Tucker SL, Buchholz TA, et al. Cyclin E and survival in patients with breast cancer. *N Engl J Med* 2002;347(20):1566-1575.

Khatri S, Yepiskoposyan H, Gallo CA, et al. FOXO3a regulates glycolysis via transcriptional control of tumor suppressor TSC1. *J Biol Chem* 2010;285(21):15960-15965.

Kim KH, Sederstrom JM. Assaying cell cycle status using flow cytometry. *Curr Protoc Mol Biol* 2015;111:28.6.1-28.6.11.

Kim RH, Peters M, Jang Y, et al. DJ-1, a novel regulator of the tumor suppressor PTEN. *Cancer Cell* 2005;7(3):263-273.

King A, Selak MA, Gottlieb E. Succinate dehydrogenase and fumarate hydratase: linking mitochondrial dysfunction and cancer. *Oncogene* 2006;25(34):4675-4682.

Koritzinsky M, Wouters BG. The roles of reactive oxygen species and autophagy in mediating the tolerance of tumor cells to cycling hypoxia. *Semin Radiat Oncol* 2013;23(4):252-261.

Krzywinska E, Stockmann C. Hypoxia, metabolism and immune cell function. *Biomedicines* 2018;6(2).

LaGory EL, Giaccia AJ. The ever-expanding role of hif in tumour and stromal biology. *Nat Cell Biol* 2016;18(4):356-365.

Lee K, Esselman WJ. Inhibition of PTPs by H(2)O(2) regulates the activation of distinct MAPK pathways. *Free Radic Biol Med* 2002;33:1121-1132.

Levy JMM, Towers CG, Thorburn A. Targeting autophagy in cancer. *Nat Rev Cancer* 2017;17(9):528-542.

Li B, Gordon GM, Du CH, et al. Specific killing of Rb mutant cancer cells by inactivating TSC2. *Cancer Cell* 2010;17(5):469-480.

Li Y, Patel SP, Roszik J, Qin Y. Hypoxia-driven immunosuppressive metabolites in the tumor microenvironment: new approaches for combinational immunotherapy. *Front Immunol* 2018;9:1591.

Lin A, Maity A. Molecular pathways: a novel approach to targeting hypoxia and improving radiotherapy efficacy via reduction in oxygen demand. *Clin Cancer Res* 2015;21(9):1995-2000.

Linge A, Löck S, Gudziol V, et al. Low cancer stem cell marker expression and low hypoxia identify good prognosis subgroups in HPV(-) HNSCC after postoperative radiochemotherapy: a multicenter study of the DKTK-ROG. *Clin Cancer Res* 2016;22(11):2639-2649.

Löfstedt T, Fredlund E, Holmquist-Mengelbier L, et al. Hypoxia inducible factor-2alpha in cancer. *Cell Cycle* 2007;6(8):919-926.

Lunt SJ, Fyles A, Hill RP, Milosevic M. Interstitial fluid pressure in tumors: therapeutic barrier and biomarker of angiogenesis. *Future Oncol* 2008;4(6):793-802.

Luoto KR, Kumareswaran R, Bristow RG. Tumor hypoxia as a driving force in genetic instability. *Genome Integr* 2013;4(1):5.

Majmundar AJ, Wong WJ, Simon MC. Hypoxia-inducible factors and the response to hypoxic stress. *Mol Cell* 2010;40(2):294-309.

Marie-Egyptienne DT, Lohse I, Hill RP. Cancer stem cells, the epithelial to mesenchymal transition (EMT) and radioresistance: potential role of hypoxia. *Cancer Lett* 2013;341(1):63-72.

Matoba S, Kang JG, Patino WD, et al. p53 regulates mitochondrial respiration. *Science* 2006;312(5780):1650-1653.

Maxwell PH, Wiesener MS, Chang GW, et al. The tumour suppressor protein VHL targets hypoxia-inducible factors for oxygen-dependent proteolysis. *Nature* 1999;399(6733):271-275.

Mazurek S, Boschek CB, Hugo F, et al. Pyruvate kinase type M2 and its role in tumor growth and spreading. *Semin Cancer Biol* 2005;15(4):300-308.

Metran-Nascente C, Yeung I, Vines DC, et al. Measurement of tumor hypoxia in patients with advanced pancreatic cancer based on ^{18}F-fluoroazamyin arabinoside uptake. *J Nucl Med* 2016;57(3):361-366.

Minchinton AI, Tannock IF. Drug penetration in solid tumours. *Nat Rev Cancer* 2006;6(8):583-592.

Miranda-Gonçalves V, Lameirinhas A, Henrique R, Jerónimo C. Metabolism and epigenetic interplay in cancer: regulation and putative therapeutic targets. *Front Genet* 2018;9:427.

Moreno-Sánchez R, Rodríguez-Enríquez S, Marín-Hernández A, et al. Energy metabolism in tumor cells. *FEBS J* 2007;274:1393-1418.

Morita M, Gravel SP, Hulea L, et al. mTOR coordinates protein synthesis, mitochondrial activity and proliferation. *Cell Cycle* 2015;14(4):473-480.

Mortensen LS, Johansen J, Kallehauge J, et al. FAZA PET/CT hypoxia imaging in patients with squamous cell carcinoma of the head and neck treated with radiotherapy: results from the DAHANCA 24 trial. *Radiother Oncol* 2012;105(1):14-20.

Newsholme EA, Crabtree B, Ardawi MS. The role of high rates of glycolysis and glutamine utilization in rapidly dividing cells. *Biosci Rep* 1985;5(5):393-400.

Nogueira V, Park Y, Chen CC, et al. Akt determines replicative senescence and oxidative or oncogenic premature senescence and sensitizes cells to oxidative apoptosis. *Cancer Cell* 2008;14(6):458-470.

Noman MZ, Hasmim M, Messai Y, et al. Hypoxia: a key player in antitumor immune response. A review in the theme: cellular responses to hypoxia. *Am J Physiol Cell Physiol* 2015;309(9):569-579.

Nordsmark M, Bentzen SM, Rudat V, et al. Prognostic value of tumor oxygenation in 397 head and neck tumors after primary radiation therapy. An international multi-center study. *Radiother Oncol* 2005;77(1):18-24.

Nordsmark M, Loncaster J, Aquino-Parsons C, et al. The prognostic value of pimonidazole and tumour pO_2 in human cervix carcinomas after radiation therapy: a prospective international multi-center study. *Radiother Oncol* 2006;80(2):123-131.

Overgaard J. Hypoxic modification of radiotherapy in squamous cell carcinoma of the head and neck—a systematic review and meta-analysis. *Radiother Oncol* 2011;100(1):22-32.

Ozcan U, Ozcan L, Yilmaz E, et al. Loss of the tuberous sclerosis complex tumor suppressors triggers the unfolded protein response to regulate insulin signaling and apoptosis. *Mol Cell* 2008;29(5):541-551.

Pagès F, Galon J, Dieu-Nosjean MC, Tartour E, Sautès-Fridman C, Fridman WH. Immune infiltration in human tumors: a prognostic factor that should not be ignored. *Oncogene* 2010;29(8):1093-1102.

Papandreou I, Cairns RA, Fontana L, et al. HIF-1 mediates adaptation to hypoxia by actively downregulating mitochondrial oxygen consumption. *Cell Metab* 2006;3:187-197.

Park S, Chang CY, Safi R, et al. ERRα-regulated lactate metabolism contributes to resistance to targeted therapies in breast cancer. *Cell Rep* 2016;15(2):323-335.

Paulsson J, Micke P. Prognostic relevance of cancer-associated fibroblasts in human cancer. *Semin Cancer Biol* 2014;25:61-68.

Pugh CW. Modulation of the hypoxic response. *Adv Exp Med Biol* 2016;903:259-271.

Rankin EB, Giaccia AJ. Hypoxic control of metastasis. *Science* 2016;352(6282):175-180.

Robey RB, Hay N. Is Akt the "Warburg kinase"? Akt-energy metabolism interactions and oncogenesis. *Semin Cancer Biol* 2009;19(1):25-31.

Roostaee A, Benoit YD, Boudjadi S, Beaulieu JF. Epigenetics in intestinal epithelial cell renewal. *J Cell Physiol* 2016;231(11):2361-2367.

Rouschop KM, Wouters BG. Regulation of autophagy through multiple independent hypoxic signaling pathways. *Curr Mol Med* 2009;9(4):417-424.

Schito L, Rey S. Cell-autonomous metabolic reprogramming in hypoxia. *Trends Cell Biol* 2018;28(2):128-142.

Segard T, Robins OD, Yusoff IF, et al. Detection of hypoxia with ^{18}F-fluoromisonidazole (18F-FMISO) in suspected or proven pancreatic cancer. *Clin Nucl Med* 2013;38(1):1-6.

Selak MA, Armour SM, MacKenzie ED, et al. Succinate links TCA cycle dysfunction to oncogenesis by inhibiting HIF-alpha prolyl hydroxylase. *Cancer Cell* 2005;7(1):77-85.

Semenza GL. HIF-1: upstream and downstream of cancer metabolism. *Curr Opin Genet Dev* 2010;20(1):51-56.

Shackelford DB, Shaw RJ. The LKB1-AMPK pathway: metabolism and growth control in tumour suppression. *Nat Rev Cancer* 2009;9(8):563-575.

Shannon AM, Bouchier-Hayes DJ, Condron CM, et al. Tumour hypoxia, chemotherapeutic resistance and hypoxia-related therapies. *Cancer Treat Rev* 2003;29(4):297-307.

Sharma M, Astekar M, Soi S, Manjunatha BS, Shetty DC, Radhakrishnan R. pH gradient reversal: an emerging hallmark of cancers. *Recent Pat Anticancer Drug Discov* 2015;10(3):244-258.

Stambolic V, MacPherson D, Sas D, et al. Regulation of PTEN transcription by p53. *Mol Cell* 2001;8(2):317-325.

Steel GG. *Growth Kinetics of Tumours: Cell Population Kinetics in Relation to the Growth and Treatment of Cancer*. Oxford: Clarendon Press; 1977.

Suzuki S, Tanaka T, Poyurovsky MV, et al. Phosphate-activated glutaminase (GLS2), a p53-inducible regulator of glutamine metabolism and reactive oxygen species. *Proc Natl Acad Sci U S A* 2010;107(16):7461-7466.

Tannock IF. Biology of tumor growth. *Hosp Pract* 1983;18(4):81-93.

Tharmalingham H, Hoskin P. Clinical trials targeting hypoxia. *Br J Radiol* 2019;92(1093):20170966.

Thomlinson RH, Gray LH. The histological structure of some human lung cancers and the possible implications for radiotherapy. *Br J Cancer* 1955;9(4):539-549.

Trachootham D, Alexandre J, Huang P. Targeting cancer cells by ROS-mediated mechanisms: a radical therapeutic approach? *Nat Rev Drug Discov* 2009;8(7):579-591.

Van der Heiden MG, Cantley LC, Thompson CB. Understanding the Warburg effect: the metabolic requirements of cell proliferation. *Science* 2009;324(5930):1029-1033.

Vaupel P, Mayer A. Tumor hypoxia: causative mechanisms, microregional heterogeneities, and the role of tissue-based hypoxia markers. *Adv Exp Med Biol* 2016;923:77-86.

Von Ahrens D, Bhagat T, Nagrath D, Maitra A, Verma A. The role of stromal cancer-associated fibroblasts in pancreatic cancer. *J Hematol Oncol* 2017;10(1):76.

Vousden KH, Ryan KM. p53 and metabolism. *Nat Rev Cancer* 2009;9(10):691-700.

Waitkus MS, Diplas BH, Yan H. Biological role and therapeutic potential of IDH mutations in cancer. *Cancer Cell* 2018;34(2):186-195.

Warburg O. On the origin of cancer cells. *Science* 1956;123(3191):309-314.

White E, Mehnert JM, Chan CS. Autophagy, metabolism, and cancer. *Clin Cancer Res* 2015;21(22):5037-5046.

Williams GH, Stoeber K. The cell cycle and cancer. *J Pathol* 2012;226:352-364.

Wilson W, Hay M. Targeting hypoxia in cancer therapy. *Nat Rev Cancer* 2011;11(6):393-410.

Wise DR, DeBerardinis RJ, Mancuso A, et al. Myc regulates a transcriptional program that stimulates mitochondrial glutaminolysis and leads to glutamine addiction. *Proc Natl Acad Sci U S A* 2008;105(48):18782-18787.

Wong KK, Engelman JA, Cantley LC. Targeting the PI3K signaling pathway in cancer. *Curr Opin Genet Dev* 2010;20(1):87-90.

Wouters BG, Koritzinsky M. Hypoxia signalling through mTOR and the unfolded protein response in cancer. *Nat Rev Cancer* 2008;8(11):851-864.

Yang L, Roberts D, Takhar M, et al. Development and validation of a 28-gene hypoxia-related prognostic signature for localized prostate cancer. *EBioMedicine* 2018;31:182-189.

Yang L, Taylor J, Eustace A, et al. A gene signature for selecting benefit from hypoxia modification of radiotherapy for high-risk bladder cancer patients. *Clin Cancer Res* 2017;23(16):4761-4768.

Zips D, Zöphel K, Abolmaali N, et al. Exploratory prospective trial of hypoxia-specific PET imaging during radiochemotherapy in patients with locally advanced head-and-neck cancer. *Radiother Oncol* 2012;105(1):21-28.

Cancer Heterogeneity

Craig Gedye

Chapter Outline

- 13.1 **Introduction**
- 13.2 **Heterogeneity in Cancer**
  - 13.2.1 Methods used to Study Tumor Heterogeneity
  - 13.2.2 Stromal Heterogeneity in Cancer
  - 13.2.3 Genetic Heterogeneity in Tumors
- 13.3 **Epigenetic Heterogeneity in Cancer**
  - 13.3.1 Epithelial-Mesenchymal Transition
  - 13.3.2 Cancer Stem Cells
  - 13.3.3 Phenotypic Plasticity
  - 13.3.4 Models of Epigenetic Heterogeneity May Be Facets of the Same Process
  - 13.3.5 Genetic and Epigenetic Heterogeneity in Cancer are Interdependent
- 13.4 **Clinical Implications of Cancer Heterogeneity**
  - 13.4.1 Prognostic and Predictive Relevance of Cancer Heterogeneity
  - 13.4.2 Exploring Cancer Heterogeneity in Clinical Practice
  - 13.4.3 Implications of Cancer Heterogeneity for Treatment
- **Summary**
- **References**

13.1 INTRODUCTION

Every patient's cancer is different. Cancers arising from the same organ may have different histology and metastatic potential, may be indolent or aggressive, and may have different response to therapy. Cells within a cancer are also different. Within individual tumors, some cells are genetically normal stromal cells and some are somatically-mutated malignant cells. And within the malignant cell pool, related but differently evolved malignant clones vie for survival, exploiting different epigenetic strategies, within different microenvironments within each tumor (Fig. 13–1; see Chap. 12, Sec. 12.2).

Understanding this complexity and heterogeneity is daunting, but has been appreciated pragmatically for decades, with clinicians combining different chemotherapy agents or different treatment modalities (eg, chemotherapy with radiation) in an effort to overcome treatment failure and improve patient survival. Modern scientific technologies are expanding our knowledge of heterogeneity, and this rapidly unfolding area offers opportunities to better understand the mechanisms of tumor recurrence, distant metastasis, and resistance to cancer treatment.

Paget's recognition that metastases "seed" into organs that provide a fertile "soil" provided the conceptual framework that tumor cells must interact with their microenvironment, and that some tumor cells may be more fit than others for this process (Paget, 1889). Pierce and colleagues demonstrated that teratocarcinomas and mouse squamous cell carcinomas contained highly tumorigenic cells that could differentiate into morphologically differentiated cell types that were unable to form tumors when transplanted in mice (Pierce and Wallace, 1971). They described cancers as a "caricature" of normal tissue renewal, whereby tumor stem cells divide and differentiate giving rise to terminal postmitotic differentiated cells.

Till and McCulloch (1961) provided the first experimental evidence of normal tissue stem cells by injecting tiny numbers of bone marrow cells into lethally irradiated mice (Till and McCulloch, 1961). They observed the formation of colonies of cells from all 3 blood lineages. When transplanted into secondary recipient mice, some clones could again give rise to blood cells from multiple lineages. Pierce and Speers demonstrated in clonogenic assays that only a fraction of cells from freshly excised human tumors could form colonies in tissue culture (including myeloma, lymphoma, neuroblastoma, ovarian carcinoma, chronic lymphocytic leukemia, small cell lung cancer, and melanoma), although this capability may be limited by the imperfect nature of the tissue culture medium (Pierce and Speers, 1988). This result led the authors to speculate that these rare clonogenic cells had been tumor stem cells in vivo. These early observations of a rare population of cells that possess tumor-repopulating potential raised the critical

306 CHAPTER 13

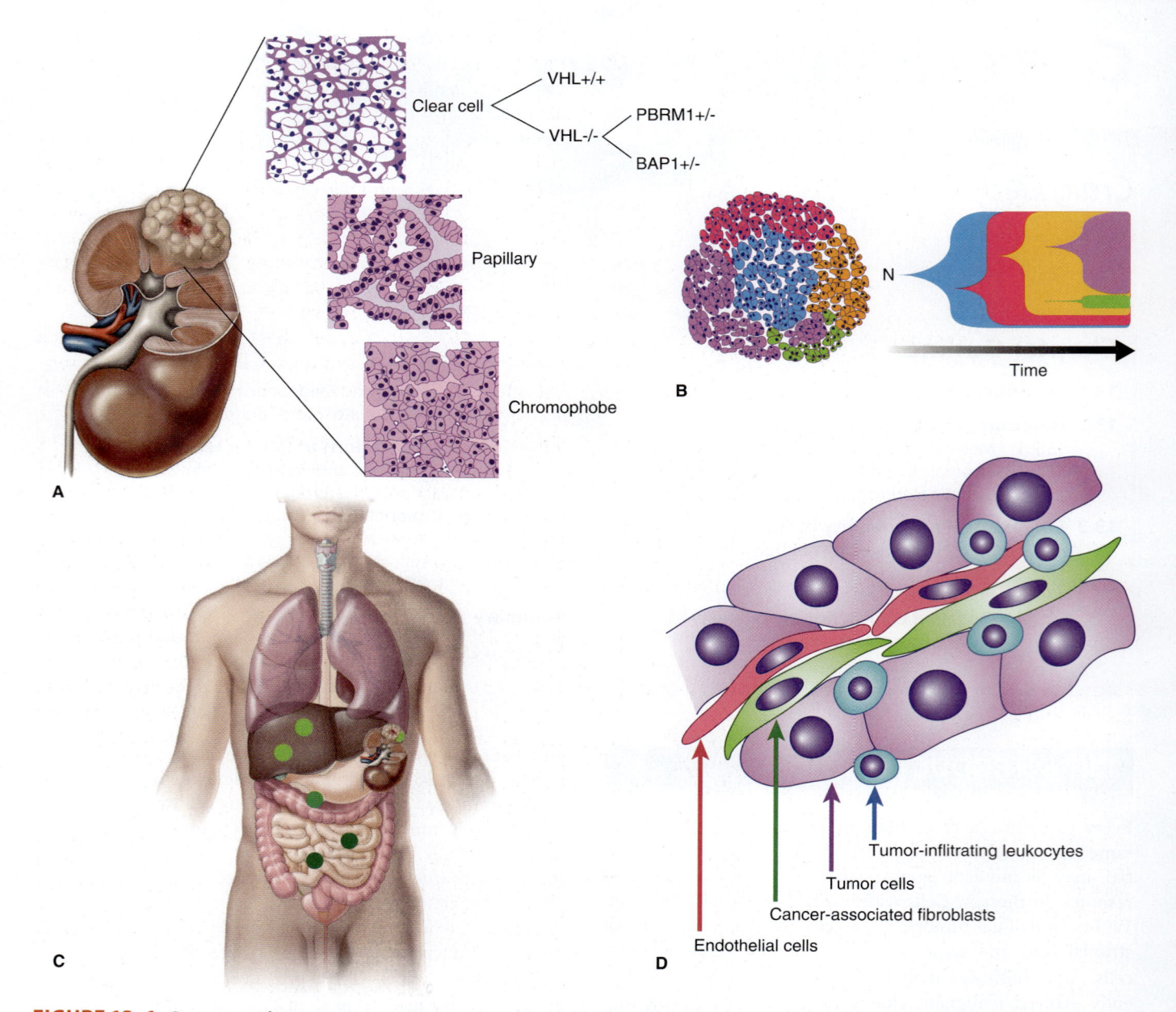

FIGURE 13–1 Cancers are heterogeneous. This heterogeneity can be considered in many interdependent dimensions. For example, **A)** cancers from the same organ vary markedly in histology and genetic driver mutations between different individuals. **B)** Within a primary cancer, there can be widespread clonal genetic diversity as the primary cancer evolves from a normal (N) cell. **C)** Cancer cells that metastasize distant to the primary lesion often have a different genomic sequence to primary cancers and may show different epigenetic phenotypes, sometimes as a result of being in different microenvironments. **D)** Finally, cancers show stromal heterogeneity as many cells within cancers are nonmalignant (eg, endothelial cells, leucocytes, and fibroblasts).

question of whether genetic or epigenetic factors were at play, and whether there was a "special" population of cells with intrinsic properties causing tumor repopulation (ie, cancer stem cells [CSCs]), or whether this was a general property of all cancer cells, under the influence of extrinsic factors.

This chapter attempts to address our evolving understanding of different but complementary models proposed to account for genetic and epigenetic heterogeneity of human cancers. Although our understanding of this process has in large part been driven by studies to understand CSCs, there are multiple overlapping mechanisms contributing to cancer heterogeneity.

13.2 HETEROGENEITY IN CANCER

13.2.1 Methods Used to Study Tumor Heterogeneity

Interpatient heterogeneity is obvious in all cancers, with some patients having very different clinical outcomes and possessing distinct driver mutations, which imply that different patients might benefit from different therapies. For example, in melanoma, 50% of patients have cancers driven by BRAF

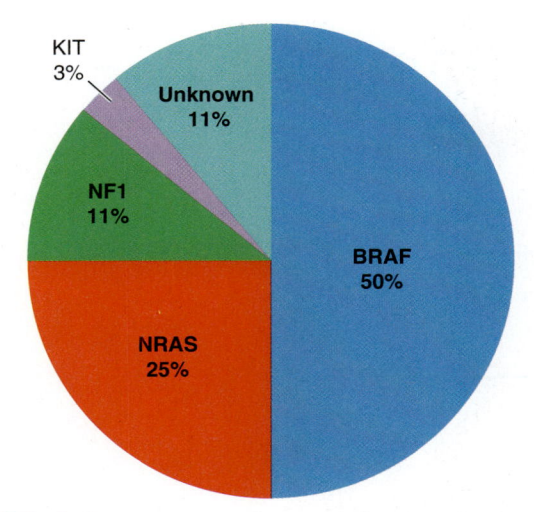

FIGURE 13–2 Dimensions of cancer heterogeneity. Inter-patient heterogeneity is demonstrable for all cancers, with some patients having different clinical outcomes, and where different driver mutations can identify patients that might benefit from different therapies. For example, in melanoma ~50% of patients have cancers driven by *BRAF* (blue), 25% with *NRAS* mutations (red), 11% with *NF1* mutations (green), 3% with KIT mutations (purple), and 11% have a mixture of rarer driver mutations (aqua). Only *BRAF* mutations are routinely "actionable".

mutations, 25% by NRAS mutations, 11% with NF1 mutations, and 3% with KIT mutations (Fig. 13–2).

To study the diversity of cells within cancers, a wide variety of methods are used to determine the genetic origins and epigenetic states of cancer cells; differences in their morphology; variability arising from microenvironmental, autocrine, and paracrine signaling; and stochastic plasticity that allows cells to modify their phenotype. Molecular techniques to study genetic variation in DNA include Sanger sequencing, in situ hybridization, and next-generation DNA sequencing (NGS). Investigation of variation in protein expression among cancer cells employs techniques such as Western blotting, flow cytometry, immunohistochemistry, immunofluorescence, mass cytometry, and mass spectroscopy. Analysis of cell phenotypes by mRNA expression can employ polymerase chain reaction (PCR), gene expression microarrays, or RNA sequencing. Newer techniques to study epigenetic regulation that are providing mechanistic insights into cancer heterogeneity include whole-genome methylation arrays, bisulfite sequencing, histone modification analysis, and microRNA and noncoding RNA arrays. These techniques are becoming increasingly comprehensive and suitable for samples available in small quantities, especially when studying isolated populations of cells obtained directly from human tumors. These methods are discussed in Chapter 2.

Flow-assisted cell sorting, tissue microdissection, and isolation of circulating tumor cells can be used to perform analysis of small cell populations from tumors, and even single cells. These methods use a variety of markers to separate cancer and normal cells (eg, cell surface proteins and markers of metabolic or cellular function such as aldehyde dehydrogenase).

Individual cancer cells are usually obtained from solid human tumors immediately after their surgical removal. Tumors are usually mechanically disaggregated, then digested to a single cell suspension by use of enzymes such as collagenase, hyaluronidase, and DNase. These processes can cause considerable cellular damage and may alter the cell surface phenotype of cells. The resulting single cell suspension can be examined by flow cytometry, cultured in vitro, or injected into immunocompromised mice (see Fig. 13–3). Viable cells can be sorted by fluorescence-activated cell sorting (FACS; Alexander et al, 2009) or isolated by magnetic cell separation using antibodies conjugated to tiny paramagnetic beads, which allow cells to be physically separated in a high magnetic field (Palmon et al, 2012). Stromal cells in tumors can be obtained by sorting cancer-associated fibroblasts, CD45+ hematopoietic cells or CD31+ endothelial cells. From the remaining cancer cells, one may then identify a population of cells suspected of being CSCs (see Sec. 13.3.2), for example, by selecting CD133+ cells.

Phenotypic analysis of individual cells is now possible with technologies such as mass cytometry and single-cell transcriptomics (see Chap. 2, Sec. 2.4). For example, mass cytometry or CyTOF can be applied to tumor-derived single-cell suspensions, identifying and characterizing broad populations of immune cells within individual patients' tumors (Chevrier et al, 2017). With improvements in nucleic acid purification, amplification, sequencing, and bioinformatics, genetic, transcriptional, and epigenetic information can be acquired from single cells or nuclei. For example, single-cell genome-wide bisulfite sequencing can be performed to examine the "methylome" in individual cells (Smallwood et al, 2014). "Multiomics" analysis (eg, genome, methylome, transcriptome) is possible from the same single cell (Macaulay et al, 2017).

The functional tumor forming capacity of isolated cancer cells is assessed by their ability to generate tumors on serial transplantation in immune-deficient animals and their ability to recapitulate the genetic and phenotypic heterogeneity of the original tumor (Fig. 13–3). Early experiments in stem cell biology used lethally irradiated mice as recipients of transplanted bone marrow cells (Till and McCulloch, 1961), but investigation of human cancer cell biology requires genetically immunocompromised mice. Athymic nude mice have been superseded by severe combined immunodeficiency (SCID) mice that lack T and B lymphocytes. Improved engraftment is seen when SCID mice are crossed with diabetic NOD mice, yielding NOD/SCID mice, which have been refined further, using mice that have mutations in the Rag2 or interleukin-2 receptor gamma chain (IL2Rγ$^{-/-}$) genes (NOD/SCID/ IL2Rγ$^{-/-}$ or NSG mice; Ito et al, 2002). Injections into NOD/SCID or NSG mice are often performed in conjunction with Matrigel, a heterogeneous mixture of basement membrane proteins secreted by mouse sarcoma cells, which enhances tumor transplantability. Mouse xenograft experiments are being further refined using various forms of "humanization," either via incorporation of human tissue such as fetal bone or adult skin, the addition of human growth factors, and by the engraftment of human hematopoietic stem cells to reconstitute immunocompromised mice with human immune cells (Verma et al, 2001).

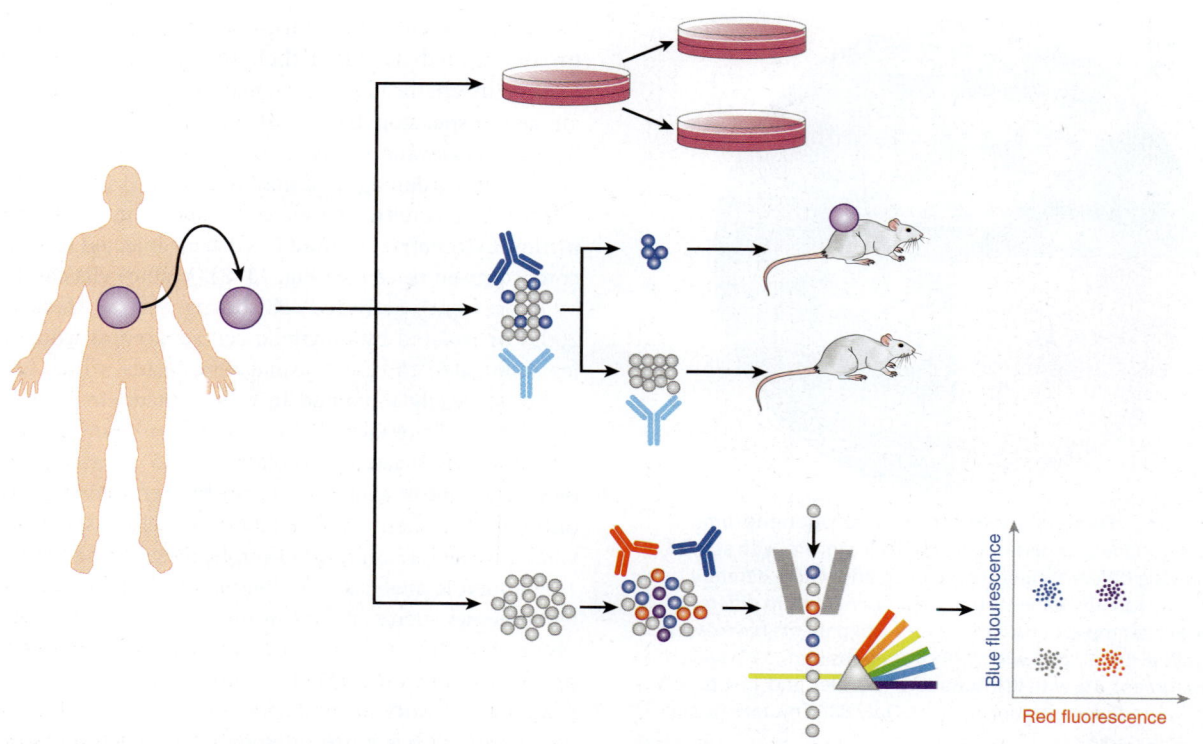

FIGURE 13–3 Methods used to study tumor heterogeneity. Cancer samples from patients can be mechanically dissociated and then enzymatically digested and filtered to generate a suspension of single cells. This single-cell suspension can be used to establish new cancer cell lines, to measure the tumor-forming ability of these cancer cells (or subsets of them) by injection into immunocompromised mice, or can be analyzed by flow cytometry (cells are labeled with fluorescent-labeled antibodies [eg, red, blue] and depending on target protein expression have different fluorescence when exposed to laser light). Finally, cells can be saved for later use by cryogenic freezing.

Although these various hosts for xenografts provide useful biological tools, they provide an artificial environment and the results obtained may not reflect the behavior of tumor cells in their original environment.

Although in vivo methods are viewed as the gold standard, in vitro assays of cancer complexity may allow for rapid screening of drug activity and interrogation of signaling pathways in the context of heterogeneity. Recent improvements in methodology have addressed criticisms of cell culture models, particularly that the microenvironment for cancer cells growing in a culture dish is very different from that within the primary tumor. For example glioblastoma cells grown in bovine serum acquire mutations in vitro that distort their genotypes and phenotypes such that they are not representative of the patient's tumor (Lee et al, 2006). Human tumor cells cultured de novo as "tumor-spheres" in defined serum-free media (Brewer et al, 1993) can generate cell lines with morphologic heterogeneity that express markers of a primitive stemlike phenotype, and form xenografts that are invasive and maintain the phenotype of the original tumor. Cell lines grown in defined media have been employed to demonstrate the efficacy of targeting glioblastoma stem cells by various stem cell–signaling pathways, but most of these in vitro models are not well validated as representing properties of CSCs (van Staveren et al, 2009), nor benchmarked against in vivo models or as surrogates of patient response. However, if a patient's cancer can be successfully xenografted, this portends a worse prognosis for several cancers including non–small cell lung carcinoma (John et al, 2011).

Once tumors or cell lines have formed, their genotype, phenotype, and differentiation status must be studied to ascertain if it remains constant with each subsequent passage, and for how long it represents an accurate reproduction of the original patient's tumor. Some studies have shown that the phenotype of human cancers rapidly destabilizes in xenograft models (Stewart et al, 2011).

13.2.2 Stromal Heterogeneity in Cancer

Every seed needs appropriate soil to germinate and grow. All cancers contain stromal cells that support and may protect malignant cells. Cancer cells in turn recruit, manipulate, and nurture this stromal microenvironment to establish and maintain their nutrition and survival. Stromal cells include endothelial cells that line tumor blood vessels and lymphatics; pericytes to support mature endothelium in larger vessels (Fig. 13–4; see Chap. 11, Sec. 11.5); cancer-associated fibroblasts that both provide physical scaffolding (extracellular matrix [ECM] consisting of collagen, fibronectin, and various other macromolecules) and interact with and influence malignant cells; and tumor-associated macrophages, lymphocytes, and other hematopoietic cells (see Chap. 12, Sec. 12.2). The stromal component of a tumor can be sparse, for example, in melanoma or large cell lymphomas where the malignant population dominates, or it can be profuse,

Mesenchymal lineage cells are likely derived from fibroblasts, perivascular pericytes, and circulating mesenchymal stem cells. By producing ECM (like collagen), they support blood vessels, the influx and efflux of leukocytes, and the physical structure of the tumor. Cancer-associated fibroblasts (CAFs) can also have profound pro-tumorigenic effects on the immune microenvironment in cancers, by acting to engage and educate regulatory T cells (Pommier and Fearon, 2016; see Chap. 21, Sec. 21.3.4).

The fibroblast component of cancer is very pronounced in pancreatic carcinoma, where a dense desmoplastic stroma intermingles with nests of cancer cells. There are distinct populations of CAFs within tumors. CAFs with high expression of α-smooth muscle actin (αSMA) were found located immediately adjacent to neoplastic cells in mouse and human pancreatic carcinoma: these CAFs probably function like myofibroblasts, providing stiff, structural support (Öhlund et al, 2017). In the same patients, a distinct subpopulation of CAFs was found distant from cancer cells, which lacked the myofibroblast phenotype and instead secreted IL6 and other inflammatory mediators, and thus likely had an immunomodulatory and proangiogenic role.

Like the structural and supportive fibroblasts, the blood vessels supporting tumors are also heterogeneous. These vascular structures are sometimes co-opted from adjacent normal blood vessels, or can be newly formed from cells recruited from the adjacent normal tissues, circulating endothelial cells from bone marrow, or from within the tumor itself (see Chap. 11, Sec. 11.5). Some studies have identified different subsets of microvessels in cancers such as clear cell renal cell carcinoma (ccRCC) where undifferentiated (CD31$^+$/CD34$^-$) and differentiated (CD34$^+$) vessels were found. In patients with high-grade, aggressive cancers with a shorter survival, there were some larger, well-formed differentiated blood vessels, but also many smaller, poorly supported undifferentiated blood vessels. Patients with lower-grade cancers and better overall survival had mostly the larger, more mature, stable, differentiated blood vessels (Yao et al, 2007).

The diversity of hematopoietic lineage cells in cancer is also becoming apparent. Limited flow cytometry experiments could capture the diversity of specific subsets (eg, tumor-infiltrating lymphocytes), but high-dimensional techniques are now allowing a comprehensive overview of immune cells in the tumor microenvironment. A recent study provides an atlas of the extraordinary diversity of lymphocyte and macrophage populations in clear cell renal cell carcinoma, showing differentiation of myeloid cells in the tumor microenvironment and the interrelationship between different populations of immune cells and their association with clinical outcome (Chevrier et al, 2017).

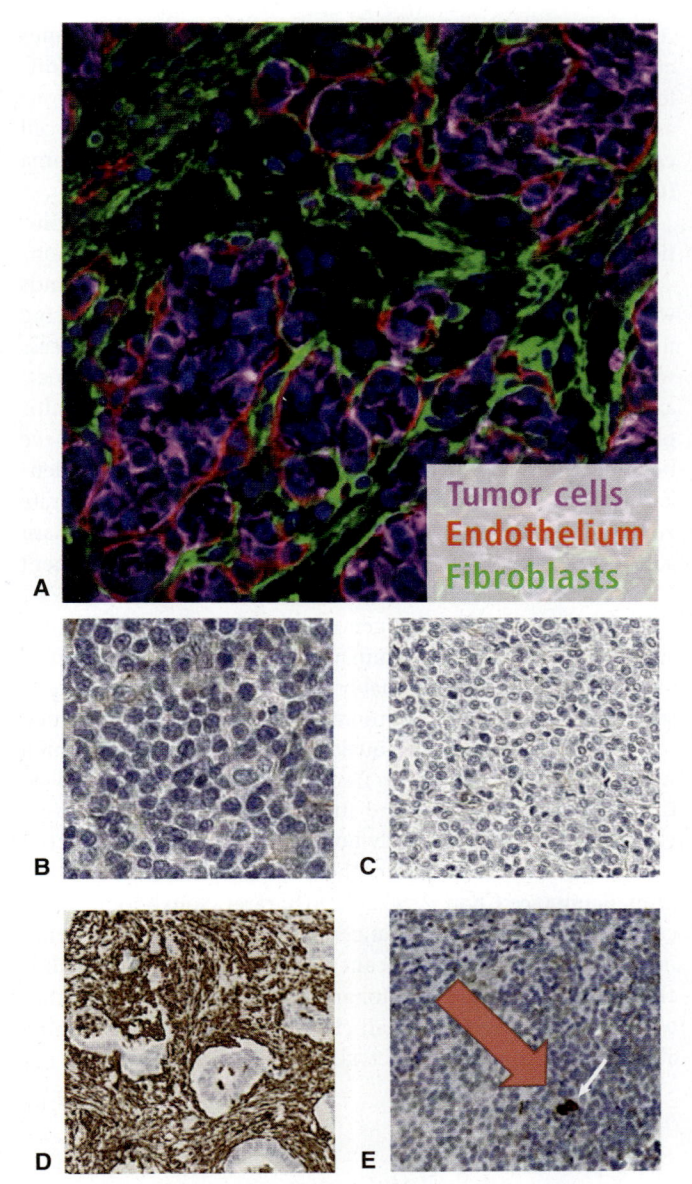

FIGURE 13–4 Different cancers have different stromal microenvironments. **A)** Clear cell renal cell carcinoma is often arranged as nests of cancer cells (magenta, staining the epithelial marker cytokeratin) within a network of endothelial cells (red) and cancer-associated fibroblasts (green; cell nuclei in blue). In large cell lymphoma (**B**) and melanoma (**C**), the cancer exists as sheets of tumor cells, with very few stromal cells (brown) present. In contrast, some cancers have a dense infiltrate of genetically normal fibroblasts or leukocytes: (**D**) pancreatic adenocarcinoma (with stroma stained brown) and (**E**) Hodgkin lymphoma, with only rare malignant Reed-Sternberg cells stained for the cell surface marker CD15 (arrow). (Reproduced with permission from Human Protein Atlas available at http://www.proteinatlas.org).

such as in pancreatic adenocarcinoma, which is dominated typically by a thick fibrous stroma. At the extreme of this spectrum is Hodgkin lymphoma, where rare malignant Reed-Sternberg cells sit isolated in a sea of reactive inflammatory cells (Fig. 13–4). This variability in the tumor microenvironment influences the effectiveness of cancer treatments and may itself be a legitimate target of cancer treatment (see Chap. 18, Sec. 18.4.7).

13.2.3 Genetic Heterogeneity in Tumors

Cancers are driven by somatic alterations in their DNA. Genetic heterogeneity between different patients' cancers is a major determinant of diversity in histology and clinical behavior. For example, approximately 15% of colorectal carcinomas have microsatellite instability, and they have more mutations than other colorectal cancers (The Cancer Genome Atlas, 2012). MSI-high colorectal cancers might have a poorer response to chemotherapy but are associated with a higher chance of response to checkpoint immunotherapy. A higher tumor mutational burden might offer a more adaptable genetic repertoire that can lead to early resistance to chemotherapy, but conversely exposes the tumor to better immune surveillance through expression of more neoantigens.

The different driver mutations (see Chap. 7, Sec. 7.4) found in individual patients' cancers are increasingly important in treatment selection: examples include the selective use of hormonal agents and HER2-targeted therapies in subgroups of women with breast cancer, and the use of BRAF and c-KIT inhibitors in different subsets of melanoma (see Chap. 19). Evolving evidence shows that the genetic heritage of each cancer is also critical. If a mutation occurs early in the evolution of a cancer (eg, *BRAF* in melanoma), then it is much more likely to be relevant for targeted therapies (ie, it is an "actionable" mutation) or for checkpoint immunotherapy (McGranahan et al, 2016).

Whether cancer progression, treatment resistance, and clinical failure are due to properties inherent in the dominant clone, or due to outgrowth and rapid selection of rarer subclones, is likely to be variable but of critical importance to the management of an individual's cancer. Cancers are now well recognized as comprising related but variable subclones that appear to arise from the sequential acquisition of multiple mutations, each in turn conferring a survival advantage to a clonal population of cells (see Chap. 10, Sec. 10.1). This was proposed as a stepwise process in colorectal cancer where macroscopic transition from adenoma to dysplastic adenoma to carcinoma to invasive and metastatic carcinoma has been shown to parallel the acquisition of mutations in genes such as *APC*, *KRAS*, *PIK3CA*, and *TP53* (Vogelstein et al, 1988; Jones et al, 2008). More often this process is stochastic, as many different genetic clones can be identified in premalignant lesions associated with cancers, for example, in melanoma, renal cell carcinoma, colorectal carcinoma, and pancreatic carcinoma (Campbell et al, 2008, 2010).

An alternative model proposes simultaneous parallel evolution in cancer. This theory for carcinogenesis was also demonstrated in colorectal cancer (Sottoriva et al, 2015) where glands within tumors were found to have evolved in parallel producing numerous intermixed subclones. A stringent selection process was not seen, and both clonal (shared) and private (subclonal) alterations arose early during carcinogenesis. Similarly, multiple genetically distinct leukemia-initiating cell subclones have been demonstrated in children with acute lymphoblastic leukemia. These diverse clones have differing abilities to generate xenografts and there is a poor clinical outcome if the dominant subclone is capable of growth in the mouse microenvironment (Notta et al, 2011).

Earlier lower-definition genomic studies suggested that a single clone usually predominates within the primary tumor and in metastases, presumably due to a process of genetic selection. For example, examination of the genome performed by DNA microarray single-nucleotide polymorphisms in men with metastatic hormone-refractory prostate cancer showed that the in situ primary and multiple bone metastases were clonally related and relatively homogeneous (Liu et al, 2009).

With the advent of faster, cheaper, and thus deeper DNA sequencing (see Chap. 2, Sec. 2.2.10), rarer clonal populations can be identified in many cancers (Fig. 13–5). Rapid sequencing of thousands of single cancer cells has identified various clonal and subclonal evolutionary patterns in breast and other cancers, including very small clonal populations with highly aberrant genomes (Wang et al, 2014; Lan et al, 2017). For

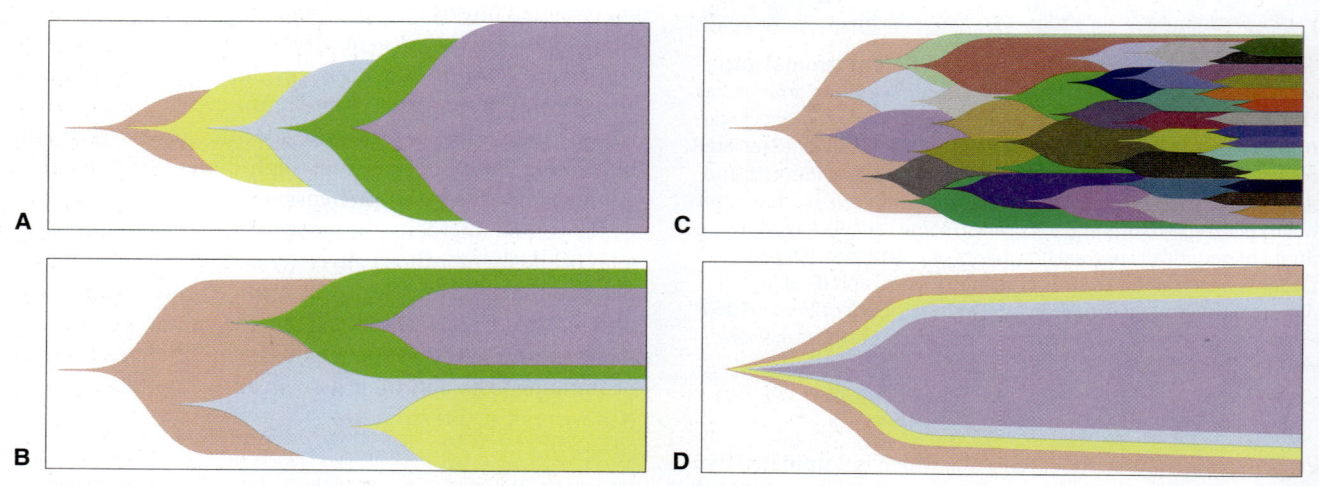

FIGURE 13–5 Intratumoral heterogeneity. Different models of clonal evolution are proposed to occur in cancers. **A)** Linear evolution proposes that precancerous lesions might be dominated by a single driver mutation, which is replaced with dominance of subsequently acquired mutations. **B)** Coevolution of different clones from an original driver clone gives a branching evolution model. **C)** A neutral evolution model supposes that there is no specific selection of clones, a pattern that might be seen when DNA repair genes are damaged, for example, hypermutator phenotype. **D)** Rapid development of a stable population of clones that cooperate can come from a punctuated evolution model (Modified with permission from Davis A, Gao R, Navin N. Tumor evolution: Linear, branching, neutral or punctuated? *Biochim Biophys Acta Rev Cancer* 2017 Apr;1867(2):151-161.)

example, deeper sequencing technologies have allowed study of genomic rearrangements in the hypervariable region of the Ig heavy chain locus showing that chronic lymphocytic leukemia becomes more complex and diverse over time, and after treatment (Campbell et al, 2008). This clonal evolution had long been suspected in solid tumors, and a landmark series of studies documented the diversity and complexity of genetic evolution in clear cell renal cell carcinoma. The clonal evolution of ccRCC was mapped in multiple fragments from 5 patients' primary cancers, and from a variety of metastatic lesions. The founding mutation in the *VHL* gene was found in all cells within a tumor, with physically distant parts of the cancer acquiring additional sets of mutations as the cancer populations diverged and evolved. At an early point, however, one clone within the cancer branched out, acquiring sufficient functional complexity for the cancer cells to disseminate and metastasize, and all metastatic lesions were phylogenetically related to this small part of the primary cancer (Gerlinger et al, 2012). Subsequently, more patients' samples were subjected to similar analysis, and confirmed the branched clonal evolution of ccRCC (Gerlinger et al, 2014) but also revealed that the extent of clonal diversity in each patient's cancer was similar in magnitude to the genomic differences between different patients' cancers. That is, intratumoral heterogeneity is similar in evolutionary distance to intertumoral heterogeneity; the cancer cells in a single person's cancer are as diverse as different people's cancers are from each other (Martinez et al, 2013). Studies of many other types of solid tumors have shown marked genetic heterogeneity with multiple subclones being present in the primary tumor and in different metastases that can evolve over time and after exposure to treatments (McGranahan and Swanton, 2017; Fig. 13–5).

Our growing understanding of the evolutionary histories of each person's cancer is expanding to reveal the mechanisms by which these lineages arise. Small-scale genomic alterations (eg, single nucleotide alterations; see Chap. 2, Sec. 2.2.9) are important, but large-scale genomic events can dominate the evolutionary history in some patients. Newly recognized mechanisms such as "chromothripsis" where the genome of a cell shatters, re-forms, and the cell retains viability can give rise to highly aggressive cancers (Rode et al, 2016), whereas coordinated genomic changes such as DNA translocations and deletions can occur in an interdependent fashion in cancers such as prostate cancer (Baca et al, 2013). This "chromoplexy" may account for the dysregulation and disruption of prostate cancer genes that occur in a seemingly coordinated manner, and has been termed "punctuated evolution," where an early explosion of evolution rapidly leads to a stable population of clones.

Understanding the mechanisms for genomic evolution within a cancer has major implications for treatment and cancer control. For example, the long-held theory that cancer genetic evolution is stepwise and clonal in cancers like pancreatic carcinoma suggested that lesions like pancreatic intraepithelial neoplasm (PIN) evolved in a stepwise fashion, and were precursors to invasive cancers. However recent evidence challenges this assumption, showing that generation of pancreatic cancer is neither gradual nor sequential. Up to two-thirds of pancreatic carcinomas harbor complex rearrangement patterns associated with mitotic errors, which enables an early and rapid evolutionary explosion that gives rise quickly to an environmentally competitive population of clones, a cancer that has quickly adapted for invasive growth and metastatic spread, that is, the "punctuated evolution" model (Notta et al, 2016). In patients with these cancers, attempts at early detection are likely to be futile, as there is a fully adapted cancer poised for local invasion and disseminated metastasis.

Genomic clonal complexity develops more slowly in some cancers, and metastases and recurrences can occur late in the course of disease. An example is breast carcinoma, where locally recurrent tumors and metastatic lesions contain most of the original drivers of disease (mutations in cancer genes such as *TP53*, *GATA3*, *PIK3CA*, *AKT1*, and *ERBB2*), but have also acquired further variants that confer additional survival advantages (eg, SWI/SNF and JAK-STAT mutations) or alterations that enable drug resistance, for example, ESR1 mutations (Yates et al, 2017) (Fig. 13–6). Mutational processes were found to be similar in primary tumors and after relapse, but genotoxic interventions such as radiotherapy and chemotherapy can damage the genome, paradoxically enabling further genetic diversification.

In another study (Jamal-Hanjani et al, 2017), non–small cell lung cancer was found to have widespread intratumoral heterogeneity with both small and large genetic variations. Core driver mutations in genes such as *EGFR*, *MET*, *RAF*, and *TP53* were identified as clonal, but additional driver alterations were heterogeneously distributed in different cancer cell populations, indicating that they occurred later in evolution in more than 75% of patients. When large-scale instability occurred (eg, in tumors with DNA repair defects), it resulted in parallel evolution of different cancer cell populations and up to 5 times increased risk of death or tumor recurrence.

An understanding of the different evolutionary patterns of cancer can inform our understanding of their clinical behavior (Sansregret et al, 2018). Although competing models suggested both sequential and parallel acquisition of mutations in colorectal cancer, a recent study shows that in a minority of patients, lymphatic and distant metastases share an evolutionary trajectory, whereas in approximately two-thirds of patients, parallel evolution has occurred and more distant metastases have a different genomic pedigree to lymphatic metastases (Naxerova et al, 2017). Thus, multiple metastatic lesions might need to be characterized in order to guide targeted therapy. A bioinformatic analysis across many cancers from the Cancer Genome Atlas project found that the majority of patients' cancers (86%) had at least 2 clones of at least 10% abundance, which was associated with worse patient survival, particularly if a driver mutation was detected in the minor clone (Andor et al, 2015). Finally, by tracking individual cancer cells within populations, clones of cancer cells that are resistant to treatments can be present in very small numbers prior to drug treatment exposure. This has been shown in models of lung cancer and leukemia that respond to treatment with targeted therapies but then develop treatment resistance (Bhang et al, 2015). Thus, by combining our understanding of

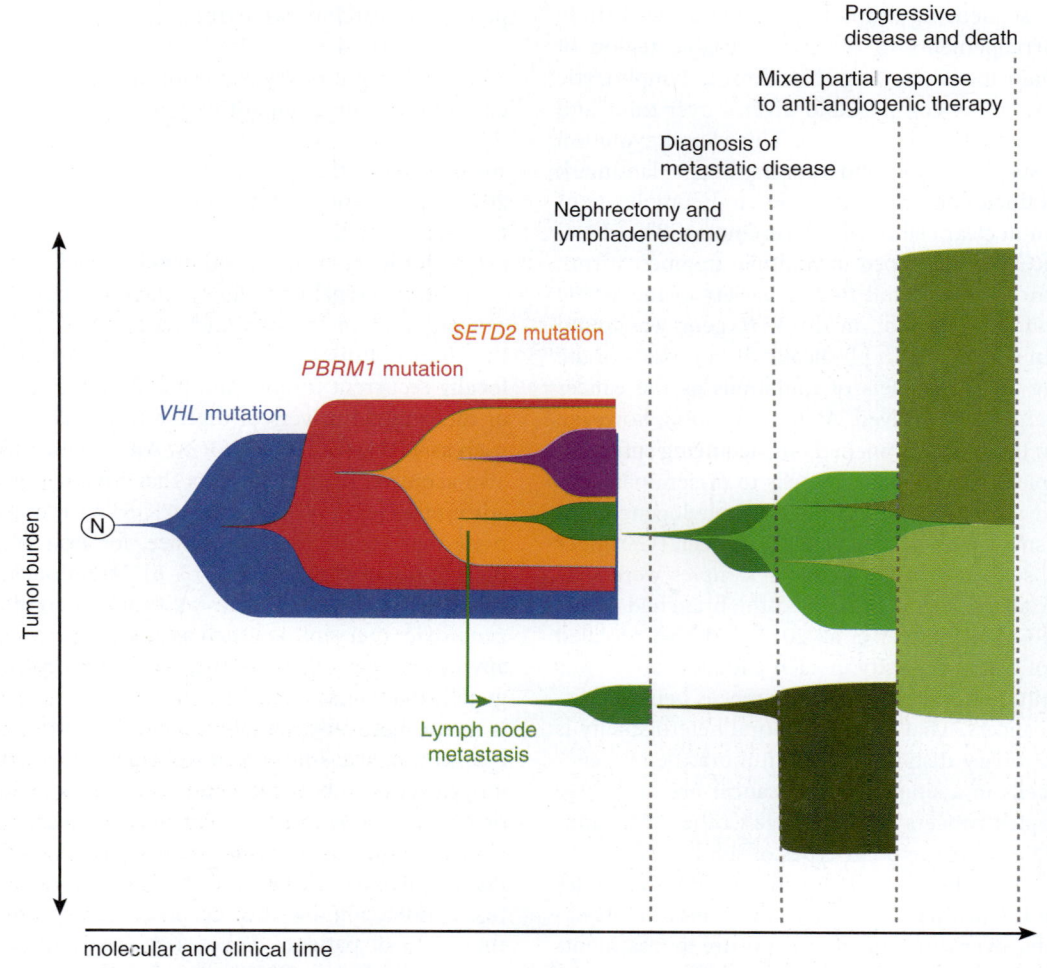

FIGURE 13–6 Increasingly detailed genomic data from next-generation DNA sequencing technology reveals the evolutionary genomic and genetic structure of cancer cell populations. "Deep" sequencing detects rare clones (represented in different colors here to show their outgrowth and evolution from previous clones) within tumor cell populations. New mutations confer new abilities on cancer populations, including local recurrence, distant metastasis, and treatment resistance. In this example, a primary renal cancer begins with a founder *VHL* mutation, acquires *PBRM1* and *SETD2* mutations, and develops locoregional lymph node metastases treated with surgery. Systemic treatment of metastatic disease is partially successful, but resistant distant metastasis progresses and causes treatment failure and the patient's death.

the clonal genetic structure of cancers with evolutionary principles, we may begin to reveal the mechanisms of resistance and treatment failure.

13.3 EPIGENETIC HETEROGENEITY IN CANCER

Although mature cancers often contain a dominant clone of malignant cells, the properties of individual malignant cells in this clone will be variable; this heterogeneity is also true for cells in the multiple subclones that may occur in tumors. These properties are governed by epigenetic changes that influence the expression of genes within the common genome (see Chap. 3) and are often driven by microenvironmental influences.

Clinically apparent malignancies represent a relatively late stage in the evolution of a cancer. Each gram of cancer may contain half-a-billion cancer cells, and may shed large numbers of cancer cells into the circulation each day. Evidence that only a small proportion of these mobilized tumor cells leads to clinical metastases (see Chap. 10, Sec. 10.4.2) poses the question whether all cancer cells have equivalent potential to form metastases (ie, is it a stochastic process), or whether different cancer cells have intrinsically different self-renewal and differentiation potentials (ie, whether there is an intratumoral hierarchy). Several theories have been proposed to account for epigenetic tumor heterogeneity; 3 common models are reviewed below: (1) stochastic production of tumor cells with different properties, often linked with evidence of epithelial-mesenchymal transition (EMT); (2) the hierarchical CSC hypothesis; and (3) phenotypic plasticity. These models are not mutually exclusive and may coexist.

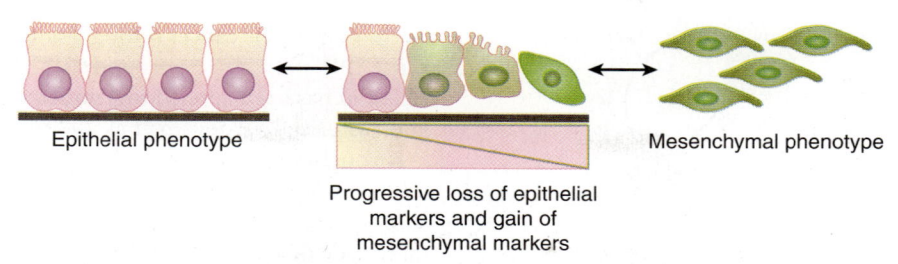

FIGURE 13–7 Epithelial to mesenchymal transition. Every cancer cell might have the potential to self-renew to maintain the primary tumor or form a new metastasis if a cell becomes mobile and finds the correct microenvironment. According to this theory, tumor maintenance or dissemination is a random or stochastic process, and variation between different behaviors may involve transition to and from epithelial to mesenchymal transition (EMT) phenotypes. The EMT describes the process of transformation of cells with a polarized, epithelial phenotype to cells with a motile, mesenchymal phenotype.

13.3.1 Epithelial-Mesenchymal Transition

The epithelial-mesenchymal transition is a process that describes the ability of cells to trans-differentiate from a polarized epithelial phenotype to a motile, mesenchymal cell phenotype (Brabletz et al, 2018; Fig. 13–7). The reverse of this process is termed mesenchymal-epithelial (MET) transition, and both processes are proposed to occur in embryogenesis, wound healing, and cancer.

EMT has been studied in in vitro and other model systems and involves molecular events that give rise to morphologic and functional alterations of cell behavior. Through the influence of extracellular signals from molecules such as TGF-β, Wnt, and PDGF (see Chap. 6, Sec. 6.4), cells with a polarized epithelial phenotype upregulate the expression of proteins and molecules that drive the cell to reorganize its cytoskeleton (eg, desmin), disconnect from underlying extracellular matrix (eg, metalloproteinases), downregulate adhesion molecules such as E-cadherin, and migrate through the local environment or more distally via vascular channels. EMT might occur in cancer because mutated cancer cells may be more easily influenced by microenvironmental signals, as receptors for these molecules may be overexpressed, and downstream signaling pathways may be constitutively activated by the acquisition of further mutations. Many aspects of EMT have been translated from developmental biology and wound healing to cancer biology. To date, evidence that an EMT contributes to malignancy is based primarily on mouse models, in vitro studies, or correlative pathologic studies (Shibue and Weinberg, 2017). A number of genes and signaling pathways are frequently invoked in describing EMT, but these processes have also been invoked in other models of epigenetic heterogeneity in cancer; for example, the *BMI1* gene has been reported relevant in EMT (Yang et al, 2010), but it is also studied in CSCs (see below).

Evidence for EMT in cancer includes the observation that cultured human epithelial cancer cells can express markers of EMT, such as loss of E-cadherin expression, and upregulation of expression of N-cadherin, smooth-muscle actin, vimentin, TWIST, SNAIL, and S100A4. Cancer cells expressing these markers can be identified at the "leading edge" of human tumors by histopathology, and are thus hypothesized to account for the population of cancer cells that can be shed into the circulation and become metastatic (Brabletz et al, 2018; see Chap. 10, Sec. 10.3.2). This phenomenon has also been observed in xenograft models (Kalluri and Weinberg, 2009).

There is clinical evidence for the relevance of EMT in human cancers. For example, markers of EMT are associated with poor prognosis in gastric carcinoma (Ryu et al, 2012), renal cell carcinoma (Mikami et al, 2011), breast carcinoma (Nes et al, 2012), and non–small cell lung carcinoma (Hung et al, 2009). Expression of EMT markers in cancer cells is also associated with resistance to treatment, including cytotoxic chemotherapy, hormonal agents, and drugs targeting growth factor signaling pathways such as EGF and HER2. It is unclear if EMT can be targeted to improve cancer management, but several preclinical studies suggest that targeting microRNAs (see Chap. 2, Sec. 2.3.3) associated with EMT (such as the miR-200 family) may lead to differentiation of mesenchymal-phenotype cancer cells to epithelial-phenotype cells, which might then be more susceptible to chemotherapy (Mikami et al, 2011).

13.3.2 Cancer Stem Cells

The CSC hypothesis states that only a minority of cancer cells has the potential to self-renew, proliferate indefinitely, and differentiate to give rise to more differentiated tumor cells (Fig. 13–8; Reya et al, 2001). Although cancer "nonstem cells" may retain limited proliferative potential, they are proposed as unable to propagate local recurrence or seed distant metastases. The CSC model represents tumors as caricatures of renewing tissues, such as the bone marrow, intestine, and skin, where a limited number of stem cells has the capacity to self-renew and to produce progeny that differentiate and carry out the normal function of that tissue (see Chap. 12, Sec. 12.1.3). Conceptually, this model suggests that in contrast to an infection, where all bacteria must be eliminated to cure the disease, cancer could be viewed rather like the organizational hierarchy of a beehive, with a queen bee, workers, and drones; only "queen bees" are able to propagate or reestablish the colony (Shlush et al, 2017).

To identify a CSC subpopulation, one should demonstrate tumor initiation when a limited number of such cancer cells are injected. Evidence for CSC self-renewal is obtained by observing xenograft formation after serially transplanting reisolated CSCs into secondary and tertiary recipient mice. Proposed

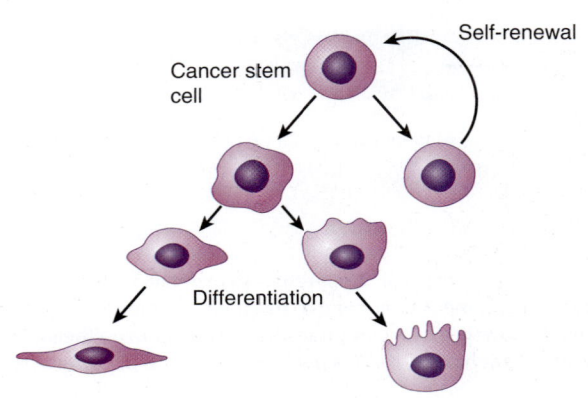

FIGURE 13-8 Cancer stem cells (CSCs) hypothesis. The cancer stem cells (CSCs) hypothesis posits that cancers are organized hierarchically in a parody of normal stem cell hierarchies, where only a subpopulation of CSCs has the potential to self-renew, extensively proliferate, and differentiate to form the bulk of the tumor consisting of non–stem cancer cells with a terminally differentiated phenotype. According to this hypothesis, terminally differentiated non–stem cancer cells do not necessarily possess the capability to dedifferentiate back to CSC.

CSCs must differentiate and recapitulate the phenotype of the tumor from which they were derived. Based on the above properties, CSCs are defined functionally as tumor-initiating cells (TICs), xenograft-initiating cells, or cancer-initiating cells (Ailles and Weissman, 2007).

Proposed CSC markers have been discovered by trial and error, but have frequently been translated from normal stem cell biology to the cancer setting. For example, CD133 (prominin-1, PROM1) has been used as a marker for neural stem cells and has been applied to neuroectodermal tumors such as glioblastoma (Lenkiewicz et al, 2009).

An ongoing question relates to the origin of tumor-initiating cells or CSCs. In some cancers, CSCs may be derived from somatic stem and progenitor cells of normal tissues, and there is evidence for this in leukemia (Lapidot et al, 1994) and medulloblastoma (Singh et al, 2004). However, terminally differentiated cells can be long-lived (Rawlins and Hogan, 2008), and may have sufficient time to acquire oncogenic mutations that allow them to evade apoptosis and senescence, proliferate independently of microenvironmental signals, and reactivate their self-renewal potential. The variation in histology, differentiation, and phenotype in cancers arising from a single tissue may be due in part to different cells of origin. The expression in cancer of genes and pathways that are expressed and active in embryonic stem cells and normal somatic stem cells, such as OCT4, NANOG, BMI1, and the Hedgehog, NOTCH, and WNT signaling networks (see Chap. 6, Sec. 6.4) should not be taken as proof of the existence of "cancer stem cells." Their re-expression in cancer most likely reflects the activation of molecular programs useful for self-renewal, asymmetric cell division, dormancy, migration/metastasis, proliferation, and differentiation, which are properties of both somatic stem cells and cancer cells (Table 13–1).

13.3.2.1 CSCs in Hematologic Malignancies

The first study in support of the CSC hypothesis in human cancers demonstrated the isolation of leukemia-initiating cells from

TABLE 13-1 Similar signaling pathways are used by somatic stem cells, cancer cells undergoing EMT, and cancer stem cells.

Pathway	Normal Stem Cell	Cancer Cell	Cancer Stem Cell
BMI1	Self-renewal of HSC and neural stem cells	Upregulated in AML and overexpressed in medulloblastoma	Overexpressed in, and induces self-renewal of, leukemic stem cells (Raaphorst, 2003)
Hedgehog pathway	Maintenance of HSC, development of skin, and postnatal and adult brain	Implicated in pancreatic carcinoma, basal cell carcinoma, and medulloblastoma	Regulates self-renewal and tumorigenicity in glioma and myeloma (Merchant and Matsui, 2010)
WNT signaling pathway	Maintenance of HSC and normal intestinal epithelial cells	WNT overexpressed in many human cancers	β-Catenin loss reduces self-renewal of normal and CML stem cells (Zhao et al, 2007)
NOTCH signaling pathway	Self-renewal of HSC and neural stem cells	Mutation or aberrant activation of NOTCH1 cause T-ALL in humans	Notch pathway inhibition depletes stem-like cells in glioblastoma (Fan et al, 2006)
HOX gene family	Self-renewal, proliferation, and differentiation of HSC	Prognostic marker in AML, described in T-ALL and drives leukemogenesis in a murine model	MEIS1 regulates MLL leukemia stem cell potential and hierarchy (Somervaille et al, 2009)
SOX gene family	Pivotal regulators of developmental programs such as fate determination and differentiation	Expressed in many cancers	Epigenetic switch between SOX2 and SOX9 regulates cancer cell plasticity (Lin et al, 2016)
NANOG	Regulator of self-renewal in embryonic stem cells	Expressed in many cancers	Promotes stem-like behavior in castrate-resistant prostate cancer stem cells (Kregel et al, 2014)
TGF-β	ACTIVIN and NODAL necessary for pluripotency	Accelerator to break cell-cycle regulation; pivotal to EMT and metastasis	Inhibition of differentiation and tumorigenesis (Strizzi et al, 2008)

AML, acute myeloid leukemia; *BMI1*, BMI1 polycomb ring finger oncogene; *CML*, chronic myeloid leukemia; *EMT*, epithelial-mesenchymal transition; *HOX*, homeobox genes; *HSC*, hematopoietic stem cells; *T-ALL*, T-cell acute lymphocytic leukemia; *TGF-β*, transforming growth factor beta.

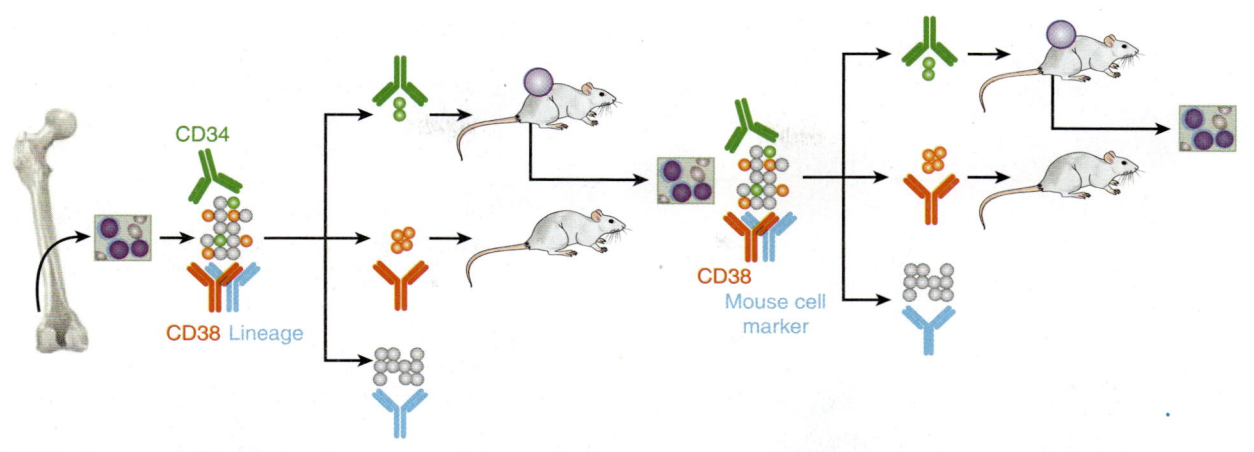

FIGURE 13-9 CSC in hematologic cancers. Leukemic stem cells were identified using cell-surface markers established from normal hematopoietic stem cell biology; these leukemic cells were negative for the progenitor cell marker CD38 but expressed the normal stem cell marker CD34. To identify and separate the "stem" and "nonstem" cancer cells, other antibodies (in blue) are used to identify and segregate non-cancerous cells (eg, lymphocytes and macrophages) from the human sample (the "lineage" cells) and mouse cells from the xenografted leukemia sample. Mice that engraft the leukemia are represented here with a green rectangle. Cells could be serially passaged through several generations of mice and maintained the same phenotype and morphology as the leukemia from the original patient.

people with acute myeloid leukemia (AML) (Lapidot et al, 1994; Fig. 13–9). Leukemic cells from the bone marrow and peripheral blood of patients with AML could be engrafted in severe combined immunodeficiency (SCID) mice supplemented with human stem cell factor (SCF) and a human granulocyte macrophage colony-stimulating factor (GM-CSF) interleukin-3 (IL-3) fusion protein. Some mice developed a morphologic and histochemical disease reminiscent of the original patient. Large numbers of AML cells were required for engraftment. In vitro clonogenic assays showed rare frequencies (0.3%–0.9%) of AML colony-forming units (CFUs) in primary patient samples or from AML cells extracted in bone marrow aspirates from transplanted mice, suggesting that the potential to engraft leukemia into SCID mice was a property of only a few, rare cells. AML cells expressing a phenotype similar to normal human hematopoietic stem cells (CD34^{++}/CD38^{neg}) were found to be more likely to engraft in SCID mice than CD34$^+$/CD38$^+$ or CD34$^-$ cells. In more immunocompromised NOD/SCID mice, which have far fewer natural killer cells (Chap. 21, Sec. 21.5.2), AML cells could engraft following injection of 10-20-fold lower numbers of AML cells, although there was wide variation in the serial leukemia-initiating cell frequency from different patients, suggesting underlying differences between their leukemias. Subsets of AML cells were again isolated by flow cytometry and injected into NOD/SCID mice. CD34$^+$ cells were able to engraft whereas CD34^{neg} cells did not engraft. The CD34^{++}/CD38^{neg} AML subsets were highly enriched for serial leukemia-initiating cells: as few as 5000 of these cells could engraft a NOD/SCID mouse, whereas 5×10^5 CD34^{low}/CD38$^+$ could not engraft. AML cells isolated from mice injected with CD34^{++}/CD38^{neg} cells showed a similar pattern of cell surface markers (immunophenotype) and similar morphology compared to the original cancer, implying in vivo differentiation of engrafted leukemia stem cells (LSC). CD34^{++}/CD38^{neg} cells could be isolated from primary xenografted animals and transplanted into secondary recipients with similar efficiencies of engraftment and recapitulation of ex vivo phenotype showing evidence of in vivo self-renewal of these cells (Lapidot et al, 1994). Bonnet and Dick (1997) extended these findings by tracking fluorescent AML cells through multiple generations. Long-term LSCs gave rise to short-term LSCs, and quiescent long-term LSCs gave rise to both short-term and long-term LSCs, demonstrating a "hierarchy within the hierarchy" of LSCs within AML. The similarity of this hierarchy to normal hematopoiesis suggested that the cell of origin for AML may be a normal hematopoietic stem cell (Lapidot et al. 1994).

CSCs have proven more challenging to study in other hematologic malignancies, such as lymphomas and myeloma. This apparent difficulty may be related to the broad spectrum of histologic, immunohistochemical, and clinical subtypes in lymphoma, and perhaps also due to a higher dependence on the microenvironment. Addition of human bone fragments improves engraftment and growth of human myeloma in immunocompromised mice, by providing an appropriate niche and/or bone marrow stromal cells that can secrete supportive human cytokines (Hope et al, 2004).

13.3.2.2 CSCs in Solid Tumors

CSCs have been identified in many solid cancers, including squamous cell carcinoma of the head and neck (Prince et al, 2007), colorectal cancer (Dalerba et al, 2007), pancreatic carcinoma (Hermann et al, 2007), hepatocellular carcinoma (Yang et al, 2008), ovarian carcinoma (Stewart et al, 2011), and prostate carcinoma (Collins et al, 2005). Cancers of the brain, breast, melanoma, and colorectal carcinoma are discussed in detail below (Fig. 13–10).

1. *Brain tumors:* CSCs were characterized in glioblastomas and medulloblastomas (Singh et al, 2004). Freshly excised tumors from adults and children were cultured in serum-free

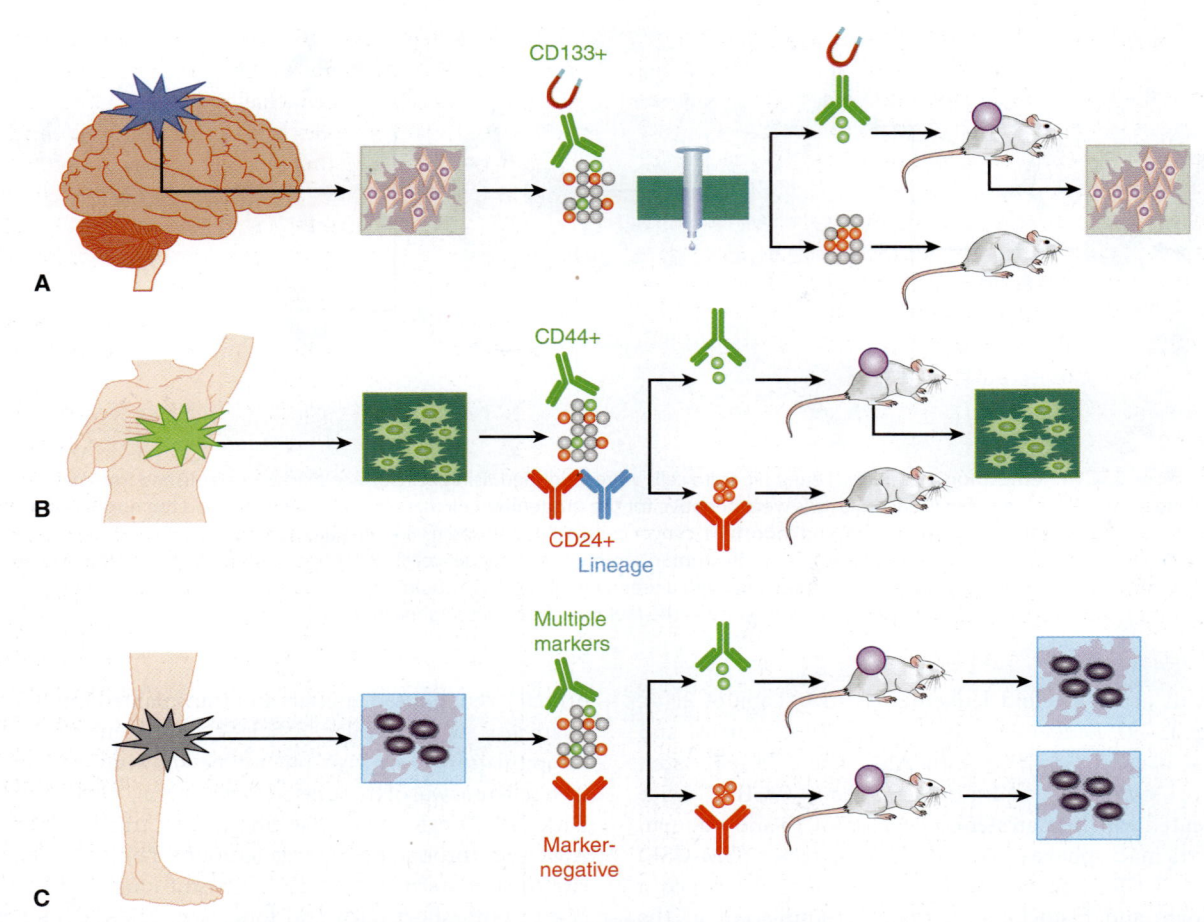

FIGURE 13–10 Cancer stem cells (CSCs) in solid tumors. **A)** Magnetically separated CD133⁺ glioma stem cells orthotopically implanted into mouse brain can recapitulate human glioma xenograft complexity; CD133⁻ cells cannot. **B)** Lineage-negative, epithelial marker-positive, CD44⁺, and CD24⁻ breast cancer stem cells can form xenografts in the mouse mammary fat pad. **C)** Although several CSC markers had been proposed in melanoma, a systematic examination of 22 heterogeneously expressed markers in melanoma failed to discover a marker that could enrich the already very frequent tumorigenic cells in melanoma; almost all malignant cells in melanoma appear to be CSCs.

media supplemented with various growth factors; all tumors grew nonadherently as neurosphere-like clusters. In vitro self-renewal was measured by assessing the rate of secondary sphere formation in a limiting dilution assay. CD133 was selected as a putative marker for brain CSCs as it had been used as a marker to select normal brain stem cells (Uchida et al, 2000). CD133⁺ cells were highly clonogenic compared to CD133ⁿᵉᵍ cells and showed higher proliferation and sphere formation at limiting dilutions of cells. In primary tumor specimens, CD133⁺ cells accounted for between 6% and 45% of all cells. Sphere-forming cells matched the differentiation profile of the primary tumor under controlled conditions.

CD133⁺ and CD133ⁿᵉᵍ cells isolated directly from freshly excised human medulloblastomas and glioblastomas were injected orthotopically into the brains of NOD/SCID mice at decreasing doses of cells. Tumors developed in most mice injected with as few as 100 CD133⁺ cells. Injections of up to 100,000 CD133ⁿᵉᵍ cells did not form tumors, but the cells did survive at the injection sites. Self-renewal of CD133⁺ cells was demonstrated in vivo by serial transplantation of CD133⁺ xenograft cells into secondary mice (Singh et al, 2004).

Other studies indicate that CD133 may not be an essential marker for CSC in brain cancer. Two groups reported that some glioma cell lines were completely negative for CD133 expression (Beier et al, 2007; Gunther et al, 2008). CD133-negative glioma lines tended to grow more slowly in vitro and in vivo and had a different gene expression profile compared to CD133⁺ glioma lines. Primary cells depleted of CD133⁺ cells from ex vivo patient glioblastoma specimens were tumorigenic and re-expressed CD133 (Wang et al, 2008).

A detailed functional analysis in a larger group of primary tumor samples, and de novo cultured glioblastoma samples, provided some unification of these conflicting observations: it showed that CD133-negative tumor cells were able to form tumors but that this property was largely dependent on CD133 reactivation. This plasticity (see below) suggests that although CD133 may not be a hierarchical marker for CSC in glioblastoma, it may still be critical for tumor formation (Brescia et al, 2013).

2. Breast cancer: Breast CSCs were the first to be identified in a solid malignancy (Al-Hajj et al, 2003). Cells from metastatic pleural effusions from 8 patients and cells from 1 primary breast cancer were either sorted by flow cytometry or passaged through mice and sorted from xenografts. These sorted cell populations were implanted orthotopically (in the mammary fat pad) in female, estrogen-supplemented NOD/SCID mice that had been further immunocompromised by treatment with etoposide. Flow cytometry was used to sort the cells, allowing exclusion of mouse cells and dead human cells, and identification and exclusion of human stromal cells like leucocytes (Fig. 13–10). Tumor cells with a CD44$^+$/CD24^{neg} phenotype were found in all of the xenografts (CD44$^+$/CD24^{neg} represented 11%-35% of all tumor cells) and these were enriched (10-50-fold) for tumor-forming ability versus CD44^{neg}/CD24$^+$ cells. As few as 200 EpCAM$^+$/CD44$^+$/CD24^{neg}/Lineage^{neg} cells could form a tumor when injected into immunocompromised mice. The authors demonstrated that tumor-forming potential was not related to cell cycle (ruling out brisker proliferation) and showed that cells gave rise to heterogeneous xenografts with similar characteristics and cellular markers to the primary human tumor. Thus, the identity of CSCs in breast cancer was narrowed to being included in this EpCAM$^+$/CD44$^+$/CD24^{neg}/Lineage^{neg} population of cells.

3. *Melanoma:* Evidence of CSCs from human melanoma samples was obtained using the CD133 and ABCB5 cell surface markers (Schatton et al, 2008). ABCB5 staining was found in fresh melanoma biopsies that were transplanted to form xenografts, and ABCB5 tended to stain areas of xenografts with less melanin. In a very small number of melanoma samples, ABCB5$^+$ cells were marginally enriched for malignant melanoma–initiating cells (MMICs; CSC frequency of ~1/111,000, vs 1 in ~1,000,000 unsorted melanoma cells). CD133$^+$ cells from melanoma were found to have greater ability to form colonies in tissue culture and were associated with patient-specific expression of cancer-testis antigens (Gedye et al, 2009).

Quintana et al (2008) have challenged the hypothesis that there is a subpopulation of CSCs in melanoma. This group injected melanoma cells with Matrigel into more severely immunocompromised NOD/SCID/IL2Rγ$^{-/-}$ (NSG) mice, which lack NK cell activity and found that xenograft-forming cells were extremely common in melanoma: up to 30% of unselected individual melanoma cells implanted subcutaneously could form a xenograft. A large panel of cell surface markers was tested in a second study, but none could discriminate for enriching tumor-forming cells (Quintana et al, 2010). Thus, it appears that no selection by a particular marker, no hierarchy, and no CSCs have yet been demonstrated in melanoma.

4. *Colorectal carcinoma:* Similar complexities have evolved in our understanding of cancer heterogeneity in colorectal carcinoma. CSCs were identified variously as being CD133$^+$, or CD44$^+$, and most recently LGR5$^+$. However, 2 recent reports (Melo et al, 2017; Shimokawa et al, 2017) have shown that human and murine colorectal cancer can survive and propagate without LGR5+ cells, although the pattern of growth is altered. LGR5-negative cells were able to replenish LGR5+ cell populations, suggesting again that the concept of a hierarchical model for cancer heterogeneity is unnecessary and a model incorporating phenotypic plasticity is more appropriate.

13.3.2.3 Criticisms of the CSC Hypothesis

The observation that a xenograft could grow from almost any single unselected melanoma cell challenged the CSC hypothesis, and spurred further research into conceptual, technical, and analytical criticisms of the concept. Lander pointed out that complex, seemingly hierarchical phenomena can arise as a result of simple stochastic rules (Lander, 2009). Following the report that a high proportion of melanoma cells could generate tumors when implanted with Matrigel in severely immunocompromised NSG mice, many groups transplanted other types of tumor cells into NSG mice and found that tumor-initiating cells remain rare in epithelial cancers (Ishizawa et al, 2010) and leukemia (Vargaftig et al, 2012). There are technical problems with xenograft experiments, although addressing them is helping to advance the field (Fig. 13–11): these include the loss of CSC marker expression during tumor digestion, failure to account numerically and functionally for stromal cells such as fibroblasts, and the interspecies difference in tumor microenvironment between mice and humans. Mathematical analysis shows that the absolute number of CSCs appears to vary depending on the context; for example, in some data sets, the absolute number of CSCs in the "negative" cell population outweighs the number in the selected "cancer stem cell marker positive" fraction (Hill, 2006). Our group has examined the influences of experimental methodology while studying the CSC hypothesis in clear cell renal cell carcinoma (Gedye et al, 2016). At every step of the experimental process (Fig. 13–11), we discovered biases that substantially alter our interpretation of the source and number of cancer cells, their processing, their viability, appropriate stromal support, and the difference between human and murine cell signaling. We concluded that the proportion of cells in clear cell renal carcinoma with stem cell properties is grossly underestimated by standard experimental methods. These studies highlight functional limitations of the models that support the CSC hypothesis.

Intense scrutiny of the CSC model has the positive effect of improving the experimental models used to study human cancer. For example, human tumor cells cultured de novo as "tumorspheres" in defined serum-free media can generate cell lines with morphologic heterogeneity that express markers of a primitive stem-like phenotype. They also form xenografts that are invasive and maintain the genotype of the original tumor and can be employed to demonstrate the efficacy of targeting glioblastoma stem cells by targeting various stem cell–signaling pathways (Pollard et al, 2009).

13.3.3 Phenotypic Plasticity

A third model for epigenetic heterogeneity is phenotypic plasticity, where cancer cell populations are in a dynamic equilibrium controlled by epigenetic mechanisms allowing the cells to switch between different cell phenotypes in response to microenvironmental stimuli. In melanoma cell lines, the histone demethylase JARID1B was found to be expressed in slowly cycling cells (that lacked expression of the proliferation marker Ki-67, and retained a dye stain showing an absence

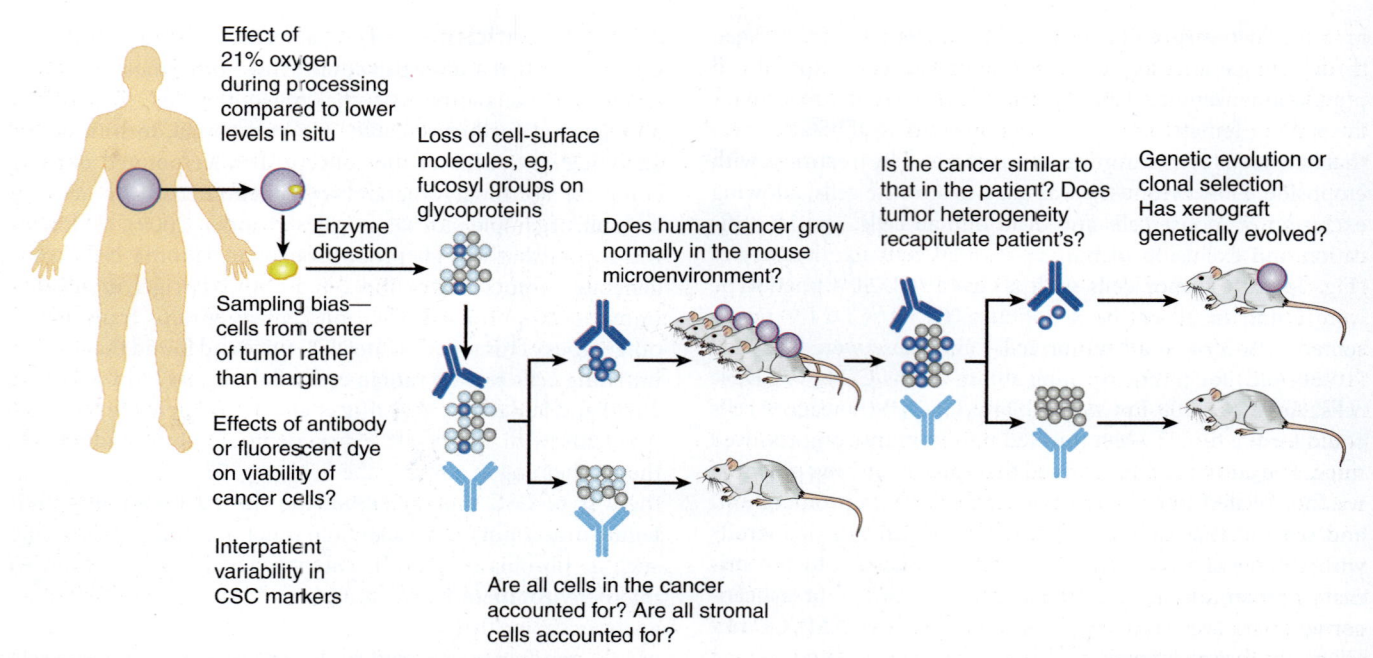

FIGURE 13–11 Experimental bias confounds analysis of cancer heterogeneity. Cancer cells are strongly influenced by the microenvironment and context, which complicates and challenges experimental investigation of models of heterogeneity, in particular the CSC hypothesis. Biases that might influence in vitro and xenograft experiments include the source of cancer cells, the way they are processed, evaluation of their viability, appropriate stromal support, and the difference between human and murine cell signaling proteins (eg, murine HGF does not stimulate human c-MET). Because many of these variables fail to recapitulate the in situ tumor microenvironment, analysis of heterogeneity is likely to be heavily biased. *CSC*, cancer stem cell; *HGF*, hepatocyte growth factor.

of cell division), and this cell population showed evidence of stem cell–like properties such as self-renewal (Roesch et al, 2010). Knockdown of *JARID1B* was associated initially with an increase in proliferation, followed by eventual exhaustion of cell growth, suggesting that JARID1B+ cells were necessary for maintenance of the cell population. The expression of JARID1B was not hierarchal; JARID1B+ cells could be derived from JARID1B− cells suggesting a dynamic plasticity between cell phenotypes rather than a hierarchical CSC organization. A similar dynamic plasticity of CD133+ to CD133− cells has been described in glioblastoma (Brescia et al, 2013).

Sharma et al found in cancer cell lines exposed to gefitinib an inhibitor of the epidermal growth factor receptor (EGFR) tyrosine kinase (see Chap. 19, Sec. 19.4.1), that while most cancer cells died rapidly, a tiny (~0.3%) quiescent subpopulation of "drug-tolerant persister" (DTP) cells survived and gradually began to proliferate (Sharma et al, 2010). Cell lines could become drug-sensitive after growth in the absence of drug, suggesting plasticity in the drug-tolerant phenotype. DTP cells expressed high levels of the histone demethylase JARID1A. Knockdown of *JARID1A* in these cell lines prevented the epigenetic mechanism of chromatin remodeling and modification and abrogated completely the survival of the DTP cells. Inhibition of chromatin remodeling by inhibition of histone deacetylation also inhibited DTP cell survival. Liau et al showed similar results in primary glioblastoma and early-passage glioblastoma cell lines, suggesting that this mechanism is active in vivo and is not limited to cancer cell lines (Liau et al, 2017). Another histone demethylase (KDM6A) was found responsible for reversible maintenance of drug-resistant stem cells, demonstrating how a process of phenotypic plasticity can underpin survival of cells with a stem cell phenotype (Liau et al, 2017).

For example, in genetically normal mouse embryonic stem cell cultures an examination of phenotypes (eg, presence or absence of the markers Oct4, Sox2, and Nanog) has shown the presence of cells in a so-called super state, where only a small (~0.2%–1.5%) fraction of cells were "totipotent," that is, capable of generating all cells in the body including germ cells, rather than simply "pluripotent," that is, able to generate all somatic tissues but not germ cells (Macfarlan et al, 2012). Epigenetic modification of histones (eg, methylation of histone 3 lysine 4 (H3K4) and acetylation of H3 and H4) was shown to partially control these changes between cell states, demonstrating an epigenetic basis for this phenotypic plasticity. By using fluorescent stains to track every cell in culture, it was found that all cells within the culture had the potential to enter the totipotent state. Although demonstrated for embryonic cells, similar processes may take place in tumors.

13.3.4 Models of Epigenetic Heterogeneity May Be Facets of the Same Process

As described above, there are several competing models to account for epigenetic heterogeneity in cancer, including EMT, CSCs, and plasticity. Most biological models have uncertainties and exceptions, and rather than one model being "right" or "wrong," there is evidence that the studies supporting these models may reflect aspects of the same biology, and that the experimental evidence for each model has been approached from different conceptual directions. This can be exemplified by studies examining breast cancer cells that express the CD44$^+$/CD24^{neg} phenotype.

CD44$^+$/CD24^{neg} breast cancer cells were described initially as breast CSCs (Al-Hajj et al, 2003). Subsequently, breast cancer cells expressing CD44$^+$/CD24^{neg} phenotype have also been reported as breast cancer cells that have become resistant to hormonal therapy (Creighton et al, 2009), resistant to chemotherapy (Li et al, 2008), resistant to radiation therapy (Lagadec et al, 2010), had become immune-evasive (Reim et al, 2009), or had undergone EMT (Mani et al, 2008). Thus, the models most commonly proposed to account for epigenetic heterogeneity, EMT and CSCs may have considerable overlap (Shibue and Weinberg, 2017), and the proposed CD44$^+$/CD24^{neg} phenotype may be describing cancer cells that survive or adapt to therapeutic targeting using epigenetic mechanisms. Thus, the distinction between these models (EMT, CSC, plasticity) may be less important than recognizing that these overlapping features may define a common mechanism for cancer to evade treatment.

13.3.5 Genetic and Epigenetic Heterogeneity in Cancer Are Interdependent

Genetic and epigenetic complexity evolves simultaneously, and can be interrelated. For example, a study of glioblastoma multiforme demonstrated genetic variation in different clonal populations derived from single cancer cells from different patients' tumors. Within each tumor were clones with different gene mutations associated with each clonal phenotype, and within each clonal population, genetically identical cells had a wide variation in their phenotypes, in the degree of aggressiveness of their behavior, and in their ability to resist drug treatments (Meyer et al, 2015). Furthermore, exposure to treatment can influence this process either by selection of subclones or by treatment-related mutation that generates diverse novel genomic structures in resistant cancer cells (Kim et al, 2015).

The relationships of genetic and epigenetic heterogeneity were also shown in tumor samples from patients with esophageal carcinoma (Hao et al, 2016). By using DNA exome sequencing to examine genetic evolution, and bisulfite sequencing to examine epigenetic variation in DNA methylation, it was shown that the cancers evolved over space and over time, and different parts of the cancer acquired different mutations and clonal architectures. Within each clonal subpopulation, the epigenetic DNA methylation patterns remain conserved, suggesting that genetic populations carried conserved epigenetic signatures.

How these complementary but distinct mechanisms of heterogeneity interact mechanistically is slowly becoming apparent. When yeast cells take on different phenotypes to adapt to their local conditions and environment, this adaptation gives these populations different opportunities for genetic evolution and thus longer-term survival (Bódi et al, 2017). This behavior

has been demonstrated in lung cancer cell lines (Frank and Rosner, 2012) and also in experimental and primary human breast cancers. Cancer cells at the leading boundary of the tumor possess a different phenotype from cells in the tumor core, suggesting that at least some intratumoral heterogeneity in the molecular properties of cancer cells is governed by predictable regional variations in environmental selection forces, and that evolution is not simply driven by random accumulation of mutations (Lloyd et al, 2016). Recent data suggest that constitutive activation of the TGF-β pathway in CD44$^+$/CD24^{neg} breast cancer cells was necessary and sufficient to impair DNA damage repair mechanisms, allowing an increased accumulation of DNA copy number alterations, greater genetic diversity, and improved adaptability to drug treatment (Pal et al, 2017).

13.4 CLINICAL IMPLICATIONS OF CANCER HETEROGENEITY

13.4.1 Prognostic and Predictive Relevance of Cancer Heterogeneity

Although one may debate the relative merits of different epigenetic heterogeneity models, the EMT/CSC phenotype has been associated with markers of poor patient outcome such as progression, survival, and distant metastasis. Increased expression of the stem cell marker CD133 predicts poor survival of patients with glioblastoma (Kong et al, 2008) and is associated with increased risk of progression, poorer survival, and poorer response to therapy of colorectal carcinoma (Sanders and Majumdar, 2011). Liu et al compared the gene-expression profile of CD44$^+$/CD24^{neg} breast EMT/CSC-like cells with that of normal breast epithelium, deriving a 186-gene "invasiveness" gene signature (IGS) that was associated with both overall and metastasis-free survival in women with breast cancer (Liu et al, 2007). Although there are many other prognostic gene signatures for breast cancer, the IGS was also associated with prognosis in medulloblastoma, lung cancer, and prostate cancer, implying more general relevance. Gene expression profiling of leukemic stem cell populations also yielded a signature of "stemness" associated with poor prognosis (Eppert et al, 2011). In this study, multiple different phenotypes of leukemic stem cell subsets (eg, CD34$^+$, CD34$^+$/CD38^{neg}) in multiple patients' samples were engrafted into mice, Different subpopulations of cells engrafted from different patients, but a core gene expression signature, were found in the subset of engrafting leukemic stem cells. Finally, as noted above, if cancers had at least 2 detectable clones, this was associated with worse patient survival, particularly if a driver mutation appeared in the less abundant clone (Andor et al, 2015).

Cancer heterogeneity can also provide insights into the failure of cancer therapy. Some tumors recur at the site of resection despite apparently adequate surgical margins; Prince et al demonstrated that the putative CSCs defined by CD44$^+$/BMI1$^+$ expression in head and neck squamous carcinomas are most often positioned at the edge of the tumor, abutting connective tissue, and may be the cause of recurrence (Prince et al, 2007).

Calabrese et al showed that glioblastoma stem cells are located in a perivascular location, perhaps accounting for the propensity of glioma to extend beyond the apparent tumor margin, leading to frequent disease relapse following attempted curative surgery (Calabrese et al, 2007).

An appreciation of cancer heterogeneity also informs our understanding of resistance to chemotherapy (see Chap. 18, Sec. 18.4). Putative CSCs expressing CD133 in de novo glioblastoma cell lines are intrinsically more chemoresistant than more differentiated cells (Liu et al, 2006), and intrinsically resistant breast cancer cells bear CSC markers (Li et al, 2008). Colorectal cancer cells with CSC markers are also more likely to survive treatment with oxaliplatin chemotherapy (Dylla et al, 2008). Preclinical studies have also demonstrated a link between EMT and chemoresistance in mouse models of breast and pancreatic cancer (Wang et al, 2016).

Resistance to radiation treatment has been shown to be an intrinsic property of cells with CSC markers in human glioblastoma (Bao et al, 2006) and breast cancer (Diehn et al, 2009), possibly because of lower levels of reactive oxygen species in their environment compared with more differentiated cancer cells (Brunner et al, 2012). In human breast cancer, expression of HOXB9 has been demonstrated to contribute to EMT-related radioresistance by accelerating DNA damage responses (Chiba et al, 2012).

13.4.2 Exploring Cancer Heterogeneity in Clinical Practice

Several groups have studied cancer heterogeneity and clonal evolution in biopsies taken at different times from individual patients' tumors, thereby revealing the importance of heterogeneity in clinical practice. For example, a detailed genomic investigation of women with advanced breast cancer showed that the cancer cells that had the genetic fitness to metastasize had occurred late in the evolution of the primary breast cancer, but continued to evolve after dissemination (Yates et al, 2017; see Fig. 13–6). Further mutations included clinically actionable alterations such as changes in the SWI/SNF and JAK2-STAT3 pathways. Similarly, deep sequencing has suggested that brain metastases may exhibit private mutations, that is, genetic and genomic changes that are restricted to cancers lesions in the brain that are not in the primary cancer, or in other metastases. This "branched" evolution may explain differential metastatic fitness, and may also reveal novel therapeutic targets (Brastianos et al, 2015).

Evolving technologies allow liquid biopsy for the diagnosis and monitoring of cancer heterogeneity in clinical practice. The detection of specific mutations in circulating tumor DNA (ctDNA), such as the BRAF^{V600E} mutation in melanoma can be used to select patients for treatment with BRAF/MEK inhibitors and monitor both their response and tumor heterogeneity during treatment (Haselmann et al, 2018). ctDNA can also be analyzed in patients with non–small cell lung cancer to predict resistance to first-generation inhibitors of EGFR in those with EGFR mutations (Sacher et al, 2016). Detection of highly prevalent DNA mutations in blood samples will likely soon deliver an effective way of monitoring outcomes in some patients, but this technique may have a more limited application for a deeper understanding of cancer heterogeneity.

Circulating tumor cells (CTCs) are found in the blood of patients with a wide spectrum of cancers, but usually not in healthy control subjects. CTCs have been shown to provide a surrogate biomarker for the presence or absence of some types of tumor, for semiquantitative assessment of tumor burden, and for monitoring response to treatment. CTCs may also permit real-time study of cancer complexity and heterogeneity.

In CTCs derived from patients with multiple myeloma, the mutational profile mirrored the changes found in cells in bone marrow biopsies, with a high concordance in somatic copy number alterations (Mishima et al, 2017). Women with ovarian cancer undergoing surgery and chemotherapy were found to have different kinds of CTCs, including those with an epithelial phenotype (~20%) or EMT-like CTCs (~30%). After platinum-based chemotherapy, the frequency of EMT-like CTCs increased up to 50%, and a new population of PI3Kα$^+$/Twist$^+$ EMT-like CTCs was observed. A higher proportion of these potentially more adaptive EMT-like CTCs was associated with poorer survival (Chebouti et al, 2017).

CTCs may be used to help to direct treatment. The phenotypic heterogeneity of circulating prostate cancer cells in the blood of men with castrate-resistant prostate cancer has been revealed by high-resolution imaging, thereby quantifying the physical diversity of cell types in individual patient samples (Scher et al, 2017). Low diversity was associated with better overall survival in patients treated with hormonal agents such as abiraterone or enzalutamide (see Chap. 20, Sec. 20.5), whereas greater heterogeneity was associated with better survival in men taking chemotherapy.

The fidelity of whole-genome sequencing of single cells has improved, and it allows the identification of distinct clones within a cancer, to identify driver mutations, and to pinpoint the tissue of origin of the cancer (Gulbahce et al, 2017). Whole-genome sequencing of CTCs may soon lead to high-resolution analysis of cancers that can diagnose, prognosticate, and guide personalized therapy. However, this activity must continue to occur in the context of prospective clinical trials. The strategy of using "precision oncology" to discover "actionable" mutations has so far had mixed results in delivering "personalized cancer medicine" (Tannock and Hickman, 2016).

Much work needs to occur before liquid biopsy biomarkers can become routine diagnostic tests. Only one CTC platform is FDA approved (CellSearch) and then only in the context of enumerating potential CTCs as a prognostic biomarker. Commercially available gene mutation platforms promoted to give a broad overview of mutations within an individual patient's cancer have been FDA approved but show poor concordance (~20%) between testing tumor DNA and ctDNA (Kuderer et al, 2017).

13.4.3 Implications of Cancer Heterogeneity for Treatment

The multidimensional heterogeneity of cancer presents a challenge to improving the treatment of established and disseminated cancers. The most effective treatment for a localized cancer remains local therapy, such as surgery or external beam radiotherapy; although there may be some differences in radiosensitivity among heterogeneous cell populations in the primary tumor, the main problem is that microscopic spread may have occurred. Adjuvant systemic therapy is given with local treatment of many primary tumors and its effectiveness will depend on responsiveness of micrometastases and will be limited by heterogeneity of tumor cell populations within them. This problem of heterogeneity dominates treatment of metastatic cancer, where there may be initial response to drug therapy followed by relapse as resistant subpopulations are either selected or develop because of adaptation (see Chap. 18, Sec. 18.4). Most solid tumors of adults are not curable once they have metastasized.

Immune checkpoint inhibitors (ICIs) used in cancer immunotherapy might offer one approach to mitigating the effects of tumor heterogeneity. Such therapy is more effective in tumors that have a high number of mutations, cancers caused by carcinogens such as tobacco or ultraviolet radiation, or those with a hypermutator phenotype (eg, microsatellite instability). This increased mutation burden leads to higher expression of neoantigens (see Chap. 21, Sec. 21.5), which presumably gives more targets to the immune system. However these mutations are likely to be diverse and to increase the degree of tumor heterogeneity, so effective treatment will require immune effector cells against multiple targets. However, some tumors may contain neoantigens created as a consequence of a critical driver mutation that occurred early in the life history of the cancer's evolution, leading to a clonal (or truncal) mutation that is shared in every cancer cell. A neoantigen present in every cell in the cancer (despite heterogeneity in other cellular properties) might be associated with an increased chance of a highly effective response to treatment (McGranahan et al, 2016). Supporting this concept, a recent study showed that the emergence of acquired resistance to immune checkpoint inhibitors (anti–PD-1 or anti–PD-1/anti–CTLA-4) in patients with non–small cell lung cancer after an initial response was frequently associated with genomic changes resulting in loss of mutation-associated neoantigens in resistant cancer clones (Anagnostou et al, 2017). This result also suggests that one strategy to improve cancer control is to expand immune responses to unrecognized cancer clones. For example, vaccination of immunocompetent mice with murine embryonic stem cells generated a "stem cell"–focused immune response that rendered these mice strongly resistant to subsequent engraftment with murine cancer cell lines (Kooreman et al, 2018), whereas treatment with anti-CTLA4 checkpoint antibodies appears to work in large part by increasing the breadth of the immune response (Robert et al, 2014; Fig. 13–12).

The concept of "precision medicine" is based on sequencing each person's cancer, and finding a molecularly defined treatment option for every patient (see Chap. 22, Sec. 22.3.2). Intratumoral heterogeneity is a barrier to the effectiveness of small molecules targeting driver mutations, as resistant subclones can be selected and outcompete sensitive tumor clones. One strategy to limit this resistance is by combining agents targeting genes in the same pathway, for example, by targeting BRAF and MEK in BRAF mutant melanoma (Fig. 13–12), but this has proven difficult to generalize because synergistic combinations have not been identified in most cancers, and because of the toxicity of targeted agents when used in combination (see also Chap. 19). Although the combination of BRAF and MEK inhibitors is associated with improved overall survival of people with melanoma (Flaherty et al, 2012), resistance and relapse is inevitable and occurs by multiple mechanisms, and sometimes by different mechanisms in an individual patient (Shi et al, 2014).

Another strategy that might constrain heterogeneity is differentiation therapy, using agents that cause differentiation of EMT/CSC-like cancer cells to make them more susceptible to standard therapies. A clinical example is the use of all-trans-retinoic acid (ATRA) and arsenic trioxide in the treatment of M3 acute promyelocytic leukemia (APML). ATRA and arsenic trioxide act by different mechanisms to destabilize the PML-RARα fusion translocation oncogene that is the molecular driver in most cases of APML. These agents cause differentiation and loss of self-renewal in the leukemic promyelocytes, and when combined, clinical trials have shown durable complete remissions in patients without the need for cytotoxic chemotherapy (Diehn and Clarke, 2006).

Efforts to overcome resistance to chemotherapy associated with CSC in other cancers are being tested in preclinical models and early-phase clinical trials, but with less success. The notch and hedgehog signaling pathways have been shown to regulate stem cells in many cancers (see Chap. 6, Sec. 6.4). Gamma-secretase inhibitors of the Notch pathway such as DAPT are active in preclinical models of head and neck cancer (Zhao et al, 2016), but clinical trials have shown little benefit for NOTCH inhibitors in diverse cancers. The Hedgehog signaling network was shown to be critical to CSC self-renewal, migration, and proliferation in pancreatic carcinoma (Mueller et al, 2009) but evaluation of inhibitors such as vismodegib to target pancreatic CSCs has been clinically unsuccessful (Kim et al, 2014) despite showing substantial biologic changes.

Finally as cancer cell populations respond to environmental cues, they can be envisioned as members of an ecosystem, and cancer can be viewed from the perspective of evolutionary ecology (Aktipis et al, 2015). Interruptions in drug dosing (taking away an ecological selection pressure) might allow populations of cancer cells to rebalance between resistant/dormant and sensitive/active populations (Fig. 13–12). This notion is based on the counterintuitive idea that stopping a drug while it is still working and then reintroducing the same agent on disease progression will extend the overall duration of benefit of that drug (Jansen et al, 2015). Computer modeling suggests that this strategy might extend the duration of benefit up to 5-fold (Hansen et al, 2017). The strategy of adaptive therapy uses patient-specific tumor dynamics to inform on/off treatment decisions, with the goal of suppressing proliferation of treatment-resistant cells, while extending the duration of therapy while lowering cumulative drug exposure. A pilot study using this strategy has been reported for prostate cancer (Zhang et al, 2017).

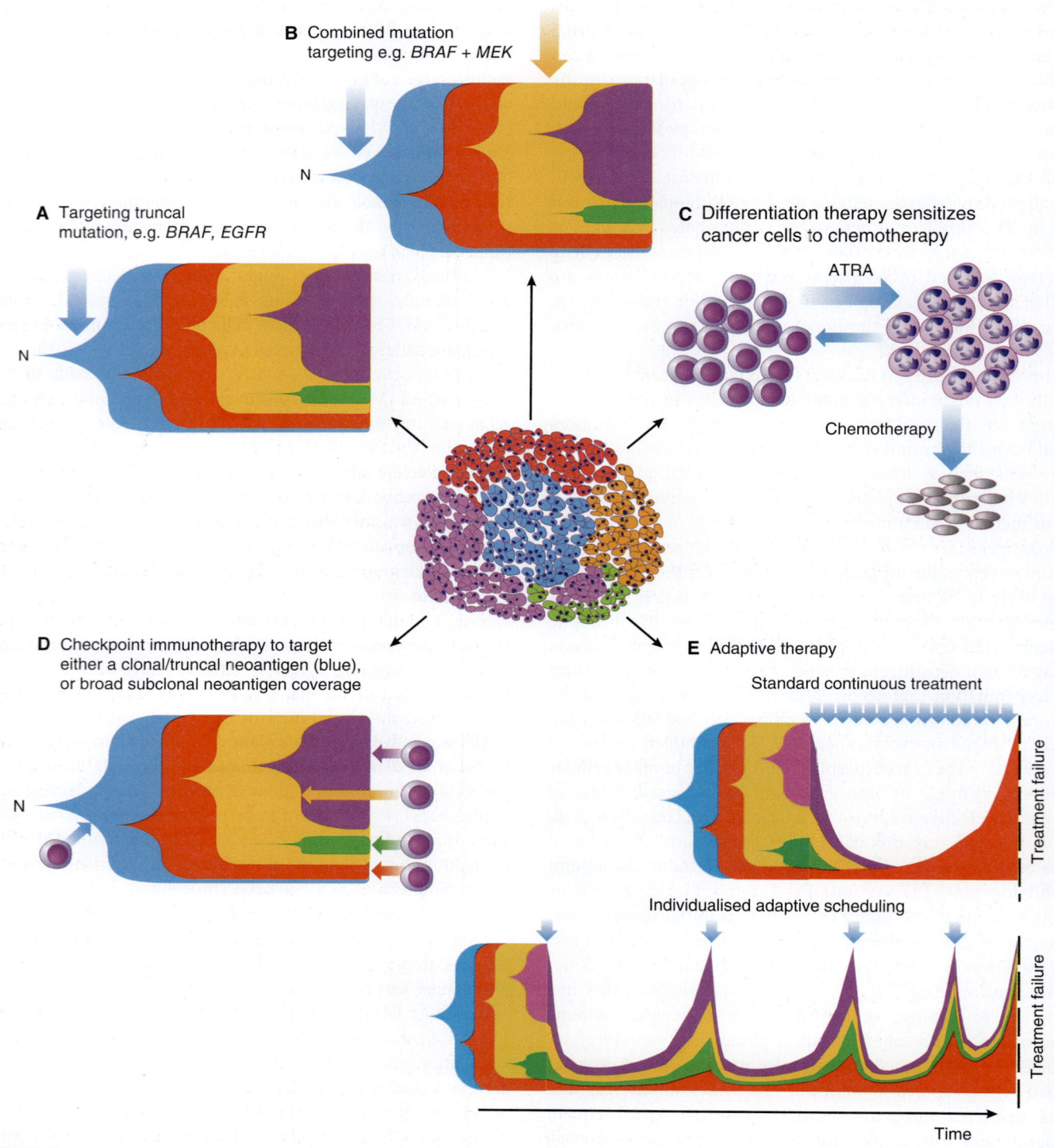

FIGURE 13-12 Strategies to overcome cancer heterogeneity. A) Treatments that can address a clonal/truncal mutation allows treatment of all cancer cells in a population. Examples include epidermal growth factor receptor (EGFR) tyrosine kinase inhibitors in *EGFR*-mutant non–small cell lung cancer. **B)** Combination of agents that inhibit the same signaling pathway (eg, BRAF and MEK inhibitors) can improve patient outcomes, though few cancers have these combinatorial treatments available. **C)** Differentiation of stemlike cells can prevent self-renewal and give rise to cells that are more vulnerable to cytotoxic chemotherapy (eg, all-trans retinoic acid [ATRA] in M3 acute promyelocytic leukemia); again there are few treatments in the clinic but agents are being tested against different pathways in different cancers. **D)** Checkpoint immunotherapy can control and seemingly cure cancer in a small number of patients; this might occur when there is immune recognition of a clonal neoantigen (McGranahan et al, 2016), or more comprehensive immune recognition delivering disease control across a broader population of tumor clones, eg, due to addition of anti-CTLA4 inhibition, which can expand the immune repertoire. **E)** Adaptive therapy employs evolutionary ecology principles to monitor tumor burden and use a therapy when disease progression is symptomatic, but once clinical control is established, treatment is withdrawn to limit outgrowth of treatment resistant clones (red). Treatment is recommenced when tumor burden increases again, and while resistance eventually develops, cancer control is prolonged compared with standard continuous dosing.

In summary, cancer heterogeneity represents an important reason for treatment failure, morbidity, and mortality from cancer, but improved understanding of the genetic and epigenetic mechanisms underlying heterogeneity is allowing development of strategies to combat it.

SUMMARY

- All cancers are heterogeneous.
- Genome-wide sequencing has greatly enhanced our ability to track the dynamics and origins of genetic cancer heterogeneity.
- Cancer heterogeneity is multidimensional and involves malignant cells and stromal cells, with clonal and epigenetic heterogeneity within the malignant cell population, which together with the variable local and metabolic environment lead to phenotypic heterogeneity.
- Genetic heterogeneity is a major driver of tumor relapse, recurrence, and treatment failure.
- Epigenetic heterogeneity may be hierarchical or stochastic. In a hierarchical model, only a subset of "cancer stem cells" has the potential to self-renew, proliferate indefinitely, and differentiate to nonstem cells. In a stochastic model, every cell has the potential to self-renew and recapitulate the tumor; epithelial-mesenchymal transition and phenotypic plasticity models may explain this stochastic model.
- Models of epigenetic heterogeneity are likely facets of the same process, as experimental evidence supporting plasticity, EMT, and the CSC hypothesis identifies similar markers and similar behaviors.
- EMT/CSC-like cancer cells have phenotypes predictive of poor patient prognosis and resistance to conventional cancer treatment.
- Adapting therapy to genetic and epigenetic diversity in cancer will require new types of therapy that are dependent on an understanding of the mechanisms underlying tumor heterogeneity.

REFERENCES

Ailles LE, Weissman IL. Cancer stem cells in solid tumors. *Curr Opin Biotechnol* 2007;18(5):460-466.

Aktipis CA, Boddy AM, Jansen G, et al. Cancer across the tree of life: cooperation and cheating in multicellularity. *Philos Trans R Soc Lond B Biol Sci* 2015;370(1673).

Al-Hajj M, Wicha MS, Benito-Hernandez A, Morrison SJ, Clarke MF. Prospective identification of tumorigenic breast cancer cells. *Proc Natl Acad Sci U S A* 2003;100(7):3983-3988.

Alexander CM, Puchalski J, Klos KS, et al. Separating stem cells by flow cytometry: reducing variability for solid tissues. *Cell Stem Cell* 2009;5(6):579-583.

Amirouchene-Angelozzi N, Swanton C, Bardelli A. Tumor evolution as a therapeutic target. *Cancer Discov* 2017;7(8):805-817.

Anagnostou V, Smith KN, Forde PM, et al. Evolution of neoantigen landscape during immune checkpoint blockade in non–small cell lung cancer. *Cancer Discov* 2017;7(3):264-276.

Andor N, Graham TA, Jansen M, et al. Pan-cancer analysis of the extent and consequences of intratumor heterogeneity. *Nat Med* 2015;22(1):105.

Baca Sylvan C, Prandi D, Lawrence Michael S, et al. Punctuated evolution of prostate cancer genomes. *Cell*. 2013;153(3):666-677.

Bao S, Wu Q, McLendon RE, et al. Glioma stem cells promote radioresistance by preferential activation of the DNA damage response. *Nature* 2006;444(7120):756-60.

Beier D, Hau P, Proescholdt M, et al. CD133(+) and CD133(−) glioblastoma-derived cancer stem cells show differential growth characteristics and molecular profiles. *Cancer Res* 2007;67(9):4010-4015.

Bhang H-eC, Ruddy DA, Krishnamurthy Radhakrishna V, et al. Studying clonal dynamics in response to cancer therapy using high-complexity barcoding. *Nat Med* 2015;21(5):440.

Bódi Z, Farkas Z, Nevozhay D, et al. Phenotypic heterogeneity promotes adaptive evolution. *PLOS Biol* 2017;15(5):e2000644.

Bonnet D, Dick JE. Human acute myeloid leukemia is organized as a hierarchy that originates from a primitive hematopoietic cell. *Nat Med* 1997;3(7):730-737.

Brabletz T, Kalluri R, Nieto MA, Weinberg RA. EMT in cancer. *Nat Rev Cancer* 2018;18(2):128.

Brastianos PK, Carter SL, Santagata S, et al. Genomic characterization of brain metastases reveals branched evolution and potential therapeutic targets. *Cancer Discov* 2015;5(11):1164-1177.

Brescia P, Ortensi B, Fornasari L, Levi D, Broggi G, Pelicci G. CD133 is essential for glioblastoma stem cell maintenance. *Stem Cells* 2013;31(5):857-869.

Brewer GJ, Torricelli JR, Evege EK, Price PJ. Optimized survival of hippocampal neurons in B27-supplemented neurobasal, a new serum-free medium combination. *J Neurosci Res* 1993;35(5):567-576.

Brunner TB, Kunz-Schughart LA, Grosse-Gehling P, Baumann M. Cancer stem cells as a predictive factor in radiotherapy. *Semin Radiat Oncol* 2012;22(2):151-174.

Calabrese C, Poppleton H, Kocak M, et al. A perivascular niche for brain tumor stem cells. *Cancer Cell* 2007;11(1):69-82.

Campbell PJ, Pleasance ED, Stephens PJ, et al. Subclonal phylogenetic structures in cancer revealed by ultra-deep sequencing. *Proc Natl Acad Sci U S A* 2008;105(35):13081-13086.

Campbell PJ, Yachida S, Mudie LJ, et al. The patterns and dynamics of genomic instability in metastatic pancreatic cancer. *Nature* 2010;467(7319):1109-1113.

Chebouti I, Kasimir-Bauer S, Buderath P, et al. EMT-like circulating tumor cells in ovarian cancer patients are enriched by platinum-based chemotherapy. *Oncotarget*. 2017;8(30):48820-48831.

Chevrier S, Levine JH, Zanotelli VRT, et al. An immune atlas of clear cell renal cell carcinoma. *Cell* 2017;169(4):736-749. e718.

Chiba N, Comaills V, Shiotani B, et al. Homeobox B9 induces epithelial-to-mesenchymal transition-associated radioresistance by accelerating DNA damage responses. *Proc Natl Acad Sci U S A* 2012;109(8):2760-2765.

Collins AT, Berry PA, Hyde C, Stower MJ, Maitland NJ. Prospective identification of tumorigenic prostate cancer stem cells. *Cancer Res* 2005;65(23):10946-10951.

Creighton CJ, Li X, Landis M, et al. Residual breast cancers after conventional therapy display mesenchymal as well as tumor-initiating features. *Proc Natl Acad Sci U S A* 2009;106(33):13820-13825.

Dalerba P, Dylla SJ, Park IK, et al. Phenotypic characterization of human colorectal cancer stem cells. *Proc Natl Acad Sci U S A* 2007;104(24):10158-10163.

Davis A, Gao R, Navin N. Tumor evolution: linear, branching, neutral or punctuated? *Biochim Biophys Acta Rev Cancer* 2017;1867(2):151-161.

Diehn M, Cho RW, Lobo NA, et al. Association of reactive oxygen species levels and radioresistance in cancer stem cells. *Nature* 2009;458(7239):780-783.

Diehn M, Clarke MF. Cancer stem cells and radiotherapy: new insights into tumor radioresistance. *J Natl Cancer Inst* 2006;98(24):1755-1757.

Dylla SJ, Beviglia L, Park IK, et al. Colorectal cancer stem cells are enriched in xenogeneic tumors following chemotherapy. *PLoS One* 2008;3(6):e2428.

Eppert K, Takenaka K, Lechman ER, et al. Stem cell gene expression programs influence clinical outcome in human leukemia. *Nat Med* 2011;17(9):1086-1093.

Fan X, Matsui W, Khaki L, et al. Notch pathway inhibition depletes stem-like cells and blocks engraftment in embryonal brain tumors. *Cancer Res* 2006;66(15):7445-7452.

Flaherty KT, Infante JR, Daud A, et al. Combined BRAF and MEK inhibition in melanoma with BRAF V600 mutations. *N Engl J Med* 2012;367(18):1694-1703.

Frank SA, Rosner MR. Nonheritable cellular variability accelerates the evolutionary processes of cancer. *PLoS Biol.* 2012;10(4):e1001296.

Gedye C, Quirk J, Browning J, et al. Cancer/testis antigens can be immunological targets in clonogenic CD133+ melanoma cells. *Cancer Immunol Immunother* 2009;58(10):1635-1646.

Gedye C, Sirskyj D, Lobo NC, et al. Cancer stem cells are underestimated by standard experimental methods in clear cell renal cell carcinoma. *Sci Rep* 2016;6:25220.

Gerlinger M, Horswell S, Larkin J, et al. Genomic architecture and evolution of clear cell renal cell carcinomas defined by multiregion sequencing. *Nat Genet* 2014;46(3):225-233.

Gerlinger M, Rowan AJ, Horswell S, et al. Intratumor heterogeneity and branched evolution revealed by multiregion sequencing. *N Engl J Med* 2012;366(10):883-892.

Gulbahce N, Magbanua MJM, Chin R, et al. Quantitative whole genome sequencing of circulating tumor cells enables personalized combination therapy of metastatic cancer. *Cancer Res* 2017;77(16):4530-4541.

Gunther HS, Schmidt NO, Phillips HS, et al. Glioblastoma-derived stem cell-enriched cultures form distinct subgroups according to molecular and phenotypic criteria. *Oncogene* 2008;27(20):2897-2909.

Hansen E, Woods RJ, Read AF. How to use a chemotherapeutic agent when resistance to it threatens the patient. *PLoS Biol* 2017;15(2):e2001110.

Hao J-J, Lin D-C, Dinh HQ, et al. Spatial intratumoral heterogeneity and temporal clonal evolution in esophageal squamous cell carcinoma. *Nat Genet* 2016;48(12):1500-1507.

Haselmann V, Gebhardt C, Brechtel I, et al. Liquid profiling of circulating tumor DNA in plasma of melanoma patients for companion diagnostics and monitoring of BRAF inhibitor therapy. *Clin Chem* 2018;64(5):830-842.

Hermann PC, Huber SL, Herrler T, et al. Distinct populations of cancer stem cells determine tumor growth and metastatic activity in human pancreatic cancer. *Cell Stem Cell* 2007; 1(3):313-323.

Hill RP. Identifying cancer stem cells in solid tumors: case not proven. *Cancer Res* 2006;66(4):1891-1895; discussion 1890.

Hope KJ, Jin L, Dick JE. Acute myeloid leukemia originates from a hierarchy of leukemic stem cell classes that differ in self-renewal capacity. *Nat Immunol* 2004;5(7):738-743.

Hung JJ, Yang MH, Hsu HS, Hsu WH, Liu JS, Wu KJ. Prognostic significance of hypoxia-inducible factor-1alpha, TWIST1 and Snail expression in resectable non-small cell lung cancer. *Thorax* 2009;64(12):1082-1089.

Ishizawa K, Rasheed ZA, Karisch R, et al. Tumor-initiating cells are rare in many human tumors. *Cell Stem Cell* 2010; 7(3):279-282.

Ito M, Hiramatsu H, Kobayashi K, et al. NOD/SCID/γc-null mouse: an excellent recipient mouse model for engraftment of human cells. *Blood* 2002;100(9):3175-3182.

Jamal-Hanjani M, Wilson GA, McGranahan N, et al. Tracking the evolution of non–small-cell lung cancer. *N Engl J Med* 2017;376(22):2109-2121.

Jansen G, Gatenby R, Aktipis CA. Opinion: control vs. eradication: applying infectious disease treatment strategies to cancer. *Proc Natl Acad Sci U S A* 2015;112(4):937-938.

John T, Kohler D, Pintilie M, et al. The ability to form primary tumor xenografts is predictive of increased risk of disease recurrence in early-stage non–small cell lung cancer. *Clinical Cancer Res* 2011;17(1):134-141.

Jones S, Chen WD, Parmigiani G, et al. Comparative lesion sequencing provides insights into tumor evolution. *Proc Natl Acad Sci U S A* 2008;105(11):4283-4288.

Kalluri R, Weinberg RA. The basics of epithelial-mesenchymal transition. *The Journal of Clinical Investigation.* 2009;119(6): 1420-1428.

Kim EJ, Sahai V, Abel EV, et al. Pilot clinical trial of hedgehog pathway inhibitor GDC-0449 (Vismodegib) in combination with gemcitabine in patients with metastatic pancreatic adenocarcinoma. *Clinical Cancer Res* 2014;20(23):5937-5945.

Kim H, Zheng S, Amini SS, et al. Whole-genome and multisector exome sequencing of primary and post-treatment glioblastoma reveals patterns of tumor evolution. *Genome Research.* 2015;25(3):316-327.

Kong DS, Kim MH, Park WY, et al. The progression of gliomas is associated with cancer stem cell phenotype. *Oncology reports*. 2008;19(3):639-643.

Kooreman NG, Kim Y, de Almeida PE, et al. Autologous iPSC-based vaccines elicit anti-tumor responses in vivo. *Cell Stem Cell* 2018;22(4):501-513.

Kregel S, Szmulewitz RZ, Vander Griend DJ. The pluripotency factor NANOG is directly upregulated by the androgen receptor in prostate cancer cells. *The Prostate*. 2014;74(15): 1530-1543.

Kuderer NM, Burton KA, Blau S, et al. Comparison of 2 commercially available next-generation sequencing platforms in oncology. *JAMA Oncol* 2017;3(7):996-998.

Kusnoor SV, Koonce TY, Levy MA, et al. My cancer genome: evaluating an educational model to introduce patients and caregivers to precision medicine information. *AMIA Jt Summits Transl Sci Proc* 2016;2016:112-121.

Lagadec C, Vlashi E, Della Donna L, et al. Survival and self-renewing capacity of breast cancer initiating cells during fractionated radiation treatment. *Breast Cancer Res* 2010; 12(1):R13.

Lan X, Jörg DJ, Cavalli FMG, et al. Fate mapping of human glioblastoma reveals an invariant stem cell hierarchy. *Nature* 2017;549(7671):227-232.

Lander A. The "stem cell" concept: is it holding us back? *J Biol* 2009;8(8):70.

Lapidot T, Sirard C, Vormoor J, et al. A cell initiating human acute myeloid leukaemia after transplantation into SCID mice. *Nature* 1994;367(6464):645-648.

Lee J, Kotliarova S, Kotliarov Y, et al. Tumor stem cells derived from glioblastomas cultured in bFGF and EGF more closely mirror the phenotype and genotype of primary tumors than do serum-cultured cell lines. *Cancer Cell* 2006;9(5):391-403.

Lenkiewicz M, Li N, Singh SK. Culture and isolation of brain tumor initiating cells. *Curr Protoc Stem Cell Biol* 2009; 3:Unit 3.3.1-3.3.10.

Li X, Lewis MT, Huang J, et al. Intrinsic resistance of tumorigenic breast cancer cells to chemotherapy. *J Natl Cancer Inst* 2008;100(9):672-679.

Liau BB, Sievers C, Donohue LK, et al. Adaptive chromatin remodeling drives glioblastoma stem cell plasticity and drug tolerance. *Cell Stem Cell* 2017;20(2):233-246.e7.

Lin S-C, Chou Y-T, Jiang SS, et al. Epigenetic switch between SOX2 and SOX9 regulates cancer cell plasticity. *Cancer Res* 2016;76(23):7036.

Liu G, Yuan X, Zeng Z, et al. Analysis of gene expression and chemoresistance of CD133+ cancer stem cells in glioblastoma. *Mol Cancer* 2006;5:67.

Liu R, Wang X, Chen GY, et al. The prognostic role of a gene signature from tumorigenic breast-cancer cells. *N Engl J Med* 2007;356(3):217-226.

Liu W, Laitinen S, Khan S, et al. Copy number analysis indicates monoclonal origin of lethal metastatic prostate cancer. *Nat Med* 2009;15(5):559-565.

Lloyd MC, Cunningham JJ, Bui MM, Gillies RJ, Brown JS, Gatenby RA. Darwinian dynamics of intratumoral heterogeneity: not solely random mutations but also variable environmental selection forces. *Cancer Res* 2016;76(11): 3136-3144.

Macaulay IC, Ponting CP, Voet T. Single-cell multiomics: multiple measurements from single cells. *Trends Genet* 2017; 33(2):155-168.

Macfarlan TS, Gifford WD, Driscoll S, et al. Embryonic stem cell potency fluctuates with endogenous retrovirus activity. *Nature* 2012;487(7405):57-63.

Mani SA, Guo W, Liao M-J, et al. The epithelial-mesenchymal transition generates cells with properties of stem cells. *Cell* 2008;133(4):704-715.

Martinez P, Birkbak NJ, Gerlinger M, et al. Parallel evolution of tumour subclones mimics diversity between tumours. *J Pathol* 2013;230(4):356-364.

McGranahan N, Furness AJS, Rosenthal R, et al. Clonal neoantigens elicit T cell immunoreactivity and sensitivity to immune checkpoint blockade. *Science* 2016;351(6280):1463-1469.

McGranahan N, Swanton C. Clonal heterogeneity and tumor evolution: past, present, and the future. *Cell* 2017; 168(4):613-628.

Melo FdSe, Kurtova AV, Harnoss JM, et al. A distinct role for Lgr5+ stem cells in primary and metastatic colon cancer. *Nature* 2017;543(7647):676-680.

Merchant AA, Matsui W. Targeting hedgehog—a cancer stem cell pathway. *Clin Cancer Res* 2010;16(12):3130-3140.

Meyer M, Reimand J, Lan X, et al. Single cell-derived clonal analysis of human glioblastoma links functional and genomic heterogeneity. *Proc Natl Acad Sci U S A* 2015;112(3):851-856.

Mikami S, Katsube K, Oya M, et al. Expression of Snail and Slug in renal cell carcinoma: E-cadherin repressor Snail is associated with cancer invasion and prognosis. *Lab Invest*. 2011;91(10):1443-1458.

Mishima Y, Paiva B, Shi J, et al. The mutational landscape of circulating tumor cells in multiple myeloma. *Cell Rep* 2017;19(1):218-224.

Mueller MT, Hermann PC, Witthauer J, et al. Combined targeted treatment to eliminate tumorigenic cancer stem cells in human pancreatic cancer. *Gastroenterology* 2009; 137(3):1102-1113.

Naxerova K, Reiter JG, Brachtel E, et al. Origins of lymphatic and distant metastases in human colorectal cancer. *Science* 2017;357(6346):55-60.

Nes JH, Kruijf E, Putter H, et al. Co-expression of SNAIL and TWIST determines prognosis in estrogen receptor-positive early breast cancer patients. *Breast Cancer Res Treat* 2012; 133(1):49-59.

Notta F, Chan-Seng-Yue M, Lemire M, et al. A renewed model of pancreatic cancer evolution based on genomic rearrangement patterns. *Nature* 2016;538(7625):378-382.

Notta F, Mulligan CG, Wang JCY, et al. Evolution of human BCR-ABL1 lymphoblastic leukaemia-initiating cells. *Nature* 2011;469(7330):362-367.

Öhlund D, Handly-Santana A, Biffi G, et al. Distinct populations of inflammatory fibroblasts and myofibroblasts in pancreatic cancer. *J Exp Med* 2017;214(3):579-596.

Paget S. The distribution of secondary growths in cancer of the breast. *Lancet* 1889;1:571-573.

Pal D, Pertot A, Shirole NH, et al. TGF-β reduces DNA ds-break repair mechanisms to heighten genetic diversity and adaptability of CD44+/CD24- cancer cells. *eLife* 2017;6:e21615.

Palmon A, David R, Neumann Y, Stiubea-Cohen R, Krief G, Aframian DJ. High-efficiency immunomagnetic isolation of solid tissue-originated integrin-expressing adult stem cells. *Methods* 2012;56(2):305-309.

Pierce GB, Speers WC. Tumors as caricatures of the process of tissue renewal: prospects for therapy by directing differentiation. *Cancer Res* 1988;48(8):1996-2004.

Pierce GB, Wallace C. Differentiation of malignant to benign cells. *Cancer Res* 1971;31(2):127-134.

Pollard SM, Yoshikawa K, Clarke ID, et al. Glioma stem cell lines expanded in adherent culture have tumor-specific phenotypes and are suitable for chemical and genetic screens. *Cell Stem Cell* 2009;4(6):568-580.

Pommier A, Fearon DT. Disruption of anti-tumor T cell responses by cancer-associated fibroblasts. In: Donnadieu E, ed. *Defects in T Cell Trafficking and Resistance to Cancer Immunotherapy*. Cham, Switzerland: Springer International Publishing; 2016:77-98.

Prince ME, Sivanandan R, Kaczorowski A, et al. Identification of a subpopulation of cells with cancer stem cell properties in head and neck squamous cell carcinoma. *Proc Natl Acad Sci U S A* 2007;104(3):973-978.

Quintana E, Shackleton M, Foster HR, et al. Phenotypic heterogeneity among tumorigenic melanoma cells from patients that is reversible and not hierarchically organized. *Cancer Cell* 2010;18(5):510-523.

Quintana E, Shackleton M, Sabel MS, Fullen DR, Johnson TM, Morrison SJ. Efficient tumour formation by single human melanoma cells. *Nature* 2008;456(7222):593-598.

Raaphorst FM. Self-renewal of hematopoietic and leukemic stem cells: a central role for the Polycomb-group gene, Bmi-1. *Trends Immunol* 2003;24(10):522-524.

Rawlins EL, Hogan BLM. Ciliated epithelial cell lifespan in the mouse trachea and lung. *Am J Physiol Lung Cell Mol Physiol* 2008;295(1):L231-L234.

Reim F, Dombrowski Y, Ritter C, et al. Immunoselection of breast and ovarian cancer cells with trastuzumab and natural killer cells: selective escape of CD44high/CD24low/HER2low breast cancer stem cells. *Cancer Res* 2009;69(20):8058-8066.

Reya T, Morrison SJ, Clarke MF, Weissman IL. Stem cells, cancer, and cancer stem cells. *Nature* 2001;414(6859):105-111.

Robert L, Tsoi J, Wang X, et al. CTLA4 blockade broadens the peripheral T-cell receptor repertoire. *Clin Cancer Res* 2014;20(9):2424-2432.

Rode A, Maass KK, Willmund KV, Lichter P, Ernst A. Chromothripsis in cancer cells: an update. *Int J Cancer* 2016;138(10):2322-2333.

Roesch A, Fukunaga-Kalabis M, Schmidt EC, et al. A temporarily distinct subpopulation of slow-cycling melanoma cells is required for continuous tumor growth. *Cell* 2010;141(4):583-594.

Ryu HS, Park DJ, Kim HH, Kim WH, Lee HS. Combination of epithelial-mesenchymal transition and cancer stem cell-like phenotypes has independent prognostic value in gastric cancer. *Hum Pathol* 2012;43(4):520-528.

Sacher AG, Paweletz C, Dahlberg SE, et al. Prospective validation of rapid plasma genotyping for the detection of EGFR and KRAS mutations in advanced lung cancer. *JAMA Oncol* 2016;2(8):1014-1022.

Sanders MA, Majumdar AP. Colon cancer stem cells: implications in carcinogenesis. *Front Biosci* 2011;16:1651-1662.

Sansregret L, Vanhaesebroeck B, Swanton C. Determinants and clinical implications of chromosomal instability in cancer. *Nat Rev Clin Oncol* 2018;15(3):139.

Schatton T, Murphy GF, Frank NY, et al. Identification of cells initiating human melanomas. *Nature* 2008;451(7176):345-349.

Scher HI, Graf RP, Schreiber NA, et al. Phenotypic heterogeneity of circulating tumor cells informs clinical decisions between ar signaling inhibitors and taxanes in metastatic prostate cancer. *Cancer Res* 2017;77(20):5687-5698.

Sharma SV, Lee DY, Li B, et al. A chromatin-mediated reversible drug-tolerant state in cancer cell subpopulations. *Cell* 2010;141(1):69-80.

Shi H, Hugo W, Kong X, et al. Acquired resistance and clonal evolution in melanoma during BRAF inhibitor therapy. *Cancer Discov* 2014;4(1):80-93.

Shibue T, Weinberg RA. EMT, CSCs, and drug resistance: the mechanistic link and clinical implications. *Nat Rev Clin Oncol* 2017;14(10):611.

Shimokawa M, Ohta Y, Nishikori S, et al. Visualization and targeting of LGR5+ human colon cancer stem cells. *Nature* 2017;545(7653):187-192.

Shlush LI, Mitchell A, Heisler L, et al. Tracing the origins of relapse in acute myeloid leukaemia to stem cells. *Nature* 2017;547:104.

Singh S, Hawkins C, Clarke I, et al. Identification of human brain tumour initiating cells. *Nature* 2004;432(7015):396-401.

Smallwood SA, Lee HJ, Angermueller C, et al. Single-cell genome-wide bisulfite sequencing for assessing epigenetic heterogeneity. *Nat Methods* 2014;11(8):817.

Somervaille TC, Matheny CJ, Spencer GJ, et al. Hierarchical maintenance of MLL myeloid leukemia stem cells employs a transcriptional program shared with embryonic rather than adult stem cells. *Cell Stem Cell* 2009;4(2):129-140.

Sottoriva A, Kang H, Ma Z, et al. A Big Bang model of human colorectal tumor growth. *Nat Genet* 2015;47(3):209-216.

Stewart JM, Shaw PA, Gedye C, Bernardini MQ, Neel BG, Ailles LE. Phenotypic heterogeneity and instability of human ovarian tumor-initiating cells. *Proc Natl Acad Sci U S A* 2011;108(16):6468-6473.

Strizzi L, Abbott DE, Salomon DS, Hendrix MJ. Potential for cripto-1 in defining stem cell-like characteristics in human malignant melanoma. *Cell Cycle* 2008;7(13):1931-1935.

Tannock IF, Hickman JA. Limits to personalized cancer medicine. *N Engl J Med* 2016;375(13):1289-1294.

The Cancer Genome Atlas N. Comprehensive molecular characterization of human colon and rectal cancer. *Nature* 2012;487(7407):330.

Till JE, McCulloch EA. A direct measurement of the radiation sensitivity of normal mouse bone marrow cells. *Radiat Res* 1961;14:213-222.

Uchida N, Buck DW, He D, et al. Direct isolation of human central nervous system stem cells. *Proc Natl Acad Sci U S A* 2000;97(26):14720-14725.

van Staveren WC, Solis DY, Hebrant A, Detours V, Dumont JE, Maenhaut C. Human cancer cell lines: experimental models for cancer cells in situ? For cancer stem cells? *Biochim Biophys Acta* 2009;1795(2):92-103.

Vargaftig J, Taussig DC, Griessinger E, et al. Frequency of leukemic initiating cells does not depend on the xenotransplantation model used. *Leukemia* 2012;26(4):858-860.

Verma B, Ritchie M, Mancini M. Development and applications of patient-derived xenograft models in humanized mice for oncology and immune-oncology drug discovery. *Curr Protocol Pharmacol* 2017;78:14.41.1-14.41.12.

Vogelstein B, Fearon ER, Hamilton SR, et al. Genetic alterations during colorectal-tumor development. *N Engl J Med* 1988;319(9):525-532.

Wang J, Sakariassen PO, Tsinkalovsky O, et al. CD133 negative glioma cells form tumors in nude rats and give rise to CD133 positive cells. *Int J Cancer* 2008;122(4):761-768.

Wang J, Wei Q, Wang X, et al. Transition to resistance: an unexpected role of the EMT in cancer chemoresistance. *Genes Dis* 2016;3(1):3-6.

Wang Y, Waters J, Leung ML, et al. Clonal evolution in breast cancer revealed by single nucleus genome sequencing. *Nature* 2014;512(7513):155-160.

Yang M-H, Hsu DS-S, Wang H-W, et al. Bmi1 is essential in Twist1-induced epithelial-mesenchymal transition. *Nat Cell Biol* 2010;12(10):982-992.

Yang ZF, Ngai P, Ho DW, et al. Identification of local and circulating cancer stem cells in human liver cancer. *Hepatology* 2008;47(3):919-928.

Yao X, Qian C-N, Zhang Z-F, et al. Two distinct types of blood vessels in clear cell renal cell carcinoma have contrasting prognostic implications. *Clinical Cancer Res* 2007;13(1):161-169.

Yates LR, Knappskog S, Wedge D, et al. Genomic evolution of breast cancer metastasis and relapse. *Cancer Cell* 2017;32(2):169-184.e167.

Zhang J, Cunningham JJ, Brown JS, Gatenby RA. Integrating evolutionary dynamics into treatment of metastatic castrate-resistant prostate cancer. *Nat Commun* 2017;8(1):1816.

Zhao C, Blum J, Chen A, et al. Loss of [beta]-catenin impairs the renewal of normal and CML stem cells in vivo. *Cancer Cell* 2007;12(6):528-541.

Zhao Z-L, Zhang L, Huang C-F, et al. NOTCH1 inhibition enhances the efficacy of conventional chemotherapeutic agents by targeting head neck cancer stem cell. *Sci Rep* 2016;6:24704.

Imaging in Oncology

Mattea L. Welch and David A. Jaffray

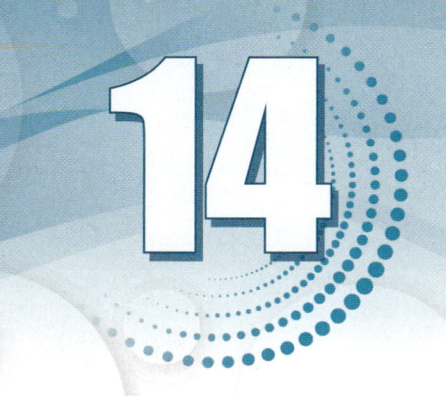

Chapter Outline

14.1 Introduction
14.2 General Concepts Relating to Cancer Imaging
14.3 Imaging Technologies
    14.3.1 X-ray–Based Systems: Radiography and Computed Tomography
    14.3.2 Magnetic Resonance Imaging
    14.3.3 Single-Photon and Positron Emission Tomography
    14.3.4 Ultrasound Imaging
    14.3.5 Optical Imaging
14.4 Imaging of Animal Models in Oncology
14.5 New Directions in Oncologic Imaging
    14.5.1 Quantitative Methods and Quality Assurance
    14.5.2 Improving on RECIST Criteria
    14.5.3 Images and Biological Information Combined for Discovery
    14.5.4 Image Guidance in Cancer Treatment
    14.5.5 Machine Learning for Image Reconstruction, Prognostics and Predictions
Summary
References

14.1 INTRODUCTION

The need to detect and characterize cancer in an individual has resulted in a dramatic increase in the use of imaging. Clinical imaging is a routine part of diagnosis, staging, guiding localized therapy, and assessing response to treatment. Cancers occur anatomically among surrounding normal tissues, including critical structures, such as major organs, vessels, and nerves, and delineation of the extent of malignant and nonmalignant tissues is essential for planning surgery and radiation therapy. Cancers also have morphologic, physiologic, and biochemical heterogeneity (see Chap. 13), which is important in understanding their biology and potential response to treatment. The ability to explore and define this heterogeneity with modern imaging methods, as well as serum and tissue-derived metrics, will enable more precise cancer treatments.

Imaging is diverse in that it offers multiple different representations of disease information. For example, computed tomography (CT) or magnetic resonance (MR) imaging provides an "anatomical image" of the malignant tissue among nonmalignant tissue; positron emission tomography (PET) images generate a "functional image" of disease status related to tissue function such as glucose metabolism (see Chap. 12) or hypoxic fraction (see Chap. 12); and optical imaging can be used to generate a "microscopic image" used during classification of histologic type and grade. Imaging is applied at these multiple levels to help characterize, understand, and plan the treatment of cancers (Fig. 14–1). Advances in imaging are central in the fight against cancer. This chapter introduces the rapidly evolving field of oncologic imaging by presenting both the physical principles underlying the most common imaging modalities and their clinical and research applications in oncology.

14.2 GENERAL CONCEPTS RELATING TO CANCER IMAGING

Imaging is a broad science that encompasses the design, development, evaluation, and application of technologies that allow spatial and temporal characterization of an object; ideally, with minimal invasion. When using imaging, it is important to understand what *signal* is detected and how this signal relates to the underlying *biological processes* or *structural elements*. Imaging signals can be broadly classified as *endogenous or exogenous*. *Endogenous signals* are those associated with the intrinsic characteristics of the body and how these characteristics affect the imaging modality. For example, a chest radiograph detects a lung lesion because of the intrinsic difference in x-ray attenuation by the lung and tumor tissue (see Fig. 14–1D). *Exogenous signals* are those that arise from the introduction of an imaging agent (eg, injecting an iodinated x-ray–absorbing contrast agent for CT scanning or a positron-emitting tracer such as ^{18}F-fluorodeoxyglucose [FDG] for PET imaging) that alters or generates the image

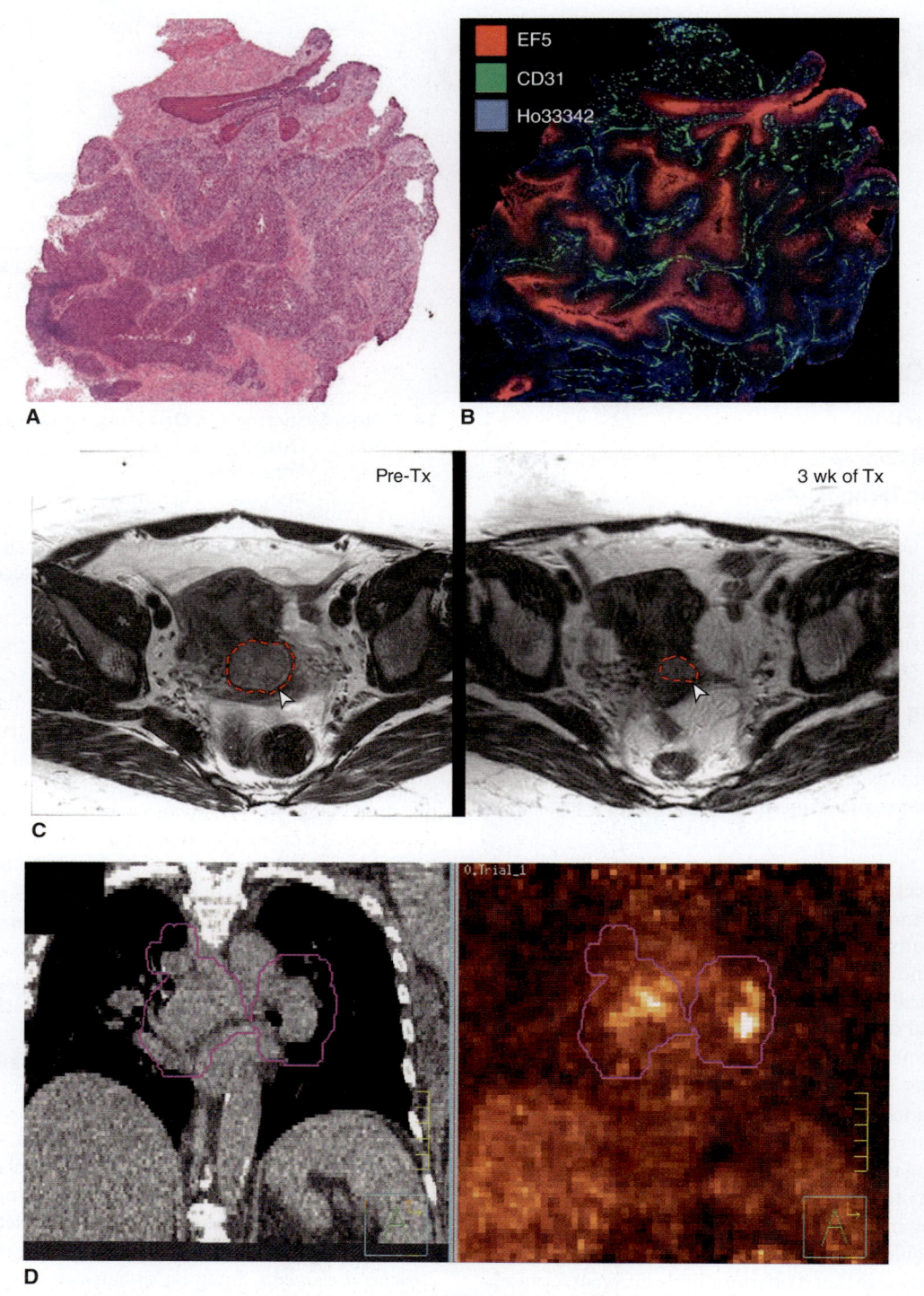

FIGURE 14-1 Different visual representations of cancer at different spatial scales and time points. **A)** Traditional hematoxylin and eosin (H&E) staining of a cervix cancer xenograft. These stains highlight the cellular architecture and are used to assess histologic type and grade of cancer. **B)** More advanced immunohistochemical staining of the same tumor demonstrating the complex microenvironment with the tumor. Substantial variation in microvasculature (CD31, green) and oxygen tension (EF5, red) are seen despite the evidence that the tumor is perfused (indicated by the injected Hoechst 33342 dye, blue). **C)** T_2-weighted MR image of a cancer of the cervix before (left) and during (right) radiotherapy (after 25 × 1.8-Gy fractions) showing regression of the tumor as outlined in red. **D)** Slice taken from a CT image of a lung cancer patient being planned for radiation therapy. The corresponding fluorodeoxyglucose (FDG)-PET image is on the right. Functional and anatomical information are often complementary in describing the extent and nature of the cancer. The purple outlines demonstrate the volume to be irradiated as part of the radiation treatment, where the radiation target delineation has been refined by the functional information provided by the PET image.

signal in a manner that can be distinguished from normal, endogenous signals (see Fig. 14–1D).

Molecular imaging exploits advances in molecular biology pertaining to the development of a variety of targeted molecular imaging agents. The distribution of these agents in the body reflects the regional differences in biological activity or expression of the targets to which they bind. Furthermore, these molecules can also be used as drug delivery vehicles to treat cancerous tissue. Multimodal imaging procedures, hybrid imaging devices, and probes that allow the use of many different imaging signals to be acquired and coregistered may also be used to provide a more complete characterization of the cancer. The development of combination PET and CT scanners highlights the value of combining two modalities wherein the specificity of disease detection is improved through the combination of anatomical and functional information in a single representation (see Fig. 14–1). The complexity of biological, structural, and microenvironmental factors (eg, stroma, blood vessels, hypoxia, interstitial fluid pressure) within solid cancers (see Chap. 12) is likely to require the use of many imaging modalities to fully characterize the multiple biological states of an individual's cancer (see Fig. 14–1).

Modern imaging systems are largely digital and allow separation of the image signals into many adjacent spatial compartments called *pixels* (2-dimensional [2D]) or *voxels* (3-dimensional [3D]) (see PET image in Fig. 14–1D for a "pixelated" image). Systems capable of generating images with smaller pixels or voxels do not necessarily have higher resolution. The *limiting spatial resolution* of a system is determined by its ability to resolve the spatial details of the underlying image signal and is determined by the physics of signal formation. For example, in chest radiography machines, x-rays emanate from a focal spot that can range in size. A large x-ray focal spot causes blurring because x-rays originating from different positions on the focal spot will take slightly different angles through the chest before hitting the detector, thus creating an image of the same anatomic structure at slightly different positions. This limits the spatial resolution or detail contained in the resulting chest radiograph. In addition to spatial resolution, the underlying signal needs to be detected in each voxel with a sufficient level of precision to make the image of value. The ratio of the signal in a voxel to the variation in signal found in its neighbors (or to itself over time) is a metric referred to as the *signal-to-noise ratio (SNR)*. This is an important metric in characterizing the performance of an imaging system. Although it is almost always desirable to increase the SNR, this typically comes at a cost of either increased imaging time, increased radiation exposure, a loss in resolution, or, when using exogenous imaging agents, toxicity associated with a larger quantity of the imaging agent injected.

14.3 IMAGING TECHNOLOGIES

Imaging methods employ different forms of energy to probe and detect anatomy and biological processes. Figure 14–2 presents these energy forms together with an overlay of exogenous imaging agents. In the following sections, the dominant imaging modalities used in cancer are reviewed in terms of the process of signal formation, as well as a synopsis of their more interesting applications in oncology.

14.3.1 X-Ray–Based Systems: Radiography and Computed Tomography

X-ray imaging is based on the attenuation of x-rays within different tissues in the body. The discovery of x-rays by Roentgen in 1895 revealed the value of noninvasive imaging, and its clinical applications were immediate. Despite 100 years in advancing this technology, the main methods of x-ray generation and detection have not changed substantially: a vacuum x-ray tube and a 2D detector on either side of the subject remain the central elements. Although the chest radiograph is still a useful tool, x-ray–based CT has become a standard technology to detect and stage cancer since its invention in the 1960s by Hounsfield and Cormack. The basic process for image generation is shown in Figure 14–3A, where a 2D array of x-ray detectors is located opposite a powerful x-ray tube operating in excess of 100,000 volts (~120 kVp). The gantry rotates the tube and detectors through 360 degrees over a period of less than 0.5 seconds while acquiring hundreds of 2D digital radiographs of the patient. A computerized image reconstruction process of digital filtering and back-projection allows an estimate of the x-ray attenuation coefficient of each voxel in a "slice" (1-5 mm thick) through the patient to be estimated (Kak et al, 1988), generating a 3D image. Modern CT scanners can acquire multiple slices simultaneously (by virtue of having multiple rings of detectors), and images of the entire body can be acquired by moving the patient through the CT scanner during rotation. Computerized postprocessing of the individual voxels then allows reconstruction of an image in any plane desired.

The CT image signal is quantified by Hounsfield units (HU), a linear measure of the attenuation coefficient of the tissue relative to water (water is 0 HU and air is –1000 HU). Images formed at typical imaging doses would have approximately 1% noise (10 HU) and percentage differences in HU between tissues such as fat and muscle are only approximately 5% (corresponding to a differential of ~50 HU). The lack of specificity of the CT signal has prevented it from being used to differentiate between some normal and cancerous tissues. However, the recent development of dual-energy CT imaging provides a much higher fidelity in characterizing tissues, and it is anticipated that these systems will revitalize the concept of tissue classification (Kuno et al, 2012), tumor delineation (Toepker et al, 2013), and radiotherapy treatment (van Elmpt et al, 2016). High-atomic-number contrast agents (e.g., iodinated molecules) are used routinely in CT imaging to increase the contrast-to-noise ratio of various structures and are used in bolus studies with fast (2-3 images per second) repetitive scanning to study tissue perfusion (Ippolito et al, 2017).

CT has the advantage that it achieves high spatial resolution (<1 mm), soft-tissue discrimination, is highly reproducible, and can be employed quantitatively for measuring tumor

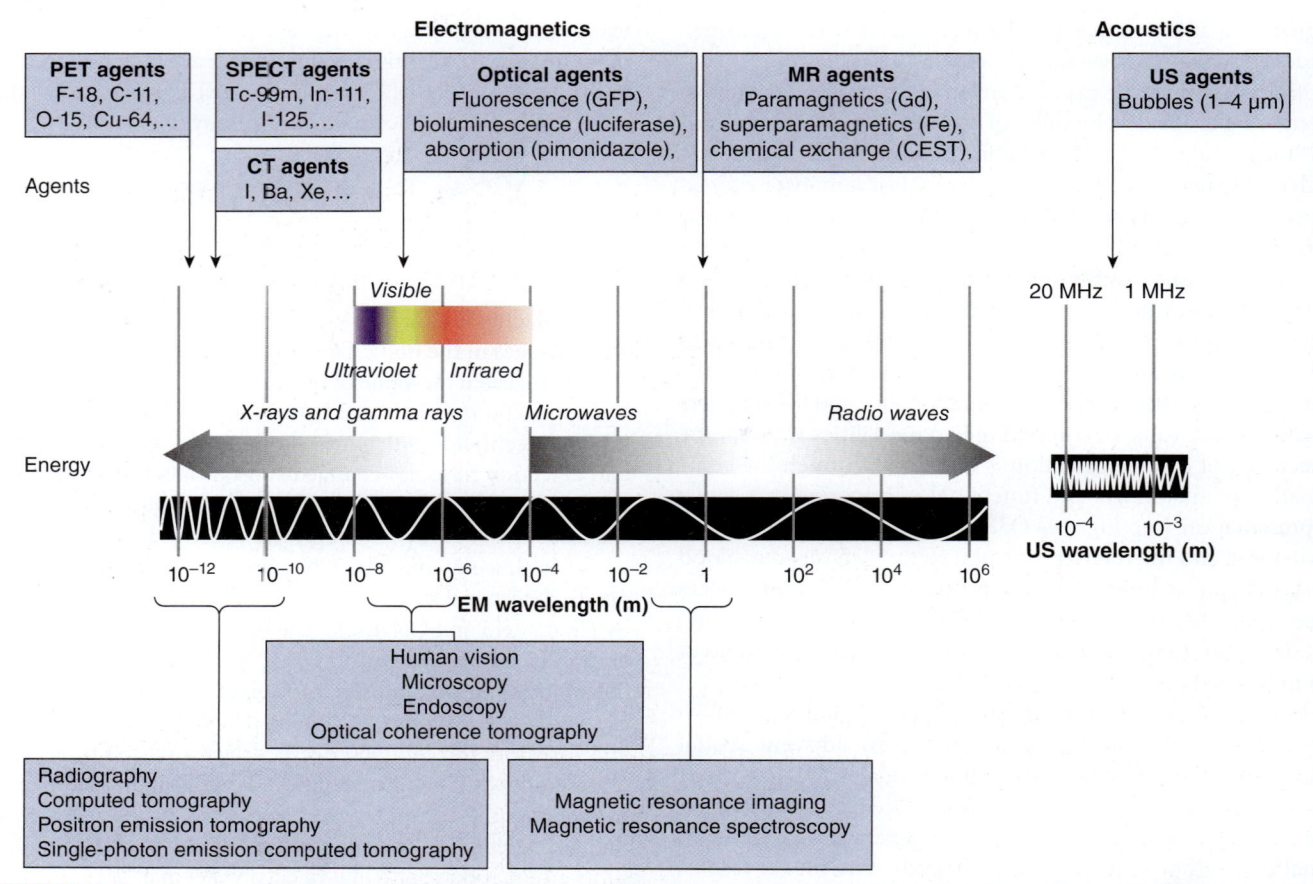

FIGURE 14–2 **Images can be developed from endogenous signals or from exogenous signals induced by the introduction of contrast agents or molecular probes.** The detection of these signals is through either electromagnetic or acoustic energy transfer. Imaging agents are designed to either produce the detected signal (eg, radiolabeled PET/single-photon emission computed tomography [SPECT]) or to alter the interaction between the object and the applied energy (eg, high atomic number materials such as iodine, barium, or xenon in radiography and CT, paramagnetic agents in MR, bubbles in ultrasound). Optical imaging operates at energies corresponding to biological processes and can therefore provide insight into active biological processes (eg, detection of bioluminescent signals). Similarly, MR offers insight into the chemical activity in the body by exploiting effects related to the impact of chemical milieu on nuclear magnetic resonance to create imagelike maps of these effects. This is referred to as MR spectroscopy imaging (MRSI). Chemical milieu can also be probed through the exchange of protons between specific chemical species (CEST).

size and detecting response. The SNR and image quality are related to the applied dose of ionizing radiation—typical CT imaging doses range from 1 to 10 cGy (see Chap. 15, Sec. 15.2, for definition of radiation dose). CT imaging is used routinely for detection, staging, and post-treatment follow-up of cancer (eg, its role in noninvasive cancer staging has led to a reduction in the frequency of exploratory laparoscopic surgery). Characterization of the regional extent of disease is undertaken using pretreatment, posttreatment, and follow-up CT imaging. CT has a major role in directing therapy, including its use in planning surgical and radiation fields, and providing guidance in interventional radiology for biopsy of tumor tissue and for radiofrequency ablation of liver metastases.

Dynamic CT imaging (with multiple slices/volumes per second) can be used to characterize the vascularity and permeability of blood vessels in tumors; CT scanning is undertaken after a bolus intravenous (IV) injection of a low-molecular-weight iodinated agent. This is referred to as *perfusion CT*, *functional CT*, or, more recently, *dynamic contrast-enhanced computed tomography (DCE-CT)*. DCE-CT is sensitive to vascular changes that occur before conventional size-related measures of tumor response and can provide early prognostic information (Ng et al, 2017). New targeted and nontargeted contrast agents composed of micelle and lipoprotein-based nanoparticles are also being developed to improve imaging patients with renal impairment (Cormode et al, 2014).

CT is also used to screen for lung cancer in higher-risk populations (see Chap. 22, Sec. 22.4), and randomized clinical trials have demonstrated its ability to improve outcome for people with lung cancer (Field et al, 2015). However, the value of CT screening for cancer in other sites has not been established, and there are concerns about potential health effects and secondary malignancies relating to the radiation exposure from CT-based screening of the general public (Huang et al, 2014).

14.3.2 Magnetic Resonance Imaging

The MR image signal arises from the interaction of electromagnetic fields with tissue following 5 concepts (see Fig. 14–3B):

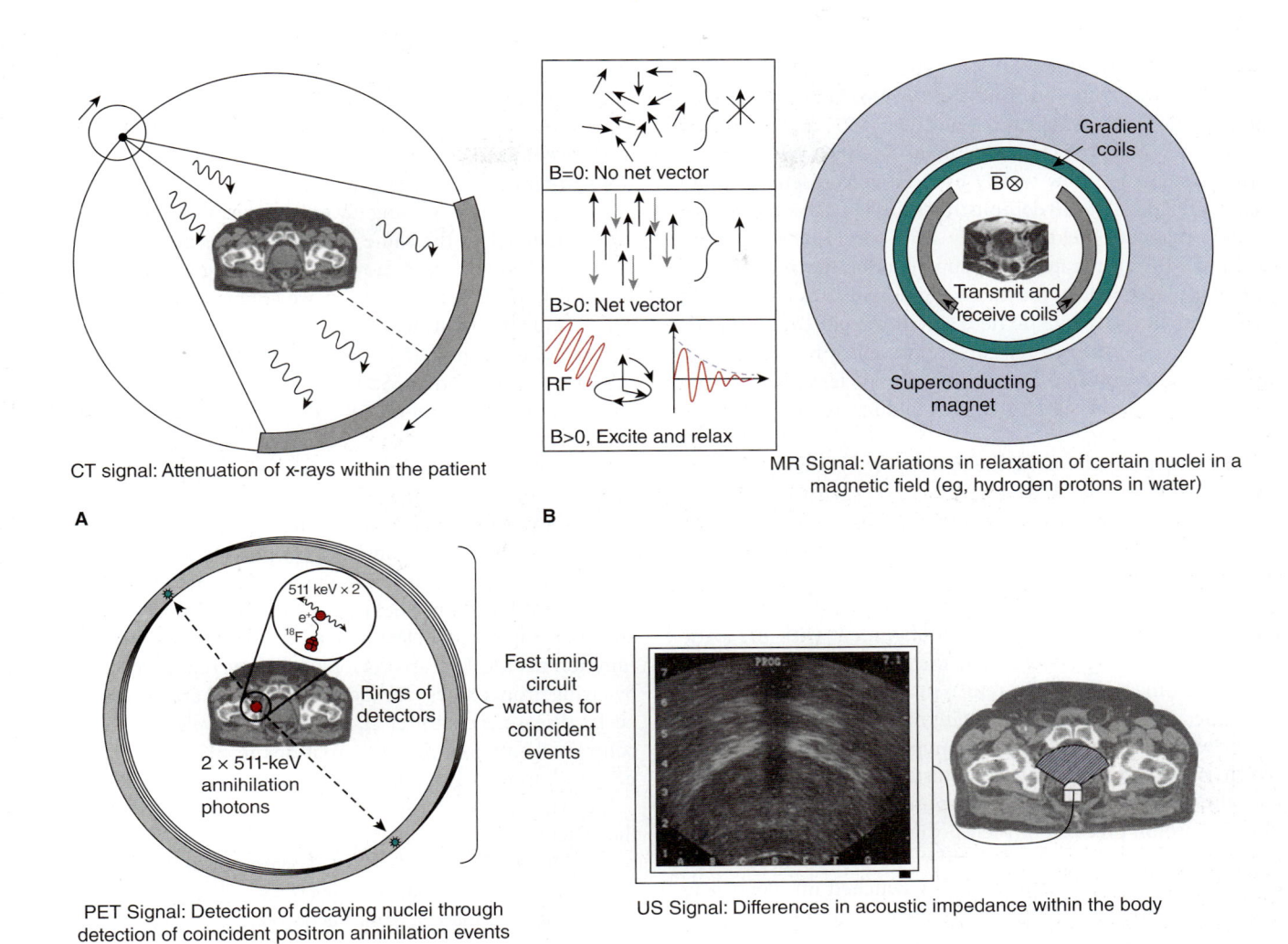

FIGURE 14–3 Imaging technologies used in oncology. A) In a modern CT imaging system, a multirow detector and high-power x-ray source rotate about the patient at high speed (>2 revolutions per second). Thousands of "projections" are collected as the patient advances through the scanner, and computers are used to "reconstruct" multiple imaged slices representing the attenuation characteristics of the patient. This is presented in grayscale form as the CT image. **B)** An MR image signal has many forms, but relies largely on the excitation and relaxation of a population of field-aligned magnetic dipoles associated with protons (hydrogen nuclei) in water. MR imaging systems consist of a large superconducting magnet that maintains the static field (typically 1.5 T), that causes the field alignment of the magnetic dipoles of hydrogen nuclei of the water molecules, and a set of gradient-inducing coils that manipulate the magnetic field throughout the volume. The radiofrequency transmit and receive coils are responsible for perturbing the hydrogen nuclei and then recording their relaxation back to the ground state in the presence of the magnetic field. **C)** PET imaging is often used in conjunction with a CT system (called a PET-CT scanner). PET image formation is achieved through detection of positron-emitting decay events that ultimately produce pairs of 511-keV photons at approximately 180 degrees from each other. This image is then superimposed on the CT image generated at the same time by the dual-purpose scanner. **D)** Ultrasonographic (US) imaging systems exploit variations in acoustic impedance within the body to generate images. Ultrasound waves are reflected at boundaries between tissues of differential impedance (eg, fat, muscle, bladder wall). In this figure, an axial ultrasonographic image of the prostate is shown as generated by a transrectal ultrasound probe (see illustration).

(1) the human body contains a large number of hydrogen nuclei (ie, protons) in water, which act as "tiny bar magnets"; (2) an applied, static magnetic field (eg, 1.5 tesla [T]) sets a slight bias in the orientation of the protons, aligning them along a common axis (ie, the static field)—the higher the field, the larger the bias; (3) the application of an external radiofrequency field by an antenna perturbs the protons, changing their orientation; (4) the surrounding chemical and physical microenvironment impacts the time (T1) required for the protons to return to alignment (relax) with the static field; and (5) the relaxation of the hydrogen nuclei back to alignment with the static field induces a current that is measured by a detecting antenna (conducting loop) exterior to the object.

Damadian (1971) first proposed that the rate of relaxation of protons in water could distinguish normal from tumor tissue and demonstrated that tumors (sarcomas and hepatomas) had differing T1 relaxation times that were 1.5 to 2 times longer than in normal tissues in the same animal. These differences in relaxation times are due to the different environments in which the protons relax to alignment with the static field—the presence of cancer alters this environment compared to that found in normal tissue.

The development of methods to generate images of nominal relaxation times followed from the work of Lauterbur (1973) and Mansfield (Mansfield and Maudsley, 1977) for which they received the Nobel Prize in Medicine in 2003. MR imaging (MRI) systems are now widely used in cancer detection and diagnosis. Figure 14–3B demonstrates the central components: A static magnetic field (typically 1.5 T or 15,000 times the earth's field) is generated by a superconducting magnet; the patient is placed within the magnet; gradient coils create slight differences in the magnetic field across the patient to encode for location in 3 orthogonal directions; and, finally, a pair of antennae is responsible for exciting the nuclei and detecting the electromagnetic signal that they induce as they return to their ground states.

In a 1.5-T magnetic field, the precession frequency of water protons (rate of rotation around its axis, similar to a spinning top) is 64 MHz. Radiofrequency (RF) pulses of energy applied at this frequency excite the protons and alter the angle at which they are precessing around the magnetic field lines (Fig. 3B). Once a 90-degree pulse is switched off, the protons gradually relax to their lower-energy state in alignment with the static field by exchanging energy with their surrounding environment. The time taken for the return to alignment (the T_1 signal, also called the *spin-lattice relaxation time*) is one metric of the local chemical and physiological environment of the protons, which varies between tissues, as disease evolves, and before and after treatment, therefore providing tissue contrast. The phase of proton precession (their position around the spinning top) can be synchronized within the transverse plane (through a 180-degree pulse). When the RF is switched off, dephasing gradually occurs and the time to reduce the transverse magnetization is referred to as T_2, or *spin-spin relaxation time*. This dephasing is caused by the same processes as T_1 relaxation; however, it is also impacted by magnetic field inhomogeneities and local static field disturbances. The additional susceptibilities of T_2 results in consistently shorter relaxation times than T_1.

Because complete isolation of T_1 and T_2 signals is challenging, images are typically T_1 or T_2 "weighted" depending on the RF pulse sequence applied. By varying the time between RF pulses (repetition time [TR]) and the time to sample the resulting signal (echo time [TE]), it is possible to "weight" the image. There are 3 basic weightings used in clinical practice: T_1, T_2, and proton-density weighting. In general, T_1 weighting provides anatomic detail, whereas T_2-weighted images are used to distinguish soft tissues. Proton density simply reflects the density of water protons available for signal production in the voxel.

MR can also be used to explore other tissue parameters, such as changes in local transport of water in tissue that may reflect cellular sensitivity to treatment. This can be characterized by exposing excited nuclei in tissue to variations in a magnetic field and examining the rate of signal loss; this is referred to as apparent diffusion coefficient (ADC) imaging (Le Bihan et al, 1986). Figure 14–4A illustrates the process used in MR to estimate the diffusion of water within a voxel (Hagmann et al, 2006). In brief, a conventional spin-echo sequence is modified by applying 2 gradient pulses across the tissue before and after the 180-degree pulse. These gradient pulses, and resulting proton precession phase shifts, encode the degree of proton mobility in the applied gradient plane (ie, diffusion) into a loss of recovered signal as a result of transport-induced imperfections in rephasing of the spins. In other words, by applying a gradient and then reversing it we can determine which protons have remained in the same location (ie, no net phase shift), and which protons have moved (ie, resulting in a phase shift). Figure 14–4B presents diffusion-weighted images of a patient before and after treatment for lymphoma.

Exogenous agents can be applied to alter the MR signal and increase image contrast. Spin-lattice relaxation time (T_1) and spin-spin relaxation time (T_2) may be shortened considerably in the presence of paramagnetic species (eg, gadolinium) because of their unpaired electrons, which produce a strong magnetic moment that induces magnetic relaxation of surrounding protons. Stable agents that contain gadolinium are used in the clinical setting (eg, gadopentate dimeglumine or gadolinium-diethylenetriamine pentaacetic acid [Gd-DPTA]; gadoteridol [Gd-HP-D03A]), but they lack tumor specificity and their rapid renal clearance puts patients with poor renal function at risk. Research is looking to overcome these issues by using iron oxides, for detection and characterization of nodal disease (Fortuin et al, 2018), and developing new MR contrast agents that rely on variations in pH between malignant and nonmalignant tissue (Wei et al, 2017).

Magnetic resonance spectroscopy imaging (MRSI) involves the extension of nuclear magnetic resonance (NMR) techniques employed in chemistry. Spectra associated with the chemical shift in resonance peaks for various biomolecules in small regions of interest can be acquired on MRI systems. Collecting a number of spectra in adjacent regions in a rectilinear array (Fig. 14–5A) and generating a coarse image is referred to as *MRSI* or *chemical shift imaging* (CSI). MRSI can be applied to protons in water, as well as other nuclei with a magnetic moment such as ^{31}P, ^{13}C, and ^{19}F. Figure 14–5B illustrates the nature of the spectra produced on a clinical 1.5-T MR scanner when performing proton imaging of the prostate; the poorly resolved spectra are reduced to ratios of peaks to form a color-coded image of disease burden. Adoption of higher field (3-T) MR scanners will lead to greater spectral separation of the peaks and improved differentiation of recurrent versus stable disease.

The excellent soft-tissue discrimination of MR makes it well suited to oncology, and MRI has a role in the diagnosis, staging, and management of many solid cancers. For example, MR has become the dominant imaging method for cancers of the central nervous system where the high T_1 contrast and sensitivity of T_2 to changes in edema (caused by increased water content, and therefore altered surrounding environment) delineate the extent of disease and allow understanding of the patterns of spread. Its role in evaluating metastatic lesions in the spinal column, including those requiring urgent treatment because of spinal cord compression, is definitive. Although use of MR in breast screening or directing surgery is controversial, it is useful as a method of breast imaging for screening women with a personal or strong family history of breast cancer

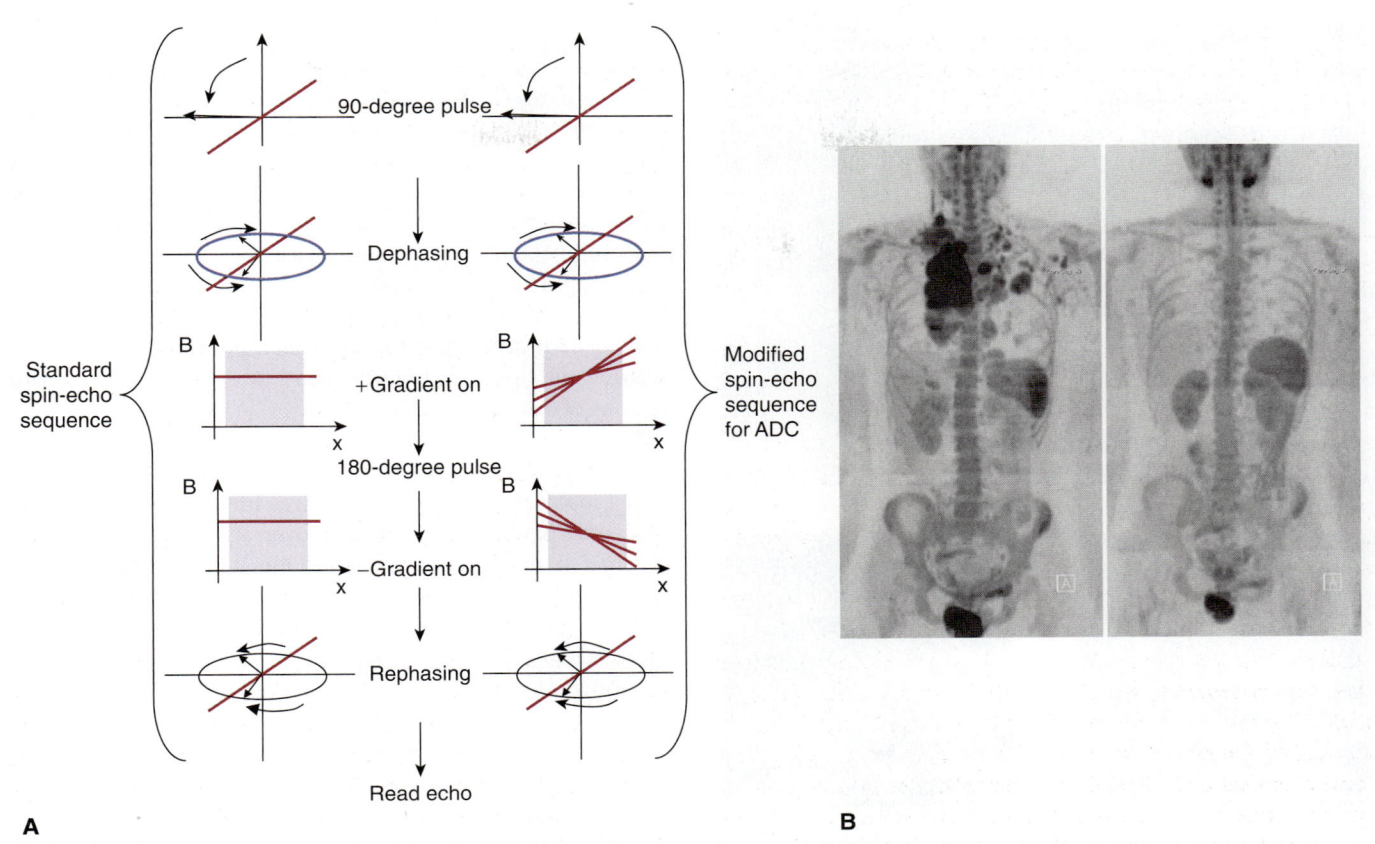

FIGURE 14–4 **A)** The ADC (or diffusion-weighted imaging [DWI]) imaging technique seeks to measure the diffusion of water within a voxel by exposing the excited water protons to a spatial gradient during their dephasing to encode for their diffusive transport. This exposure is done before and after a 180-degree spin-echo pulse. Voxels that contain spins exposed to differential fields because of diffusive transport will have a reduced echo following the 180-degree rephasing pulse. Those that are stationary will be refocused to within normal T_2 losses. **B)** DWI is also of interest in assessing total cancer burden, as these techniques can also be used to image the entire body. In their review of DWI in oncology, demonstrate DWI in the assessment of pretreatment disease burden and its response to chemotherapy in a patient with Hodgkin lymphoma. The 2 panels show pre-and post-RT treatment DWI images. The dark regions present in the post-RT panel correspond to tracer that is accumulated naturally in the body (eg, in the bladder). (B. Reproduced with permission from Padhani AR, Koh DM, Collins DJ. Whole-body diffusion-weighted MR imaging in cancer: current status and research directions. *Radiology* 2011 Dec;261(3):700-718.)

(Lehman et al, 2018). Dynamic contrast-enhanced magnetic resonance (DCE-MR) (conceptually equivalent to DCE-CT) is emerging as a biomarker to predict patient prognosis and the biologic aggressiveness of a tumor (Li et al, 2015).

14.3.3 Single-Photon and Positron Emission Tomography

Radiotracer molecules that emit high-energy gamma-rays or positrons, and are analogs of metabolites or bind to molecular targets in tissue, can be injected into the body where they can reflect different aspects of the disease. These accumulated radiotracers emit exogenous signals that reflect the nature of the cancer and contribute to its management (eg, a radiolabeled sugar analog will accumulate in areas of high metabolism) (see Chap. 12).

Single-photon emission computed tomography (SPECT) imaging depends on emission of gamma-rays in the range of 100 keV that are detected by a gamma camera, which is then used to reconstruct an estimate of the distribution of the gamma-ray emitters in the body. SPECT is utilized in cancer for the staging and assessment of cancer progression in the form of a "bone scan." In this technique, the patient is injected with a small amount of radioactive technetium-99m (^{99m}Tc)-labeled medronic acid (a bisphosphonate) and then scanned with a gamma or 3-dimensional (3D) SPECT camera. The accumulation of the medronic acid in regions of bone remodeling is a sensitive detector of metastasis to bone.

In contrast to SPECT, PET employs radioisotopes that emit a positron on decay. For example, a radioactive isotope of fluorine (^{18}F) emits a positron that annihilates through interaction with an electron in the body to produce a pair of photons (511 keV each), which are emitted at approximately 180 degrees to each other. Figure 14–3C illustrates the coincident detection of the event in detectors distributed on multiple rings around the patient. Large numbers of these coincident events are then used to generate an image of the spatial distribution of the annihilation events, which represents the

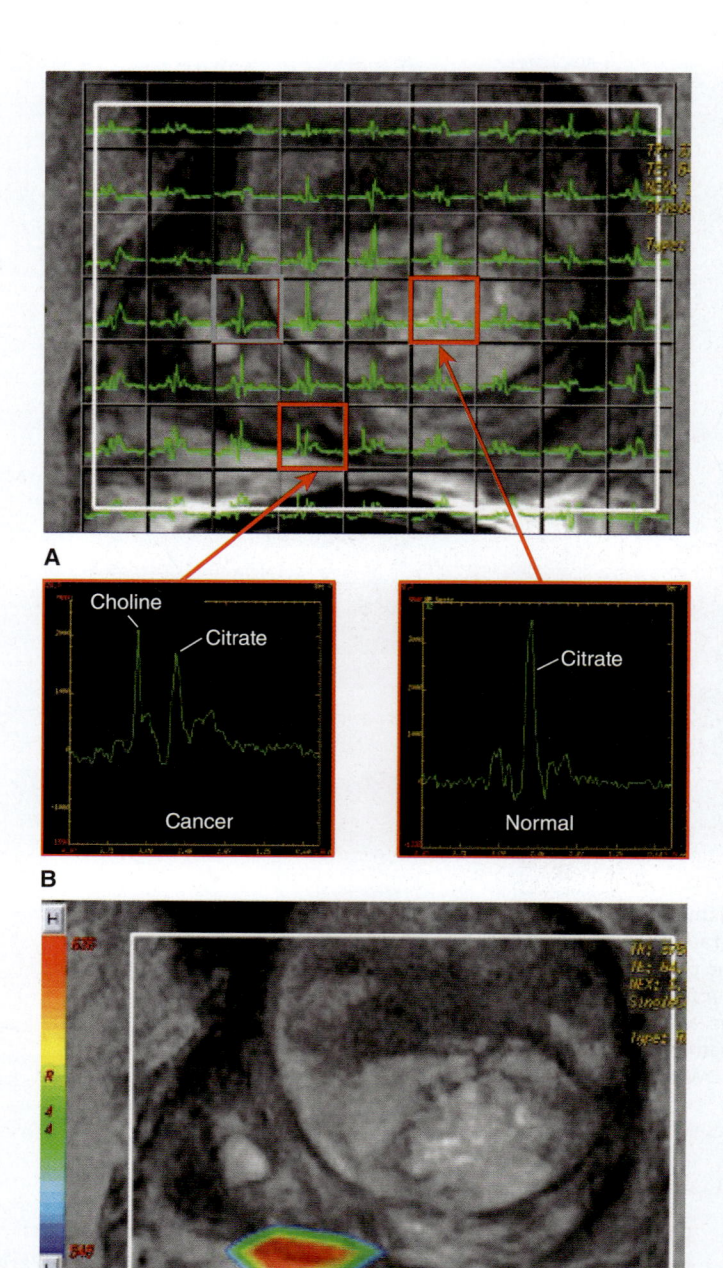

FIGURE 14–5 Magnetic resonance spectroscopy (MRS) offers the potential for metabolic imaging by detecting molecular environment–induced frequency shifts in the resonance of nuclei. **A)** A set of MR spectra acquired in a rectilinear array and overlaid on the conventional MR image of the prostate (1.5 T with endorectal coil). The spectra contain a citrate peak present in normal and disease tissues, whereas the elevated choline peak corresponds to disease (**B**). **C)** Spectral analysis in these studies consists of calculating ratios of signal over specific frequency intervals or peak heights estimated from peak-fitting algorithms (eg, Cho/Cit ratios). These ratios are then converted to a color-coded pattern and overlaid on the MR image to identify regions of elevated disease burden.

distribution of the ^{18}F-labeled agent. The standardized uptake value (SUV) is a metric used in PET imaging to quantify the ratio of image-derived radioactivity concentration to whole body injected radioactivity concentration, and is corrected for patient size and time of imaging. The most widely used PET agent is the radiolabeled sugar ^{18}F-fluorodeoxyglucose (FDG), which becomes trapped within cells that have active glucose metabolism, as is the case for malignant tumors (see Chap. 13, Sec. 12.3.1). FDG is injected intravenously into the body and allowed to circulate and metabolize for approximately 45 minutes; the patient is then positioned in the PET scanner and images of the whole body are collected to evaluate regions of elevated uptake.

There are advantages and disadvantages to the SPECT and PET approaches. The ability to integrate radioisotopes directly into a molecule of interest minimizes impact on the pharmacokinetics of the agent itself. Moreover, agents can be designed to target many aspects of tumor cell metabolism and the tumor microenvironment. However, the half-life of the probe needs to be selected for the specific objective: the radioactive half-life needs to be longer than the half-life of the physical process that one is interested in characterizing, but it should not be much longer, or the radiation dose delivered would be excessive. Some positron-emitting radioisotopes (^{15}O, ^{11}C) can be integrated into various molecules but have very short half-lives and require production in a cyclotron that is adjacent to the radiochemistry laboratory and the imaging suite. ^{18}F, the most commonly used positron-emitting radioisotope, has a half-life of 110 minutes and can be shipped from remote sources within a few hours with sufficient activity for imaging purposes. ^{99m}Tc is the most commonly used SPECT isotope and is a daughter product of a molybdenum generator that can be located within the local SPECT laboratory, it has a half-life of 6 hours.

The development of combined PET-CT and SPECT-CT systems was motivated by the advantages of using CT to correct for attenuation by the patient's anatomy in reconstruction of the image (Townsend et al, 2003), but the additional imaging information provided from the CT is also beneficial. Combined PET and SPECT-MRI systems have also been introduced to provide improved soft-tissue and temporal resolution over CT. Additionally, PET and SPECT-MRI have the advantage that the images can be acquired simultaneously (Rosales, 2014).

PET tracers are designed to collect a diverse array of information about a patient's disease. For example, FDG-PET provides information about tumor metabolism, but also increases accuracy of staging and treatment in cervix cancer because of decreased interobserver variability in gross tumor volume (GTV) delineation (Han et al, 2016). Numerous other cancer-related PET agents are currently in development, but are not yet established in clinical use. For example, ^{18}F-misonidazole (FMISO)-PET and ^{18}F-fluoroazomycin arabinoside (FAZA)-PET are hypoxia-localizing agents that become trapped in cells as a result of reduction in the absence of oxygen, so that accumulation occurs only in cells that have low oxygen concentration (see Chap. 12, Chap. 16, Sec. 16.4; Krohn et al, 2008). Imaging of hypoxic regions within tumors

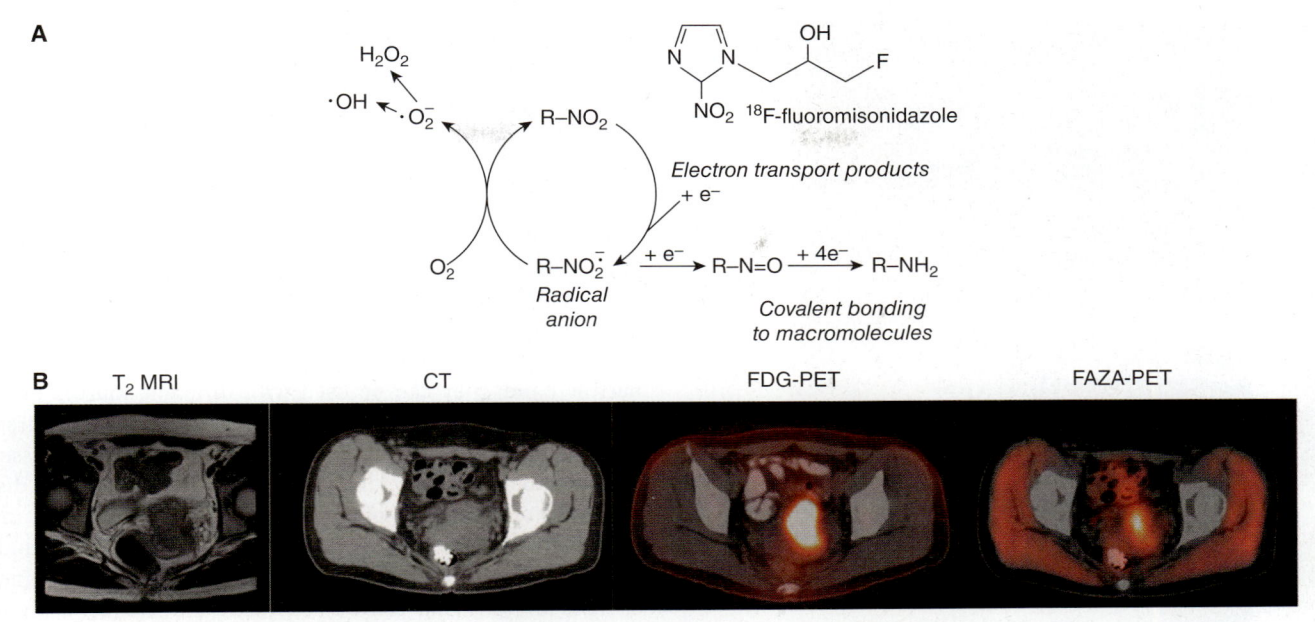

FIGURE 14–6 PET tracers accumulate in cells based upon metabolic activity and oxygen content. A) FMISO is a hypoxia PET-tracer that is accumulated in the cell through a process that is dependent on reduction of the nitro (NO$_2$) group by 1 e− nitroreductases. If O$_2$ is not present, the tracer is sequentially further reduced to an alkylating agent and is bound in the cell. In the presence of oxygen, the initial reduction step is back-oxidized to re-create the original molecule, which can diffuse out of the cell again. B) MRI, CT, and fused FDG-PET and FAZA-PET images of a patient with locally advanced cervical cancer demonstrate the diverse information that can be collected using different imaging modalities and tracers. The fused PET-CT images are at a similar level of the tumor and indicate the metabolic and hypoxic information that can be collected using FDG and FAZA tracers, respectively. (A) Reproduced with permission from Krohn KA, Link JM, Mason RP. Molecular imaging of hypoxia. *J Nucl Med* 2008 Jun;49 Suppl 2:129S-148S.; B) Used with permission from Dr. Kathy Han, Princess Margaret Cancer Centre.)

provides an opportunity for dose escalation protocols to improve control of tumors with substantial regions of hypoxia (Welz et al, 2017), as well as monitoring of hypoxia-activated prodrugs, radiosensitizers, and hypoxia-selective gene therapy (Rey et al, 2017).

14.3.4 Ultrasound Imaging

Ultrasound imaging utilizes the variations in acoustic impedance (ie, resistance encountered by an ultrasound beam) in the different tissues of the body to generate anatomic images. Figure 14–3D illustrates an ultrasound probe configuration for transrectal ultrasonography of the prostate. Piezoelectric crystals are capable of generating very high-frequency acoustic waves (ultrasonic) in the range of 1 to 20 MHz (inaudible to humans). The ultrasound image is formed through manipulation of the acoustic source and detection of the reflected acoustic pressure wave. Although ultrasound is limited in its depth of penetration (1-15 cm), it has advantages including low cost, adaptability to small probes for directing minimally invasive biopsy procedures (eg, endobronchial ultrasound, prostate biopsy), and use in tissues that are relatively homogenous (eg, liver imaging). In addition to structural information, ultrasound offers accurate assessment of flow rates in large blood vessels using the Doppler phenomenon, in which the relative motion of the blood induces frequency shifts in the reflected sound waves; Doppler ultrasonography is the standard technique for detecting deep vein thrombosis in veins of the leg, a common phenomenon in people with cancer. Ultrasound can also be applied with contrast agents such as microbubbles (Wilson and Burns, 2001) that reflect the sound waves and produce high-contrast signals. This technique has been used to measure perfusion of parenchymatous organs, aiding in the differentiation of benign and malignant tumors, and can predict tumor response to chemotherapy (Fröhlich et al, 2015).

In the clinic, ultrasonography is used in the detection, diagnosis, clinical staging, and treatment of cancer, and can be overlaid on MRI to improve accuracy and provide complementary information (Siddiqui et al, 2015). Ultrasonography has proven useful in the characterization of lesions in the breast, liver, and kidney, and use of ultrasonic contrast agents, such as microbubbles, has improved this performance substantially. Ultrasonography is used for directing biopsies, providing information in the surgical management of prostate or pancreatic lesions, and is also employed for localizing structures during radiation therapy. For example, during brachytherapy of prostate cancer using permanent radioactive seed implants, transrectal ultrasonography is used to localize both the gland and the seeds as they are placed in the gland by the oncologist. Ultrasonographic techniques are also undergoing evaluation as a possible method for blood-brain barrier disruption to improve administration of drugs (Carpentier et al, 2016). These methods are not currently standard clinical practice because of procedural invasiveness and adverse effects, but show great promise (Huang et al, 2017).

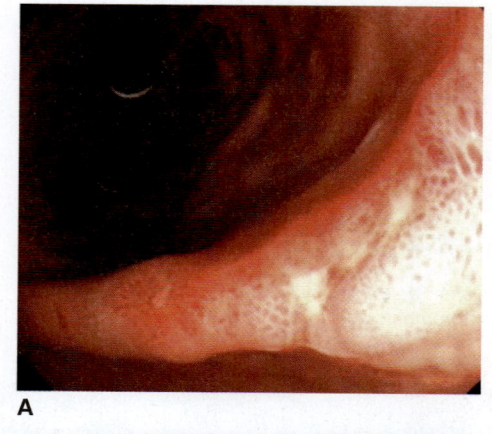

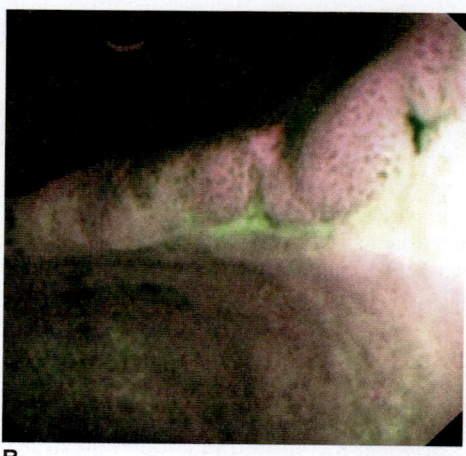

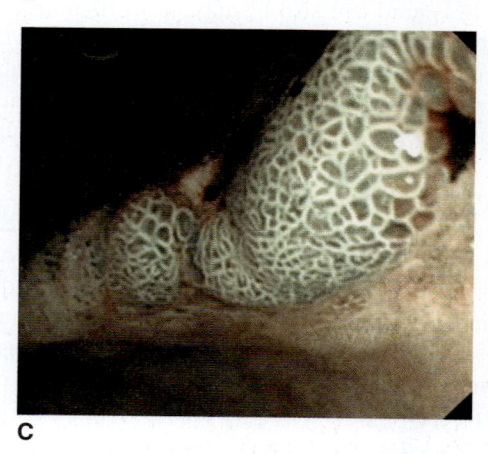

FIGURE 14–7 Endoscopic techniques continue to evolve as demonstrated in this series of images from Filip et al (2011). Endoscopy of an early gastric adenocarcinoma at the level of the gastric angle reveals (**A**) an irregular ulcer visualized in white-light endoscopy and (**B**) autofluorescence images showing in magenta the neoplastic margins and a larger lesion extension, as compared with white-light endoscopy. Further advances in resolution and selection of a narrow wavelength band (**C**) shows a modified pit pattern of the colonic mucosa according to standard classification measures, with irregular and distorted vascular pattern in the center suggesting high-grade dysplasia/early cancer. (Reproduced with permission from Filip M, Iordache S, Săftoiu A, et al: Autofluorescence imaging and magnification endoscopy. *World J Gastroentero*l 2011 Jan 7;17(1):9-14.)

14.3.5 Optical Imaging

Optical imaging has an expanding role in characterization and management of cancer. Advances in fiberoptic and camera technologies that permit high-quality optical imaging to be applied within the body's orifices, cavities, and luminal structures (eg, colonoscopy, bronchoscopy, and cystoscopy) has accelerated the development of endoscopic systems. High-definition video capture and the integration of channels for improved guidance of biopsy/resection is increasing the application of these systems. Sensors can collect light over a wide spectrum from near infrared to blue or operate on a narrow band; they can be used with different sources ranging from white light to higher-frequency sources to generate fluorescence. The endogenous absorption of light in tissue provides the signal for detection and characterization of disease. Although optical imaging suffers from scattering and absorption within the body, it has several advantages, including the high efficiency of optical detectors, the abundance of light photons that can be generated and interact without harm to tissue, and the ability to support molecular imaging. Optical imaging is used to detect lesions on luminal structures (eg, colon, glottis, esophagus), and autofluorescence detection has shown promise for early diagnosis of oral squamous cell carcinoma and other premalignant and malignant disorders (Luo et al, 2016). Figure 14–7 illustrates how white light, autofluorescence, and narrowband imaging each provide increasing detail in the characterization of a gastric adenocarcinoma.

Endoscopic imaging is used widely for cancer detection, and colonoscopy is now a recommended procedure to screen for colorectal cancer in people older than 50 years (Bacchus et al, 2016). The same tools are used to biopsy and remove suspicious lesions. Challenges persist in the characterization of flat lesions and the introduction of optical imaging techniques beyond that of white light is undergoing evaluation (Backes et al, 2017). Endoscopy is also a routine part of cancer management of many sites including cancer of the head and neck, lung, and esophagus. The low cost and adaptability of endoscopes have resulted in other uses, including the design of radiation therapy treatments (Weersink et al, 2011) and the assessment of the response of tissue to cancer therapeutics. Georg et al (2009) have correlated a scoring system for rectal damage evaluated by endoscopy with the volume of rectal tissue receiving elevated doses during radiation therapy of the cervix. The continued advances in endoscope technology and in optical imaging probes make this a promising area of development for cancer imaging.

14.4 IMAGING OF ANIMAL MODELS IN ONCOLOGY

Small animal imaging systems are designed to characterize cancer in animal models and its response to novel therapies. Imaging is forming an effective bridge between the clinical and preclinical domains as investigators relate image-based observations from the clinic to the biological basis of the disease

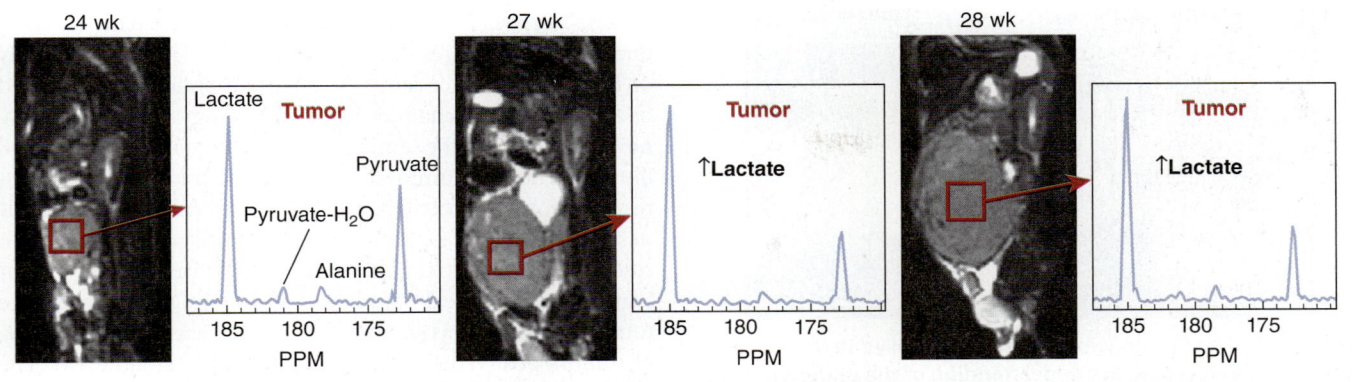

FIGURE 14-8 **The development of 3D MRSI with hyperpolarized ^{13}C is an exciting development for oncology imaging.** Postinjection rapid MR spectroscopy (14 seconds/spectrum over a 0.135-cm³ region within the tumor) can be used to monitor the signal from injected ^{13}C-pyruvate and its metabolic derivatives, including lactate and alanine. In this transgenic model of prostate cancer (TRAMP), Kurhanewicz et al (2008) demonstrate high levels of lactate were produced from hyperpolarized ^{13}C-pyruvate and that lactate production (relative to the pyruvate signal) in the tumor increased as the tumor progressed in a transgenic prostate cancer model. (Reproduced with permission from Kurhanewicz J, Bok R, Nelson SJ, et al: Current and potential applications of clinical ^{13}C MR spectroscopy. *J Nucl Med* 2008 Mar;49(3):341-344.)

in pertinent genetically engineered animals or human tumor xenografts (see Chap. 17, Sec. 17.4). Preclinical models of cancer typically include human tumor xenografts (primary or serially transplanted) and genetically engineered murine or rat models. The use of imaging technologies (micro-MRI, PET, CT, SPECT, and optical imaging) can interrogate local tumor growth, metastatic progression, tumor metabolism, and treatment response to allow for the design and testing of novel clinical regimens.

The scaling of CT systems from man to mouse was made possible by the creation of high-resolution digital detectors (~0.1-mm resolution) for radiography and fluoroscopy, because conventional CT detectors (~1-mm resolution) would not adequately visualize the mouse model structures. In addition to the challenges of achieving high resolution, a high radiation dose is necessary to maintain a good signal-to-noise ratio (SNR). In CT, the SNR in a cubic voxel depends on the square of the voxel dimension. Thus, achieving 50-μm images with an SNR comparable to that found in human CT imaging (500-μm images) would require the imaging dose to be increased 100-fold. This technology has been applied with a compromise between noise and acceptable imaging doses (~5-30 cGy), and preclinical micro-CT systems with spatial resolution as low as 3.7 μm are available (Hu et al, 2014). Preclinical CT systems have been used to measure tumor growth, assess bone injury in metastatic models of disease, and even to mimic the DCE-CT techniques used in clinical oncology. For example, rat brain CT perfusion imaging has been studied as an early biomarker for response to stereotactic radiosurgery of malignant rat gliomas (Yeung et al, 2014). Robotic systems directed under preclinical CT can achieve targeted biopsies with mean errors of less than 100 μm. Also, cone-beam CT systems have been integrated with irradiation systems to direct small radiation beams (<5 mm in diameter) to treat xenograft tumors in mice (Clarkson et al, 2011; Yang et al, 2015).

The powerful soft-tissue imaging capability of MR has driven the development of high-magnetic-field (eg, 7-T) MR scanners to enable high-resolution, low-noise imaging of small animals. For example, DCE-MR methods have been adapted to these platforms for quantitative, multiparametric evaluation of response to treatment. This has been of particular interest to those examining the optimization of treatment protocols that employ antivascular agents (see Chap. 11, Sec. 11.7). The creation of a "preclinical mimic" of clinical imaging techniques is an attractive development to allow preclinical evaluation of therapies that would benefit from an image-based biomarker of response.

The ability to monitor noninvasively chemical interactions within the body has the potential to reveal a great deal about cancer biology. Concentrations of highly polarized ^{13}C and ^{129}Xe nuclei produce sufficient signal to map molecular distributions of injected ^{13}C and ^{129}Xe within organs for several seconds after injection (Santyr et al, 2014) and have demonstrated their capabilities as indicators of tumor perfusion (Park et al, 2016). Additionally, hyperpolarized ^{129}Xe gas MRI has demonstrated promise as a method to assess regional radiation-induced lung injury (Zanette et al, 2018). Metabolic species can also be monitored using ^{13}C-labeled metabolites with frequency selection and careful design of pulse sequences. Figure 14-8 demonstrates the capabilities of MRI techniques when combined with high-contrast metabolically active agents (Kurhanewicz et al, 2008). These techniques bring a perspective for understanding cancer metabolism and are being tested in clinics (Wang et al, 2017).

Preclinical SPECT and PET imaging systems are routinely employed in oncologic research. Figure 14-9 illustrates the result of an FDG-PET imaging study in a mouse tumor model. The close proximity of the detectors to the animal permits higher resolution imaging than can be achieved in clinical systems and illustrates heterogeneity in FDG uptake across the tumor. PET and SPECT systems are very useful in tracking accumulation and delivery of radiolabeled therapeutic agents (Xiao et al, 2012) and for probing molecular markers of cancer during therapy (Vaidyanathan et al, 2016). Preclinical systems can be used to evaluate novel PET probes, such as hypoxia agents, which need to be cross-calibrated

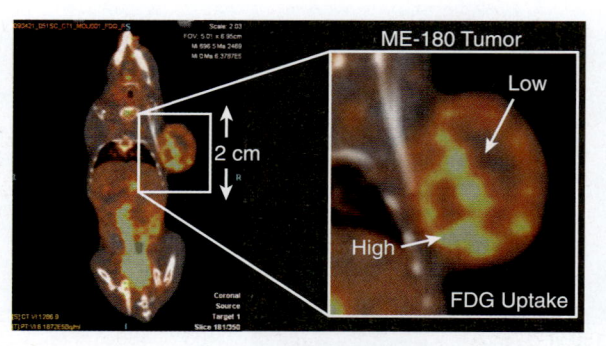

FIGURE 14–9 PET imaging can also be applied in the preclinical setting to increase our understanding of the underlying biology, as well as inform the design of clinical imaging studies. In this example, an FDG-PET image is acquired of a subcutaneous tumor (ME-180, cancer cervix model). The accumulation of FDG is seen to be quite heterogeneous within the mass. The generation of such a high-resolution image would be challenging on a clinical PET scanner because of the detector geometry. The use of a preclinical system helps to inform our understanding of a clinical FDG image and how it relates to the very-high-resolution microscopy demonstrated in Figure 14–1A. (Used with permission from STTARR Facility, Toronto, Canada.)

against other measures of the partial pressure of oxygen (pO$_2$) (Huizing et al, 2017).

Ultrasonographic systems have also been adapted to support very-high-frequency probes for preclinical studies and ultrasound microscopy (Foster et al, 2009). Ultrasonography is being employed to characterize growth delay in tumor models following therapy, predict the response of tumors to antiangiogenic therapies (Zhou et al, 2016), and measure cellular responses to treatment, such as apoptosis (Tadayyon et al, 2017). Preclinical ultrasonography is used to evaluate the development of novel ultrasound contrast agents that are actively and/or passively targeted, or can be used with therapeutic agents (Gao et al, 2017).

Development of preclinical optical imaging technologies includes flat-field bioluminescent and fluorescent imaging systems, as well as the development of 3D systems to allow quantitative measures (Graves et al, 2004). These systems rely on high-performance cameras that incorporate charge-coupled devices and multichannel plate technology to achieve low-noise images of the emitted optical signal. Figure 14–10 illustrates how bioluminescence from the transfection of fluorescent proteins or luciferase into cells can enhance the usefulness of these devices. Endoscopic confocal microscopes with resolutions of approximately 5 μm allow visualization of biologic processes in real time (Lin et al, 2008). Optical coherence tomography systems are able to track vascular remodeling of tumors post-radiation therapy (Demidov et al, 2018). The development of these preclinical tools has spurred the initiation of research in optical tracers and probes, such as nano agents designed for multimodal image guidance with CT and near-infrared fluorescence for preoperative and intraoperative imaging, respectively (Zheng et al, 2015).

14.5 NEW DIRECTIONS IN ONCOLOGIC IMAGING

14.5.1 Quantitative Methods and Quality Assurance

Use of imaging for noninvasive characterization of disease requires that the measurement systems are accurate and provide fidelity of the spatial distribution. For example, the relatively low resolution of the FDG-PET imaging system reduced the geometrical sampling of the injected radioactive tracers, this in turn reduces the accuracy of the SUV estimation since the image-derived concentration of the tracer cannot be captured in detail; however, this knowledge is not routinely applied in assessing clinical response. Similar issues are found in MRI, wherein changes to an imaging sequence or modification of the MR scanner can introduce spurious results into longitudinal imaging studies designed to monitor response. It

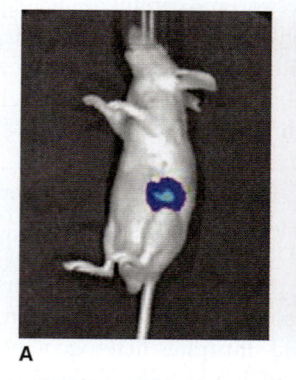

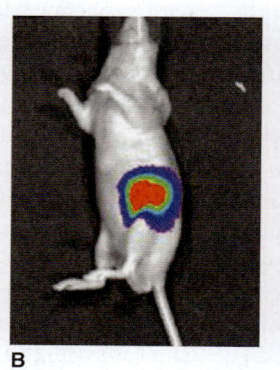

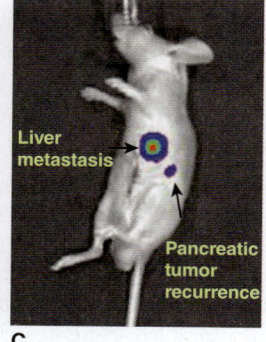

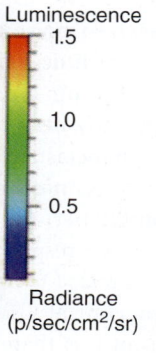

FIGURE 14–10 Bioluminescence of fluorescent proteins or luciferase can increase utility of optical imaging. Chai et al (2013) demonstrated how luciferase could increase visualization of orthotopic pancreatic models using optical imaging for non-invasive tracking of disease progression. Visualization of the pancreatic tumor (**A**) 10 days after injection of cancer cells, and (**B**) 31 days after injection. Luciferase can also visualize liver metastasis and pancreatic tumor recurrence after resection as seen in panel **C**. (Reproduced with permission from Chai MG, Kim-Fuchs C, Angst E, Sloan EK. Bioluminescent orthotopic model of pancreatic cancer progression. *J Vis Exp* 2013 Jun 28;(76):50395.)

was recognized nearly 10 years ago by The National Institutes of Health in the United States that increased effort to improve quantitative performance of clinical imaging was needed (Clarke et al, 2009). The Quantitative Imaging Network (QIN) was formed with aims to "promote research and development of quantitative imaging methods for the measurement of tumor response to therapies in clinical trial settings, with the overall goal of facilitating clinical decision making" (NCI/NIH, 2009 and Clarke et al, 2014). Many QIN teams are solving technical questions such as the effects of respiratory gating in ^{18}F-FAZA PET-CT on hypoxic fractions in lung patients (Vines et al, 2016), whereas others are beginning large multicenter clinical trials (Kurland et al, 2016). This program for coordinated imaging in clinical trials is also establishing a qualification program that includes standardized operating procedures for quality assurance, patient preparation, imaging, and image analysis. In conjunction with these efforts, there has been an increased use of test phantoms for evaluating both static and dynamic imaging sequences, as well as evaluating the dose delivered during CT imaging. QIN defined a data sharing policy and facilitated its usage through a partnership with The Cancer Imaging Archive (TCIA). In turn, these data sets have been used in multiple data analysis challenges and competitions facilitated by QIN (Kalpathy-Cramer et al, 2014). These efforts are helping to transform clinical CT, MR, and PET scanners from simply being "imaging systems" into quantitative measurement tools that can be used to make certified measurements to direct cancer care.

14.5.2 Improving on RECIST Criteria

Although the generation of the image is often the focus of imaging research, the extraction of relevant information for use in directing therapy or correlative studies is of equivalent importance. For example, the Response Evaluation Criteria in Solid Tumors (RECIST) was published in 2000 as a consensus among European, American, and Canadian cancer research groups and revised in 2009 (Eisenhauer et al, 2009). The fundamental measure in RECIST is the longest diameter of the target lesion(s) and its change during therapy (ie, 30% decrease for response, 20% increase for progressive disease). Given the wealth of information collected by imaging methods described in this chapter, the RECIST measure is a remarkable condensation of information. Nevertheless, RECIST criteria are used widely in clinical trials. The development of quantitative imaging metrics beyond tumor size and burden should allow more advanced analysis of tumor response to treatment. One example of this is the Immune-Related Response Criteria (irRC) that were developed to account for potential increased tumor burden after immunotherapy that is not always indicative of treatment failure (Wolchok et al, 2009; see Chap. 21, Sec. 21.5). In this case, RECIST would recommend cessation of treatment despite responses that do occur due to immunotherapeutic agents after disease progression. The introduction of functional measures such as FDG-PET, the use of contrast agents, the broader use of MRI in assessment of response (eg, DCE-MR), and the development of computer-assisted response evaluation measures has raised concerns about the relevance and effectiveness of the RECIST criteria (Tuma 2006; Allen et al, 2017). The continued growth of uni- and multimodal image sets will require automated algorithms to assist in observer-independent interpretation and efficient reporting if the impact of imaging on cancer is going to reach its full potential.

14.5.3 Images and Biological Information Combined for Discovery

There has been a substantial shift in the past decade toward using multiple modalities for the characterization of cancer. The combination of molecular and anatomical imaging, such as PET and CT, allows 3D quantitative analysis of a molecular imaging signal and improved understanding of disease heterogeneity. Although PET-CT images were initially motivated by the advantages of using CT for correction of attenuation, they have proven to be even more valuable as a result of improved accuracy in determining the anatomical location of abnormal metabolic activity when both images, perfectly registered, are available to the nuclear medicine physician. Research groups are now developing combined MR-PET imaging systems with the expectation of further gains in reduced radiation exposure, shortened imaging times, and increased soft-tissue delineation (Partovi et al, 2014). There are also ongoing efforts to integrate optical, CT, and MRI systems in the preclinical domain to allow optical systems to be more quantitative (Wang et al, 2015). Fusion of technologies such as imaging mass spectrometry (low spatial resolution with high chemical information) and optical microscopy will permit exploration of molecular distributions with high spatial resolution and chemical specificity (Van de Plas et al, 2015). Challenges for multimodal imaging in the clinical domain are stimulating development of software to allow images collected at various time points and by various modalities to be integrated, and corrected for variations in anatomical position (Brock and Dawson, 2014). Opportunities to combine biologic and imaging information have also been enabled by large field of view microscopes, registration/deformation software algorithms, and standardized tissue-handling protocols. The combination of this information allows histopathologic validation of imaging signals. For example, Heijblom et al (2015) explored photoacoustic imaging in breast cancer as a method of vascular imaging, and compared the resulting tumor shape and size to those obtained by MRI and histopathology (Fig. 14-11).

14.5.4 Image Guidance in Cancer Treatment

Integrated cone-beam CT imaging is used to guide radiotherapy, and dedicated MRI systems are being designed to guide these treatments with better visualization of soft-tissues (Mutic and Dempsey, 2014). In addition to designing MR-guided

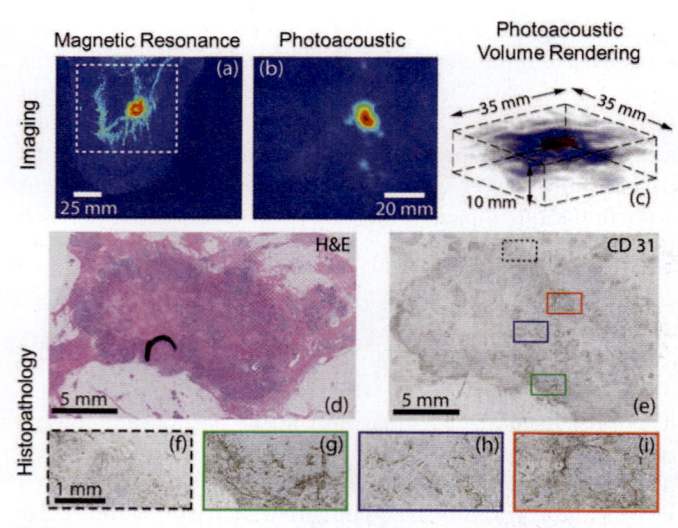

FIGURE 14-11 Comprehensive characterization of cancer heterogeneity requires integration of multiple imaging modalities and biological information. Information extracted from the various techniques can be used to find complementary information that leads to a greater understanding of disease heterogeneity (eg, PET-CT imaging), or to define correlative relationships. Heijblom et al (2015) examined the utility of photoacoustic imaging (PA) as a method of vascular imaging in breast cancer, and compared it to descriptors extracted from MRI and histopathologic staining. Average intensity projections of (**A**) MRI and (**B**) PA showed good correspondence regarding lesion location, size, and shape. Furthermore, PA-derived sizes and shapes showed similarities to those derived from histopathologic investigation of a core needle biopsy, as seen in panels **D** and **E**. The highlighted sections (**F-I**) indicate spread of the vascularity over the tumor. In this study, Heijblom et al were able to show how methods can be complementary (PA vs histopathologic investigation) or correlative (PA vs MRI) to gain greater insight into the disease. (Reproduced with permission from Heijblom M, Piras D, Brinkhuis M, et al. Photoacoustic image patterns of breast carcinoma and comparisons with Magnetic Resonance Imaging and vascular stained histopathology. *Sci Rep* 2015 Jul 10;5:11778.)

radiotherapy systems, MR systems capable of guiding high-intensity focused ultrasound (HIFU) for a variety of cancers are also under evaluation (Harding et al, 2018). The relatively slow acquisition times have limited the use of MRI in sites influenced by motion (eg, chest), but this is changing rapidly with the development of faster imaging techniques that employ multiple channels. Additionally, the progression to higher field strength magnets (3 T) offers increases in SNR and spatial resolution. Challenges including RF shielding, lack of relationship between MR relaxation times and electron densities, and altered dose distributions are being explored and met by researchers and manufacturers.

Molecular imaging initiatives that combine diagnostic, therapeutic, and monitoring applications are providing new opportunities for treatment of neuroendocrine and prostate tumors. Theranostics is one such initiative that exploits biological pathways in the body by using molecules targeted to specific cell markers; these molecules can be used as exogenous agents for diagnostic imaging, and later as delivery vehicles for radiopharmaceuticals. This process can be repeated after the initial treatment to observe whether there is still a positive uptake of the molecule, indicating the need for more treatment. A recent Theranostic clinical trial demonstrated longer progression-free survival and higher response rate in somatostatin receptor–positive midgut neuroendocrine tumors targeted using ^{177}Lu (Strosberg et al, 2017). Ongoing studies are evaluating the targeting of prostate-specific membrane antigen (PSMA) for imaging of recurrent and metastatic lesions using PET. PSMA-PET imaging is capable of detection of lesions as small as 4 mm (Dietlein et al, 2015), thereby facilitating ablative therapies with curative intent.

Recent developments of multifunctional nanoparticles are expanding the ability to observe and target tumors using a single particle. Intentionally manipulated nano-sized particles can be loaded with (all-in-one) or assembled from (one-for-all) various drug, imaging, and targeting agent building blocks (Huynh and Zheng, 2013). These nanoparticles leverage the strengths of imaging to optimize drug therapy through focused energy disruption of the nanoparticles, thereby influencing drug biodistribution and release (Patel et al, 2012). Additionally, Jin et al (2016) demonstrated how nanoparticles could increase prostate tumor selectively in mice using MRI-guided focal photothermal therapy (Fig. 14–12). However, complex toxicity studies, synthesis, and scalability need to be considered for development and clinical application of such nanoparticles. Despite these challenges, there is a clear potential for nanoparticles to revolutionize combined imaging and treatment in cancer (Cui et al, 2017).

14.5.5 Machine Learning for Image Reconstruction, Prognostics, and Predictions

Machine learning has the potential to reduce cognitive burden of physicians using models trained in performing medical exercises (e.g. segmentation (Dou et al 2017 and Milletari et al 2016)) and will free up their time for more complicated tasks. Machine learning also has the ability to perform CT image reconstruction with reduced radiation dose (Wang, 2017), detect and reduce CT metal artifacts (Gjesteby et al, 2017 and Welch et al 2020) generated by dental implants or joint replacements, and improve interpretability of intermediate steps (Choy, 2016).

Machine learning techniques applied to imaging have developed as an area of discovery-driven cancer research. The studies apply bioinformatics methods to quantified image signals to predict prognosis and outcomes of various treatments, as well as linkages to genomic information. Such machine learning techniques applied to medical images are referred to as "radiomics" and have shown potential for utilizing otherwise ignored imaging data. Figure 14–13 demonstrates one of the original radiomics studies that links radiologist classification of MR images of brain tumors with various tissue-derived microarray signatures. The largest automated radiomics study to date was completed by Aerts et al in 2014 and demonstrated the ability of quantified CT imaging features to predict patient

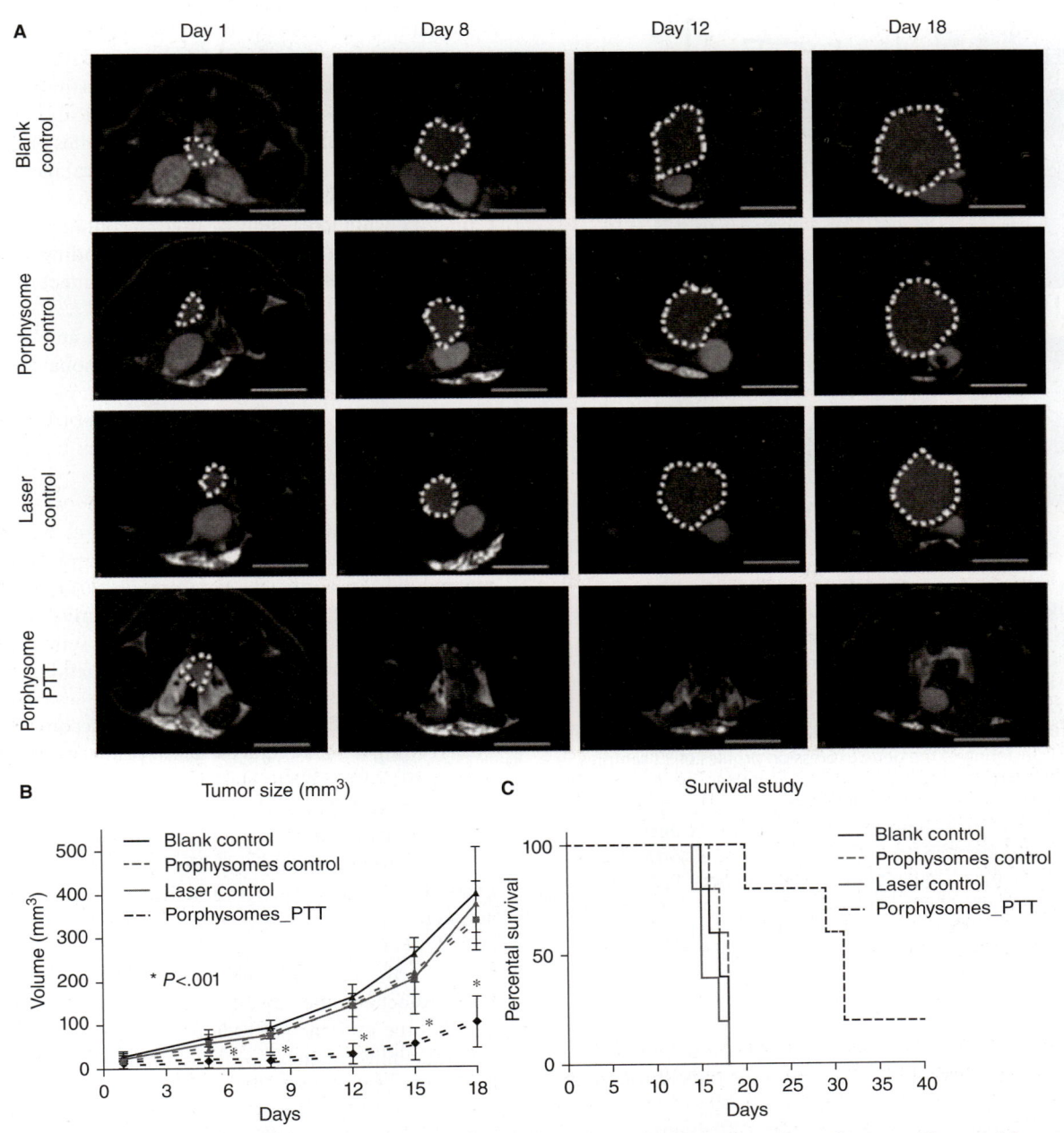

FIGURE 14-12 Nanoparticles are single particles designed to improve imaging and treatment of tumors. The particles are customizable and can be built from, or loaded with, a variety of agents. Jin et al (2016) utilized a nanoparticle to determine if it could increase selectivity of orthotopic prostate tumors during MRI-guided focal photothermal ablation therapy (PTT), thereby increasing survival. (**A**) MR images of post-treatment tumor growth comparing PTT to 3 control groups: blank, porphysome alone, and laser alone. Porphysome PTT resulted in greater suppression of tumor growth (**A**) and improved overall survival (**B**). These results demonstrated the potential utility of nanoparticles to improve selectivity of tumor over normal tissue during PTT, thereby providing a potential safe and effective treatment for localized prostate cancer. (Reproduced with permission from Jin CS, Overchuk M, Cui L, et al. Nanoparticle-Enabled Selective Destruction of Prostate Tumor Using MRI-Guided Focal Photothermal Therapy. *Prostate* 2016 Sep;76(13):1169-1181.)

outcomes in lung and head and neck patients. These methods have also been applied to PET images to explore radiomics feature implementation (Bogowicz et al, 2017), risk assessment of head and neck cancer failure using more sophisticated modeling techniques (Vallières et al, 2017), and MR images for diagnosis of pediatric brain tumors (Fetit et al, 2018). However, care must be taken when developing and interpreting complex models to ensure accurate reporting of robustness and added benefit over current methods (Welch et al, 2019). With proper consideration of automated techniques, the ability to analyze patient images using machine learning methods has the potential to provide opportunities for decision support systems to improve patient treatments, reduce side effects, and enhance outcomes. Radiomics may result in impactful models and signatures that change standard decision-making protocols. However, more importantly, radiomics is representing a

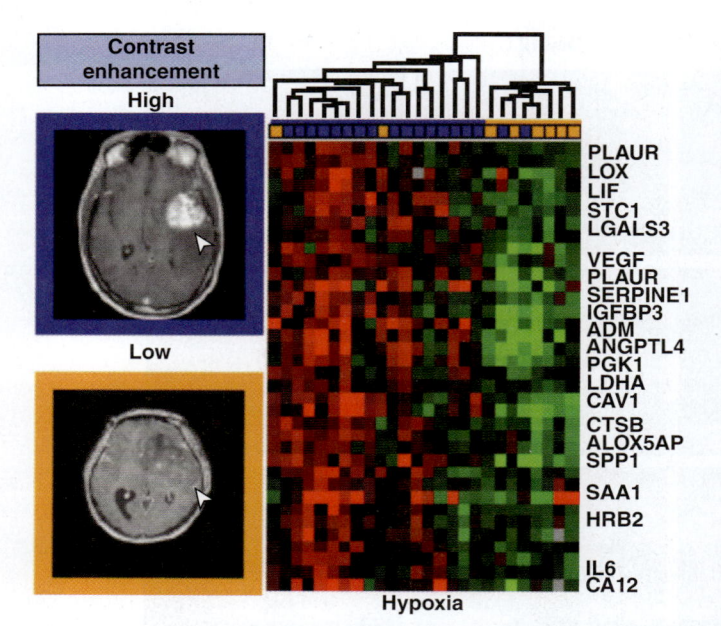

FIGURE 14-13 Radiomics involves the integration of imaging signals or "image-based biomarkers" into the bioinformatics framework being developed for genetic profiling and correlations with outcome. Imaging also brings distinct spatial information, such as size, invasiveness, and texture, and can be remeasured during the course of therapy. Diehn et al (2008) examined the gene-expression surrogates for traits in MR images. MR image signal phenotypes (10 types defined by expert radiologists) were defined, and hierarchical clustering of the gene expression profiles of 32 samples, including glioblastoma multiforme and normal brain specimens, was performed and tested for statistical significance. The results specific to contrast accumulation in the brain and hypoxia have been selected and shown here where the box color above the expression map corresponds to image trait values for the different tumors. (Reproduced with permission from Diehn M, Nardini C, Wang DS, et al. Identification of noninvasive imaging surrogates for brain tumor gene-expression modules. *Proc Natl Acad Sci* USA 2008 Apr 1;105(13):5213-5218.)

shift within cancer research and care toward more automated approaches that will improve efficiency of high-throughput techniques.

SUMMARY

- Imaging provides a means to characterize the dynamic, heterogeneous nature of cancer through morphological and biological signals.
- Advances in CT, MR, and ultrasonographic imaging technologies allow detection and delineation of disease for screening, staging, design of treatment, and assessment of response to therapy.
- Injecting exogenous agents that interact with specific biological processes enables "molecular imaging" of cancer. These approaches require highly sensitive imaging such as positron emission tomography (PET) and single-photon emission computed tomography (SPECT) systems or novel approaches to MR.
- Substantial effort is required to validate and quantify the measured image signals, to develop standards for their consistent deployment across multiple institutions, and to bring them to evaluation through clinical trials.
- Research is establishing image-based studies of cancer biology, and linking preclinical and clinical models to accelerate translation.
- Imaging will increasingly be used in conjunction with other measures to advance our understanding of the heterogeneity of cancers and the development of new treatment options.
- The potential to use these comprehensive and automated imaging measures in the "personalized cancer medicine" paradigm to target each patient's treatment is an exciting prospect in cancer treatment.

REFERENCES

Aerts HJ, Velazquez ER, Leijenaar RTH, et al. Decoding tumour phenotype by noninvasive imaging using a quantitative radiomics approach. *Nat Commun* 2014;5:4006.

Allen BC, Florex E, Sirous R, et al. Comparative effectiveness of tumor response assessment methods: standard of care versus computer-assisted response evaluation. *JCO Clin Cancer Informa* 2017;1:1-16.

Bacchus CM, Dunfield L, Gorber SC, et al. Recommendations on screening for colorectal cancer in primary care. *Can Med Assoc J* 2016;188(5):340-348.

Backes Y, Moss A, Hons M, Reitsma JB, Siersema PD, Moons LMG. Narrow band imaging, magnifying chromoendoscopy, and gross morphological features for the optical diagnosis of T1 colorectal cancer and deep submucosal invasion: a systematic review and meta-analysis. *Am J Gastroenterol* 2016;112(1):54-64.

Bogowicz M, Leijenaar RTH, Tanadini-Lang S, et al. Post-radiochemotherapy PET radiomics in head and neck cancer—the influence of radiomics implementation on the reproducibility of local control tumor models. *Radiother Oncol* 2017;125(3):385-391.

Brock KK, Dawson LA. Point: principles of magnetic resonance imaging integration in a computed tomography–based radiotherapy work flow. *Semin Radiat Oncol* 2014;169-174.

Carpentier A, Canney M, Vignot A, et al. Clinical trial of blood-brain barrier disruption by pulsed ultrasound. *Sci Transl Med* 2016;8(343):343re2.

Chai MG, Kin-Fuchs C, Angst E, Sloan EK. Bioluminescent orthotopic model of pancreatic cancer progression. *J Vis Exp* 2013;76:1-5.

Choy CB, Xu D, Gwak J, Chen K, Savarese S. 3D-R2N2: a unified approach for single and multi-view 3D object reconstruction. arXiv: 160400449v1. 2016;1:1-17.

Clarke LP, Nordstrom RJ, Zhang H, et al. Quantitative imaging network: NCI's historical perspective and planned goals. *Transl Oncol* 2014;7(1):1-4.

Clarkson R, Lindsay PE, Ansell S, et al. Characterization of image quality and image-guidance performance of a preclinical microirradiator. *Med Phys* 2011;38(2):845-856.

Cormode DP, Naha PC, Fayad ZA. Nanoparticle contrast agents for computed tomography: a focus on micelles. *Contrast Media Mol Imaging* 2014;9(1):37-52.

Cui L, Her S, Borst G, Bristow R, Jaffray DA, Allen C. Radiosensitization by gold nanoparticles: will they ever make it to the clinic? *Radiother Oncol* 2017;124(3):344–56.

Damadian R. Tumor detection by nuclear magnetic resonance. *Science* 1971;181:1151-1153.

Demidov V, Maeda A, Sugita M, et al. Preclinical longitudinal imaging of tumor microvascular radiobiological response with functional optical coherence tomography. *Sci Rep* 2018;(October 2017):1-12.

Diehn M, Nardini C, Wang DS, et al. Identification of noninvasive imaging surrogates for brain tumor gene-expression modules. *Proc Natl Acad Sci U S A* 2008;105(13):5213-5218.

Dietlein M, Kobe C, Kuhnert G, et al. Comparison of [^{18}F] DCFPyL and [^{68}Ga] Ga- PSMA-HBED-CC for PSMA-PET imaging in patients with relapsed prostate cancer. *Mol Imaging Biol* 2015;17(May):575-584.

Dou Q, Yu L, Chen H, et al. 3D deeply supervised network for automated segmentation of volumetric medical images. *Med Image Anal* 2017;41:40-54.

van Elmpt W, Landry G, Das M, Verhaegen F. Dual energy CT in radiotherapy: current applications and future outlook. *Radiother Oncol* 2016;119(1):137-144.

Fetit AE, Novak J, Rodriguez D, et al. Radiomics in pediatric neuro-oncology: a multicentre study on MRI texture analysis. *NMR Biomed* 2018;31(1):1-13.

Field JK, Duffy SW, Baldwin DR, et al. UK Lung Cancer RCT Pilot Screening Trial: baseline findings from the screening arm provide evidence for the potential implementation of lung cancer screening. *Thorax* 2016;71(2):161-170.

Filip M, Iordache S, Saftoiu A, et al. Autofluorescence imaging and magnification endoscopy. *World J Gastroenterol* 2011;17(1):9-14.

Fortuin AS, Brüggemann R, Linden Van Der, et al. Iron oxides for metastatic lymph node detection: back on the block. *WIREs Nanomed Nanobiotechnol* 2018;10(1):e1471.

Foster FS, Mehi J, Lukacs M, et al. A new 15-50 MHz array-based micro-ultrasound scanner for preclinical imaging. *Ultrasound Med Biol* 2009;35(10):1700-1708.

Fröhlich E, Muller R, Cui X, Schreiber-dietrich D, Dietrich CF. Dynamic contrast-enhanced ultrasound for quantification of tissue perfusion. *J Ultrasound Med* 2015;34(2):179-196.

Gao S, Wang G, Qin Z, Wang X, Zhao G. Biomaterials oxygen-generating hybrid nanoparticles to enhance fluorescent/photoacoustic/ultrasound imaging guided tumor photodynamic therapy. *Biomaterials* 2017;112:324-335.

Georg P, Kirisits C, Goldner G, et al. Correlation of dose-volume parameters, endoscopic and clinical rectal side effects in cervix cancer patients treated with definitive radiotherapy including MRI-based brachytherapy. *Radiother Oncol* 2009;91(2):173-180.

Gjesteby L, Yang Q, Xi Y, Zhou Y, Zhang J, Wang G. Deep learning methods to guide CT image reconstruction and reduce metal artifacts. Proc SPIE 10132, Med Imaging 2017 Phys Med Imaging. 2018;(March 2017).

Graves EE, Weissleder R, Ntziachristos V. Fluorescence molecular imaging of small animal tumor models. *Curr Mol Med* 2004;4(4):419-430.

Hagmann P, Jonasson L, Maeder P, et al. Understanding diffusion MR imaging techniques: from scalar diffusion-weighted imaging to diffusion tensor imaging and beyond. *Radiographics* 2006;26(suppl 1):S205-S223.

Han K, Croke J, Foltz W, et al. A prospective study of DWI, DCE-MRI and FDG PET imaging for target delineation in brachytherapy for cervical cancer. *Radiother Oncol* 2016;120(3):519-525.

Harding D, Giles SL, Brown MRD, et al. Evaluation of quality of life outcomes following palliative treatment of bone metastases with magnetic resonance-guided high intensity focused ultrasound: an international multicentre study. *Clin Oncol* 2018;30(4):233-242.

Heijblom M, Piras D, Brinkhuis M, et al. Photoacoustic image patterns of breast carcinoma and comparisons with magnetic resonance imaging and vascular stained histopathology. *Sci Rep* 2015;5:11778.

Hu J, Cao Y, Wu T, Li D, Lu H. High-resolution three-dimensional visualization of the rat spinal cord microvasculature by synchrotron radiation micro-CT. *Med Phys* 2014;41(10):101904.

Huang W, Muo C, Lin C, et al. Paediatric head CT scan and subsequent risk of malignancy and benign brain tumour: a nation-wide population-based cohort study. *Br J Cancer* 2014;110(9):2354-2360.

Huang Y, Alkins R, Schwarz M, Hynynen K. Opening the blood-brain barrier with MR imaging–guided focused ultrasound: preclinical testing on a trans–human skull. *Radiology* 2017;282(1):123-130.

Huizing FJ, Hoeben BAW, Franssen G, et al. Preclinical validation of ^{111}In-girentuximab-F (ab 0) 2 as a tracer to image hypoxia related marker CAIX expression in head and neck cancer xenografts. *Radiother Oncol* 2017;124(3):521-525.

Huynh E, Zheng G. Engineering multifunctional nanoparticles: all-in-one versus one-for-all. *Wiley Interdiscip Rev Nanomed Nanobiotechnol* 2013;5(3):250-265.

Ippolito D, Querques G, Okolicsanyi S, Talei Franzesi C, Strazzabosco M, Sironi S. Diagnostic value of dynamic contrast-enhanced CT with perfusion imaging in the quantitative assessment of tumor response to sorafenib in patients with advanced hepatocellular carcinoma: a feasibility study. *Eur J Radiol* 2017;90:34-41.

Jin CS, Overchuk M, Cui L, et al. Nanoparticle-enabled selective destruction of prostate tumor using MRI-guided focal photothermal therapy. *Prostate* 2016;76(13):1169-1181.

Kak AC, Slaney M. *Principles of Computerized Tomographic Imaging*. New York, NY: IEEE Press; 1988.

Kalpathy-Cramer J, Freymann JB, Kirby JS, Kinahan PE, Prior FW. Quantitative imaging network: data sharing and competitive algorithm validation leveraging the Cancer Imaging Archive 1. *Transl Oncol* 2014;7(1):147-152.

Krohn KA, Link JM, Mason RP. Molecular imaging of hypoxia. *J Nucl Med* 2008;49(suppl 2):129S-148S.

Kuno H, Onaya H, Iwata R, Kobayashi T, Fuji S, Hayashi R, et al. Evaluation of cartilage invasion by laryngeal and hypopharyngeal squamous cell carcinoma dual-energy CT. *Radiology* 2012;265(2):488-496.

Kurhanewicz J, Bok R, Nelson SJ, et al. Current and potential applications of clinical ^{13}C MR spectroscopy. *J Nucl Med* 2008;49(3):341-344.

Kurland BF, Muzi M, Peterson LM, et al. Multicenter clinical trials using ^{18}F-FDG PET to measure early response to oncologic therapy: effects of injection-to-acquisition time variability on required sample size. *J Nucl Med* 2016;57(2):226-231.

Lauterbur P. Image formation by induced local interactions: examples employing nuclear magnet resonance. *Nature* 1973;242:190-191.

Le Bihan D, Breton E, Lallemand D, et al. MR imaging of intravoxel incoherent motions: application to diffusion and perfusion in neurologic disorders. *Radiology* 1986;161(2):401-407.

Lehman CD, Lee JM, Demartini WB, et al. Screening MRI in women with a personal history of breast cancer. *J Natl Cancer Inst* 2018;108(March):1-8.

Li L, Wang K. Parameters of dynamic contrast-enhanced MRI as imaging markers for angiogenesis and proliferation in human breast cancer. *Med Sci Mont* 2015;21:376-382.

Lin KY, Maricevich M, Bardeesy N, et al. In vivo quantitative microvasculature phenotype imaging of healthy and malignant tissues using a fiber-optic confocal laser microprobe. *Transl Oncol* 2008;1(2):84-94.

Luo X, Xu H, He M, et al. Accuracy of autofluorescence in diagnosing oral squamous cell carcinoma and oral potentially malignant disorders: a comparative study with aerodigestive lesions. *Sci Rep* 2016;6:29943.

Mansfield P, Maudsley AA. Medical imaging by NMR. *Br J Radiol* 1977;50(591):188-194.

Mason RP, Zhao D, Pacheco-Torres J, et al. Multimodality imaging of hypoxia in preclinical settings. *Q J Nucl Med Mol Imaging* 2010;54(3):259-280.

Milletari F, Navab N, Ahmadi SA. V-net: fully convolutional neural networks for volumetric medical image segmentation. *IEEE Conf 3D Vis* 2016;567-573.

Mutic S, Dempsey JF. The ViewRay System: magnetic resonance–guided and controlled radiotherapy. *Semin Radiat Oncol* 2014;24(3):196-199.

NCI/NIH. *Quantitative Imaging for Evaluation of Responses to Cancer Therapies (U01)*. http://imaging.cancer.gov/programsandresources/SpecializedInitiatives/qin.

Ng CS, Zhang Z, Lee SI, Marques HS, Burgers K, Su F, et al. CT perfusion as an early biomarker of treatment Efficacy in advanced ovarian cancer: an ACRIN and GOG Study. *Clin Cancer Res* 2017;23(14):3684-3692.

Padhani AR, Koh DM, Collins DJ. Whole-body diffusion-weighted MR imaging in cancer: current status and research directions. *Radiology* 2011;261(3):700-718.

Park I, von Morze C, Lupo JM, et al. Investigating tumor perfusion by hyperpolarized ^{13}C MRI with comparison to conventional gadolinium contrast-enhanced MRI and pathology in orthotopic human GBM xenografts. *Magn Reson Med* 2017;77(2):841-847.

Partovi S, Robbin MR, Steinbach OC, et al. Initial experience of MR/PET in a clinical cancer. *J Magn Reson Imaging* 2014;39(4):768-780.

Patel RH, Wadajkar AS, Patel NL, Kavuri VC, Nguyen KT, Liu H. Multifunctionality of indocy anine green-loaded biodegradable nanoparticles for enhanced optical imaging and hyperther mia intervention of cancer. *J Biomed Opt* 2012;17(4):046003.

Rey S, Schito L, Koritzinsky M, Wouters BG. Molecular targeting of hypoxia in radiotherapy. *Adv Drug Deliv Rev* 2017;109:45-62.

Rosales RTM De. Potential clinical applications of bimodal PET-MRI or SPECT-MRI agents. *J Label Compd Radiopharm* 2014;57(4):298-303.

Santyr G, Fox M, Thind K, Hegarty E, et al. Anatomical, functional and metabolic imaging of radiation-induced lung injury using hyperpolarized MRI. *NMR Biomed.* 2014;27(12):1515-1524.

Siddiqui MM, Rais-Bahrami S, Turkbey B. Comparison of MR/ultrasound fusion–guided biopsy with ultrasound-guided biopsy for the diagnosis of prostate cancer. *JAMA* 2015;313(4):390-397.

Strosberg J, El-Haddad G, Wolin E, et al. Phase 3 trial of 177 Lu-Dotatate for midgut neuroendocrine tumors. *N Engl J Med* 2018;(2011):125-135.

Tadayyon H, Gangeh MJ, Vlad R, Kolion MC, Czarnota GJ. Ultrasound imaging of apoptosis: spectroscopic detection of DNA-damage effects in vivo. In *Methods of Molecular Biology: Fast Detection of DNA Damage*, 1644th ed. New York, NY: Humana Press. https://doi.org/https://doi.org/10.1007/978-1-4939-7187-9_4.

Toepker M, Czerny C, Ringl H, et al. Can dual-energy CT improve the assessment of tumor margins in oral cancer? *Oral Oncol* 2014;50(3):221-227.

Townsend DW, Beyer T, Blodgett TM. PET/CT scanners: a hardware approach to image fusion. *Semin Nucl Med* 2003;33(3):193-204.

Tuma RS. Sometimes size doesn't matter: reevaluating RECIST and tumor response rate endpoints. *J Natl Cancer Inst* 2006;98(18):1272-1274.

Vaidyanathan G, Mcdougald D, Choi J, et al. Preclinical evaluation of ^{18}F-labeled anti-HER2 nanobody conjugates for imaging HER2 receptor expression by immuno-PET. *J Nucl Med* 2016;57(6):967-973.

Vallières M, Kay-rivest E, Perrin LJ, et al. Radiomics strategies for risk assessment of tumour failure in head-and-neck cancer. *Sci Rep* 2017;7(1):10117.

Van De Plas R, Yang J, Spraggins J, Caprioli RM. Image fusion of mass spectrometry and microscopy: a multimodality paradigm for molecular tissue mapping. *Nat Methods* 2015;12(4):4-6.

Vines DC, Driscoll BD, Yeung I, Publicover J, Sun A, Jaffray DA. Effects of respiratory gated ^{18}F-FAZA PET-CT on hypoxic fraction in patients and phantom. Paper presented at: 14th ImNO Annual Meeting (p. 157). 2016.

Wang K, Chi C, Hu Z, et al. Optical molecular imaging frontiers in oncology: the pursuit of accuracy and sensitivity. *Engineering* 2015;1(3):309-323.

Wang J, Wright AJ, Hu D, Hesketh R, Brindle KM. Single shot three-dimensional pulse sequence for hyperpolarized. *Magn Reson Med* 2017;752:740-752.

Weersink RA, Qiu J, Hope AJ, et al. Improving superficial target delineation in radiation therapy with endoscopic tracking and registration. *Med Phys* 2011;38(12):6458-6468.

Wei Y, Liao R, Ahmed A, Xu H, Zhou Q. pH-responsive pHLIP (pH low insertion peptide) nanoclusters of superparamagnetic iron oxide nanoparticles as a tumor-selective MRI contrast agent. *Acta Biomater* 2017;55:194-203.

Welch ML, McIntosh C, Haibe-Kains B, Milosevic MF, Wee L, Dekker A, Hui Huang S, Purdie TG, O'Sullivan B, Aerts HJWL, Jaffray DA. Vulnerabilities of radiomic signature development: The need for safeguards. *Radiotherapy and Oncology* 2019;130:P2-P9.

Welch ML, McIntosh C, Traverso A, Wee L, Purdie TG, Dekker A, Haibe-Kains B, Jaffray DA. External validation and transfer learning of convolutional neural networks for computed tomography in dental artifact classification. *PMB* 2020;65:3.

Welz S, Monnich D, Pfannenberg C, et al. Prognostic value of dynamic hypoxia PET in head and neck cancer: results from a planned interim analysis of randomixed phase II hypoxia-image guided dose escalation trial. *Radiother Oncol* 2017;124(3):526-532.

Wilson SR, Burns PN. Liver mass evaluation with ultrasound: the impact of microbubble contrast agents and pulse inversion imaging. *Semin Liver Dis* 2001;21(2):147-159.

Wolchok JD, Hoos A, Day SO, et al. Guidelines for the evaluation of immune therapy activity in solid tumors: immune-related response criteria. *Cancer Ther Clin* 2009;15(23):7412-7421.

Xiao Y, Hong H, Matson VZ, et al. Gold nanorods conjugated with doxorubicin and cRGD for combined anti-cancer drug delivery and PET imaging. *Theranostics* 2012;2(8):757-768.

Yang Y, Armour M, Wang KK. Evaluation of a cone beam computed tomography geometry for image guided small animal irradiation Evaluation of a cone beam computed tomography geometry for image guided small animal irradiation. *Phys Med Biol* 2015;60(13):5163-5177.

Yeung TP, Kurdi M, Wang Y, et al. CT perfusion imaging as an early biomarker of differential response to stereotactic radiosurgery in C6 rat gliomas. *PLoS One* 2014;9(10):e109781.

Zanette B, Stirrat E, Jelveh S, Hope A, Santyr G. Physiological gas exchange mapping of hyperpolarized 19Xe using spiral-IDEAL and MOXE in a model of regional radiation-induced lung injury. *Med Phys* 2018;45:2.

Zheng J, Muhanna N, Souza R De, et al. Biomaterials A multimodal nano agent for image-guided cancer surgery. *Biomaterials*. 2015;67:160-168.

Zhou J, Wang H, Zhang H, Lutz AM, Tian L, Willmann K. VEGFR2-targeted three-dimensional ultrasound imaging can predict responses to antiangiogenic therapy in preclinical models of colon cancer. *Cancer Res* 2016;76(14):4081-4089.

Molecular and Cellular Basis of Radiotherapy

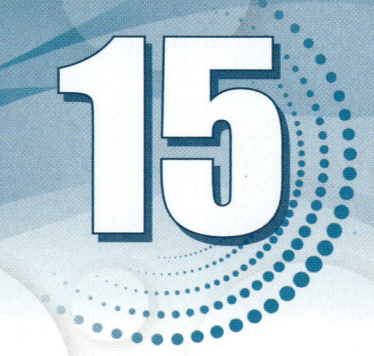

Marianne Koritzinsky and Scott V. Bratman

Chapter Outline

- 15.1 Introduction
- 15.2 Interaction of Radiation with Matter
  - 15.2.1 Types of Radiation, Energy Deposition, and Measurements of Radiation Dose
  - 15.2.2 Linear Energy Transfer and Energy Absorption
  - 15.2.3 Radiation Damage Within the Cell
- 15.3 Cell Death After Ionizing Radiation
  - 15.3.1 Mechanisms of Cell Death
  - 15.3.2 In Vitro and In Vivo Assays for Radiation Cell Survival
- 15.4 Molecular and Cellular Responses to Ionizing Radiation
  - 15.4.1 Genetic Instability
  - 15.4.2 Cell-Cycle Sensitivity and DNA Damage Checkpoints
  - 15.4.3 Cellular and Molecular Repair
  - 15.4.4 Intracellular Signaling following Ionizing Radiation
  - 15.4.5 Intercellular Responses to Ionizing Radiation
- Summary
- References
- Appendix 15.1 Mathematical Models Used to Characterize Radiation Cell Survival

15.1 INTRODUCTION

Since their discovery by Roentgen more than a century ago, x-rays have played a major role in modern medicine. The first recorded use of x-rays for the treatment of cancer occurred within 1 year of their discovery. Subsequently, there has been intensive study of x-rays and other ionizing radiations, and their clinical application to cancer treatment has become increasingly sophisticated. This chapter and Chapter 16 review the biological effects of ionizing radiation and the application of that knowledge to cancer treatment.

The present chapter begins with a review of the physical properties of ionizing radiations and the effects of energy deposition in cells. The molecular and cellular processes that ensue will be described, as well as response pathways that influence radiosensitivity and proliferation.

15.2 INTERACTION OF RADIATION WITH MATTER

15.2.1 Types of Radiation, Energy Deposition, and Measurements of Radiation Dose

X- and γ-rays constitute part of the continuous spectrum of electromagnetic (EM) radiation that includes radio waves, infrared (heat), ultraviolet (UV), and visible light (Fig. 15–1). All types of EM radiation can be considered as moving packets (quanta) of energy called *photons*. The amount of energy in each individual photon defines its position in the EM spectrum. For example, x- or γ-ray photons carry more energy than heat or light photons and are therefore at the high-energy

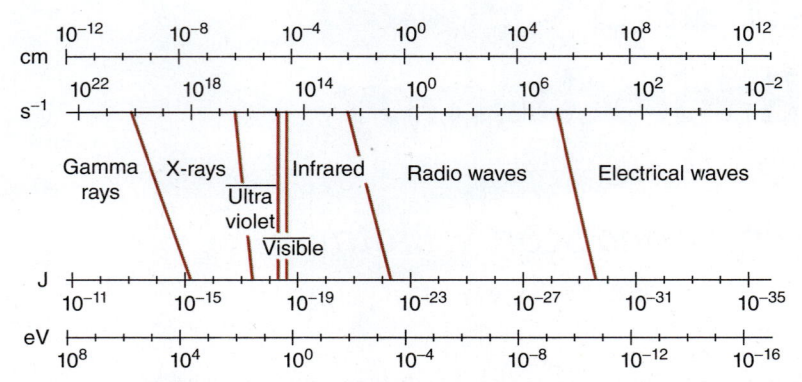

FIGURE 15–1 EM spectrum showing the relationship of photon wavelength in centimeters (cm) to its frequency in inverse seconds (s⁻¹) and to its energy in joules (J) and electron volts (eV). The various bands in the spectrum are indicated. Slanted lines between bands indicate the degree of overlap in the definition of the various bands.

end of the EM spectrum. Individual photons of x- or γ-rays are sufficiently energetic that their interaction with matter can result in the complete displacement of an electron from its orbit around the nucleus of an atom. Such an atom (or molecule) is left with a net (positive) charge and is thus an ion; hence the term *ionizing radiation*. Typical binding energies for electrons in biological material are in the neighborhood of 10 eV (electron volts). Thus, photons with energies greater than 10 eV (ie, x- or γ-rays) are considered to be ionizing radiation, whereas photons with energies of 2 to 10 eV are in the UV range and are nonionizing. An interaction that transfers energy, but does not completely displace an electron, is called an *excitation* because it leaves the atom or molecule in a higher-energy state.

UV radiation is split into 3 general classes, UV-C, UV-B, and UV-A, corresponding to wavelengths of 200 to 290 nm, 290 to 320 nm, and greater than 320 nm, respectively. UV-C and UV-B irradiation can be absorbed by DNA in cells leading to the production of various photoproducts, such as covalent bonds between pyrimidine rings (6-4 photoproducts [6-4 PPs] or cyclobutane pyrimidine dimers [CPDs]) that disrupt the normal base-pairing in the DNA helix. Such lesions may be repaired by processes such as nucleotide excision repair (see Chap. 9, Sec. 9.3.3). If not repaired, they can give rise to mutations during replication. Because of the limited penetration of UV radiation through tissue, its effects in humans are primarily associated with the skin (see Chap. 9, Sec. 9.2.2.1).

X-rays are produced when accelerated electrons hit a tungsten target and then decelerate, emitting a spectrum of *Bremsstrahlung* radiation. The resulting spectrum of radiation energies is filtered to produce a clinically useful beam of x-rays with the desired energy and collimated to narrow the beam to the desired shape. When x-ray photons interact with tissue, they give up energy by 1 of 3 processes: the photoelectric effect, the Compton effect, or pair production. In the energy range most widely used in radiotherapy (4-18 MeV), the Compton effect is the most important mechanism leading to deposition of energy in tissue. This energy transfer involves a collision between a photon and an outer orbital electron of an atom, with partial transfer of energy to the electron and scattering of the photon into a new direction. The electron (and the photon) can then undergo further interactions, causing more ionizations and excitations, until its energy is dissipated. All 3 of the interaction processes result in the production of energetic electrons that, in turn, lose energy by exciting and ionizing target atoms and molecules thereby setting more electrons in motion. In the end, most of the energy that is absorbed by tissue irradiated with x-rays or γ-rays comes from the interactions caused by this cascade of secondary electrons.

Modern clinical radiotherapy uses ionizing radiation to treat people with cancer. The radiation can be delivered to tissues by external beam radiotherapy using linear accelerators that produce high-energy x-rays or electron beams, ^{60}Co sources that emit γ-rays by radioactive decay, or particle accelerators that produce protons or carbon ions. Clinical radiotherapy can also be given using brachytherapy, which delivers a localized radiation dose from within an organ or tissue using γ-rays emitted by implanted isotopes such as ^{131}I, ^{125}I, ^{192}Ir, and ^{103}Pd (see Chap. 16, Sec. 16.2.3). Particles used for clinical radiotherapy include electrons, *light particles* such as protons and neutrons, and *heavy particles* such as carbon ions. Charged particles such as protons and carbon ions deposit energy by interactions with electrons causing ionization and excitation. In contrast, neutrons deposit energy by collisions with nuclei, particularly hydrogen nuclei (protons), thereby transferring their energy to create moving charged particles capable of both ionization and excitation. The choice of the type of delivery of radiotherapy depends on tumor type and location within the body (see Chap. 16, Sec. 16.2.4), as well as the availability of resources. The vast majority of radiotherapy is delivered by x-rays produced by linear accelerators or by γ-rays.

Radiation dose is measured by the energy (joules, J) absorbed per unit mass (kg) and the standard unit is the gray (Gy, 1Gy is equivalent to 1 J/kg). Radiation dose is a critical factor that contributes to the biological effect of ionizing radiation, but biological effects also depend on the location and volume of tissue over which the dose is distributed. For example, a whole-body dose of 8 Gy would result in the death (by bone marrow failure) of many animals, including humans, yet the amount of energy deposited, if evenly distributed, would cause a temperature rise of only about 2×10^{-3} °C (about 100× less than drinking a cup of coffee). It is the size and clustered nature of the individual energy-deposition events caused by ionizing radiations that is the reason for their efficacy in damaging biological systems.

15.2.2 Linear Energy Transfer and Energy Absorption

The deposition of energy in matter (eg, a tumor or normal tissue) by charged particles (including secondary electrons) is chiefly a result of electrical field interactions. As a charged particle moves through matter, the particle's energy loss dE, along a portion of its track dx, is proportional to its charge Z and the electron density of the target ρ, and inversely proportional to its velocity v, as indicated by the mathematical relationship in Equation 15.1:

$$\frac{dE}{dx} \alpha \frac{Z^2 \rho}{v^2} \quad (15.1)$$

Although photons, charged particles, and neutrons all cause dose deposition by setting electrons in motion, they do so with varying effectiveness and patterns, resulting in differences in the dose deposition. The important difference between various types of radiation is the average *density* of energy loss *along* the track of the particle. The average energy lost by a particle over a given track length is known as the *linear energy transfer* (LET). The units of LET represent energy lost per unit path-length, for example, keV/μm. Table 15–1 provides some early track values of LET for different particles. Because the energy of a particle depends on its mass (m) and velocity (E = mv^2), it can be seen from Equation 15.1 that as a particle slows down, for instance, as it traverses a tumor or normal tissue, it loses energy more rapidly and reaches a maximum rate of energy loss just before it reaches the end of its path (Fig. 15–2). The LET of an individual charged particle thus varies along the length of its track, and the maximum LET at

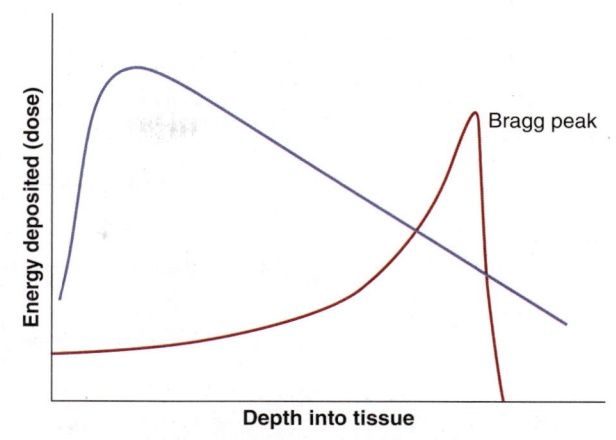

FIGURE 15–2 Schematic of energy deposition by photons (blue) versus charged particles (red) along their track in tissue. Photons result in absorbed dose that falls off exponentially after a shallow build-up phase. A charged particle deposits limited energy until it slows down and reaches the end of its track, resulting in high levels of absorbed dose in the region of the Bragg peak.

the end of the path is referred to as the Bragg peak. A Bragg peak is not observed when photons are used to irradiate tissue, because the secondary electrons that are set in motion are easily deflected and their track through the tissue is tortuous. Their initiation and termination points occur at random in the tissue, averaging out the variation in LET along individual tracks. Clinically, one can take advantage of the Bragg peak from heavier charged particles to maximize dose deposition at a target at specified depth such as a tumor (see Chapter 16, Sec. 16.2.4). In addition to this advantage in shaping the dose distribution, high-LET radiation also has a higher relative biologic effectiveness, as described below.

15.2.3 Radiation Damage Within the Cell

The interactions leading to energy deposition in tissue occur very rapidly and generate chemically reactive free electrons and free radicals (molecules with unpaired electrons). Cellular molecules are altered either as a result of *direct* energy absorption or as a result of energy transfer from one molecule to another, giving rise to *indirect* effects (Fig. 15–3A). Most of the energy deposited in cells is absorbed initially in water (because the cell is approximately 80% water), leading to the rapid (ie, within 10^{-14} to 10^{-4} seconds) production of reactive intermediates (oxidizing and reducing radicals), which, in turn, can interact with other molecules in the cell (indirect effect). The hydroxyl [OH·] radical, an oxidizing agent, is probably the most damaging. The cell contains naturally occurring thiol compounds such as glutathione, cysteine, cysteamine, and metallothionein, whose sulfhydryl (SH) group(s) can react chemically with the free radicals to decrease their damaging effects. Other antioxidant non-sulfhydryl metabolites include the vitamins C and E and intracellular enzymes such as manganese superoxide dismutase (MnSOD) and catalase that metabolize the reactive superoxide [O_2^-] and hydrogen peroxide [H_2O_2] respectively. Because of this scavenging effect, the intracellular levels of

TABLE 15–1 Linear energy transfer of various radiations.

Radiation	LET (keV/μm)
Photons	
^{60}Co(~1.2 MeV)	0.3
200-keV x-ray	2.5
Electrons	
1 Mev	0.2
100 keV	0.5
10 keV	2
1 keV	10
Charged particles	
Proton 2 MeV	17
Alpha 5 MeV	90
Carbon 100 MeV	160
Neutrons	
2.5 MeV	15 to 80
14.1 MeV	3 to 30

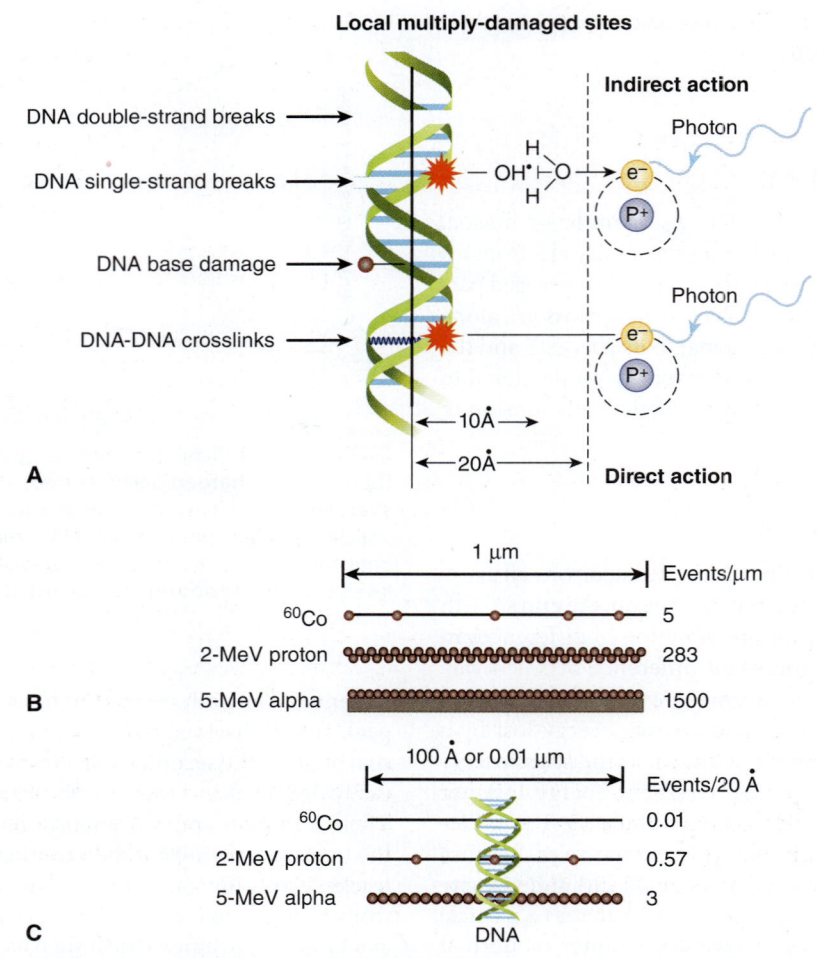

FIGURE 15–3 **A)** Direct and indirect effects of ionizing radiation on DNA. In the indirect model, chemically reactive free radicals are produced during ionization of water molecules in close proximity (ie, 10-20 angstroms [Å]) to the DNA helix. These free radicals, such as the hydroxyl radical, OH·, can react chemically with DNA to produce DNA damage. In the direct model, absorption of the energetic electron occurs directly within the DNA causing localized damage without an intermediate free radical step. Indirect and direct damage can lead to clusters of DNA single-strand and double-strand breaks, DNA base damage, DNA–DNA or DNA–protein crosslinks. These can occur as local multiply-damaged sites (LMDS). **B)** and **C)** The frequency of primary energy-loss events along the tracks of various radiations of widely differing linear energy transfer. **B)** Schematic of primary energy-loss events over a distance of 1 μm. **C)** Primary energy-loss events over 0.01 μm or 100 Å, depending on type of radiation. The dimensions of a DNA double helix are illustrated. (Part A Modified with permission from Hall EJ. Radiobiology for the Radiologist, 5th ed. Philadelphia, PA: Lippincott, Williams & Wilkins; 2000.)

thiols and antioxidative molecules contribute to the response of cells and tissues to radiation (Zhang and Martin, 2014).

The random nature of energy-deposition events means that radiation-induced changes can occur in any molecule in a cell. The most important consequences of ionizing radiation result from lesions in DNA: DNA damage persists and is propagated over cell generations if not repaired, whereas damaged proteins, RNA, and lipids are removed by routine turnover. Even relatively small amounts of DNA damage can lead to cell lethality. Approximately, 10^5 ionizations can occur within a diploid cell per gray of absorbed radiation dose, leading to about 1000 to 3000 DNA–DNA or DNA–protein crosslinks, 1000 damaged DNA bases, 500 to 1000 single-strand and 25 to 50 double-strand DNA breaks (Fig. 15–3). Focal areas of DNA damage can arise because of the clustering of ionizations within a few nanometers of the DNA (Ward, 1994; Lomax et al, 2013). These "local multiply damaged sites" (LMDSs) include combinations of single- or double-strand breaks in the sugar-phosphate backbone of the molecule, alteration, or loss of DNA bases, and formation of crosslinks between the DNA strands or between DNA and chromosomal proteins. Most types of DNA lesions can be repaired by DNA repair pathways (see Chap. 9). However, coordinating DNA repair pathways to repair clustered LMDS-associated lesions is difficult in cells, resulting in the high efficacy of ionizing radiation in causing cell death (Lomax et al, 2013). High LET irradiation causes an increase in both the number and complexity of DNA clustered lesions that are more difficult to repair, and therefore causes more cell death per gray.

Although ionizing radiation causes many types of DNA damage, most studies suggest that cell death following radiation is correlated with either initial or residual levels of DNA double-strand breaks (Jeggo and Lavin, 2009). Table 15–2 outlines evidence to support the role of damage to DNA as crucial in causing cell death.

TABLE 15-2 Evidence supporting DNA as a critical target for radiation-induced lethality.

1. Microbeam irradiation demonstrates the cell nucleus to be much more sensitive than the cytoplasm.
2. Radioisotopes with short-range emissions (eg, ^{2}H, ^{125}I) incorporated into DNA cause cell killing at much lower absorbed doses than those incorporated into the cellular cytoplasm.
3. Incorporation of thymidine analogs (eg, iododeoxyuridine [IUdR] or bromodeoxyuridine [BUdR]) into DNA modifies cellular radiosensitivity.
4. The level of chromatid and chromosomal aberrations following ionizing radiation correlates with cell lethality.
5. The number of unrepaired DNA double-strand breaks correlates with cell lethality following ionizing radiation in many cells.
6. For different types of radiation, cell lethality correlates best with the level of radiation-induced DNA double-strand breaks rather than with other types of damage.
7. The extreme radiosensitivity of some mutant cells is a result of defects in DNA repair (see Chap. 9, Secs. 9.3 and 9.5).

Although DNA is the most important cellular target in most cells, reactive oxygen species (ROS) induced by ionizing radiation can interact with proteins in the cell membrane, some of which may be involved in signal transduction. This can lead to apoptosis in certain cell types (eg, endothelial cells) by activation of the ceramide-sphingomyelin pathway. Therefore, preincubation of cells with agents capable of altering either protein function or lipid peroxidation within the cell membrane, including ceramide antibodies, can modify the level of radiation-induced apoptosis (Corre et al, 2013). As such, the cellular response to ionizing radiation is mediated both by damage to DNA and a complex interaction between proteins located within the plasma membrane, cytoplasm, and nucleus of the cell (see Sec. 15.4), although DNA damage is the dominant factor in most situations. Ultimately, this leads to activation of the DNA damage response (DDR) (Chap. 9, Sec 9.3) and other cellular signaling cascades that regulate DNA repair, cell proliferation, and cell death.

15.3 CELL DEATH AFTER IONIZING RADIATION

15.3.1 Mechanisms of Cell Death

The fate of a cell after radiation depends on 2 factors: (1) whether radiation triggers pathways to initiate apoptosis, and (2) the success of DNA repair. A few cell types, typically those of hematopoietic origin or from testes, initiate apoptosis rapidly (within hours) after radiation. In these cases, cell death is a direct consequence of signaling occurring in response to the initial DNA damage (Aldridge and Radford, 1998; Brown and Wouters, 1999). These cell types have low survival after radiation, rendering cancers like lymphoma and testicular cancer highly radiosensitive. Most cell types, however, do not initiate apoptosis rapidly after radiation, and their survival is instead dependent on whether or not the DNA is sufficiently restored (Fig. 15-4).

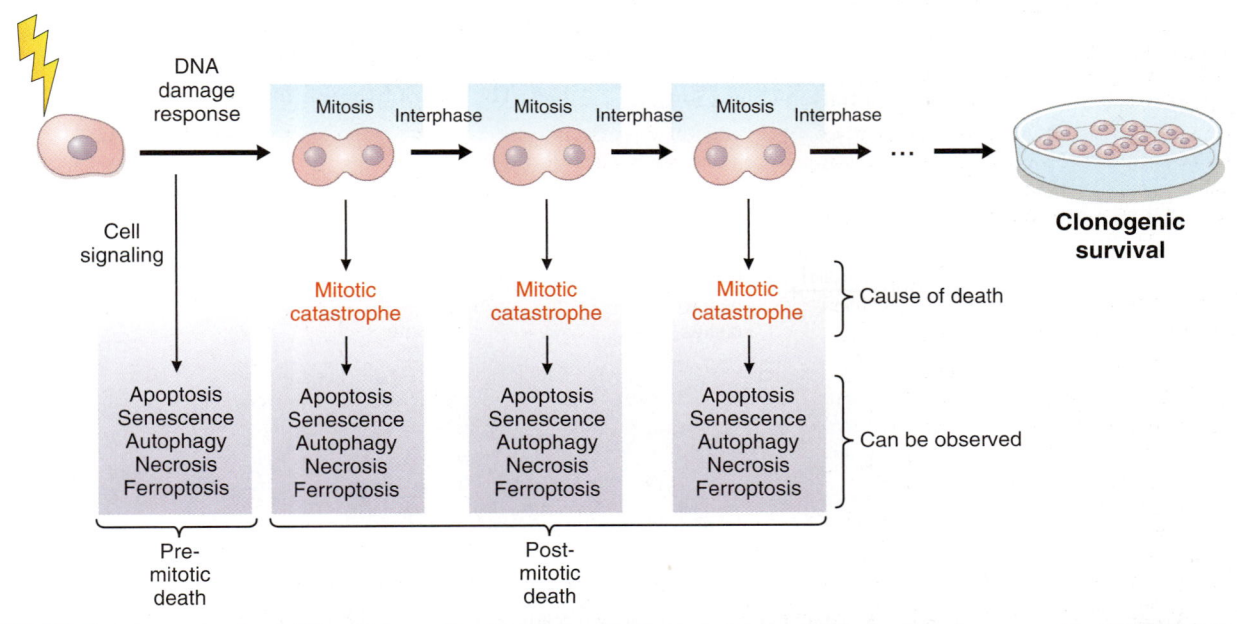

FIGURE 15-4 Schematic of possible cell fates after irradiation. Radiation induces cell signaling largely governed by the DNA damage response. In a minority of cell types, this can result in early pre-mitotic death owing to the activation of cell death pathways such as apoptosis. More commonly, cells will undergo mitotic catastrophe during the first mitosis after radiation, or even after several successful cell divisions. Numerous cell death pathways can be observed as a consequence of the mitotic catastrophe. The redundancy of cell death pathways and the wide time frame over which they are activated renders accurate quantification of overall cell death in response a difficult task. Usually, radiobiologists quantify clonogenic survival at long time points (eg, 2 weeks) after radiation, which reflects the cumulative effect of all cell death pathways occurring at all earlier time points. (Joiner et al 2018.)

Misrepair of DNA can lead to inactivation, mutation, truncation, or hyperactivation of specific genes, but in most cases, these kinds of permanent DNA alterations are not toxic. It is typically larger chromosome aberrations that interfere with DNA segregation in mitosis that are deadly. Double-strand DNA breaks followed by DNA repair can sometimes lead to chromosome fragments without a centromere that will lead to substantial DNA loss in one daughter cell and micronuclei outside of the nucleus in another, both of which can be toxic. Other times, chromosomes can end up with 2 or more centromeres, which renders the sister chromatids impossible to segregate in mitosis. Forces on the centromeres eventually cause such chromosomes to break, leading to cell death or further exacerbation of chromosomal aberrations that are increasingly incompatible with successful mitosis. Such *mitotic catastrophe* is the most common *cause* of cell death after ionizing radiation (Fig. 15–4). Therefore, many types of cells do not show morphologic evidence of radiation damage until they attempt to divide. Some cells may even successfully go through 1 or more mitoses and interphases before finally experiencing a mitotic catastrophe. Secondary to mitotic catastrophe, cells can initiate senescence, or die by apoptosis, ferroptosis, necrosis, or other cell death pathways. Some biochemical and morphologic differences between cell death pathways are reviewed in Chapter 8, Section 8.4. Regardless of which pathway is initiated, the cell is destined to die because of the mitotic catastrophe. Because cells can initiate many different cell death pathways at various time points within the first few cell cycles after radiation, it is difficult to use specific cell death assays as endpoints to reflect overall cell toxicity. It is more meaningful to instead measure cell *survival* after several cell divisions. Measuring long-term survival takes into account the cumulative effect of all types of cell death integrated over the time after irradiation (Fig. 15–4).

15.3.2 In Vitro and In Vivo Assays for Radiation Cell Survival

Inhibition of the continued reproductive ability of cells is an important consequence of the molecular and cellular responses to radiation, as it occurs at relatively low doses (a few grays) and it is the major aim of clinical radiotherapy. A tumor is controlled if its stem cells (see Chap. 13, Sec. 13.3.2) are prevented from continued proliferation. A cell that retains unlimited proliferative capacity after radiation treatment is regarded as having *survived* the treatment. In contrast, a cell that has lost the ability to generate a "clone" or *colony* is regarded as having been "killed," even though it may undergo a few divisions or remain intact and metabolically active for a substantial period after irradiation. Colony formation following irradiation is thus an important end point, because it relates to a cell's ability to repopulate normal or tumor tissues following exposure to ionizing radiation (see also Chap. 16, Secs. 16.3 and 16.5). In an assay that is used to assess colony formation, cells grown in culture are irradiated either before or after preparation of a suspension of single cells and plated at low concentration in tissue-culture dishes. Following irradiation, the cells are incubated for a number of days, and those that retain proliferative capacity divide repeatedly to form discrete colonies of cells (Fig. 15–5). After incubation, the colonies are fixed and stained so that they can be counted.

Cells that do not retain proliferative capacity following irradiation (ie, are killed) may divide a few times, but form only very small "abortive" colonies. If a colony contains more than 50 cells (ie, derived from a single cell by at least 6 division cycles), it is assumed that it arose from a surviving cell that retained unlimited replicative potential. The plating efficiency (PE) of the cell population is calculated by dividing the number of colonies formed by the number of cells seeded—or plated. The ratio of the PE for the irradiated cells to the PE

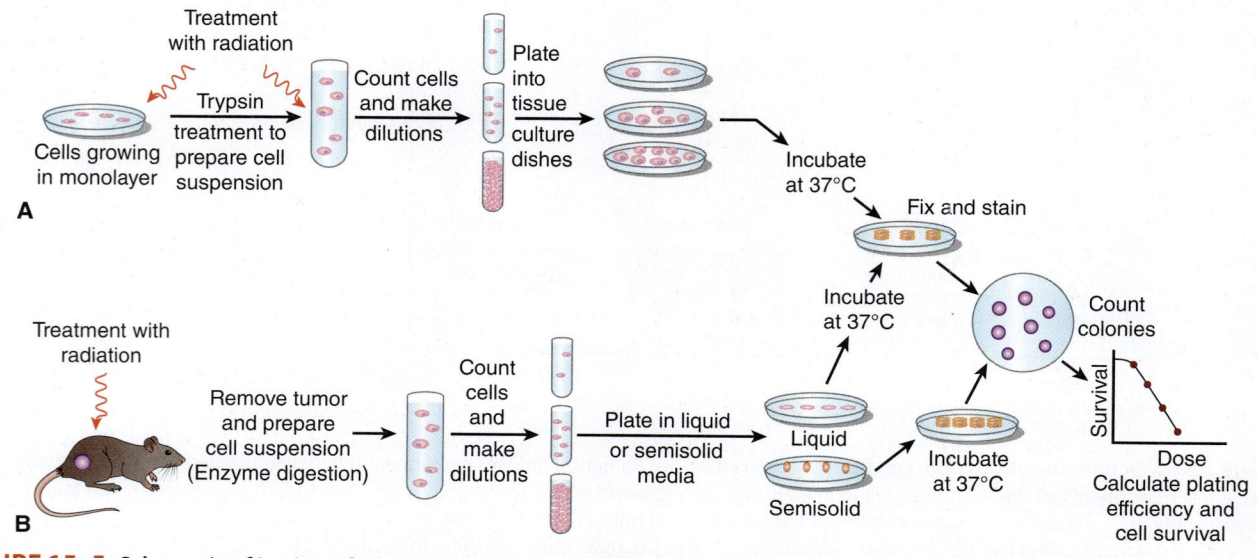

FIGURE 15–5 Schematic of in vitro plating assays to assess cell survival. **A)** Assay for the radiation sensitivity of cells growing in culture. **B)** In vivo–in vitro assay for the sensitivity of tumor cells grown and irradiated in vivo.

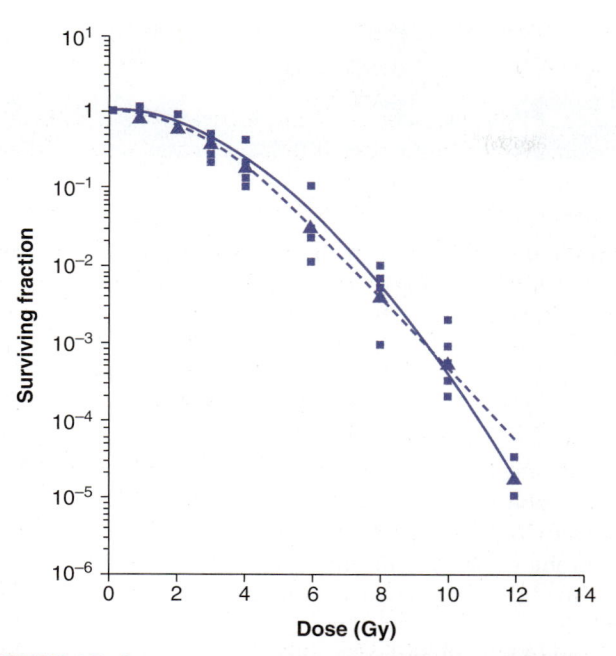

FIGURE 15-6 Survival data for a murine melanoma cell line treated with low-LET (γ-rays) radiation. The surviving fraction is plotted on a logarithmic scale against dose plotted on a linear scale. The data from 5 independent survival experiments are shown as the squares, with the geometric mean value at each dose shown as the triangles. The survival curves shown are the result of fitting the data to target theory (dashed line) or linear-quadratic (solid line) models (Appendix 15.1). (Reproduced with permission from Bristow RG, Hardy PA, Hill RP. Comparison between in vitro radiosensitivity and in vivo radioresponse of murine tumor cell lines. I: Parameters of in vitro radiosensitivity and endogenous cellular glutathione levels. *Int J Radiat Oncol Biol Phys* 1990 Jan;18(1):133-145.)

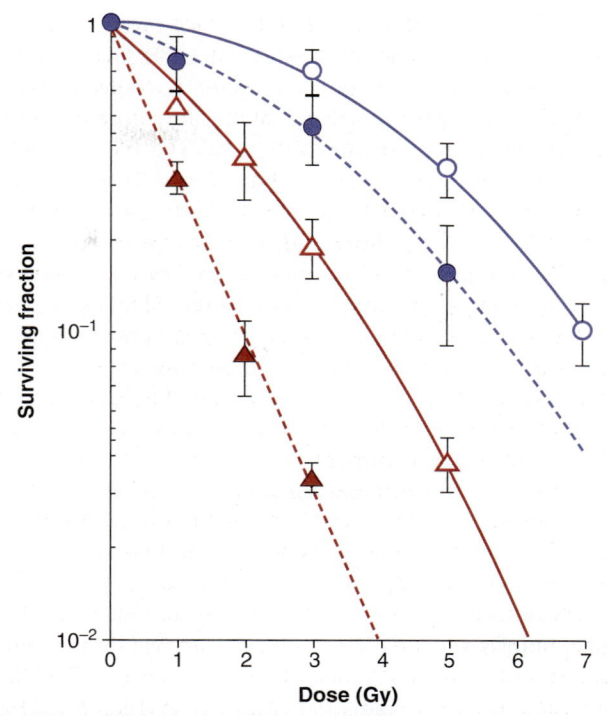

FIGURE 15-7 Survival curves for a canine osteosarcoma cell line treated with gamma rays, protons, or carbon or iron ions. White circles indicate γ-rays (LET 0.2 keV/μm); blue circles indicate protons (LET 1 keV/μm); white triangles indicate carbon ions (LET 50 keV/μm). Red triangles indicate iron ions (LET 200 keV/μm). (Reproduced with permission from Maeda J, Cartwright IM, Haskins JS, et al. Relative biological effectiveness in canine osteosarcoma cells irradiated with accelerated charged particles. *Oncol Lett* 2016 Aug;12(2):1597-1601.)

for control cells is calculated to give the fraction of cells surviving the treatment (*cell survival* or *surviving fraction*). If a range of radiation doses is used, then these cell-survival values can be plotted to give a *survival curve*, such as the ones shown in Figures 15–6 and 15–7. Cells taken directly from animal or human tumors can also be grown in culture, allowing the in vitro assay to be extended to study the radiation sensitivity of tumor cells treated in vivo (see Fig. 15–5).

The techniques described above have been used to obtain survival curves for a wide range of malignant and normal cell populations. In general, for low-LET radiation (eg, x- or γ-rays), these curves have the shape(s) illustrated in Figure 15–6, when the surviving fraction of the cell population is plotted on a log scale as a function of dose plotted on a linear scale. At low doses, there is evidence of a "shoulder" region; but at higher doses, the curve either becomes steeper or straight so that survival decreases exponentially with dose (dotted line in Fig. 15–6) or appears to be continually bending downward on the semilogarithmic plot (solid line in Fig. 15–6). There is greater variation in the low-dose or shoulder region of the radiation survival curves obtained for mammalian cells as compared to the variation in the slopes of the high-dose region of the curves (see Chap. 16, Sec. 16.3.2).

Figure 15–7 illustrates the difference in survival curves for x- or γ-rays (low-LET) and for protons, carbon ions, and iron ions (increasing-LET as indicated) irradiation. In general, the shoulder of the survival curve is reduced for higher-LET radiation and the curve is steeper. The (radio) biological effectiveness (RBE) of different types of radiation can be defined as the ratio of the dose of a standard type of radiation to that of the test radiation that gives the same biological effect. The standard type of radiation was originally taken as 200- or 250-kVp (peak kilovoltage) x-rays. Cobalt-60 γ-rays are also used as a standard for comparison studies, although their RBE relative to 250-kVp x-rays is approximately 0.9. Because the shoulder of the survival curve is reduced for high-LET radiation, the RBE varies with the dose or the survival level at which it is determined.

Cell kill after radiation is a stochastic process. For a given radiation dose, each individual cell has a certain probability to survive, which translates into the surviving fraction of a large population of such cells. Many different mathematical models have been used to produce equations that can fit survival curves to data within the limits of experimental error. Given the stochastic nature of cell kill, these models are all derivatives of the equation for a Poisson distribution.

Two commonly used models are the *target-theory* and *linear-quadratic* models of cell survival (explained in Appendix 15.1) from which parameters (D_0, n, or α and β, respectively) can be used to describe the shape of the low-dose and high-dose regions of the cell survival curve. The accuracy of the data is usually such that either shape could fit the data adequately over the first few decades of survival, as illustrated in Figure 15–6. Such descriptions are useful when comparing cellular radiosensitivity among a variety of cell types or when the shape of the survival curve is altered following treatment with drugs or changes in the environment (eg, hypoxia; see Chap. 12, Sec. 12.4 and Chap. 16, Sec. 16.4).

Clonogenic survival remains the gold standard for determining the radiosensitivity of cells in vitro. However, it is time-consuming and difficult to scale for high throughput. Moreover, not all cell types form colonies in vitro. Because cells often die by mitotic catastrophe after several cell divisions, assays that measure short-term proliferation rates or programmed cell death/apoptosis often do not correlate with long-term survival and the clonogenic assay. One exception is that apoptosis may predict clonogenic survival for lymphoma and testicular cancer cell lines, as these cell types tend to die by apoptosis following irradiation (Aldridge and Radford, 1998; Brown and Wouters, 1999). Some high-throughput assays measuring surrogate endpoints of proliferation rates at longer times (eg, 9 days) after irradiation have been shown to correlate well with clonogenic survival within a limited dose range if careful cell line–specific optimization is first carried out (Abazeed et al, 2013). Assays that evaluate cellular growth for a short period (eg, 1–5 days) following radiation, such as the MTT (3-[4,5-dimethylthiazol-2-yl]-2,5 diphenyl tetrazolium bromide) (or similar) assay that determines cellular viability by colorimetric assessment of the reduction of a tetrazolium compound, are generally not appropriate for radiosensitivity studies of other cell types because they do not reflect the later death (following a few cell divisions) that is detected with a colony-forming assay. Such assays also have a limited range, and it is rarely possible to assess more than 90% cell kill. At present, clonogenic survival remains the most accepted method for determining the radiosensitivity of cells in vitro.

Methods have also been developed for assessing the ability of cells to form colonies in vivo. One of these is the spleen-colony method, which has been used to assess both the radiation and drug sensitivity of specific bone marrow (stem) cells (McCulloch and Till, 1962). In this assay, bone marrow from treated animals is injected into irradiated new hosts, and colonies from surviving bone marrow (spleen colony-forming) cells can be then counted in the spleen. Initially, these cells were thought to be hematopoietic stem cells but it is now known that they are downstream of the true hematopoietic stem cells in the maturation hierarchy. In an analogous method, the lung-colony assay, tumor cells from treated animals are injected intravenously and form colonies in the lungs of syngeneic mice (Hill and Bush, 1969). Other colony-forming assays have been developed to study the radiation response of stem cells in situ in certain proliferative tissues, including skin, and the gastro-intestinal tract (Withers, 1967; Tucker et al, 1991).

15.4 MOLECULAR AND CELLULAR RESPONSES TO IONIZING RADIATION

15.4.1 Genetic Instability

Many human cancers contain cells with chromosomal rearrangements, including chromosomal translocations, deletions, and amplifications. Chromosome rearrangements can also be observed in cells after irradiation, and if nonlethal, may contribute to the carcinogenic properties of ionizing radiation. Chromosomal instability following irradiation has been demonstrated using a variety of techniques including spectral karyotyping (SKY), fluorescence in situ hybridization (FISH), inverse polymerase chain reaction (PCR), and DNA sequencing (see Chap. 2, Sec. 2.2). DNA double-strand breaks can lead to chromosomal rearrangements at the first mitosis after exposure to ionizing radiation and the type of aberration (ie, chromosomal vs chromatid types of rearrangements; Fig. 15–8) can reflect the cell-cycle phase at the time of irradiation. Chromosomal rearrangements in irradiated cells often contain chromosomal fragments from other sites of DNA damage in the same cell (see Chap. 9, Sec, 9.2).

If a cell survives and proliferates after irradiation, delayed chromosomal instability can be observed in the descendants of the exposed cell. Such radiation-induced chromosomal instability may be secondary to a breakage-fusion-bridge cycle or to *epigenetic effects*, which perpetuate the unstable phenotype in irradiated cells (Huang et al, 2003). In some instances, chromosomal aberrations that result from radiation exposure can contribute directly to secondary carcinogenesis (see Chap. 9, Sec 9.5).

15.4.2 Cell-Cycle Sensitivity and DNA Damage Checkpoints

Mammalian cells have evolved to protect against accumulation of mutations. A crucial component of how cells achieve this is through a series of checkpoints that delay progression through the cell cycle in the presence of DNA damage such as that caused by ionizing radiation. Such delays allow for the repair of DNA damage in cells prior to undergoing either DNA replication or mitosis and are thought to prevent genetic instability in future cell generations. Radiation-induced cell-cycle checkpoints exist at the G1/S-phase transition, during S phase and in G_2 phase (Kastan and Bartek, 2004).

Cells in different phases of the cell cycle have different radiosensitivity (Terasima and Tolmach, 1961; Wilson, 2004). If a single radiation dose is given to cells in different phases, then usually it is found that cells in late S phase have the highest probability of survival after radiation (ie, are the most resistant), and that cells in mitosis (M phase) are the most sensitive (see Fig. 15–9). Although many cell lines appear to have a resistant period in S phase following irradiation in vitro, cell lines have variability in sensitivity just before mitosis in the G_2 phase of the cell cycle (Wilson, 2004).

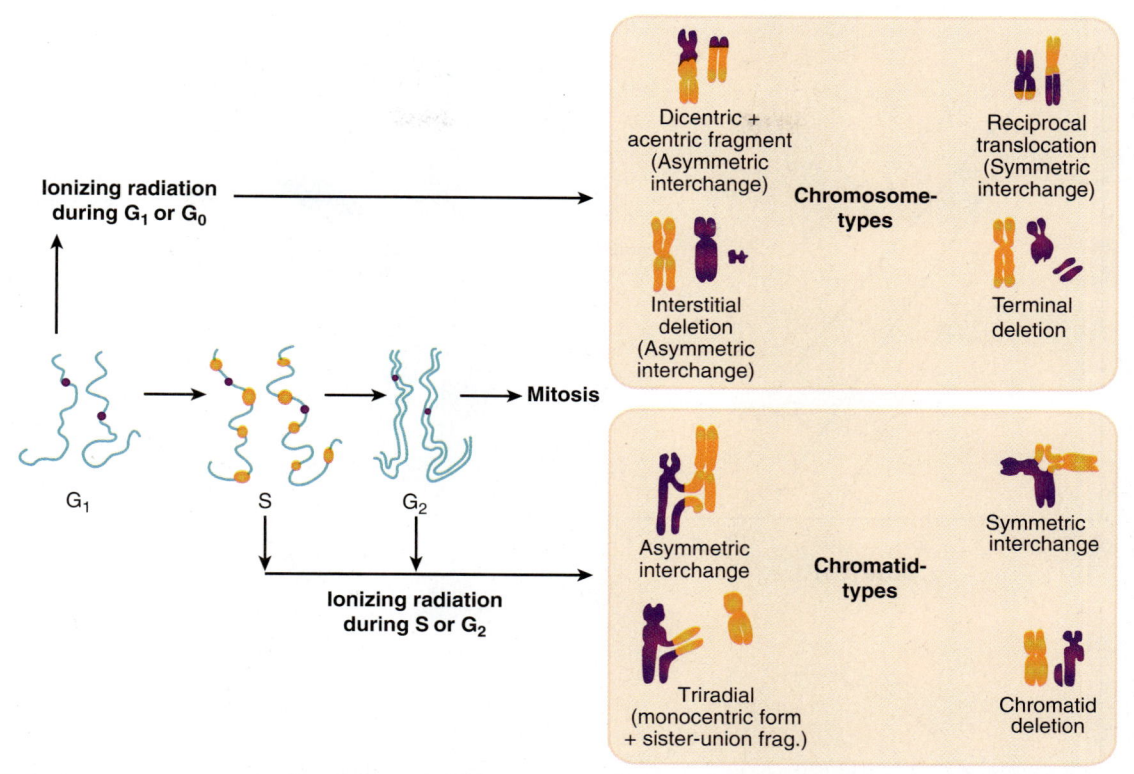

FIGURE 15–8 Chromosomal versus chromatid types of radiation-induced damage as a function of cell-cycle phase during irradiation. If a cell is irradiated during the G_1 or early S phase when only 1 chromosomal homolog exists, a nonrepaired DNA-DSB (double-strand break) can lead to dicentrics, reciprocal translocations, and acentric fragments. During irradiation in late S and G_2 phases, sister chromatids have duplicated and the DNA-DSB gives rise to interchanges, triradials, or a chromatid deletion. Consequently, the type of chromosomal damage observed may reflect the relative ability of cells to use the nonhomologous end-joining (optimally used during G_1) or homologous recombination (optimal in S and G_2) repair pathways to correct the DNA-DSB. (Modified with permission from Nagasawa H, Brogan JR, Peng Y, Little JB, Bedford JS. Some unsolved problems and unresolved issues in radiation cytogenetics: a review and new data on roles of homologous recombination and non-homologous end joining. *Mutat Res* 2010 Aug 14;701(1):12-22.)

The molecular signaling governing the mammalian cell cycle and its response to DNA damage (including that of ionizing radiation) is discussed in detail in Chaps. 8 and 9. The ATM (ataxia-telangiectasia mutated) and ATR (ataxia-telangiectasia and Rad3 related) proteins initiate checkpoint pathways (Shiloh, 2003). The *G1/S checkpoint* is controlled by ATM-mediated phosphorylation of p53 and regulatory factors that lead to stabilization and activation of p53. P53 activation leads to transcriptional upregulation of p21 that inhibits the CDK2/cyclinA and CDK4/cyclinD complexes that are required for transition into S-phase. ATM also phosphorylates proteins that contribute to slowing down DNA replication and cell-cycle progression in S phase, such as BRCA1, NBS1, FANCD2, and CHK2 (see Chap. 8). CHK2 in turn phosphorylates CDC25A, which marks it for degradation, leading to deactivation of the CDC25A-dependent CDK1 and CDK2 driving S-phase progression (Shiloh, 2003). The G1/S checkpoint is dose-dependent, reflecting the observation that increased radiation dose leads to a longer cell cycle delay.

Two separate molecular mechanisms govern checkpoints in *G2/M*, allowing damaged DNA to be repaired prior to mitosis (Nagasawa et al, 1994; Kao et al, 2001). A transient, ATM-dependent and dose-independent (between 1 and 10 Gy) checkpoint occurs early after irradiation of cells in the G_2 phase. In contrast, the "G_2 accumulation checkpoint" is ATR- and dose-dependent and occurs in cells that reach G_2 after being exposed to radiation in earlier cell-cycle phases (Xu et al, 2002). The G_2 checkpoints are engaged as a result of ATM- or ATR-dependent phosphorylation of CHK2 and CHK1 that in turn phosphorylate CDC25C and Wee1, eventually resulting in inhibition of the mitosis promoting CDK1/cyclin B factor (Xu et al, 2002; Shiloh, 2003) (see Chap. 8 Sec. 8.3.2.4).

Cells lacking either of the proteins critical for activating cell cycle checkpoints demonstrate aberrant cell cycle progression after radiation. Tumor cells often exhibit a disrupted G_1/S checkpoint because of inactivating mutations and/or deletion of the tumor suppressor protein p53. All the cell cycle checkpoints protect cells against propagation of genetic alterations. The ATR-dependent G_2/M checkpoint is additionally important for cell survival after radiation. There are therefore ongoing attempts to develop drugs that abrogate the G_2/M checkpoint in tumor cells to potentiate the cytotoxicity of ionizing radiation over that of normal cells (Dillon et al, 2014). These drugs may target ATR, CHK1, or Wee1, leading to the induction of premature mitosis and mitotic catastrophe in the treated cells.

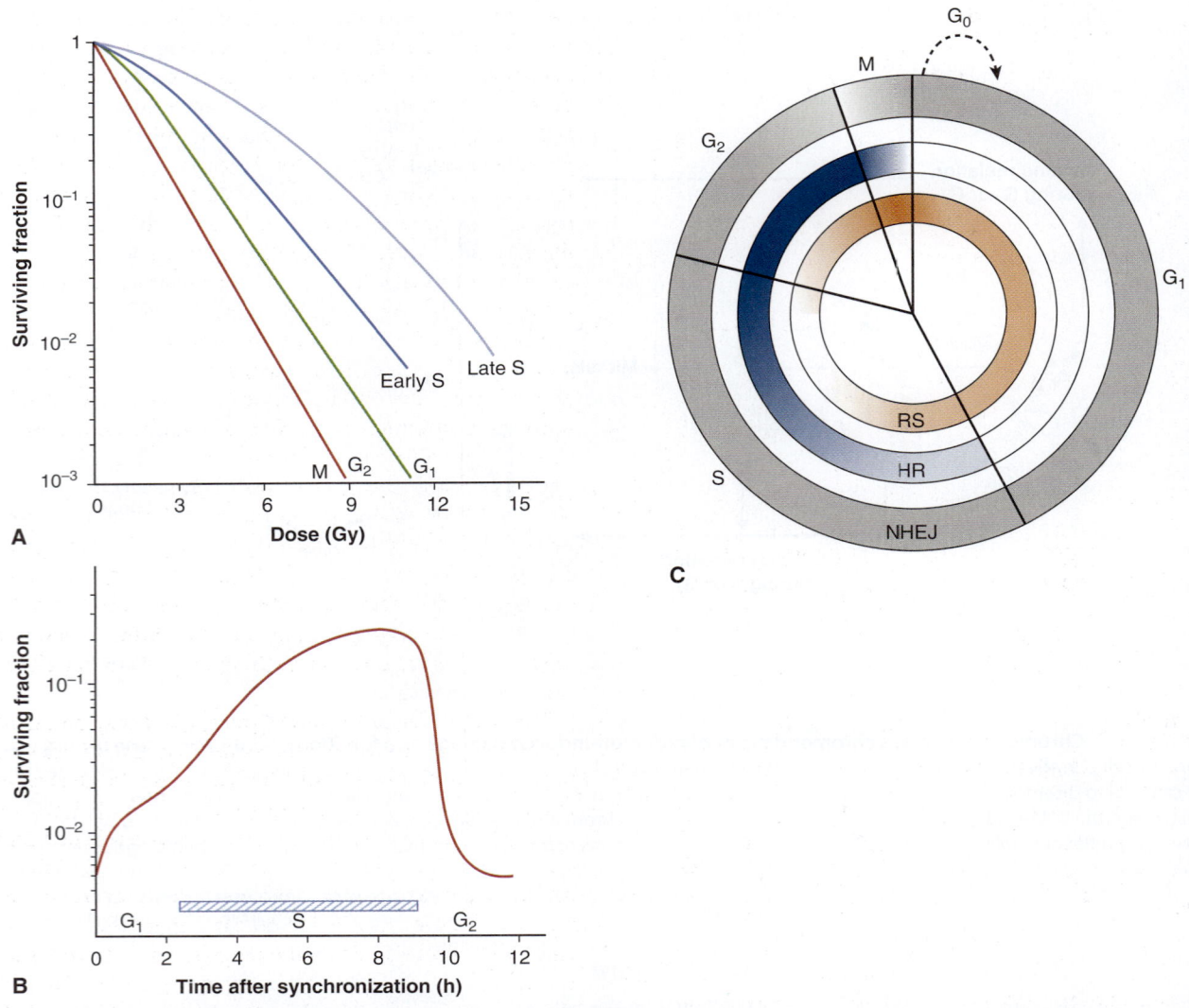

FIGURE 15-9 The effect of position in the cell cycle on cellular radiosensitivity. **A)** Survival curves for Chinese hamster cells irradiated in different phases of the cell cycle. **B)** Cells were selected in mitosis and irradiated with a fixed dose as a function of time of incubation after synchronization. The pattern of cell survival reflects the changing cellular sensitivity as the cells move through the cell cycle. **C)** Diagram indicating radiation-induced cell-cycle checkpoints, the active repair mechanisms during the various cell-cycle phases, and relative radiosensitivity. There is a radiation-induced cell-cycle checkpoint at the end of G_1 phase, a general slow-down in S, a second check point at the end of G_2 phase. *HR*, Homologous recombination which occurs during the S and G_2 phases of the cell cycle; *NHEJ*, nonhomologous end-joining recombination that occurs in all phases of the cell cycle; *RS*, relative radiosensitivity. Dark shading indicates activity of the particular repair pathway. Dark red shading indicates most radiosensitive portions of the cell cycle.

15.4.3 Cellular and Molecular Repair

The repair of cellular damage between radiation doses is the major mechanism underlying the clinical observation that a larger total dose can be tolerated when the radiation dose is fractionated. The shoulder of the survival curve reflects accumulation of *sublethal damage* that can be repaired (Elkind and Sutton, 1960) (Fig. 15–10). When Chinese hamster cells were incubated at 37°C for 2.5 hours between the first and second radiation treatments, the original shoulder of the survival curve was partially regenerated, and it was completely regenerated when the cells were incubated for 23 hours between the treatments (Fig. 15–10A). When the interval between 2 fixed doses of radiation was varied (Fig. 15–10B), there was a rapid rise in survival as the interval was increased from zero (single dose) to about 2 hours. This was followed by a decrease before the survival rose again to a maximum level after about 12 hours. This pattern of recovery is a result of 2 processes. *Repair of sublethal damage (SLDR)* accounts for the early rise in survival. Because cells that survive radiation tend to be synchronized in the more resistant phases of the cell cycle, their subsequent progression (inevitably into more sensitive phases) leads to a reduction in survival at 4 hours. Continued repair and repopulation explain the increases in survival at later

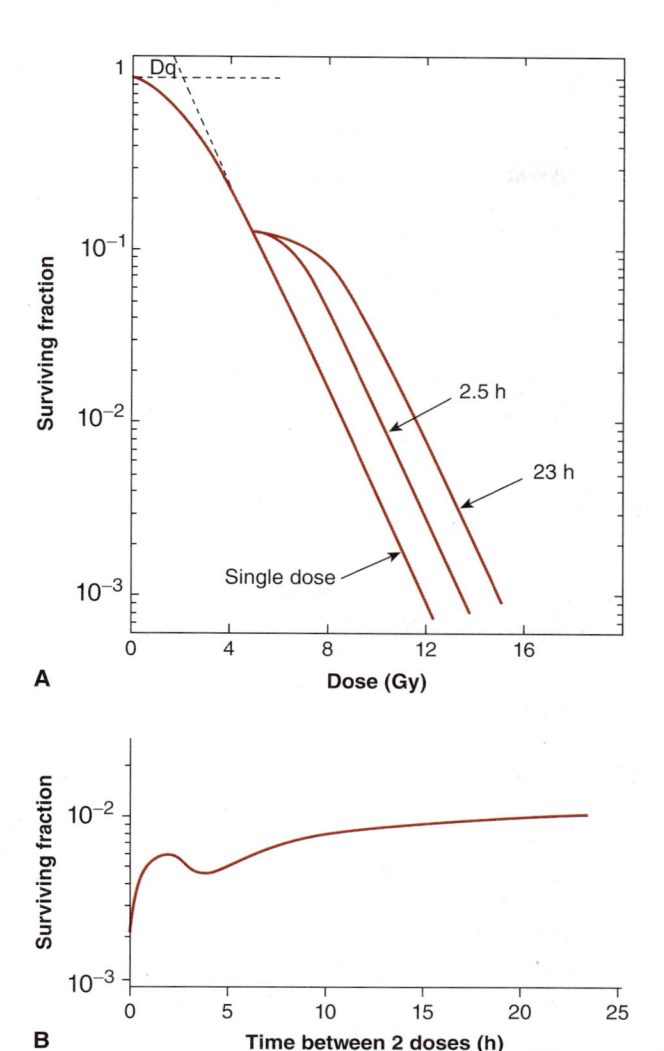

FIGURE 15–10 Illustration of the repair of sublethal damage that occurs between 2 radiation treatments. **A)** Survival curves for a single-dose treatment or for treatments involving a fixed first dose followed, after 2.5 or 23 hours of incubation (at 37°C), by a range of second doses. Dq is a measure of the shoulder width, see Appendix 15.1. **B)** Pattern of survival observed when 2 fixed doses of irradiation are given with a varying time interval of incubation (at 37°C) between them.

times (see Chap. 16, Sec. 16.6). This pattern of *SLDR* has been demonstrated for a wide range of cell lines.

The repair capacity of the cells of many tissues has been demonstrated using cell survival and functional assays in vivo (eg, Withers and Mason, 1974). An increase in total dose is required to give the same level of biological damage when a single dose (D_1) is split into 2 doses (total dose D_2) with a time interval between them (Fig. 15–11). The difference in dose ($D_2 - D_1$) is a measure of the repair by the cells in the tissue.

The capacity of different cell populations to undergo *SLDR* is reflected by the width of the shoulder on their survival curve—that is, the D_q or $D_2 - D_1$ value. Survival curves for bone marrow cells have little to no shoulder, possibly because of their propensity to undergo radiation-induced apoptosis. Cells that demonstrate little or no evidence of cellular repair and that do not undergo radiation-induced apoptosis (such as fibroblasts derived from the radiosensitive disorders AT and Nijmegen breakage syndrome [NBS]; (see Chap. 9, Sec. 9.5) also lack a shoulder to their survival curve and accumulate increased levels of DNA breaks (Shiloh, 2003; Jeggo and Lavin, 2009). The increased radiosensitivity associated with an increased accumulation of residual and lethal DNA double-strand breaks is illustrated in Figure 15–12. Other cells (eg, jejunal crypt cells) can demonstrate a large *SLDR* for repair capacity ($D_2 - D_1$ value of 4 to 5 Gy; see Fig. 15–11A).

The effect of a given dose of radiation on human tissues and cells differs widely for exposures given over a short time (acute irradiation) and over an extended period of time (chronic irradiation given at a low-dose rate). Dose rates above approximately 1 Gy/min can be regarded as acute (single-dose) treatment and result in survival curves similar to that in Figure 15–6. As the total dose of x- or γ-rays is delivered at decreasing dose rates, the DNA damage in the cell diminishes progressively because of repair of the damage during the treatment. As a result, the shape of the radiation survival curve changes from one exhibiting a shoulder at high dose rates to one approaching linearity at low dose rates (Fig. 15–13A, B).

The magnitude of the *dose-sparing effect* may be calculated as the relative survival for the same dose given under conditions of low-dose rate irradiation compared to survival under conditions of acute-dose rate irradiation. Cell lines with a greater capacity to repair sublethal damage will demonstrate a large dose-sparing effect relative to those cells that have limited capacity to repair the damage. In addition to cellular repair, low-dose rate irradiation can trigger the G_1, S, and G_2 checkpoints, slowing down the progression of the cells through the cycle, but if the dose rate is low enough, the cells will continue to divide and repopulate. Because cells in late S phase are often the most radioresistant, they will preferentially survive, but eventually will move into the more sensitive phases of the cell cycle during radiation, a process termed *redistribution*. The process of repopulation leads to relative radioresistance of the cell population, whereas cell-cycle redistribution leads to relative radiosensitization. Most of the effect of cellular repair occurs in the range of dose rates of 1.0 to 0.01 Gy/min. Below approximately 0.1 Gy/min, the effects of cell-cycle progression (redistribution and the G_2 block; see Sec. 15.4.2) become apparent; below approximately 0.01 Gy/min, the effects of cell repopulation will start to become evident as the radiation damage is not severe enough to trigger cell-cycle arrest. Repair, repopulation, and redistribution are important for understanding dose fractionation in clinical radiotherapy, as described in Chapter 16, Section 16.6.

Cell survival can be increased by holding cells after irradiation under conditions of suboptimal growth, such as low temperature, nutrient deprivation, or high cell density. The latter conditions may reflect those experienced by G_0-G_1 populations of cells in growth-deprived regions of tumors (Malaise et al, 1989) (see Chap. 12, Sec. 12.1). The property is a result of

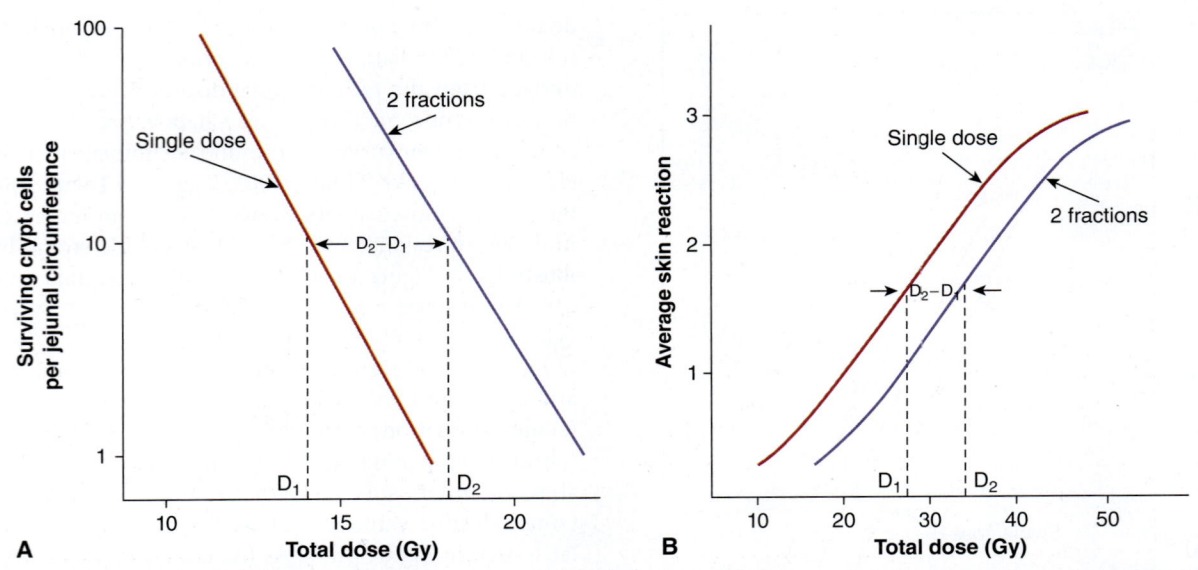

FIGURE 15-11 Repair of radiation damage in vivo. **A)** Survival curves for murine intestinal crypt cells γ-irradiated in situ with a single dose (red line) or with 2 equal fractions given 3 hours apart (blue line). **B)** Average skin reaction following x-irradiation of mouse skin with a single dose (red line) or 2 fractions given 24 hours apart (blue line). In both cases, an increase in total dose is required to give the same level of biological damage when a single dose (D_1) is split into 2 doses (total dose D_2) with a time interval between them. The difference in dose ($D_2 - D_1$) is a measure of the repair by the cells in the tissue.

the repair of *potentially lethal damage* (PLDR), which usually results in a change in the slope of the cell-survival curve. Such repair may contribute to increased radiation survival observed in vivo for some transplantable cell lines when compared to the radiosensitivity of the same cells growing in vitro.

The molecular components of DNA repair pathway(s) are described in Chapter 9, Section 9.3. Multiple studies indicate that double-strand breaks (DSBs) are responsible for most lethal damage induced by ionizing radiation (Jeggo and Lavin, 2009). The main pathways of repair of DNA-DSBs include

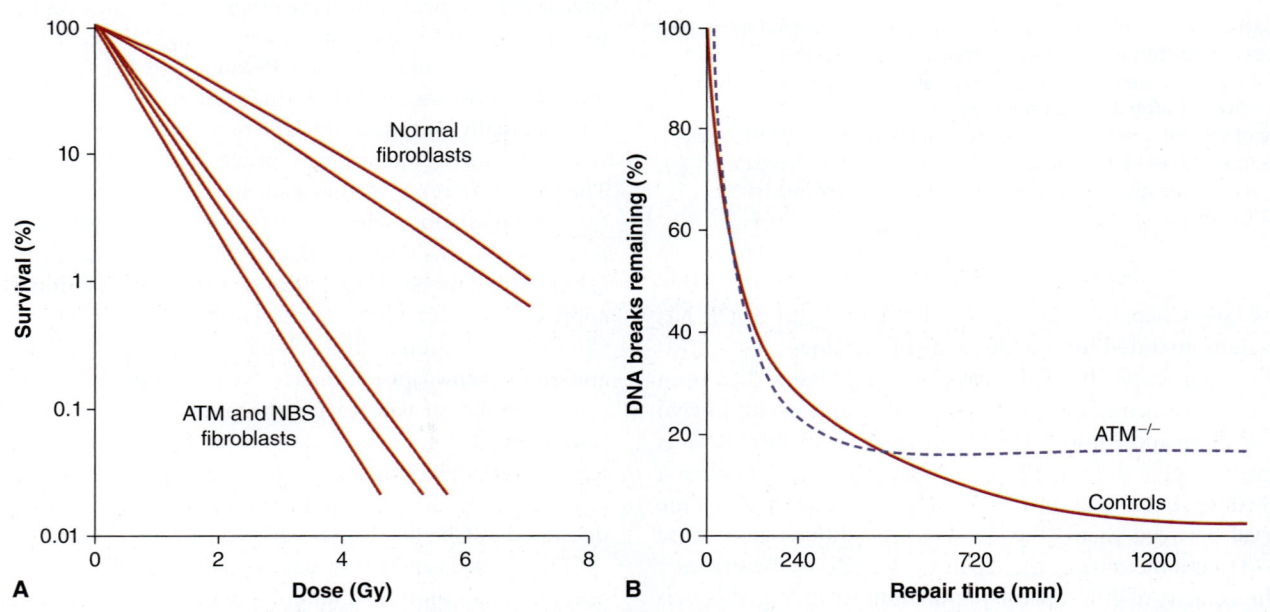

FIGURE 15-12 **The relationship between radiosensitivity and DNA double-strand breaks.** In addition to aberrant cell-cycle checkpoints, increased radiosensitivity and subtle DNA double-strand break repair defects are associated with the ATM and NBS disorders. Shown in **(A)** is the relative radiation survival for normal diploid fibroblasts versus that of ATM or NBS fibroblasts. Shown in **(B)** are the DNA double-strand break rejoining curves (based on pulse-field gel electrophoresis) for AT cells relative to normal cells. The number of DNA double-strand breaks remaining is plotted against time following irradiation. Although the 2 sets of data initially have similar rates of DNA rejoining, the AT cells have increased numbers of residual DNA double-strand breaks relative to controls at later times post-irradiation.

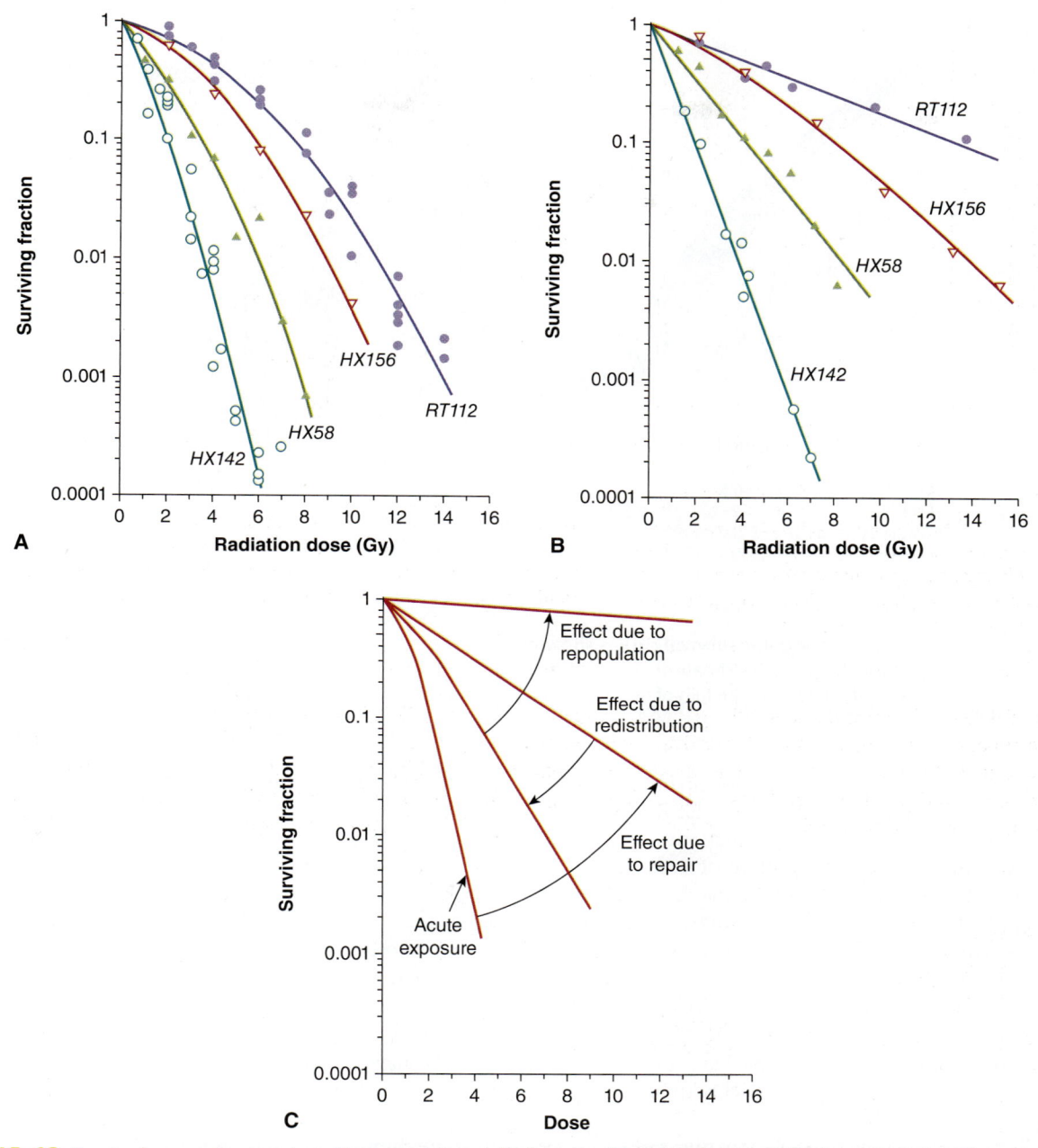

FIGURE 15-13 Survival curves for a series of human cancer cells lines irradiated under acute (high; >1 Gy/min) (A) or continuously (low; ~1 Gy/h) (B) dose rates. C) Schematic to illustrate the influence on the survival curve following continuous low-dose rate irradiation, of the processes of cellular repair, redistribution, and repopulation. (Part A & B Modified with permission from Steel GG. The ESTRO Breur lecture. Cellular sensitivity to low dose-rate irradiation focuses the problem of tumour radioresistance. *Radiother Oncol* 1991 Feb;20(2):71-83.; Part C Data from Dr. JD Chapman, Fox Chase Cancer Center, Philadelphia.)

homologous recombination (HR), which is maximally operational during S- and G_2-phases, and nonhomologous end joining (NHEJ), which is operational throughout the cell cycle (Rothkamm et al, 2003; Valerie and Povirk, 2003), as diagrammed in Figure 15-9C.

DNA repair capacity influences cellular radiosensitivity. Cells from patients with DNA repair deficiency syndromes such as AT and NBS are exquisitely radiosensitive (see Fig. 15-12 and Chap. 9, Sec. 9.5). Radiosensitivity has also been observed among cells from mice in which NHEJ is deficient, for example, as a result of mutations in the DNA-PKcs or Ku70 genes (see Chap. 9, Sec. 9.4.1). Cells deficient in HR-related repair (eg, *BRCA1* or *BRCA2* mutant cells) may also be radiosensitive (Powell and Kachnic, 2003), but not nearly to the extent as cells that are deficient in NHEJ. This can be attributed to the ability of NHEJ to act throughout the cell cycle whereas HR is only active in a portion of the cell cycle.

Broadly, cells fall into 3 categories of sensitivity to ionizing radiation (Fig. 15-14A): Group I includes "normal" cells, Li-Fraumeni cells with p53-mutations, and cells from patients

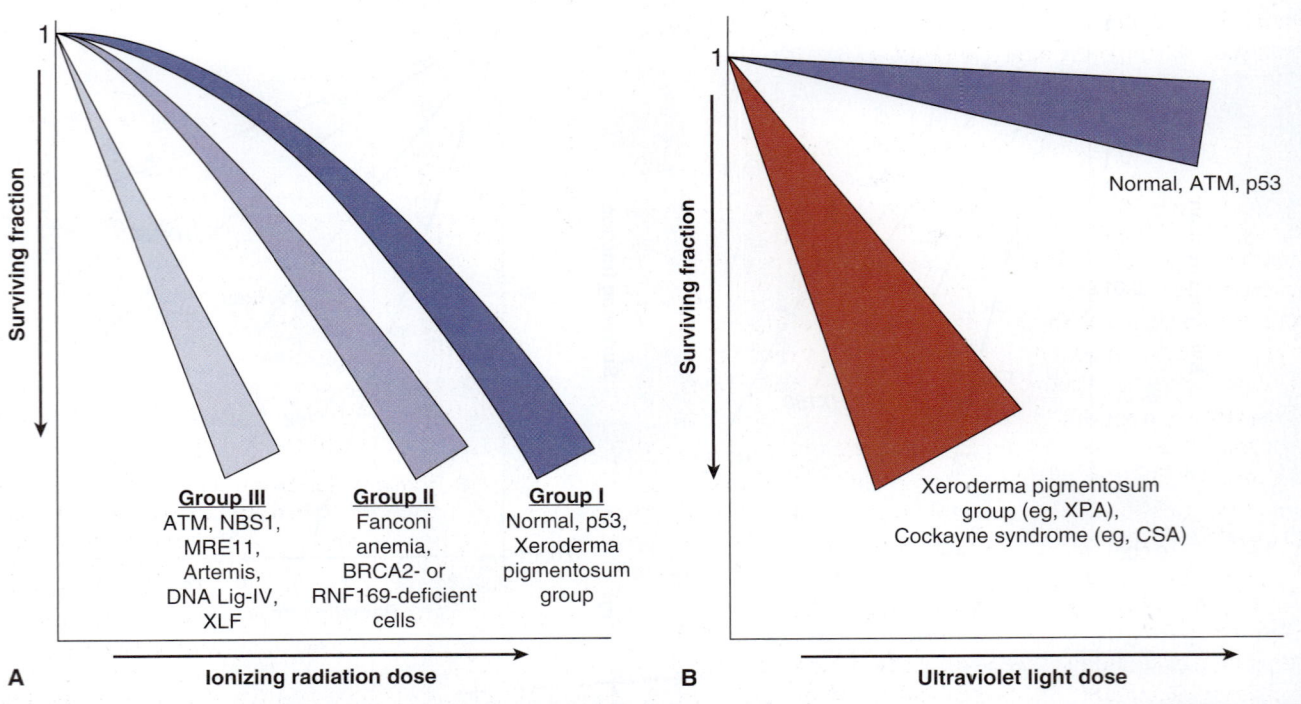

FIGURE 15–14 Schematic of clonogenic survival curves showing differences in survival following ionizing (A) and UV (B) radiation for cells deficient in genes involved in DNA repair or DNA damage signaling. These data are derived from experiments using DNA repair–deficient cells from DNA instability syndromes (details of these syndromes are as discussed in Chap. 9, Secs. 9.3 and 9.5).

with defects in DNA repair pathways not involved in DSB repair, such as nucleotide excision repair (NER). The G_1/S checkpoint may be lost owing to p53-mutations, but this has little effect on the radiosensitivity of most cells. Group II includes cells that have defects in HR proteins, such as RNF168 (see Chap. 9, Sec. 9.3). Group III is the most radiosensitive and includes cells with defects in NHEJ and with mutations in genes from DNA repair disorders such as NBS1, ATM or DNA ligase IV (Girard et al, 2000). These cells are sensitive as a consequence of errors in end-processing and end-joining of DSB, defects in chromatin modifications that prevent efficient rejoining of DSBs, and inefficient G_2/M-checkpoint (Beucher et al, 2009) (see Chap. 9, Sec. 9.5).

Most cells that show sensitivity to ionizing radiation are not sensitive to UV radiation. Cells derived from people with Cockayne syndrome or xeroderma pigmentosum patients with NER defects are exquisitely sensitive to UV irradiation (Fig. 15–14B). This is consistent with the different types of damage caused by ionizing versus UV radiation and the different DNA repair pathways that are used (eg, DNA DSBs and single-strand breaks, repaired by HR and NHEJ vs cyclobutane pyrimidine dimers [CPDs] and 6-4PPs repaired by NER, respectively). It also highlights the repair of DSBs as the primary determinant of survival following ionizing radiation.

Greater understanding of the relationship between deficient DNA repair and radiosensitivity may lead to strategies designed to radiosensitize tumor cells. For example, genetic/epigenetic-mediated targeting or small molecule inhibitors that decrease the activity of DNA-PKcs or ATM would result in defective DSB repair and increased radiation cell killing (Thoms and Bristow, 2010). Inhibiting the repair of DNA base damage and single-strand DNA breaks with inhibitors of poly (ADP-ribose) polymerase (PARP; see Chap. 19, Sec. 19.6.2) can also lead to radiosensitization (Chalmers et al, 2010), but the degree of radiosensitization and DSB repair differs in vitro and in vivo because of the effects of the microenvironment, which may lead to differential DSB induction and altered expression and function of DSB repair pathways (Chan et al, 2009; Jamal et al, 2010).

There may be a therapeutic advantage to targeting DNA repair in combination with radiotherapy if cell kill in tumor cells can be increased relative to cell kill in normal tissues. In some tumor cells, DNA repair pathways may be nonfunctional so that the tumor cells are radiosensitized if there are tumor-specific defects in HR or NHEJ. Furthermore, some drugs, such as PARP inhibitors, may be selectively toxic to HR-defective tumor cells based on synthetic lethality (see Chap. 19, Sec. 19.6.2), which could be used to decrease the number of target tumor cells prior to or during radiotherapy.

DNA repair capacity of cancer cells may be variable within a given tumor. Cancer stem cells, the subset of cancer cells that are most capable of repopulating a tumor and driving recurrence (see Chap. 13, Sec. 13.3.2), have been reported to be less susceptible to DNA damage and to more readily undergo DNA repair following radiation (Bao et al, 2006; Diehn et al, 2009). Only a subset of tumors may have a clear cellular hierarchy reminiscent of normal tissues with stem cells that display resistance to radiation. Nonetheless, there are ongoing efforts to address this proposed relative radioresistance of cancer stem cells through therapeutic targeting (Park et al, 2018).

15.4.4 Intracellular Signaling Following Ionizing Radiation

Cellular and molecular repair pathways triggered by ionizing radiation set off a cascade of intracellular signaling events that impact cell cycling, proliferation, and survival. The main effects of radiation that are responsible for intracellular signaling are (1) DNA damage and (2) plasma membrane damage.

The DNA damage response, once initiated by ionizing radiation, activates cell cycle checkpoints and multifaceted DNA repair mechanisms as described in Sections 15.4.2 and 15.4.3. Activation of DNA damage response proteins also leads to large shifts in gene expression and downstream signaling, causing alterations in cellular processes such as metabolism and secretion.

Plasma membrane damage can produce signaling cascades within irradiated cells. High doses of radiation can initiate a sphingomyelin/ceramide-dependent signaling pathway within the plasma membrane, which can induce apoptosis in the absence of DNA damage (Ruiter et al, 1999; Kolesnick and Fuks, 2003). Sphingomyelin/ceramide-mediated apoptosis may be particularly important in endothelial, lymphoid, and hematopoietic cells and may have a greater impact on radiation-induced toxicity than on solid tumor response to radiation (Moding et al, 2015).

Multiple intracellular signaling pathways have been proposed as therapeutic targets to potentiate radiation-induced cell death. These include the receptor tyrosine kinase pathways such as those downstream of epidermal growth factor receptor (EGFR) and the phosphatidylinositol-3 kinase (PI3K)-AKT/mTOR pathway (Bristow et al, 2018). These pathways can enhance DNA repair capacity, and also stimulate proliferation which diminishes efficacy of clinical radiotherapy schedules (see Chap. 16, Sec. 16.3). Although studies have demonstrated possible radiosensitizing effects using preclinical tumor models, more work is needed to evaluate their benefits in a clinical setting (see Chap. 16, Sec. 16.2.5).

15.4.5 Intercellular Responses to Ionizing Radiation

Irradiated cells can influence the behavior and survival of neighboring cells and tissues. The concept of a *bystander effect* has been illustrated by the transfer of media from irradiated cells to an unirradiated cell population, which can lead to cell death in the nonirradiated cells. Similarly, targeting 10% to 30% of a cell population with high LET irradiation using a focused microbeam can lead to cell death in the nontargeted surrounding cells within the culture dish (Fig. 15–15). *Abscopal effects* may also occur, in which there is shrinkage of nontargeted metastatic tumor sites following treatment of a localized tumor. The mechanisms underlying these effects

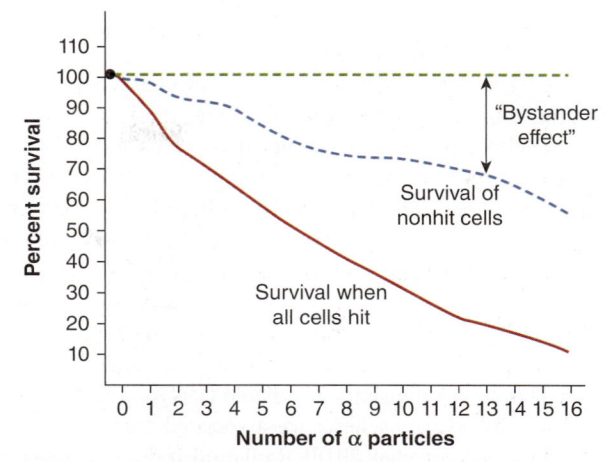

FIGURE 15–15 The radiation bystander effect. Direct single-cell irradiation of V79 cells with α particles can be accomplished using a specialized targeting microbeam in which the irradiation and fate of single cells can be tracked postirradiation. It was observed that cells that were not targeted by the α particles can also be killed (ie, they do not form colonies). This *radiation bystander effect* may be secondary to factors released by irradiated cells into the surrounding media. In the plot shown, direct cell kill increases with increasing α-particle dose following single-cell irradiation. However, the death of nonirradiated cells also increases as a function of dose. The difference between an expected survival of 100% for nonirradiated cells and the actual survival observed, reflects the extent of cell kill by the bystander effect.

and their importance for radiation effects in vivo are still being elucidated and may have important implications for the efficacy and risks/toxicity of radiotherapy (Rodriguez-Ruiz et al, 2018; Yahyapour et al, 2018). The mechanisms of intercellular responses to ionizing radiation can be grouped according to 3 attributes: (1) the types of intercellular signaling molecules/pathways; (2) the types of neighboring cells/tissues; and (3) the timing of the effect. These mechanisms are discussed below.

Irradiated cells can produce a wide range of molecules with the potential to exert effects on neighboring cells and tissues (Sokolov and Neumann, 2018; Yahyapour et al, 2018). DNA has emerged as a critical messenger that is released following ionizing radiation. As a result of DNA damage, DNA fragments can enter the cytoplasm or extracellular space, often contained within small nuclear remnants (ie, micronuclei) or extracellular vesicles (exosomes). This DNA can influence many cell types to produce bystander and abscopal effects. For example, proinflammatory responses in neighboring cancer cells can occur as a result of pattern recognition receptor (PRR) binding, for instance to toll-like receptor 9 (TLR9) (Yahyapour et al, 2018). PRR binding by DNA can also drive a proinflammatory response in a cell autonomous fashion; nuclear DNA that escapes into the cytoplasm or micronuclei can activate the PRR, cGAS, resulting in inflammatory signaling via activation of STING and expression of interferons (Harding et al, 2017; Mackenzie et al, 2017). Signaling effects can also be triggered within antigen-presenting cells in the tumor microenvironment upon uptake of extracellular DNA released by irradiated cells (Deng et al, 2014; Woo et al, 2014), which could contribute to an antitumor immune response.

Intercellular responses to ionizing radiation can be observed over variable amounts of time. Transfer of effectors from irradiated cells to neighboring cells and tissues may start almost immediately after irradiation. For instance, reactive oxygen and nitrogen species, which are produced immediately in cells exposed to ionizing radiation can be transferred to neighboring cells. In contrast, intercellular responses that depend on DNA damage and/or cell death can be delayed. For example, mitotic catastrophe, which produces DNA chromosomal breaks and micronuclei leading to cGAS/STING activation, is often the result of multiple cycles of flawed cell divisions. Irradiated cells may also undergo senescence and adopt a senescence-associated secretory phenotype (SASP) (Nguyen et al, 2018). Radiation-induced senescence has been observed in irradiated fibroblasts, endothelial cells, epithelial cells, and immune cells. Once established, SASP can contribute to longstanding changes in immune cell recruitment and can affect angiogenesis, fibroblast function, and extracellular matrix remodeling over months-to-years. These effects are mediated by numerous endocrine/paracrine signaling molecules released by senescent cells, including IL-1, TNF-α, and TGF-β (Nguyen et al, 2018). Compared with the direct effects of ionizing radiation on cancer cells, indirect effects on intercellular signaling and phenotypes are poorly understood. Future studies that seek to elucidate these effects and their underlying mechanisms may allow for greater exploitation of the efficacy and toxicities of radiotherapy in patients.

SUMMARY

- Ionizing radiation causes damage to cells and tissues by depositing energy as a series of discrete events.
- Different types of radiation have different abilities to cause biologic damage because of the different densities of the energy deposition events produced.
- The RBE of densely ionizing (high-LET) radiation is greater than that of low-LET radiation. Radiation can cause damage to any molecule in a cell, but for most cells, damage to DNA is most crucial in causing cell lethality expressed by loss of proliferative potential.
- Certain cell types can undergo radiation-induced apoptosis as a result of plasma membrane damage and sphingomyelin/ceramide-dependent signaling.
- Depending on cell type, cells may die by a permanent (terminal) growth arrest, undergo interphase death or lysis during radiation-induced apoptosis, or undergo up to 4 abortive mitotic cycles before mitotic catastrophe.
- Several assays have been developed for assessing the clonogenic capacity of both normal and malignant cells, and these have been used to obtain radiation survival curves for a wide range of cell types.
- For x- and γ-rays, survival curves for most mammalian cells have a shoulder region at low doses, whereas at higher doses, the survival decreases approximately exponentially with dose.
- Following treatment with low-LET radiation, cells can repair some of their damage over a period of a few hours; thus, if the treatment is prolonged or fractionated, it is less effective than if given as a single acute dose.
- Cells in S phase are often more resistant than cells in the G_2/M phases, but there is variability between cell types.
- The accurate and timely rejoining of DNA DSBs are correlated to the relative radiation survival of both normal and tumor cells. Defects in the DNA repair pathways in tumor cells may be useful in targeting repair-defective cancer cells using synthetic lethality or molecular-targeting treatment strategies.
- Cell-cycle checkpoints in cells are activated following irradiation (to allow time for DNA repair) and the molecular events relating to cell-cycle arrest involve ATM, p53, and CYCLIN-CDK complexes that are associated with cell-cycle regulation.
- Molecular-targeted drugs that interfere with cell-cycle checkpoints or modify intracellular signaling following DNA damage may increase radiosensitivity.
- Irradiated cells can influence the survival and behavior of neighboring cells and tissues. Targeting these indirect effects of radiation may impact the efficacy and toxicity of radiotherapy.

REFERENCES

Abazeed ME, Adams DJ, Hurov KE, et al. Integrative radiogenomic profiling of squamous cell lung cancer. *Cancer Res* 2013;73(20):6289-6298.

Aldridge DR, Radford IR. Explaining differences in sensitivity to killing by ionizing radiation between human lymphoid cell lines. *Cancer Res* 1998;58(13):2817-2824.

Bao S, Wu Q, McLendon RE, et al. Glioma stem cells promote radioresistance by preferential activation of the DNA damage response. *Nature* 2006;444(7120):756-760.

Beucher A, Birraux J, Tchouandong L, et al. ATM and Artemis promote homologous recombination of radiation-induced DNA double-strand breaks in G2. *EMBO J* 2009;28(21):3413-3427.

Bristow RG, Alexander B, Baumann M, et al. Combining precision radiotherapy with molecular targeting and immunomodulatory agents: a guideline by the American Society for Radiation Oncology. *Lancet Oncol* 2018;19(5):e240-e251.

Bristow RG, Hardy PA, Hill RP. Comparison between in vitro radiosensitivity and in vivo radioresponse of murine tumor cell lines. I: parameters of in vitro radiosensitivity and endogenous cellular glutathione levels. *Int J Radiat Oncol Biol Phys* 1990;18(1):133-145.

Brown JM, Wouters BG. Apoptosis, p53, and tumor cell sensitivity to anticancer agents. *Cancer Res* 1999;59(7):1391-1399.

Chalmers AJ, Lakshman M, Chan N, Bristow RG. Poly(ADP-ribose) polymerase inhibition as a model for synthetic lethality in developing radiation oncology targets. *Semin Radiat Oncol* 2010;20(4):274-281.

Chan N, Koch CJ, Bristow RG. Tumor hypoxia as a modifier of DNA strand break and cross-link repair. *Curr Mol Med* 2009;9(4):401-410.

Corre I, Guillonneau M, Paris F. Membrane signaling induced by high doses of ionizing radiation in the endothelial compartment. Relevance in radiation toxicity. *Int J Mol Sci* 2013;14(11):22678-22696.

Deng L, Liang H, Xu M, et al. STING-dependent cytosolic DNA sensing promotes radiation-induced type I interferon-dependent antitumor immunity in immunogenic tumors. *Immunity* 2014;41(5):843-852.

Diehn M, Cho RW, Lobo NA, et al. Association of reactive oxygen species levels and radioresistance in cancer stem cells. *Nature* 2009;458(7239):780-783.

Dillon MT, Good JS, Harrington KJ. Selective targeting of the G2/M cell cycle checkpoint to improve the therapeutic index of radiotherapy. *Clin Oncol (R Coll Radiol)* 2014;26(5):257-265.

Elkind MM, Sutton H. Radiation response of mammalian cells grown in culture. 1. Repair of X-ray damage in surviving Chinese hamster cells. *Radiat Res* 1960;13:556-593.

Foray N, Badie C, Alsbeih G, Fertil B, Malaise EP. A new model describing the curves for repair of both DNA double-strand breaks and chromosome damage. *Radiat Res* 1996;146(1):53-60.

Girard PM, Foray N, Stumm M, et al. Radiosensitivity in Nijmegen Breakage Syndrome cells is attributable to a repair defect and not cell cycle checkpoint defects. *Cancer Res* 2000;60(17):4881-4888.

Hall EJ. *Radiobiology for the Radiologist*. 5th ed. Philadelphia: Lippencott, Williams & Wilkins; 2000.

Hall EJ, Hei TK. Genomic instability and bystander effects induced by high-LET radiation. *Oncogene* 2003;22(45):7034-7042.

Harding SM, Benci JL, Irianto J, Discher DE, Minn AJ, Greenberg RA. Mitotic progression following DNA damage enables pattern recognition within micronuclei. *Nature* 2017;548(7668):466-470.

Hill RP, Bush RS. A lung-colony assay to determine the radiosensitivity of cells of a solid tumour. *Int J Radiat Biol Relat Stud Phys Chem Med* 1969;15(5):435-444.

Huang L, Snyder AR, Morgan WF. Radiation-induced genomic instability and its implications for radiation carcinogenesis. *Oncogene* 2003;22(37):5848-5854.

Jamal M, Rath BH, Williams ES, Camphausen K, Tofilon PJ. Microenvironmental regulation of glioblastoma radioresponse. *Clin Cancer Res* 2010;16(24):6049-6059.

Jeggo P, Lavin MF. Cellular radiosensitivity: how much better do we understand it? *Int J Radiat Biol* 2009;85(12):1061-1081.

Joiner M, Van der Kogel A. *Basic Clinical Radiobiology*. Boca Raton, FL: CRC Press/Taylor & Francis Group; 2018.

Kao GD, McKenna WG, Yen TJ. Detection of repair activity during the DNA damage-induced G2 delay in human cancer cells. *Oncogene* 2001;20(27):3486-3496.

Kastan MB, Bartek J. Cell-cycle checkpoints and cancer. *Nature* 2004;432(7015):316-323.

Kolesnick R, Fuks Z. Radiation and ceramide-induced apoptosis. *Oncogene* 2003;22(37):5897-5906.

Lomax ME, Folkes LK, O'Neill P. Biological consequences of radiation-induced DNA damage: relevance to radiotherapy. *Clin Oncol (R Coll Radiol)* 2013;25(10):578-585.

Mackenzie KJ, Carroll P, Martin CA, et al. cGAS surveillance of micronuclei links genome instability to innate immunity. *Nature* 2017;548(7668):461-465.

Maeda J, Cartwright IM, Haskins JS, et al. Relative biological effectiveness in canine osteosarcoma cells irradiated with accelerated charged particles. *Oncol Lett* 2016;12(2):1597-1601.

Malaise EP, Deschavanne PJ, Fertil B. The relationship between potentially lethal damage repair and intrinsic radiosensitivity of human cells. *Int J Radiat Biol* 1989;56(5):597-604.

McCulloch EA, Till JE. The sensitivity of cells from normal mouse bone marrow to gamma radiation in vitro and in vivo. *Radiat Res* 1962;16:822-832.

Moding EJ, Castle KD, Perez BA, et al. Tumor cells, but not endothelial cells, mediate eradication of primary sarcomas by stereotactic body radiation therapy. *Sci Transl Med* 2015;7(278):278ra234.

Nagasawa H, Brogan JR, Peng Y, Little JB, Bedford JS. Some unsolved problems and unresolved issues in radiation cytogenetics: a review and new data on roles of homologous recombination and non-homologous end joining. *Mutat Res* 2010;701(1):12-22.

Nagasawa H, Keng P, Harley R, Dahlberg W, Little JB. Relationship between gamma-ray-induced G2/M delay and cellular radiosensitivity. *Int J Radiat Biol* 1994;66(4):373-379.

Nguyen HQ, To NH, Zadigue P, et al. Ionizing radiation-induced cellular senescence promotes tissue fibrosis after radiotherapy. A review. *Crit Rev Oncol Hematol* 2018;129:13-26.

Park SY, Kim JY, Jun Y, Nam JS. Strategies to tackle radiation resistance by penetrating cancer stem cell line of scrimmage. *Recent Pat Anticancer Drug Discov* 2018;13(1):18-39.

Powell SN, Kachnic LA. Roles of BRCA1 and BRCA2 in homologous recombination, DNA replication fidelity and the cellular response to ionizing radiation. *Oncogene* 2003;22(37):5784-5791.

Rodriguez-Ruiz ME, Vanpouille-Box C, Melero I, Formenti SC, Demaria S. Immunological mechanisms responsible for radiation-induced abscopal effect. *Trends Immunol* 2018;39(8):644-655.

Rothkamm K, Kruger I, Thompson LH, Lobrich M. Pathways of DNA double-strand break repair during the mammalian cell cycle. *Mol Cell Biol* 2003;23(16):5706-5715.

Ruiter GA, Zerp SF, Bartelink H, van Blitterswijk WJ, Verheij M. Alkyl-lysophospholipids activate the SAPK/JNK pathway and enhance radiation-induced apoptosis. *Cancer Res* 1999;59(10):2457-2463.

Shiloh, Y. ATM and related protein kinases: safeguarding genome integrity. *Nat Rev Cancer* 2003;3(3):155-168.

Sokolov M, Neumann R. Changes in gene expression as one of the key mechanisms involved in radiation-induced bystander effect. *Biomed Rep* 2018;9(2):99-111.

Steel GG. The ESTRO Breur lecture. Cellular sensitivity to low dose-rate irradiation focuses the problem of tumour radioresistance. *Radiother Oncol* 1991;20(2):71-83.

Terasima T, Tolmach LJ. Changes in x-ray sensitivity of HeLa cells during the division cycle. *Nature* 1961;190:1210-1211.

Thoms, J, Bristow RG. DNA repair targeting and radiotherapy: a focus on the therapeutic ratio. *Semin Radiat Oncol* 2010;20(4):217-222.

Tucker SL, Thames HD, Brown BW, Mason KA, Hunter NR, Withers HR. Direct analyses of in vivo colony survival after single and fractionated doses of radiation. *Int J Radiat Biol* 1991;59(3):777-795.

Valerie K, Povirk LF. Regulation and mechanisms of mammalian double-strand break repair. *Oncogene* 2003;22(37):5792-5812.

Ward JF. The complexity of DNA damage: relevance to biological consequences. *Int J Radiat Biol* 1994;66(5):427-432.

Wilson GD. Radiation and the cell cycle, revisited. *Cancer Metastasis Rev* 2004;23(3-4):209-225.

Withers HR. The dose-survival relationship for irradiation of epithelial cells of mouse skin. *Br J Radiol* 1967;40(471):187-194.

Withers HR, Mason KA. The kinetics of recovery in irradiated colonic mucosa of the mouse. *Cancer* 1974;34(3):suppl:896-903.

Woo SR, Fuertes MB, Corrales L, et al. STING-dependent cytosolic DNA sensing mediates innate immune recognition of immunogenic tumors. *Immunity* 2014;41(5):830-842.

Xu B, Kim ST, Lim DS, Kastan MB. Two molecularly distinct G(2)/M checkpoints are induced by ionizing irradiation. *Mol Cell Biol* 2002;22(4):1049-1059.

Yahyapour R, Motevaseli E, Rezaeyan A, et al. Mechanisms of radiation bystander and non-targeted effects: implications to radiation carcinogenesis and radiotherapy. *Curr Radiopharm* 2018;11(1):34-45.

Zhang Y, Martin SG. Redox proteins and radiotherapy. *Clin Oncol (R Coll Radiol)* 2014;26(5):289-300.

APPENDIX 15.1 MATHEMATICAL MODELS USED TO CHARACTERIZE RADIATION CELL SURVIVAL

Appendix 15.1.1 Target Theory

The target-theory model was based on the hypothesis that a number of critical targets had to be inactivated for cells to be killed. Cell killing by radiation is now recognized to be more complex, but the equation and parameters derived from the model are still used to describe the shape of cell survival curves. The number of targets (dN) inactivated by a small dose of radiation (dD) should be proportional to the initial number of targets N and dD, so that

$$dN \propto N \cdot dD \quad \text{or} \quad dN = \frac{N \cdot dD}{D_0}, \quad \text{[Appendix Eq. 15.1]}$$

where $1/D_0$ is a constant of proportionality because the number of active targets N decreases with increasing dose. Then, a negative sign is introduced because the number of active targets N decreases with increasing dose, and the equation can be integrated to give

$$N = N_0 \cdot e^{-D/D_0}, \quad \text{[Appendix Eq. 15.2]}$$

where N_0 is the number of active targets present at zero dose. If it is assumed that cells contain only a single target that must be inactivated for them to be killed, then the fractional survival (S) of a population of cells is represented by

$$S = \frac{N}{N_0} = e^{-D/D_0} \quad \text{[Appendix Eq. 15.3]}$$

where N_0 and N are the initial and final number of cells surviving a radiation dose D. This also represents the probability that any individual cell will survive the radiation dose D. Appendix Equation 15.3 gives a *single-hit, single-target* survival curve that is a straight line on a semilogarithmic plot originating at a surviving fraction of 1 at zero dose (Appendix Fig. 15–1, *line a*). Survival curves of this shape have been obtained for viruses and bacteria, for radiosensitive normal and malignant cells (ie, cells in the bone marrow or lymphoma cells), and for many types of cells treated with high-LET radiation. The term D_0 represents the dose required to reduce the surviving fraction to 0.37 and is a measure of the slope of *line a* in Appendix Figure 15–1. It can be shown mathematically that the radiation dose required to kill 90% of the initial number of cells, termed the D_{10} value, is equivalent to $2.3 \times D_0$ (where 2.3 is the natural logarithm of 10).

If, instead of one target, it is assumed that a cell contains n identical targets, *each of which* must be inactivated (by a single hit) to cause cell death, then the *multitarget, single-hit* cell survival equation can be represented by

$$S = \frac{N}{N_0} = 1 - (1 - e^{-D/D_0})^n \quad \text{[Appendix Eq. 15.4]}$$

Again, this equation represents the probability that any individual cell will survive a dose D. A plot of this equation leads to a survival curve with a shoulder at low doses and a straight-line section on a semilogarithmic plot, as shown in Appendix Figure 15–1, *line b*. The parameters D_0, n, and D_q can be determined for this curve as shown. At doses that are large compared to D_0 (ie, $D \gg D_0$), Appendix Equation 15.4 reduces to $S = n \exp - (D/D_0)$, which is similar to Appendix Equation 15.3. The straight-line part of the survival curve thus extrapolates to a value n at zero dose and has a slope defined by D_0. As indicated previously, the D_0 value is the dose required to reduce cell survival from S to $0.37S$ in the *straight-line region* of the survival curve. The quasi-threshold dose D_q, is the dose at which the extrapolated straight-line section of the survival curve crosses the dose axis (survival = 1) and quantitatively describes the size of the shoulder. It can be calculated by $D_q = D_0 \ln n$. For this model, the size of the shoulder is regarded as giving an indication of the repair capacity of cells.

One limitation of Appendix Equation 15.4 is that it predicts that a certain amount of damage must be accumulated in a cell before it is killed—that is, at very low doses, the

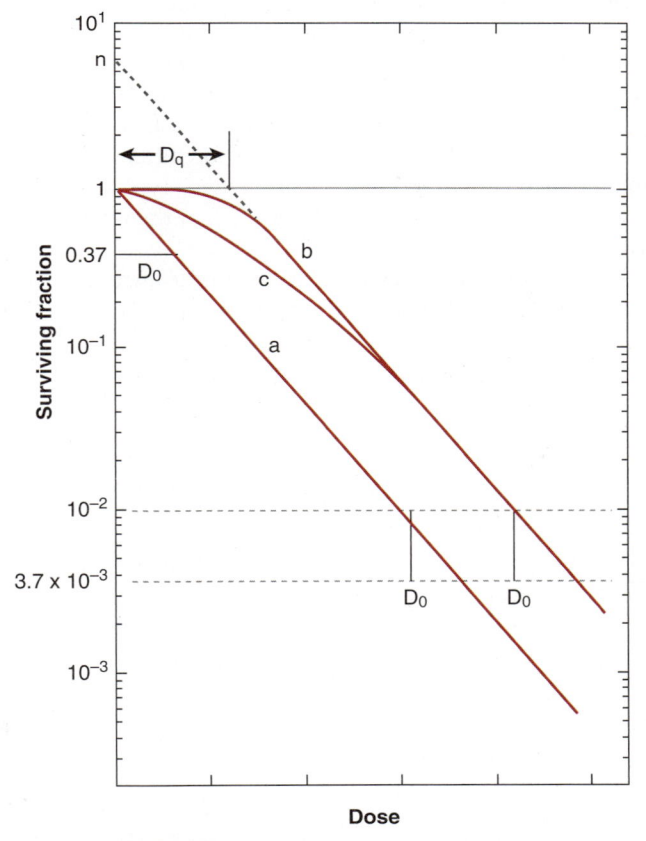

APPENDIX FIGURE 15–1 Survival curves defined by the single-hit and multitarget models of cell killing discussed in the text. Curve a. Single-hit (single-target) survival curve defined by Appendix Equation 15.3. Curve b. Multitarget survival curve defined by Appendix Equation 15.4. Curve c. Composite (2-component) survival curve resulting from both multitarget and single-hit components. Also shown is how the parameters D_0, n, and D_q can be derived from the survival curves.

survival curve should be parallel to the dose axis or have an initial slope of zero. This is contrary to much experimental data, which indicate that, for cell populations irradiated with x- or γ-rays, the survival curve often has a finite initial slope (Appendix Fig. 15–1, *line c*).

Appendix 15.1.2 The Linear-Quadratic Model

The linear-quadratic model is based on the concept that multiple lesions, induced by radiation, interact in the cell to cause cell killing. The assumption that 2 lesions can interact to cause cell killing gives an equation that can fit most experimental survival curves, at least over the first few decades of survival, and is given by

$$S = \frac{N}{N_0} = e^{-(\alpha D + \beta D^2)}$$ **[Appendix Eq. 15.5]**

The linear-quadratic equation defines a survival curve that is concave downward on a semilogarithmic plot and never becomes strictly exponential (see Appendix Fig. 15–2, red line). However, the curvature is usually small at high doses. The α component describes the initial slope of the survival curve at low doses, whereas the β component describes the interaction of lesions that become increasingly probable at higher doses (Appendix Fig. 15–2, blue dashed lines). The values for α and β vary considerably for different types of mammalian cells both in vitro and in vivo. Typical values of α are in the range 1 to 10^{-1} Gy^{-1} and of β in the range 10^{-1} to 10^{-2} Gy^{-2}.

Alternative equations similar to the linear-quadratic equation can be derived by making various biological assumptions,

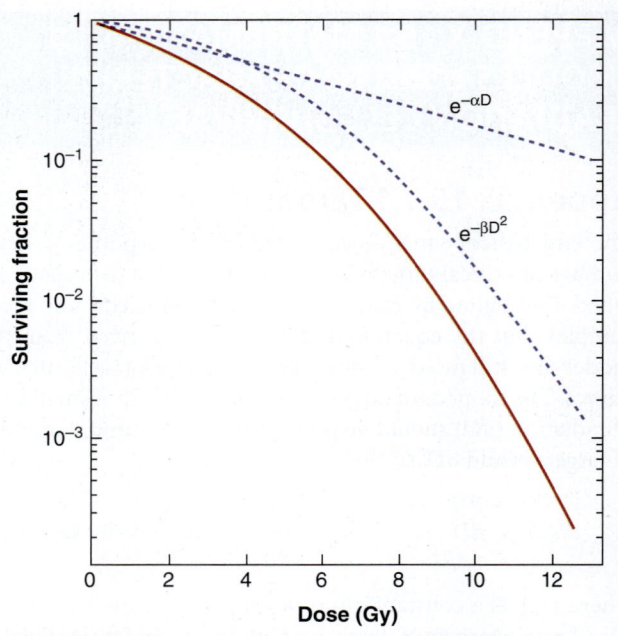

APPENDIX FIGURE 15–2 Survival curve (*red line*) as defined by the linear-quadratic model of cell killing, Appendix Equation 15.5. The curves defined by the 2 components of the equation are shown separately as the blue dashed lines.

for example, concerning the capacity of cells to repair radiation damage and the effect of radiation treatment on that capacity (Foray et al, 1996). It should be stressed that a good fit of a given equation to the survival data does not validate the underlying biological assumptions of the model. However, these modeling approaches can be useful in altering radiotherapy fractionation schedules (discussed in Chap. 16, Sec. 16.7.3).

Tumor and Normal Tissue Response to Radiotherapy

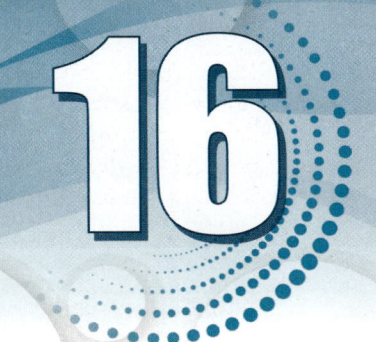

16

Scott V. Bratman and Marianne Koritzinsky

Chapter Outline

16.1 Introduction
16.2 Principles of Clinical Radiotherapy
    16.2.1 Radiotherapy Dose
    16.2.2 External Beam Radiotherapy Planning and Dose Delivery
    16.2.3 Brachytherapy, Radionucleotides, and Radioimmunotherapy
    16.2.4 Particle Therapy
    16.2.5 Combining Radiotherapy With Other Cancer Treatments
16.3 Tumor Control Following Radiotherapy
    16.3.1 Dose Response and Tumor Control Relationships
    16.3.2 Predicting the Response of Tumors
16.4 Hypoxia and Radiation Response
    16.4.1 The Oxygen Effect and Radiosensitivity
    16.4.2 Tumor Hypoxia
    16.4.3 Prognostic Significance of Hypoxia Measured in Tumors
    16.4.4 Targeting Hypoxic Cells in Tumors

16.5 Normal Tissue Response to Radiotherapy
    16.5.1 Cellular and Tissue Responses
    16.5.2 Acute Tissue Responses
    16.5.3 Late Tissue Responses
    16.5.4 Whole-Body Irradiation
    16.5.5 Retreatment Tolerance
    16.5.6 Predicting Normal Tissue Response
    16.5.7 Radioprotection
    16.5.8 Therapeutic Ratio
16.6 Radiotherapy Fractionation
    16.6.1 Repair
    16.6.2 Repopulation
    16.6.3 Redistribution
    16.6.4 Reoxygenation
16.7 Modeling the Effects of Fractionation
    16.7.1 Time and Dose Relationships
    16.7.2 Isoeffect Curves
    16.7.3 The Linear Quadratic Equation and Models for Isoeffect
    16.7.4 Altered Fractionation Schedules
Summary
References

16.1 INTRODUCTION

The purpose of clinical radiotherapy for cancer is to control tumor growth, the likelihood of which depends on the dose of radiation delivered. However, this dose is limited by the damage caused to surrounding normal tissues and the consequent risk of complications. Whether a certain risk of developing complications is regarded as acceptable depends both on the function of the tissue(s) and the severity of the damage involved. This risk must be compared to the probability of benefit (ie, eradicating the tumor) to determine the overall gain from the treatment. This gain can be estimated for an average group of patients, but it may vary for individual patients, depending on the particular characteristics of their tumors and the normal tissues at risk. The balance between the probabilities for tumor control and normal tissue complications gives a measure of the therapeutic ratio of a treatment (see Sec. 16.5.8). The therapeutic ratio can be improved either by increasing the effective radiation dose delivered to the tumor relative to that given to surrounding normal tissues, or by increasing the biologic response of the tumor relative to that of the surrounding normal tissues.

External beam radiation therapy is usually delivered in relatively small daily doses over the course of several weeks. The empiric development of such multifractionated treatments, which involve giving fractions of approximately 1.8 to 3 Gy daily for 5-8 weeks, is an example of exploiting biologic factors to improve the therapeutic ratio. More recently, technical improvements in the physical aspects of radiation therapy have allowed an increase in the effective dose of radiation to deep-seated tumors without increasing the dose to normal

Treatment head for delivering high-energy photons

CT scanner for image guidance during radiotherapy

Conventional RT
Uniform intensity across radiation beam; square or rectangular field

↓

3D-CRT
Uniform intensity across the fields; irregular shapes of field

↓

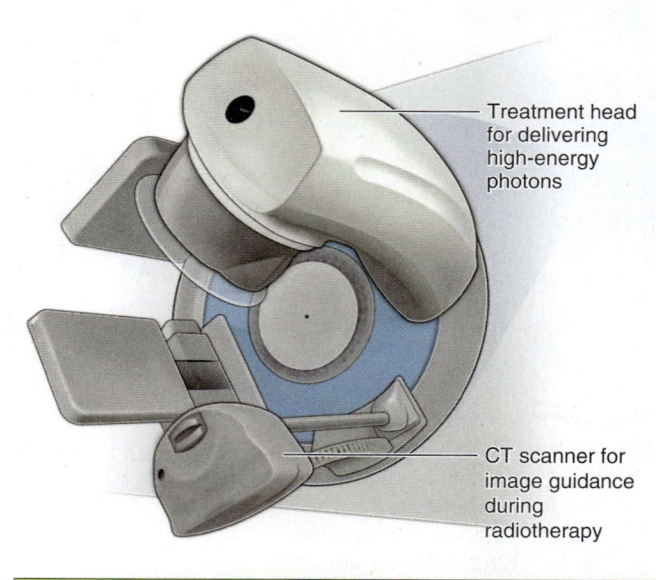

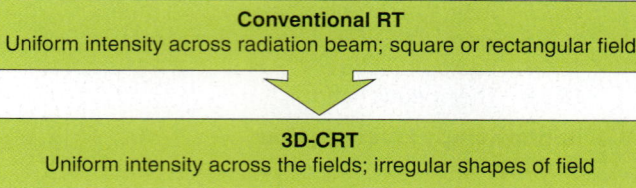

IMRT
Varying intensity of beam; irregular shapes and higher conformity

↓

IGRT
IMRT that changes to follow changes in size, shape, and location of tumor and other organs

FIGURE 16–1 The evolution of modern radiotherapy planning techniques from conventional radiotherapy (RT) to 3-dimensional conformal radiotherapy (3D-CRT), to IMRT, and, finally, to image-guided radiotherapy (IGRT). For many tumor sites, IMRT and IGRT improve the therapeutic ratio by allowing for increased radiotherapy dose to tumor and decreased dose to normal tissues. *IMRT*, intensity-modulated radiation therapy; *IGRT*, image-guided radiation therapy.

tissues. Some of these sophisticated treatment planning methods include *3-dimensional conformal radiotherapy* (3D-CRT), *intensity-modulated radiation therapy* (IMRT), *image-guided radiation therapy* (IGRT), and *stereotactic radiosurgery* (SRS) / *stereotactic body radiation therapy* (SBRT) (Fig. 16–1). These new methods limit the volume of normal tissues irradiated to high doses and allow escalated doses to the tumor. Alternatively, low-dose-rate and high-dose-rate brachytherapy can deliver a highly localized dose by placing radioactive sources directly within or adjacent to tumors (see Fig. 16–2). Although these newer treatment strategies improve the efficiency of radiation therapy delivery, biologic factors may also provide opportunities to improve the therapeutic ratio. Biologic factors

that may influence the outcome of radiation therapy and their exploitation to improve therapy are discussed in this chapter.

16.2 PRINCIPLES OF CLINICAL RADIOTHERAPY

16.2.1 Radiotherapy Dose

As noted above, clinical radiotherapy includes both external-beam radiotherapy and brachytherapy; treatment choice depends on the type of tumor and location within the body. The dose of radiation is determined by the intent of the therapy (ie, curative or palliative), the volume of tumor, the expected relative radiosensitivity of the tumor cells, and the expected toxicity to the surrounding normal tissues. Other factors relate to the condition of the patient, including age and health problems that might increase the side effects of radiotherapy (eg, inflammatory and connective tissue disorders). The acute and chronic side effects that may occur following local radiotherapy are linked to the normal structures and tissues within the irradiated volume (Table 16–1); these effects increase with the volume of the irradiated field and with the size of the dose fractions. For example, head and neck irradiation can lead to altered swallowing or a dry mouth (xerostomia), whereas irradiation of pelvic structures may lead to a change in bladder and bowel function. Total-body radiotherapy, which is sometimes given in addition to chemotherapy during bone marrow transplantation (Wong et al, 2018), can lead to nausea and vomiting, decreased blood counts, and altered humoral and cell-mediated immune responses (see Sec. 16.5.4; Chap. 21, Secs. 21.2 and 21.3).

The intent of curative radiotherapy is to achieve local control of the tumor, thereby preventing local tissue destruction, organ failure, and the seeding of secondary metastases. Most curative radiotherapy regimens have consisted of daily treatments, or fractions, in the range of 1.8 to 3 Gy per day over a period of 5-8 weeks (5 days/wk). More recently, curative radiotherapy regimens have also included SRS/SBRT, in which much larger fraction sizes are employed (≥5 Gy per fraction), with the entire course of treatment delivered in typically 1-5 fractions. There are substantial data to indicate that increased radiotherapy dose is associated with increased local control (Tamponi et al, 2019). Typically, the dose to normal tissues is limited so that severe complications occur in no more than 5% of the surviving patients after a period of 5 years (known as the $TD5/5$ value). However, this dose limit may be increased in order to increase the likelihood of cure, especially if radiotherapy is the only curative treatment option for the patient.

Radiotherapy is also often given in order to palliate symptoms without an expectation of achieving cure. Palliative radiotherapy is given to achieve better pain control, to control bleeding, or to prevent tissue destruction or ulceration. These radiotherapy treatments are usually of short duration and

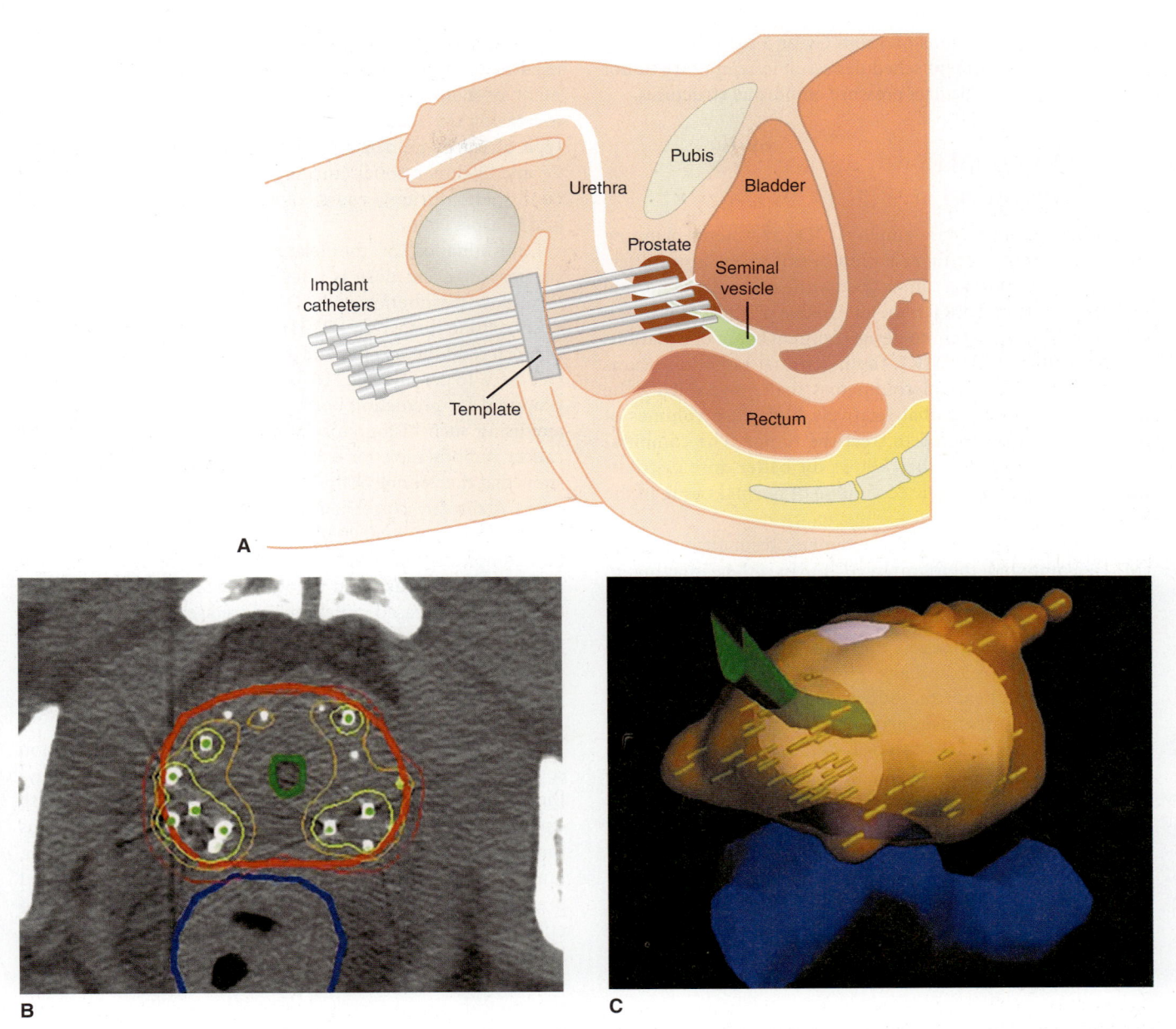

Tumor and Normal Tissue Response to Radiotherapy   371

FIGURE 16–2 Images of a prostate gland treated with high-dose rate radiotherapy using catheters placed into the prostate gland (**A**) through the patient's perineum. **B)** CT image near middle of prostate overlaid with contours delineating prostate (red), urethra (green), and rectum (dark blue). Also shown are isodose lines corresponding to 100% (red), 150% (orange), and 200% (yellow) of the prescribed dose of 145 Gy. **C)** 3D rendering of the 145-Gy isodose surface (translucent orange) covering the prostate.

TABLE 16–1 Severe acute and chronic side effects of radiotherapy.*

Irradiation Site	Tissues at Risk	Acute Effect	Chronic Effect[†]
Brain	Brain; neural structures (eye, brainstem)	Drowsiness, hair loss	Cognitive dysfunction and decreased visual acuity
Head and neck	Oral mucosa, salivary glands, skin	Oral inflammation (mucositis), xerostomia (dry mouth), erythema (skin redness)	Permanent xerostomia, decreased ability to open mouth (trismus), dental caries, skin fibrosis
Thorax	Esophageal mucosa, lung, skin	Esophagitis, pneumonitis	Lung fibrosis, esophageal stricture, skin fibrosis
Abdomen	Intestine, pancreas, liver, spleen, kidneys	Nausea, hepatitis, diarrhea	Renal compromise, liver fibrosis, intestinal obstruction
Pelvis	Bladder, rectum, prostate	Increased frequency and dysuria, diarrhea	Bladder or rectal bleeding or rectal ulceration, impotence

*Acute and chronic (late) effects will be idiosyncratic to the patient, the total dose, the dose fractionation, and the irradiation volume.
[†]Severe chronic effects observed in less than 5% of population at 5 years.

consist of 1 to 4 fractions of 5 to 8 Gy or 5 to 10 fractions of 3 to 4 Gy. Such treatment schedules result in temporary tumor shrinkage that can alleviate pressure on normal structures.

16.2.2 External Beam Radiotherapy Planning and Dose Delivery

Conformal radiotherapy employs 3D treatment planning using a series of specific radiation beams given from different angles to maximize tumor dose while minimizing normal tissue irradiation. IMRT is an alternative method that uses a computerized algorithm to design optimal beam orientations and intensities. With IMRT, the individual radiation beams are shaped using special collimators that move during the time of irradiation, so that relatively high-dose volumes of irradiation are contoured to treat the tumor. The combination of multiple beams then allows for better dose distributions resulting in a decreased volume of normal tissue in the high-dose region.

Both types of planning use magnetic resonance imaging (MRI), computed tomography (CT), or other imaging to localize the tumor and critical normal tissues (see Chap. 14, Sec. 14.3). The photon energy (see Chap. 15, Sec. 15.2) and number of radiation beams and their orientation are then chosen (see Fig. 16.3, and also Fig. 16.4*B*). The typical dose rate for external beam radiotherapy is 1 to 6 Gy/min. Successful delivery is tracked during treatment using verification images. The extent of the tumor is defined as the *gross tumor volume* (GTV) detected by the imaging and physical exam. The surrounding region suspected to harbor cancer cells is defined as the *clinical target volume* (CTV). The final radiation plan is designed to treat a region encompassing the GTV and CTV called the *planning target volume* (PTV). The PTV *adds a margin around the CTV to* account for body or organ movement and daily uncertainties in positioning the patient for treatment. Special techniques and markers are sometimes used to track organ movement within the body (eg, movement of a lung tumor during normal breathing), thereby increasing the accurate targeting of the radiation dose. This type of image-guided radiation therapy (IGRT) uses serial 2- and 3-dimensional imaging to optimize the treatment coordinates during a course of radiation treatment (Dawson and Sharpe, 2006).

Determination of the relationship between normal tissue response and dose is often confounded by the nonuniform dose distribution within the normal organs. However, a dose-volume histogram (DVH) can be generated as part of a modern radiotherapy plan for each exposed organ in a patient (see Sec. 16.2.4 and Fig. 16–4*C*). Several models have been proposed for predicting normal tissue response to radiotherapy using such histograms (Marks et al, 2010b). In prostate cancer radiotherapy, for example, DVH plots can be used to show that the volume of the anterior rectum irradiated to high doses is directly correlated to late complications within the rectum (Bauman et al, 2012; Budaus et al, 2012). One important complexity with IMRT plans is that increased volumes of normal tissue are exposed to lower doses and this raises concerns about increased radiation-induced second malignancies.

16.2.3 Brachytherapy, Radionucleotides, and Radioimmunotherapy

Low-dose-rate (LDR; dose rates of up to ~2 Gy/h) radiation sources placed into or beside the tumor (known as brachytherapy) can be used, either alone or in combination with external beam radiotherapy, to treat accessible tumors such as those of the cervix, prostate, head and neck, breast, bladder, lung, esophagus, and some sarcomas. Close to the implanted brachytherapy source, the radiation dose is high, leading to effective killing of tumor cells, whereas normal cell killing is less at increasing distances from the source as a result of lower doses (and dose rates). Computer-controlled brachytherapy systems can also deliver radiation doses as short high-dose pulses (pulsed-dose brachytherapy) or with a high-dose rate (HDR brachytherapy; rate of dose delivery exceeds 12 Gy/h). HDR brachytherapy uses a relatively intense source of radiation (eg, iridium 192) delivered through temporarily placed applicators. The applicators are first placed into the tumor, and then their positions are precisely detected by CT scan for treatment planning. A computer-generated plan then measures the optimal dwell times of the radiation source along the path of the applicators. Thus, HDR brachytherapy can provide a sculpted dose cloud to conform to the shape of the target (see Fig. 16–2). With HDR brachytherapy, the patient typically receives the total dose in a series of 1 to 10 treatments. Clinical experience has demonstrated that HDR brachytherapy can be safely delivered with similar side effect profiles to other radiotherapy modalities (Morton et al, 2017).

The use of injected radionucleotides to treat cancer is based on the selective uptake by tumors or adjacent normal tissues, so that local irradiation may lead to death of the tumor cells. Examples are ^{131}I to treat well-differentiated thyroid cancer,

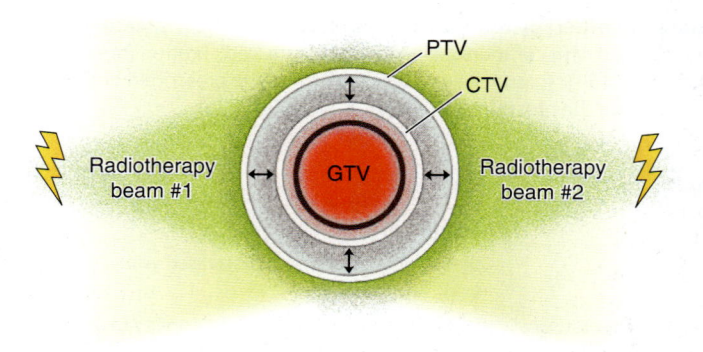

FIGURE 16–3 Schematic representation of target volumes used for modern external beam radiotherapy. The gross tumor volume (GTV) denotes the visible tumor evident on medical imaging and physical examination. A region surrounding the GTV that is suspected to harbor cancer cells is defined as the clinical target volume (CTV). A margin around the CTV is added to create the planning target volume (PTV). The PTV margin accounts for movement and uncertainties in patient positioning and is used to design radiation fields.

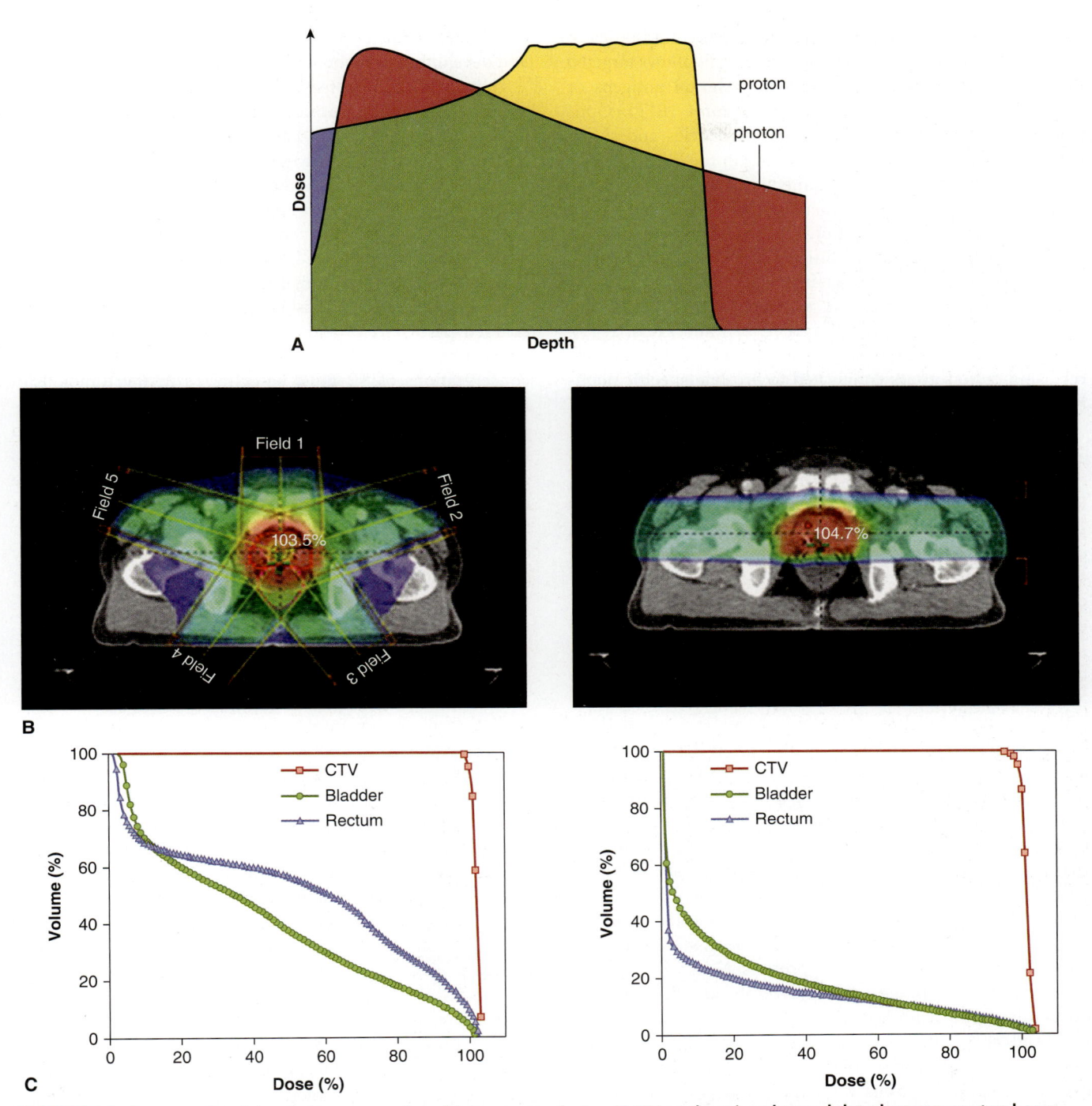

FIGURE 16–4 Generalized depth dose curves for a high-energy photon (6 MV or above) and a modulated-energy proton beam. (**A**) The proton beam delivers its dose at increased depth as compared to a high-energy photon beam. Colors illustrate differences between photon and proton depth dose distribution (red, dose delivered by the photon beam that is greater than that delivered by the proton beam; green, same dose from both photon and proton beams; blue, dose delivered by proton beam but not photon beam; gold, dose delivered to defined target by protons but not by photons). (**B**) Comparison of isodose distributions and **C**) dose volume histograms (DVH) for photons versus protons for a typical prostate cancer radiotherapy plan. The 5-beam photon plan (left) shows increased volumes (y-axis on plot) of bladder and rectum being irradiated for increasing percentage of the total dose delivered (x-axis on plot) when compared to the use of a 2-beam proton plan (right). *CTV*, clinical tumor volume to be treated with the total radiotherapy dose.

radiolabeled somatostatin analogs for the treatment of neuroendocrine tumors, and ^{89}Sr or ^{223}Ra to treat bone metastases, mainly in prostate cancer (Autio et al, 2012; Parker et al, 2013). The latter isotopes are chemically similar to calcium and thus taken up selectively into bone metastases that are undergoing osteoblastic remodeling; once incorporated into the bone lesion, these radioisotopes deposit their energy into neighboring cancer cells, causing cell death.

The conjugation of radioisotopes to specific antibodies or to agents that bind to receptors on cancer cells allows targeted radiotherapy to tumors expressing the relevant antigens or receptors and is termed *radioimmunotherapy* (RIT). Optimal radioisotopes are those emitting a-particles and short-range electrons (ie, β-particles) resulting in the killing of cells within a radius of 1 to 3 cell diameters of the bound isotope (eg, ^{111}Indium). Clinical implementation of RIT has some challenges, including the difficulty of accurate dosimetry and treatment planning. Nonetheless, clinical benefit has been observed for radiolabeled antibodies against CD20 (^{131}I-tositumomab and ^{90}Y-ibritumomab) for the treatment of CD20$^+$ follicular B-cell non-Hodgkin lymphoma (Green and Press, 2017). Ongoing studies are exploring the use of RIT for prostate cancer using radioisotopes conjugated to prostate-specific membrane antigen (PSMA) (Kulkarni et al, 2018).

16.2.4 Particle Therapy

Particle therapy is a form of external-beam radiotherapy using beams of energetic protons, neutrons, or positive (eg, carbon) ions for cancer treatment. The most common type of particle therapy is proton therapy. Particle therapies may contribute to improvements in the therapeutic ratio in several ways. First, such particles have higher linear energy transfer (LET) that leads to an increase in the (radio)biological effectiveness (RBE) of the radiation (see Chap. 15, Sec. 15.3.2) because the damage caused is more difficult for cells to repair. When less of the damage can be repaired, there is reduced variability in response between different cells and also reduced variation in radiosensitivity with position in the cell cycle. Deposition of more irreparable damage also results in less protection for hypoxic (ie, poorly oxygenated) tumor cells (see below). Another advantage of particle therapies is that much of the energy is deposited in tissue at the end of particle tracks (Fig. 16–4A) (ie, in the region of the Bragg peak; see Chap. 15, Sec. 15.2.2). This can be exploited to give improved depth-dose distributions for deep-seated tumors, and is of benefit particularly for protons. Neutron beams do not demonstrate a Bragg peak, and depth-dose distributions are similar to those for low-LET radiation. Carbon ions have the disadvantage that beyond the Bragg peak, the dose does not decrease to zero, because nuclear reactions between the carbon ions and the atoms of the tissue lead to production of lighter ions that have a significant range.

One potential disadvantage of high-LET radiation is that the high repair capacity of some (late-responding) normal tissues (see Secs. 16.7.1 and 16.7.2) cannot be leveraged because of the complex nature of the radiation damage. However, the ability to deliver dose in a finely focused manner using protons or heavy ions reduces the volume of normal tissue exposed to high doses, limiting this concern. Protons may be advantageous for treatment of some tumors, such as choroidal melanomas and skull-base tumors that require precise treatment of a highly localized lesion, and in pediatric tumors where the dose to normal structures needs to be decreased as much as possible to avoid developmental side effects during growth and development (Weber et al, 2018).

There have been extensive clinical studies using high-energy neutrons, but such treatments have been associated with an increase in complications, particularly subcutaneous fibrosis, and randomized trials have not demonstrated therapeutic gain (Fowler, 1988; Raju, 1996); thus, there is limited current use of such therapy. An alternative approach is boron neutron capture therapy (BNCT), in which compounds enriched with ^{10}B are administered prior to irradiation with a lower-energy (thermal) neutron beam. Thermal neutrons interact preferentially with the ^{10}B atoms, and a fission reaction produces high-energy charged particles (^{7}Li and ^{4}He), resulting in cell killing. For an improved therapeutic ratio with BNCT, relatively high concentrations of ^{10}B must be achieved in the tumor, with low concentrations in normal tissues. New boronated compounds and new strategies for delivering them are needed to improve the differential concentrations achievable in tumors and surrounding normal tissues, but encouraging results have been obtained, particularly for the treatment of brain tumors (Yamamoto et al, 2008; Barth et al, 2018). However, the depth-dose distribution for the thermal neutron beam is relatively poor and this remains a serious limitation in the clinical use of this treatment for deep-seated tumors.

16.2.5 Combining Radiotherapy With Other Cancer Treatments

Radiotherapy is commonly used in combination with other cancer treatments, including surgery and drug therapy with hormones, chemotherapy, or molecular targeted agents. Radiotherapy can be given prior to surgery to reduce the tumor volume, or after surgery to sterilize microscopic or residual disease within, and just beyond, the surgical bed. Alternatively, surgery can be used as salvage therapy in patients where the use of radiotherapy alone was not sufficient to control the tumor locally. Concomitant chemotherapy is used for treatment of locally advanced head and neck, brain, bladder, lung, pancreatic, esophageal, and cervical cancers to increase the probability of cure or local control by radiotherapy, and concomitant hormone therapy is used to improve survival of men with locally advanced and high-risk localized prostate cancer. Results from preclinical local tumor control experiments suggest that multiple radiobiologic mechanisms might contribute to an improved therapeutic ratio with this approach, including the prevention of tumor cell repopulation (proliferation during therapy), decreased number of clonogenic tumor cells, increased cellular radiation sensitivity, improved reoxygenation of (previously hypoxic) clonogenic tumor cells during the combined treatment, and modulation of infiltrating immune cells (Zips et al, 2008; Ahn et al, 2010; Begg et al, 2011; Derer et al, 2016). Important interactions between radiation and chemotherapy in tumor and normal tissues are reviewed in Chapter 17, Section 17.6.4.

Increasingly, molecular-targeted agents that can synergize with radiotherapy are being tested in clinical settings.

The first agent to experience widespread clinical implementation was the EGFR inhibitor, cetuximab. When given concomitantly with radiotherapy for head and neck cancer, cetuximab demonstrated improved locoregional control and overall survival compared with radiotherapy alone (Bonner et al, 2010). However, subsequent studies have failed to confirm a benefit for adding cetuximab or other EGFR-targeted agents to the combination of radiotherapy and cisplatin in patients with head and neck or lung cancer (Juergens et al, 2017), and cetuximab was shown to be inferior to cisplatin in combination with radiotherapy for human papillomavirus (HPV)–positive head and neck cancer (Fig. 16–5) (Gillison et al, 2019; Mehanna et al, 2019). The use of an EGFR inhibitor was thought to combat tumor cell repopulation during radiotherapy as the basis for the improved therapeutic ratio for this combination (Zips et al, 2008). Other agents that improve cellular radiosensitivity by targeting DNA repair pathways are undergoing active study in preclinical and clinical settings (Chap. 15, Sec. 15.4) (Bristow and Hill, 2008). Agents that target tumor hypoxia in combination with radiotherapy are described below in Section 16.4.4.

Immunotherapy has recently become an important component of cancer therapeutics (see Chap. 21). There are 2 principal ways in which immunotherapy agents are being combined with radiotherapy. First, in the curative setting in which high-dose radiotherapy is used as a definitive treatment, immunotherapy agents are being explored as neoadjuvant or adjuvant treatments to improve the likelihood of cure. For example, delivery of the PD-L1 targeted antibody, durvalumab, following chemoradiotherapy for stage III non–small cell lung cancer resulted in improved outcomes (Antonia et al, 2017). Second, in the metastatic and palliative setting, radiotherapy is being explored as an "in situ tumor vaccine" that could improve responses to immunotherapy by modulating the local tumor microenvironment to enhance immune mechanisms and/or by triggering abscopal effects that could act against tumors not in the radiation field (Rodriguez-Ruiz et al, 2018). Possible molecular mechanisms of abscopal effects associated with radiotherapy are addressed in Chapter 15, Section 15.4.5.

16.3 TUMOR CONTROL FOLLOWING RADIOTHERAPY

16.3.1 Dose Response and Tumor Control Relationships

The emphasis in Chapter 15 on the molecular and cellular effects of radiation treatment reflects a view that the response of tumors can be understood largely in terms of the sensitivity of the cancer cells within those tumors. However, there is increasing evidence that the extracellular environment in tumors can play a substantial role in their response to treatment (Hanahan and Weinberg, 2011). For radiation, hypoxia is known to play an important role in tumor response (see Sec. 16.4.2; Chap. 12, Sec. 12.4). Likewise, an intact immune system is important for response to radiotherapy (Schaue, 2017). Consequently, experimental techniques that assess tumor response in situ rather than measuring the survival of tumor cells after removing and dissociating the tumor are important (Fig. 16–6). The size of untreated and irradiated tumors can be measured as a function of time to allow the generation of growth curves (Fig. 16–6A). The delay in growth is the difference in time for treated and untreated tumors to grow to a defined size. At higher radiation doses, some tumors will be permanently controlled. If groups of animals receive different radiation doses to their tumors, the percentage of controlled tumors can be plotted as a function of dose to give a curve as shown in Figure 16–6B.

The concept that tumors contain a fraction of cells that have unlimited proliferative capacity (ie, cancer stem cells [CSCs]) was introduced in Chapter 13. As discussed in that chapter, there are uncertainties about the properties of such cells and about the plasticity of the CSC phenotype during or following treatment (Vlashi and Pajonk, 2015), but because cells expressing a CSC phenotype are the ones that can regenerate the tumor after treatment, their radiosensitivity is critical to achieving tumor control. For a simple model, which assumes that the response of a tumor to radiation depends on the individual responses of the cells within it, the dose of radiation required to control a tumor would only depend on (1) the radiation sensitivity of the CSCs and (2) their number. From a knowledge of the sensitivity of the CSCs in a tumor, it would be possible to predict the expected level of survival following a given single radiation dose. A simple calculation, using Appendix 15.1, Equation 15.4 (see Chap. 15), and typical survival curve parameters for well-oxygenated cells (D_0 = 1.3 Gy, D_q = 2.1 Gy), indicates that a single radiation dose of 26 Gy might be expected to reduce the probability of survival of an individual cell to approximately 10^{-8}. For a tumor containing 10^8 CSCs, this dose would thus leave, on average, 1 surviving CSC. Because of the random nature of radiation damage, there will be statistical fluctuation around this value. The statistical fluctuation expected from random cell killing by radiation follows a Poisson distribution; the probability (P_n) of a tumor having n surviving CSCs when the average number of CSCs surviving is a is given by

$$P_n = \frac{(a^n e^{-a})}{n!} \quad \text{[Eq. 16.1]}$$

For tumor control, the important parameter is P_0, which is the probability that a tumor will contain no surviving CSCs (ie, n = 0). From Equation 16.1,

$$P_0 = e^{-a} \quad \text{[Eq. 16.2]}$$

For a = 1, as in the example above, the probability of control would be e^{-1} = 0.37. Different radiation doses will, of course, result in different values of a, and it is possible to construct a theoretical curve relating the probability of tumor control with dose, which shows a sigmoid relationship (Fig. 16–7, solid lines).

The central red curve in Figure 16–7 represents a group of identical tumors each containing 10^8 CSCs. For tumors

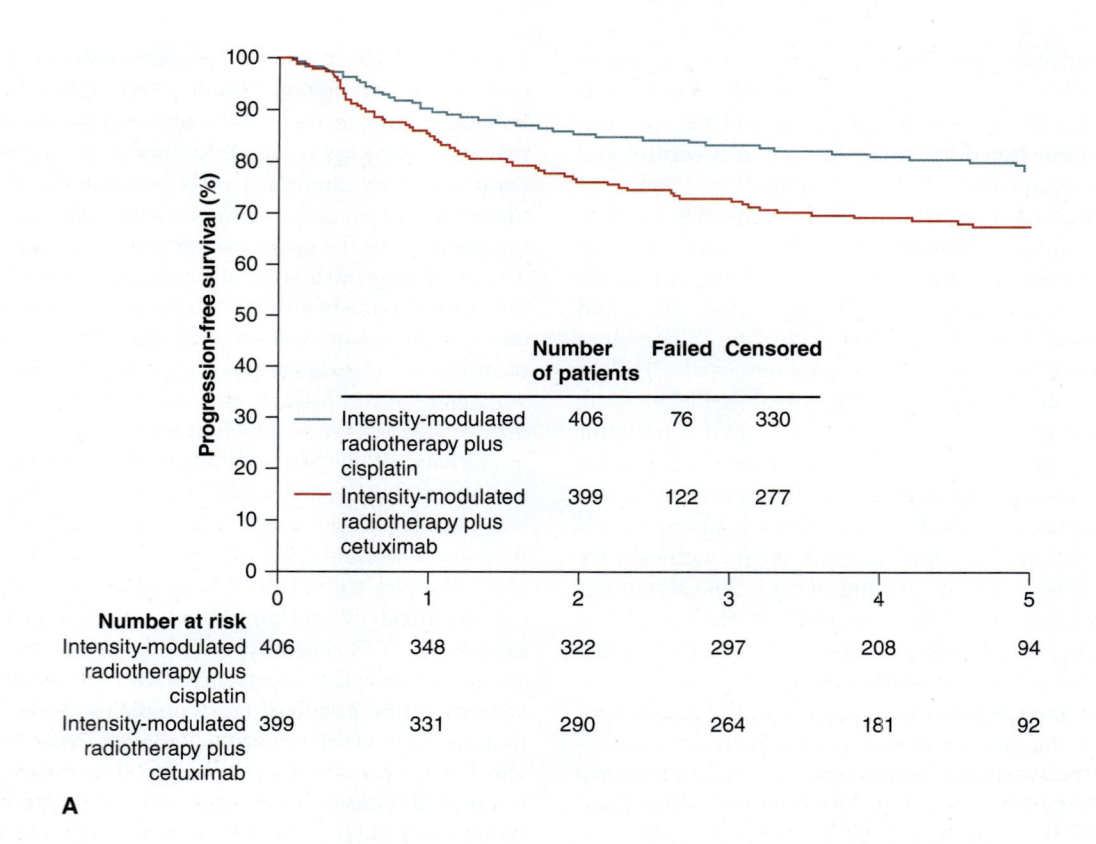

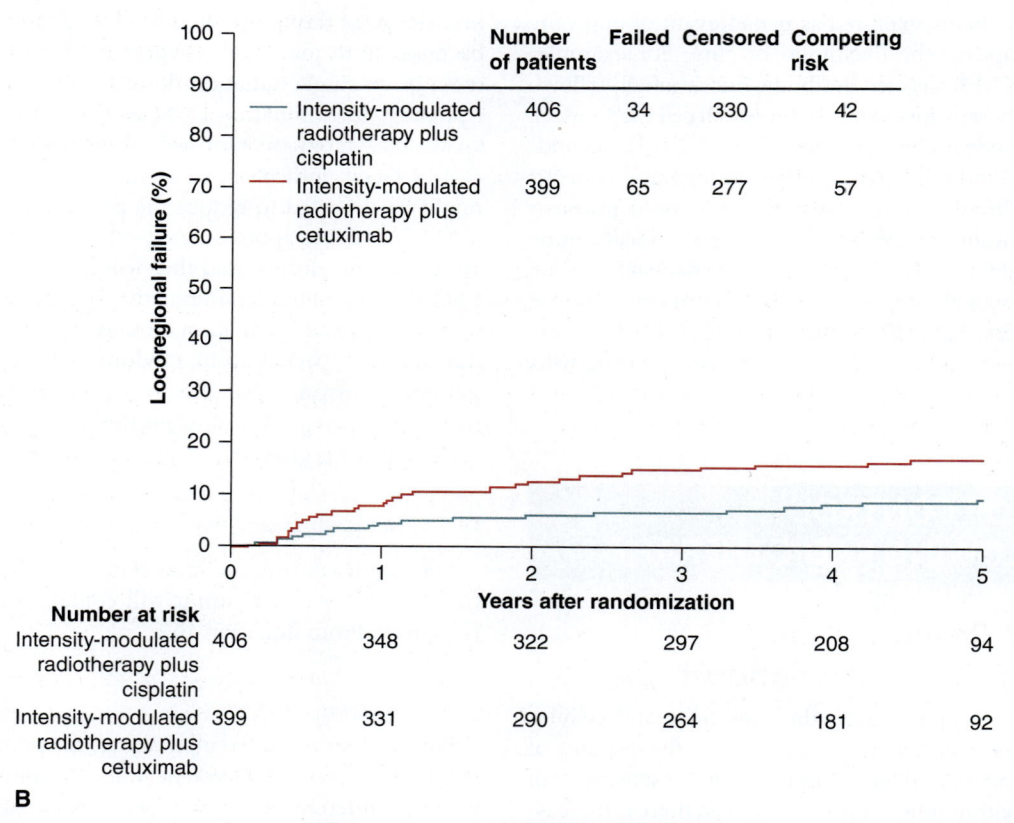

FIGURE 16–5 Kaplan-Meier estimates of (A) progression-free survival and (B) locoregional control among all patients randomly assigned to radiotherapy plus cisplatin or radiotherapy plus cetuximab. (Reproduced with permission from Gillison ML, Trotti AM, Harris J, et al. Radiotherapy plus cetuximab or cisplatin in human papillomavirus-positive oropharyngeal cancer (NRG Oncology RTOG 1016): a randomised, multicentre, non-inferiority trial. *Lancet* 2019 Jan 5;393(10166):40-50.)

The above discussion also assumes that the CSCs exhibit a uniform radiosensitivity within a tumor. Some studies have suggested the possibility that CSCs may be more resistant to radiation than other (progenitor) cell populations in a tumor (Krause et al, 2011). Also, the microenvironment of the CSCs in the tumor can affect their sensitivity to radiation, and there may also be differences as a result of genetic or epigenetic heterogeneity among the tumor cells. The role of hypoxia is well documented (see Sec. 16.4.2), but there may also be interactions of the cells with the extracellular matrix (ECM) and/or interactions with growth factors, such as transforming growth factor β1 (TGF-β1), which may influence cellular sensitivity and tumor response (Bouquet et al, 2011). Interactions between the tumor cells and the ECM can also influence cellular signaling, such as the EGFR/MEK/ERK (extracellular signal regulated kinase) or phosphatidylinositol-3 kinase (PI3K)/AKT pathways (see Chap. 7, Sec. 7.5) that can affect cellular sensitivity to radiation (see Chap. 15, Sec. 15.4.4). Knowledge of the role that such factors may play in tumor response to radiation is limited, but there is evidence that cell contact and expression of certain integrins can affect the radiation sensitivity of cells (Eke and Cordes, 2011). Also, vascular damage and radiation-induced apoptosis of endothelial cells in tumors may play a role in response to radiation treatment (Garcia-Barros et al, 2010) through (opposing) effects of death of tumor cells from nutrient deprivation or increase in hypoxia and radioresistance of surviving tumor cells. Bone marrow–derived myeloid populations of cells, particularly monocytes/macrophages, may also enhance repair of the vasculature in tumors, and/or induce immunity mechanisms, thereby increasing their resistance to irradiation (Kioi et al, 2010; Zaleska et al, 2011).

16.3.2 Predicting the Response of Tumors

Even tumors of the same size and histopathologic type are likely to vary in their proportion of CSCs. Thus, a dose-control curve for a group of human tumors will be a composite of the simple ones shown in Figure 16–7; the slope of the composite dose-control curve will be less than that for the individual simple curves (see Fig. 16–7, dashed line). Fractionation of the radiation treatment (see Sec. 16.6) and heterogeneity in the radiosensitivity of CSCs (either intrinsic or as a result of their microenvironment) will also result in a decrease in the slope of the dose-control curve. Thus, the slope of the dose-control curve derived from a clinical study is likely to be quite shallow. It is therefore desirable to seek a way of assigning the tumors to more homogeneous groups, so that patients with differences in prognosis can be identified. This is a major motivation for attempts to develop predictive assays. In vitro studies of a wide range of cell lines derived from human tumors have shown intrinsic variations in radiation sensitivity. Survival curves can vary considerably even for cells of similar histopathologic types, particularly in the width of the shoulder region (Fig. 16–8). Even small differences in the shoulder region can be important because they are magnified during the multiple fractionated daily doses of 1.8 to 2 Gy given in clinical radiotherapy.

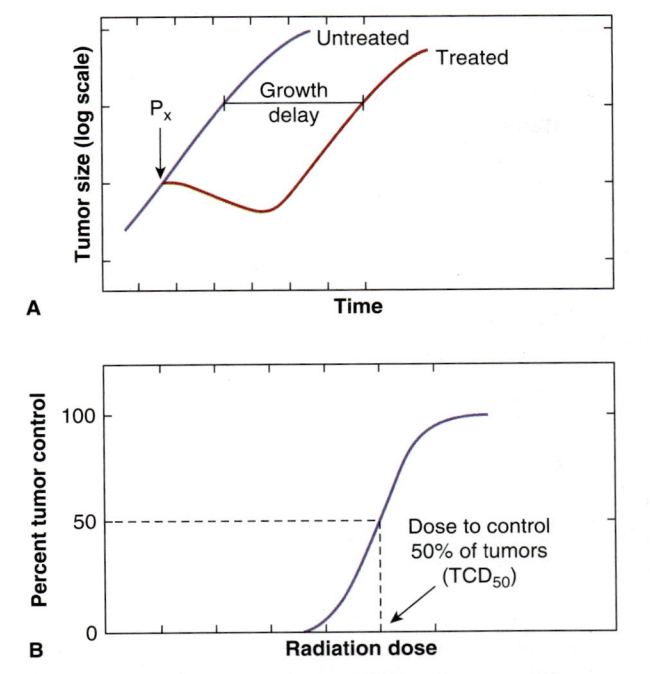

FIGURE 16–6 Illustration of 2 assays for tumor response. In (**A**), growth curves for groups of treated and untreated tumors are shown and the measurement of growth delay indicated. At large doses, some of the tumors may not regrow and the percentage of controlled tumors can be plotted as a function of dose as in (**B**).

containing 10^7 or 10^9 CSCs, the curves will be displaced (to smaller [blue] or larger [green] doses, respectively) by a dose sufficient to reduce survival by a factor of 10. These dose-control curves illustrate the concept that the dose of radiation required to control a tumor depends on the number of CSCs that it contains, although as noted above, the uncertainties about the identification of such cells and the plasticity of their phenotype may make it difficult to determine the effective number of cells with CSC potential in an individual tumor.

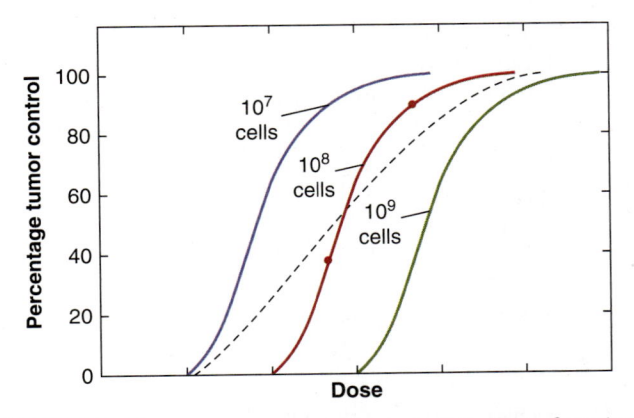

FIGURE 16–7 Percentage tumor control plotted as a function of dose for single-radiation treatments. Theoretical curves for groups of tumors containing different numbers of tumor stem cells are shown. The points on the red curve labeled "10^8 cells" are derived as discussed in the text. The composite curve (dashed) was obtained for a group containing equal proportions from the 3 individual groups.

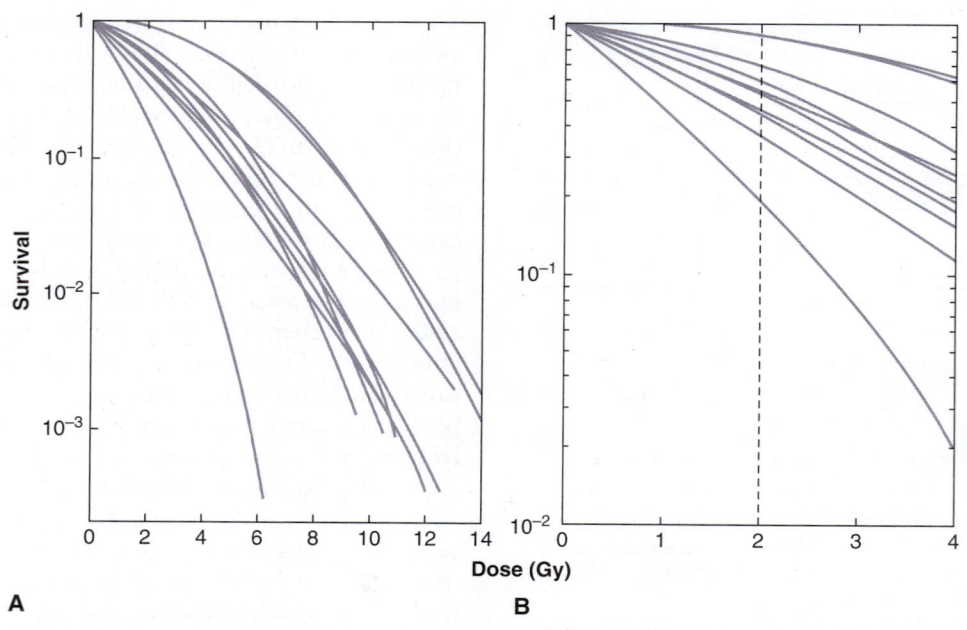

FIGURE 16-8 **A) Survival curves for a number of different human melanoma cell lines.** The lines were drawn to be continuously curving and conform to the linear-quadratic model (see Chap. 15, Appendix 15.1). **B)** The low-dose region of the curves is illustrated, demonstrating the range of cell survival values at 2 Gy.

Estimates of the surviving fraction following a dose of 2 Gy for different human tumor cell lines growing in culture may be grouped according to histopathologic type and compared with the likelihood that such tumors will be controlled by radiation treatment (Table 16–2). There is a trend toward higher levels of survival at 2 Gy for the cells from tumor groups that have been found less radiocurable.

TABLE 16–2 Values of the surviving fraction (cell survival) at 2 Gy for human tumor cell lines.

Tumor Cell Type*	Number of Lines	Mean Survival at 2 Gy (Range)

1. Lymphoma
   Neuroblastoma
   Myeloma
   Small-cell lung cancer
   Medulloblastoma
	14	0.20 (0.08-0.37)

2. Breast cancer
   Squamous-cell cancer
   Pancreatic cancer
   Colorectal cancer
   Non-small-cell lung cancer
	12	0.43 (0.14-0.75)

3. Melanoma
   Osteosarcoma
   Glioblastoma
   Hypernephroma
	25	0.52 (0.20-0.86)

*Tumor types are grouped (1 to 3) approximately in decreasing order of their likelihood of local control by radiation treatment.

The concept that tumor response for an individual patient can be predicted has been tested using the survival following 2 Gy (SF2) for cells from primary human cervix tumor biopsies grown in soft agar. West et al (1997) found that patients with tumors containing radioresistant cells (SF2 > median) had significantly worse local control and survival than those with tumors containing more radiosensitive cells (SF2 < median; Fig. 16–9) and similar results were reported for head and neck cancers (Bjork-Eriksson et al, 2000). However, other groups have had difficulty confirming the generality of these findings. Furthermore, the widespread application of such assays has been limited by technical problems; for example, the soft agar assay requires 5-6 weeks before scoring, and measurements could not be obtained in 25% to 30% of tumors. Other potential limitations of such assays are as follows: (1) they do not account for microenvironmental factors influencing radiosensitivity; (2) tumors may contain clonogenic (CSC) subpopulations of different intrinsic radiosensitivity; (3) the assay relies on colony formation in agarose to identify CSCs, and some of them may not proliferate in this artificial environment; and (4) if other (progenitor) tumor cells can also form small colonies, the assay may not be measuring the radiosensitivity of the CSCs alone.

Genetic profiling is being investigated as an approach to prediction of treatment response and identification of possible therapeutic targets to enhance response (Tan et al, 2017; Bristow et al, 2018). Mutations associated with DNA repair (such as ataxia-telangiectasis mutated [ATM]) can affect radiation sensitivity, and as discussed in Chapter 9, Section 9.5, inhibitors of DNA repair in combination with radiotherapy might be used to take advantage of inherent defects in DNA

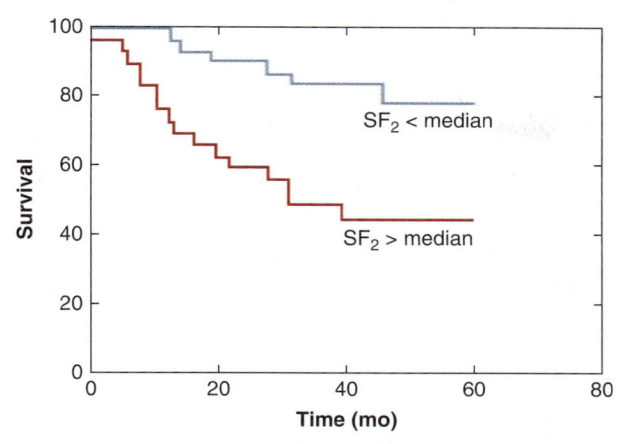

FIGURE 16-9 Actuarial survival in patients with cervical cancer treated by radical radiotherapy as a function of intrinsic radiosensitivity of tumors stratified as above (red line) or below (blue line) the median survival following 2 Gy (SF2) of 0.41. Overall survival and local control (not shown) are significantly worse for patients with SF2 >0.41. (Reproduced with permission from Levine EL, Renehan A, Gossiel R, et al. Apoptosis, intrinsic radiosensitivity and prediction of radiotherapy response in cervical carcinoma. *Radiother Oncol* 1995 Oct;37(1):1-9.)

repair in tumor cells. This field is evolving rapidly with powerful techniques for profiling tumor genetic material now making their way into the clinic.

16.4 HYPOXIA AND RADIATION RESPONSE

16.4.1 The Oxygen Effect and Radiosensitivity

The biologic effects of radiation on cells are enhanced by oxygen. The primary mechanism (called the *oxygen fixation hypothesis*) is believed to be that oxygen can interact with (secondary) radicals on cellular molecules such as DNA, formed by their interaction with the (primary) hydroxyl radicals produced by radiation effects on water in the cell (Fig. 16–10A). These interactions result in damage to DNA that is permanent or "fixed" and must be repaired by the cell enzymatically. For this effect, oxygen must be present in the cells at the time of or within a few milliseconds of the radiation exposure (because of the short lifetime of the radicals). At low levels of oxygen, free sulfhydryls in the cells can effectively compete with oxygen to interact with the radicals and can cause an immediate chemical restitution. Cells irradiated under conditions of severe acute hypoxia require about 3 times more dose to achieve the same probability of cell kill as cells irradiated in air (Fig. 16–10B). The sensitizing effect of different concentrations of oxygen is shown in Figure 16–10C. At very low levels of oxygen, the cells are resistant but, as the level of oxygen increases, their sensitivity rises rapidly to almost maximal levels at oxygen concentrations above approximately 35 µmol/L (equivalent oxygen partial pressure ~25 mm of mercury [mm Hg]). The oxygen concentration at which the sensitizing effect is one-half of maximum (the Km value) varies among cell lines (probably as a result of free sulfhydryl levels in the cells) but is usually in the region 5 to 15 µmol/L (4-12 mm Hg equivalent partial pressure).

The degree of sensitization afforded by oxygen is characterized by the oxygen enhancement ratio (OER), which is defined (see Fig. 16–10B) as the ratio of doses required to give the same biologic effect in the absence or the presence of oxygen. For doses of x- or γ-radiation greater than approximately 3 Gy, the OER for a wide range of cell lines in vitro, and for most tissues in vivo, is in the range of 2.5 to 3.3. For x- or γ-ray doses less than approximately 3 Gy (ie, in the shoulder region of the survival curve), the OER is reduced in a dose-dependent manner. A reduction of the OER at low doses is clinically important because the individual treatments of a fractionated course of treatment are usually 2 Gy or less. The OER is also dependent on the type of radiation, declining to a value of 1 (ie, no enhancement by oxygen) for radiation with LET values greater than approximately 200 kiloelectron volts per micrometer (keV/µm) (see Fig. 16–10D). This is because high LET radiation is dominated by direct action, which results in more complex damage that cannot be chemically restituted. The competition between sulfhydryls and oxygen therefore becomes irrelevant.

16.4.2 Tumor Hypoxia

The oxygen effect is relevant for the treatment of cancer with radiotherapy because cancer cells in human tumors often experience low oxygen levels (hypoxia; see also Chap 12, Sec. 12.4). The oxygen level (pO_2) in most normal tissues ranges between approximately 20 and 80 mm Hg, whereas tumors often contain regions where the pO_2 is less than 5 mm Hg. These conditions in solid tumors are primarily caused by the abnormal vasculature that develops during tumor angiogenesis (see Chap. 11, Sec. 11.5). The blood vessels in solid tumors have highly irregular architecture and are more widely separated than in normal tissues. Tumor cells consume the oxygen delivered, resulting in a gradual decline in oxygen tension as a function of distance from the vessel. The diffusion distance of oxygen in tissue depends on the oxygen consumption rate, and is typically in the order of 150 µm (Fig. 16–11; see also Chap. 12, Fig. 12–14). Tumor cells beyond this distance from vessels experience severe chronic hypoxia and are radiation resistant. Although the cells would eventually die from chronic lack of oxygen, they may survive for days in such harsh environments (Ljungkvist et al, 2005).

Tumor cells may also be exposed to shorter (often fluctuating) periods (minutes to a few hours) of acute hypoxia as a result of intermittent flow in individual blood vessels (see Fig. 16–11). If such an episode of poor perfusion occurred simultaneously with a radiation fraction, cells surrounding that vessel would be radiation resistant. Tumor hypoxia has been observed in a majority of tumors both human and

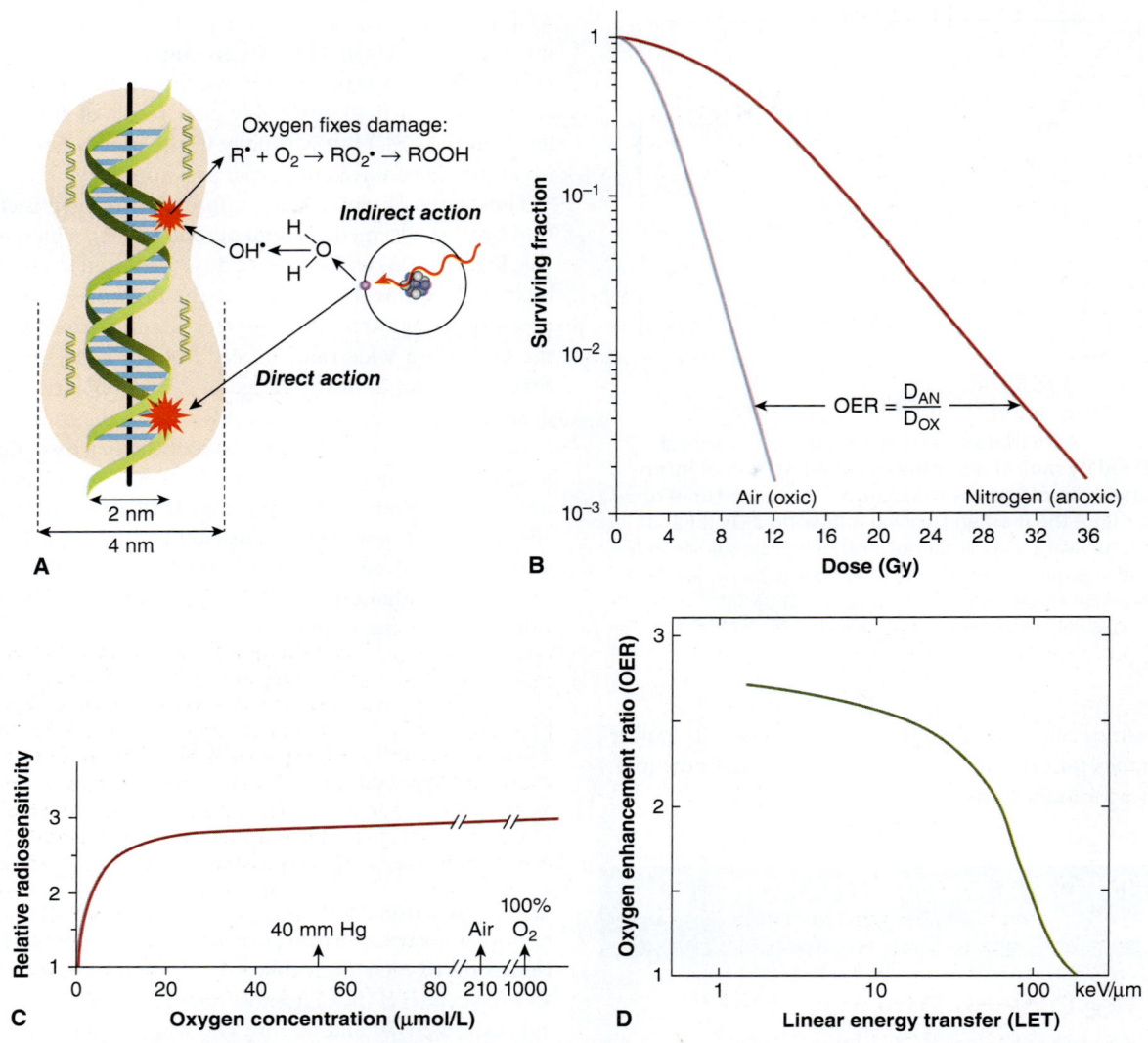

FIGURE 16–10 Effect of oxygen as a radiosensitizer. **A)** Illustration of oxygen interacting with damage to DNA caused by hydroxyl (OH) radicals created by the effects of radiation on water molecules. **B)** Survival curves obtained when cells are treated with low-LET radiation in the presence (air) or absence (nitrogen) of oxygen. The OER is calculated as indicated (D_{OX} = dose in air, D_{AN} = dose in nitrogen) and as described in the text. **C)** The relative radiosensitivity of cells is plotted as a function of oxygen concentration in the surrounding medium to illustrate the dependence of the sensitizing effect on oxygen concentration. **D)** Illustration of the dependence of the OER on the LET of the radiation. (Part (A) Modified with permission from Hall EJ: Radiobiology from the Radiologist, 3rd ed. Philadelphia, PA: Lippincott; 1998.)

experimental (see Sec. 16.4.3 and Chap. 12, Sec. 12.4), but has been found to be very heterogeneous both within and among tumors, even those of similar histopathologic type, and it does not correlate simply with standard prognostic factors such as tumor size, stage, and grade (Vaupel et al, 2001). Acute and chronic hypoxia can coexist in the same tumor and hypoxic regions in tumors are often diffusely distributed throughout the tumor (see Fig. 16–11) and are rarely concentrated only around a central core of necrosis.

Evidence that cells in the hypoxic regions of tumors growing in experimental animals are viable and capable of regrowing the tumor is provided by analysis of cell survival curves generated by irradiating the tumor in situ and then plating the cells in vitro. For most tumors, the terminal slope of such curves is characteristic of that for hypoxic cells (Fig. 16–12). The proportion of viable hypoxic cells in tumors can be estimated (Fig. 16–12) from the ratio (S_{Air}/S_{Anox}) of the cell survival obtained for tumors in air-breathing animals irradiated with a large dose to the cell survival obtained for tumors irradiated with the same dose under anoxic conditions (eg, tumor blood supply clamped). As discussed below, substantial levels of hypoxia in human tumors have been shown to be a poor prognostic indicator. However, cells exposed to acute versus chronic hypoxia in the tumor may exhibit different degrees of resistance. Cells exposed to longer periods of severe (chronic) hypoxia can accumulate in the G1 phase of the cell cycle and reduce expression of DNA repair proteins (see Chap. 12, Sec. 12.4), both effects contributing to making the cells more

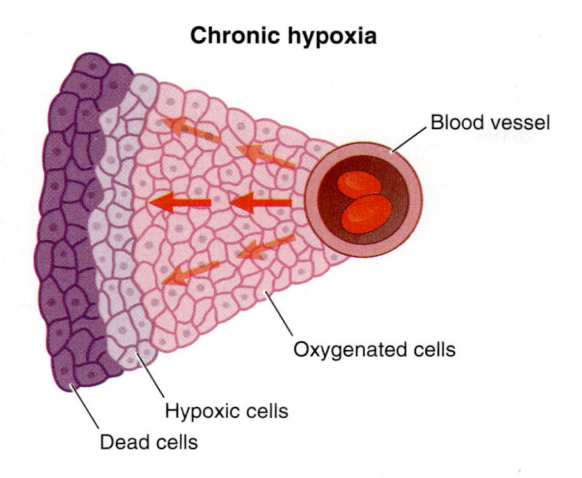

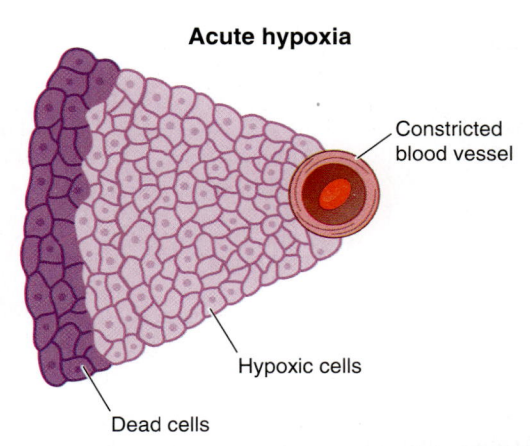

FIGURE 16-11 Schematic of 2 models for the development of hypoxia in tumors. Hypoxia may arise as a result of short term constriction or fluctuating blood flow (as illustrated in the lower diagram (acute hypoxia) or as a result of diffusion limitations in the tumor cord model (outward diffusion from vessels) as illustrated in the upper diagram (chronic hypoxia).

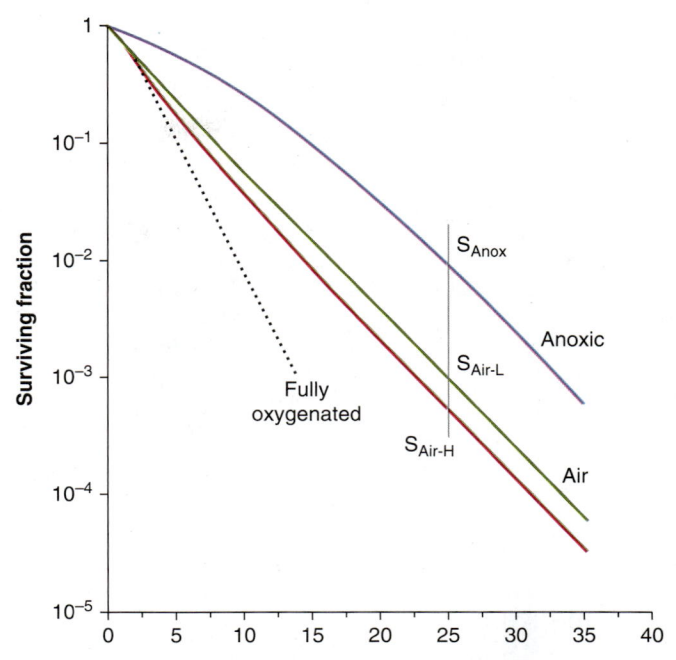

FIGURE 16-12 The influence of a subpopulation of hypoxic cells on the survival curve obtained for an irradiated tumor. The 4 curves shown are for a well-oxygenated population of cells (dotted line), 2 curves derived from tumors irradiated under air-breathing conditions, and a curve for tumors irradiated under anoxic conditions (blue line). The 2 curves for irradiation under air-breathing conditions are for tumors in animals with high (H-red line) or low (L-green line) hemoglobin levels. The hypoxic fraction can be estimated by taking the ratio of the survival obtained under air-breathing conditions (S_{Air}) to that obtained under anoxic conditions (S_{Anox}) at a dose level where the survival curves are parallel, as illustrated. For the tumors in animals with a high hemoglobin level, this value is approximately 0.06 (6%), and for the tumors in animals with low hemoglobin, it is approximately 0.12 (12%).

radiosensitive. The chronically hypoxic tumor cell populations are in consequence slightly less radioresistant than the acutely hypoxic cell populations. In addition to being radiation resistant, hypoxic tumor cells may be protected from the effects of cycle-active chemotherapy because of slow proliferation as well as poor drug delivery (see Chap 18, Sec 18.4.7). Hypoxia also stimulates adaptation through numerous molecular signaling mechanisms that stimulate the metastatic ability of the cancer cells (see Chap. 10, Sec. 10.2.4). Hypoxia may therefore play an important role in treatment outcome for many tumor types through several mechanisms (Bristow and Hill, 2008; Marie-Egyptienne et al, 2013).

16.4.3 Prognostic Significance of Hypoxia Measured in Tumors

Techniques used to determine oxygenation status in individual tumors are reviewed in Chapter 12 (Sec. 12.4.1 and Table 12-3). Wide pO_2 variations exist within and between tumors (Fig. 16–13A, B). Since the mid-1990s, a large body of literature has accumulated supporting the negative prognostic value of tumor hypoxia in many disease sites. For instance, among prostate cancer, cervix cancer, and head and neck cancer patients treated with radiotherapy, those with hypoxic tumors have a worse prognosis (see Fig. 16–13C, D) (Toustrup et al, 2011; Milosevic et al, 2012; Hill et al, 2015). Hypoxic cervix tumors treated by surgery also had a worse prognosis (Hockel et al, 1996), consistent with the fact that hypoxic tumors also tend to be more aggressive and have increased metastasis (Lunt et al, 2009).

More recently, data have emerged to suggest that the prognostic value of hypoxia is highly dependent on tumor etiology. For example, both HPV positive and negative head and neck cancers can be hypoxic, but hypoxia is only a prognostic factor in patients carrying HPV-negative tumors (Toustrup et al, 2011). Likewise, hypoxia is only a negative prognostic factor in prostate cancer if the tumor has a high level of genome instability (Lalonde et al, 2014). The exact reasons for these

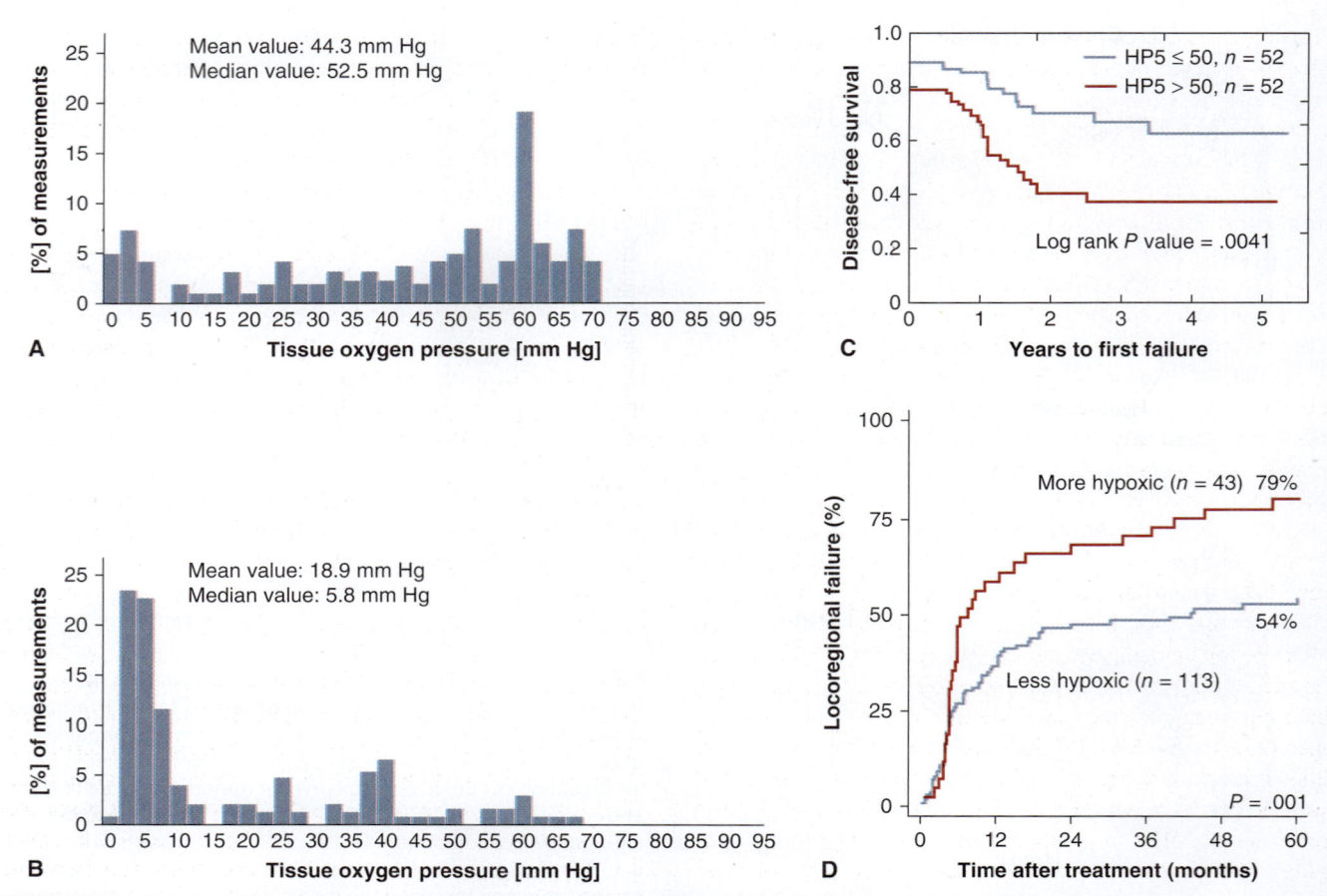

FIGURE 16-13 Distribution of tumor pO$_2$ in 2 human cervix carcinomas as measured by the Eppendorf oxygen electrode and treatment outcome for patients with high/low levels of hypoxia in their tumors. **A, B)** Each distribution represents 160 individual measurement points in the tumor. Tumor in (**A**) is less hypoxic and shows fewer regions with low pO$_2$ measurements than tumor in (**B**). Panel (**C**) shows results for cancer of the cervix treated with radiotherapy and demonstrates that patients with tumors with a higher degree of hypoxia (HP5 > 50%) have poorer disease-free survival. HP5 is the percentage of pO$_2$ measurements in the tumor that were below 5 mm Hg. Panel (**D**) shows the cumulative incidence of locoregional tumor failure in head and neck cancer patients treated with conventional radiotherapy alone and separated into "more" and "less" hypoxic tumors by a 15-gene hypoxia signature. (Panel (B) Used with permission from Fyles, unpublished.; Panel (D) Reproduced with permission from Toustrup K, Sørensen BS, Nordsmark M, et al. Development of a hypoxia gene expression classifier with predictive impact for hypoxic modification of radiotherapy in head and neck cancer. *Cancer Res* 2011 Sep 1;71(17):5923-5931.)

differences remain unknown, but the observations may be of importance for patient selection to receive interventions targeting hypoxia.

16.4.4 Targeting Hypoxic Cells in Tumors

Because hypoxic cells represent a radiation-resistant subpopulation in tumors that is not present in most normal tissues, the therapeutic ratio might be improved by techniques to reduce the influence of hypoxic cells on tumor response. Various approaches have been investigated over the last 50 years, including (1) attempts to increase oxygen delivery to tumors; (2) use of drugs to modify oxygen consumption of the tumor cells to increase oxygen diffusion distances in the tumor; (3) use of drugs that mimic the radiosensitizing properties of oxygen; (4) use of drugs that are specifically toxic to hypoxic cells; (5) use of high-LET radiations that have a reduced OER (see Sec. 16.4.1 and Fig. 16-10D); and (6) use of drugs that exploit the reduced DNA repair capacity of chronically hypoxic cells. Some of these approaches are discussed in this section.

16.4.4.1 Increasing Oxygen Delivery Clinical studies demonstrate the negative effect of anemia on prognosis (Fu et al, 2000; Fyles et al, 2000; Hoff et al, 2011), and blood transfusions have been used to maintain patients at normal hemoglobin levels during radiotherapy. A small randomized study in patients with carcinoma of the cervix showed improvement of local control with blood transfusions (Bush, 1986) but this was not observed in head and neck cancers (Hoff et al, 2011). Transfusions are therefore not employed currently as a general strategy to improve radiation response. The administration of erythropoietin has also been used to correct anemia (Seidenfeld et al, 2001), but there is little evidence that it can improve local control or disease-free survival following radiotherapy (Henke et al, 2003). Furthermore, there have been concerns about the use of erythropoietin-stimulating agents in the context of cancer because it can cause thrombosis, and malignant cells may express erythropoietin receptors leading to stimulation of growth and inferior patient outcomes (Debeljak et al, 2014). Experimental studies suggest that carbon monoxide in cigarette smoke, which can reduce the oxygen-carrying and unloading capacity of the blood, may result in reduced tumor oxygenation. Patients with head and neck cancer who continue to smoke during radiotherapy have decreased local control and survival after radiation treatment (Hoff et al, 2012), although effects in women with cervix cancer were not significant (Fyles et al, 2002).

Oxygen delivery to tumor cells may be increased by giving animals or patients oxygen under hyperbaric conditions (200-300 kPa) during radiation treatment and early clinical studies with high-pressure oxygen (HPO) as an adjuvant to radiation therapy did demonstrate significant improvement in local tumor control and survival for patients with cancers of the head and neck and cervix, but this has not been observed in the limited studies of tumors at other sites (Overgaard and Horsman, 1996). The technical difficulties of giving modern radiation treatments with the patient in an HPO chamber have led to this technique being abandoned in favor of other strategies. One such strategy is the use of a combination of nicotinamide, which has been shown to increase tumor perfusion, and carbogen (95% O_2 and 5% CO_2) breathing. Randomized trials have demonstrated improved regional control in laryngeal cancer and improved overall survival in bladder cancer (Hoskin et al, 2010; Janssens et al, 2012). In laryngeal cancer, benefit from nicotinamide in combination with carbogen breathing can be predicted from intrinsic markers of hypoxia or low hemoglobin levels (Rademakers et al, 2013; Janssens et al, 2014). Although these trials were promising, the strategy is not widely adopted due to the practical challenges of implementing carbogen breathing and the relatively modest benefit demonstrated. Tumor perfusion, oxygenation, and radiation response can also be improved with antiangiogenic agents in animal tumor models, possibly as a result of regularization of the vasculature (Goel et al, 2011), but this has not yet been translated to the clinic.

Another strategy to increase tumor oxygenation, which is complementary to that of increasing oxygen supply, is to decrease cellular oxygen consumption. Inhibiting oxygen consumption allows oxygen to diffuse further into the tumor tissue, thereby decreasing tumor hypoxia. Several drugs approved for other indications have been demonstrated to exert this effect in experimental models, and the ability of a few of these drugs to improve tumor oxygenation in human tumors are being evaluated in clinical trials (Zannella et al, 2013; Ashton et al, 2016).

16.4.4.2 Hypoxic Cell Sensitizers and Cytotoxins The development of drugs that mimic the radiosensitizing properties of oxygen, known as *hypoxic cell radiosensitizers*, was based on the idea that the radiosensitizing properties of oxygen are a consequence of its electron affinity and that other electron affinic compounds might act as sensitizers. Certain nitroimidazoles, such as nimorazole, are able to sensitize hypoxic cells both in vitro and in animal tumors. The extent of the sensitization can be assessed in terms of a sensitizer enhancement ratio (SER) that is analogous to the OER discussed in Section 16.4.1. Nimorazole was associated with improved tumor control in head and neck cancer in a trial from the Danish Head and Neck Cancer Study (DAHANCA) group (Overgaard et al, 1998). Furthermore, a meta-analysis of results for patients with head and neck cancer treated in randomized trials, using radiotherapy with HPO or hypoxic cell sensitizers (see Fig. 16–14) has

Head and Neck Cancer Metaanalysis: Hypoxic Modification of Radiotherapy

End Point	Hypoxic Modification (Events/Total)	Control (Events/Total)	Odds Ratio and 95% CI	Odds Ratio	Risk Reduction
Locoregional control	1203/2406	1383/2399		0.71 (0.63 to 0.80)*	8% (5% to 10%)*
Disease-specific survival	1175/2335	1347/2329		0.73 (0.64 to 0.82)*	7% (5% to 10%)*
Overall Survival	1450/2312	1519/2305		0.87 (0.77 to 0.98)*	3% (0% to 6%)*
Distant metastasis	159/1427	179/1391		0.87 (0.69 to 1.09)*	2% (−1% to 4%)*
Radiotherapy complications	307/1864	297/1822		1.00 (0.82 to 1.23)*	0% (−3% to 2%)*

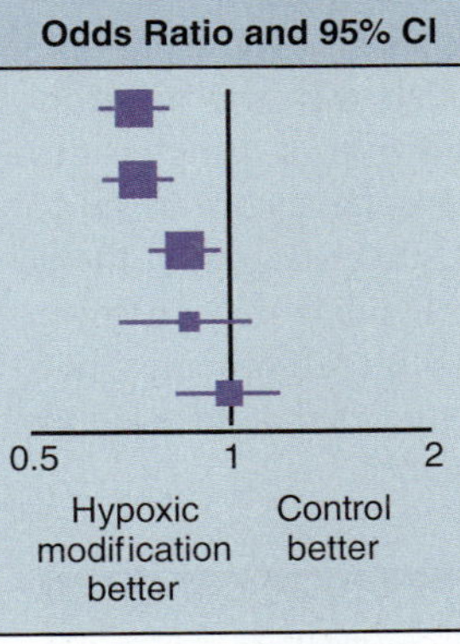

*95% CI.

FIGURE 16–14 Clinical outcomes from hypoxic modification with radiotherapy in head and neck cancer. The meta-analysis of 32 randomized trials demonstrates statistically significant improvements in tumor locoregional control, disease-specific survival, and overall survival, but no significant differences in distant metastasis or radiotherapy complications. The forest plot denotes the summary odds ratio and 95% confidence interval, with the size of the squares being proportional to the total number of patients for each endpoint. (Reproduced with permission from Overgaard J. Hypoxic modification of radiotherapy in squamous cell carcinoma of the head and neck--a systematic review and meta-analysis. *Radiother Oncol* 2011 Jul;100(1):22-32.)

indicated a small but significant improvement in local control and survival (Overgaard, 2011). Greater benefits might have been observed if there had been selection of patients with high levels of hypoxia in their tumors; reanalysis of the clinical samples from this trial showed that a 15-gene hypoxia classifier was predictive for benefit from nimorazole (Toustrup et al, 2012). The benefit of nimorazole in HPV-negative head and neck cancer and the predictive value of tumor hypoxia determined by the gene signature and/or FAZA-PET imaging is being evaluated prospectively in a multicenter international randomized clinical trial (Christiaens et al, 2017).

Another approach to reducing the influence of hypoxia on the radiation response of tumors has been to use (bioreductive) drugs that are toxic under hypoxic conditions (see Chap. 18, Sec. 18.4.7.2). The most extensively studied of these drugs in the context of radiotherapy is tirapazamine, which is cytotoxic to hypoxic cells at oxygen concentrations up to approximately 10 μmol/L (equivalent partial pressure of approximately 7 mm Hg) (Brown, 1999). Under hypoxia, tirapazamine is metabolized to an agent that produces DNA damage, including double-strand breaks, probably by interacting with topoisomerases. In the presence of oxygen, the active form is converted (by oxidation) back to the parent compound. Tirapazamine has shown efficacy in some clinical trials, but a large randomized Phase III trial of tirapazamine with chemoradiotherapy for head and neck cancers failed to show significant benefit, although this may have been related to the quality of the radiotherapy delivered (Peters et al, 2010; Rischin et al, 2010). This trial did not select for patients with more hypoxic tumors, and analysis of a small subset in whom hypoxia imaging was performed suggested benefit only for those with the most hypoxic tumors (Rischin et al, 2006), similar to the retrospective analysis for nimorazole described above. This has important implications for clinical studies of other hypoxic cytotoxins currently under development (Bonnet et al, 2018). One such drug is TH-302 (known also as evofosfamide), a 2-nitroimidazole with a bromoisophosphoramide mustard side chain that is released following reduction under hypoxic conditions to give a diffusible toxic product that can kill less hypoxic (bystander) cells as well as the producing cell. Although studies in animal tumor models with this agent in combination with radiotherapy have shown promising results (eg, Peeters et al, 2015; Nytko et al, 2017), large clinical studies using this combination are lacking. Taken together, there is some clinical evidence that targeting hypoxia may enhance the therapeutic ratio in patients treated with radiotherapy, but to date, there have been few landmark studies that have led to hypoxia targeting in routine clinical practice.

16.5 NORMAL TISSUE RESPONSE TO RADIOTHERAPY

16.5.1 Cellular and Tissue Responses

Radiation treatment can cause loss of function in normal tissues. In renewal tissues, such as skin, bone marrow, and the gastrointestinal mucosa, loss of function may be correlated with loss of proliferative activity of stem cells. In these and other tissues, loss of function may also occur through damage to more mature cells and/or through damage to supporting stroma and vasculature, and through the induction of potentially damaging inflammatory responses (Stewart and Dorr, 2009). Traditionally, the effects of radiation treatment on normal tissues have been divided, based largely on directly observable functional and histopathologic end points, into early (or acute) responses, which occur within 3 months of radiation treatment, and late responses that may take many months or years to develop. Such endpoints do not assess early changes in gene expression associated with irradiation that occur in all tissues (see below).

Acute responses occur primarily in tissues where rapid cell renewal is required to maintain the function of the organ. Because many cells express radiation damage during mitosis, there is early death and loss of cells killed by the radiation treatment. Late responses tend to occur in organs whose parenchymal cells divide infrequently (eg, liver or kidney) or rarely (eg, central nervous system or muscle) under normal conditions. Depletion of the parenchymal cell population as a result of entry of cells into mitosis, with the resulting expression of radiation damage and cell death, will thus be slow. Secondary organ dysfunction can also result from progressive damage to the connective tissue and vasculature of the organ, leading to fibrotic change and impairment in vasculature. The loss of functional cells may induce other parenchymal cells to divide, causing further cell death as they express their radiation damage, leading eventually to functional failure of the organ. Consequential late effects may also occur where severe early reactions have led to impaired tissue recovery and/or development of infection.

Several systems for documenting normal tissue responses (side effects) to irradiation in patients have been developed to facilitate cross-comparisons between investigators and institutions. These include the Radiation Therapy Oncology Group (RTOG) / European Organization for Research and Treatment of Cancer (EORTC) classification, the Common Terminology Criteria for Adverse Events (CTCAE v5) scale devised by the National Cancer Institute (Basch et al, 2014), and the Late Effects Normal Tissue Task Force Subjective, Objective, Management, and Analytic (LENT/SOMA) system, designed specifically to score late reactions (Hoeller et al, 2003).

The radiosensitivity of the cells of some normal tissues can be determined directly using in situ assays that allow the observation of proliferation from single surviving cells in vivo. One such assay determines the fraction of regenerating crypts in the small intestine following radiation doses sufficient to reduce the number of surviving stem cells per crypt to one or less, and analysis of the results allows the generation of a survival curve (Tucker et al, 1991). Survival curves obtained for the cells of different normal tissues in mice and rats are shown in Figure 16–15. Considerable variability in sensitivity is apparent, and as with tumor cells, most of the difference appears to be in the shoulder region of the survival curve, suggesting differences in repair capacity (see below).

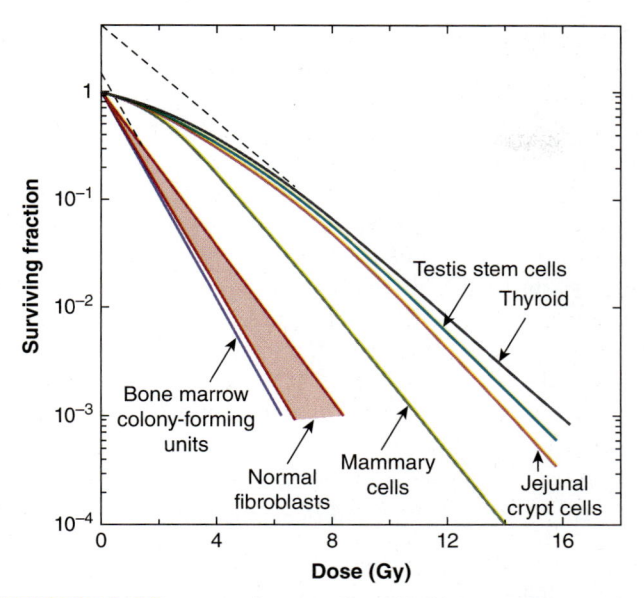

FIGURE 16-15 Survival curves for cells from some normal tissues. Most of the curves are for cells from rodent tissues, and the curves were produced using in vivo or in situ clonogenic assays. Survival curves for normal human fibroblasts are for cultured cell strains. (Data from Dr. JD Chapman, Fox Chase Cancer Center, Philadelphia.)

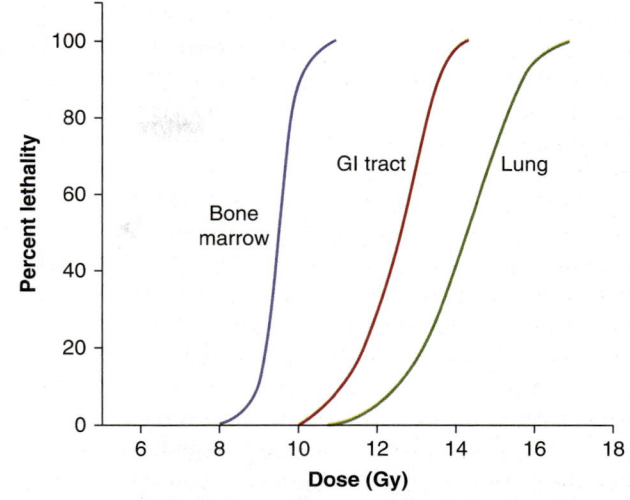

FIGURE 16-16 Three different curves indicating percentage lethality plotted as a function of radiation dose for the same strain of mouse. The "bone marrow" (blue) and "GI tract" (red) curves were obtained using whole-body irradiation and assessing lethality prior to day 30 or prior to day 7, respectively, because death as a result of damage to the gastrointestinal tract occurs earlier than that as a result of bone marrow failure. The green curve labeled "lung" was obtained by assessing lethality 180 days after local irradiation to the thorax.

Alternative experimental analyses of normal tissue radiation damage most often use functional assays. The crudest functional assay is the determination of the dose of radiation given either to the whole body or to a specific organ that will cause lethality in 50% of the treated animals within a specified time (LD_{50}). The relationship between lethality and single radiation dose is usually sigmoidal in shape, and some experimentally derived relationships for different normal tissues in mice are shown in Figure 16-16.

For individual organs, a level of functional deficit can be defined and the percentage of irradiated subjects that express at least this level of damage following different radiation doses is plotted as a function of dose. A tolerance dose for a specific organ can then be defined as the dose above which more than 5% of patients express that level of functional deficit (TD5). In animal models, complete dose-response curves have been obtained and an example for the rat spinal cord using forelimb paralysis as the end point is shown in Figure 16-17. These curves are sigmoidal in shape and generally quite steep. Similar results have been reported for specific functional deficits in many other tissues (eg, Brush et al, 2007).

An influx of immune cells (macrophages, lymphocytes, and neutrophils) into irradiated tissue, and increased cytokine and chemokine expression, has been observed within hours after irradiation (potentially before functional changes have occurred within irradiated organs due to cell death), and aspects of this inflammatory response may persist over months as the irradiated tissue transits to regeneration and repair (McKelvey et al, 2018). Early increases in cytokine expression can occur after low doses of radiation (~1 Gy), but longer-term changes have been observed after larger doses (5-25 Gy). A wide range of cytokines is involved including pro- and anti-inflammatory factors, such as tumor necrosis factor alpha (TNF-α), interleukin 1 (IL-1α and IL-1β), and TGF-β. In specific tissues, the response to radiation may include release of other growth factors that are associated with collagen deposition, fibrosis, inflammation, and aberrant vascular growth. These inflammatory factors may induce production of damaging radicals, such as reactive oxygen species, independently of those caused directly by the radiation treatment. The interplay between cell killing, cell repopulation, cytokine production,

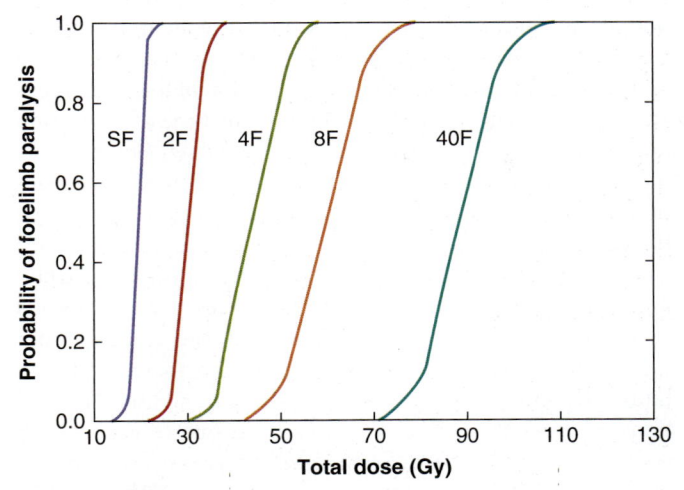

FIGURE 16-17 Dose-response curves for forelimb paralysis following fractionated radiation treatments to the rat spinal cord. The fractions (F) were given once daily to allow for repair of radiation damage between fractions. SF, Single fraction.

vascular damage, and immune cell infiltrates in producing the overall tissue damage remains poorly understood and is likely to vary from one organ to another (McKelvey et al, 2018).

16.5.2 Acute Tissue Responses

Acute radiation responses occur mainly in renewal tissues and have been related to death of critical cell populations such as the stem cells in the crypts of the small intestine, in the bone marrow, or in the basal layer of the skin. These responses occur within 3 months of the start of radiotherapy (in humans) but are not usually limiting for fractionated radiotherapy because of the ability of the stem cells in the tissue to undergo rapid repopulation to regenerate the tissue. Nevertheless, acute responses can be challenging for patients and may need clinical intervention (see below). Radiation-induced cell death in normal tissues generally occurs when the cells attempt mitosis; thus the tissue tends to respond on a time scale similar to the normal rate of loss of functional cells in that tissue and the demand for proliferation of the supporting stem cells. Radiation-induced apoptosis can also be detected in many tissues, but is usually a minor factor in overall radiation-induced cell death, except in lymphoid and myeloid tissue.

Endothelial cells in the vasculature supporting the crypts and villi of the small intestine of mice have been reported to be prone to radiation-induced apoptosis. Prevention of this effect can protect the animals against radiation-induced gastrointestinal injury, suggesting that dysfunction of the vasculature can reduce the ability of the crypts to regenerate (Paris et al, 2001; Rotolo et al, 2012). Endothelial cell death may be more prominent following larger radiation doses (>10 Gy) such as those used in SBRT than at the doses more commonly used for fractionated radiation therapy (~2 Gy).

Following irradiation of mucosa (and skin), there is early erythema within a few days of irradiation as a result of increased vascular permeability related to the release of 5-hydroxytryptamine by mast cells. Similar mechanisms may lead to early nausea and vomiting observed following irradiation of the intestine. Expression of further acute mucositis (or moist desquamation in skin) and ulceration depends on the relative rates of cell loss and cell proliferation of the transit cells and the (basal) stem cells in the tissue. The time of expression for this damage depends on the time over which (intensity of) the dose is received (Fig. 16-18), and the extent of these reactions and the length of time for recovery is dependent on the total dose received and the volume (area) of mucosa (or skin) irradiated. Early recovery depends on the number of surviving basal stem cells present in hair follicles that are needed to repopulate the tissue, and these cells can migrate from undamaged areas into the irradiated area. Erythema occurs in humans at single doses greater than about 24 Gy in 2-Gy fractions, whereas mucositis occurs after fractionated doses above approximately 50 Gy in 2-Gy fractions. Severe skin reactions in patients are relatively uncommon as high-energy photon radiation beams have a build-up region that results in a reduced dose at the skin surface (see Sec. 16.2.4 and Fig. 16-4A), but

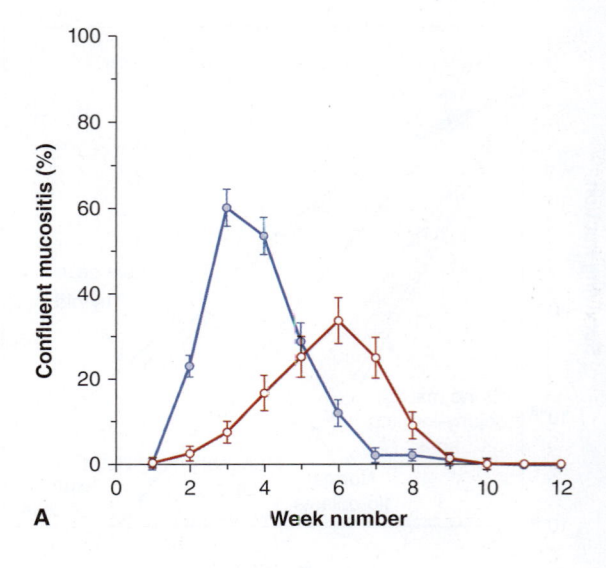

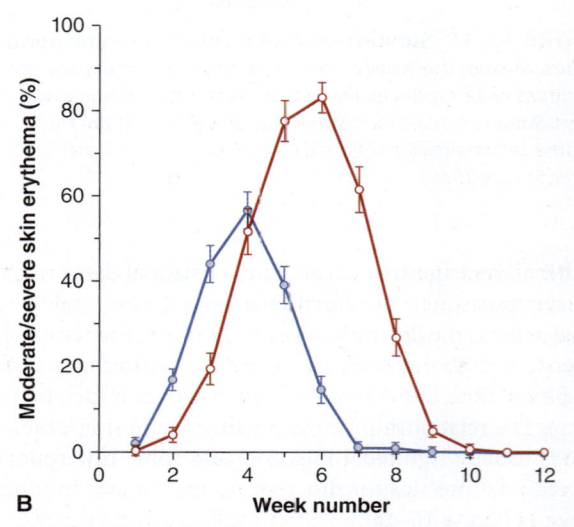

FIGURE 16–18 Estimated prevalence of confluent mucositis (**A**) or moderate to severe skin reactions (**B**) in patients following conventional radiotherapy over 5-6 weeks (red lines) or accelerated radiotherapy in less than 2 weeks (blue lines) in the CHART (Continuous Hyperfractionated Accelerated Radiotherapy) study. (Modified with permission from Bentzen SM, Saunders MI, Dische S, Bond SJ. Radiotherapy-related early morbidity in head and neck cancer: quantitative clinical radiobiology as deduced from the CHART trial. *Radiother Oncol* 2001 Aug;60(2):123-135.)

oral mucositis is prevalent during radiation treatment of head and neck cancers.

16.5.3 Late Tissue Responses

Late tissue responses occur in organs whose parenchymal cells normally divide infrequently and hence do not express mitosis-linked death until later times when called on to divide. They also occur in tissues that manifest early reactions, such as skin/subcutaneous tissue and intestine, but these reactions (subcutaneous fibrosis, vascular damage [eg, telangiectasia],

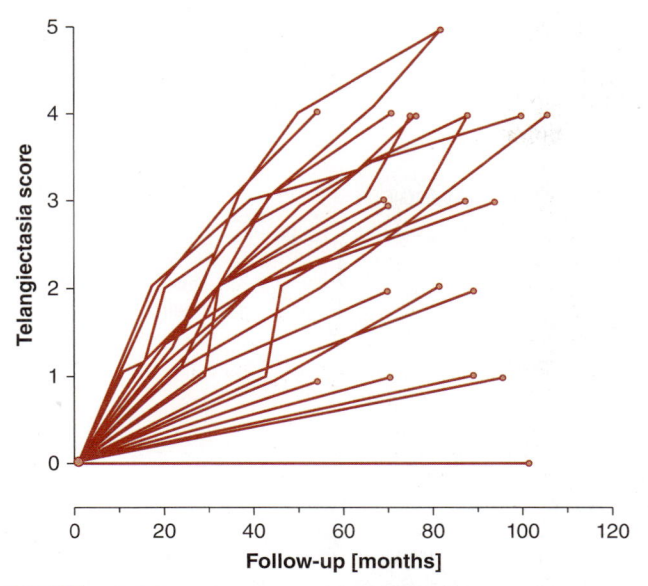

FIGURE 16–19 Clinical manifestations of skin telangiectasis. Progression of telangiectasia in individual patients treated with 5 fractions of 1.8 Gy/wk to a total of 35 fractions. (Modified with permission from Turesson I. Individual variation and dose dependency in the progression rate of skin telangiectasia. *Int J Radiat Oncol Biol Phys* 1990 Dec;19(6):1569-1574.)

intestinal stenosis) are quite different from the early reactions. Late responses (usually regarded as those that occur more than 3 months after treatment) usually limit the dose of radiation that can be delivered to a patient during radiotherapy. Damage can be expressed as diminished organ function, such as radiation-induced nephropathy (with symptoms of hypertension or increased serum creatinine) or myelopathy (with symptoms of paralysis) following spinal cord damage, as illustrated in Figure 16–17. Late responses generally are dependent on fraction size in addition to dose (Fig. 16–17) and are usually progressive over time (Fig. 16–19). As discussed below, the nature and timing of late responses depend on the tissue involved.

One common late response is the slow development of tissue fibrosis that occurs in many tissues (eg, subcutaneous tissue, muscle, lung, gastrointestinal tract), often several years after radiation treatment. Radiation-induced fibrosis is associated with a chronic inflammatory response following irradiation, the aberrant and prolonged expression of the growth factor TGF-β, radiation-induced differentiation of fibroblasts into fibrocytes that produce collagen, and metabolic reprogramming toward an anabolic and glycolytic state (Zhao et al, 2019). Transforming growth factor-β also plays a major role in wound healing and the development of radiation fibrosis has similarities to the healing of chronic wounds (Denham and Hauer-Jensen, 2002). Another common late reaction is progressive vascular damage, including telangiectasia that can be observed in skin and mucosa, and loss of microvasculature leading to atrophy (and fibrosis) that is manifested in skin and other tissues. Figure 16–19 shows the development of telangiectasia in patients following fractionated treatment and illustrates that heterogeneity in response between different patients is not limited to tumors but can also occur with normal tissue effects (Turesson, 1990).

The lung is an important site of late radiation damage. There are 2 types of reactions: pneumonitis that occurs 2-6 months after irradiation, and fibrosis that usually occurs more than 1 year after irradiation. These reactions can cause increases in tissue density on CT scans (see Chap. 14, Sec. 14.3.1) and increases in breathing rate if severe. Measuring changes in breathing rate has been used extensively to assay the dose–response relationship for radiation-induced lung damage in rats and mice, particularly the development of pneumonitis. Studies in rodents have documented that inflammatory cells and inflammatory cytokines play a major role in lung response to radiation injury (Fig. 16–20), but the relationship between this inflammatory response and the later development of functional symptoms is unclear. Studies in lung cancer patients suggest that increased levels of TGF-β and other cytokines in plasma following radiotherapy can contribute to the likelihood of developing lung complications (Kainthola et al, 2017).

The dose required to cause functional impairment in lung depends on the volume irradiated, with small volumes being able to tolerate quite large doses (Marks et al, 2010a); this is a result of the functional reserve of the remaining lung because the irradiated region will develop fibrosis. Studies in rodents, using the dose required to cause an increased breathing frequency in 50% of animals (ED_{50}) as an end point, have defined a relationship between ED_{50} and lung volume irradiated, which indicates that the base of the lung is more sensitive than the apex (Travis et al, 1997). The underlying mechanisms may relate to the functional reserve in different regions of the lung and/or to the extent of cytokine production following irradiation of different regions of the lung. There is also evidence for regional effects following irradiation of human lung (Marks et al, 2010a). Genetic variability may also underlie differences in fibrotic responses to radiation (Edvardsen et al, 2013; Kainthola et al, 2017).

A theoretical framework introduced by (Withers et al, 1988) suggests that late responding tissues can be considered as arrays of functional subunits (FSUs) containing groups of cells that are critical for function (eg, bronchioli in lung, nephrons in the kidney). These FSU were postulated to be able to be regenerated from a single surviving tissue stem cell. Furthermore, tissues were considered to have these FSUs operating in parallel to achieve overall tissue function (such as occurs in lung, kidney, liver) or in series (such as in spinal cord or intestine) in analogy with electrical circuits. Tissues with a parallel structure of FSUs have substantial reserve capacity and, although damage to a small volume may completely inactivate this volume, the remaining regions can maintain function and/or may undergo hypertrophy to replace any loss of function (eg, kidney and liver). Tissues with a series structure of FSUs may cease to function if even a small region of the tissue is irreparably damaged, such as may occur in the spinal cord where localized injury can cause complete tissue dysfunction and myelopathy, or in the intestine if severe stenosis causes

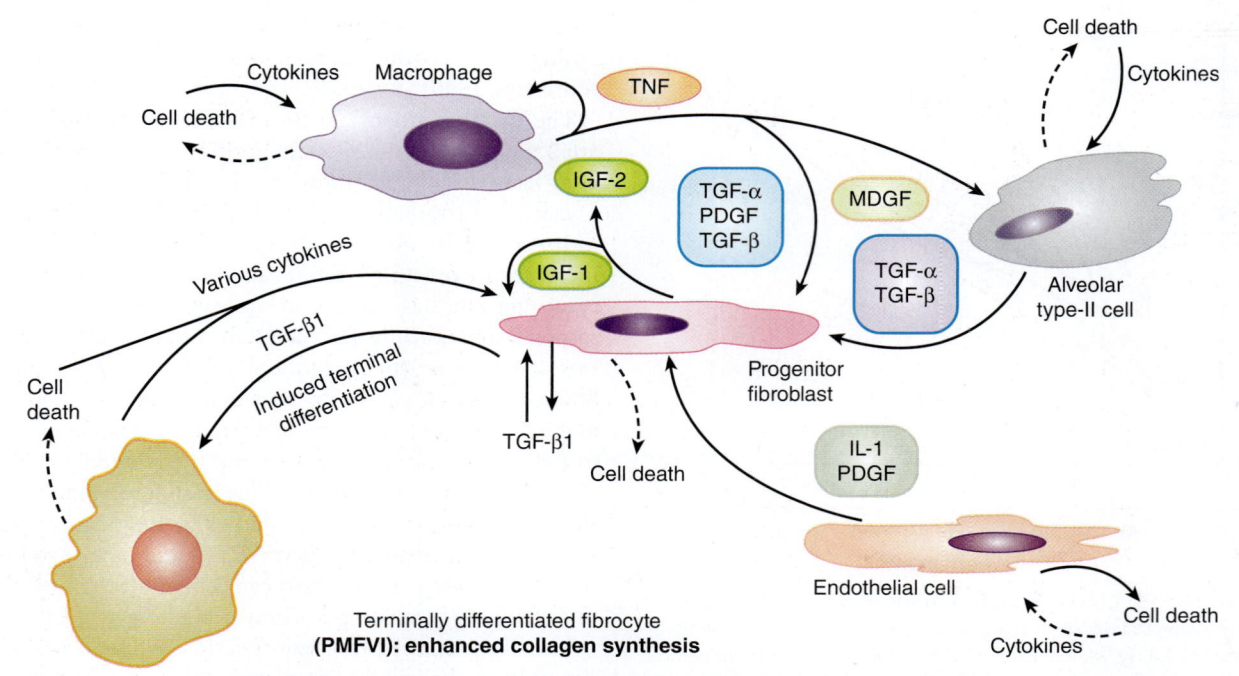

IGF = Insulin-like growth factor, PDGF = Platelet-derived growth factor, MDGF = Macrophage/monocyte-derived growth factor, TGF = Transforming growth factor, TNF = Tumor necrosis factor, IL = Interleukin.

FIGURE 16–20 Potential cellular interactions and cytokine induction after irradiation of lung tissue. The various cell populations and some of the cytokines induced potentially leading to fibrosis (increased collagen levels) are illustrated. (Modified with permission from Rodemann HP, Bamberg M. Cellular basis of radiation-induced fibrosis. *Radiother Oncol* 1995 May;35(2):83-90.)

obstruction. In practice, tissues do not fall neatly into these 2 categories for various reasons, including the common role of the vasculature, the development of inflammatory responses that may extend beyond the treatment field, because FSUs may require more than one type of undamaged stem cells for repair and these stem cells may migrate into areas of damage either locally or via the circulation. However, the concept that the volume irradiated to high dose is critical to tissue response and that this varies for different organs is well established and used in mathematical models designed to predict normal tissue complication probabilities (NTCP) (Bentzen et al, 2010; Marks et al, 2010b).

16.5.4 Whole-Body Irradiation

Normal tissue damage due to radiotherapy is confined spatially to the tissues directly surrounding the tumor that are irradiated to high doses. Radiation accidents can result in whole-body irradiation where the damage is manifested as a result of radiation to large volumes of sensitive organs. The response of animals to single-dose whole-body irradiation can be divided into 3 separate syndromes (hematologic, gastrointestinal, and neurovascular) that manifest following different doses and at different times after irradiation (Mettler and Voelz, 2002; Dainiak et al, 2003). The neurovascular syndrome occurs following large doses of radiation (>20 Gy) and usually results in rapid death (hours to days) as a consequence of cardiovascular and neurologic dysfunction. The gastrointestinal syndrome occurs after doses greater than approximately 5 to 15 Gy and, in rodents, doses at the upper end of this range usually result in death at about 1 week after irradiation as a consequence of severe damage to the mucosal lining of the gastrointestinal tract; this causes a loss of the protective barrier with consequent infection, loss of electrolytes, and fluid imbalance. Intensive nursing with antibiotics, fluid, and electrolyte replacement can prevent early death from this syndrome in human victims of radiation accidents, but these patients may die later as a result of damage to other organs, particularly skin, if large areas are exposed.

The hematopoietic syndrome occurs at doses in the range of 2 to 8 Gy in humans (3-10 Gy in rodents) and is caused by severe depletion of blood elements as a result of killing of precursor cells in the bone marrow. This syndrome causes death in rodents (at the higher dose levels) between approximately 12 and 30 days after irradiation, and somewhat later in larger animals, including humans. Death can sometimes be prevented by bone marrow transplantation (BMT) and cytokine therapy (eg, granulocyte-macrophage colony-stimulating factor [GM-CSF], granulocyte colony-stimulating factor [G-CSF], stem cell factor) provided that the radiation exposure is not too high such that damage to other organs may become lethal. Following the Chernobyl accident, 31 of the emergency workers (of 104 identified as showing symptoms of acute radiation syndrome) died within 4 months. Most of these workers received bone marrow doses greater than 4 Gy, with much higher doses to the skin (10-30 times). Bone marrow failure was the primary cause of death, particularly for those dying within the first 2 months. Although 13 of these patients had BMT, most died, probably because of serious radiation damage to the skin (UNSCEAR, 2008). There are substantial differences in the doses required to induce death from the hematopoietic syndrome (ie, LD_{50} value) between different species of animals and even between different strains of the same species. The LD_{50} value for humans has been estimated at 4 to 7 Gy, depending on the available level of supportive care (excluding BMT). Following doses greater than approximately 2 Gy, humans will develop early nausea and vomiting within hours of irradiation (prodromal syndrome), which may be controlled with 5-hydroxytryptamine antagonists.

16.5.5 Retreatment Tolerance

In the event that a tumor recurs or the patient has a new primary tumor, there may be a need to further irradiate normal tissues that have been irradiated previously. Although tissues may repair damage and regenerate after irradiation, previously irradiated tissues may have a reduced tolerance for subsequent radiation treatments, indicating the presence of residual injury. For tissues that undergo only an early response to radiation, there is almost complete recovery in a few months, so that a second high dose of radiation can be tolerated. For late-responding tissue damage, the extent of the residual injury depends on the level of the initial damage and is tissue dependent. There is substantial recovery in skin, mucosa, spinal cord, and lung over a period of 3-6 months, but kidney and bladder show little evidence of recovery (Stewart and Dorr, 2009). Clinical studies have demonstrated that retreatment to high doses with curative intent is possible depending on the tissues involved but usually entails increased risk of normal tissue damage.

16.5.6 Predicting Normal Tissue Response

Patients receiving identical radiation treatments may experience differing levels of normal tissue injury (see, eg, Fig. 16–19). Thus, predictive assays might be useful in identifying those patients who are at greater risk of experiencing the side effects of radiotherapy. The enhanced radiosensitivity of patients with ataxia telangiectasia (AT) and other DNA repair–deficiency syndromes (see Chap. 9, Sec. 9.5) supports a genetic contribution to individual variability in radiosensitivity. Large-scale genetic studies are underway to uncover additional genetic variants that are associated with radiation-related side effects (West et al, 2010; Herskind et al, 2016). Many other factors, such as diet or environment, could also play a role. Several studies have quantified the in vitro radiosensitivity of fibroblasts and peripheral lymphocytes as a potential predictive assay for normal tissue damage. These studies show variations in the radiosensitivity of fibroblasts from individual patients, but are inconsistent in predicting late radiation fibrosis (Russell and Begg, 2002). Thus, although cellular sensitivity is an important contributor to normal tissue damage, other factors, such as cytokine induction and the response of the tissue stroma and vasculature, likely also play an important role in normal tissue injury.

16.5.7 Radioprotection

Protection against radiation damage can be achieved by reducing the physical dose of radiation delivered to an organ. For instance, injected rectal spacers can reduce the dose to the rectal wall in men treated with prostate brachytherapy (Serrano et al, 2017). Likewise, salivary gland toxicity can be reduced in head and neck cancer patients by surgically transferring the submandibular gland outside the radiation field (Jensen et al, 2010).

When physical separation of an organ is not sufficient/possible, drug treatments may achieve some degree of radioprotection (Weiss and Landauer, 2009). Examples include agents that can scavenge radiation-produced radicals, such as superoxide dismutase enzymes, or sulfhydryl-containing compounds, such as glutathione and cysteine. Because of the short lifetimes of radiation-induced radicals, exogenously added agents have to be present in the cell at the time of the irradiation. They are equally effective for tumor and normal cells in vitro; thus, specificity for therapeutic application in vivo depends largely on preferential uptake of such agents into the normal tissue. One agent that appears to fulfill this criterion is amifostine, a prodrug that is converted into a sulfhydryl-containing compound in vivo by the action of alkaline phosphatases. The selective activity of this compound in normal tissue is believed to be a result of poor tumor distribution from tumor blood vessels and reduced levels of alkaline phosphatase in tumors. Amifostine was shown to protect a variety of normal tissues with variable, mostly small, protection of tumors in animal models (for review, see Lindegaard and Grau, 2000). Studies in patients with head and neck and lung cancers showed substantial protection of normal tissue, including salivary gland, lung, and mucosa, without detectable change in tumor response (Brizel et al, 2000; Antonadou et al, 2003); however, the compound is not widely used clinically because of unrelated toxicities.

Another strategy for protection of normal tissue is to block the development of late radiation effects with treatment given after the end of the radiation. Various strategies, including anti-inflammatory agents and antioxidants, are being studied in patients to determine whether they can reverse the progressive nature of radiation-induced fibrosis (Westbury and Yarnold, 2012; Straub et al, 2015).

16.5.8 Therapeutic Ratio

The concept of therapeutic ratio is illustrated in Figure 16–21, which shows theoretical dose–response curves for tumor control and normal tissue complications as described in Sections 16.3.1 and 16.5.1 (see also similar curves for systemic therapy in Chap. 17, Sec. 17.5.1 and Fig 17.9). Tumor-control curves (red lines) tend to be shallower than those for normal tissue response (blue lines) because of the extensive heterogeneity among tumors, as discussed in Section 16.3.1. The therapeutic ratio is often defined as the percentage of tumor cures that are obtained at a given level of normal tissue complications (ie, by taking a vertical cut through the 2 curves at a tolerance dose, eg, at 5% complications after 5 years). In experimental

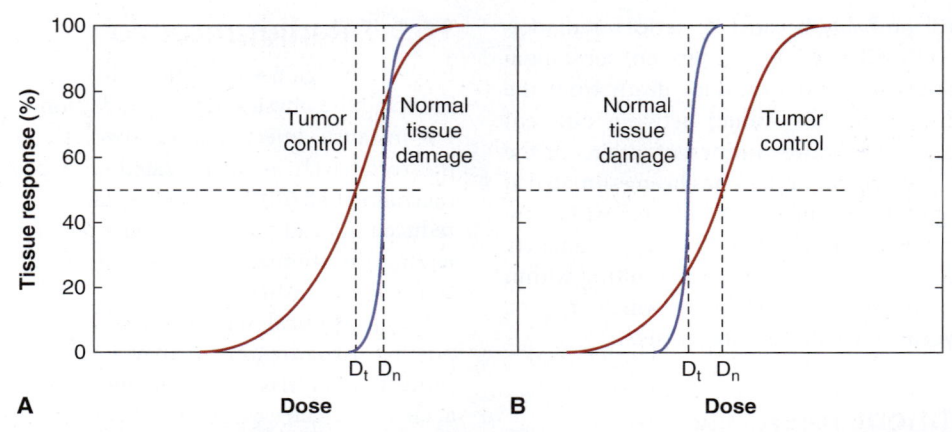

FIGURE 16–21 Illustration of the concept of a therapeutic ratio in terms of dose–response relationships for tumor control and normal tissue damage. The red curves represent dose response for tumor control, and the blue curves represent dose response for critical normal tissue damage. See the text for specific discussion of the 2 parts of the figure.

studies, an alternative approach is to define the therapeutic ratio as the ratio of radiation doses D_n/D_t required to produce a given percentage of complications and tumor control (usually 50%). It is then a measure of the horizontal displacement between the 2 curves. It remains imprecise, however, because it depends on the shape of the dose–response curves for tumor control and normal tissue complications. The curves shown in Figure 16–21A depict a situation in which the therapeutic ratio is favorable because the tumor-control curve is displaced to the left of that for normal tissue damage. The greater this displacement, the more radiocurable the tumor. Because the tumor-control curve is shallower than that for normal tissue damage, the therapeutic ratio tends to be favorable only for low and intermediate tumor-control levels. If the 2 curves are close together or the curve for tumor control is displaced to the right of that for complications (Fig. 16–21B), the therapeutic ratio is unfavorable because a high level of complications must be accepted to achieve even a minimal level of tumor control.

16.6 RADIOTHERAPY FRACTIONATION

The therapeutic ratio is improved in many clinical disease sites by fractionating the radiation treatment, that is, by delivering the radiation dose in many small amounts over several days or weeks. Many of the biologic effects that contribute to improving the therapeutic ratio by fractionation have been identified. The most important biologic factors influencing the responses of tumors and normal tissues to fractionated treatment are often called the "four Rs": repair, repopulation, redistribution, and reoxygenation. Some of these biologic factors were introduced in Chapter 15, and here they are discussed further in the context of fractionated irradiation.

16.6.1 Repair

When a single dose of radiation is divided in two with time in between, it will typically lose some efficacy. This is because cells have time to repair some of the initial damage before more damage is imparted. If all of the radiation is given at once, a larger proportion of it will be irreparable. The shoulder on a survival curve after single radiation doses is usually indicative of the capacity of the cells to repair radiation damage. If multiple doses are given with sufficient time between the fractions for repair to occur (6-24 hours, depending on the cells or tissue involved), the shoulder repeats and survival curves for cells treated with fractionated irradiation will be similar to those illustrated in Figure 16–22. The dashed lines in this figure represent the effective survival curves for different fractionated treatments. The effective slope depends on the size of the individual dose fractions, becoming shallower as the fraction size is reduced (eg, dashed red curve vs dashed green curve). This effect is also illustrated by the dose-response curves shown in Figure 16–17 for forelimb paralysis of rats following irradiation with different numbers of fractions to the spinal cord, where the curves for higher numbers of (smaller) fractions are displaced to higher total doses.

In cell culture, the repair is largely associated with capacity for enzymatic DNA damage repair. In tissues, other factors could also contribute to the recovery between fractions. Although fractionation results in reduced radiation efficacy for both tumors and normal tissues, the sparing effect tends to be larger for normal tissue effects than for tumor control. Fractionation therefore increases the therapeutic ratio. The loss of efficacy on the tumor can be compensated for by giving a higher total dose before reaching normal tissue tolerance.

16.6.2 Repopulation

In both tumors and normal tissues, proliferation of surviving cells may occur during the course of fractionated treatment. Furthermore, as cellular damage and cell death occur during the course of the treatment, the tissue may respond with an increased rate of proliferation of the surviving cells, termed *accelerated repopulation*. Tumor cell repopulation results in increased numbers of surviving cells during the course of the treatment and reduced overall response to irradiation. This effect is most important in early-responding normal tissues (eg, skin, gastrointestinal tract)

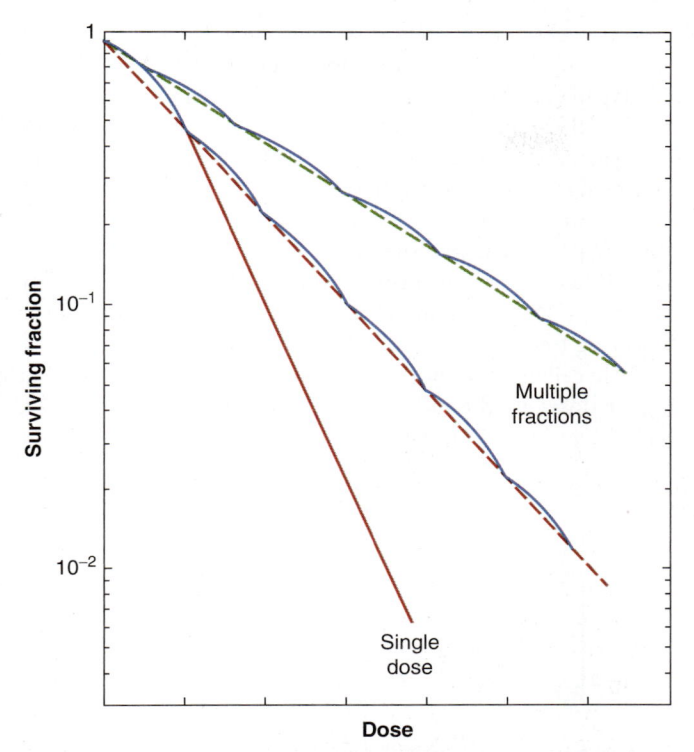

FIGURE 16-22 **The influence of fractionating the radiation treatment on the shape of cell-survival curves.** The cell-survival curve for single-dose radiation (red solid curve) displays a shoulder at lower doses due to the influence of damage repair. For multifraction radiation (dashed curves), repair that occurs between fractions causes the shoulder of the survival curve to repeat for each fraction; this results in curves that are shallower for smaller fraction sizes (eg, green vs red dashed curves).

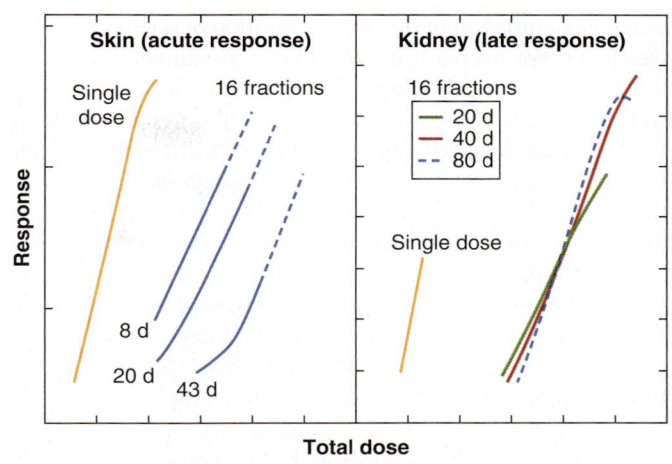

FIGURE 16-23 **Illustration of the effect of repopulation during fractionated treatment of skin or kidney.** Treatment was a single dose or 16 equal fractions given in different overall times as indicated. Acute skin response was assessed using a numerical scoring technique, and kidney response was determined by reduction in ethylenediaminetetraacetic acid (EDTA) clearance. For both tissues, the fractionated treatment results in the curves moving to the right (higher doses) because of repair. For the acute skin reactions, extending the time over which a course of 16 fractions is given (from 8 to 43 days) results in a further increase in the total dose required for a given level of response (isoeffective dose). In contrast, for late response of kidney there is no change in the isoeffective dose for 16 fractions regardless of whether the treatment is given over 20 or 80 days.

or in tumors whose stem cells are capable of rapid proliferation. In contrast, it will be of little consequence in late-responding, slowly proliferating tissues (eg, kidney, liver, spinal cord), which do not suffer much early cell death and hence do not produce an early proliferative response to the radiation treatment. Figure 16-23 illustrates the effect of repopulation for early skin reactions versus (lack of repopulation) for late kidney response. Repopulation responses are particularly important in reducing acute normal tissue responses during prolonged treatments, such as those involving a period without irradiation (split-course treatment), but this effect can also be important in decreasing tumor response as discussed below.

Repopulation is likely to be more important toward the end of a course of treatment, when sufficient damage has accumulated (and cell death occurred) to induce a robust regenerative response. This is consistent with clinical observations that oral mucosa can start to heal toward the end of a 6- to 7-week course of therapy, despite the continued treatment, because of rapid proliferation of basal (stem) cells in the mucosa. Similar increases in proliferation of surviving (stem) cells can also occur in tumors. Evidence that accelerated repopulation can occur in human tumors during a course of fractionated therapy is shown in Figure 16-24. Here the (normalized) total dose required to give 50% control of head and neck cancers is

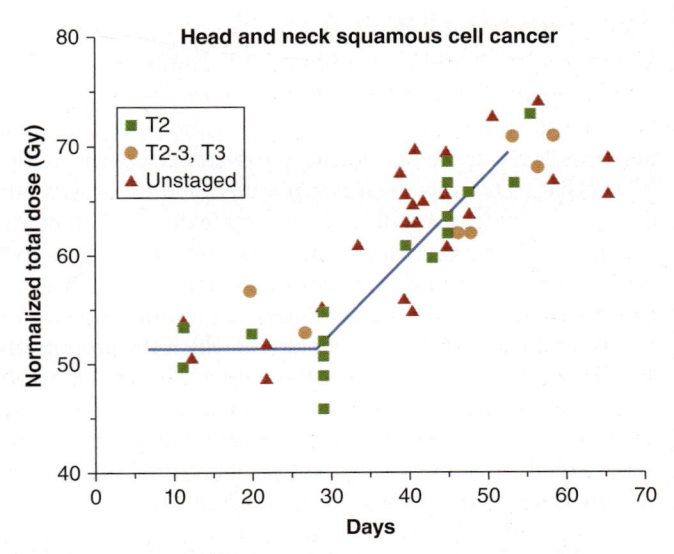

FIGURE 16-24 **Estimated total doses of fractionated irradiation required to achieve 50% probability of tumor control for squamous cell carcinomas of the head and neck (various stages) plotted as a function of the overall treatment time.** Each point is for a different group of patients and is obtained from published results. The actual doses used to treat the different groups of patients were normalized to a standard schedule of 2 Gy per fraction using the technique described in Section 16.7.3.

plotted as a function of the overall duration of the fractionated treatment. For overall times less than approximately 4 weeks, there is little change in the dose required for 50% tumor control; at longer times, however, there is a substantial increase in the total dose required as the duration of treatment increases (Withers et al, 1988). This observation suggests that the initial part of the fractionated therapy has resulted in increased proliferation of the surviving tumor stem cells, which for head and neck tumors becomes apparent at about 4 weeks after the start of the treatment. The data are consistent with an (accelerated) doubling time of approximately 4 days for the clonogenic tumor cells, compared with a median volume doubling time of approximately 2 to 3 months for unperturbed tumor growth (see Chap. 12, Sec. 12.1). Repopulation of tumor cells during a conventional course of radiotherapy is an important factor influencing local tumor control in patients with rapidly growing tumors and is the reason why it is preferable to avoid treatment delays during therapy. Repopulation provides the biologic rationale for accelerated fractionated radiation therapy (see Sec. 16.7.4). Overall treatment time would be expected to be less important for slower-growing tumors such as prostate or breast cancer. Whether repopulation has a positive or negative effect on the therapeutic ratio during fractionated radiotherapy therefore depends on the tumor and the relevant normal tissues.

New approaches to directly measure tumor stem cell proliferation might help to identify which patients have tumors needing accelerated therapy. An alternative approach may be combination with systemic therapy (see Sec. 16.2.5 and Chap. 17, Sec. 17.6.4) to reduce repopulation during treatment, although this may exacerbate early normal tissue reactions.

16.6.3 Redistribution

Variation in the radiosensitivity of cells in different phases of the cell cycle results in the cells in the more resistant phases being more likely to survive a dose of radiation (see Chap. 15, Sec. 15.4.2). In addition, radiation activates cell-cycle checkpoints that transiently prevent replication and division. Both effects contribute to a shift in the cell-cycle distribution of the viable cell population, which will affect the response to a second dose of radiation. The redistribution effect is not likely to have much influence on late responses, as these occur predominantly as a result of injury to tissues in which the proportion of cells in proliferative phases of the cell cycle is low. Although there might be relevant redistribution effects in tumors, these are difficult to manipulate, and take advantage of, given the rather small cell cycle–specific differences in radiosensitivity and the heterogeneous nature of human tumors.

16.6.4 Reoxygenation

The response of tumors to large single doses of radiation is dominated by the presence of hypoxic cells within them, even if only a very small fraction of the tumor stem cells is hypoxic (see Sec. 16.4). However, with time, some of the surviving hypoxic cells may gain access to oxygen (*reoxygenate*) and become more sensitive to a subsequent radiation treatment. Reoxygenation can occur naturally between fractions as a result of fluctuating perfusion of blood vessels (see Sec. 16.4.2). Reoxygenation can also be due to reduced oxygen consumption by damaged or dying cells, which allows oxygen to reach the previously hypoxic cells. Removal of dead cells will also allow hypoxic cells to move closer to the blood vessels. Reoxygenation can result in a substantial increase in the sensitivity of tumors during fractionated treatment. The survival curve following fractionated irradiation for a tumor containing 10% hypoxic cells that do not reoxygenate would be dominated at higher doses by the radioresistant hypoxic cells (Fig. 16–25, blue (b) and green (a) dashed lines), whereas that for a tumor

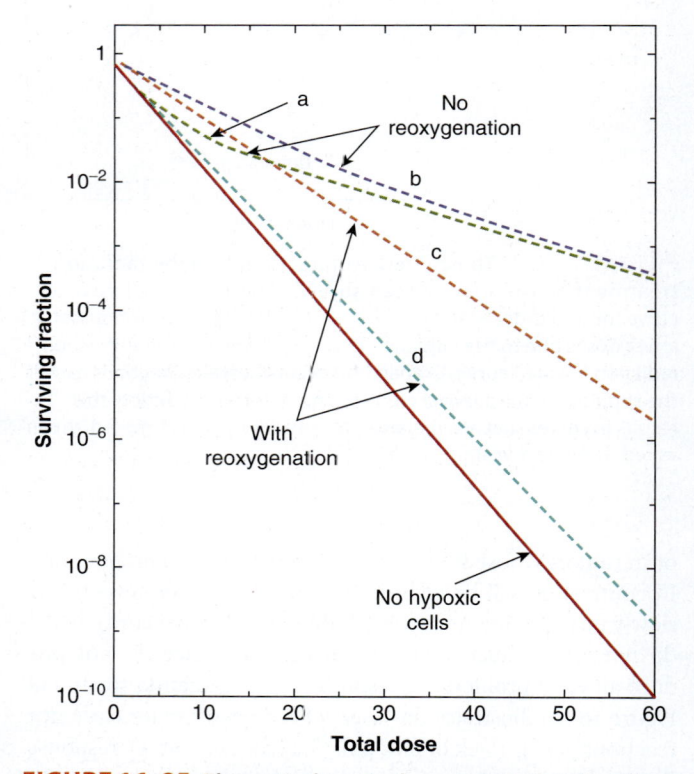

FIGURE 16–25 Theoretical survival curves calculated to illustrate the influence of reoxygenation on the level of cell killing in a tumor following treatment with 2-Gy fractions. The solid red line illustrates the expected survival curve for a tumor with no hypoxic cells. For a tumor with hypoxic cells, it was assumed that the tumor initially had 10% hypoxic cells and either 90% well-oxygenated cells (green [a] and turquoise [d] dashed lines representing survival without and with reoxygenation respectively) or a proportion of well-oxygenated cells and cells at intermediate oxygen concentrations calculated using a radial diffusion model (blue [b] and orange [c] dashed lines representing survival without and with reoxygenation respectively). It was assumed that reoxygenation was sufficient to maintain the same proportions of hypoxic cells among the surviving cells during the fractionated treatment. (Reproduced with permission from Wouters BG, Brown JM. Cells at intermediate oxygen levels can be more important than the "hypoxic fraction" in determining tumor response to fractionated radiotherapy. *Radiat Res* 1997 May;147(5):541-550.)

cell population that has complete reoxygenation between dose fractions (Fig. 16–25, turquoise (d) dashed line) lies close to the curve for a fully oxygenated population. In practice, there will also be many cells at intermediate oxygen levels in tumors, and as seen in Figure 16–25 (orange (c) dashed line) these cells will likely dominate the survival curve when reoxygenation occurs during fractionated treatment (Wouters and Brown, 1997). Reoxygenation has been shown to occur in almost all rodent tumors that have been studied, but the extent and timing of reoxygenation are variable.

Reoxygenation is probably a major reason why fractionating treatment leads to an improvement in therapeutic ratio (as compared to a few large doses) in clinical radiotherapy, given that this sensitizing effect is limited to tumors. There is limited direct information about reoxygenation of cells in human tumors during treatment, but measurements of the pO_2 in human tumors using Eppendorf oxygen electrodes (see Sec. 12.4.1) during fractionated radiotherapy have demonstrated increasing oxygen levels in some tumors (Dunst et al, 1999). Although this is consistent with reoxygenation, these measurements do not distinguish between oxygen levels of surviving cells and those of cells already inactivated by the treatment. Evidence that the oxygen status of tumors can predict treatment outcome following radiation therapy (see Sec. 16.4.3) suggests that reoxygenation is inadequate to eliminate the effects of hypoxia during standard fractionated treatment in all tumors in humans. Indeed, studies imaging hypoxia with MISO-PET in head and neck cancer have suggested that the presence of hypoxia is most prognostic a few weeks into a fractionated treatment schedule, perhaps reflecting the importance of hypoxia specifically in tumors where treatment does not induce complete reoxygenation (Lock et al, 2017). Shortened treatment schedules as in SBRT (see Sec. 16.2.1) may limit the chance for tumors to reoxygenate, consistent with data from animal models that demonstrate a larger protection for hypoxic tumors when using larger fraction sizes. Administration of hypoxic cell sensitizers might be particularly relevant in this clinical setting.

16.7 MODELING THE EFFECTS OF FRACTIONATION

16.7.1 Time and Dose Relationships

Repair and repopulation increase the total dose required to achieve a given level of biologic damage (an isoeffect) from a course of fractionated radiation treatment. In contrast, redistribution and reoxygenation would be expected to reduce the total dose required for an isoeffect. It is often difficult to dissect the influence of these factors, but reoxygenation applies mostly to tumors (because they contain hypoxic cells), whereas repopulation and redistribution apply both to tumors and proliferating normal tissues. Repair is an important factor in the response of virtually all tissues. Experimental studies from many decades ago, examining acute reactions in pig skin, established that fraction number (reflecting repair of sublethal damage between fractions) was a more important factor than overall treatment time (reflecting repopulation) in determining isoeffect in fractionation schedules extending out to 4 weeks (Fowler and Stern, 1963). Further studies established that fraction size (which is linked to fraction number in therapy regimes) is the critical parameter regarding normal tissue response, as illustrated for cell killing in Figure 16–22. For tumors and early normal tissue reactions, the contribution of repopulation increases as the fractionated treatment is extended to longer times, as illustrated in Figures 16–23 and 16–24. Repopulation makes a lesser contribution for late normal tissue reactions but repair plays the major role, as illustrated in Figure 16–23 and discussed in Sections 16.6.1 and 16.6.2. Redistribution reduces the effect of repopulation, but is probably a minor factor affecting tissue response to fractionated treatment, as discussed in Section 16.6.3.

That the biologic effect of radiation depends on the fractionation schedule has important clinical implications for the planning of therapy. To obtain the maximum dose to a tumor while minimizing dose to surrounding normal tissue, modern radiotherapy will often use a number of overlapping radiation beams. The dose at any given location will be calculated by summing the doses given by the various individual beams, and the dose distribution will be represented by a series of isodose curves (like elevations on a topographic map) joining points that are expected to receive equal radiation dose levels. In clinical practice, the total treatment time for delivery of the multiple beams is an important consideration and should be kept relatively short (eg, <0.5 hours).

16.7.2 Isoeffect Curves

Different fractionation schedules that give the same level of biologic effect can be presented in the form of an isoeffect curve. Isoeffect curves are generated by plotting the total radiation dose to give a certain biologic effect against the overall treatment time, fraction number, or fraction size, as illustrated in Figure 16–26. Experimental studies, performed mainly in rodents, have established isoeffect curves for different normal tissues using end points of either early or late radiation damage. Some of these isoeffect curves are shown in Figure 16–27, with the dashed blue lines representing early tissue responses and the red solid lines late responses. The isoeffect lines for late responses are steeper than those for early responses, meaning that a larger increase in total dose is required to give the same level of late toxicity as the dose per fraction is reduced and the number of fractions increased. This implies a greater capacity for the repair of damage in late-responding tissues, resulting in a larger sparing effect of fractionation. Although the observation that late-responding normal tissues demonstrate greater repair capacity than early-responding normal tissues was made decades ago, the responsible biologic mechanisms remain poorly understood. Nevertheless, this is a fundamental radiobiologic principle underlying altered fractionation schedules using multiple daily fractions in clinical radiotherapy. This is discussed in more detail in Section 16.7.4.

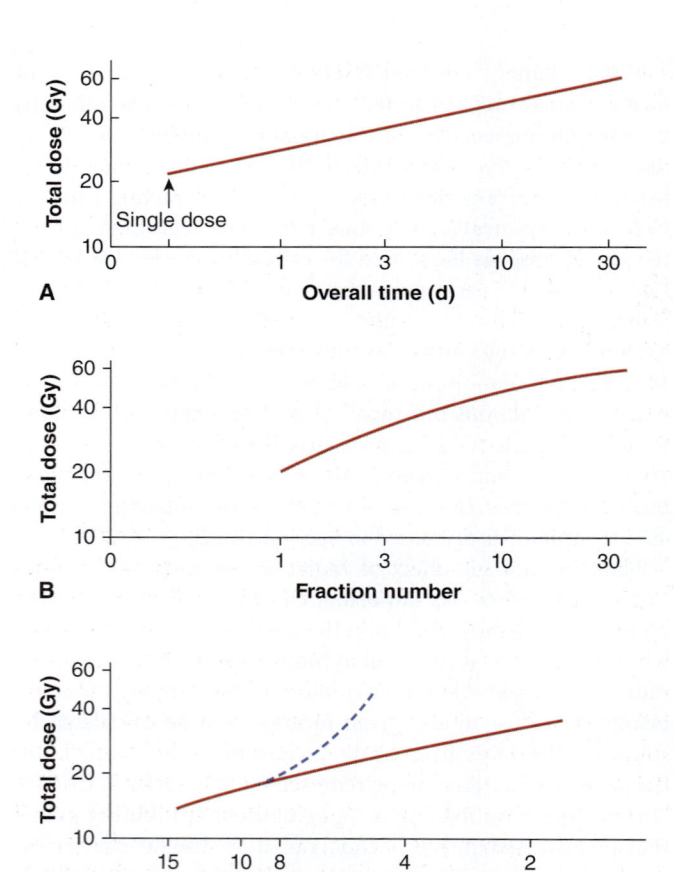

FIGURE 16–26 Isoeffect curves for fractionated treatments plotted in 3 different formats. A) Line plotted by Strandqvist (1944) to define normal tissue tolerance and control of carcinoma of the skin and lip using the axes of total dose and overall treatment time. **B)** Isoeffect curve for damage to pig skin plotted as total dose versus number of fractions (adapted from Fowler, 1971.) **C)** Isoeffect curve for the crypt cells of the mouse intestine plotted as total dose versus fraction size using an inverted scale. The solid (red) line is for fractions given 3 hours apart and the dashed (blue) line for fractions given 24 hours apart. All 3 curves illustrate that the total (isoeffective) dose increases with fractionated treatment.

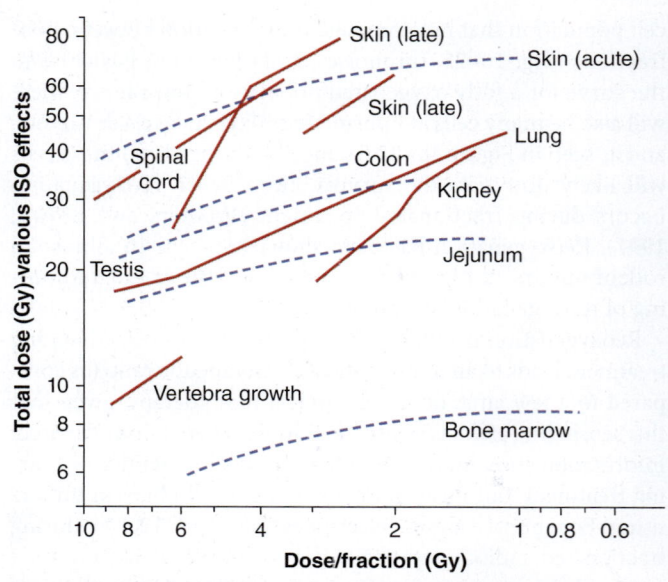

FIGURE 16–27 Isoeffect curves for a number of rodent tissues obtained using a variety of different cell survival or functional assays. The total dose required to obtain a fixed level of tissue damage is plotted as a function of the dose/fraction. The displacement of the curves on the vertical axis is a result of the fact that different isoeffective end points were used for the different tissues.

16.7.3 The Linear Quadratic Equation and Models for Isoeffect

Modeling isoeffect relationships (particularly for normal tissues) can allow appropriate choice of dose and schedule when changing fractionation schedules. Several models have been proposed, but most modeling is currently based on the linear-quadratic (LQ) equation (see Chap. 15, Appendix 15.1). In using the LQ model, it is assumed that each fraction has an equal effect; thus, for a fractionated regime (n fractions of size d), the surviving fraction of cells (SF) is

$$SF = e^{-n(\alpha d + \beta d^2)} \quad \text{[Eq. 16.3]}$$

This reduces to

$$-\ln SF = n(\alpha d + \beta d^2) \quad \text{[Eq. 16.4]}$$

It is further assumed that if different fractionation regimes (eg, n_1 fractions of size d_1 and n_2 fractions of size d_2) are isoeffective for a given tissue, they lead to the same SF. Thus, we have

$$\text{Isoeffect } (E) = -\ln SF = n_1(\alpha d_1 + \beta d_1^2)$$
$$= n_2(\alpha d_2 + \beta d_2^2) \quad \text{[Eq. 16.5]}$$

Equation (16.5) can then be simplified to give

$$\frac{n_1 d_1}{n_2 d_2} = \frac{(\alpha + \beta d_2)}{(\alpha + \beta d_1)} \quad \text{[Eq. 16.6]}$$

or

$$\frac{n_1 d_1}{n_2 d_2} = \frac{\left(\frac{\alpha}{\beta} + d_2\right)}{\left(\frac{\alpha}{\beta} + d_1\right)} \quad \text{[Eq. 16.7]}$$

From this relationship and knowing the values of n_1, d_1, n_2, and d_2 in isoeffect schedules, the constant α/β can be determined for a particular tissue. This constant can then be used in the equation to predict other isoeffective treatment schedules. The α/β ratio for a tumor type or tissue reflects the sensitivity of the tissue to fractionation. We can see from Eq. 16.7 that as α/β increases, the fraction size d becomes less significant and the effect is determined by the total dose nd. Hence, fractionation has a smaller sparing effect in tissues with large α/β than in tissue with low α/β. The therapeutic ratio hence favors fractionation when the α/β of the tumor is higher than that of the limiting normal tissue.

Data similar to those shown in Figure 16–27 have been used to estimate α/β values for different normal tissues in rodents. In general, late-responding normal tissues have α/β values in the range of 2 to 5 Gy, whereas early-responding normal tissues have α/β values in the range of 8 to 12 Gy. Tumors generally have values similar to or greater than early-responding normal tissues. The available data for human tissues suggest values in the same ranges, but confidence limits are large and grouping the responses of different tissues as described above is an oversimplification. Similarly, there are exceptions to the general rule that all tumors have α/β values similar to or greater than those for early-responding tissues, particularly for some slowly growing tumors. For example, studies suggest that prostate and breast cancers may have low α/β values between 1 and 4 Gy, suggesting a large repair capacity (eg, Owen et al, 2006).

Critical to the original derivation of the LQ model was the assumption that the primary factor underlying normal tissue responses to irradiation was killing of the relevant parenchymal cell population. As discussed in Section 16.5, normal tissue response to irradiation is now recognized as multifactorial, and this simplifying assumption is unlikely to be correct. Nevertheless, the model has proven to be valuable in the clinic provided that it is not extrapolated to predict the effects of fractionation schedules that are very different from clinical experience (eg, fraction sizes outside the range of 1-5 Gy). There is controversy as to whether the model can be used to predict responses to schedules with larger doses per fraction (Brown et al, 2014).

In the original LQ model, there was no consideration of the effect of treatment time: this is a limitation that applies primarily to early normal tissue (and tumor) responses, where repopulation plays a substantial role. Also, it was assumed that there is complete repair between the fractions, which is incorrect when the interfraction interval is too short or where repair of sublethal damage is slow, as occurs in some late-responding tissues, such as neural tissues. Modifications to the model allow corrections to be made for these factors, but there remains uncertainty in their ability to predict outcomes when dose and schedule are modified. More detailed discussion can be found in Joiner and van der Kogel (2018) and Hall and Giaccia (2018).

16.7.4 Altered Fractionation Schedules

The possibility of obtaining a therapeutic gain by exploiting the higher capacity for repair of radiation damage in late-responding normal tissues, as compared with early-responding normal tissues and many tumors, has been investigated by reducing the fraction size below that used conventionally (from approximately 2 Gy to 1-1.5 Gy) and increasing the number of fractions. The increase in dose that can be tolerated at the isoeffective level of late normal tissue damage should be greater than that required to maintain the same level of tumor control, meaning that the tumor would receive a larger biologically effective dose and hence the control rate should be higher.

The larger number of fractions required must be given more than once per day (or over weekends) if the treatment time is not to be prolonged. Such a treatment protocol is termed *hyperfractionation*. Clinical trials for patients with head and neck cancers evaluating a larger total dose delivered by hyperfractionation (2 fractions per day with 4- to 6-hour intervals) have reported an increase in local control with no difference in late normal tissue damage (see Horiot et al, 1992), although others (Fu et al, 2000) reported increased late effects as well as improved tumor control in their study.

The intent of hyperfractionation is to reduce late effects while achieving the same or better tumor control and the same or slightly increased early effects. The time interval between the fractions must be sufficiently long to allow for complete repair to occur. Repair kinetics have been estimated in normal rodent tissues, and half-times for repair ranged from 0.5 hours in jejunum to 1 to 2 hours in skin, lung, and kidney, so that repair will be complete in most normal tissues after an interfraction interval of 6 to 8 hours. However, for some late-responding tissues in humans, including nervous tissue, estimated repair half-times are in the range of 3 to 5 hours, so repair may not be complete even with an interfraction interval of 8 hours (Bentzen et al, 1999; Lee et al, 1999). Thus, an increase in late morbidity would be expected when multiple fractions per day are given to fields that include the spinal cord, as was observed in the CHART (Continuous Hyperfractionated Accelerated Radiotherapy) trials in which patients were given 3 fractions per day (Dische and Saunders, 1989). An increase in early normal tissue reactions would be expected with hyperfractionation because the larger α/β value for early-responding tissues implies a smaller change in the amount of repair as fraction size is reduced relative to that occurring in late-responding tissues (that have smaller α/β values). Severe mucositis was observed in the CHART trial (see Fig. 16–18), but the very short total treatment time limited the possibility for repopulation to occur in the mucosa and this was likely also a contributing factor.

Shortening of the overall treatment time has also been investigated as an approach to improving the therapeutic ratio because it reduces the time for repopulation to occur in the tumor during treatment (see Sec. 16.6.2). A similar effect might be achieved by blocking growth factors or their receptors, which are required for tumor cell proliferation. The tolerance of late-responding normal tissues should be little affected because cell proliferation is slow within them. Reduced treatment time is achieved by giving more than 1 fraction per day with standard dose fractions of 1.8 to 2.5 Gy, usually given 6 to 8 hours apart to allow for repair (although these time intervals may be insufficient to allow full repair in some late-responding tissues, as discussed above). This strategy is called *accelerated fractionation*. Randomized trials of accelerated compared with conventional fractionation for treatment of head and neck cancer have provided evidence supporting the importance of repopulation as a cause of treatment failure. A CHART study gave a reduced total dose in the experimental arm of the study, but maintained the same tumor control level,

TABLE 16–3 Summary of normal tissue responses to altered schedules of fractionated radiation.

Normal Tissue Reaction*	Acute	Late	Consequential
Tissues	Skin, oral mucosa, GI mucosa	Liver, kidney, spinal cord, lung or skin fibrosis, muscle	Skin, mucosa
Time of onset	<3 mo	>6 mo	>6 mo
α/β values	~8-12 Gy	~2-4 Gy	??
Fractionation response	Hyperfractionated ⇔ Accelerated ⇑	Hyperfractionated ⇓ Accelerated ⇔	Hyperfractionated ⇓ Accelerated ⇑

*See Sec. 16.5.1 for definition of normal tissue reactions.

with a slight reduction in late morbidity (Dische et al, 1997). A second study, which gave a similar total dose in both arms, reported increased tumor control in the accelerated fractionation arm, but there was also increased late toxicity (Horiot et al, 1997). This increased toxicity was likely a result of the short (4-hour) interfraction interval, which was probably not sufficient to allow for complete repair between the fractions. Table 16–3 outlines factors relating to altered fractionation schedules and their effects on acute, late, and consequential normal tissue reactions. A meta-analysis of studies of altered fractionation regimes in head and neck squamous cell cancers concluded that hyperfractionation resulted in less acute and late toxic effects compared with accelerated fractionation (Lacas et al, 2017).

A more extreme form of accelerated therapy involves SBRT to treat some tumors, including those in the brain, in which large single doses or a few large fractions are given (3-5 fractions of 8-20 Gy each). This technique has been applied for localized treatments of small primary lesions and isolated metastases, particularly in the lung (Timmerman et al, 2014). Such treatments are expected to cause complete loss of normal tissue function in the high-dose region of the beam, and tolerability of such treatments depends on the small volume irradiated, its location, and the reserve capacity of the unirradiated normal tissues involved (see Sec. 16.5.3).

SUMMARY

- Radiotherapy for cancer has developed empirically and usually involves giving 25 to 40 individual dose fractions of approximately 2 Gy once daily, over a period of 5-8 weeks.
- Improvements in technology have led to the introduction of conformal and intensity-modulated radiotherapy, allowing a decrease in normal tissue dose (and, hence, side effects) with dose escalation to tumor tissues.
- Other radiotherapy technologies that have improved the therapeutic ratio through physical means for some types of tumors include high-LET irradiation, brachytherapy, and changes in fractionation.
- Four biologic factors (the "4 Rs") influence response to fractionated treatment and the therapeutic ratio. These are repair of radiation damage, repopulation of damaged tissues by proliferation of surviving cells, redistribution of proliferating cells through the cell cycle, and reoxygenation of hypoxic cells. Repair and repopulation are the reasons why normal tissues can tolerate a larger total dose when it is fractionated, and repair is the main process influencing late radiation damage that is often dose limiting. Repopulation by tumor cells during the latter part of conventional (5- to 7-week) fractionated treatments increases the dose required for tumor control. Reoxygenation in tumors contributes to the improved therapeutic ratio obtained with fractionated treatment.
- Both tumor and normal tissue responses to irradiation are complex. Radiation can kill individual tumor and normal cells directly, and this can be expressed as mitosis-linked cell death or, in a few tissues, as early apoptosis. Damage to vasculature may lead to secondary death of cells. Particularly in normal tissues, there are other indirect effects, such as the induction of cytokines and inflammation that can influence early and late tissue responses.
- Tumor control requires the killing of all the tumor stem cells but there is heterogeneity in cellular radiosensitivity in tumors as a result of genetic and microenvironmental factors.
- Different fractionated schedules that give an equal level of normal tissue response or tumor control can be expressed in the form of isoeffect relationships described by the parameter α/β of the LQ model. Late-responding tissues tend to have smaller α/β values than early-responding tissues, implying greater capacity for repair of damage that leads to late effects, but there is uncertainty about values for specific tissues and endpoints.
- A therapeutic gain can be achieved by using hyperfractionation, where treatment with smaller dose fractions is given 2 or 3 times per day, but if the time between fractions is too short, increased late normal tissue damage may occur.
- Giving treatments more than once per day with the aim of reducing overall treatment time (accelerated fractionation) can also lead to a therapeutic gain if repopulation occurs more rapidly in the tumors than in the dose-limiting normal tissues and sufficient time is allowed between the fractions for full repair to occur.

▶ Factors predicting for response to fractionated radiotherapy include genomic instability, HPV status, mutations in DNA repair machinery and tumor hypoxia. Genetic analyses of tumors and normal cells of patients may lead to better predictive assays.

REFERENCES

Ahn GO, Tseng D, Liao CH, Dorie MJ, Czechowicz A, Brown JM. Inhibition of Mac-1 (CD11b/CD18) enhances tumor response to radiation by reducing myeloid cell recruitment. *Proc Natl Acad Sci U S A* 2010;107(18):8363-8368.

Antonadou D, Throuvalas N, Petridis A, Bolanos N, Sagriotis A, Synodinou M. Effect of amifostine on toxicities associated with radiochemotherapy in patients with locally advanced non-small-cell lung cancer. *Int J Radiat Oncol Biol Phys* 2003;57(2):402-408.

Antonia SJ, Villegas A, Daniel D, et al. Durvalumab after chemoradiotherapy in stage III non-small-cell lung cancer. *N Engl J Med* 2017;377(20):1919-1929.

Ashton TM, Fokas E, Kunz-Schughart LA, et al. The antimalarial atovaquone increases radiosensitivity by alleviating tumour hypoxia. *Nat Commun* 2016;7:12308.

Autio KA, Scher HI, Morris MJ. Therapeutic strategies for bone metastases and their clinical sequelae in prostate cancer. *Curr Treat Options Oncol* 2012;13(2):174-188.

Barth RF, Mi P, Yang W. Boron delivery agents for neutron capture therapy of cancer. *Cancer Commun (Lond)* 2018; 38(1):35.

Basch E, Reeve BB, Mitchell SA, et al. Development of the National Cancer Institute's patient-reported outcomes version of the common terminology criteria for adverse events (PRO-CTCAE). *J Natl Cancer Inst* 2014 Sep 29;106(9).

Bauman G, Rumble RB, Chen J, Loblaw A, Warde P. Intensity-modulated radiotherapy in the treatment of prostate cancer. *Clin Oncol (R Coll Radiol)* 2012;24(7):461-473.

Begg AC, Stewart FA, Vens C. Strategies to improve radiotherapy with targeted drugs. *Nat Rev Cancer* 2011;11(4):239-253.

Bentzen SM, Constine LS, Deasy JO, et al. Quantitative Analyses of Normal Tissue Effects in the Clinic (QUANTEC): an introduction to the scientific issues. *Int J Radiat Oncol Biol Phys* 2010;76(3)(suppl):S3-S9.

Bentzen SM, Saunders MI, Dische S. Repair halftimes estimated from observations of treatment-related morbidity after CHART or conventional radiotherapy in head and neck cancer. *Radiother Oncol* 1999;53(3):219-226.

Bentzen SM, Saunders MI, Dische S, Bond SJ. Radiotherapy-related early morbidity in head and neck cancer: quantitative clinical radiobiology as deduced from the CHART trial. *Radiother Oncol* 2001;60(2):123-135.

Bjork-Eriksson T, West C, Karlsson E, Mercke C. Tumor radiosensitivity (SF2) is a prognostic factor for local control in head and neck cancers. *Int J Radiat Oncol Biol Phys* 2000;46(1):13-19.

Bonner JA, Harari PM, Giralt J, et al. Radiotherapy plus cetuximab for locoregionally advanced head and neck cancer: 5-year survival data from a phase 3 randomised trial, and relation between cetuximab-induced rash and survival. *Lancet Oncol* 2010;11(1):21-28.

Bonnet M, Hong CR, Wong WW, et al. Next-generation hypoxic cell radiosensitizers: nitroimidazole alkylsulfonamides. *J Med Chem* 2018;61(3):1241-1254.

Bouquet F, Pal A, Pilones KA, et al. TGFβ1 inhibition increases the radiosensitivity of breast cancer cells in vitro and promotes tumor control by radiation in vivo. *Clin Cancer Res* 2011;17(21):6754-6765.

Bristow RG, Hill RP. Hypoxia and metabolism. Hypoxia, DNA repair and genetic instability. *Nat Rev Cancer* 2008;8(3): 180-192.

Bristow RG, Alexander B, Baumann M, et al. Combining precision radiotherapy with molecular targeting and immunomodulatory agents: a guideline by the American Society for Radiation Oncology. *Lancet Oncol* 2018;19(5):e240-e251.

Brizel DM, Wasserman, TH, Henke M, et al. Phase III randomized trial of amifostine as a radioprotector in head and neck cancer. *J Clin Oncol* 2000;18(19):3339-3345.

Brown JM. The hypoxic cell: a target for selective cancer therapy—Eighteenth Bruce F. Cain Memorial Award lecture. *Cancer Res* 1999;59(23):5863-5870.

Brown JM, Carlson DJ, Brenner DJ. The tumor radiobiology of SRS and SBRT: are more than the 5 Rs involved? *Int J Radiat Oncol Biol Phys* 2014;88(2):254-262.

Brush J, Lipnick SL, Phillips T, Sitko J, McDonald JT, McBride WH. Molecular mechanisms of late normal tissue injury. *Semin Radiat Oncol* 2007;17(2):121-130.

Budaus L, Bolla M, Bossi A, et al. Functional outcomes and complications following radiation therapy for prostate cancer: a critical analysis of the literature. *Eur Urol* 2012;61(1): 112-127.

Bush RS. The significance of anemia in clinical radiation therapy. *Int J Radiat Oncol Biol Phys* 1986;12(11):2047-2050.

Chapman JD, Dugle DL, Reuvers AP, Meeker BE, Borsa J. Letter: studies on the radiosensitizing effect of oxygen in Chinese hamster cells. *Int J Radiat Biol Relat Stud Phys Chem Med* 1974;26(4):383-389.

Christiaens M, Collette S, Overgaard J, et al. Quality assurance of radiotherapy in the ongoing EORTC 1219-DAHANCA-29 trial for HPV/p16 negative squamous cell carcinoma of the head and neck: results of the benchmark case procedure. *Radiother Oncol* 2017;123(3):424-430.

Dainiak N, Waselenko JK, Armitage JO, MacVittie TJ, Farese AM. The hematologist and radiation casualties. *Hematology Am Soc Hematol Educ Program* 2003;473-496.

Dawson LA, Sharpe MB. Image-guided radiotherapy: rationale, benefits, and limitations. *Lancet Oncol* 2006;7(10): 848-858.

Deacon J, Peckham MJ, Steel GG. The radioresponsiveness of human tumours and the initial slope of the cell survival curve. *Radiother Oncol* 1984;2(4):317-323.

Debeljak N, Solar P, Sytkowski AJ. Erythropoietin and cancer: the unintended consequences of anemia correction. *Front Immunol* 2014;5:563.

Denekamp J. Cell kinetics and radiation biology. *Int J Radiat Biol Relat Stud Phys Chem Med* 1986;49(2):357-380.

Denham JW, Hauer-Jensen M. The radiotherapeutic injury—a complex "wound." *Radiother Oncol* 2002;63(2):129-145.

Derer A, Frey B, Fietkau R, Gaipl US. Immune-modulating properties of ionizing radiation: rationale for the treatment of cancer by combination radiotherapy and immune checkpoint inhibitors. *Cancer Immunol Immunother* 2016;65(7):779-786.

Dische S, Saunders M, Barrett A, Harvey A, Gibson D, Parmar M. A randomised multicentre trial of CHART versus conventional radiotherapy in head and neck cancer. *Radiother Oncol* 1997;44(2):123-136.

Dische S, Saunders MI. Continuous, hyperfractionated, accelerated radiotherapy (CHART): an interim report upon late morbidity. *Radiother Oncol* 1989;16(1):65-72.

Dunst J, Hansgen G, Lautenschlager C, Fuchsel G, Becker A. Oxygenation of cervical cancers during radiotherapy and radiotherapy + cis-retinoic acid/interferon. *Int J Radiat Oncol Biol Phys* 1999;43(2):367-373.

Edvardsen H, Landmark-Hoyvik H, Reinertsen KV, et al. SNP in TXNRD2 associated with radiation-induced fibrosis: a study of genetic variation in reactive oxygen species metabolism and signaling. *Int J Radiat Oncol Biol Phys* 2013;86(4):791-799.

Eke I, Cordes N. Radiobiology goes 3D: how ECM and cell morphology impact on cell survival after irradiation. *Radiother Oncol* 2011;99(3):271-278.

Fertil B, Malaise EP. Inherent cellular radiosensitivity as a basic concept for human tumor radiotherapy. *Int J Radiat Oncol Biol Phys* 1981;7(5):621-629.

Fowler JF. Experimental animal results relating to time-dose relationships in radiotherapy and the "ret" concept. *Br J Radiol* 1971;44(518):81-90.

Fowler JF. What to do with neutrons in radiotherapy: a suggestion. *Radiother Oncol* 1988;13(3):233-235.

Fowler JF, Stern BE. Fractionation and dose-rate. II. Dose-time relationships in radiotherapy and the validity of cell survival curve models. *Br J Radiol* 1963;36:163-173.

Fu KK, Pajak TF, Trotti A, et al. A Radiation Therapy Oncology Group (RTOG) phase III randomized study to compare hyperfractionation and two variants of accelerated fractionation to standard fractionation radiotherapy for head and neck squamous cell carcinomas: first report of RTOG 9003. *Int J Radiat Oncol Biol Phys* 2000;48(1):7-16.

Fyles A, Milosevic M, Hedley D, et al. Tumor hypoxia has independent predictor impact only in patients with node-negative cervix cancer. *J Clin Oncol* 2002;20(3):680-687.

Fyles AW, Milosevic M, Pintilie M, Syed A, Hill RP. Anemia, hypoxia and transfusion in patients with cervix cancer: a review. *Radiother Oncol* 2000;57(1):13-19.

Garcia-Barros M, Thin TH, Maj J, et al. Impact of stromal sensitivity on radiation response of tumors implanted in SCID hosts revisited. *Cancer Res* 2010;70(20):8179-8186.

Gillison ML, Trotti AM, Harris J, et al. Radiotherapy plus cetuximab or cisplatin in human papillomavirus-positive oropharyngeal cancer (NRG Oncology RTOG 1016): a randomised, multicentre, non-inferiority trial. *Lancet* 2019;393(10166):40-50.

Goel S, Duda DG, Xu L, et al. Normalization of the vasculature for treatment of cancer and other diseases. *Physiol Rev* 2011;91(3):1071-1121.

Green DJ, Press OW. Whither radioimmunotherapy: to be or not to be? *Cancer Res* 2017;77(9):2191-2196.

Hall EJ, Giaccia AJ. *Radiobiology from the Radiologist*. 8th ed. Philadelphia, PA: Lippincott; 2018.

Hanahan D, Weinberg RA. Hallmarks of cancer: the next generation. *Cell* 2011;144(5):646-674.

Henke M, Laszig R, Rube C, et al. Erythropoietin to treat head and neck cancer patients with anaemia undergoing radiotherapy: randomised, double-blind, placebo-controlled trial. *Lancet* 2003;362(9392):1255-1260.

Herskind C, Talbot CJ, Kerns SL, Veldwijk MR, Rosenstein BS, West CM. Radiogenomics: a systems biology approach to understanding genetic risk factors for radiotherapy toxicity? *Cancer Lett* 2016;382(1):95-109.

Hill RP, Bristow RG, Fyles A, Koritzinsky M, Milosevic M, Wouters BG. Hypoxia and predicting radiation response. *Semin Radiat Oncol* 2015;25(4):260-272.

Hill RP, Bush RS, Yeung P. The effect of anaemia on the fraction of hypoxic cells in an experimental tumour. *Br J Radiol* 1971;44(520):299-304.

Hockel M, Schlenger K, Aral B, Mitze M, Schaffer U, Vaupel P. Association between tumor hypoxia and malignant progression in advanced cancer of the uterine cervix. *Cancer Res* 1996;56(19):4509-4515.

Hoeller U, Tribius S, Kuhlmey A, Grader K, Fehlauer F, Alberti W. Increasing the rate of late toxicity by changing the score? A comparison of RTOG/EORTC and LENT/SOMA scores. *Int J Radiat Oncol Biol Phys* 2003;55(4):1013-1018.

Hoff CM, Grau C, Overgaard J. Effect of smoking on oxygen delivery and outcome in patients treated with radiotherapy for head and neck squamous cell carcinoma—a prospective study. *Radiother Oncol* 2012;103(1):38-44.

Hoff CM, Lassen P, Eriksen JG, et al. Does transfusion improve the outcome for HNSCC patients treated with radiotherapy?—results from the randomized DAHANCA 5 and 7 trials. *Acta Oncol* 2011;50(7):1006-1014.

Horiot JC, Bontemps P, van den Bogaert W, et al. Accelerated fractionation (AF) compared to conventional fractionation (CF) improves loco-regional control in the radiotherapy of advanced head and neck cancers: results of the EORTC 22851 randomized trial. *Radiother Oncol* 1997;44(2):111-121.

Horiot JC, Le Fur R, N'Guyen T, et al. Hyperfractionation versus conventional fractionation in oropharyngeal carcinoma: final analysis of a randomized trial of the EORTC cooperative group of radiotherapy. *Radiother Oncol* 1992;25(4):231-241.

Hoskin PJ, Rojas AM, Bentzen SM, Saunders MI. Radiotherapy with concurrent carbogen and nicotinamide in bladder carcinoma. *J Clin Oncol* 2010;28(33):4912-4918.

Janssens GO, Rademakers SE, Terhaard CH, et al. Accelerated radiotherapy with carbogen and nicotinamide for laryngeal cancer: results of a phase III randomized trial. *J Clin Oncol* 2012;30(15):1777-1783.

Janssens GO, Rademakers SE, Terhaard CH, et al. Improved recurrence-free survival with ARCON for anemic patients with laryngeal cancer. *Clin Cancer Res* 2014;20(5):1345-1354.

Jensen SB, Pedersen AM, Vissink A, et al. A systematic review of salivary gland hypofunction and xerostomia induced by cancer therapies: management strategies and economic impact. *Support Care Cancer* 2010;18(8):1061-1079.

Joiner MC, van der Kogel AJ. *Basic Clinical Radiobiology*. Boca Raton, FL: CRC Press/Taylor and Francis Group; 2018.

Juergens RA, Bratman SV, Tsao MS, et al. Biology and patterns of response to EGFR-inhibition in squamous cell cancers of the lung and head & neck. *Cancer Treat Rev* 2017;54:43-57.

Kainthola A, Haritwal T, Tiwari M, et al. Immunological aspect of radiation-induced pneumonitis, current treatment strategies, and future prospects. *Front Immunol* 2017;8:506.

Kioi M, Vogel H, Schultz G, et al. Inhibition of vasculogenesis, but not angiogenesis, prevents the recurrence of glioblastoma after irradiation in mice. *J Clin Invest* 2010;120(3):694-705.

Krause M, Yaromina A, Eicheler W, Koch U, Baumann M. Cancer stem cells: targets and potential biomarkers for radiotherapy. *Clin Cancer Res* 2011;17(23):7224-7229.

Kulkarni HR, Singh A, Langbein T, et al. Theranostics of prostate cancer: from molecular imaging to precision molecular radiotherapy targeting the prostate specific membrane antigen. *Br J Radiol* 2018;91(1091):20180308.

Lacas B, Bourhis J, Overgaard, et al. Role of radiotherapy fractionation in head and neck cancers (MARCH): an updated meta-analysis. *Lancet Oncol* 2017;18(9):1221-1237.

Lalonde E, Ishkanian AS, Sykes J, et al. Tumour genomic and microenvironmental heterogeneity for integrated prediction of 5-year biochemical recurrence of prostate cancer: a retrospective cohort study. *Lancet Oncol* 2014;15(13):1521-1532.

Lee AW, Sze WM, Fowler JF, Chappell R, Leung SF, Teo P. Caution on the use of altered fractionation for nasopharyngeal carcinoma. *Radiother Oncol* 1999;52(3):207-211.

Levine EL, Renehan A, Gossiel R, et al. Apoptosis, intrinsic radiosensitivity and prediction of radiotherapy response in cervical carcinoma. *Radiother Oncol* 1995;37(1):1-9.

Lindegaard JC, Grau C. Has the outlook improved for amifostine as a clinical radioprotector? *Radiother Oncol* 2000;57(2):113-118.

Ljungkvist AS, Bussink J, Kaanders JH, et al. Hypoxic cell turnover in different solid tumor lines. *Int J Radiat Oncol Biol Phys* 2005;62(4):1157-1168.

Lock S, Perrin R, Seidlitz A, et al. Residual tumour hypoxia in head-and-neck cancer patients undergoing primary radiochemotherapy, final results of a prospective trial on repeat FMISO-PET imaging. *Radiother Oncol* 2017;124(3):533-540.

Lunt SJ, Chaudary N, Hill RP. The tumor microenvironment and metastatic disease. *Clin Exp Metastasis* 2009;26(1):19-34.

Marie-Egyptienne DT, Lohse I, Hill RP. Cancer stem cells, the epithelial to mesenchymal transition (EMT) and radioresistance: potential role of hypoxia. *Cancer Lett* 2013;341(1):63-72.

Marks LB, Bentzen SM, Deasy JO, et al. Radiation dose-volume effects in the lung. *Int J Radiat Oncol Biol Phys* 2010a;76(3)(suppl):S70-S76.

Marks LB, Yorke ED, Jackson A, et al. Use of normal tissue complication probability models in the clinic. *Int J Radiat Oncol Biol Phys* 2010b;76(3)(suppl):S10-S19.

McKelvey KJ, Hudson AL, Back M, Eade T, Diakos CI. Radiation, inflammation and the immune response in cancer. *Mamm Genome* 2018;29(11-12):843-865.

Mehanna H, Robinson M, Hartley A, et al. Radiotherapy plus cisplatin or cetuximab in low-risk human papillomavirus-positive oropharyngeal cancer (De-ESCALaTE HPV): an open-label randomised controlled phase 3 trial. *Lancet* 2019;393(10166):51-60.

Mettler FA, Jr, Voelz GL. Major radiation exposure—what to expect and how to respond. *N Engl J Med* 2002;346(20):1554-1561.

Milosevic M, Warde P, Menard C, et al. Tumor hypoxia predicts biochemical failure following radiotherapy for clinically localized prostate cancer. *Clin Cancer Res* 2012;18(7):2108-2114.

Morton G, Chung HT, McGuffin M, et al. Prostate high dose-rate brachytherapy as monotherapy for low and intermediate risk prostate cancer: early toxicity and quality-of life results from a randomized phase II clinical trial of one fraction of 19Gy or two fractions of 13.5Gy. *Radiother Oncol* 2017;122(1):87-92.

Nytko KJ, Grgic I, Bender S, et al. The hypoxia-activated prodrug evofosfamide in combination with multiple regimens of radiotherapy. *Oncotarget* 2017;8(14):23702-23712.

Overgaard J. Hypoxic modification of radiotherapy in squamous cell carcinoma of the head and neck—a systematic review and meta-analysis. *Radiother Oncol* 2011;100(1):22-32.

Overgaard J, Hansen HS, Overgaard M, et al. A randomized double-blind phase III study of nimorazole as a hypoxic radiosensitizer of primary radiotherapy in supraglottic larynx and pharynx carcinoma. Results of the Danish Head and Neck Cancer Study (DAHANCA) Protocol 5-85. *Radiother Oncol* 1998;46(2):135-146.

Overgaard J, Horsman MR. Modification of hypoxia-induced radioresistance in tumors by the use of oxygen and sensitizers. *Semin Radiat Oncol* 1996;6(1):10-21.

Owen JR, Ashton A, Bliss JM, et al. Effect of radiotherapy fraction size on tumour control in patients with early-stage breast cancer after local tumour excision: long-term results of a randomised trial. *Lancet Oncol* 2006;7(6):467-471.

Paris F, Fuks Z, Kang A, et al. Endothelial apoptosis as the primary lesion initiating intestinal radiation damage in mice. *Science* 2001;293(5528):293-297.

Parker C, Nilsson S, Heinrich D, et al. Alpha emitter radium-223 and survival in metastatic prostate cancer. *N Engl J Med* 2013;369(3):213-223.

Peeters SG, Zegers CM, Biemans R, et al. TH-302 in combination with radiotherapy enhances the therapeutic outcome and is associated with pretreatment [18F]HX4 hypoxia PET imaging. *Clin Cancer Res* 2015;21(13):2984-2992.

Peters LJ, O'Sullivan B, Giralt J, et al. Critical impact of radiotherapy protocol compliance and quality in the treatment of advanced head and neck cancer: results from TROG 02.02. *J Clin Oncol* 2010;28(18):2996-3001.

Rademakers SE, Hoogsteen IJ, Rijken PF, et al. Pattern of CAIX expression is prognostic for outcome and predicts response to ARCON in patients with laryngeal cancer treated in a phase III randomized trial. *Radiother Oncol* 2013;108(3):517-522.

Raju MR. Particle radiotherapy: historical developments and current status. *Radiat Res* 1996;145(4):391-407.

Rischin D, Hicks RJ, Fisher R, et al. Prognostic significance of [18F]-misonidazole positron emission tomography-detected tumor hypoxia in patients with advanced head and neck cancer randomly assigned to chemoradiation with or without tirapazamine: a substudy of Trans-Tasman Radiation Oncology Group Study 98.02. *J Clin Oncol* 2006;24(13):2098-2104.

Rischin D, Peters LJ, O'Sullivan B, et al. Tirapazamine, cisplatin, and radiation versus cisplatin and radiation for advanced squamous cell carcinoma of the head and neck (TROG 02.02, HeadSTART): a phase III trial of the Trans-Tasman Radiation Oncology Group. *J Clin Oncol* 2010;28(18):2989-2995.

Rodemann HP, Bamberg M. Cellular basis of radiation-induced fibrosis. *Radiother Oncol* 1995;35(2):83-90.

Rodriguez-Ruiz ME, Vanpouille-Box C, Melero I, Formenti SC, Demaria S. Immunological mechanisms responsible for radiation-induced abscopal effect. *Trends Immunol* 2018;39(8):644-655.

Rotolo J, Stancevic B, Zhang J, et al. Anti-ceramide antibody prevents the radiation gastrointestinal syndrome in mice. *J Clin Invest* 2012;122(5):1786-1790.

Russell NS, Begg AC. Editorial radiotherapy and oncology 2002: predictive assays for normal tissue damage. *Radiother Oncol* 2002;64(2):125-129.

Schaue D. A century of radiation therapy and adaptive immunity. *Front Immunol* 2017;8:431.

Seidenfeld J, Piper M, Flamm C, et al. Epoetin treatment of anemia associated with cancer therapy: a systematic review and meta-analysis of controlled clinical trials. *J Natl Cancer Inst* 2001;93(16):1204-1214.

Serrano NA, Kalman NS, Anscher MS. Reducing rectal injury in men receiving prostate cancer radiation therapy: current perspectives. *Cancer Manag Res* 2017;9:339-350.

Stewart FA, Dorr W. Milestones in normal tissue radiation biology over the past 50 years: from clonogenic cell survival to cytokine networks and back to stem cell recovery. *Int J Radiat Biol* 2009;85(7):574-586.

Strandqvist M. Studien Uber die kumulative Wirkung der Rontgenstrahlen bei Fracktionierung. *Acta Radiologica, Suppl LV*. 1944.

Straub JM, New J, Hamilton CD, Lominska C, Shnayder Y, Thomas SM. Radiation-induced fibrosis: mechanisms and implications for therapy. *J Cancer Res Clin Oncol* 2015;141(11):1985-1994.

Tamponi M, Gabriele D, Maggio, A, et al. Prostate cancer dose-response, fractionation sensitivity and repopulation parameters evaluation from 25 international radiotherapy outcome data sets. *Br J Radiol* 2019;92(1098):20180823.

Tan JSH, Lin X, Chua KLM, Lam PY, Soo KC, Chua MLK. Exploiting molecular genomics in precision radiation oncology: a marriage of biological and physical precision. *Chin Clin Oncol* 2017;6(suppl 2):S19.

Thames HD Jr, Withers HR, Peters LJ, Fletcher GH. Changes in early and late radiation responses with altered dose fractionation: implications for dose-survival relationships. *Int J Radiat Oncol Biol Phys* 1982;8(2):219-226.

Timmerman RD, Herman J, Cho LC. Emergence of stereotactic body radiation therapy and its impact on current and future clinical practice. *J Clin Oncol* 2014;32(26):2847-2854.

Toustrup K, Sorensen BS, Lassen P, et al. Gene expression classifier predicts for hypoxic modification of radiotherapy with nimorazole in squamous cell carcinomas of the head and neck. *Radiother Oncol* 2012;102(1):122-129.

Toustrup K, Sorensen BS, Nordsmark M, et al. Development of a hypoxia gene expression classifier with predictive impact for hypoxic modification of radiotherapy in head and neck cancer. *Cancer Res* 2011;71(17):5923-5931.

Travis EL, Liao ZX, Tucker SL. Spatial heterogeneity of the volume effect for radiation pneumonitis in mouse lung. *Int J Radiat Oncol Biol Phys* 1997;38(5):1045-1054.

Tucker SL, Thames HD, Brown BW, Mason KA, Hunter NR, Withers HR. Direct analyses of in vivo colony survival after single and fractionated doses of radiation. *Int J Radiat Biol* 1991;59(3):777-795.

Turesson, I. Individual variation and dose dependency in the progression rate of skin telangiectasia. *Int J Radiat Oncol Biol Phys* 1990;19(6):1569-1574.

UNSCEAR. *Sources and Effects of Ionizing Radiation Report to the General Assembly: Volume II: Annex D: Health Effects due to Radiation from the Chernobyl Accident*. New York, NY: United Nations; 2008.

Vaupel P, Kelleher DK, Hockel M. Oxygen status of malignant tumors: pathogenesis of hypoxia and significance for tumor therapy. *Semin Oncol* 2001;28(2)(suppl 8):29-35.

Vlashi E, Pajonk F. Cancer stem cells, cancer cell plasticity and radiation therapy. *Semin Cancer Biol* 2015;31:28-35.

Weber DC, Habrand JL, Hoppe BS, et al. Proton therapy for pediatric malignancies: Fact, figures and costs. A joint consensus statement from the pediatric subcommittee of PTCOG, PROS and EPTN. *Radiother Oncol* 2018;128(1):44-55.

Weiss JF, Landauer MR. History and development of radiation-protective agents. *Int J Radiat Biol* 2009;85(7):539-573.

West C, Rosenstein BS, Alsner J, et al. Establishment of a radiogenomics consortium. *Int J Radiat Oncol Biol Phys* 2010;76(5):1295-1296.

West CM, Davidson SE, Roberts SA, Hunter RD. The independence of intrinsic radiosensitivity as a prognostic factor for patient response to radiotherapy of carcinoma of the cervix. *Br J Cancer* 1997;76(9):1184-1190.

Westbury CB, Yarnold JR. Radiation fibrosis—current clinical and therapeutic perspectives. *Clin Oncol (R Coll Radiol)* 2012;24(10):657-672.

Withers HR, Mason KA. The kinetics of recovery in irradiated colonic mucosa of the mouse. *Cancer* 1974;34(3)(suppl):896-903.

Withers HR, Taylor JM, Maciejewski B. The hazard of accelerated tumor clonogen repopulation during radiotherapy. *Acta Oncol* 1988;27(2):131-146.

Wong CS, Minkin S, Hill RP. Linear-quadratic model underestimates sparing effect of small doses per fraction in rat spinal cord. *Radiother Oncol* 1992;23(3):176-184.

Wong JYC, Filippi AR, Dabaja BS, Yahalom J, Specht L. Total body irradiation: Guidelines from the International Lymphoma Radiation Oncology Group (ILROG). *Int J Radiat Oncol Biol Phys* 2018;101(3):521-529.

Wouters BG, Brown JM. Cells at intermediate oxygen levels can be more important than the "hypoxic fraction" in determining tumor response to fractionated radiotherapy. *Radiat Res* 1997;147(5):541-550.

Yamamoto T, Nakai K, Matsumura A. Boron neutron capture therapy for glioblastoma. *Cancer Lett* 2008;262(2):143-152.

Zaleska K, Bruechner K, Baumann M, Zips D, Yaromina A. Tumour-infiltrating CD11b+ myelomonocytes and response to fractionated irradiation of human squamous cell carcinoma (hSCC) xenografts. *Radiother Oncol* 2011;101(1):80-85.

Zhao X, Psarianos P, Ghoraie LS, et al. Metabolic regulation of dermal fibroblasts contributes to skin extracellular matrix homeostasis and fibrosis. *Nat Metab* 2019;1(1):147-157.

Zannella VE, Dal Pra A, Muaddi H, et al. Reprogramming metabolism with metformin improves tumor oxygenation and radiotherapy response. *Clin Cancer Res* 2013;19(24):6741-6750.

Zips D, Krause M, Yaromina A, et al. Epidermal growth factor receptor inhibitors for radiotherapy: biological rationale and preclinical results. *J Pharm Pharmacol* 2008;60(8):1019-1028.

Discovery and Evaluation of Anticancer Drugs

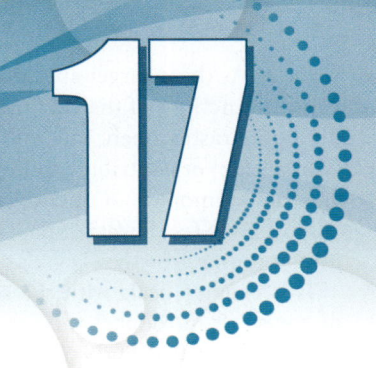

Kyaw Lwin Aung, David W. Cescon, and Aaron D. Schimmer

Chapter Outline

- 17.1 Introduction
- 17.2 Strategies to Develop Anticancer Drugs
  - 17.2.1 High Throughput DNA Sequencing
  - 17.2.2 Gene Expression and Identification of Potential Targets for Anticancer Drugs
  - 17.2.3 Functional Genomic Screens
  - 17.2.4 Identification of Active Drugs
- 17.3 New Strategies for Cancer Treatment
  - 17.3.1 Small Molecule Tyrosine Kinase Inhibitors (TKIs)
  - 17.3.2 Enzyme Inhibitors
  - 17.3.3 Antibody-Based Anticancer Therapies
  - 17.3.4 Disrupters of Protein-Protein Interactions
  - 17.3.5 Antisense Oligonucleotides and RNAi
  - 17.3.6 Directed Drug Delivery
- 17.4 Preclinical Evaluation of Potential Anticancer Drugs
  - 17.4.1 Evaluation for Activity Against Cultured Cells
  - 17.4.2 Evaluation of Potential Anticancer Drugs In vivo
- 17.5 Toxicity of Anticancer Drugs
  - 17.5.1 The Concept of Therapeutic Index
  - 17.5.2 Toxicity to Bone Marrow and Scheduling of Treatment
  - 17.5.3 Toxicity of Drugs to Other Proliferative Tissues
  - 17.5.4 Nausea, Vomiting, and Other Common Toxicities
  - 17.5.5 Drugs as Carcinogens
  - 17.5.6 Determinants of Normal-Tissue Toxicity
  - 17.5.7 Preclinical Data Needed to Support First in Human Trials
- 17.6 Treatment With Multiple Agents
  - 17.6.1 Influence on Therapeutic Index
  - 17.6.2 Synergy and Additivity
  - 17.6.3 Modifiers of Drug Activity or Toxicity
  - 17.6.4 Drugs and Radiation
  - 17.6.5 Relationship Between Tumor Remission and Cure
- Summary
- References

17.1 INTRODUCTION

Drug-based systemic therapy is used primarily as (1) the major treatment modality for a few types of curable malignancies, such as Hodgkin disease and other hematopoietic cancers, acute leukemia in children, and testicular cancer in men; (2) palliative treatment for many types of advanced cancers; and (3) adjuvant treatment before, during, or after local treatment (surgery and/or radiotherapy) with the dual aims of both eradicating occult micrometastases and of improving local control of the primary tumor. Such treatments usually involve a combination of drugs. The most important factors underlying the successful use of drugs in combination are (1) the ability to combine drugs at close to full tolerated doses with additive effects against tumors and less than additive toxicities to normal tissues and (2) the expectation that drug combinations will include at least 1 drug to which the tumor is sensitive. Since the first documented clinical use of chemotherapy in 1942, when the alkylating agent nitrogen mustard was used to obtain a brief clinical remission in a patient with lymphoma, there have been continuous efforts to develop new, effective anticancer therapies. Initially focused on cytotoxic chemotherapies (the pharmacology of which are described in Chap. 18), the number and range of cancer drugs has expanded, with more than 200 drugs or biologic agents licensed for use in North America, and many more undergoing clinical trials. New types of anticancer agents that have emerged include monoclonal antibodies (such as trastuzumab, cetuximab, bevacizumab, and blinatumomab) that target cell surface receptors, and small molecules that interact with various cell signaling or survival pathways (eg, imatinib, erlotinib, afatinib, venetoclax). These newer "targeted" agents (reviewed in Chap. 19) represent a substantial shift in emphasis in anticancer drug therapy. In contrast to conventional cytotoxic agents, which usually target proliferating cells and interact with DNA, these target specific pathways that interfere with various functions of the cell including those that promote cell division (trastuzumab, imatinib), cell survival, and apoptosis (venetoclax) or contribute to immune-mediated cellular damage (blinatumomab). Other agents, such as those that inhibit angiogenesis (eg, bevacizumab; see Chap. 11) act indirectly to inhibit tumor growth.

This chapter deals with the scientific basis of cancer drug discovery. It introduces the concepts of how cancer drug targets are identified and some of the approaches used to discover and design new drugs. The chapter also discusses the biologic properties of important anticancer drugs, experimental methods used to determine their activity, their toxicity to normal tissues, the concept of therapeutic index, and the biologic basis of using drugs in combination and with radiotherapy. The many causes of drug resistance are addressed in Chapters 18 and 19.

17.2 STRATEGIES TO DEVELOP ANTICANCER DRUGS

17.2.1 High Throughput DNA Sequencing

Although many chemotherapy drugs were developed by observing effects of compounds on cancer cells in culture and in experimental animals without knowledge of a specific molecular target, modern drug discovery begins with the identification of a therapeutic target. To identify novel targets, a variety of strategies can be employed, including surveying the mutations or expression of genes within a cancer cell to identify dysregulated genes, gene families, or pathways.

Improvements in the speed of DNA sequencing and reductions in cost have increased the ability to sequence the exomes of primary cancer samples and normal tissues from multiple patients, and to generate comprehensive molecular portraits of many tumor types (Bailey et al, 2018; see Chap. 2, Sec. 2.2.1.0). Through these studies, mutations in oncogenes or tumor suppressor genes that are potential therapeutic targets have been identified. For example, through a focused sequencing effort in patients with melanoma, BRAF V600E somatic mutations were identified in 52% of patients with melanoma (Davies et al, 2002). These mutations lead to constitutive activation of this kinase and signaling through the downstream MAP kinase pathway (see Chap. 6, Sec. 6.2.4). Based on the discovery of BRAF mutations in melanoma, the selective BRAF V600E inhibitor, vemurafenib, was developed. Vemurafenib produces clinical responses in patients with metastatic melanoma and improves survival when used as a single agent or in combination with other targeted therapies (Sosman et al, 2012; Larkin et al, 2014).

Subsequently, whole-exome sequencing of primary samples from patients with hairy cell leukemia identified the same BRAF V600E mutation in all tested samples. On the basis of this recognized "actionable alteration," vemurafenib was tested in patients with hairy cell leukemia, and responses in more than 95% of patients with relapsed or refractory disease were observed (Tiacci et al, 2015). However, vemurafenib is not universally active in all types of cancer with BRAF mutations, highlighting that other factors influence tumor dependencies and vulnerability to targeting.

One of the challenges in identifying drug targets through DNA sequencing is distinguishing between mutations that contribute to (and are critical for) cancer development and/or growth, known as "driver mutations," and mutations not associated with cancer development or growth, known as "passenger mutations." Driver mutations are potentially valuable drug targets, whereas inhibiting "passenger" mutations is not expected to have the same therapeutic effect. Differentiating between drivers and passengers is a complex process and can require use of advanced statistical analysis, structural studies to investigate the impact of the mutation on the protein structure, and molecular studies to demonstrate transformation as a result of overexpression of the mutant gene. However, the availability of increasingly large sequencing data sets of human cancers permits the development of computational tools to classify most commonly recurrent mutations as drivers or passengers (Bailey et al, 2018).

17.2.2 Gene Expression and Identification of Potential Targets for Anticancer Drugs

Similar to DNA sequencing that focuses on DNA mutations, messenger RNA (mRNA) derived from primary tumor and normal cells can be sequenced. RNA sequencing (described in Chap. 2, Sec. 2.2.12) provides a quantitative measure of expression of mRNA and can also identify alterations including oncogenic gene fusions (Fig. 17–1). Using bioinformatics, computer algorithms, and advanced statistical analysis, patterns of dysregulated genes and pathways that occur in a given cancer, or cancer subtype, can be identified. These may be targeted or may suggest pathways or targets of interest to inform the development of new cancer drugs or therapeutic strategies. RNA sequencing can also identify gene fusions and mutations that may be targets for new anticancer drugs. Oncogenic gene fusions have been successfully exploited in chronic myelogenous leukemia (CML; BCR-ABL fusion) (Hochhaus et al, 2017) and lung cancer (ALK fusions) (Solomon et al, 2014). The recent approval of Larotrectinib in solid cancers with fusions in NTRK genes is an example of a rare but recurrent driver alteration that occurs across a wide range of cancer histologies (Drilon et al, 2018). By using quantitative mRNA expression analysis together with DNA copy number analyses, amplification of oncogenes that are critical for tumor initiation and progression can also be identified or confirmed as potential drug targets. For example, by using large-scale genome sequencing data sets (eg, The Cancer Genome Atlas), wild-type *KRAS* amplification without coding mutations was found in 13% of CIN (chromosomal instability) variant gastric cancer, and this was confirmed by the high mRNA expression level of *KRAS* using TCGA expression data (Wong et al, 2018).

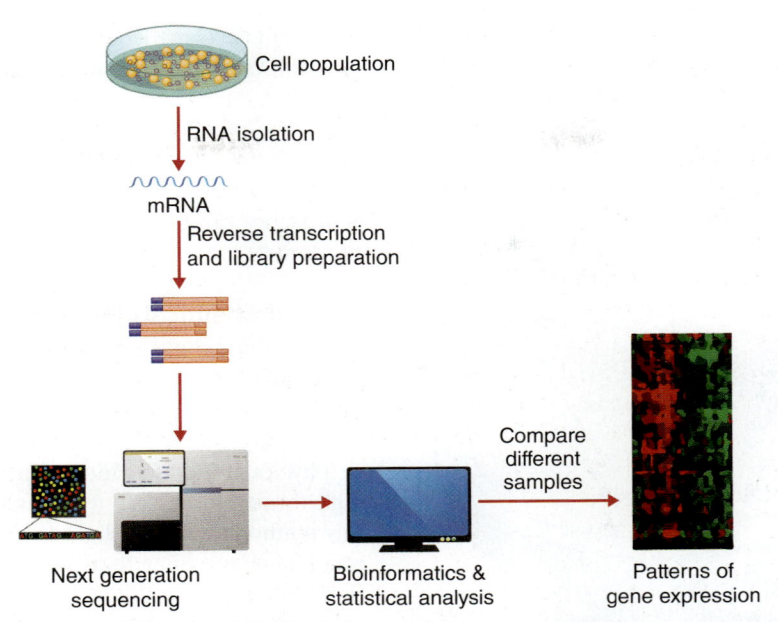

FIGURE 17–1 RNA sequencing to study gene expression. To study gene expression, mRNA is isolated from cells and converted to cDNA, which is then prepared for and subjected to next generation sequencing (see Chap. 2). Using bioinformatics, computer algorithms, and advanced statistical analysis, the abundance of mRNA sequences can be compared between groups of cells. These groups of cells can represent different cell lines, tissues, or treatments.

17.2.3 Functional Genomic Screens

Potential targets of anticancer drugs can also be identified through functional genomic screens using RNAi (RNA interference) or CRISPR/Cas9 (see Chap. 2, Secs. 2.3.3 and 2.3.6) in the absence of a selective drug or molecular probe. RNAi exploits endogenous cellular gene-silencing mechanisms and leads to degradation of host mRNA sequences with subsequent reductions in expression levels of the target protein (Fig. 17–2). Using this approach, the functional importance of individual gene knockdown can be ascertained, based on reduction in cell proliferation or survival, or other phenotypic changes of interest. When combined with high throughput screening, the functional significance of knocking down thousands of individual genes in the human genome can be evaluated. For example, high-throughput shRNA (short hairpin RNA) screens identified mitochondrial proteases critical for the growth of acute myelogenous leukemia (AML) cell lines such as ClpP (Cole et al, 2015): inhibitors of such proteases can then be developed and evaluated in clinical trials for patients with AML.

CRISPR (Clustered Regularly Interspaced Short Palindromic Repeats) is based on endogenous sequences in prokaryotes that can be used to functionally delete, mutate, or modulate the expression of a gene of interest. In the original and most commonly applied form of CRISPR, RNA guide sequences direct the Cas9 nuclease to specific sites in the genome where the Cas9 nuclease cleaves the gene of interest, leading to protein-terminating deletions or mutations. Compared to RNAi, CRISPR has less off-target effects and can achieve complete target knockout or produce single-point mutations.

Libraries of guide RNAs can be introduced into Cas9 nuclease–expressing cells to screen for genes essential for cell function. For example, using this approach, Wnt and FZD5 signaling (see Chap. 6, Sec. 6.4.1) were shown to be required for the survival of RNF43-mutated pancreatic cancer cells, suggesting a potential therapy for this subgroup of patients with pancreatic cancer (Steinhart et al, 2017).

Similar approaches can be used to identify drug combination strategies. Here, combinations of drug and RNAi or CRISPR can identify genes whose mutation, knockout, or knockdown can sensitize cells to the drug of interest. These approaches are based on the concept of synthetic lethality, which describes a situation where single gene defects are compatible with cell viability but a combination of gene defects causes cell death or impairment of cell fitness (Iglehart and Silver, 2009; Fig. 17–3). Synthetic lethality screening provides a novel way to target loss of function mutations in tumor suppressor genes that cannot be targeted directly (Ashworth et al, 2011). The classic example of this is inhibition of poly(ADP-ribose) polymerase (PARP) enzyme in patients with *BRCA1* or *BRCA2* loss of function germ-line mutations (Ashworth and Lord 2018). The main function of PARP is to recognize the sites of single-stranded DNA breaks and recruit DNA repair proteins to these sites. Loss of PARP function usually causes unrepaired single-stranded DNA breaks that in turn give rise to stalled DNA replication forks. These forks, if unrepaired, can result in DNA double-strand breaks leading to cell death. In tumor cells with normally functioning BRCA proteins, PARP inhibition is not lethal as BRCA proteins repair these stalled replication forks using homologous recombination (see Chap. 9, Sec. 9.3.4). However, in tumor cells with loss of BRCA

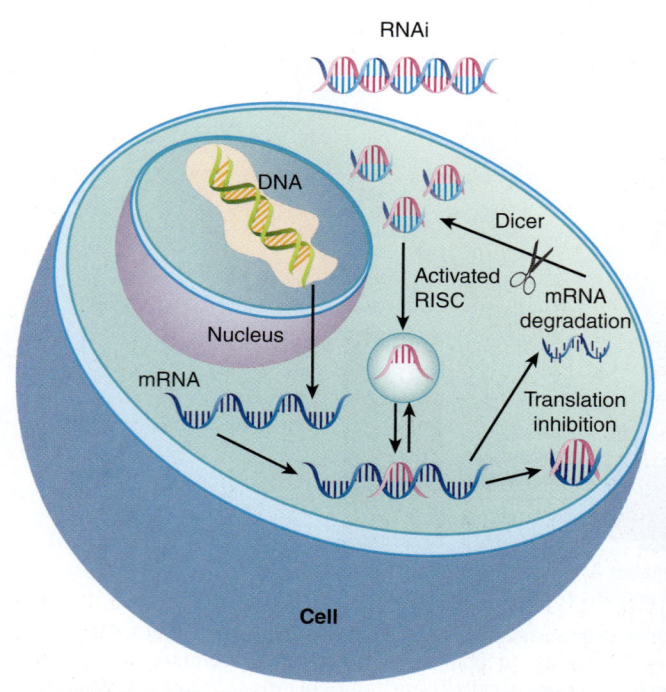

FIGURE 17–2 Proposed mechanism of action of RNAi to silence gene expression. On entry of double-stranded RNA into the cytoplasm, the endogenous enzyme Dicer cleaves the RNA into short sequences of approximately 21 nucleotides. These short sequences then interact with the RISC (RNA-inducing silencing complex) that matches these sequences to complementary endogenous mRNA. On binding, the endogenous mRNA target is degraded, leading to eventual reduction in target protein levels or its translation inhibited by complementary base pairing.

function, DNA damage induced by PARP inhibition is left unrepaired and is lethal. As such, PARP inhibitors cause selective cell death in *BRCA* mutant (functional loss of both alleles) cancer cells. This concept has been clinically validated in *BRCA* mutant breast, ovarian, prostate, and pancreatic cancers (the development of PARP inhibitors is discussed in Chap. 19, Sec. 19.6.2).

Large-scale functional genomic data sets now enable the identification of cancer dependencies, including those linked to specific molecular alterations or acting in a synthetic lethal fashion, within or across tumor histologies (Tsherniak et al, 2017).

17.2.4 Identification of Active Drugs

Once a therapeutic target has been identified, several approaches can be used to develop or select for inhibitors of this target.

17.2.4.1 Chemical Libraries *Chemical libraries* can be used for high throughput screening of large libraries of compounds to identify small molecule leads for novel anticancer drugs. These screens can identify chemical compounds that inhibit the desired target in cell-free assays, by using enzymatic methods or physical binding. Fluorescent polarization is a common high-throughput assay to evaluate drug-target binding: in this method, polarized light is used to measure the speed of rotation or "tumbling time" of a fluorescently labeled molecule (Lea and Simeonov, 2011). Under fluorescent polarization, the speed of rotation of the molecule is coupled to the emission of light in a polarized plane; small molecules rotate faster and larger molecules rotate slower. When the fluorescently labeled molecule (probe) interacts with its target protein, the molecule tumbles more slowly. Drug screening assays search for chemicals that disrupt the interaction between the fluorescently labeled probe and target protein, thereby increasing the tumbling of the fluorescent probe. The lead compounds are then investigated for their effects on intact cells.

Alternatively, cell-based screens can be conducted to identify chemical compounds that alter a cancer-associated cellular phenotype such as viability, or the ability to migrate or invade in tissue culture models. Follow-up studies are then required to identify the targets and mechanisms of the lead compounds. The chemicals present in these large libraries are usually synthetic compounds that represent diverse types of chemical structures. Smaller and more focused chemical libraries can also be developed to provide more in-depth coverage of a specific type of chemical structure. These focused libraries are useful to help identify more active analogs of compounds identified from a larger screen.

Newer technology has coupled novel chemical libraries with DNA barcoding and sequencing. By creating combinatorial libraries of chemical compounds coupled to a unique DNA sequence, it is possible to generate libraries of more than 5 million compounds. These molecules can be incubated with a protein drug target of interest and the bound chemicals identified through PCR amplification of the DNA tag and sequencing. This technology offers the opportunity to increase dramatically the chemical space surveyed by high throughput screening (Goodnow et al, 2017).

17.2.4.2 Natural Product Libraries *Natural product libraries* can be fruitful sources of leads for novel therapeutic agents. Natural products isolated from plants, marine life, herbs, etc are isolated initially as extracts containing multiple compounds. Later, the individual chemical compounds are

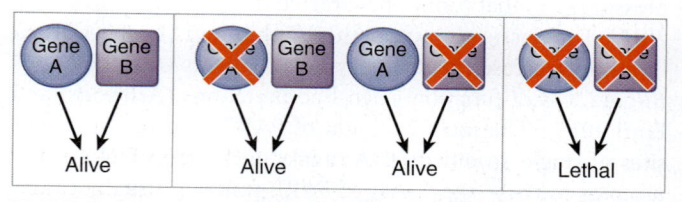

FIGURE 17–3 The concept of synthetic lethality. Cells with BRCA1 or BRCA2 deficiency lack the ability to repair DNA lesions by homologous recombination. Application of a PARP inhibitor, which inhibits the alternative pathway of base excision repair is then selectively lethal to such cells that are dependent on this pathway, especially after application of an agent that induces lesions in DNA such as chemotherapy with platinum-containing drugs.

isolated and purified, and methods to isolate individual compounds from extracts have improved. In addition, advances in medicinal and synthetic chemistry permit modification of natural products to improve their utility as anticancer agents. Natural products offer some potential advantages over synthetic chemical compounds. For example, they may have unique physical and chemical structures that cannot easily be synthesized. Some extracts from natural products may be sufficiently active to permit their direct evaluation in clinical trials. Multiple chemotherapeutic agents in clinical use are natural products or are derived from them: for example, paclitaxel is a chemotherapeutic agent isolated from the bark of the yew tree. Eribulin, which is approved for the treatment of breast cancer and sarcomas, is an antimicrotubule chemotherapy originally derived from a marine sponge. Its total chemical synthesis requires a >60-step process (Ledford, 2010).

17.2.4.3 Libraries of Known Drugs

Libraries of known drugs are a potential source of new anticancer agents. Old drugs with previously unrecognized anticancer activity can be rapidly incorporated in cancer treatments by relying on their prior safety, pharmacokinetic, solubility, and stability data. A classic example is the development of thalidomide as a novel antimyeloma therapy. Thalidomide was developed as a therapy for nausea during pregnancy, but withdrawn from the market in 1961 due to teratogenicity. In 1999, thalidomide was reported to be active in multiple myeloma and produced a 32% response rate in patients with refractory disease. Subsequently, thalidomide in combination with melphalan and prednisone was shown to prolong survival of older patients when compared to melphalan and prednisone alone (Palumbo et al, 2006). The success of thalidomide led to the development of the second-generation analog lenalidomide that also improves outcomes in patients with multiple myeloma as well as other hematologic malignancies such as myelodysplasia (Dimopoulos et al, 2007). Metformin, the most widely used oral hypoglycemic agent worldwide, that inhibits complex I in mitochondria, is being investigated for its anticancer activity in multiple clinical trials (Pernicova and Korbonits, 2014). The identification of old drugs with unrecognized anticancer activity has been largely serendipitous, but more recently, academic as well as commercial investigators have taken a systematic approach to their identification by compiling libraries of on-patent and off-patent drugs and screening these libraries for unrecognized anticancer activity.

17.2.4.4 Rational Drug Design

Rational drug design can be used to develop therapeutic agents if the 3-dimensional structure of a target is known. These structure-based studies can be used to follow up on screens of available molecules or can be the starting point to develop the initial lead compounds. Guided by the crystal structure of a protein target, small molecules that bind the active site of the target can be synthesized. These initial compounds are then tested for activity in cell-free and cell-based assays, and refinements are made to the chemical structure to improve potency,

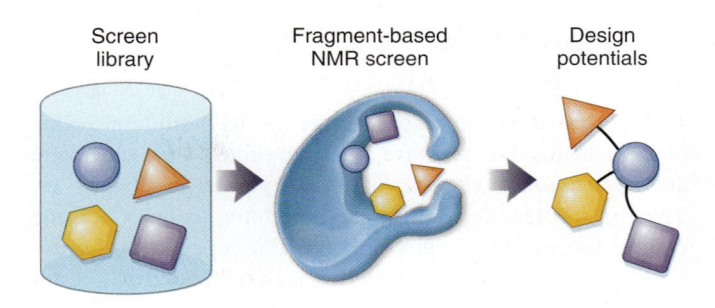

FIGURE 17-4 NMR binding studies can aid in the development of novel therapeutic agents for cancer. Using NMR, small fragment-based chemical libraries can be screened searching for small molecules that bind with micromolar affinity. When such fragments bind the target protein in close proximity, the molecules can be linked together chemically to create a new molecule that binds much more avidly with nanomolar affinity.

stability, specificity, and solubility. Thus, through an iterative process, potent and selective drugs are developed. Often, the selection of compounds can be aided by virtual modeling where chemical structures are docked into target proteins using computer software that re-creates 3-dimensional images of the molecule and its protein target. Million-compound libraries can be screened in virtual docking studies to identify "hits," which can be validated in physical binding studies.

Binding assays using nuclear magnetic resonance (NMR) can evaluate interactions between drugs and targets, and can identify compounds that bind with low affinity. Small libraries of approximately 10,000 low-molecular-weight compounds are incubated with isotopically labeled target proteins. Binding of fragments is assessed by NMR, which can detect weak interactions that require concentrations of the 2 components in the 20-100 µM range. By chemically linking 2 binding fragments, a molecule with much higher (nM) affinity can be generated (Fig. 17-4). Through this approach, small molecule inhibitors of bcl-2 were developed to promote apoptosis (see Chap. 8, Sec. 8.4); they were shown to be capable of inducing regression in experimental models of cancer and one of them (venetoclax) has subsequently been approved for the treatment of chronic lymphocytic leukemia (CLL) (Seymour et al, 2018).

17.3 NEW STRATEGIES FOR CANCER TREATMENT

Newer anticancer agents entering clinical use tend to be targeted to specific molecular targets in the cancer cell: they include small molecules targeting transmembrane and intracellular kinases, small molecules targeting other intracellular enzymes, antibodies that inhibit or activate cell surface proteins, small molecules that disrupt protein-protein interactions, and gene knockdown with antisense oligonucleotides or RNAi. These agents are discussed in detail in Chapter 19 but underlying principles and properties are given below.

17.3.1 Small Molecule Tyrosine Kinase Inhibitors (TKIs)

Multiple small molecules that target the ATP-binding pocket of intracellular kinases have been developed. The repertoire and application of current TKIs are reviewed in Chapter 19. The first protein tyrosine kinase inhibitor to enter routine clinical use was imatinib, which was developed as an inhibitor of the ABL tyrosine kinase that is dysregulated as a result of the *BCR-ABL* fusion gene (Druker et al, 2001; see Chap. 7, Sec. 7.5.1, and Chap. 19, Sec. 19.6.4). This agent, therefore, has activity in tumors that carry abnormalities in this gene and found initial clinical application in the management of CML (which expresses *BCR-ABL*), where it can induce remission in a large proportion of patients. As occurs with many kinase targets, mutations in the active site of the ABL kinase can render CML cells resistant to imatinib and lead to disease progression. The recognition of this phenomenon has led to the development of subsequent generations of inhibitors that can overcome this form of acquired resistance (Cortes et al, 2012).

Imatinib also inhibits the tyrosine kinase activity of KIT, the product of the *C-KIT* oncogene, and the platelet-derived growth factor receptor (PDGFR). Consistent with this effect, imatinib has activity against gastrointestinal stromal tumors (GISTs), the majority of which express *C-KIT*, and eosinophilic syndromes that have defects in PDGFR signaling (see Chap. 19, Sec. 19.3).

Activation of the EGFR signaling pathway promotes cellular proliferation and survival through signaling via the RAS/RAF/MAPK, PI3K/AKT, and STAT pathways (see Chap. 6, Sec. 6.2). Small-molecule ATP mimics (gefitinib and erlotinib) have been developed that bind and inhibit the enzymatic site of the EGFR kinase. Likewise, humanized monoclonal antibodies (cetuximab and panitumumab) bind the EGFR receptor and inhibit signaling through this pathway (Fig. 17–5).

The development of second- and later-generation therapies to overcome drug resistance mutations and the "repurposing" of TKIs for new uses illustrate recurring themes in the development of numerous approved therapies for solid tumors.

Although drugs like imatinib highlight the attractiveness of highly specific kinase inhibitors, kinase inhibitors that inhibit multiple targets also have clinical utility. Examples of such multikinase inhibitors are sunitinib and sorafenib, which inhibit RAF, VEGF, PDGF, and cKIT kinases (see Chap. 19, Sec. 19.3). The numerous TKIs now incorporated into clinical cancer treatment are described in Chapter 19.

17.3.2 Enzyme Inhibitors

Small molecules that bind and inhibit the active sites of enzymes important for tumor growth and proliferation have been developed and are in clinical use. Proteasome inhibitors are one example of this class of agent. The 26S proteasome has as its major function the degradation of cellular proteins, including damaged, misfolded, and regulatory proteins (see Chap. 2, Sec. 2.X). Tumor cells require proteasome-dependent

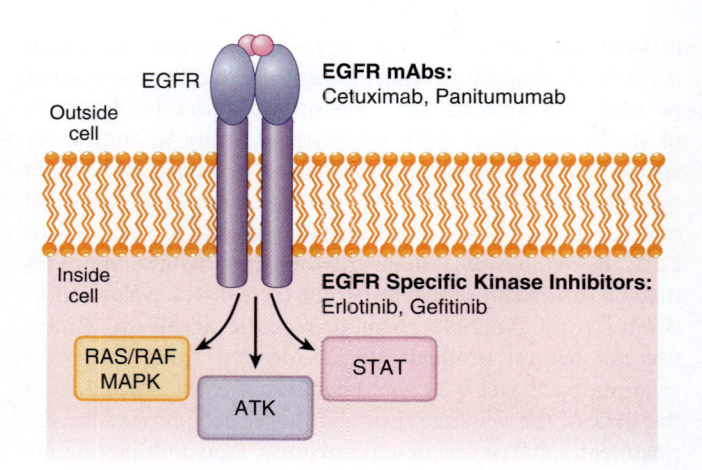

FIGURE 17–5 Targeting the EGFR signaling pathway. Activation of the EGFR signaling pathway promotes cellular proliferation and survival through signaling through the RAS/RAF/MAPK, PI3K/AKT, and STAT pathways. Small-molecule ATP mimics (gefitinib and erlotinib) have been developed that bind and inhibit the enzymatic site of the EGFR kinase. Likewise, humanized monoclonal antibodies (cetuximab and panitumumab) bind the EGFR receptor and inhibit signaling through this pathway.

turnover of many cell-cycle proteins in order to successfully complete mitosis (see Chap. 8, Sec. 8.Y). Proteasome inhibitors can lead to induction of endoplasmic reticulum (ER) stress with activation of the unfolded protein response, inhibition of the NF kappa B inflammatory pathway, increased generation of reactive oxygen species, and activation of caspase-8 leading to death by apoptosis (Hideshima et al, 2009; Moreau et al, 2012). Bortezomib is a covalently bound but reversible inhibitor of the β5-subunit of the proteasome that is used for the treatment of relapsed multiple myeloma and mantle cell lymphoma. Newer proteasome inhibitors, such as carfilzomib, inhibit the active site of the proteasome irreversibly: this drug is more potent than bortezomib and can produce clinical responses in bortezomib-resistant patients (see Chap. 19, Sec. 19.7.11; Tzogani et al, 2017).

Histone deacetylase (HDAC) catalyzes the removal of acetyl groups from lysine residues of nucleosomal histones. The acetylation status of histones influences the regulation of transcriptional activity of some genes, and aberrant activity of HDAC is associated with the development of some malignancies. Histone deacetylase inhibitors have been developed that bind the zinc ion in the active site of HDAC, thereby inhibiting its enzymatic function. Several HDAC inhibitors are approved for the treatment of cutaneous T-cell lymphoma and multiple myeloma (see Chap. 19, Sec. 19.6.3.1).

Inhibition of the enzyme PARP, which is involved in DNA repair, has been described in Section 17.2.3 as an example of synthetic lethality, because its activity is greatest against tumors that have other defects in DNA repair, such as breast and ovarian cancers with mutations in BRCA1 and BRCA2 (see Chap. 19, Sec. 19.6.2)

Clinical success has been achieved in the targeting of isocitrate dehydrogenase (IDH), an enzyme involved in cancer metabolism, where mutant forms have been identified in both hematologic and solid tumors. These mutant "neomorphic" enzymes differ in structure and catalyze distinct reactions from the wild-type proteins and thus provide opportunities to selectively target their oncogenic activity (Dang et al, 2016; DiNardo et al, 2018). Molecular targeted agents such as enasidenib, which is a potent selective inhibitor of mutant IDH2, have been shown to be effective in treating patients with relapsed or refractory AML that harbor IDH2 mutations (Stein et al, 2017). These drugs are described in more detail in Chapter 19, Section 19.6.3.2.

17.3.3 Antibody-Based Anticancer Therapies

Antibodies and their derivatives represent a major class of clinically used cancer therapies, and are discussed in Chapter 19, Section 19.1.3, and Chapter 21, Section 21.5.2. Specific inactivating antibodies against the extracellular portion of a membrane-based receptor tyrosine kinase provide an alternative to small molecule kinase inhibitors to inhibit signaling pathways. One such receptor is human epidermal growth factor receptor 2 (HER-2), which does not have a known growth factor ligand, but whose constitutive activity provides intracellular signals leading to cell proliferation. Antibody therapies targeting HER-2, including trastuzumab and pertuzumab, have improved the treatment and outcomes in the ~20% of breast cancers where HER-2 is amplified or overexpressed, which historically had very poor outcomes.

Other antibody-based therapies target cell surface proteins that are overexpressed by the tumor cell but do not activate or inhibit the targets. For example, rituximab is a chimeric monoclonal antibody that binds to the CD20 protein found on the surface of CLL and lymphoma cells and has clinical benefit when used as a single agent or in combination with chemotherapy. Binding of rituximab to CD20 does not impact the function of this protein, but rather leads to elimination of the malignant cells through mechanisms including promotion of antibody- and complement-mediated cytotoxicity and induction of apoptosis. Antibodies directed against other cell surface proteins have been developed including alemtuzumab that targets CD52, which is approved for the treatment of T-cell lymphoma and CLL.

Antibody drug conjugates (ADC) are also used as anticancer therapy (Lambert and Morris 2017). An example is trastuzumab-emtansine for HER2-overexpressing breast cancer: the recombinant HER2 monoclonal antibody (trastuzumab) conjugated with a microtubule disrupting agent, using a nonreducible thioether link. Binding of the antibody to HER2 results in tumor cell uptake and cleavage of the linker to provide intracellular, tumor-targeted delivery of DM1. This drug is active in women with HER2 overexpressing breast cancer, who are resistant to trastuzumab-based therapy (see Chap. 19, Sec. 19.4.2; Verma et al, 2012). Conjugating a monoclonal antibody with a cytotoxic agent allows simultaneous inhibition of a signaling pathway and selective delivery of a cytotoxic drug to the cancer cell: multiple ADCs are in development.

BiTes (Bi-specific T-cell engagers) are another novel class of antibody therapies. BiTe antibodies are bispecific monoclonal antibodies that are fused in order to engage the tumor cell on one end and T cells at the CD3 receptor on the other end. BiTe antibodies direct the T cell to the tumor cells and facilitate T cell–mediated cytotoxicity against the tumor. The BiTe antibody blinatumomab is directed against the CD19 cell surface antigen on B cells. In patients with relapsed B-ALL, blinatumomab produces higher rates of remission and longer survival compared with reinduction chemotherapy (Kantarjian et al, 2017).

17.3.4 Disrupters of Protein-Protein Interactions

Protein-protein interactions play a critical role in most cellular functions, and developing inhibitors of these interactions is an attractive therapeutic strategy. Vinblastine and vincristine are established cancer therapies that work by this mechanism as they disrupt the interaction between α and β tubulin. The relatively large surface area involved in protein-protein interactions has made the development of specific inhibitors challenging but when critical contacts can be localized to small areas of the protein, the development of these inhibitors can be successful. For example, the small molecule venetoclax (see Sec. 17.2.4 and Chap. 19, Sec. 19.7.3) selectively binds Bcl-2 in the BH3 pocket and prevents this antiapoptotic protein from binding to and inhibiting its proapoptotic binding partners (see Chap. 8; Kang and Reynolds, 2009). Venetoclax is approved for refractory CLL with high-risk genetic changes (Roberts et al, 2016) and is being evaluated in additional malignancies.

Another example includes the small-molecule inhibitors that disrupt the MDM2-TP53 protein-protein interaction, such as idasanutlin and DS-3032b. MDM2, a negative regulator of wild-type TP53, is oncogenic when overexpressed in TP53 wild-type cells providing a rationale for targeting interaction between MDM2 and TP53. There are 3 well-defined TP53-binding pockets on the surface of MDM2, making it possible to disrupt the interaction between these 2 proteins using small-molecule inhibitors. Agents that disrupt this interaction, which are potentially relevant to the large fraction of cancers where wild-type TP53 expression is retained, are under investigation (Wang et al, 2017).

17.3.5 Antisense Oligonucleotides and RNAi

Antisense oligonucleotides and RNAi (see Chap. 2, Sec. 2.3.3) act by binding to specific target mRNAs in cancer cells and promoting their degradation. Although RNAi is more effective than antisense oligonucleotides at knocking down protein expression, antisense technology was discovered first and is more advanced in clinical development. Antisense therapies have been approved for noncancer conditions such as Familial

Hypercholesterolemia where the antisense agent mipomersen inhibits apolipoprotein B synthesis to lower LDL cholesterol (Stein and Castanotto, 2017). Antisense molecules directed against multiple cancer targets are under investigation in clinical trials (MacLeod and Crooke, 2017).

17.3.6 Directed Drug Delivery

A major limitation to the use of nontargeted chemotherapy is lack of selectivity for tumor cells. As new targets that are expressed selectively on tumor cells are characterized, a potential method for increasing the therapeutic index of conventional drugs is to link them to a carrier that may be targeted to tumor cells. Such carriers may include liposomes and other types of nanoparticles as well as monoclonal antibodies (as described in Sec. 17.3.3 for trastuzumab-emtansine).

A large body of preclinical research relates to the entrapment of anticancer drugs in nanoparticles (Petros and DeSimone 2010), and some agents have been approved for clinical use. For example, pegylated liposomal doxorubicin improved the outcome of patients with Kaposi sarcoma compared with conventional chemotherapy, and reduced cardiac toxicity when compared with conventional doxorubicin for treatment of metastatic breast cancer (Duggan and Keating 2011). Liposomal vincristine is effective as monotherapy in patients with relapsed and refractory Philadelphia chromosome-negative ALL (O'Brien et al, 2013). Recently, the encapsulation of fixed molar ratios of cytarabine and daunorubicin into a liposome was shown to improve rates of remission and survival of older patients with secondary and poor-risk AML (Lancet et al, 2018). These agents are not targeted specifically against molecules expressed selectively on cancer cells, but there are several mechanisms whereby drugs associated with liposomes or other nanoparticles might lead to improvement in therapeutic index relative to free drug: (1) slow, continuous release of the anticancer drug into the circulation; this may protect against organ-specific toxicity (eg, cardiotoxicity due to doxorubicin) and/or lead to improvement in antitumor effects; (2) fusion of liposomes with cell membranes, leading to efficient internal delivery of drugs; this may overcome drug resistance because of impaired uptake of free drug; (3) selective deposition of nanoparticles in tumor tissue, because of their enhanced permeability and retention as a result of the abnormal vasculature of tumors (see Chap. 11). Development of clinically useful targeted nanocarriers remains an active area of research (Rosenblum et al, 2018).

17.4 PRECLINICAL EVALUATION OF POTENTIAL ANTICANCER DRUGS

Compounds identified through drug discovery platforms need to be evaluated in preclinical studies both for their ability to inhibit their putative targets and for their potential anticancer effects. There are multiple steps in the evaluation of a potential anticancer drug, and only a small proportion of such agents will eventually enter clinical trials (Fig. 17–6); these steps involve identification and verification of the target and mechanism of action, evaluation for activity against cultured tumor cells, and evaluation of activity and toxicity in in vivo models. It is important to verify the specificity of the target molecule or pathway in animal models and in early clinical trials, as putative targeted agents may sometimes have unexpected

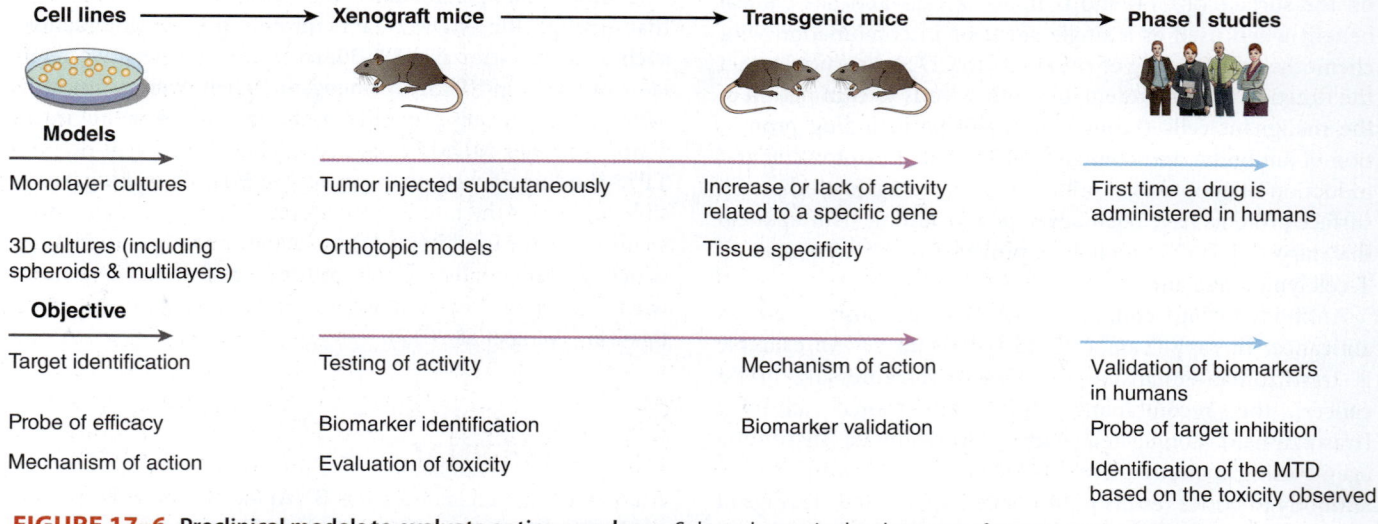

FIGURE 17–6 Preclinical models to evaluate anticancer drugs. Selected steps in development of anticancer drugs. Drugs are usually evaluated first for activity against cultured cells, and solid tumor models should be encouraged to reflect the microenvironment of solid tumors. This is usually followed by demonstration of activity against xenografts generated from implantation of selected human tumor cell lines into immune-deficient mice; xenografts better reflect the properties of the corresponding human tumor if grown in the same tissue of origin (ie, implanted orthotopically). Use of genetically modified (transgenic) mice allows information about the relation between drug activity and expression of potential target genes. Finally the drug is evaluated in phase I studies in humans; these are expanding from simple evaluation of tolerance and pharmacokinetics to provide further information about the molecular target and to identify and validate biomarkers correlating with drug activity.

toxic effects that are independent of inhibition of the target for which they were designed.

17.4.1 Evaluation for Activity Against Cultured Cells

An important phase of preclinical testing involves evaluating whether the candidate agent can either kill or inhibit the proliferation of cancer cells. Screening of candidate drugs requires an initial assay of activity that is rapid and can be automated, and such approaches have been used to evaluate large panels of anticancer drugs in hundreds of cancer cell lines in parallel. Some measures of cell damage that have been used employ dyes such as methyl thiazole tetrazolium (MTT), which depends on the reduction of a tetrazolium-based compound to a blue formazan product by living but not dead cells. The amount of reduced product is quantified in an automated system using multiple tissue-culture wells in which cells have been exposed to a range of doses of the drugs under test. Another dye that is useful in quantifying cell number is sulforhodamine B, a pink anionic dye that binds to basic amino acids of fixed cells such that dye intensity is linearly related to the number of cells. These tests assess the number of metabolically active cells in the culture at the time of analysis and hence largely track the effects of the treatment to induce rapid cell death (eg, apoptosis) and/or reduced proliferation. In general, they are useful for assessing changes in the number of metabolically active cells over a range of 100% to about 5%.

Following treatment with drugs, tumor cells may undergo programmed cell death or apoptosis, which can be quantified by various methods (eg, by Annexin V and TUNEL staining) to provide an estimate of the number of cells undergoing apoptosis or an apoptotic index (see Chap. 8, Sec. 8.4.1). This index generally increases after drug treatment of tumors, and the proportion of cells undergoing apoptosis may give a broad indication of drug effectiveness. However, there is evidence that radiation and many drugs often kill cancer cells by mechanisms other than apoptosis (see also Chap. 15, Sec. 15.3), and that assays of apoptosis correlate poorly with cell killing assessed by colony-forming assays (Brown and Attardi, 2005). Even where apoptosis is an important mechanism leading to drug-induced cell death, it is a dynamic process whose assessment can be very dependent on the time after treatment when measurements are made.

The important activity of an effective anticancer drug is to cause tumor cells with high proliferative capacity to lose their capacity for indefinite proliferation, and therefore the ability to regenerate the tumor. The above assays, as well as other short-term methods for evaluation of drug effects including induced morphologic changes or other properties of cancer cells such as changes in DNA, RNA or protein synthesis all suffer from the fundamental limitation that they apply to an unselected population of cells, and may have limited correlation with loss of reproductive potential of the cells.

Colony-forming assays can be performed following exposure to potential anticancer drugs of established cell lines derived from tumors, primary malignant cells derived from patient samples, or normal hematopoietic and other cells. In such assays, candidate cells are exposed to various doses of the agent of interest for a fixed time, or to a fixed dose (that is expected to be achievable in vivo) for varying times. The drug is then washed out, and different numbers of cells are evaluated for colony formation in a new environment (see also Chap. 15, Sec. 15.3.2). If the assay is performed in tissue culture, the number of colonies per cell plated is called the plating efficiency, and the ratio of the plating efficiency from drug-treated cells to untreated cells is the surviving fraction. Surviving fraction (plotted on a logarithmic scale) can then be plotted against drug dose (for a fixed time exposure) or against time (for exposure to a fixed drug concentration) to produce a survival curve. This assay can usually assess cell survival over at least 3-4 decades of survival.

An example of a survival curve is shown in Fig 17-7; it is analogous to survival curves generated to describe the dose response to radiation (see Chap. 15, Sec. 15.3), although there is rarely an exponential decrease in cell survival with increasing drug dose as may be observed for radiation. Many chemotherapy drugs (eg, antimetabolites such as cytosine arabinoside and methotrexate) are relatively specific in killing cells in a given phase of the cell cycle (usually S-phase), so there is an initial steep fall in survival as the sensitive cells are killed, but then a flattening of the survival curve. Survival may be further decreased by more prolonged exposure to the drug, although such drugs often also retard entry of cells into the drug-sensitive phase. Most drugs, including molecular targeted agents, are more active against rapidly proliferating cells, even if they are not cell cycle phase–specific. For these drugs also, there will be a trend for cell survival curves to be concave upward, as in Figure 17-7, as higher doses interact with progressively more resistant slowly proliferating cells.

Drug activity may depend critically on cell-cell interactions, and such interactions are lost when potential drugs are evaluated against dispersed cells in culture. In vitro co-culture models may permit characterization of the microenvironment's contribution to drug response. Other models that include in vitro–generated blood vessels, or coincubation with immune cells, may offer clues as to antiangiogenic or immunomodulatory properties of the compound of interest. The tumor microenvironment is particularly important for development of drugs with activity against solid tumors. Contact between cells in solid tumors can mediate drug resistance, although to be effective the drugs must penetrate tissue from blood vessels to reach all of the target tumor cells in a toxic concentration and should be active under microenvironmental conditions (hypoxia, acidity) that inhibit tumor cell proliferation (see Chap. 12, Sec. 12.4; Minchinton and Tannock, 2006).

Although evaluation of drugs in monolayer cell cultures has limited ability to predict responsiveness in solid tumors, in vitro models including tumor spheroids and multilayered cell cultures can reproduce important properties of solid tumors such as cellular contact and an extracellular matrix, as well as gradients of nutrient distribution, cell proliferation, and drug access. Substantial effort has been invested in developing 3-dimensional culture systems for growing

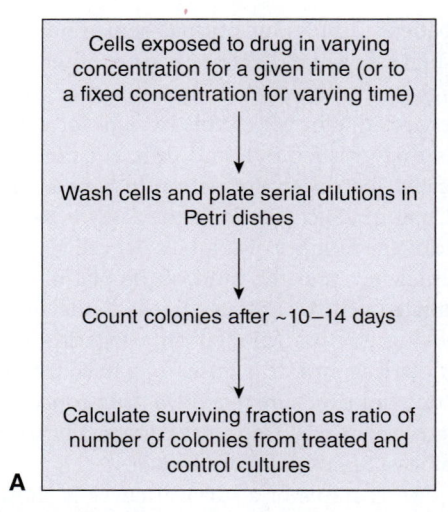

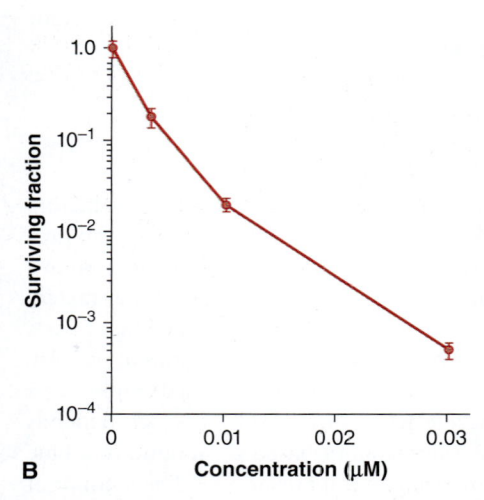

FIGURE 17-7 Cell survival curves. A) Cells are exposed either in monolayer or in suspension culture to different doses of a drug for a given time, or to a single dose of the drug for a variable time. The cells are then washed in fresh medium, and serial dilutions are plated in Petri dishes; colonies formed from surviving cells are counted, usually 10-14 days later. **B)** Experimentally determined cell survival curve for murine EMT6 cells exposed to the drug mitoxantrone. Note that surviving fraction is plotted using a logarithmic scale against dose on a linear scale.

patient-derived tumor cells (or normal cells, which can be used to assess tumor cell–specific killing), called "organoids" (Drost and Clevers, 2018). The degree to which these may better predict antitumor activity in patients as compared to 2-dimensional culture of cell lines remains an active area of investigation.

If a potential drug shows activity as assessed by 1 or more of the above assays, it is important to determine its target and mechanism of action. If the agent is designed to target a certain molecule, such as a receptor tyrosine kinase, it is important to show that the agent does in fact bind to its target, and that it inhibits downstream signaling from that target at a concentration that could be achieved in in vivo studies. Helpful strategies might include comparing the sensitivity of cells selected for the presence of, and/or dependence on, a particular target or pathway, and evaluation against genetically modified cells that are not dependent on the target or pathway. Likewise, selecting populations of cells resistant to the drug and using genetic approaches, including gene expression profiling or genetic sequencing, to identify mechanism of resistance, can derive insights into mechanism of action. Unfortunately, there has been inconsistency and nonreproducibility in many claims of target inhibition, and more thorough evaluation and coordination between laboratories is required to ensure accurate target identification (Prinz et al, 2011; Begley and Ellis, 2012).

17.4.2 Evaluation of Potential Anticancer Drugs In vivo

The in vitro assays described in the preceding sections assess directly the sensitivity of cultured tumor cells to drug treatment, but they do not assess the impact of the drug's pharmacokinetics or its toxicity for normal cells, both of which are important determinants of the clinical efficacy of a cancer drug. Assays that have been used to assess the effects of drugs on tumors in animals include drug-induced delay in tumor growth and evaluation of colony formation in vitro following treatment of tumors and excision and plating of the tumor cells. Comparison of tumor growth in treated and untreated animals is used most frequently to evaluate drug effects against solid tumors that are transplanted into animals (Fig. 17–8). Tumor shrinkage and delay of regrowth model the clinical assessment of tumor remission. Drugs that appear promising in in vitro screens are usually evaluated against xenografts where human tumor cell lines are implanted into immune-deficient mice. Syngeneic murine tumors, which can be transplanted into inbred immune competent mice, are also used for in vivo testing, and are particularly relevant for the evaluation of immunotherapy agents (Day et al, 2015).

Historically, the most widely used host for xenografting of human tumors has been the congenitally athymic nude mouse (so called because they lack fur). The nude mouse is not a perfect host because it may produce antibodies and also has large numbers of natural killer cells that may inhibit tumor growth (see Chap. 21, Sec. 21.3). Alternative hosts include mice with severe combined immune deficiency carrying the NOD mutation (NOD/SCID). These mice are better recipients for transplanted human tissues and have allowed the establishment of grafts of lymphoid and hemopoietic tissues, as well as of solid tumors. Even more immunocompromised mice have been developed (NOD/SCID mice also carrying a null mutation in the IL2 receptor common gamma chain [NSG]), which permit high engraftment rates of primary patient tissues, facilitating the generation of patient-derived xenografts (PDXs). These models, discussed below, are now widely viewed as a gold standard for preclinical testing of anticancer therapies, as they can better capture the heterogeneity and spectrum of clinical tumors (Dobrolecki et al, 2016).

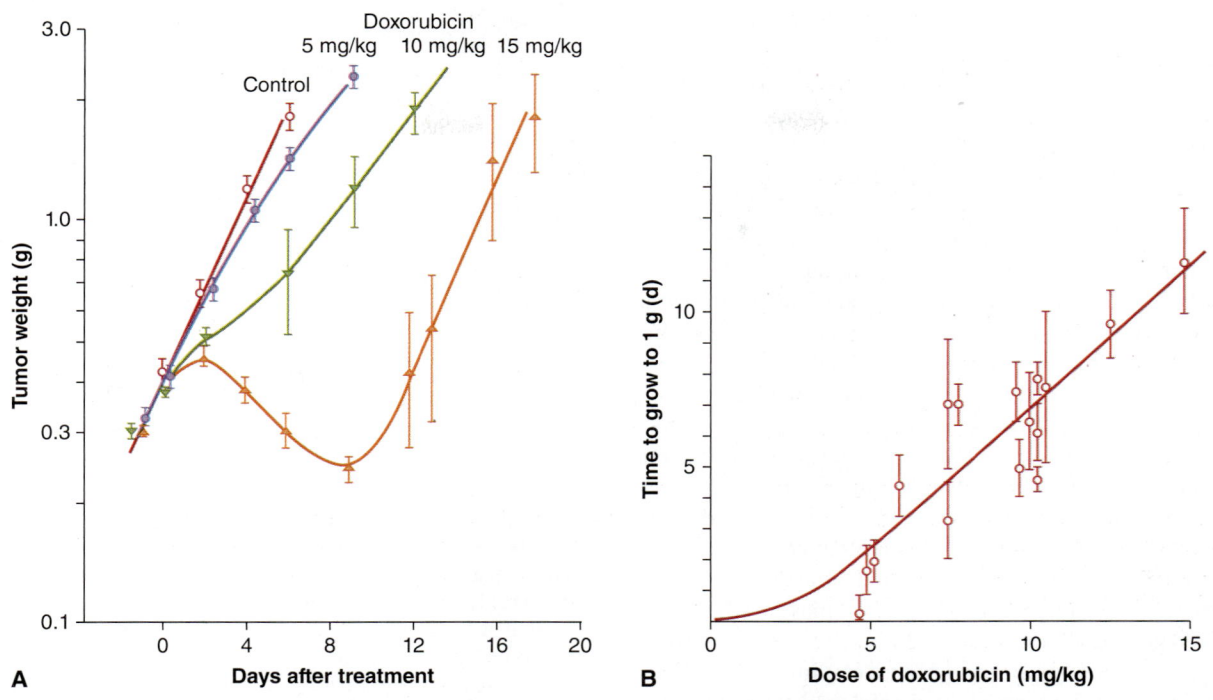

FIGURE 17-8 A) Illustration of tumor growth curves for treatment of an experimental tumor with doxorubicin. Tumor weight was estimated by prior calibration with measurements of tumor diameter and is plotted on a logarithmic scale against time on a linear scale. Straight lines then represent exponential growth, and tumor doubling time can be determined from the slope. Note that growth curves after drug treatment are not always parallel to the growth curve for controls and that inter-animal variation may lead to large standard errors. **B)** Dose-response curve relating drug dose to the time for tumors to grow from size at treatment (~0.4 g) to 1 g.

Xenografts possess the advantage that they may have characteristics more similar to those of the human tumors from which they are derived (eg, enzyme activities) as compared to tumors of murine origin. However, xenograft models have several limitations for evaluation of potential new drugs. The stromal component of a xenograft is not human, so it is difficult to evaluate the effect of the microenvironment on drug response, or to evaluate drugs such as monoclonal antibodies that may target only human proteins (eg, bevacizumab, which targets human VEGF and does not recognize murine VEGF). Second, the rate of growth of xenografts derived from serially transplanted human tumor cell lines is often rapid (typical doubling times of a few days) compared with that of primary human tumors (typical doubling times of 1-3 months), and they are more likely to respond to antiproliferative agents. Third, the animal is immune-compromised, so testing of agents with immunomodulatory effects is difficult or impossible. Finally, it may be difficult to select for resistance to drugs using cell line xenograft models, thereby limiting the use of these in vivo models in studying mechanisms of drug resistance. Xenografts derived directly from patient tumors, without prior development of cell growth in vitro, can reduce some but not all of these limitations (Dobrolecki et al, 2016).

Transplantation of tumor cells into subcutaneous sites of mice allows easy evaluation of tumor size, but there is evidence that the molecular profile and microenvironment of the tumors is more similar to their human counterpart if they are transplanted orthotopically (eg, mammary tumors are implanted in the mammary fat-pad of female mice, or pancreatic tumors are transplanted into the pancreas of mice) (Day et al, 2015). Humanized mouse models have also been developed; for example, human mammary cells and/or fibroblasts have been transplanted into a cleared mouse mammary gland. Evaluation of tumor growth (or shrinkage after treatment) is more difficult in orthotopic than subcutaneous sites but is facilitated by a variety of methods for imaging of small animals. Also, a gene encoding a marker such as green fluorescent protein (GFP) or luciferase may be introduced and stably expressed in the malignant cells, allowing them to be detected and quantified by optical imaging in the whole animal, permitting assessment of not only the primary site but also assessment of metastatic spread and the influence of treatment.

Genetically engineered mouse models (GEMMs), in which the expression of a protein is temporally and/or spatially controlled by genetic manipulation to cause tumor development, are being used to better assess transformation events and potential anticancer activity (including prevention strategies) related to their inhibition (Day et al, 2015). These transgenic mouse models (see Chap. 2, Sec. 2.3.5) can simulate some aspects of human cancer by introducing alterations in oncogenes or tumor suppressor genes in germ-lines of mice. GEMM can be used in 2 ways in the evaluation of preclinical agents: the treatment of an established tumor or their effects on tumor prevention. For example, administration of the anti-EGFR/HER-2 tyrosine kinase inhibitor lapatinib prevents tumor initiation in MMTV-erbB2 transgenic mice (Strecker et al, 2009). Evidence of activity of a drug to prevent or delay tumor formation in GEMM can give important insight into mechanisms of activity, and may indicate molecular properties of a tumor (ie, biomarkers) that may correlate with increased likelihood of activity. However, activity of a drug in GEMM does not necessarily imply that the drug will also be active in treating tumors with similar types of genetic changes in humans.

Benefits of GEMM for preclinical evaluation of potential anticancer drugs include the following: (1) the tumor has developed in an immune-competent animal, and (2) genetic alterations can be modified in a time- and tissue-specific manner (Day et al, 2015). However, GEMM are imperfect models for human tumors where there are often multiple genetic abnormalities (including both drivers and passengers), because the initial molecular alterations in the mice are limited to the ones that have been introduced, which often consist of strong oncogenic drivers. Also the stroma and other normal tissue elements are derived from the rodent, and may have the same engineered genetic alteration as the tumor. To avoid this, tissue or cell type–specific engineering can be employed, or the generated tumors can be transplanted into wild-type syngeneic mice. Transplantation also offers the possibility of shortcutting the long latency for appearance of spontaneous tumors and the possibility of treating genetically similar transplants with different drugs. Thus far, GEMM have been used more often for the study of the transformation process than for evaluation of novel drugs, but are increasingly relevant to permit the evaluation of cancer immunotherapies.

PDXs involve the direct implantation of primary tumors from patients into mice without subjecting them to cell culture conditions. In parallel, these tumors are often extensively characterized for their gene expression and mutation profiles. PDX models offer the opportunity to create mouse models of tumors that better recapitulate the patient's tumor, and are more representative of the spectrum of genomic alterations seen clinically than the existing cancer cell lines. The evaluation of new therapies and biomarkers of response in PDX models may provide a better indication of the likelihood that a treatment will be successful in patients.

A limitation of most of the above in vitro and in vivo assays of drug activity is that they evaluate relatively short-term effects against cells that have been selected to grow in culture or in mice. As discussed in Chapter 13, Section 13.3.2, some tumors may contain a small population of cells with indefinite potential for proliferation, or *tumor stem cells*, and in such cases, elimination of these cells would be necessary to achieve long-term remission or cure (Nassar and Blanpain, 2016).

17.5 TOXICITY OF ANTICANCER DRUGS

17.5.1 The Concept of Therapeutic Index

In addition to their antitumor effects, all anticancer drugs are toxic to normal tissues, and it is this toxicity that limits the

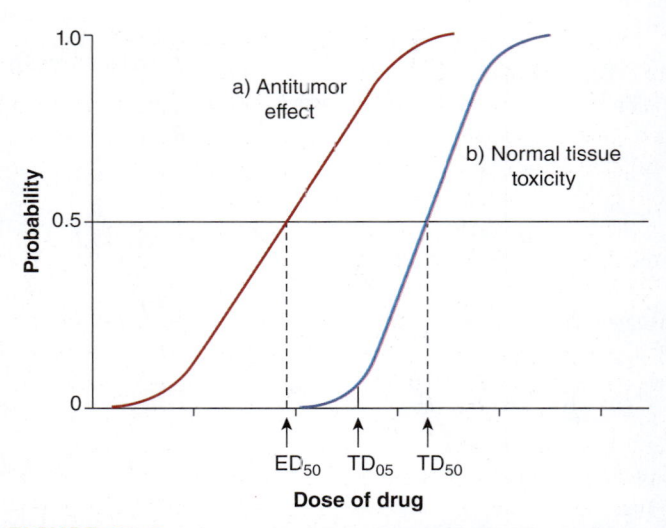

FIGURE 17–9 Schematic relationships between dose of a drug and the probability of a given measure of antitumor effect (curve a), and the probability of a given measure of normal-tissue toxicity (curve b). Heterogeneity among tumors often leads to a shallower slope of the line representing tumors as shown. The therapeutic index might be defined as the ratio of doses to give 50% probabilities of normal-tissue damage and antitumor effects. However, if the endpoint for toxicity is severe (eg, sepsis due to bone marrow suppression), it would be more appropriate to define the therapeutic index at a lower probability of toxicity (eg, TD-05/ED-50).

dose of drugs that can be given to patients. The relationship between the probability of a biologic effect of a drug and the administered dose is usually described by a sigmoid curve (Fig. 17–9), although it is possible for targeted agents that there is an optimal dose where the target is completely inhibited and using higher doses only adds toxicity. If the drug is to be useful, the curve describing the probability of antitumor effect (eg, complete clinical remission) must be displaced toward lower doses as compared with the curve describing the probability of major toxicity to normal tissues (eg, myelosuppression leading to infection). *Therapeutic Index* (or *Therapeutic Ratio*) may be defined from such curves as the ratio of the dose required to produce a given probability of toxicity and the dose required to give a defined effect against the tumor. The therapeutic index in Figure 17–9 might be represented by the ratio of the drug dose required for a 5% level of probability of severe toxicity (sometimes referred to as toxic dose–05 or TD-05) to that required for 50% probability of antitumor effect (ie, effective dose–50 or ED-50). Any stated levels of probability might be used. The appropriate end points of tumor response and toxicity will depend on the limiting toxicity of the drug and the intent of treatment (ie, cure vs palliation). Improvement in the therapeutic index is the goal of systemic treatment. However, although dose-response curves similar to those of Figure 17–9 have been defined in animals, they have been obtained rarely for drug effects in humans. They emphasize the important concept that any modification in treatment that leads to increased killing of tumor cells in tissue culture or animals must be assessed for its effects on critical normal tissues prior to therapeutic trials.

Toxicity to normal tissues limits both the dose and frequency of drug administration. Many drugs cause toxicity because of their preferential activity against rapidly proliferating cells, and this is especially true for chemotherapy, but also for some targeted agents: normal adult tissues that maintain a high rate of cellular proliferation include the bone marrow, intestinal mucosa, hair follicles, and gonads. Nausea, vomiting, fatigue, and carcinogenic effects are also common side effects of many drugs. In addition, several drug-specific toxicities to other tissues of the body may be observed. The biologic basis for toxic damage to normal tissues that may occur through a common mechanism is discussed below, whereas toxic effects specific for individual drugs are described in Chapters 18 and 19. Targeted agents, in particular, may cause side effects that are not specific to rapidly proliferating tissues; these drugs are often given continuously, and although they may target molecular pathways that are deranged in tumors, they often have effects to inhibit the corresponding normal pathways, thus leading to toxic effects on the host.

17.5.2 Toxicity to Bone Marrow and Scheduling of Treatment

Within the bone marrow, there is evidence for a pluripotent stem cell that under normal conditions proliferates slowly to replenish cells in the myelocytic, erythroid, and megakaryocytic lineages (Fig. 17–10A). Lineage-specific precursors proliferate more rapidly than stem cells, whereas the morphologically recognizable but immature precursor cells (eg, myeloblasts) have a very rapid rate of cell proliferation. Beyond a certain stage of maturation, proliferation ceases and the cells mature into circulating blood cells. The relationship between proliferation and maturation in bone-marrow precursor cells provides a plausible explanation for the observed fall and recovery

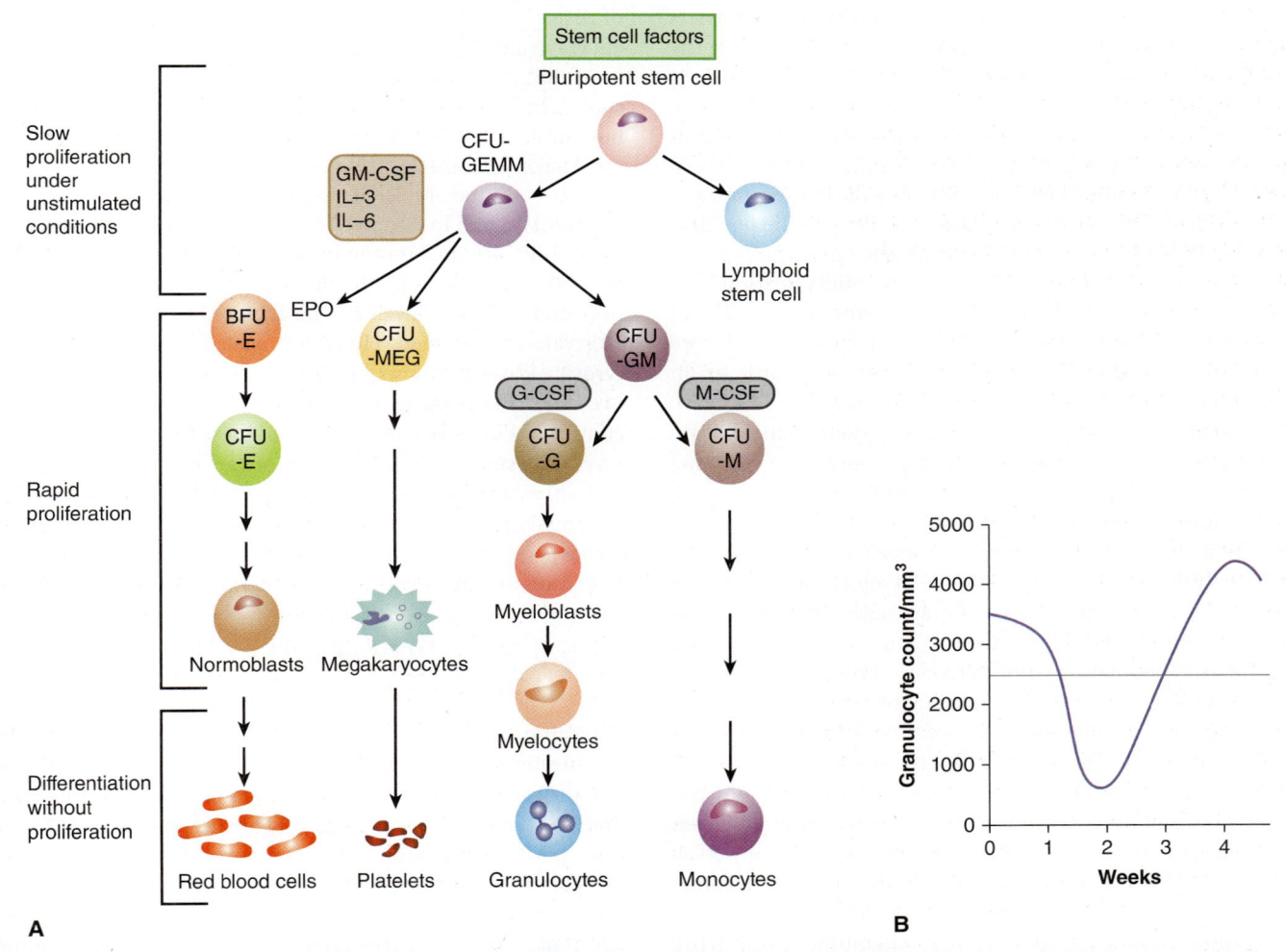

FIGURE 17–10 A) Schematic diagram of the differentiation of hemopoietic precursor cells in the bone marrow, leading to the production of red blood cells, platelets, granulocytes, and monocytes. Various cells are stimulated to proliferate and/or differentiate by the growth factors IL-3, GM-CSF, G-CSF, M-CSF, erythropoietin (EPO), stem cell factor, and others; only their main target cells are indicated here. Under normal conditions, the early precursor cells proliferate slowly, intermediate precursors proliferate rapidly (in the megakaryocytic series, there is nuclear replication without cell division) to expand the population, and later precursors of the functional cells differentiate without further cell division. B) Fall and recovery of the peripheral granulocyte count after chemotherapy. For most drugs, the count falls to a nadir at 10-14 days after treatment, with complete recovery by 3-4 weeks.

of blood granulocytes (and more rarely of platelets) that follows treatment with most chemotherapy drugs (Fig. 17–10B). Proliferation-dependent cytotoxic drugs deplete the rapidly proliferating cells in the earlier part of the maturation series, with minimal effects against the more mature nonproliferating cells and against slowly proliferating stem cells. Blood counts may remain in the normal range while the more mature surviving cells continue to differentiate but will then fall rapidly at a time when the depleted cells would normally have completed maturation. A substantial decrease in the number of mature cells is common for granulocytes because their lifetime is only 1-2 days, less common for platelets (lifetime of a few days), and rare for red blood cells (mean lifetime of about 120 days), but it may also be influenced by differences in the intrinsic sensitivities of their precursor cells for different drugs. The number of mature granulocytes usually decreases at 8-10 days after treatment with drugs such as cyclophosphamide, doxorubicin, or paclitaxel but may do so earlier for other drugs (eg, vinblastine). The variation in time from treatment to the fall in peripheral blood counts for different drugs probably reflects their different effects on the rate of cell maturation. When the peripheral granulocyte count falls, proliferation of stem cells is mediated by release of growth factors, with subsequent recovery of the entire bone marrow population. Administration of growth factors (eg, granulocyte colony stimulating factor, or G-CSF) after chemotherapy can accelerate the reappearance of mature cells in the peripheral blood and decrease the possibility of infection that can occur in the absence of mature granulocytes. For many drugs (eg, cyclophosphamide, doxorubicin, taxanes), recovery of peripheral blood counts is complete at ~3 weeks after therapy (or at ~2 weeks if growth factors are given), and further treatment may be given with little or no evidence of residual damage to bone marrow.

Following treatment with some drugs, such as melphalan, or with wide-field radiation to a high proportion of the bone marrow, recovery of mature granulocytes and platelets to normal levels is slower, usually requiring about 6 weeks after treatment. Drugs that produce prolonged myelosuppression tend to show only a small difference in effects against slowly and rapidly proliferating cells and may cause direct damage to slowly or nonproliferating stem cells. Thus, recovery is delayed because of repopulation from a smaller number of bone marrow stem cells, and some damage may be permanent because of incomplete repopulation of the stem-cell pool.

Recovery of blood counts after treatment with anticancer drugs is the usual determinant of the interval between courses of chemotherapy. If myelosuppressive drugs are given when peripheral blood counts are low, they will not only delay recovery and increase the chance of infection and bleeding, but will also have a higher chance of depleting the stem-cell population, because it is likely to be proliferating rapidly. Drug administration can be repeated up to 1 week after initial treatment, before the decrease in mature granulocytes and platelets is observed; this schedule has been incorporated into several drug regimens where anticancer drugs are given on days 1 and 8 of a 21- or 28-day cycle. Some drugs (eg, bleomycin, vincristine, and many of the newer targeted agents) cause only minimal toxicity to bone marrow, probably because of intrinsic resistance of the precursor cells; they can be given when peripheral granulocyte and platelet counts are low following the use of myelosuppressive agents.

Red blood cells have a long lifetime, which usually prevents the rapid development of anemia following initiation of chemotherapy. However, repeated courses of chemotherapy cause repeated interruptions of red cell production so that the serum level of hemoglobin tends to decrease slowly, leading to anemia and contributing to fatigue. This effect can occur with all types of drug therapy, but occurs rapidly following the use of cisplatin and its analogs. Injection of erythroid stimulating agents, which are analogs of the growth factor erythropoietin, can be used to stimulate production of red blood cells, but the use of these agents in patients with solid tumors is discouraged, because they may cause thrombosis.

Chemotherapy is scheduled most often using intermittent large doses, but continuous daily administration of low doses of drugs (known as metronomic therapy) can give superior effects in animal models, perhaps because of additional effects to inhibit angiogenesis (Kerbel and Kamen, 2004). Although such schedules have activity (and low toxicity) against some human tumors, there is no evidence that they provide better long-term outcomes.

Many of the molecular targeted agents described in Section 17.3 and in Chapter 19 require chronic administration to provide sustained inhibition of their target receptor or pathway. Monoclonal antibodies have long half-lives in the circulation, and sustained levels can be achieved by dosing at weekly intervals or less often. However, most inhibitors of receptor tyrosine kinases are small molecules with relatively short half-lives, and these agents are most often given by mouth on a continuous daily schedule. Many of these agents inhibit pathways that stimulate proliferation of cancer (and other cells), and although used alone, they do not usually lead to myelosuppression; they can add substantially to this and other toxicities when used in combination with chemotherapy, and dose reduction of both agents is then generally required.

17.5.3 Toxicity of Drugs to Other Proliferative Tissues

Ulceration of the mucosa in the mouth, throat, esophagus, or intestine may occur after treatment with antiproliferative drugs, and can lead to soreness, intestinal bleeding, and diarrhea. It is due to interruption of the production of new cells that normally replace the mature cells continually being sloughed into gastrointestinal tract. Damage to bone marrow is more commonly dose-limiting in humans, but mucosal ulceration may occur after treatment with several drugs, including methotrexate, 5-fluorouracil, bleomycin, oxaliplatin, and cytosine arabinoside; it may also occur after treatment with several targeted agents (eg, mTOR inhibitors and multitargeted TKIs), presumably because they inhibit proliferation and maturation in mucosal epithelium. Mucosal damage usually begins about

5 days after treatment, and its duration increases with the severity. Full recovery is usually possible if the patient can be supported through this period; recovery is analogous to that in the bone marrow, with repopulation from slowly proliferating stem cells.

Some drugs can also produce diarrhea without directly damaging the intestinal mucosa. For example, irinotecan can produce diarrhea soon after administration as a consequence of a direct cholinergic effect on the cells of the intestinal mucosa. This type of diarrhea may be prevented through the use of anticholinergic drugs. A second form of diarrhea, secretory in nature, may occur several days following administration of irinotecan, and may be due to damage to the mucosa coupled with cytokine release causing fluid secretion (see Chap. 18, Sec. 18.3.3).

Partial or complete hair loss is common after treatment with many anticancer drugs and is due to lethal effects of drugs against proliferating cells in hair follicles; this usually begins about 2 weeks after treatment. Full recovery usually occurs after cessation of treatment, suggesting the presence of slowly proliferating precursor cells (Dunnill et al, 2018). In some patients, regrowth of hair is observed despite continued treatment with the agent that initially caused its loss. Regrowth of hair might reflect a compensating proliferative process that increases the number of stem cells or may represent the development of drug resistance in a normal tissue akin to that which occurs in tumors.

Spermatogenesis in men and formation of ovarian follicles in women both involve rapid cellular proliferation and are susceptible to the toxic effects of many anticancer drugs. Men who receive chemotherapy often have decreased production of sperm and consequent infertility. Testicular biopsy demonstrates a loss of germinal cells within the seminiferous tubules, presumably because of drug effects against these rapidly proliferating cells. Anti-spermatogenic effects may be reversible after lower doses of chemotherapy, but some men remain permanently infertile. Chemotherapy given to premenopausal women often leads to temporary or permanent cessation of menstrual periods and to menopausal symptoms, and is accompanied by a fall in serum levels of estrogen. Reversibility of this effect depends on age, the types of drug used, and the duration and intensity of chemotherapy. Biopsies taken from the ovaries have shown failure of formation of ovarian follicles, sometimes with ovarian fibrosis. The pathologic findings are consistent with a primary effect of drugs against the proliferating germinal epithelium. Sperm, oocyte, and embryo cryopreservation are standard approaches employed for fertility preservation in young men and women prior to chemotherapy treatment for curable malignancies.

17.5.4 Nausea, Vomiting, and Other Common Toxicities

Nausea and vomiting are frequent during the first few hours after treatment with many types of chemotherapy, but occur less commonly after use of targeted agents. Drug-induced vomiting may occur because of direct stimulation of chemoreceptors in the brainstem, which then emit signals via connecting nerves to the neighboring vomiting center, thus eliciting the vomiting reflex. Major evidence for this mechanism comes from studies in animals, where induction of vomiting by chemotherapy is prevented by removal of the chemoreceptor zone. In addition to a central mechanism, some chemotherapeutic agents exert direct effects on the gastrointestinal tract that may contribute to nausea and vomiting. Several neurotransmitters, such as serotonin (5HT3) and substance P are involved in transmitting signals involved in producing nausea and vomiting. Medications have been developed that inhibit nausea and vomiting after chemotherapy. The most effective of these are the serotonin antagonists (such as ondansetron), which block 5HT3 receptors, and the NK-1 receptor antagonists (such as aprepitant), which block substance P.

Fatigue is a common side effect of both the presence of cancer and its treatment, and several types of chemotherapy as well as many targeted agents can cause profound fatigue. Unfortunately there are no pharmacologic treatments that relieve fatigue, and the only strategy of proven benefit is exercise, possible only for select patients with metastatic cancer (Mustian et al, 2017).

The hand-foot syndrome (or palmar-plantar erythrodysesthesia) may occur during treatment with several types of chemotherapy (eg, capecitabine) and with targeted agents such as sunitinib and sorafenib (Miller et al, 2014). Patients have redness and pain on the palms of the hands and soles of the feet, sometimes with blistering and desquamation, which can be quite disabling. The condition responds to interruption and reduction of dose of the anticancer drug. The cause of this condition is uncertain, although it might relate in part to sensitivity of proliferating cells in the basal layer of the skin in these sites.

Subtle cognitive dysfunction has also been identified as a side effect of chemotherapy, especially in women who are receiving adjuvant chemotherapy for breast cancer (Vardy et al, 2007; Moore, 2014). The mechanisms underlying these effects are unknown; they may be mediated in part by changes in the levels of sex hormones and induction of menopausal symptoms, but are probably also due to direct effects of anticancer drugs on the brain.

17.5.5 Drugs as Carcinogens

Many anticancer drugs cause toxic damage through effects on DNA; they can also cause mutations and chromosomal damage. These properties are shared with known carcinogens (see Chap. 5, Sec. 5.2), and patients who are long-term survivors of such chemotherapy may be at an increased risk for developing a second malignancy. This effect has become apparent only under conditions where chemotherapy has resulted in long-term survival for some patients with drug-sensitive diseases (eg, Hodgkin disease, other lymphomas, testicular cancer) or where it is used as an adjuvant to decrease the probability of recurrence of disease following local treatment (eg, breast cancer). Many of the second malignancies are acute leukemias, and their most common time of presentation is 2-6 years after initiation of chemotherapy. Increased incidence of solid tumors may also be observed after longer periods of follow-up. Alkylating agents are the drugs most commonly implicated as the cause of second malignancy, and there is increased risk if patients also receive radiation. It is often difficult to separate an increase in the probability of second malignancy due to treatment with that associated with the primary neoplasm (eg, in a patient with lymphoma) or with a shared etiologic factor, either environmental or due to genetic predisposition.

Comparisons of the incidence of leukemia and other malignancies in clinical trials that randomize patients to receive adjuvant chemotherapy, or no chemotherapy after primary treatment, have provided conclusive evidence of the carcinogenic potential of some drugs. The relative risk of myeloid neoplasms (leukemia and myelodysplastic syndrome [MDS]) in drug-treated, as compared with control patients, was increased in women receiving adjuvant therapy for breast cancer that included an alkylating agent (especially when melphalan was used) but for modern regimens that include conventional dose cyclophosphamide, the risk is small. Drugs that target topoisomerase II (eg, doxorubicin, epirubicin, mitoxantrone, and etoposide; see Chap. 18, Sec. 18.3.3) have also been identified as causes of treatment-related leukemia compared with those not receiving this treatment. For women receiving adjuvant treatment for early breast cancer, an increased risk of marrow neoplasm compared to those treated with surgery alone was identified with a hazard ratio of 6.8, and a rate of 0.46 cases per 1,000 patient-years (Wolff et al, 2015). Leukemias that occur following treatment with topoisomerase inhibitors have characteristic chromosomal translocations that distinguish them from those that occur following alkylating agents, and they tend to occur after a shorter latent period of 1-3 years after treatment of the primary cancer (Mistry et al, 2005).

The risk of second solid tumors following treatment with chemotherapy is far lower than the risk of developing leukemia. Nonetheless, a 4.5-fold increase in the risk of transitional cell carcinoma of the urothelium has been demonstrated in patients who had received cyclophosphamide for the treatment of non-Hodgkin lymphoma (Travis et al, 1995), and there is an increased risk of breast and other cancers in patients who are treated for Hodgkin lymphoma with radiotherapy or chemotherapy, and especially in those receiving both treatments. The absolute risk of second malignancy is small compared with the potential benefits in treating curable cancers, but care is needed in using carcinogenic drugs as adjuvant chemotherapy for malignancies where benefit is minimal.

Some nonchemotherapy drugs are also associated with increased risks of other cancers. Endometrial cancer risk is increased 2- to 3-fold with the use of adjuvant tamoxifen to prevent recurrences of breast cancer, but the absolute risk is below 1% and most are curable by surgery (Matesich and Shapiro, 2003). AML and MDS have been observed in small numbers of patients treated with PARP inhibitors; the contributions of patient genetics (these agents are often used in patients with germline BRCA1 or BRCA2 mutations), prior chemotherapy exposure and use of the PARP inhibitor remain to be elucidated. BRAF inhibitors, used mainly in the treatment of melanoma, are associated with the development of squamous cell carcinomas, through the paradoxical activation of RAS (Su et al, 2012). These therapy-induced cancers are not observed when BRAF-inhibitors are combined with MEK-inhibitors.

17.5.6 Determinants of Normal-Tissue Toxicity

When chemotherapy is given to a patient, a drug dose is selected on the basis of early-phase clinical trials that have determined the *average* dose (often per unit of body surface area) that gives some toxicity, but at an acceptable level. At this dose, there may be a small proportion of patients, who experience severe, potentially lethal, toxicity. Multiple factors influence the distribution of drugs to tissues in the body (see Chap. 18, Sec. 18.2.1) and the response of normal cells to these drugs. Some patients have genetically determined traits that influence drug metabolism or excretion, and the study of genetically determined factors that influence the probability of drug toxicity is known as pharmacogenetics (see Chap. 4, Sec. 4.6.3, and Chap. 18, Sec. 18.2.3). For example, patients who lack the enzyme dihydropyrimidine dehydrogenase (DPD), which catabolizes 5-fluorouracil, show extreme sensitivity to this drug. Genetic abnormalities that give rise to the DPD-deficient phenotype have been identified, and screening tests can identify susceptible individuals (Meulendijks et al, 2015). Changes in the activity of enzymes that metabolize other drugs, either genetically determined or induced by concomitant medications, may also have a profound effect on drug-induced toxicity (Scripture and Figg, 2006).

Because lethal damage due to chemotherapy results most often from interaction of drugs with DNA, patients with deficiencies in DNA repair (see Chap. 9, Sec. 9.5) are very sensitive to anticancer drugs, as they are to radiation. People who are heterozygous for some DNA repair gene mutations (eg, xeroderma pigmentosum or ataxia telangiectasia) may be at high risk for severe toxicity if treated with chemotherapy.

17.5.7 Preclinical Data Needed to Support First in Human Trials

Before a new drug is tested in a first-in-human phase I trial, preliminary characterization of its pharmacology and toxicology must be undertaken. Preliminary characterization includes determination of the mechanism(s) of action and schedule dependencies, antitumor activity, evaluation of limited pharmacokinetic parameters (eg, peak plasma/serum levels, area under the concentration vs time curve, and half-life; see Chap. 18, Sec. 18.2.1) in animal species, and assessment of its ability to inhibit its putative molecular target. The safety pharmacology studies should have been conducted in animals to assess the effect of the drug on vital organ functions including cardiovascular, respiratory, and central nervous systems before the initiation of clinical studies in humans. The general toxicology testing is usually performed in rodents as well as nonrodents. In scenarios where specific concerns have been identified, appropriate safety pharmacology studies should be conducted in animals before human trials. The severity and potential reversibility of the identified toxicities need to be assessed, and this assessment should include the regenerative capacity of the organ system affected. Data from embryo-fetal toxicity studies are not needed for initiating first-in-human trials, where pregnant cancer patients are typically excluded. Other specific toxicity studies such as genotoxicity, carcinogenicity, immunotoxicity, and assessment of phototoxic potential are considered based on mechanism of action as well as chemical properties of the drug tested and information of its related members in the class.

Usually, for small-molecule anticancer drugs, the starting dose for first-in-human studies is set at 1/10th the Severely Toxic Dose in 10% of the animals (STD 10) when evaluated in rodents or at one-sixth the Highest Non-Severely Toxic Dose (HNSTD) when evaluated in nonrodent species. For some classes of drugs such as immunomodulatory monoclonal antibodies, it may be appropriate to select the starting dose based on the minimal anticipated biologic effect level (MABEL). The toxicology studies to determine a no observed adverse effect level (NOAEL) or no effect level (NOEL) are not considered essential for drugs intended for use in patients with advanced cancer. The starting dose and schedule should be selected based on scientific justifications using all the available nonclinical data including pharmacokinetics, pharmacodynamics, and toxicity. In determining the incremental dose levels in human phase I studies, caution should be exercised when a steep dose-response or exposure-response curve for severe toxicity is observed in preclinical toxicology studies.

17.6 TREATMENT WITH MULTIPLE AGENTS

17.6.1 Influence on Therapeutic Index

Patients are treated frequently with drug combinations or with drugs and radiation therapy. When 2 or more agents are combined to give an improvement in the therapeutic index, this implies that the increase in toxicity to critical normal tissues is less than the increase in damage to tumor cells. Because the dose-limiting toxicity to normal tissues may vary for different drugs and for radiation, 2 agents may often be combined with only minimal reduction in doses as compared with those that would be used if either agent were given alone. Additive effects against a tumor with less than additive toxicity for normal tissue may then lead to a therapeutic advantage. Mechanisms by which different agents may give therapeutic benefit when used in combination have been classified as follows: (1) independent toxicity, which may, for example, allow combined use of anticancer drugs at dosages similar to those used when the drugs are given alone; (2) spatial cooperation, whereby disease that is missed by one agent (eg, local radiotherapy) may be treated by another (eg, drug therapy); (3) protection of normal tissues; and (4) enhancement of tumor response, where there is selective sensitization of effects of one agent against tumor cells by another (Steel and Peckham, 1979).

The above mechanisms suggest guidelines for choosing drugs that might be given in combination. Most chemotherapy drugs exert dose-limiting toxicity for the bone marrow, but this is not the case for many targeted agents and some chemotherapy agents such as vincristine (dose-limiting neurotoxicity), cisplatin (nephrotoxicity), or bleomycin (mucositis and lung toxicity). Some of these chemotherapy drugs can be combined at close to full dosage and have contributed to the therapeutic success of drug combinations used to treat lymphoma and testicular cancer. Most trials of combined chemotherapy and targeted agents have led to increased toxicity and a requirement for dose reduction, even though the targets of the drugs are different. Most such combinations have employed concurrent treatment, which is conceptually counterintuitive: targeted agents often act initially to inhibit proliferation of target cells, which might then protect them from cycle-active chemotherapy. A more logical schedule may be to use chemotherapy and targeted agents in sequence, and might have the added advantage of inhibiting tumor cell repopulation in the intervals between chemotherapy (see Chap. 18, Sec. 18.4.8; Kim and Tannock, 2005).

17.6.2 Synergy and Additivity

Claims are made frequently that 2 agents are synergistic, implying that the 2 agents given together are more effective than would be expected from their individual activities. Confusion has arisen because of disagreement as to what constitutes an expected level of effect when 2 noninteracting agents are combined. The use of multiple agents may lead to an increase in the therapeutic index, but it is rare that a claim for synergy of effects against a single population of mammalian cells can be substantiated (Ocana et al, 2012). Several methods have been used to evaluate possible synergy, additivity, or antagonism between 2 agents, including isobologram analysis as proposed by Steel and Peckham (1979), and calculation of an "interaction index" based on the median effect principle (Chou, 2010; Foucquier and Guedj, 2015).

The above concepts require consideration of the dose-response relationship following treatment of a single population of cells either in a tumor or in a normal tissue, by either agent alone, and by their combined use. Thus, suppose a given dose of agent A gives a surviving fraction of cells (S_A), that a surviving fraction (S_B) follows treatment with a given dose of agent B, and a combination of the agents gives a surviving fraction (S_{AB}; see Fig. 17–11). Claims for synergy are often made if S_{AB} is less than the product $S_A \times S_B$. This conclusion

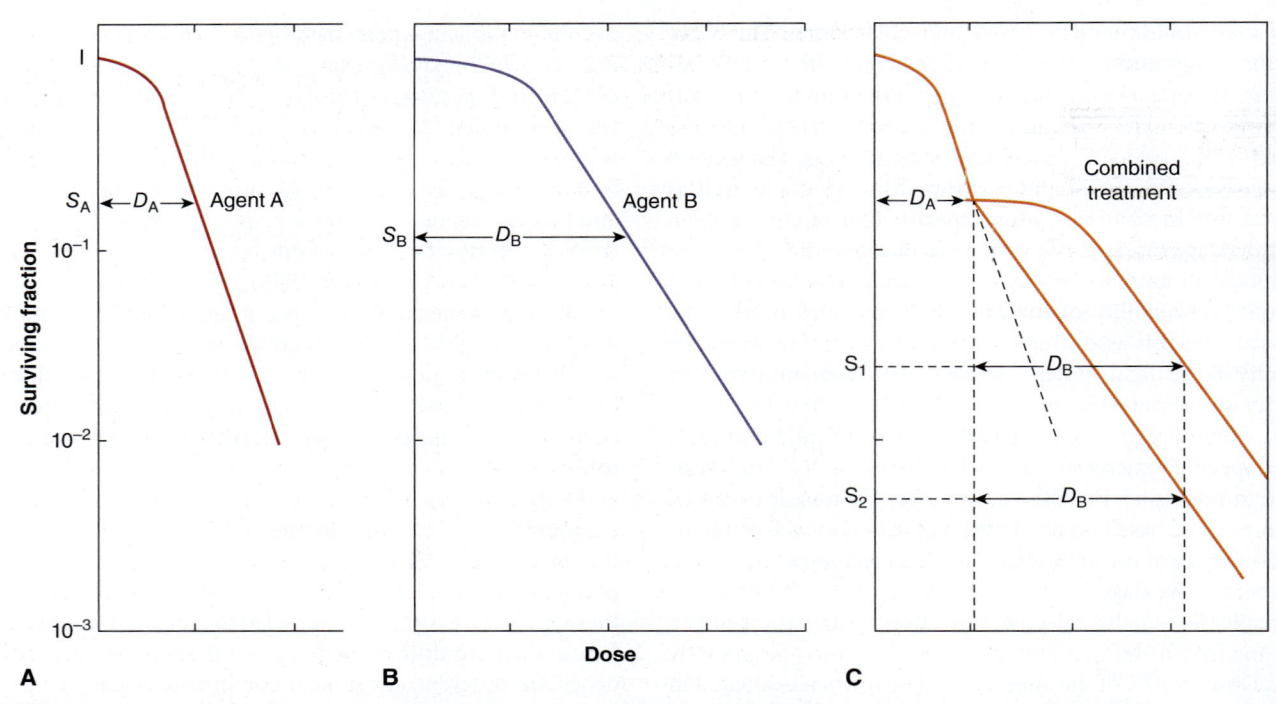

FIGURE 17-11 Interaction of 2 agents A and B. Cell survival (S_A or S_B) is indicated following treatment with either of 2 agents, A and B, each of which has a survival curve characterized by an initial shoulder followed by an exponential fall with increasing dose. **C)** Survival (S_{AB}) after combined use of dose D_A of agent A and dose D_B of agent B will be equal to S_1 ($= S_A \times S_B$) if there is no overlap of damage, and the "shoulder" representing accumulation of sublethal damage is retained for the second agent. Survival after combined treatment (S_{AB}) will be equal to S_2 if cells have accumulated maximum sublethal damage from the first agent A, and the "shoulder" of the curve is lost for the second agent B.

is correct only if cell survival is exponentially related to dose for both agents. If the survival curves have an initial shoulder, as in Figure 17–11, then combined treatment will be expected to lead to a lower level of survival if, after treatment with the first agent, A, the survival falls exponentially with dose (in the absence of a shoulder effect) for the second agent, B (Fig. 17–11). The fallacy of defining this lower level of survival as a synergistic effect can be illustrated by replacing agent B with a second, equivalent dose of agent A given immediately after the first dose: the combined survival curve then follows that for agent A (Fig. 17–11A). If agent A has a survival curve with an initial shoulder, one would then conclude erroneously that agent A was synergistic with itself.

The above discussion implies that there is a range over which 2 agents can produce additive effects. Isobologram analysis provides a method for defining this range of additivity (Steel and Peckham, 1979). Dose-response curves are first generated for each agent used alone. These dose-response curves are then used to generate isoeffect plots (known as *isobolograms*). These curves relate the dose of agent A to the dose of agent B that would be predicted, when used in combination, to give a constant level of biologic effect (eg, cell survival) for the assumptions of (1) independent damage and (2) overlapping damage (Fig. 17–12). These curves define an envelope of additivity. If, when the 2 agents are given together, the doses required to give the same level of biologic effect lie within the envelope, the interaction is said to be *additive*. If they lie between the lower

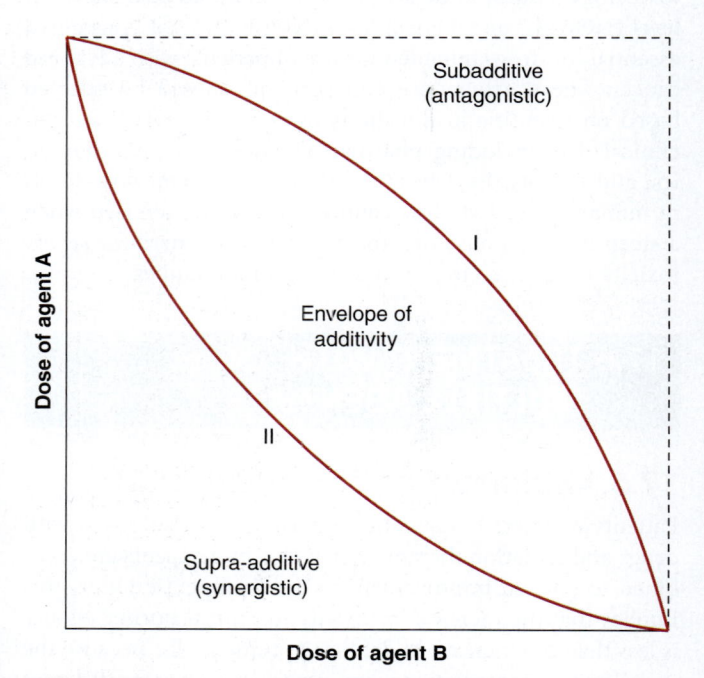

FIGURE 17-12 Isobologram relating the doses of 2 agents that would be expected to give a constant level of biologic effect when used together. It was generated from dose-response curves for each agent separately. Assumptions about overlap or nonoverlap of damage (Fig. 17–10) lead to the generation of 2 isobologram curves (I and II) that describe an envelope of additive interaction. Experimental data falling outside this envelope may indicate synergistic or antagonistic interactions, as shown.

isobologram and the axes (ie, the combined effect is caused by lower doses of the 2 agents than predicted) the interaction is *supra-additive* or synergistic. If the required doses of the 2 agents in combination lie above the envelope of additivity (ie, the effect is caused by higher doses than predicted), the interaction is *subadditive* or antagonistic (Fig. 17–12).

The median effect principle represents an alternative method of evaluating additivity or synergy between agents and a simplified explanation of the principle has been provided (Chou, 2010). The method also depends on the availability of a dose-effect relationship for each of the agents used alone, and for both agents in combination, and relies on the calculation of a "Combination Index (CI)"; a computer program is available to facilitate this. A CI of 1 represents additivity, a CI >1 synergy, and a CI <1 antagonism. The method can also be used to plot a normalized isobologram, and although the mathematical formulation is more complex, it is in conceptual agreement with the representation described in Figures 17–10 and 17–11.

Demonstration that 2 or more agents have a supra-additive or synergistic interaction has been used as a rationale for their inclusion in clinical protocols. This rationale is valid only if the interaction leads to a greater effect against the tumor as compared with that against limiting normal tissues (ie, if it leads to an improvement in therapeutic index; Sec. 17.5.1). It is theoretically possible that antagonistic agents (sub-additive interaction) could improve therapeutic index provided that there was greater antagonism of toxic effects for normal tissues as compared to toxicity for the tumor, or they have nonoverlapping toxicities.

17.6.3 Modifiers of Drug Activity or Toxicity

Some drugs with little or no toxicity for tumor cells may modify the action of anticancer drugs to produce increased antitumor effect or may protect normal tissue. One example is the use of folinic acid with 5-fluorouracil, which may provide a necessary cofactor for inhibition of the target enzyme thymidilate synthase (see Chap. 18, Sec. 18.3.2). Alternatively, reduction of the toxic effects of chemotherapy against bone marrow may be achieved by co-administration of growth factors such as granulocyte colony-stimulating factor (G-CSF), which can stimulate earlier recovery of mature granulocytes after bone marrow suppression by chemotherapy, or after stem cell transplantation (Sec. 17.5.2). G-CSF is used commonly in situations where reduction in dosage of chemotherapy might lead to a decrease in the probability of cure or long-term survival of patients.

Two other agents that may protect normal tissues from damage because of chemotherapy are dexrazoxane and amifostine. Dexrazoxane is a prodrug with an active form that chelates iron. Because complexes between iron and anthracyclines, such as doxorubicin (and the consequent formation of free radicals), appear to mediate cardiac toxicity but not antitumor effects, dexrazoxane may decrease cardiac toxicity of these drugs and increase their therapeutic index (Venturini et al, 1996). Amifostine is also a prodrug that is converted to a sulfhydryl-containing active form. Amifostine is localized selectively in normal tissues, probably because of increased activity of the activating enzyme alkaline phosphatase on the membranes of normal cells. Therefore, it may offer selective protection against a variety of drugs (and radiation) that damage cells by producing reactive intermediates, which bind to sulfhydryl groups (Kemp et al, 1996). There remain concerns, however, that these agents might also provide some protection of tumor cells from drug effects, and they are used only rarely in the clinic.

The crucial test for all modifiers is the demonstration in well-designed clinical trials that the addition of the modifier improves the therapeutic index (eg, by increasing the probability or duration of tumor response with no increase in toxicity) as compared to lower doses of chemotherapy used alone.

17.6.4 Drugs and Radiation

Improvement in therapeutic index from use of drugs and radiation requires selective effects to increase damage to tumor cells as compared to those in normal tissues. One mechanism by which combined treatment with radiation and drugs leads to therapeutic advantage arises when radiation is used to provide effective treatment for sites of bulky disease (usually the primary tumor) and drugs are used to treat metastatic sites containing smaller numbers of cells. This spatial cooperation (Sec. 17.6.1) requires no interaction of the 2 modalities but involves different dose-limiting toxicities. There are also mechanisms whereby the combined use of radiation and drugs might be used to obtain therapeutic advantage for treatment of a primary tumor. Some properties of cells that might be exploited to give therapeutic advantage for the combined use of radiation and drugs are listed in Table 17–1.

Genetic instability in tumors often leads to the presence of subclones, which coexist in the tumor with different levels of sensitivity to drugs and to radiation (see Chap. 13, Sec 13.2.3). When therapy is applied, any resistant cells that are present will have a selective survival advantage and will determine tumor response: thus, heterogeneity in therapeutic response may tend to make tumors more resistant to treatment than normal tissues. Combined treatment with radiation and drugs might then lead to improved therapeutic index if radiation can eradicate small populations of drug-resistant cells, or if drugs can eliminate populations that are relatively resistant to radiation therapy. This cooperative effect requires that mechanisms of resistance to the 2 therapeutic agents are independent. Mechanisms (other than hypoxia) that confer clinical resistance to radiotherapy remain poorly understood, but include enhanced ability to repair damage to DNA, and increased levels of SH compounds such as glutathione (or of associated GST enzymes) that scavenge free radicals (especially in hypoxic cells), and decreased ability to undergo apoptosis (see Chap. 8, Sec. 8.4.1). These mechanisms may also convey resistance to some anticancer drugs, whereas many other mechanisms of drug resistance (see Chap. 18, Sec. 18.4) are unlikely to cause resistance to radiation. Resistance to any given drug may be

TABLE 17-1 Properties of tumor cells that could be exploited to provide therapeutic advantage from the combined use of 2 drugs or of radiation and drugs.

Property	Effect of Combined Treatment
Genetic instability of tumors, leading to different mechanisms of resistance for different clones	Killing of resistant cells by one agent, and surviving cells by the second agent *if* mechanisms of resistance are independent
Two genes or pathways are in a synthetic-lethal relationship if mutations or lack of function in either of them is not lethal but mutations or lack of function in both of them produce cell death	Each agent inhibits the complementary gene or pathway—leading to synthetic lethality
DNA repair	One agent inhibits repair of DNA damage caused by the other; synthetic lethality is a special case where there is inhibition of complementary repair pathways
Differences in cell proliferation between tumor and normal tissue	Selective uptake of radiosensitizing nucleosides (eg, IUdR)
Differences in repopulation during radiation treatment for tumor and normal tissue	Inhibition of repopulation by drugs could lead to therapeutic advantage *if* repopulation were faster in the tumor
Environmental factors such as hypoxia and acidity, which are usually confined to tumors	Beneficial effects from combining radiotherapy or drugs with greater activity for cycling cells with drugs that have selective toxicity for hypoxic and/or acidic cells

caused by multiple mechanisms so that a radiation-drug combination that provides therapeutic advantage for one tumor may not do so for another if different mechanisms of drug resistance are dominant.

Mechanisms of interaction between drugs and radiation at the cellular level may be evaluated from cell survival curves for radiation obtained in the presence or absence of the drug (Fig. 17–13). Drugs may influence the survival curve in at least 3 ways: (1) the curve may be displaced downward by the amount of cell kill caused by the drug alone; (2) the shoulder on the survival curve may be lost, suggesting an inability to repair radiation damage in the presence of the drug; and (3) the slope of the exponential part of the survival curve may be changed, indicating sensitization or protection by the drug. Most drugs influence survival curves according to the first 2 patterns; this corresponds to the limits of additivity defined in Section 17.6.2, where sublethal damage may be independent or overlapping. The third pattern, leading to a change in slope of the dose-response curve, defines agents that are radiation sensitizers or protectors (see Chap. 16, Sec. 16.2.5). Sensitization of this type has been reported inconsistently for cisplatin and for prolonged exposure to 5-FU after radiation (Schürmann et al, 2018).

Proliferation of surviving cells during a course of fractionated radiation (ie, repopulation; Chap. 16, Sec. 16.6.2) acts to increase the total number of cells that must be killed (Kim and Tannock, 2005). Anticancer drugs given *during* the course of fractionated radiation might be expected to inhibit repopulation (Fig. 17–14). Combined treatment may then convey therapeutic advantage if the rate of repopulation is greater for the tumor cells than it is for normal tissues within the radiation field. Greater specificity would be expected for agents that inhibit specifically the proliferation of tumor cells, including molecular targeted agents. Improved survival of patients with head and neck cancer treated with radiotherapy and concurrent cetuximab, an inhibitor of EGFR, as compared to

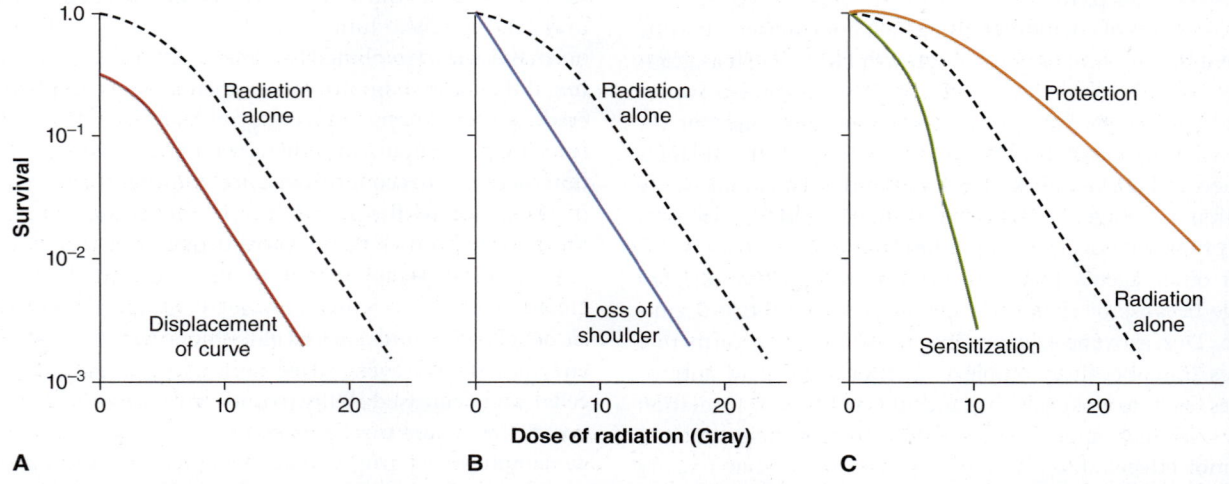

FIGURE 17–13 Possible influences of drug treatment on the relationship between radiation dose and cell survival: A) displacement of curve; B) loss of shoulder, indicating effects of drug on the repair of sublethal radiation damage; C) change in the slope of the curve, indicating sensitization or protection.

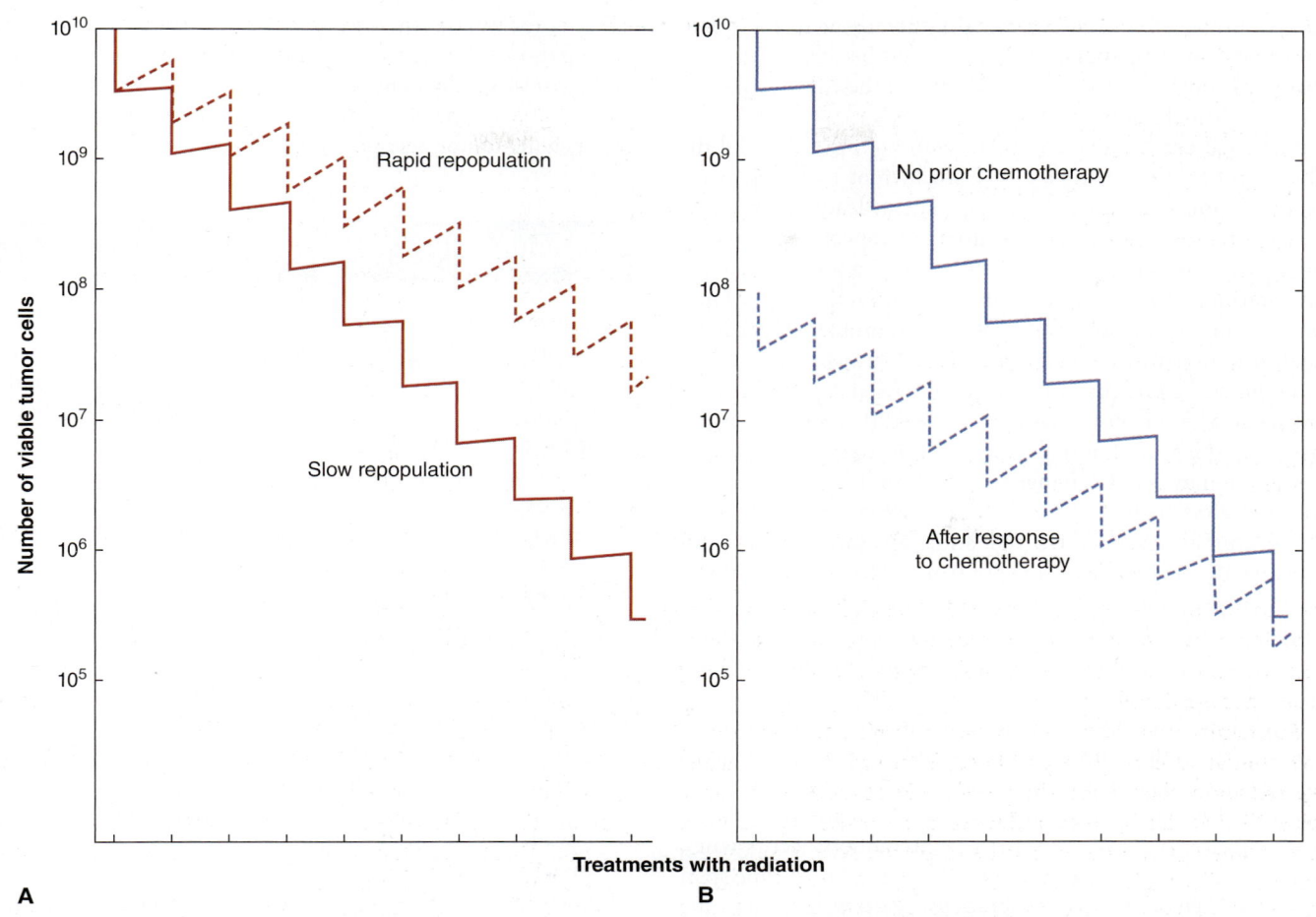

FIGURE 17–14 Schematic diagram illustrating the effect of repopulation in a tumor during a course of fractionated irradiation. Each radiation fraction is assumed to kill the same fraction of tumor cells. In **A**, the effect of different rates of repopulation is illustrated. In **B**, it is assumed that prior chemotherapy kills 99% of the cells but induces "accelerated" repopulation by the survivors. Response to radiation treatment alone (solid line) or radiation treatment following the chemotherapy (dashed line) is illustrated. The accelerated repopulation induced by the prior drug treatment rapidly negates the extra cell kill achieved by the drug treatment.

radiotherapy alone (Bonner et al, 2010), is most likely due to inhibition of repopulation of tumor cells during the course of radiotherapy, although this targeted agent does not provide better therapeutic outcome than concurrent cisplatin.

Repopulation during fractionated radiation therapy might also be influenced by prior treatment with neoadjuvant chemotherapy. Such chemotherapy may cause tumor shrinkage, followed by improved nutrition of surviving cells, with consequent stimulation of cell proliferation (Kim and Tannock, 2005). If there is increased repopulation of surviving cells during the subsequent course of fractionated radiation therapy, any advantage from initial shrinkage of the tumor caused by chemotherapy may be lost or reversed because of the decreased net effectiveness of subsequent radiation treatment (Fig. 17–14).

Regrowth of tumors following radiotherapy depends on maintenance of a vascular supply to provide nutrients to surviving cells. Clinical courses of radiotherapy are likely to lead to killing of endothelial and other cells that constitute the pre-existing vasculature and it has been proposed that tumor regeneration depends on recruitment of circulating myeloid precursors that form new blood vessels in irradiated tumors (Ahn and Brown, 2009). These circulating precursors might be killed or suppressed by chemotherapy given concurrently with radiation, or by agents that target them more specifically (Ahn et al, 2010).

A fourth mechanism that has potential for exploitation through combined use of radiation and drugs depends on the presence of a hypoxic microenvironment within solid tumors (see Chap. 12, Sec. 12.4, and Chap. 16, Sec. 16.4). A hypoxic environment conveys resistance to radiation because cell killing is dependent in part on the presence of oxygen. Several drugs have been developed that require bioreduction under hypoxic conditions for activity, and therefore have selective toxicity for hypoxic cells; effective drugs may also diffuse to influence neighboring aerobic regions (Baran and Konopleva, 2017; see also Chap. 12, Sec. 12.4.4, and Chap. 18, Sec. 18.4.7). Such drugs would be expected to have fewer effects against normal tissues, where adequate vasculature usually prevents development of a hypoxic microenvironment, although there is evidence for hypoxic regions in bone marrow and some other normal tissues (Baran and Konopleva, 2017). Hypoxia-selective drugs might augment both the effects of radiation and of conventional chemotherapy, where hypoxic cells and their neighbors might be spared because of limited drug distribution within solid tumors and their low proliferative rate (Minchinton and Tannock, 2006).

Many patients receive treatment with both drugs and radiation, and there is evidence that concurrent treatment with radiation and various chemotherapy agents leads to improvement in therapeutic index in a variety of cancer sites, including glioblastoma, head and neck, lung, esophageal, rectal, anal, and uterine cervix. In these settings, radiation therapy is a primary treatment and local failure is a major problem that can be decreased with use of concurrent chemotherapy.

Whenever radiation and drugs are used together or in sequence, there is potential for increased damage to normal tissues in the radiation field. Some of the effects of combined treatment may lead to changes in function that occur months to years after treatment. Both clinical experience and studies in animals have shown that most anticancer drugs can increase the incidence of toxicity from radiation, sometimes in organs (eg, the kidney) where the drugs alone rarely cause overt toxicity. The effect of a drug on radiation toxicity to any organ may be expressed in terms of a dose-enhancement ratio (DER), which is the dose of radiation to produce a given effect when used alone divided by the dose of radiation that gives the same effect when combined with the drug. For acute effects of radiation on normal tissues of mice, typical values of DER range from 1.0 to 1.5, depending on the drug and normal tissue; maximum interaction occurs when drug and radiation are administered within a short time span (von der Maase, 1986). The therapeutic gain factor equals the ratio of DER for the tumor to the DER for the dose-limiting normal tissue in the radiation field. In experimental systems, this may vary widely depending on the drug used, the doses of drug and radiation, and the sequence; it is difficult to predict the dose schedules that are likely to lead to therapeutic gain in patients.

Anticancer drugs may also initiate a "radiation recall" phenomenon whereby an acute inflammatory reaction is initiated in previously irradiated areas after drugs are administered to patients with cancer (Burris and Hurtig, 2010).

17.6.5 Relationship Between Tumor Remission and Cure

For most solid tumors, the limit of clinical and/or radiologic detection is about 1 gram of tissue (10^9 cells). If therapy can reduce the tumor volume below this limit of detection, the patient will be described as being in complete clinical remission. Surgical biopsy of sites that were known to be involved with tumor previously may lower the limit of detection, especially if immunohistochemistry is used to identify specific markers on tumor cells, but a pathologist is unlikely to detect sporadic tumor cells present at a frequency of less than 1 in 10,000 normal cells. Therefore, even a surgically confirmed complete remission may be compatible with the remaining presence of a large number of tumor cells (up to 10^5/g tissue). Tumor cure requires eradication of all tumor cells that have the capacity for tumor regeneration. The proportion of such cells among those of the tumor population is unknown, but clinical and even surgically confirmed complete remissions are compatible with the presence of a substantial residual population of surviving tumor-repopulating cells.

SUMMARY

- The discovery of novel anticancer drugs begins with the identification of potential therapeutic targets. Molecular characterization of events in cellular transformation and tumor progression is being used to identify new targets for anticancer agents.
- Modern approaches use high-throughput DNA and RNA sequencing, RNAi, or CRISPR technology to knockdown/knockout the genetic target and thereby determine whether it is essential for tumor growth.
- After a target is selected, drug candidates are developed using a variety of approaches including automated physical screens and structure guided rational drug design.
- Drug candidates are evaluated in preclinical models using cell culture systems and animal models. Drugs that inhibit their targets and display efficacy in preclinical models and a probable therapeutic window advance into clinical trials for definitive assessments of toxicity and efficacy.
- Characterization of molecular targets coupled with new approaches to drug discovery has generated therapeutic agents that are more selective for cancer cells as compared to normal cells. Such agents include small molecules and monoclonal antibodies that inhibit membrane-based tyrosine kinases or critical intracellular enzymes.
- Many anticancer drugs, both chemotherapy and targeted agents, act primarily to inhibit cell proliferation, and may share common toxicities against proliferating cells in normal tissues such as the bone marrow and intestine.
- Other frequent toxicities include nausea, vomiting, and fatigue and several agents can also act as carcinogens.
- Improvement in treatment requires an improvement in therapeutic index, a measure of the relative toxic effects against a tumor as compared to the dose limiting normal tissue(s).
- Anticancer drugs are used frequently in combination with each other and with radiation. Analysis of interactions between different agents is complex and claims for synergy are rarely justified.

REFERENCES

Ahn GO, Brown JM. Influence of bone marrow-derived hematopoietic cells on the tumor response to radiotherapy: experimental models and clinical perspectives. *Cell Cycle* 2009;8(7):970-976.

Ahn GO, Tseng D, Liao CH, et al. Inhibition of Mac-1 (CD11b/CD18) enhances tumor response to radiation by reducing myeloid cell recruitment. *Proc Natl Acad Sci U S A* 2010; 107(18):8363-8368.

Amir E, Seruga B, Serrano R, Ocana A. Targeting DNA repair in breast cancer: a clinical and translational update. *Cancer Treat Rev* 2010;36(7):557-565.

Ashworth A, Lord CJ. Synthetic lethal therapies for cancer: what's next after PARP inhibitors? *Nat Rev Clin Oncol* 2018;15(9):564-576.

Ashworth A, Lord CJ, Reis-Filho JS. Genetic interactions in cancer progression and treatment. *Cell* 2011;145(1):30-38.

Bailey MH, Tokheim C, Porta-Pardo E, et al. Comprehensive characterization of cancer driver genes and mutations. *Cell* 2018;174(4):1034-1035.

Baran N, Konopleva M. Molecular pathways: hypoxia-activated prodrugs in cancer therapy. *Clin Cancer Res* 2017; 23(10):2382-2390.

Begley CG, Ellis LM. Drug development: raise standards for preclinical cancer research. *Nature* 2012;483(7391):531-533.

Bonner JA, Harari PM, Giralt J, et al. Radiotherapy plus cetuximab for locoregionally advanced head and neck cancer: 5-year survival data from a phase 3 randomised trial, and relation between cetuximab-induced rash and survival. *Lancet Oncol* 2010;11(1):21-28.

Brown JM, Attardi LD. The role of apoptosis in cancer development and treatment response. *Nat Rev Cancer* 2005; 5(3):231-237.

Burris HA 3rd, Hurtig J. Radiation recall with anticancer agents. *Oncologist* 2010;15(11):1227-1237.

Chou TC. Drug combination studies and their synergy quantification using the Chou-Talalay method. *Cancer Res* 2010;70(2):440-446.

Cole A, Wang Z, Coyaud E, et al. Inhibition of the mitochondrial protease ClpP as a therapeutic strategy for human acute myeloid leukemia. *Cancer Cell* 2015;27(6):864-876.

Cortes JE, Kantarjian H, Shah NP, et al. Ponatinib in refractory Philadelphia chromosome-positive leukemias. *N Engl J Med* 2012;367(22):2075-2088.

Dang L, Yen K, Attar EC. IDH mutations in cancer and progress toward development of targeted therapeutics. *Ann Oncol* 2016;27(4):599-608.

Davies H, Bignell GR, Cox C, et al. Mutations of the BRAF gene in human cancer. *Nature* 2002;417(6892):949-954.

Day CP, Merlino G, Van Dyke T. Preclinical mouse cancer models: a maze of opportunities and challenges. *Cell* 2015; 163(1):39-53.

Dimopoulos M, Spencer A, Attal M, et al. Lenalidomide plus dexamethasone for relapsed or refractory multiple myeloma. *N Engl J Med* 2007;357(21):2123-2132.

DiNardo CD, Stein EM, de Botton S, et al. Durable remissions with Ivosidenib in IDH1-mutated relapsed or refractory AML. *N Engl J Med* 2018;378(25):2386-2398.

Dobrolecki LE, Airhart SD, Alferez DG, et al. Patient-derived xenograft (PDX) models in basic and translational breast cancer research. *Cancer Metastasis Rev* 2016;35(4): 547-573.

Drilon A, Laetsch TW, Kummar S, et al. Efficacy of Larotrectinib in TRK fusion-positive cancers in adults and children. *N Engl J Med* 2018;378(8):731-739.

Drost J, Clevers H. Organoids in cancer research. *Nat Rev Cancer* 2018;18(7):407-418.

Druker BJ, Talpaz M, Resta DJ, et al. Efficacy and safety of a specific inhibitor of the BCR-ABL tyrosine kinase in chronic myeloid leukemia. *N Engl J Med* 2001;344(14):1031-1037.

Duggan ST, Keating GM. Pegylated liposomal doxorubicin: a review of its use in metastatic breast cancer, ovarian cancer, multiple myeloma and AIDS-related Kaposi's sarcoma. *Drugs* 2011;71(18):2531-2358.

Dunnill CJ, Al-Tameemi W, Collett A, Haslam IS, Georgopoulos NT. A clinical and biological guide for understanding chemotherapy-induced alopecia and its prevention. *Oncologist* 2018;23(1):84-96.

Foucquier J, Guedj M. Analysis of drug combinations: current methodological landscape. *Pharmacol Res Perspect* 2015; 3(3):e00149.

Goodnow RA Jr, Dumelin CE, Keefe AD. DNA-encoded chemistry: enabling the deeper sampling of chemical space. *Nat Rev Drug Discov* 2017;16(2):131-147.

Hideshima T, Ikeda H, Chauhan D, et al. Bortezomib induces canonical nuclear factor-kappaB activation in multiple myeloma cells. *Blood* 2009;114(5):1046-1052.

Hochhaus A, Larson RA, Guilhot F, et al. Long-term outcomes of imatinib treatment for chronic myeloid leukemia. *N Engl J Med* 2017;376(10):917-927.

Iglehart JD, Silver DP. Synthetic lethality—a new direction in cancer-drug development. *N Engl J Med* 2009;361(2):189-191.

Kang MH, Reynolds CP. Bcl-2 inhibitors: targeting mitochondrial apoptotic pathways in cancer therapy. *Clin Cancer Res* 2009;15(4):1126-1132.

Kantarjian H, Stein A, Gökbuget N, et al. Blinatumomab versus chemotherapy for advanced acute lymphoblastic leukemia. *N Engl J Med* 2017;376(9):836-847.

Kemp G, Rose P, Lurain J, et al. Amifostine pretreatment for protection against cyclophosphamide-induced and cisplatin-induced toxicities: results of a randomized control trial in patients with advanced ovarian cancer. *J Clin Oncol* 1996;14(7):2101-2112.

Kerbel RS, Kamen BA. The anti-angiogenic basis of metronomic chemotherapy. *Nat Rev Cancer* 2004;4(6):423-436.

Kim JJ, Tannock IF. Repopulation of cancer cells during therapy: an important cause of treatment failure. *Nat Rev Cancer* 2005;5(7):516-525.

Lambert JM, Morris CQ. Antibody-drug conjugates (ADCs) for personalized treatment of solid tumors: a review. *Adv Ther* 2017;34(5):1015-1035.

Lancet JE, Uy GL, Cortes JE, et al. CPX-351 (cytarabine and daunorubicin) liposome for injection versus conventional cytarabine plus daunorubicin in older patients with newly diagnosed secondary acute myeloid leukemia. *J Clin Oncol* 2018;36(26):2684-2692.

Larkin J, Ascierto PA, Dréno B, et al. Combined vemurafenib and cobimetinib in BRAF-mutated melanoma. *N Engl J Med* 2014;371(20):1867-1876.

Lea WA, Simeonov A. Fluorescence polarization assays in small molecule screening. *Expert Opin Drug Discov* 2011;6(1):17-32.

Ledford H. Complex synthesis yields breast-cancer therapy. *Nature* 2010;468(7324):608-609.

MacLeod AR, Crooke ST. RNA therapeutics in oncology: advances, challenges, and future directions. *J Clin Pharmacol* 2017;57(Suppl 10):S43-S59.

Matesich SM, Shapiro CL Second cancers after breast cancer treatment. *Semin Oncol* 2003;30(6):740-748.

Meulendijks D, Henricks LM, Sonke GS, et al. Clinical relevance of DPYD variants c.1679T>G, c.1236G>A/HapB3, and c.1601G>A as predictors of severe fluoropyrimidine-associated toxicity: a systematic review and meta-analysis of individual patient data. *Lancet Oncol* 2015;16(16):1639-1650.

Miller KK, Gorcey L, McLellan BN. Chemotherapy-induced hand-foot syndrome and nail changes: a review of clinical presentation, etiology, pathogenesis, and management. *J Am Acad Dermatol* 2014;71(4):787-794.

Minchinton AI, Tannock IF. Drug penetration in solid tumours. *Nat Rev Cancer* 2006;6(8):583-592.

Mistry AR, Felix CA, Whitmarsh RJ, et al. DNA topoisomerase II in therapy-related acute promyelocytic leukemia. *N Engl J Med* 2005;352(15):1529-1538.

Moore HC. An overview of chemotherapy-related cognitive dysfunction, or "chemobrain." *Oncology* 2014;28(9):797-804.

Moreau P, Richardson PG, Cavo M, et al. Proteasome inhibitors in multiple myeloma: 10 years later. *Blood* 2012;120(5):947-959.

Mustian KM, Alfano CM, Heckler C, et al. Comparison of pharmaceutical, psychological, and exercise treatments for cancer-related fatigue: a meta-analysis. *JAMA Oncol* 2017;3(7):961-968.

Nassar D, Blanpain C. Cancer stem cells: basic concepts and therapeutic implications. *Annu Rev Pathol* 2016;11:47-76.

O'Brien S, Schiller G, Lister J, et al. High-dose vincristine sulfate liposome injection for advanced, relapsed, and refractory adult Philadelphia chromosome-negative acute lymphoblastic leukemia. *J Clin Oncol* 2013;31(6):676-683.

Ocana A, Amir E, Yeung C, Seruga B, Tannock IF. How valid are claims for synergy in published clinical studies? *Ann Oncol* 2012;23(8):2161-2166.

Ocana A, Pandiella A, Siu LL, Tannock IF. Preclinical development of molecular targeted agents for cancer. *Nat Revs Clin Oncol* 2010;8(4):200-209.

Palumbo A, Bringhen S, Caravita T, et al. Oral melphalan and prednisone chemotherapy plus thalidomide compared with melphalan and prednisone alone in elderly patients with multiple myeloma: randomised controlled trial. *Lancet* 2006;367(9513):825-831.

Pernicova I, Korbonits M. Metformin—mode of action and clinical implications for diabetes and cancer. *Nat Rev Endocrinol* 2014;10(3):143-156.

Petros RA, DeSimone JM. Strategies in the design of nanoparticles for therapeutic applications. *Nat Rev Drug Discov* 2010;9(8):615-627.

Prinz F, Schlange T, Asadullah K. Believe it or not: how much can we rely on published data on potential drug targets? *Nat Rev Drug Discov* 2011;10(9):712.

Roberts AW, Davids MS, Pagel JM, et al. Targeting BCL2 with venetoclax in relapsed chronic lymphocytic leukemia. *N Engl J Med* 2016;374(4):311-322.

Rosenblum D, Joshi N, Tao W, Karp JM, Peer D. Progress and challenges towards targeted delivery of cancer therapeutics. *Nat Commun* 2018;9(1):1410.

Schürmann R, Vogel S, Ebel K, Bald I. The physico-chemical basis of DNA radiosensitization: implications for cancer radiation therapy. *Chemistry* 2018;24(41):10271-10279.

Scripture D, Figg. Drug interactions in cancer therapy. *Nature Reviews Cancer* 2006;6(7):546-558.

Seymour JF, Kipps TJ, Eichhorst B, et al. Venetoclax-rituximab in relapsed or refractory chronic lymphocytic leukemia. *N Engl J Med* 2018;378(12):1107-1120.

Solomon BJ, Mok T, Kim DW, et al. First-line crizotinib versus chemotherapy in ALK-positive lung cancer. *N Engl J Med* 2014;371(23):2167-2177.

Sosman JA, Kim KB, Schuchter L, et al. Survival in BRAF V600-mutant advanced melanoma treated with vemurafenib. *N Engl J Med* 2012;366(8):707-714.

Steel GG, Peckham MJ. Exploitable mechanisms in combined radiotherapy-chemotherapy: the concept of additivity. *Int J Radiat Oncol Biol Phy* 1979;5(1):85-91.

Stein CA, Castanotto D. FDA-approved oligonucleotide therapies in 2017. *Mol Ther* 2017;25(5):1069-1075.

Stein EM, DiNardo CD, Pollyea DA, et al. Enasidenib in mutant IDH2 relapsed or refractory acute myeloid leukemia. *Blood* 2017;130(6):722-731.

Steinhart Z, Pavlovic Z, Chandrashekhar M, et al. Genome-wide CRISPR screens reveal a Wnt-FZD5 signaling circuit as a druggable vulnerability of RNF43-mutant pancreatic tumors. *Nat Med* 2017;23(1):60-68.

Strecker TE, Shen Q, Zhang Y, et al. Effect of lapatinib on the development of estrogen receptor-negative mammary tumors in mice. *J Natl Cancer Inst* 2009;101(2):107-113.

Su F, Viros A, Milagre C, et al. RAS mutations in cutaneous squamous-cell carcinomas in patients treated with BRAF inhibitors. *N Engl J Med* 2012;366(3):207-215.

Tiacci E, Park JH, De Carolis L, et al. Targeting mutant BRAF in relapsed or refractory hairy-cell leukemia. *N Engl J Med* 2015;373(18):1733-1747.

Travis LB, Curtis RE, Glimelius B, et al. Bladder and kidney cancer following cyclophosphamide therapy for non-Hodgkin's lymphoma. *J Natl Cancer Inst* 1995;87(7):524-530.

Tsherniak A, Vazquez F, Montgomery PG et al. Defining a cancer dependency map. *Cell* 2017;170(3):564-576.

Tzogani K, Camarero Jiménez J, Garcia I, et al. The European Medicines Agency review of carfilzomib for the treatment of adult patients with multiple myeloma who have received at least one prior therapy. *Oncologist* 2017;22(11):1339-1346.

Vardy J, Rourke S, Tannock IF. Evaluation of cognitive function associated with chemotherapy: a review of published studies and recommendations for future research. *J Clin Oncol* 2007;25(17):2455-2463.

Venturini M, Michelotti A, Del Mastro L, et al. Multicenter randomized controlled clinical trial to evaluate cardioprotection of desrazoxane versus no cardioprotection in women receiving epirubicin chemotherapy for advanced breast cancer. *J Clin Oncol* 1996;14(12):3112-3120.

Verma S, Miles D, Gianni L, et al. Trastuzumab emtansine for HER2-positive advanced breast cancer. *N Engl J Med* 2012;367(19):1783-1791.

von der Maase. Experimental studies on interactions of radiation and cancer chemotherapeutic drugs in normal tissues and a solid tumour. *Radiother Oncol* 1986;7(1): 47-68.

Wang S, Zhao Y, Aguilar A, Bernard D, Yang CY. Targeting the MDM2-p53 protein-protein interaction for new cancer therapy: progress and challenges. *Cold Spring Harb Perspect Med* 2017;7(5).

Wolff AC, Blackford AL, Visvanathan K, et al. Risk of marrow neoplasms after adjuvant breast cancer therapy: the national comprehensive cancer network experience. *J Clin Oncol* 2015;33(4):340-348.

Wong GS, Zhou J, Liu JB, et al. Targeting wild-type KRAS-amplified gastroesophageal cancer through combined MEK and SHP2 inhibition. *Nat Med* 2018;24(7): 968-977.

Anticancer Chemotherapy, Pharmacology, and Mechanisms of Resistance

18

Eric Chen and Ian F. Tannock

Chapter Outline

18.1 Introduction
18.2 General Principles of Pharmacology
    18.2.1 Pharmacokinetics and Pharmacodynamics
    18.2.2 Dosing of Chemotherapy in Individual Patients
    18.2.3 Pharmacogenomics
18.3 Chemotherapy Drugs
    18.3.1 Alkylating Agents
    18.3.2 Antimetabolites
    18.3.3 Topoisomerase Inhibitors
    18.3.4 Antimicrotubular Agents
    18.3.5 Miscellaneous Drugs
    18.3.6 Liposomal Drugs
18.4 Drug Resistance
    18.4.1 Molecular Mechanisms of Drug Resistance
    18.4.2 Resistance Caused By Impaired Drug Uptake
    18.4.3 Multiple Drug Resistance Caused by Enhanced Drug Efflux
    18.4.4 Resistance Caused by Decreased Drug Activation or Increased Drug Inactivation
    18.4.5 Drug Resistance and Repair of Drug-Mediated DNA Damage
    18.4.6 Apoptosis and Autophagy
    18.4.7 Drug Resistance and the Solid Tumor Environment
    18.4.8 Repopulation
Summary
References

18.1 INTRODUCTION

Although most new drugs for cancer are agents that target molecular changes that occur in tumors (described in Chap. 19), chemotherapy still provides the backbone of drug therapy for most types of cancer. Chemotherapy is used commonly to treat people with metastatic cancer, and for many common types of adult cancer can provide palliation—either by prolonging survival and/or by improving quality of life. Only for relatively rare tumors such as childhood leukemia and some other cancers affecting children, and testicular cancer in men, can chemotherapy cure metastatic disease. Chemotherapy (and other systemic treatments) are also used either before (neoadjuvant) or after (adjuvant) surgery (and sometimes before, with, or after radiotherapy) in people without overt spread of disease, and can then improve the probability of cure by eliminating undetectable micrometastases.

Principles of pharmacokinetics and pharmacodynamics of anticancer drugs are discussed in Section 18.2 of this chapter; the same principles apply also to targeted agents (described in Chap. 19). Properties of chemotherapy drugs in common clinical use are discussed in Section 18.3. The major limitation with all types of systemic treatment of cancers is the innate presence or acquired development of drug resistance of the tumor: common mechanisms of drug resistance are discussed in Section 18.4.

18.2 GENERAL PRINCIPLES OF PHARMACOLOGY

18.2.1 Pharmacokinetics and Pharmacodynamics

Pharmacokinetics is the study of the time course of drug and metabolite levels in different body fluids and tissues, including absorption, distribution, metabolism, and elimination. The study of the relationship between drug effect and its concentration is known as *pharmacodynamics*. Alterations in pharmacokinetic properties of a drug may result in different drug concentrations over time in different tissues. Understanding the pharmacodynamics of a drug can explain subsequent differences in drug effect or response.

Although most chemotherapy drugs are given by intravenous injection at discrete intervals and drug absorption is not a therapeutic concern, many newer targeted agents are given continuously by mouth. Oral drug administration is convenient for patients, but it requires patient compliance and depends on efficient absorption from the gastrointestinal tract. Only a proportion of an orally administered drug may be delivered to the systemic circulation and become available for therapeutic effects. *Absolute bioavailability* refers to the amount of a drug that is available after oral administration compared to that after intravenous administration, whereas *relative bioavailability* is the amount of a drug that is available from one formulation relative to that from another nonintravenous formulation. Factors influencing the bioavailability of a drug include patient compliance, disintegration of a capsule or a tablet and dissolution of the drug into gastrointestinal fluid, stability of the drug in the gastrointestinal tract, absorption through the gastrointestinal mucosa, and first-pass metabolism in the liver. Problems seen in cancer patients, such as changes in gastrointestinal motility, mucosal damage from cancer therapy, and the use of other medications (such as those affecting gastric pH), can affect bioavailability. Absorption of a drug may vary among patients receiving the same treatments, or within the same patient from one course of treatment to another.

Once in the blood, the distribution of a drug within the body is governed by factors such as blood flow to different organs, protein and tissue binding, lipid solubility, diffusion, and carrier-mediated transport. In general, drugs with extensive protein-tissue binding or with high lipid solubility will tend to exhibit prolonged elimination phases because the release of bound drug from tissues is slow.

Metabolism of drugs takes place primarily in the liver and consists of oxidative, reductive, and hydrolytic reactions via the superfamily of cytochrome P450 (phase I) and conjugation (phase II) enzymes. Phase I reactions can produce metabolites that retain therapeutic activity or convert an inactive prodrug (eg, cyclophosphamide) to an active moiety. Phase II reactions generally produce inactive metabolites that can be eliminated from the body by biliary or renal excretion. Many anticancer drugs have active metabolites, and this property introduces additional complexity into understanding the relationship between pharmacokinetics and pharmacodynamics. There are genetic polymorphisms that can affect the activity of many of the drug-metabolizing enzymes (Quaranta and Thomas, 2017). Acquired changes as a result of hepatic impairment or the use of other medications may affect their activity. Unfortunately, simple tests of liver function, such as serum levels of bilirubin or transaminases, have not proved useful in predicting hepatic metabolic activity because the decline in activity of metabolizing enzymes varies in the setting of hepatic dysfunction.

Most drugs are eliminated from the body by the kidney or through the biliary tract. Renal excretion can either be of the active drug or of metabolites. Impairment of renal function will influence drug clearance and may enhance toxicity for drugs that are eliminated unchanged in the urine, such as carboplatin and methotrexate. Dosage reductions proportionate to the decline in creatinine clearance (a common measure of kidney function) are usually required. Several chemotherapy drugs are also toxic to the kidney (eg, cisplatin and high-dose methotrexate), and combinations of these drugs with others that are eliminated by the kidney require extra caution and maintenance of a high urinary output.

Cancer patients frequently take multiple other medications for relief of pain, nausea, and other symptoms or for the treatment of coexisting conditions. Interaction between drugs may influence each of the processes of absorption, metabolism, distribution, and excretion. For example, patients receiving warfarin require increased monitoring if they are also receiving fluoropyrimidines because of such interactions. Possible interactions between anticancer drugs, and between such drugs and other medications, are common (Riechelmann et al, 2008).

The concentration of most anticancer drugs can be measured in the blood or in the tissue of a patient. If a drug is measured in blood or tissue over time, then a curve relating drug concentration to time can be generated. The area under the concentration-time curve (AUC) is a commonly used measure of total systemic drug exposure. For drugs like cisplatin, their effect in killing of tumor cells or toxicity to normal tissues is related directly to AUC, whereas for other drugs, such as taxanes, the duration of exposure above a threshold concentration may be more important than AUC.

The concentration-time curve (Fig. 18–1) can be modeled mathematically. Table 18–1 lists some important terms derived from such modeling. Clearance (CL) is the proportionality factor that relates the rate of elimination of a drug from the body and its plasma concentration:

$$\text{Rate of elimination} = CL \times \text{plasma concentration}$$

Clearance can be represented by a volume from which the drug is eliminated in a unit of time, such as liters per hour.

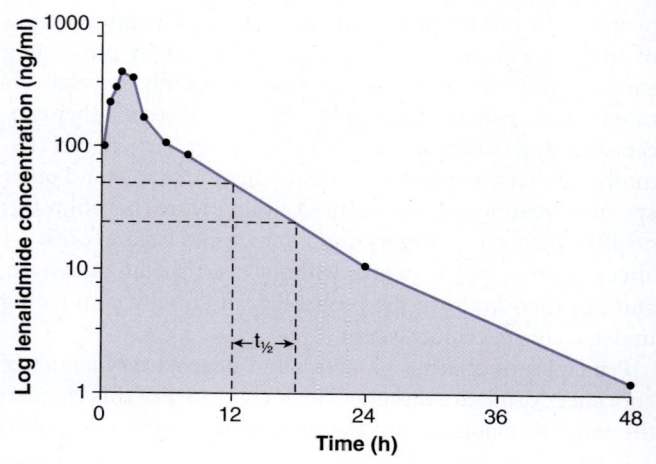

FIGURE 18–1 The plasma time-concentration curve after a single oral dose of lenalidomide.

TABLE 18–1 Glossary of terms used commonly in pharmacokinetics.

Pharmacokinetic Term	Definition
AUC	Area under the plasma concentration-time curve, either from zero to infinity (AUC_{inf}) or from zero to the last point of blood sampling (AUC_t)
$C(t)$	Drug concentration in plasma at time t
CL	Clearance, the proportionality factor that relates the rate of elimination of a drug from the body and its plasma concentration
C_{ss}	Steady-state plasma drug concentration
$t_{1/2}$	Half-life, the time required for the drug concentration to decrease by 50%
V_d	Volume of distribution, a hypothetical volume required to dissolve the total amount of drug at the same concentration as is found in blood immediately after intravenous administration

The AUC of a drug is related to the dose administered and its clearance:

$$AUC = Dose/CL$$

Thus, if the clearance of a drug declines (eg in the setting of renal or hepatic dysfunction), its AUC will increase without an adjustment in dose, resulting in increased toxicity. Similarly, individual variability in drug clearance will manifest as differences in AUC and in efficacy. Clearance is independent of dose unless there is saturation of drug-metabolizing enzymes (see also Sec. 18.2.3); the AUC will then increase at a greater rate than dose, and severe toxicity can result.

The volume of distribution (V_d) represents a hypothetical volume of body fluid that would be required to dissolve the total amount of drug at the same concentration as that found in blood immediately after intravenous administration. A large V_d (a value larger than the total volume of body water is possible) represents extensive binding of drug in tissue (eg, vinca alkaloids).

The concentration-time curves often have components that are approximately exponential (see Fig. 18–1). The half-life ($t_{1/2}$) of a drug is the time required for the drug concentration to decrease by half, and different values of $t_{1/2}$ (labeled α, β, and γ) can be used to characterize successive exponential components of the concentration-time curve; the last of these values is referred to as the terminal elimination half-life. The $t_{1/2}$ is useful in estimating the time required for a drug to reach a steady state (where the amount of drug being eliminated from the body is equal to the amount being added after multiple administrations such that the plasma concentration remains constant).

18.2.2 Dosing of Chemotherapy in Individual Patients

Most cytotoxic drugs have a narrow therapeutic index (ie, a small difference between doses that cause anticancer effects and those that cause toxicity). There is a need to reduce interindividual variability to have a consistent response and to minimize toxicity. Efforts to relate drug concentration to effects have generally been unsuccessful. Most cytotoxic agents are dosed based on body surface area (BSA) on the premise that the factors relevant in pharmacokinetics, such as cardiac output, body fat, and creatinine clearance, are all related to body size. BSA dosing is useful in interspecies comparisons, because the maximum tolerated dose (MTD) remains relatively constant between different animal species when expressed as milligrams per square meter (mg/m²), and it may have value in pediatric patients where there may be wide ranges in body size. Many reports have questioned the convention of calculating the dose of chemotherapy in adults on the basis of BSA (eg, Ratain, 1998). Multiple studies show that there is no reduction in pharmacokinetic variability when compared to a standard dose or dose based on body weight. Furthermore, BSA-based dosing makes drug administration unnecessarily complex and subject to human error.

Factors within an individual that may account for variability in pharmacokinetics and pharmacodynamics are poorly understood. The usual approach is to use a standard starting dose (in mg/m²) and then modify subsequent doses based on the observed toxicity. An exception is the dosing of carboplatin, where a relationship between kidney function and clearance of carboplatin has been demonstrated and carboplatin dose is calculated on the basis of the creatinine clearance (Calvert et al, 1989). The approach to dose modification is also influenced by the goals of therapy. Where treatment is potentially curative (eg, testicular cancer), drug doses are usually maintained despite severe toxicities, often with granulate colony stimulating factor (G-CSF) support (see Chap. 17, Sec. 17.5.2), whereas for palliation dose reductions are appropriate for even moderate toxicity. The approach to dose reduction is usually empiric, with fractional dose reductions of one or more of the drugs thought to be causing the toxicity.

Many newer anticancer drugs, especially molecular-targeted agents, are administered orally. These agents are usually initiated at a fixed dose regardless of height or weight because the therapeutic indices of these agents are wider than those of cytotoxic drugs.

18.2.3 Pharmacogenomics

Pharmacogenomics refers to the study of how genetic features of the patient (and their tumor) will influence response and toxicity, through alterations in pharmacokinetics. Pharmacogenomics seeks to explain differences in response on the basis of differences in the activity of genes that are involved in drug metabolism and are related to specific mutations or polymorphisms (Relling and Evans, 2016). The goal is to define a particular phenotype following drug exposure (eg, serious toxicity, second malignancy) and then assess changes at the genetic level that might account for this phenotype. This phenotype could be a result of determinants of drug pharmacokinetics, such as the function of drug-metabolizing enzymes, or to genetic factors that influence pharmacodynamics or even to genetic polymorphisms that might relate to the development of cancers.

An early example of the effect of pharmacogenetics on response and toxicity is the use of 5-fluorouracil (5-FU) in the treatment of colorectal cancer (see Sec. 18.3.2.2). Approximately 80% of intravenously administered 5-FU is catabolized to an inactive metabolite through the enzyme dihydropyrimidine dehydrogenase (DPD) (Henricks et al, 2015; see Fig. 18–9). Although DPD activity is present in different tissues and organs, including the gastrointestinal mucosa, the liver is the major site of 5-FU catabolism. The DPD gene is present as a single copy on chromosome 1p22, and consists of 23 exons. Mutations and polymorphism can lead to a deficiency of DPD activity. Although this deficiency does not lead to any detectable problems under normal circumstances, patients with this deficiency have increased toxicity when they are exposed to 5-FU. The most common mutation identified in patients who experienced severe 5-FU toxicity is a G-to-A mutation in the invariant GT splice donor site (DPYD*2A), which results in deletion of exon 14 and a nonfunctional DPD enzyme. It is estimated that approximately 25% of patients with grade 3/4 5-FU toxicity are homozygous or heterozygous for this mutation.

There are several other examples of genetic polymorphisms leading to alterations in drug toxicity, most of them relating to individual differences in drug-metabolizing enzymes. The topoisomerase I inhibitor irinotecan (see Sec. 18.3.3.1) is partially metabolized to SN-38, an active metabolite, through carboxylesterase. SN-38, when excreted unconjugated in the biliary tract, can cause damage to the gastrointestinal mucosa, resulting in diarrhea. Polymorphisms of uridine diphosphate glucuronosyltransferase (UGT)-1A1, the enzyme involved in conjugation of SN-38, have been identified, and those variants that result in a reduced rate of conjugation are associated with higher risk of irinotecan toxicity, such as neutropenia and diarrhea (Mathijssen et al, 2003).

Several drugs rely on enzymes to be converted to active metabolites. Reduced enzyme activity as a result of genetic polymorphism would lead to lower levels of metabolites, resulting in lower therapeutic effects. Tamoxifen, which has a major role in endocrine therapy for breast cancer, is converted to an active metabolite, endoxifen, through the cytochrome P450 family of enzymes, in particular, CYP2D6 (see also Chap. 20, Sec 20.4). So far, more than 100 genetic variants in CYP2D6 have been identified, and patients can be grouped into 4 groups based on CYP2D6 activity: ultrahigh, normal, reduced, and no activity (Schroth et al, 2009). Some, but not all, studies suggest that patients with reduced CYP2D6 activity are at higher risks of failing to respond to tamoxifen, compared to those with normal CYP2D6 activity. Other CYP enzymes are involved in metabolism of other drugs and carcinogens (Chap. 5, Sec. 5.4.2)

18.3 CHEMOTHERAPY DRUGS

18.3.1 Alkylating Agents

Alkylating agents were the first drugs introduced for the systemic therapy of cancer. They are a chemically diverse group of drugs, but they all contain alkyl groups (eg, —CH_2Cl). In vivo, the alkyl groups generate highly reactive, positively charged intermediates, which then combine with an electron-rich nucleophilic group, such as an amino, phosphate, sulfhydryl, or hydroxyl moiety, on intracellular macromolecules, such as DNA. Although nucleophilic groups occur on almost all biological molecules, alkylation of bases in DNA appears to be the major cause of lethal toxicity.

Alkylating agents may contain 1 or 2 reactive groups and are thus classified as monofunctional or bifunctional, respectively. Bifunctional alkylating agents have the ability to form cross-links between DNA strands and are the most clinically useful of these agents. Interstrand crosslinking of DNA, which prevents cell replication, unless repaired, seems to be the major mechanism of cytotoxicity for bifunctional alkylating agents, whereas the toxicity of monofunctional alkylating agents is probably related to single-strand breaks in DNA or to damaged bases.

Because alkylating agents bind directly to DNA, they lack cell-cycle specificity, although they may have greater toxicity for proliferating cells. Common toxicities include myelosuppression, immunosuppression, hair loss, nausea, and vomiting. Some alkylating agents have long-term effects, such as infertility and carcinogenesis caused by long-lasting DNA damage. Nitrogen mustard, melphalan, and nitrosoureas are associated with an increased incidence of acute myelogenous leukemia, whereas cyclophosphamide is associated with irritation of the bladder and, rarely, development of bladder cancer.

18.3.1.1 Nitrogen Mustards and Related Drugs The development of nitrogen mustard and related compounds as anticancer drugs originated from the observation of lymphoid aplasia in soldiers exposed to the more reactive, but chemically similar, sulfur mustard gas during World War II. This family of drugs, all chemically derived from nitrogen mustard (mechlorethamine), contains several drugs in common clinical use. The structures of these drugs are shown in Figure 18–2; each is bifunctional, with 2 chloroethyl groups that form the reactive electron-deficient groups responsible for alkylation of DNA.

The most common site of alkylation of DNA by nitrogen mustards is the N-7 position on the base guanine (Fig. 18–3). First, one of the chloroethyl side chains releases a chloride ion, resulting in a highly reactive, positively charged intermediate. This intermediate then binds covalently with the electronegative N-7 group on a guanine base, resulting in alkylation. Alkylation of guanine leads to mispairing with thymine or to strand breakage. The second chloroethyl side chain of nitrogen mustard may undergo a similar reaction, leading to covalent binding with another base on the opposite strand of DNA and thus to formation of an interstrand crosslink.

Mechlorethamine (nitrogen mustard) was the first anticancer drug introduced to clinical use. However, it is chemically unstable and undergoes spontaneous hydrolysis. A large number of analogs has been synthesized, and 5 of them

FIGURE 18-2 Structures of clinically used alkylating agents of the nitrogen mustard family.

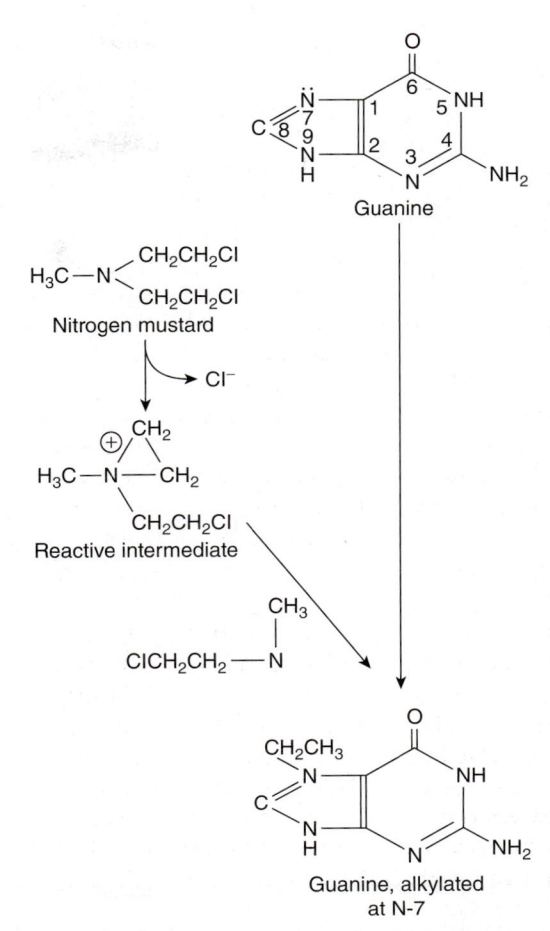

FIGURE 18-3 Reactions leading to alkylation at the N-7 position of guanine by nitrogen mustard.

(chlorambucil, melphalan, cyclophosphamide, ifosfamide, and bendamustine) have largely replaced mechlorethamine. The addition of ring structures to the nitrogen mustard molecule confers increased stability, such that these agents can be administered orally.

Chlorambucil is a well-absorbed oral drug with a narrow spectrum of activity, and is used mainly in slowly progressive neoplasms, such as low-grade lymphomas and chronic lymphocytic leukemia. Oral melphalan is used for treatment of plasma cell myeloma and in some high-dose bone marrow transplantation protocols. Absorption of melphalan is variable and unpredictable; some patients with no effect after oral administration may respond when melphalan is given intravenously. Both chlorambucil and melphalan are almost equally toxic to cycling and noncycling cells, and may lead to delayed and/or cumulative effects on bone marrow because of their toxicity to hematopoietic stem cells.

Cyclophosphamide is the alkylating agent in widest clinical use and is part of treatment protocols for breast, lymphatic, gynecologic, and pediatric tumors, in high-dose chemotherapy regimens, and for a number of autoimmune diseases. Cyclophosphamide is well absorbed after oral administration; however, the parent compound is inactive, requiring metabolism by hepatic mixed-function oxidases to form the alkylating intermediate phosphoramide mustard (Fig. 18–4). Hepatic microsomal enzymes metabolize cyclophosphamide to 4-hydroxycyclophosphamide, which exists in equilibrium with its acyclic isomer aldophosphamide. 4-hydroxycyclophosphamide enters cells and spontaneously decomposes to form phosphoramide mustard and acrolein, or it is inactivated by aldehyde dehydrogenase. Elimination of cyclophosphamide and its metabolites occurs mainly by renal excretion. Cyclophosphamide induces cytochrome P450 enzymes, and hence its own metabolism with repeated administration. This induction alters the rate but not the absolute amount of phosphoramide mustard formation, so no dose adjustment is required.

The dose of cyclophosphamide given to patients ranges from 100 to 200 mg/m^2 per day given orally, and to 600 to 1000 mg/m^2 given intravenously, every 3-4 weeks. Very high doses are used in preparation for bone marrow transplantation. The dose in this setting is limited by irreversible damage to the heart, which occurs with single doses greater than 60 mg/kg (approximately 2500 mg/m^2). The usual dose-limiting toxicity is myelosuppression, and cyclophosphamide causes a fall in granulocyte count with rapid recovery by 3-4 weeks after

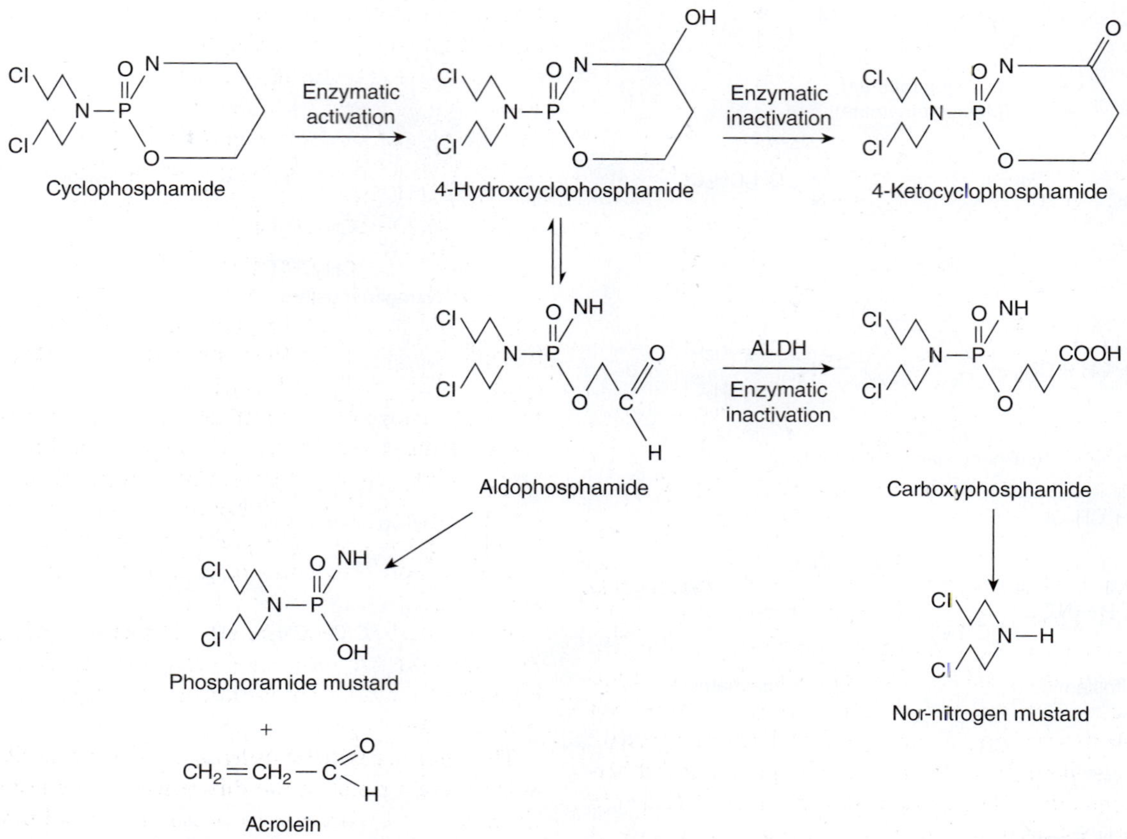

FIGURE 18–4 The metabolism of cyclophosphamide. *ALDH*, aldehyde dehydrogenase.

administration (see Chap. 17, Sec. 17.5.2). There is relative sparing of stem cells and platelets, which may be a result of the higher concentrations of aldehyde dehydrogenase in early progenitor cells. Cyclophosphamide causes hemorrhagic cystitis with chronic use or at higher doses because of the direct irritative effect of acrolein on the bladder mucosa.

Ifosfamide is an analog of cyclophosphamide that differs in the presence of only one chloroethyl group on the oxazaphosphorine ring. It is used in the treatment of testicular cancer and sarcoma. Hemorrhagic cystitis is more common as a result of increased production of acrolein, such that all patients receiving ifosfamide should be given a sulfhydryl-containing compound, such as 2-mercaptoethane sulfonate (Mesna), which conjugates with acrolein in the urinary tract and renders it inactive. As Mesna dimerizes to an inactive metabolite in blood, and is hydrolyzed to its active form only in urine, it does not affect the cytotoxicity of cyclophosphamide or ifosfamide at other sites. Neurotoxicity, manifesting as changes in mental status including confusion, hallucination, cerebellar dysfunction, seizures, and coma, may occur with higher doses of ifosfamide but not cyclophosphamide. Risks for ifosfamide neurotoxicity include low serum albumin, elevated creatinine, and prior cisplatin treatment (David and Picus, 2005).

Bendamustine is the newest bifunctional mechlorethamine derivative introduced into clinical practice. It is indicated for patients with chronic lymphocytic leukemia and indolent non-Hodgkin lymphoma.

Busulfan, an alkyl alkane sulfonate, has a different mechanism of alkylation from the nitrogen mustards. It reacts more extensively with thiol groups of amino acids and proteins, but its ability to crosslink DNA is uncertain. Busulfan has selective effects on hematopoietic stem cells, and is now used mainly as a part of myeloablative regimens for hematopoietic cell transplantation. Busulfan is eliminated via hepatic metabolism, and the higher doses of busulfan used in marrow transplantation may cause hepatic veno-occlusive disease in patients who metabolize the drug slowly.

Dacarbazine (DTIC) and temozolomide have different chemical structures from nitrogen mustards, but are also capable of forming covalent crosslink with intracellular macromolecules (Marchesi et al, 2007). DTIC was synthesized originally as an antimetabolite to inhibit purine synthesis, but is believed to function through formation of methylcarbonium ions with alkylating properties. DTIC is metabolized by CYP450 enzymes to MTIC ([methyl-triazene-1-yl]-imidazole-4-carboxamide), which alkylates DNA at the O-6 and N-7 guanine positions. DTIC is sensitive to light, but is stable in neutral solutions away from light. Temozolomide is a prodrug that is stable under acidic conditions but undergoes rapid, spontaneous, nonenzymatic conversion to MTIC at pH levels greater than 7; it is rapidly and completely absorbed after oral administration with a $t_{1/2}$ of 1 to 2 hours. Temozolomide is indicated for patients with newly diagnosed or recurrent malignant glioma, and has also shown activity in neuroendocrine tumors.

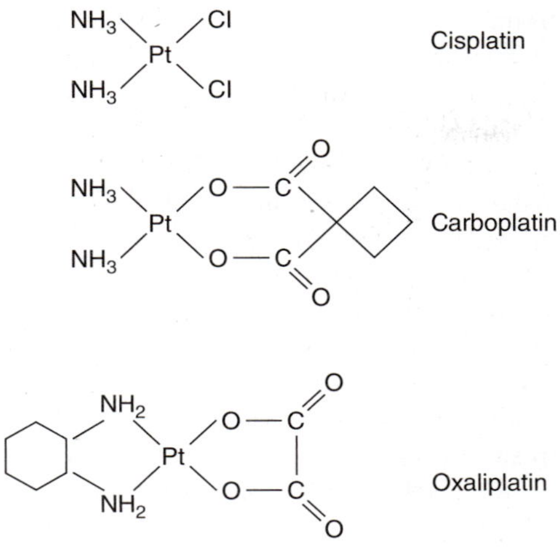

FIGURE 18-5 Structure of platinum agents.

18.3.1.2 Platinating Agents

Platinum-containing agents also exert their pharmacologic effects through alkylation. The prototype agent is cisplatin (*cis*-diamminedichloroplatinum(II); Fig. 18–5). Cisplatin was discovered following the observation that an electric current delivered to bacterial cultures via platinum electrodes led to inhibition of bacterial growth. The active compound was identified as cisplatin, and it was shown subsequently to exert broad cytotoxic activity. Cisplatin is one of the most useful anticancer agents and is part of first-line therapy for testicular, urothelial, gastroesophageal, gynecologic, and other cancers. It is also associated with substantial toxicity, which limits both the number of patients who are able to receive the drug as well as the cumulative dose that can be given. There has been a major effort to identify other platinum analogs, either to reduce the toxicity while maintaining efficacy or to expand the use of these compounds to tumors resistant to cisplatin. The 2 analogs in routine clinical use are carboplatin and oxaliplatin (Fig. 18–5).

Platinum drugs can exist in a 2+ (II) or 4+ (IV) oxidation state, with 4 or 6 bonds linking the platinum atom, respectively. All currently used platinum drugs are platinum(II) compounds that exhibit a planar structure and have 4 attached chemical groups. The nature of these groups dictates the efficacy and pharmacokinetic properties of these compounds. Two of the groups are considered carrier groups, and are chemically inert, whereas the 2 leaving groups are available for substitution and reaction with molecules such as DNA.

Cisplatin acts by a mechanism similar to that of classical alkylating agents. The chlorine atoms are leaving groups that may be compared to those of nitrogen mustards; these atoms may be displaced directly by nucleophilic groups in DNA or indirectly after chloride ions are replaced by hydroxyl groups through reaction of the drug with water. These reactions occur more readily in environments where the chloride concentration is low, such as within the cell. The preferred sites for binding of cisplatin to DNA are the 7-position of guanine and adenine bases. Because structurally similar analogs, such as transplatin, will undergo DNA binding but are devoid of cytotoxicity, the stereochemistry of the compound is critical.

Cisplatin binds to 2 sites on DNA, and 95% of the binding produces intrastrand cross-linkages, usually between 2 adjacent guanine bases or adjacent guanine and adenine sites, with the remainder that occur as interstrand guanine cross-linkages. The binding of platinum compounds to DNA is responsible for their cytotoxicity, although the mechanism by which it leads to cell death is unclear. Multiple mechanisms can lead to resistance to cisplatin (see Fig. 18–20).

Carboplatin is an analog of cisplatin with substitution of cyclobutanedicarboxylate for the chloride-leaving groups. This substitution leads to a less-reactive compound that also has less toxicity but either comparable or slightly reduced efficacy compared with cisplatin. Oxaliplatin is one of a series of analogs with a substitution of a diaminocyclohexane (DACH) for the amine carrier groups (see Fig. 18–5). The DACH analogs have a different efficacy profile from cisplatin and have shown activity in tumors resistant to cisplatin, such as colorectal cancer. Carboplatin and oxaliplatin produce the same types of DNA adducts as cisplatin, although a higher concentration of carboplatin is required to produce a comparable number of adducts to cisplatin. Adducts formed by oxaliplatin are more likely to cause cell death, probably because of the different 3-dimensional structure that results from the DACH groups.

The pharmacokinetic differences between cisplatin and its analogs are a result of the differences in the leaving groups. Cisplatin is the most reactive and, following administration, it is rapidly and irreversibly bound to plasma proteins, with more than 90% of free cisplatin lost in the first 2 hours. Total cisplatin (free and bound) disappears more slowly from plasma, with a prolonged $t_{1/2}$ of 2 to 3 days. However, recent findings indicate that cisplatin may persist for many years after treatment, and serum cisplatin levels correlate with neurotoxicity (Sprauten et al 2012). Cisplatin causes little toxicity to bone marrow as a single agent, but can add to the toxic effects of other drugs, and may lead to anemia. Its major dose-limiting toxicities are nausea and vomiting, nephrotoxicity, neurotoxicity, and ototoxicity. Vigorous intravenous hydration and maintaining a rapid urine output during and after drug administration minimize nephrotoxicity, but there is no known method for minimizing ototoxicity or neurotoxicity.

Carboplatin is more stable in vivo and is excreted primarily unchanged by the kidney, with 90% of administered dose excreted within 24 hours. The clearance of carboplatin is predicated by creatinine clearance; therefore, it is possible to determine the dose of carboplatin based on the desired carboplatin AUC and creatinine clearance (Calvert et al, 1989):

Carboplatin dose (mg) = AUC × (creatinine clearance + 25)

Carboplatin has comparable activity to cisplatin against ovarian and lung tumors but is less active against urothelial and testicular cancers. Carboplatin has a better overall toxicity profile, which may make it preferable in palliative treatment regimens. There is minimal nephrotoxicity, and the drug causes less nausea and vomiting than cisplatin, but bone marrow suppression, particularly thrombocytopenia, is the dose-limiting toxicity. Carboplatin is used in some high-dose regimens prior to stem cell transplantation because its toxicities other than myelosuppression are relatively mild.

Similar to cisplatin, oxaliplatin also binds to plasma proteins, although at a somewhat slower rate; it is also excreted primarily by the kidney. Oxaliplatin is used mainly in the treatment of gastrointestinal cancers; it has minimal renal toxicity, and causes less vomiting than cisplatin and no ototoxicity. Oxaliplatin causes a unique spectrum of sensory neurotoxicity, ranging from acute neuropathy (paresthesia, muscle spasm and fasciculations, or muscle twitching) immediately after infusion with marked sensitivity to cold, particularly in the oropharynx, to a late cumulative dose-limiting sensory neuropathy resulting in sensory ataxia and functional impairment. The late neurotoxicity is dose-dependent, leading to sensory and symmetric distal axonal neuropathy without motor involvement. It generally improves with time, but may persist up to 4 years after completion of treatment (André et al 2009).

18.3.2 Antimetabolites

18.3.2.1 Antifolates Antimetabolites are drugs that interfere with normal cellular functions, particularly the synthesis of DNA that is required for cell replication. Many of the clinically useful agents are purine or pyrimidine analogs that either inhibit the formation of the normal nucleotides or interact with DNA and prevent further extension of the new DNA strand, leading to inhibition of cell division. The antifolates (eg, methotrexate) are not nucleoside analogs; they prevent the formation of reduced folates, which are required for the synthesis of DNA.

Most antimetabolites are cell-cycle specific; their toxicity relates to effects on proliferating cells and is primarily seen in bone marrow and gastrointestinal mucosa. As they do not interact directly with DNA, they do not cause the later problems of carcinogenesis seen with alkylating agents. The effects of these drugs are dependent on the schedule of administration. For many drugs, the duration of exposure above a critical threshold required to inhibit an enzyme is more important than the peak concentration. Therefore, although large doses may be tolerated if the drug is given as a single intravenous injection, a much lower dose is required if the drug is given repeatedly or by continuous infusion.

Methotrexate is an analog of the vitamin folic acid (Fig. 18–6). Reduced folate is required for transfer of methyl groups in the biosynthesis of purines and in the conversion of deoxyuridine monophosphate (dUMP) to thymidine monophosphate (dTMP), a reaction catalyzed by thymidylate synthase. Reduced folate becomes oxidized in the latter reaction; its regeneration is dependent on the enzyme dihydrofolate reductase (DHFR) for reduction to its active form. Methotrexate competitively inhibits DHFR and prevents the formation of reduced folate (Fig. 18–7). The result of this inhibition may be cessation of DNA synthesis because of nonavailability of dTMP and/or purines, leading to cell death.

Methotrexate enters the cell primarily by active transport. However, its uptake may be by passive diffusion at high drug concentrations. Intracellular metabolism of methotrexate leads to addition of glutamic acid residues to the initial glutamate residue of the drug, a process known as *polyglutamation*. Methotrexate polyglutamates cannot be transported across the cell membrane, so their formation prevents efflux of the

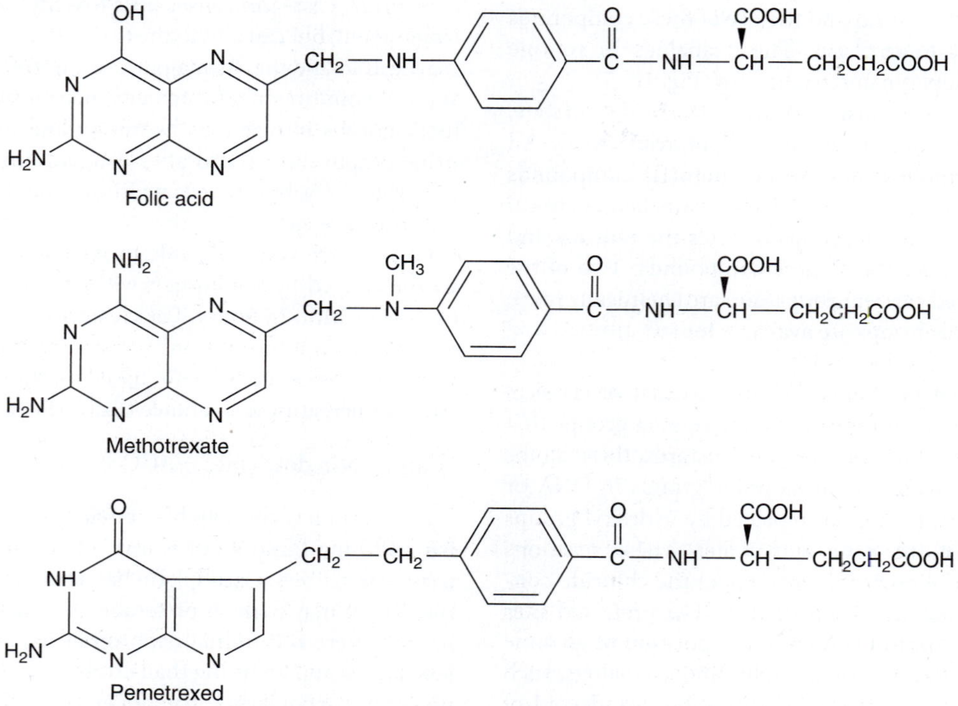

FIGURE 18–6 Structures of folic acid, methotrexate, and pemetrexed.

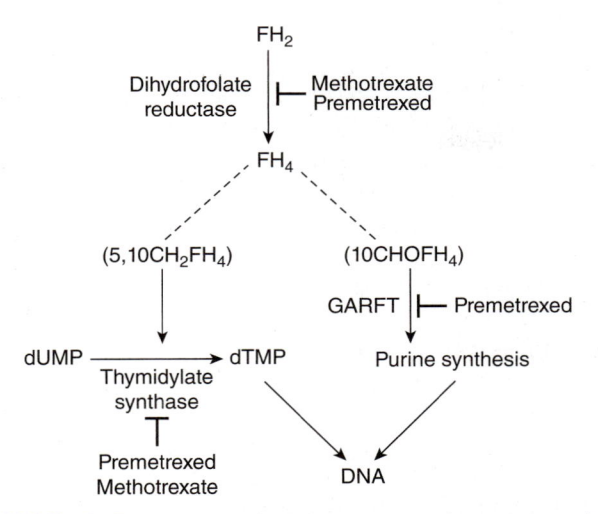

FIGURE 18-7 Influence of methotrexate and premetrexed on cellular metabolism. Methotrexate and premetrexed competitively inhibit dihydrofolate reductase (DHFR) and deplete the pools of reduced folates (FH$_4$): 5,10-methylene tetrahydrofolate (5,10CH$_2$FH$_4$) and 10-formyltetrahydrofolate (10CHOFH$_4$). Reduced folates are required in the conversion of dUMP to dTMP and for purine synthesis, respectively. Interruption of these processes leads to inhibition of DNA synthesis. Premetrexed also inhibits other steps in these pathways as shown in the figure. GARFT, glycinamide ribonucleotide formyltransferase.

drug, and they appear to be more effective than methotrexate itself in inhibiting the activity of DHFR. The cytotoxic action of methotrexate depends critically on the duration of exposure of tissue to levels of drug above a certain threshold, rather than on the peak levels of drug in the tissue. For many tissues, the threshold concentration for cytotoxicity appears to be in the range of 10^{-8} to 10^{-7} M. Methotrexate has selective toxicity for cells synthesizing DNA, and prolonged treatment with the drug may cause toxicity to more cells as they enter the S-phase of the cell cycle.

The toxicity of methotrexate may be reversed by administration of thymidine and exogenous purines or by a source of reduced folate. These agents circumvent the effects of methotrexate by restoring products of the interrupted metabolism (see Fig. 18–7). They have been used clinically to reverse the activity of methotrexate following a defined period of exposure (usually 24 to 36 hours) to methotrexate at high doses. Reduced folate in the form of 5-formyltetrahydrofolate (also known as leucovorin or folinic acid) has been used in many clinical protocols and has allowed the administration of doses of methotrexate that are increased by factors of 10 to 100 over conventional doses. The arguments put forward for such high-dose methotrexate treatment include (1) selective uptake by tumor cells, (2) better CNS penetration, and (3) lack of myelosuppression. This type of protocol allows for frequent administration of methotrexate and retained therapeutic efficacy with little or no toxicity in many patients. However, responses to treatment are observed only rarely in patients who are refractory to conventional doses of methotrexate given without leucovorin rescue. Although toxicity is often lower with the use of high doses of methotrexate and leucovorin, an occasional patient may experience life-threatening toxicity, usually as a consequence of damage to the kidney or sequestration in fluid-filled spaces (eg, ascites, pleural effusions) and consequently delayed drug clearance. Methotrexate can cause renal dysfunction during infusion as a result of precipitation of methotrexate and its metabolites in acidic urine. Therefore, most protocols of high-dose methotrexate mandate vigorous hydration and alkylation of the urine. Methotrexate infusion should not start until the urine output is more than 100 mL/h, and urine pH is 7.0 or higher.

Methotrexate can be given orally, intramuscularly, intravenously, and intrathecally (ie, into the cerebrospinal fluid that surrounds the brain and spinal cord). It crosses the blood–brain barrier but achieves cytotoxic concentrations in the CNS only with intrathecal or high-dose intravenous administration. It accumulates in fluid-filled spaces such as pleural effusions, from which it is released slowly. The parent compound and hepatic metabolites are excreted by the kidney. This excretion can be inhibited by the presence of weak organic acids such as aspirin or penicillin. Aspirin may also displace methotrexate from its binding sites on plasma albumin, and these 2 effects of aspirin can increase the toxicity of methotrexate. The methotrexate dose needs to be reduced in patients with renal dysfunction. The $t_{1/2}$ of methotrexate ranges from 3 to 10 hours.

Methotrexate has a wide spectrum of clinical activity and may be curative for women with choriocarcinoma, a tumor derived from fetal elements. Its major toxicities are myelosuppression and inflammation of the oral and gastrointestinal mucosa; these toxicities are usually observed within 5 to 7 days of administration, earlier than for many other drugs. Rarer toxicities include damage to liver, lung, and brain, the latter occurring most frequently after intrathecal administration. In general, the drug is well tolerated compared with many other anticancer drugs. Multiple mechanisms can lead to resistance to methotrexate (see Fig. 18–9).

Pemetrexed is a folate-based potent inhibitor of thymidylate synthase (TS) with glutamic acid at one end of the molecule (see Fig. 18–6). Similar to methotrexate, pemetrexed can be polyglutamated for increased retention in cells and increased potency of TS inhibition. In addition to targeting TS, pemetrexed inhibits DHFR and glycinamide ribonucleotide formyltransferase (GARFT); the latter is a folate-dependent enzyme involved in purine synthesis (see Fig. 18–7). Pemetrexed has activity in non–small cell lung cancer and mesothelioma; it is administered intravenously and renal excretion is the major route of elimination with a $t_{1/2}$ of 3 to 4 hours. The main toxicities are myelosuppression, inflammation of the oral and gastrointestinal mucosa, and skin rash. Treatment with pemetrexed requires supplementation with folic acid and vitamin B$_{12}$.

18.3.2.2 5-Fluoropyrimidines

5-Fluorouracil (5-FU) is a drug that resembles the pyrimidine bases uracil and thymine, which are components of RNA and DNA, respectively (Fig. 18-8). It penetrates rapidly into cells, where it is metabolized to nucleosides by addition of ribose or deoxyribose; these reactions are catalyzed by enzymes that normally act on uracil and thymine. Phosphorylation

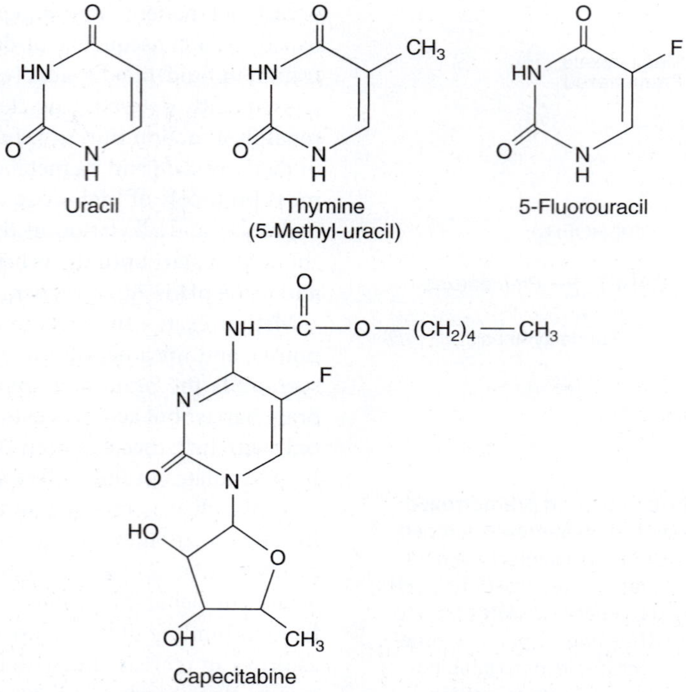

FIGURE 18-8 Structures of uracil, thymine, 5-fluorouracil (5-FU), and capecitabine.

then leads to the active fluorinated nucleotides 5-fluoro-uridine triphosphate (5-FUTP) and 5-fluoro-deoxyuridine-monophosphate (5-FdUMP) (Fig. 18–9). 5-FUTP can be incorporated into RNA in place of UTP (uridine triphosphate); this incorporation leads to inhibition of the nuclear processing of ribosomal and messenger RNA and may cause other errors of base pairing during transcription of RNA. 5-FdUMP binds irreversibly to, and inhibits, the enzyme TS, leading to depletion of dTMP (thymidine monophosphate), which is required for DNA synthesis. There is also evidence that 5-FU can cause damage to some cells via its incorporation into DNA (An et al, 2007)

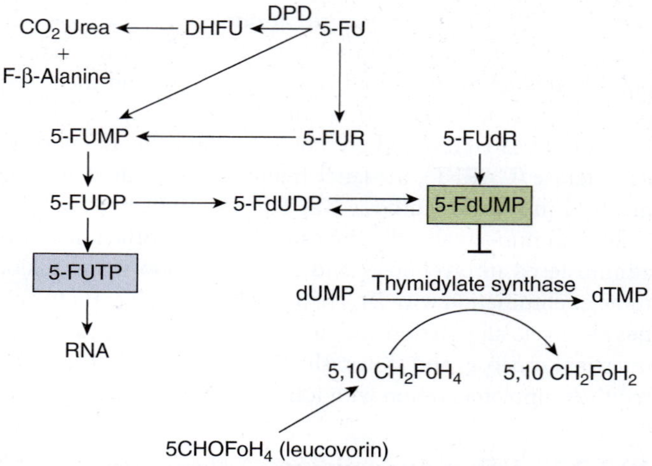

Approximately 80% of 5-FU administered is catabolized to CO_2, urea, and α-fluoro-β-alanine, mainly in the liver. The rate-limiting step in 5-FU catabolism is mediated by the enzyme DPD. The catabolism of 5-FU appears to be an important determinant of normal-tissue toxicity. Although DPD deficiency does not lead to any detectable problems in healthy individuals, patients with a partial or complete deficiency of DPD are at risk for severe toxicity from the drug.

Inhibition of TS by FdUMP is dependent on the presence of the cofactor 5,10-methyl-N-tetrahydrofolate, which combines with TS and FdUMP to form a covalent ternary complex. The dissociation rate of this complex is decreased in the presence of excess cofactor, which led to studies that established that addition of the prodrug 5-formyltetrahydrofolate (5-CHOFH$_4$, leucovorin, or folinic acid) increased the cytotoxicity of 5-FU (see Fig. 18–9). Clinical studies demonstrate that this combination has greater activity in the treatment of patients with metastatic colorectal cancer than 5-FU alone.

5-FU is used most commonly for treatment of gastrointestinal cancers. It is administered intravenously because bioavailability after oral administration is low and variable. 5-FU is eliminated rapidly from plasma with a $t_{1/2}$ of a few minutes. This agent demonstrates nonlinear pharmacokinetics because of a saturation of metabolism at higher concentrations, which may be seen when it is given by bolus injection, but not when given by infusion. This difference in pharmacokinetic behavior under these 2 conditions of administration may explain why the dose-limiting toxicity is myelosuppression for bolus

FIGURE 18-9 Metabolic pathways of 5-fluorouracil (5-FU). Fo is used here to distinguish "folate" from "F, Fluorine." DHFU, dihydrofluorouracil; DPD, dihydropyrimidine dehydrogenase; 5-FdUDP, 5-fluorodeoxyuridine diphosphate; 5-FdUMP, 5-fluorodeoxyuridine monophosphate; 5-FUDP, 5-fluorouridine diphosphate; 5-FUdR, 5-fluorodeoxyuridine; 5-FUMP, 5-fluorouridine monophosphate; 5-FUR, 5-fluorouridine.

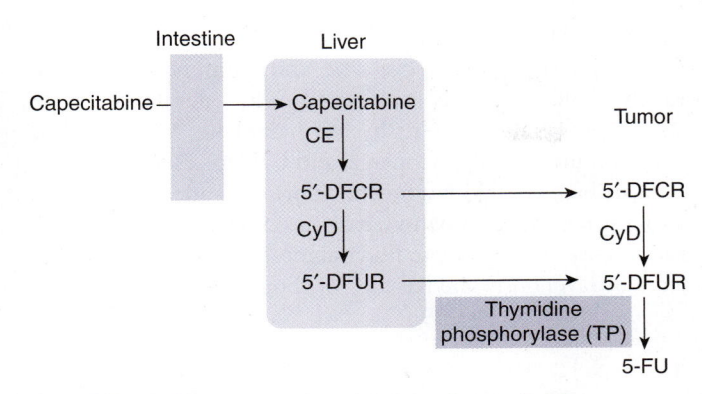

FIGURE 18–10 Enzymatic activation of capecitabine. *CE*, carboxylesterase; *CyD*, cytidine deaminase.

injection and mucositis for continuous infusion. Rarer toxicities include skin rashes, conjunctivitis, ataxia as a result of effects on the cerebellum, and cardiotoxicity. Prolonged low-dose infusion of 5-FU is associated with an increased incidence of changes in sensation as well as with redness and peeling of the skin on the palms of the hands and the soles of the feet, referred to as *palmar-plantar erythrodysesthesia* or *the hand-foot syndrome*. There is limited evidence that the prolonged 5-FU infusion improves its antitumor effects when compared with bolus injection.

Several oral fluoropyrimidine derivatives have been developed to provide a convenient route of administration and sustained drug exposure. Capecitabine is absorbed unchanged from the gastrointestinal tract, metabolized in the liver by carboxylesterase to 5'-deoxy-5-fluorocytidine (5'-DFCR), which is then converted to 5'-deoxy-5-fluorouridine (5'-DFUR) by cytidine deaminase, mainly located in the liver and tumor tissues. Further metabolism of 5'-DFUR to the cytotoxic moiety 5-FU occurs at the site of the tumor by thymidine phosphorylase, an enzyme present in higher concentrations in tumor cells, resulting in levels considerably higher in tumor tissues compared to normal tissues (Fig. 18–10; Miwa et al, 1998). The toxicity profile of capecitabine is similar to that of prolonged low-dose infusion of 5-FU, with lower frequencies of myelosuppression and stomatitis, but higher incidence of hand-foot syndrome than an intravenous bolus of 5-FU. Capecitabine has demonstrated efficacy in breast and colorectal malignancies. Randomized phase III trials comparing capecitabine to intravenous 5-FU plus leucovorin have shown equivalent efficacy in patients with metastatic colorectal cancer.

TAS-102 is a combination of trifluridine, a thymidine-based nucleoside analog, and tipiracil at a 2:1 ratio. Tipiracil inhibits thymidine phosphorylase, thereby reducing trifluridine degradation in the liver and intestine, and enabling the oral administration of trifluridine. Trifluridine monophosphate (F_3dTMP) reversibly inhibits TS. F_3dTMP can be further phosphorylated into F_3dTTP, which can be incorporated into DNA, resulting in cell death (Lenz et al 2015). TAS-102 is not metabolized by DPD; it can be safely administered to patients with suspected DPD deficiency, and it is associated with lower incidence of stomatitis and hand-foot syndrome. TAS-102 has been shown to improve survival of patients with metastatic colorectal cancer

18.3.2.3 Cytidine Analogs

Nucleoside analogs compete with their physiological counterparts for incorporation into DNA and RNA, thereby exerting their cytotoxicity. Cytosine arabinoside (*ara*-C) differs from the nucleoside deoxycytidine only by the presence of a β-hydroxyl group on the 2-position of the sugar, so that the sugar moiety is arabinose instead of deoxyribose (Fig. 18–11). *ara*-C penetrates cells rapidly by a carrier-mediated process shared with deoxycytidine and is phosphorylated to *ara*-CTP. *ara*-CTP is a competitive inhibitor of DNA polymerase, an enzyme necessary for DNA synthesis, and has similar affinity for this enzyme to the normal substrate dCTP. When *ara*-CTP binds to this enzyme, DNA synthesis is arrested and cells in S-phase may die. In addition, *ara*-CTP is incorporated into elongating DNA strands, resulting in DNA chain termination.

The availability of *ara*-CTP for cytotoxic activity depends critically on the balance between kinases that activate the drug and deaminases that degrade it. The activity of these enzymes varies greatly among different cell types, leading to different rates of generation of *ara*-CTP. Resistance to the action of *ara*-C may occur by mutations that lead to deficiency in deoxycytidine kinase or to cells with an expanded pool of

FIGURE 18–11 Structures of deoxycytidine and its analogs.

dCTP that competes with the active metabolite *ara*-CTP and regulates enzymes involved in activation and degradation of the drug. *ara*-C is specific in its activity for cells synthesizing DNA. Because it is rapidly degraded in plasma with a $t_{1/2}$ of 7 to 20 minutes, it must be given intravenously by frequent injections or by continuous infusion. The drug is used primarily for treatment of acute leukemia. Myelosuppression and gastrointestinal toxicity are the major side effects, but abnormal behavior and thought processes may also occur after high doses.

Gemcitabine (2′,2′-difluorodeoxycytidine) is a cytosine analog with structural similarities to *ara*-C (see Fig. 18–11). Unlike *ara*-C, gemcitabine has activity against a variety of solid tumors. Like *ara*-C, gemcitabine requires intracellular activation to its triphosphate derivative dFdCTP, which is then incorporated into DNA and inhibits further DNA synthesis. Although gemcitabine is less effective than *ara*-C in DNA chain termination, a favorable pharmacokinetic characteristic of gemcitabine is the prolonged retention of dFdCTP in cells, with a $t_{1/2}$ as long as 72 hours. Gemcitabine has other intracellular effects that may contribute to its cytotoxic activity including inhibition of ribonucleotide reductase, stimulation of deoxycytidine kinase, and inhibition of cytidine deaminase. Through inhibition of ribonucleoside reductase, gemcitabine affects DNA synthesis by preventing de novo synthesis of the deoxyribonucleoside triphosphate precursors. Gemcitabine has activity against non–small cell lung cancer, pancreatic cancer, breast cancer, bladder cancer, and nasopharyngeal cancer. Toxicity results primarily from myelosuppression and, especially, thrombocytopenia.

18.3.2.4 Purine Antimetabolites
There are two adenosine analogs in clinical use (Fig. 18–12). Fludarabine is a derivative that is resistant to deamination and has activity against low-grade lymphoma, chronic lymphocytic leukemia, hairy cell leukemia, and Waldenström's macroglobulinemia. After administration, fludarabine is rapidly dephosphorylated to 2-fluoro-*ara*-A, which then is transported into cells and converted to the active triphosphate derivative. Mechanisms of cytotoxicity include inhibition of DNA polymerase and termination of DNA and RNA replication. Because 2-fluoro-*ara*-A is excreted primarily unchanged in the urine, dose reduction is necessary in the setting of renal insufficiency. Fludarabine can be administered either intravenously or orally with a $t_{1/2}$ of approximately 20 hours. The major toxicity of fludarabine is myelosuppression and immunosuppression. Rarely, fludarabine is associated with development of autoimmune disease, such as hemolytic anemia and autoimmune thrombocytopenia, and CNS toxicity.

Cladribine (2CdA) is a potent chlorinated adenosine that is also resistant to deamination. It has a similar spectrum of clinical activity and toxicity to fludarabine. Cladribine is administered intravenously and has a $t_{1/2}$ of about 5 hours.

18.3.3 Topoisomerase Inhibitors
DNA topoisomerases are ubiquitous nuclear enzymes that relax supercoiled double-stranded DNA to allow DNA replication and RNA transcription. Torsional strain is relieved via the formation of a single-strand nick (topoisomerase I) or a double-strand nick (topoisomerase II), followed by swiveling of DNA at the nick(s) and subsequent relegation (Fig. 18–13). Topoisomerase inhibitors bind to and stabilize the DNA/topoisomerase cleavable complex, thus preventing the relegation of DNA strands. Irreversible damage results when an advancing DNA replication fork encounters the drug-stabilized cleavable complex, ultimately leading to lethal double-stranded breaks and cell death.

18.3.3.1 Topoisomerase I Inhibitors
Camptothecin is an extract from the wood of the Chinese tree *Camptotheca acuminata* (Fig. 18–14). Camptothecin affects only topoisomerase I activity. Cells in S-phase are very sensitive to topoisomerase I inhibition because of the essential role these enzymes play in DNA replication and the conversion of the topoisomerase-associated single-strand breaks into double-strand breaks. Initial phase I studies conducted in the early 1970s were terminated because of poor solubility and severe and unpredictable toxicity, mainly hemorrhagic cystitis and gastroenteritis. Several analogs of camptothecin have been synthesized to improve solubility and reduce toxicity after the elucidation of its mechanism of action. These analogs all have a basic heterocyclic 5-ring structure with a lactone moiety and a hydroxyl moiety on the E ring (Fig. 18–14). Substitutions on the A ring tend to increase the aqueous solubility while retaining cytotoxicity. All camptothecins can undergo a rapid, reversible, pH-dependent, nonenzymatic hydrolysis of the

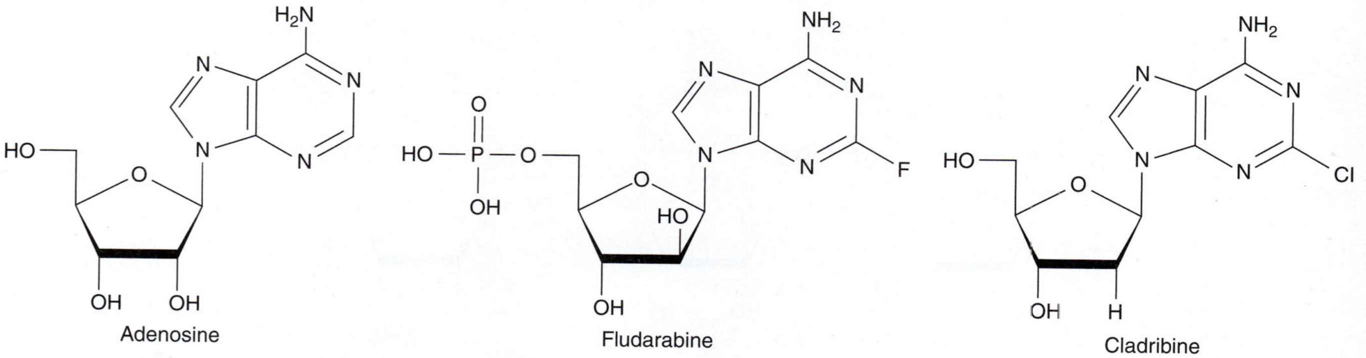

FIGURE 18–12 Structures of adenosine and analogs.

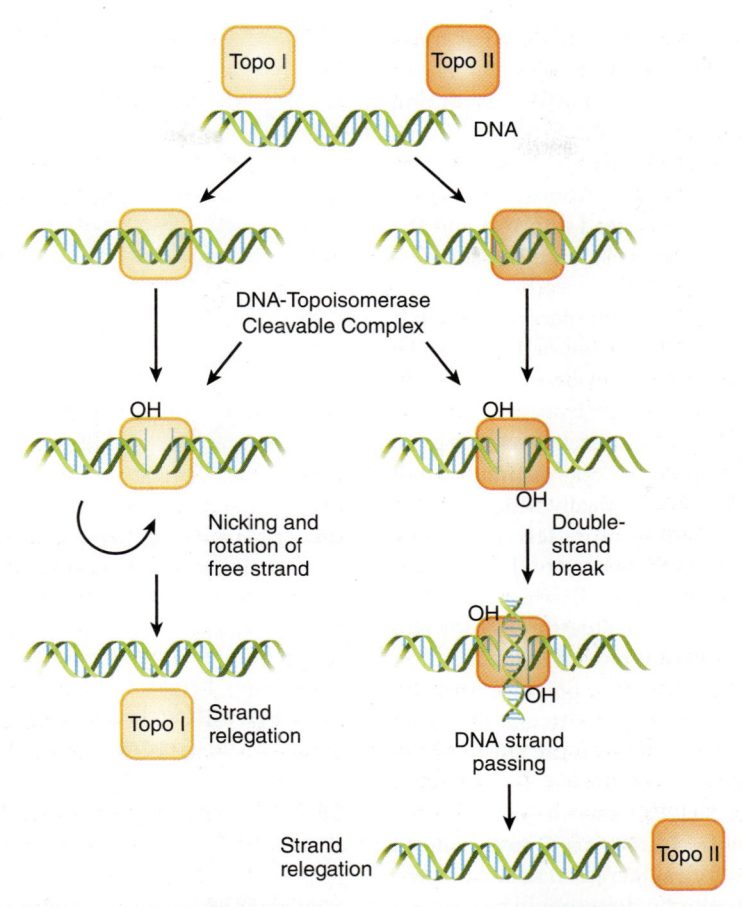

FIGURE 18-13 Topoisomerase (Topo) I and II enzymes form single-strand nicks and double-strand nicks, respectively. Swiveling of supercoiled DNA then occurs at the nick(s), followed by relegation to relieve torsional strain.

closed lactone ring to yield an open-ring carboxylate form. The carboxylate form is more water-soluble than the lactone; it predominates at physiological pH, but is much less active as an inhibitor of topoisomerase I.

Topotecan can be given orally or intravenously. It does not undergo any appreciable metabolism and is eliminated, unchanged, primarily by the kidneys. Therefore, dose reduction is required in patients with renal dysfunction. The

Compound	Molecular weight	R_1	R_2	R_3	R_4
Camptothecin	348	—H	—H	—H	—H
Topotecan	421	—H	—CH$_2$N(CH$_3$)$_2$	—OH	—H
Irinotecan	587	—CH$_2$CH$_3$	—H	O—C(=O)—N◯—N◯	—H
SN-38	392	—CH$_2$CH$_3$	—H	—OH	—H

FIGURE 18-14 Structures of camptothecin and its derivatives.

dose-limiting toxicity is myelosuppression. It is used as treatment for ovarian cancer and small cell lung cancer.

Irinotecan (CPT-11) requires esterification by serum and tissue carboxylesterases to an active metabolite SN-38. SN-38 is subsequently inactivated through glucuronidation by the enzyme uridine diphosphate (UDP)-glucuronosyltransferase 1A1 (UGT1A1) into SN-38G, and excreted into bile and the intestine. Dose-limiting toxicities consist of myelosuppression and diarrhea. Irinotecan can produce an early cholinergic syndrome consisting of abdominal cramps, diarrhea, and diaphoresis that typically occurs acutely during or immediately after infusion, and prompt resolution can be obtained with intravenous or subcutaneous atropine. Patients who experience this reaction may benefit from prophylactic atropine prior to subsequent irinotecan infusions. A second distinct type of diarrhea is associated with irinotecan, typically with a delayed onset. This type of diarrhea tends to be more severe and protracted and is believed to be a result of damage to the gastrointestinal mucosa by SN-38. Severe late-onset diarrhea, especially in the setting of myelosuppression, can be life-threatening and must be managed by aggressive hydration and high-dose loperamide (Rothenberg et al, 2001). Genetic polymorphism in the UGT1A1 gene can result in reduced activity, and increased levels of SN-38. The most common variant is the UGT1A1*28 variant, which contains 7 TA repeats in the TATA repeat box instead of the normal 6 TA repeats. Patients who are homozygous or heterozygous for the UGT1A1*28 allele have reduced UGT1A1 activity, and are therefore at increased risk of neutropenia and diarrhea, and the irinotecan dose should be reduced (Mathijssen et al, 2003). Irinotecan is approved for the treatment of advanced colorectal cancer, where it has been shown to improve survival when used in combination with 5-FU and leucovorin.

18.3.3.2 Epipodophyllotoxins

Etoposide (VP-16) and teniposide (VM-26) are semisynthetic glycoside derivatives of podophyllotoxin, an antimitotic agent derived from the mandrake plant (Fig. 18–15). Although podophyllotoxin binds to tubulin and inhibits its polymerization, etoposide and teniposide act through inhibition of DNA topoisomerase II. These agents are substrates for P-glycoprotein, and drug resistance can thus be mediated by the multidrug-resistant mechanism (see Sec. 18.4.3). Etoposide is a component of first-line treatment regimens in small cell lung cancer, testicular cancer, pediatric cancers, and malignant lymphomas. The effectiveness of etoposide is markedly schedule dependent, with repeated daily doses providing greater activity than a single intravenous administration. Etoposide can be administered orally, with a bioavailability of approximately 50% but considerable interindividual variability. Following intravenous administration, etoposide is eliminated by hepatic glucuronidation, but approximately 40% of the drug is excreted unchanged in the urine. The toxicity of etoposide at standard doses is myelosuppression and hair loss, with other side effects being uncommon. This toxicity profile makes etoposide ideal for high-dose transplantation regimens, and at these higher doses, mucositis becomes dose-limiting. An

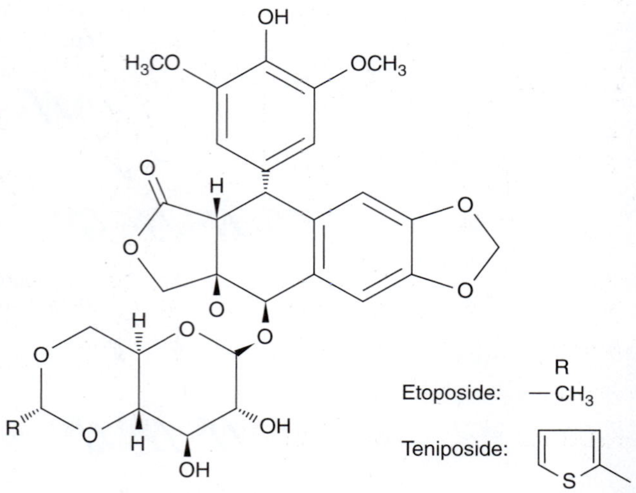

FIGURE 18–15 Structures of etoposide and teniposide. Solid and broken tapered arrows indicate bonds above and below the plane of the rest of the molecule, respectively.

association between the use of etoposide and a secondary leukemia with a characteristic 11q23 translocation has been described. In contrast to secondary leukemia arising from the use of alkylating agents, which occur with a latency of up to 10 years, those arising from etoposide tend to occur sooner, with a median latent period of approximately 2-3 years after drug administration. Most cases of etoposide-induced secondary leukemia are monocytic and myelomonocytic (FAB M-4 and M-5), with no antecedent pancytopenia before the development of frank leukemia.

Teniposide is approved for refractory pediatric acute lymphoid leukemia. Its main toxicity is myelosuppression. Teniposide is mainly eliminated through hepatic metabolism.

18.3.3.3 Anthracyclines and Anthracenediones

The original anthracycline, daunorubicin, is a product of a *Streptomyces* species isolated from an Italian soil sample in 1958. The drug remains a component of treatment protocols for acute myelogenous leukemia. Modifications of the structure of daunorubicin led to the identification of doxorubicin, an analog with greater activity against many solid tumors and one of the most active anticancer drugs in clinical use (Fig. 18–16). The success of doxorubicin led to synthesis of other analogs, but of the hundreds developed and tested, only two are used currently; both have only marginal advantages. Idarubicin can be given orally and has similar activity against acute leukemia. Epirubicin differs from doxorubicin only in its 3-dimensional configuration; it has equal activity and possibly less toxicity.

Several mechanisms may contribute to the cytocidal effect of doxorubicin and related drugs, including interaction with topoisomerase II, DNA intercalation, formation of free radicals, and effects on the cell membrane. Doxorubicin can interact with topoisomerase II by binding directly with the enzyme and preventing resealing of topoisomerase II–induced DNA cleavage, ultimately leading to cytocidal DNA breaks (see Fig. 18–13). Doxorubicin can also intercalate between base

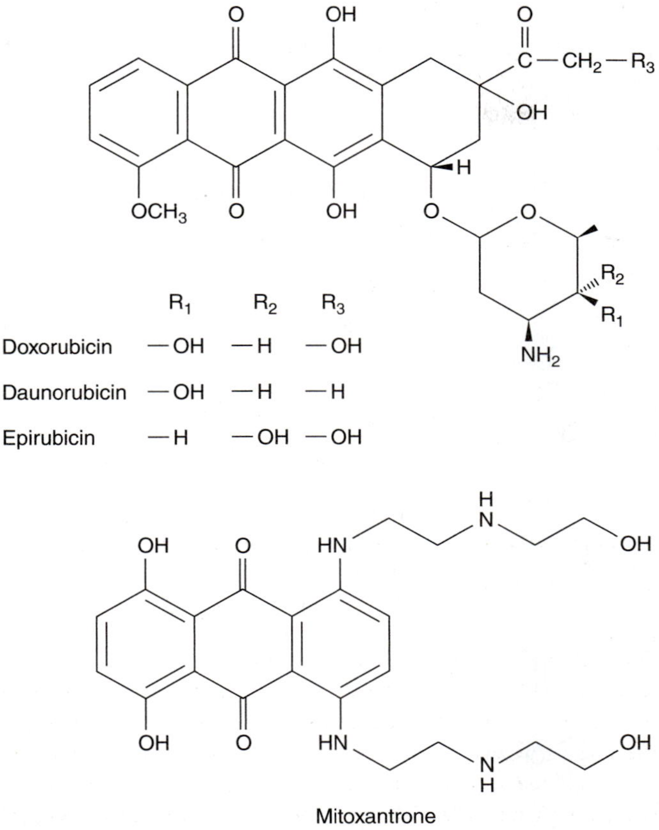

FIGURE 18–16 Structures of doxorubicin, daunorubicin, epirubicin, and mitoxantrone.

pairs perpendicular to the long axis of the double helix. However, much of the DNA is organized and folded into chromatin and may be protected from this type of drug interaction. Also the concentration of doxorubicin required to intercalate into DNA and to cause inhibition of DNA and RNA polymerase cannot be achieved in vivo without excessive toxicity.

Doxorubicin may undergo metabolism of its quinone ring to a semiquinone radical (ie, a group containing an unpaired electron) that, in turn, reacts rapidly with oxygen to yield superoxide, O_2^-. The superoxide radical is known to undergo several reactions that can lead to cell death, including oxidative damage of cell membranes and DNA (Gewirtz, 1999). There is evidence that free radical formation accounts for the cardiac toxicity of anthracyclines, but the contribution of free radicals to the killing of cancer cells is uncertain.

With the exception of idarubicin, anthracyclines are administered intravenously, because oral absorption is poor. They are widely distributed in the body, with significant binding to plasma proteins and tissue. Doxorubicin is metabolized in the liver to doxorubicinol, which retains some cytotoxic activity, and to several other metabolites; the drug and its metabolites are excreted via the bile. Thus, dosage reduction is required for patients with hepatic dysfunction or biliary obstruction.

The acute toxicities of doxorubicin include myelosuppression, total loss of hair, nausea, vomiting, mucositis, and local tissue necrosis following leakage of drug at the injection site. Repeated administration is limited by a chronic irreversible cardiomyopathy that occurs with increasing frequency once a total dose of approximately 500 mg/m² has been delivered. The mechanism of cardiotoxicity is probably related to damage to the sarcoplasmic reticulum mediated by the formation of free radicals within cardiac muscle. Patients with preexisting cardiac disease or those who have received mediastinal radiation are more likely to develop this problem. Dexrazoxane, an iron-chelating agent, reduces cardiac toxicity by binding free iron and prevents oxidative stress on cardiac tissues. Doxorubicin efficacy is not compromised when dexrazoxane is administered (Marty et al, 2006).

Mitoxantrone is less cardiotoxic compared to anthracyclines due to its reduced ability to form free radicals. Mitoxantrone is used in the treatment of advanced hormone refractory prostate cancer and acute myeloid leukemia. It is mainly eliminated through biliary excretion.

18.3.4 Antimicrotubular Agents

18.3.4.1 Vinca Alkaloids The vinca alkaloids, vinblastine, vincristine, vinorelbine, and vindesine are naturally occurring or semisynthetic derivatives from the periwinkle plant. These compounds bind to the β subunit of tubulin dimers at the vinca-binding domain and inhibit its polymerization to form microtubules. Microtubules have several important cellular functions, including formation of the mitotic spindle responsible for separation of chromosomes, and structural and transport functions in axons of nerves. Microtubules are in a state of dynamic equilibrium, with continuous formation and degradation from cytoplasmic tubulin. This process is interrupted by vinca alkaloids, and lethally damaged cells may be observed to enter an abortive metaphase and then lyse. However, experiments with synchronized cells have demonstrated that maximum lethal toxicity for vinblastine and vincristine occurs when cells are exposed during the period of DNA synthesis; presumably, the morphologic expression of that damage is observed in the attempted mitosis.

Vincristine and vinblastine are structurally similar, differing only in a substitution on the central rings (Fig. 18–17). Vinca alkaloids have large volumes of distribution, indicating a high degree of tissue binding, and are eliminated mainly by hepatic metabolism and biliary excretion. Consequently, dose reduction should be considered in patients with elevated bilirubin. The elimination half-lives of vinca alkaloids are approximately 20 hours.

Despite similarities in their structures, these drugs differ in both their clinical spectra of activity and their toxicities. Vinblastine is an important drug in combination chemotherapy of testicular cancer, whereas vincristine is a mainstay of treatment for childhood leukemia. Both drugs have been combined with other cytotoxic agents to treat lymphomas or various solid tumors. Vinorelbine has activity against non–small cell lung cancer and breast cancer.

Vinblastine causes major toxicity to bone marrow, with some risk of autonomic neuropathy, leading to constipation. The dose of vincristine is limited by its toxicity to peripheral nerves, and this damage relates to the duration of treatment as

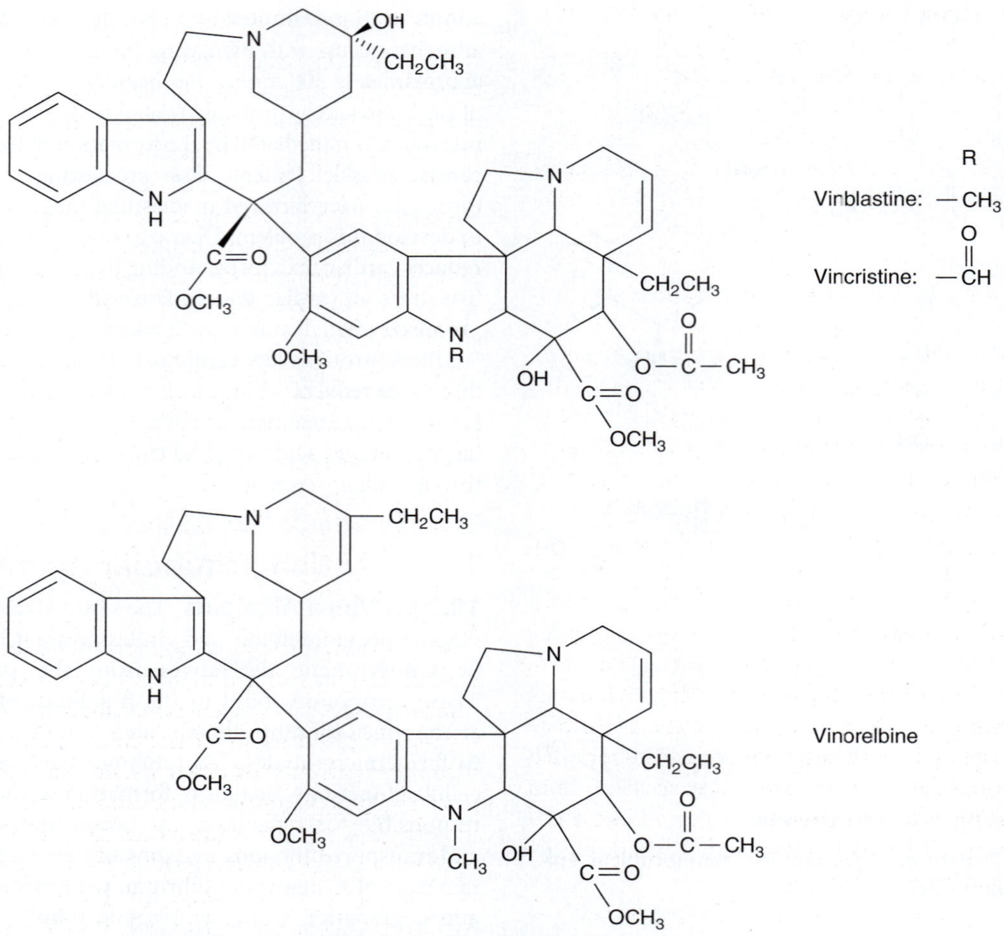

FIGURE 18-17 Structures of vinblastine, vincristine, and vinorelbine.

well as to the total dose of vincristine used. This neurotoxicity is thought to occur because of damage to the microtubules in axons. The dose-limiting toxicity of vinorelbine is myelosuppression. Neurotoxicity can occur but is less common than with vincristine, possibly because of a lower affinity for axonal microtubules. All vinca alkaloids have been associated with the syndrome of inappropriate secretion of antidiuretic hormone (SIADH).

18.3.4.2 Taxanes Paclitaxel and docetaxel are plant alkaloids derived from the bark of the Pacific yew tree *Taxus brevifolia*, and the needles of the European yew tree *Taxus baccata*, respectively (Fig. 18–18). Paclitaxel was identified as an anticancer drug more than 30 years ago, but its clinical development was hampered by a limited supply, as the Pacific yew tree is relatively rare. Subsequent discovery of an intermediary from the relatively abundant needles of the yew tree made it possible to produce large quantities for clinical evaluation and application. Docetaxel and cabazitaxel are semisynthetic derivatives of paclitaxel.

Taxanes bind to tubulin at a site different from that of the vinca alkaloids and promote microtubule stabilization through conformational changes in the β-tubulin subunit. The modulation of microtubule dynamics leads to mitotic blocking,

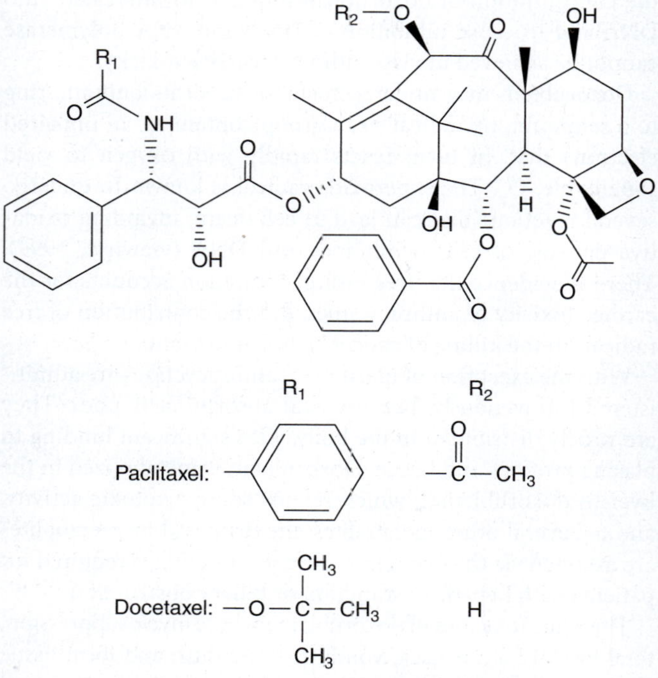

FIGURE 18-18 Structures of paclitaxel and docetaxel.

inability of dividing cancer cells to progress from metaphase into anaphase, and eventually apoptosis (Mukhtar et al, 2014).

The pharmacokinetics of paclitaxel and docetaxel are characterized by a large volume of distribution with extensive tissue binding, elimination by hepatic metabolism, and elimination half-lives of 10 to 12 hours, whereas that of cabazitaxel can be as long as 95 hours. As hepatic metabolism to inactive metabolites is mediated through cytochrome P450 enzymes, agents that influence cytochrome P450 can modify the clearance and toxicity of the taxanes; for example, patients on anticonvulsants that induce cytochrome P450 enzymes have demonstrated increased clearance and reduced toxicity of taxanes (Baker and Dorr, 2001).

Taxanes share many common toxicities. The dose-limiting toxicity is myelosuppression, mainly neutropenia. For paclitaxel, the severity of neutropenia correlates best with the duration that plasma concentration exceeds a critical threshold level ranging from 0.05 to 0.1 µmol/L. They can cause hypersensitivity reactions with bronchial constriction, allergic skin reactions such as urticaria, and hypotension. This problem has been reduced substantially by prophylactic treatment with steroids and histamine antagonists. The vehicles in which the taxanes are formulated have been implicated as possible causes of the hypersensitivity reactions, but different vehicles are used for paclitaxel (Cremophor EL) and for docetaxel (polysorbate 80). A sensory peripheral neuropathy can occur with repeated or high-dose administration. Docetaxel can also cause fluid retention manifesting as lower extremity edema and skin and nail changes over time. These drugs have activity against ovarian, breast, lung, and prostate cancers.

Nanoparticle albumin-bound paclitaxel (Nab-paclitaxel) is a solvent-free colloidal suspension of albumin-bound, 130-nm paclitaxel particles. Compared to solvent-based paclitaxel, nab-paclitaxel is associated with improved pharmacokinetic properties such as a larger volume of distribution, higher maximal concentration, and improved tumor cell penetration and accumulation. The absence of Cremophor EL reduces toxicity. It is approved for treating patients with metastatic breast cancer, non–small cell lung cancer, and pancreatic cancer.

Ixabepilone is a semisynthetic epothilone. Epothilones are initially isolated from the mycobacterium *Sporangium cellulosum*; these compounds bind to the β-subunit of tubulin, promote tubulin polymerization, and consequently mitotic arrest. Ixabepilone is indicated for patients with metastatic breast cancer. It is metabolized extensively through CYP3A4, with <10% excreted as the unchanged drug in urine and feces. Ixabepilone in combination with capecitabine is contraindicated in patients with AST or ALT >2.5 times the upper limit of normal (ULN), or bilirubin >1 × ULN due to increased risks of toxicity and neutropenia-related death.

Eribulin is a synthetic derivative of halichondrin B, which was isolated initially from marine sponge *Halichondria okadai*. It inhibits mitotic spindle formation, resulting in a block in the G2-M phase of the cell cycle. Eribulin is mainly eliminated as the unchanged drug in feces, with negligible hepatic metabolism or renal excretion. Dose reduction should be considered in patients with hepatic or renal dysfunction. Eribulin is approved for metastatic breast cancer and liposarcoma.

18.3.5 Miscellaneous Drugs

Bleomycin consists of a family of molecules with a complex structure; it is derived from fungal culture, the dominant active component being known as bleomycin A2. Bleomycin causes DNA double-stranded breaks through a complex sequence of reactions involving the binding of a bleomycin–ferrous iron complex to DNA. This binding leads to insertion of the drug between base pairs (intercalation) and unwinding of the double helix. A second step in the formation of DNA strand breaks may involve the reduction of molecular oxygen to superoxide or hydroxyl radicals, catalyzed by the bleomycin–ferrous iron complex. However, like doxorubicin, bleomycin retains some of its lethal activity under hypoxic conditions. Bleomycin may exert preferential toxicity in the G2-phase of the cycle, but also has toxicity for slowly proliferating cells in plateau-phase cell culture. Bleomycin is a large molecule that crosses cell membranes slowly. Once within the cell, it can be activated or broken down by bleomycin hydrolase; cellular sensitivity to bleomycin has been found to correlate inversely with the concentration of this enzyme.

After intravenous injection, most of the administered drug is eliminated unchanged in the urine with a $t_{1/2}$ of 4 to 8 hours. The major use of bleomycin is in combination with other drugs for the curative therapy of testicular cancer and lymphomas. Bleomycin has little toxicity to the bone marrow but may cause fever, chills, and damage to skin and mucous membranes. The most serious toxicity is interstitial fibrosis of the lung leading to shortness of breath and death of some patients; its incidence is related to cumulative dose, age, renal function, and the use of other agents that may damage the lung, such as high oxygen supplementation or radiation therapy.

Mitomycin C is derived from a *Streptomyces* species and is a quinine-containing compound that requires activation to an alkylating metabolite by reductive metabolism. Because of the requirement for reductive metabolism, the drug is more active against hypoxic than aerobic cells, at least in tissue culture. Mitomycin C causes delayed and rather unpredictable myelosuppression. More seriously, the drug can produce kidney failure through a hemolytic-uremic syndrome, which is usually fatal and is probably caused by small-vessel endothelial damage. Another potential lethal effect is interstitial lung disease with progression to pulmonary fibrosis. It is sometimes instilled into the bladder by a catheter to treat superficial bladder cancer and is also used with radiation therapy to treat cancer of the anal canal.

18.3.6 Liposomal Drugs

Liposomes consist of phospholipid bilayers enclosing an aqueous drug-containing volume. Conventional liposomes are cleared rapidly by *opsonization* (the addition of post-translational modifications that increase recognition by phagocytes or natural killer cells) of plasma components and uptake by macrophages of the reticuloendothelial system. By incorporating a layer of polyethylene glycol to its surface, liposomes can be sterically stabilized and their blood circulating time prolonged (Allen and Cullis 2013). In addition, the irregular and permeable tumor vasculature permits extravasation of liposomes, while the impaired lymphatic drainage delays clearance of liposomes from tumor microenvironments (the so-called enhanced permeability and retention effect). As a result, there is preferential uptake into tumor tissues and reduced uptake by normal tissues for liposome-encapsulated drugs.

Pegylated liposomal doxorubicin is a formulation where doxorubicin is confined in liposomes that are coated with polyethylene glycol to resist degradation by the endoreticular system. As a result, it has a long half-life, approximately 70 hours, compared with less than 10 minutes when doxorubicin alone is administered intravenously. The long circulating half-life promotes preferential uptake into tumor tissues and reduces uptake by normal tissues because of the enhanced permeability and retention effect. Pegylated liposomal doxorubicin reduces cardiac toxicity, myelosuppression, and nausea, but maintains a comparable efficacy with doxorubicin. However, pegylated liposomal doxorubicin increases the risk of skin toxicity, with 20% of patients developing grade 3 hand-foot syndrome (Gordon et al, 2001).

nal-IRI is a nanoliposomal formulation of irinotecan. Compared to the conventional irinotecan formulation, nal-IRI is associated with a higher maximum concentration (C_{max}), a larger area under the curve (AUC), slower clearance, and smaller volume of distribution (Vd), but similar side effects. nal-IRI has been approved as a second-line therapy in combination with 5-FU for pancreatic cancer following progression with gemcitabine-based therapy.

Liposomal and/or nanoparticle formulations of other anticancer drugs are under investigation with the aims of improving delivery of the drug to tumor cells and/or overcoming some mechanisms of resistance.

18.4 DRUG RESISTANCE

18.4.1 Molecular Mechanisms of Drug Resistance

Resistance to systemic therapy may have multiple causes, and the most widely studied of these are genetically determined mechanisms that lead to resistance of the individual tumor cells. The concept that drug resistance occurs via mutational events that pre-exist in a population was demonstrated in 1943 by Luria and Delbrück; their *Fluctuation Test* showed that the variation in distribution of phage-resistant bacteria among several plates could be explained only by rare mutations that pre-existed in the population.

Sensitivity to drugs may differ widely among cell populations from tumors and normal tissues and also among the cells of a single tumor. Even if drug-resistant cells are present initially only at low frequency (eg, 1 drug-resistant cell per 10^5 drug-sensitive cells), their selective advantage during drug treatment will lead to their rapid emergence as the dominant cell population, giving the clinical impression of "acquired resistance." Drug resistance may occur through mutation, deletion, or amplification of genes that influence the uptake, metabolism, and efflux of anticancer drugs from target cells. Transient changes in cellular phenotype leading to drug resistance may also occur through epigenetic mechanisms (see Chap. 3, Sec. 3.2).

A wide range of changes in the properties of tumor cells may lead to resistance to specific drugs, and Table 18–2 summarizes some of the underlying mechanisms. For example, resistance to several antimetabolite drugs (Sec. 18.3.2) can result from impaired drug uptake into cells, overproduction or reduced affinity of the drug target, upregulation of alternative metabolic pathways, impaired activation or increased inactivation of the antimetabolite, as well as increased drug (or metabolite) efflux. The folic acid analog methotrexate is an example of a drug that can be rendered ineffective by all of these mechanisms (Fig. 18–19). Similarly, resistance to cisplatin (Sec. 18.3.1) can occur because of changes in processes (drug uptake, drug efflux, and/or intracellular drug sequestration) that prevent adequate levels of the drug reaching its DNA target, or by enhanced activity of processes that repair the DNA after it has been modified by the drug (Fig. 18–20; Kelland, 2007). Because multiple mechanisms may contribute to resistance to every anticancer drug, it is not surprising that initial or acquired drug resistance is observed after treatment of most cell populations.

The following evidence indicates that many types of drug resistance are genetic in origin:

1. Characteristics of drug-resistant cells are often inherited in the absence of the selecting drug.
2. Drug-resistant cells are generated spontaneously at a rate that is consistent with known rates of genetic mutation.

TABLE 18–2 Cellular mechanisms associated with resistance to anticancer drugs.*

Mechanism	Drugs
Decreased uptake	Methotrexate, other antimetabolites, cisplatin, nitrogen mustard
Increased efflux	Anthracyclines, Vinca alkaloids, etoposide, taxanes, methotrexate, 5-FU, TKIs
Decrease in drug activation	Many antimetabolites (eg, 5-FU, *ara*-C, gemcitabine)
Increase in drug catabolism	Many antimetabolites (eg, 5-FU, *ara*-C)
Increase or decrease in target enzyme levels	Methotrexate, topoisomerase inhibitors, 5-FU, TKIs
Alterations in target protein (eg, changes in affinity)	Methotrexate, other antimetabolites, topoisomerase inhibitors, TKIs
Inactivation by binding to sulfhydryls (eg, glutathione, metallothionein)	Alkylating agents, cisplatin
Increased DNA repair	Alkylating agents, cisplatin, anthracyclines
Decreased ability to undergo apoptosis	Alkylating agents, cisplatin, anthracyclines, etoposide, anthracyclines, etc

Abbreviations: *ara*-C, Cytosine arabinoside; *5-FU*, 5-fluorouracil; *TKIs*, tyrosine kinase inhibitors.
*Additional mechanisms include those that lead to drug resistance that is expressed selectively in a solid tumor environment (see Sec. 18.3).

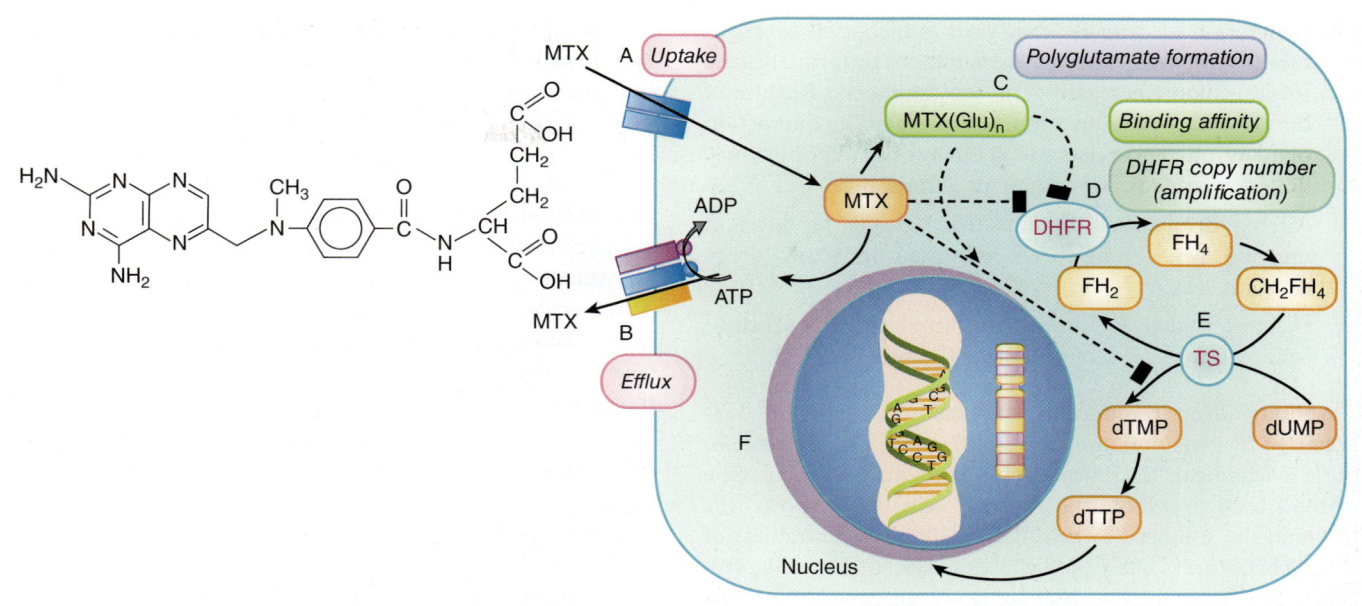

FIGURE 18–19 **Multiple molecular mechanisms underlying cellular resistance to methotrexate.** Methotrexate (MTX) uptake into cells can be limited by mutations in the reduced folate carrier (*RFC1/SLC 19A1*) (*A*). Resistance can also be observed when intracellular levels of MTX are reduced by the action of 1 or more drug efflux pumps such as P-glycoprotein or MRP1 (*B*). Changes in polyglutamylation of MTX (*C*) can reduce cellular sensitivity to this drug as MTX and its polyglutamates inhibit the enzyme dihydrofolate reductase (DHFR), causing a block in the conversion of dihydrofolate (FH$_2$) to tetrahydrofolate (FH$_4$), which ultimately results in a reduction in DNA synthesis and cell death. Binding of MTX and its polyglutamates can also be diminished by mutations in DHFR (*D*). MTX and its polyglutamates inhibit thymidylate synthesis (TS) (*E*), which also reduces DNA synthesis; drug resistance can occur because of changes in the levels or affinity of this enzyme. Finally, drug resistance may develop when the number of copies of the *DHFR* gene on chromosome 5 is increased through gene amplification (*F*).

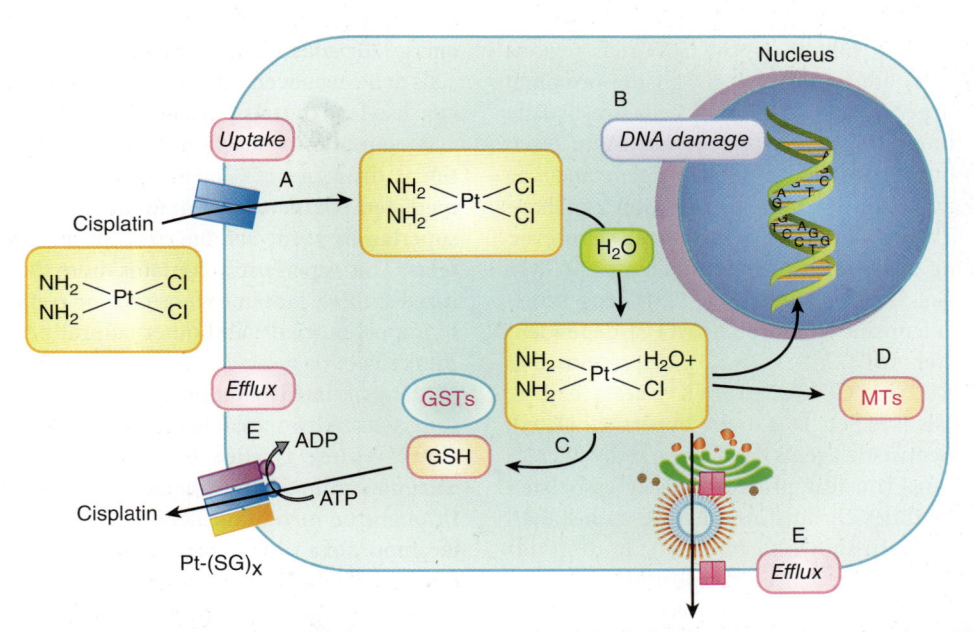

FIGURE 18–20 **Multiple molecular mechanisms underlying cellular resistance to cisplatin.** Cisplatin uptake into cells can be limited by mutations in the uptake transporter CTR1 (*SLC31A1*) resulting in drug resistance (*A*). Once inside the cell, one of the 2 Cl groups is replaced by water, producing a reactive nucleophilic species that enters the nucleus where it can covalently modify DNA (primarily by intrastrand binding to adjacent guanines) and cause cell death. Resistance can occur when the damaged DNA is repaired (eg, nucleotide excision repair) or the damaged DNA is "tolerated" (eg, loss of mismatch repair or downregulation of apoptotic pathways) (*B*). Prior to entering the nucleus, conjugation of the activated cisplatin with glutathione (GSH) by GSH *S*-transferases (GSTs) (*C*), or interaction with the sulfhydryl-containing metallothioneins (*D*) can result in reduced drug efficacy. Finally, resistance can occur if intracellular levels of cisplatin or its metabolites are reduced by the efflux activity of several membrane transporters, including the MRP2 (*ABCC2*) efflux pump and the ATP7B P-type adenosine triphosphatase (ATPase) transporter (*E*).

3. Generation of drug-resistant cells is increased by exposure to compounds that cause mutations or facilitate gene amplification (increased gene copy number). Because of the genomic instability of tumor cells and the interaction of many anticancer drugs with DNA, drug treatment may itself accelerate the development of resistance.
4. Altered drug-target proteins that are the products of mutated genes have been identified in many drug-resistant cells.
5. Drug resistance has been transferred to drug-sensitive cells by transfection of genes (see Chap. 2, Sec. 2.3).

Although drug resistance in many cultured tumor cell lines is caused by gene mutation or amplification, the relevance of these mechanisms to clinical drug treatments is variable. One method used to select drug-resistant cells is to expose cells to mutagens, followed by selection in high concentrations of drug. This process likely predisposes to selection of cells with genetically based drug resistance. However, exposure of cells to lower concentrations of drugs, without prior exposure to mutagens, can also lead to cells that show resistance that may be either stable or transient; transient resistance of some cells in the population may also occur spontaneously, without prior drug exposure.

Mechanisms underlying unstable drug resistance may include epigenetic alterations, including changes in DNA methylation and histone modifications (see Chap. 3, Sec. 3.1; Issa et al, 2017; Ronnekleiv-Kelly et al, 2017). Methylation of cytosines located within CpG dinucleotides is a frequent epigenetic modification in human DNA. CpG-rich regions (so-called CpG islands) are found typically in the proximal promoter regions of genes, and in normal cells are usually unmethylated. In tumor cells, such regions are more often methylated and transcription of the affected gene may be impaired. Gene inactivation by hypermethylation can have consequences on virtually all pathways in the cell. However, when genes encoding DNA repair enzymes (such as *MGMT* and *hMLH1*; Sec. 18.4.5; see Chap. 9, Sec. 9.3), drug transporters (such as the adenosine triphosphate [ATP]-dependent drug efflux transporter *ABCG2*; Sec. 18.3.3), or proteins that regulate the cell cycle (eg, *CDKN2/p16INK*[4a]; see Chap. 8, Sec. 8.2) and apoptosis (see Sec. 18.4.6) are hypermethylated, the response to antineoplastic agents can be markedly altered. Methylation of histones (nuclear proteins closely associated with DNA), which modifies chromatin structure, rather than DNA directly, has also been shown to contribute to drug tolerance, which may be reversible. Chronic exposure to anticancer agents has been shown to permit the selection of a small subpopulation of "drug-tolerant persister" cells via an altered chromatin state that requires histone demethylase (Sharma et al, 2010). These persister cells may go on to acquire other resistance mechanisms including genomic alterations, which may be more permanent (Ramirez et al, 2016).

Another histone modification that regulates gene expression and can influence the drug sensitivity of tumor cells is acetylation and deacetylation, (see Chap. 3, Sec. 3.1.2). Hyperacetylated histones are associated with an open chromatin configuration and are thus more permissive for gene transcription. Responses to drugs can be modulated if the gene affected is a known determinant of drug sensitivity. When combined, inhibitors of DNA methylation and histone acetylation can be effective in restoring drug sensitivity in some experimental systems, and are under investigation for a variety of solid tumors (Ronnekleiv-Kelly et al, 2017).

Genes involved in drug sensitivity and resistance can also be regulated by a process known as *RNA interference* (RNAi). This mechanism involves naturally occurring small RNA molecules, known as microRNAs (miRNAs), which can "silence" genes, typically by binding to complementary sequences in the 3′-untranslated regions of target messenger RNA (mRNA) transcripts followed by translational repression or mRNA degradation (Tekade et al, 2016; see Chap. 2, Sec. 2.3.3).

18.4.2 Resistance Caused By Impaired Drug Uptake

Drug uptake into cells occurs by one of the following mechanisms: (1) passive diffusion, in which the drug enters the cell by an energy-*independent* process without interacting with specific constituents in the cell membrane; (2) facilitated diffusion, in which the drug interacts in a chemically specific manner with a transport carrier in the cell membrane and is translocated into the cell in an energy-*independent* process; (3) binding of drug to a cell surface receptor that is then internalized; and (4) active transport, in which the drug is actively transported by a carrier-mediated process that is energy-*dependent*. All mechanisms allow for drug entry into cells down a concentration gradient, but the fourth mechanism can also lead to transport against a concentration gradient.

A common mechanism of resistance is impaired unidirectional drug influx. Cellular uptake of hydrophilic drugs is mediated commonly by members of the solute carrier (SLC) superfamily (gene symbol *SLC*) of membrane transport proteins. This superfamily contains more than 300 proteins organized into 47 families whose major physiological function is to import nutrients and other naturally occurring metabolites into cells.

Many of the SLC importers that have been implicated in the drug sensitivity of malignant and normal cells have a common core structure typified by 2 membrane-spanning domains, each containing 6 transmembrane α-helices that form a pore through the membrane. The SLC proteins mediate the cellular import of a wide range of hydrophilic anticancer drugs that often resemble the natural physiological substrates of the transporter itself. For example, methotrexate is imported across the plasma membrane primarily by an energy-dependent folic acid uptake system, the reduced folate carrier RFC1 (*SLC19A1*). Drug-resistant cells may have impaired methotrexate uptake into the cell as a result of point mutations in *RFC1/SLC19A1* (see Fig. 18–19); this mechanism of acquired resistance has been found in patients with acute leukemia (Ashton et al, 2009). Similarly, cellular uptake of purine and pyrimidine nucleoside analogs, such as gemcitabine, cladribine, fludarabine, and cytarabine (see Sec. 18.3.2), occurs primarily via membrane transport carriers such as the nucleoside transporters. Cisplatin and other platinum-containing drugs (see Sec. 18.3.1) may be taken up into cells by membrane proteins encoded by the *SLC7A11* or *CTR1/SLC31A1* genes, which normally import amino acids and copper, respectively. Cells deficient in these carrier proteins are often resistant to these drugs, at least in vitro (see Fig. 18–20; Liu et al, 2012). Naturally occurring genetic polymorphisms that result in downregulation or upregulation of these *SLC* genes in normal and/or tumor cells may also contribute to variation in systemic and intracellular levels of (and hence response to) their drug substrates.

18.4.3 Multiple Drug Resistance Caused by Enhanced Drug Efflux

The balance between drug uptake and drug efflux determines drug accumulation in cells. Many anticancer drugs, particularly natural products or their derivatives (eg, doxorubicin, vincristine, etoposide, and paclitaxel), and drug metabolites are effluxed from cells by one or more ATP-binding cassette (ABC) transporters. ABC proteins are found throughout nature, where they carry out many important functions, including the export of potential toxins from cells. Most ABC transporters move one or more molecules (which can range from ions to sugars to small peptides) across biological membranes, a process that requires energy derived from binding and hydrolysis of ATP.

The human ABC superfamily contains 48 proteins, which are organized into 7 subfamilies (*A* through *G*) based on the relative similarities of their amino acid sequences (reviewed in Robey et al, 2018). Three ABC transporters have the ability to export a wide range of structurally diverse anticancer drugs and may cause clinical drug resistance (Table 18–3). P-glycoprotein was described by Juliano and Ling (1976), and is encoded by the *ABCB1* gene (formerly known as the *MDR1* gene). Multidrug resistance protein 1 (MRP1; gene symbol *ABCC1*) was described by Cole et al. (1992), whereas the ABCG2 protein (formerly known as the breast cancer resistance protein [BCRP]) was described by Doyle et al. (1998). These 3 ABC transporters are detected consistently in drug-resistant malignant cells from patients.

In normal cells, P-glycoprotein, MRP1, ABCG2, and several other transporters are often expressed in a polarized manner and contribute to drug absorption (bioavailability), distribution (limiting drug access to so-called pharmacologic sanctuaries such as the brain, cerebral spinal fluid, and testes), and elimination (efflux into bile or urine) (Fig. 18–21). In contrast to the SLC uptake transporters, which display specificity for a single class of drugs, the clinically relevant ABC drug efflux pumps recognize and transport a structurally diverse array of molecules in addition to the anticancer drugs listed in Table 18–3.

18.4.3.1 P-Glycoprotein P-glycoprotein confers resistance against a wide spectrum of complex heterocyclic hydrophobic, antineoplastic drugs mostly derived from natural products

TABLE 18–3 ABC transporters that confer multiple drug resistance in human tumors and their specificity for individual cytotoxic anticancer drugs.

P-Glycoprotein	MRP1	ABCG2/BCRP
Doxorubicin	Doxorubicin	Doxorubicin
Daunorubicin	Daunorubicin	Daunorubicin
Epirubicin	Epirubicin	Mitoxantrone
Mitoxantrone		
Vinblastine	Vinblastine*	
Vincristine	Vincristine	
Etoposide	Etoposide	
Methotrexate	Methotrexate	Methotrexate
Paclitaxel	Paclitaxel*	
	Camptothecin derivatives	Camptothecin derivatives
	SN-38	SN-38
	Topotecan	Topotecan
	Flutamide	Gefitinib
	Hydroxyflutamide	

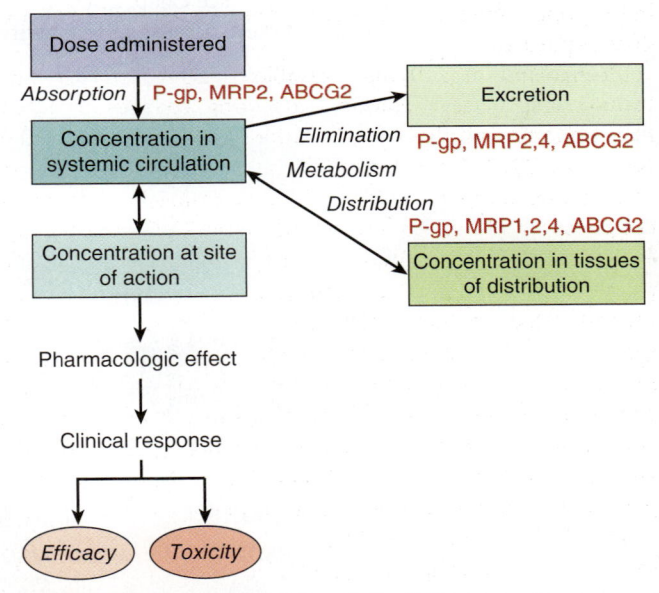

*Low level.

FIGURE 18–21 Multiple roles of the ABC transporters. Although the ABC transporters P-glycoprotein, MRP1, and ABCG2/BCRP have been widely detected in drug-resistant tumor cells, these transporters (together with MRP2 and MRP4) are also now known to affect drug sensitivity and resistance by virtue of their influence on drug absorption (P-glycoprotein, MRP2, ABCG2) and tissue distribution (P-glycoprotein, MRP1, MRP2, MRP4, ABCG2/BCRP), as well as elimination of drugs and their metabolites through the bile, kidney, or other excretory tissue. In tumor cells, the ABC transporters are all found on the plasma membrane. In normal polarized epithelial and endothelial cells in tissues such as the gut, liver, kidney, and brain that are important for drug absorption, distribution, and elimination, P-glycoprotein, MRP2, and ABCG2 are found on apical membranes whereas MRP1 is found on basolateral membranes. MRP4 is unusual in that its localization depends on the tissue in which it is expressed (eg, apical in kidney, brain; basolateral in prostate, liver). *P-gp*, P-glycoprotein. (Reproduced with permission from Slot AJ, Molinski SV, Cole SP. Mammalian multidrug-resistance proteins (MRPs). *Essays Biochem* 2011 Sep 7;50(1):179-207.)

that include the anthracycline antibiotics, the *Vinca* alkaloids, and the taxanes (Table 18–3; see Secs. 18.3.3 and 18.3.4). Other substrates include the tyrosine kinase inhibitors gefitinib and imatinib (see Chap. 19, Secs. 19.4.1 and 19.6.4). P-glycoprotein also mediates the cellular efflux of drugs such as ondansetron and granisetron, that are used with chemotherapy to control nausea and vomiting. Single–amino acid substitutions can markedly alter the substrate specificity of P-glycoprotein, and naturally occurring polymorphisms in the *ABCB1* gene affect the ability of P-glycoprotein to recognize some of its drug substrates (Robey et al, 2018).

In addition to being expressed at elevated levels in certain tumor types, P-glycoprotein is also found in normal tissues, such as the kidney and adrenal gland, as well as the lung, liver, and gastrointestinal tract. P-glycoprotein (and other ABC proteins) are localized to the apical surface of polarized cells that line the tubules or ducts or lumen of these organs, and thus provides such cells with a mechanism for extruding xenobiotic molecules that are recognized by the transporter (see Fig. 18–22; Leslie et al, 2005). P-glycoprotein is also expressed on the apical membrane of endothelial cells lining the blood–brain barrier, where it excludes toxic natural products from the central nervous system: knockout mice (see Chap. 2 Sec. 2.3.5) lacking P-glycoprotein display a marked increase in sensitivity to the neurotoxic side effects of several different drugs (Robey et al, 2018). Such animals also show enhanced oral absorption (bioavailability) of certain drugs, and this also occurs in humans when P-glycoprotein is inhibited.

Elevated levels of P-glycoprotein have been found in multiple human tumors, including sarcomas and cancers of the colon, adrenal, kidney, liver, and pancreas: these tumors tend to be resistant to chemotherapy. Elevated levels of P-glycoprotein have also been detected following relapse after chemotherapy in more drug-sensitive tumors, including multiple myeloma and cancers of the breast and ovary. These findings suggest that P-glycoprotein may contribute to clinical drug resistance. Increased P-glycoprotein has also been reported to correlate with a poor prognosis in children with neuroblastoma, rhabdomyosarcoma, and osteogenic sarcoma.

18.4.3.2 Multidrug Resistance Proteins
A second multidrug transporter, known as MRP1 (gene symbol ABCC1), was cloned from a drug-selected cell line derived from human small cell lung cancer that did not express P-glycoprotein but did contain multiple gene copies of ABCC1 (Cole et al, 1992; Fig 18–22). P-glycoprotein and MRP1 share only 15% amino acid sequence identity and differ in several structural and pharmacologic ways (Robey et al, 2018).

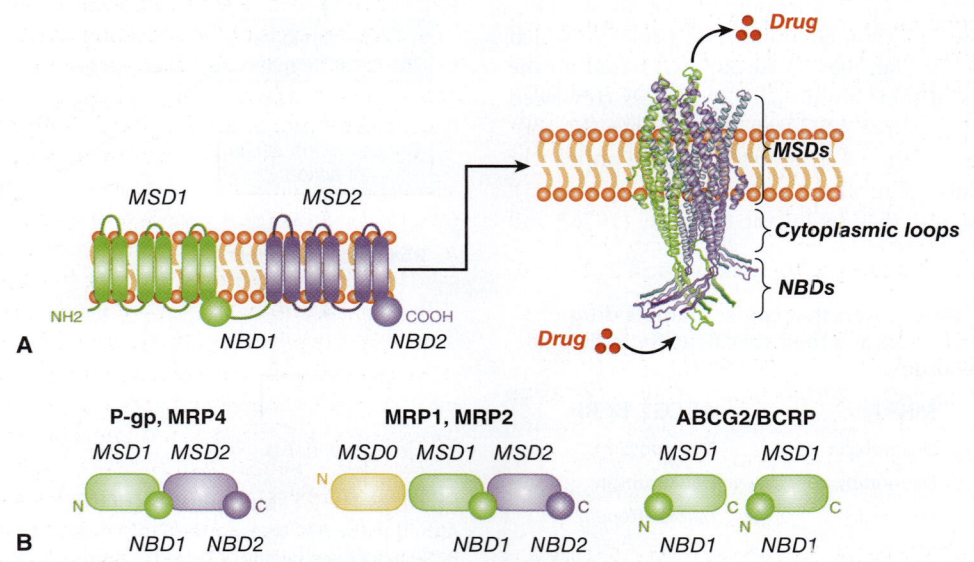

FIGURE 18–22 General structure of ABC membrane drug efflux pumps. **A)** *(left)* Shown is a linear topologic cartoon of the core structure of ABC transporters such as P-glycoprotein showing the 2 cytoplasmic nucleotide-binding domains (NBDs) and 12 transmembrane helices (here shown as cylinders) equally distributed between 2 membrane-spanning domains (MSDs). *(right)* Shown is a 3D homology model of the core structure of MRP1 generated using the crystal structure of *Staphylococcus aureus* Sav1866 as template (Hollenstein et al, 2007; DeGorter et al, 2008). The α-carbon backbone in ribbon representation of the core structure (MSD1-NBD1-MSD2-NBD2) is viewed from the plane perpendicular to the membrane bilayer (DeGorter et al, 2008). Homology models of P-glycoprotein, MRP4, and other ABC transporters look very similar. The 2 NBDs form a "sandwich" dimer for the effective binding and hydrolysis of 2 molecules of ATP, providing the energy for the transport process. Signaling between the MSDs (translocation pathway through the membrane) and the NBDs (which provide the energy for transport) is mediated by specific sequences in the cytoplasmic loops. Substrates that enter the cell by diffusion or active transport, or are formed in the cell by conjugation, are thought to be exported from the cell either directly through the pore from the cytoplasm, or in the case of hydrophobic drugs, are taken up from the inner leaflet of the membrane lipid bilayer. **B)** Domain organization of ABC transporter drug (and drug metabolite) efflux pumps implicated in drug resistance in malignant cells. P-glycoprotein and the MRPs are encoded as multidomain single polypeptides containing MSDs and NBDs in the orientations shown, whereas ABCG2/BCRP is encoded as a "half-transporter" and 2 identical subunits assemble together to form a functional transporter. Each of the MSDs contains 6 transmembrane segments (α-helices) except for MSD0 of MRP1 and MRP2, which contains just 5. *P-gp*, P-glycoprotein.

Increased expression of MRP1 leads to a net decrease in cellular accumulation of a variety of anticancer drugs, including both natural products and the folic acid analog methotrexate (see Table 18–2). Unlike P-glycoprotein, MRP1 confers at most low levels of resistance to the hydrophobic paclitaxel and vinblastine. Transport of some drugs (eg, vincristine, daunorubicin) by MRP1 depends on the presence of the antioxidant glutathione (GSH) or a tripeptide analog. In vitro, GSH causes changes in the conformation of the MRP1 protein, which increases its affinity for some of its drug substrates (Deeley and Cole, 2006), but GSH may also influence MRP1 function in other ways. In addition to anticancer drugs, MRP1 transports a broad spectrum of organic anions, the conjugated estrogens estradiol glucuronide and estrone sulfate, folic acid, GSH, and its pro-oxidant metabolite GSH disulfide (GSSG).

Increased expression of MRP1 has been observed in several types of drug-resistant human tumors, such as lung cancer and some leukemias, and in many cell lines derived from human tumors (Deeley and Cole, 2006; Robey et al, 2018). In children with neuroblastoma, expression of MRP1 was correlated with expression of the *N-MYC* oncogene and predicted poor survival. Mutations in *ABCC1* cause changes in the substrate specificity of MRP1, and in primary neuroblastoma, the naturally occurring ABCC1 polymorphism G2012T is associated with better patient outcome and altered stability of the *ABCC1* gene transcript (Pajic et al, 2011).

Although it is found rarely in tumors, MRP2 in normal cells may impact drug sensitivity because it can influence the distribution and elimination (and hence pharmacokinetics) of some anticancer drugs and their metabolites. MRP2 is structurally similar to MRP1, but unlike MRP1, it is expressed predominantly on apical membranes of the bile canaliculus, renal epithelium, and intestinal enterocytes. Thus, MRP2 plays a role in the oral bioavailability and elimination of drugs and their metabolites that are substrates of this transport protein (Nies and Keppler, 2007).

The ABCG2 protein (formerly known as the breast cancer resistance protein [BCRP]) is expressed in both leukemia and solid tumors, and frequently co-expressed with the other transporters (Robey et al, 2018). As shown in Table 18–3, the spectrum of substrate drugs is non-identical but overlaps with that recognized by P-glycoprotein or MRP1.

18.4.3.3 Reversal of Drug Resistance Mediated by ABC Transporters

Many agents have been identified that inhibit the function of ABC transporters and increase the sensitivity of drug-resistant tumor cells in culture (Robey et al, 2018). Some of these agents are themselves substrates for the transporters and inhibit competitively the efflux of anticancer drugs, but noncompetitive mechanisms have also been implicated. Multiple clinical trials have assessed the potential of P-glycoprotein antagonists to increase the sensitivity of human tumors to anticancer drugs such as doxorubicin and vinorelbine. Some patients with hematologic malignancies that were drug resistant responded to the same anticancer drugs when an inhibitor of P-glycoprotein was added to the drug regimen, but the results of studies with solid tumors have been disappointing. There are several possible reasons for the inconclusive outcomes of many of these clinical trials, including poor trial design, resistance because of mechanisms in addition to or other than P-glycoprotein, failure to select for patients with dominant expression of the transporters, and failure to achieve adequate levels of the reversing agent in the tumor tissue (Yu et al, 2012; Robey et al, 2018).

Agents such as verapamil and cyclosporine, which may reverse drug resistance as a result of P-glycoprotein in cell culture, have much less effect on drug resistance because of MRP1. Novel agents that inhibit the transport function of P-glycoprotein (as well as MRP1, MRP2, MRP4, and ABCG2) are also being investigated for their ability to improve oral absorption of antineoplastic drugs or enable better penetration of drugs into pharmacologic sanctuaries (eg, the central nervous system), tissues that are normally protected by these transporters (Matsson et al, 2009; Robey et al, 2018).

18.4.4 Resistance Caused by Decreased Drug Activation or Increased Drug Inactivation

Many antineoplastic drugs, and in particular the antimetabolites, must be converted to a pharmacologically active form after cellular uptake in order to exert their cytotoxic effects. Resistance to these agents can occur when there is a decrease in activity or levels of the activating enzyme(s), or an increase in the activity or levels of an enzyme that is responsible for detoxifying the active form of the drug. These mechanisms are discussed for individual drugs in Section 18.3.

Many anticancer drugs and carcinogens cause cellular damage by the production of chemically reactive electrophilic intermediates, especially reactive oxygen species (see Chap. 12, Sec. 12.3.4). Similar processes are involved during the interaction of ionizing radiation with tissue (see Chap. 15, Sec. 15.2.3). One mechanism by which cells protect themselves from damage is by upregulating the synthesis of sulfhydryl-containing molecules, especially the nucleophilic tripeptide glutathione (GSH), which can form conjugates with electrophilic metabolites and render them less reactive and thus nontoxic. The importance of GSH in the protection of normal cells is reflected in its widespread distribution and its relatively high intracellular concentration (>1 mM in many tissues). GSH can inactivate peroxides and free radicals, which may be produced by drugs such as etoposide and the anthracyclines (eg, doxorubicin). It can also react with positively charged electrophilic molecules, such as the active groups of cisplatin and alkylating agents, rendering them less toxic and more easily excreted. These reactions are catalyzed, respectively, by the enzymes GSH peroxidase and GSH *S*-transferase (GST) (see Fig. 18–20 and Sec. 18.3.1). By conjugating GSH to various drugs or their active metabolites, GSTs appear to play a role in the development of cellular resistance to some antineoplastic agents including alkylating and platinum-containing drugs (Sau et al, 2010; Allocati et al, 2018).

Drugs conjugated to GSH, glucuronide, or sulfate groups are negatively charged, and these conjugated organic anions are extruded from cells by an energy-dependent mechanism. This process involves GSH-conjugate export carriers (known variably as *GS-X pumps* or *multispecific organic anion transporters*), whose export function is undertaken, in large part, by the ABC transporters MRP1 and MRP2 (Deeley and Cole, 2006; Sec. 18.4.3.2). The active efflux of conjugated metabolites by the ABC transporters prevents their intracellular accumulation, thereby reducing the possibility of hydrolytic enzymes causing the regeneration of the active parent compound. However, some conjugated metabolites can be cytotoxic themselves because of their ability to inhibit enzymes important for cell viability, as well as by inhibition of the conjugating enzymes. Thus, elimination of conjugated metabolites from the cell is an important component of the detoxification process.

18.4.5 Drug Resistance and Repair of Drug-Mediated DNA Damage

Many chemotherapeutic agents cause a variety of toxic DNA lesions that lead to cell death unless the damage is repaired. Detection and repair of drug-induced DNA lesions is carried out by lesion-specific DNA repair pathways (see Chap. 9, Sec. 9.3). Resistance to DNA-damaging agents may occur because DNA repair processes in the tumor cells have become more efficient.

Cisplatin induces cell death by forming DNA-platinum adducts and interstrand DNA crosslinks, but resistance can ensue if the lesions are repaired. Repair of platinum-modified DNA often involves nucleotide excision repair (NER; see Chap. 9, Sec. 9.3.3), and variations in NER activity can be an important determinant of drug sensitivity and resistance. Elevated levels of the excision repair cross-complementation group 1 (ERCC1) enzyme, which plays a rate-limiting role in the NER pathway, have been reported to correlate with increased responsiveness to cisplatin-based adjuvant therapy in lung cancer patients, but an overview analysis failed to validate this association (Friboulet et al, 2016), possibly because of technical limitations of available antibody reagents, and it is not used in clinical practice.

Alkylating agents such as temozolomide exert their cytotoxicity, at least in part, by binding to the guanine bases in DNA (see Sec. 18.3.1). O^6-methylguanine-DNA methyltransferase (MGMT) (also known as O^6-alkylguanine DNA alkyltransferase) is one of the enzymes responsible for the repair of alkylated DNA. MGMT removes adducts from the O-6 position of guanine and transfers the alkyl group to a specific cysteine residue ("acceptor site") on the enzyme (Fig. 18–23). Because this transfer and alkylation of MGMT renders the enzyme inactive, the enzyme is considered to act by a "suicide" mechanism. Levels of MGMT or the methylation status of the *MGMT* promoter (which controls the expression of the gene) are useful predictors of the responsiveness of some tumors to alkylating agents (Barault et al 2015).

Bifunctional alkylating agents, such as cisplatin, as well as drugs targeting topoisomerase I and II, can cause the accumulation of double-strand breaks (DSBs), leading to cell death unless the breaks are repaired. Repair of DSBs can take place by either nonhomologous or homology-directed repair pathways,

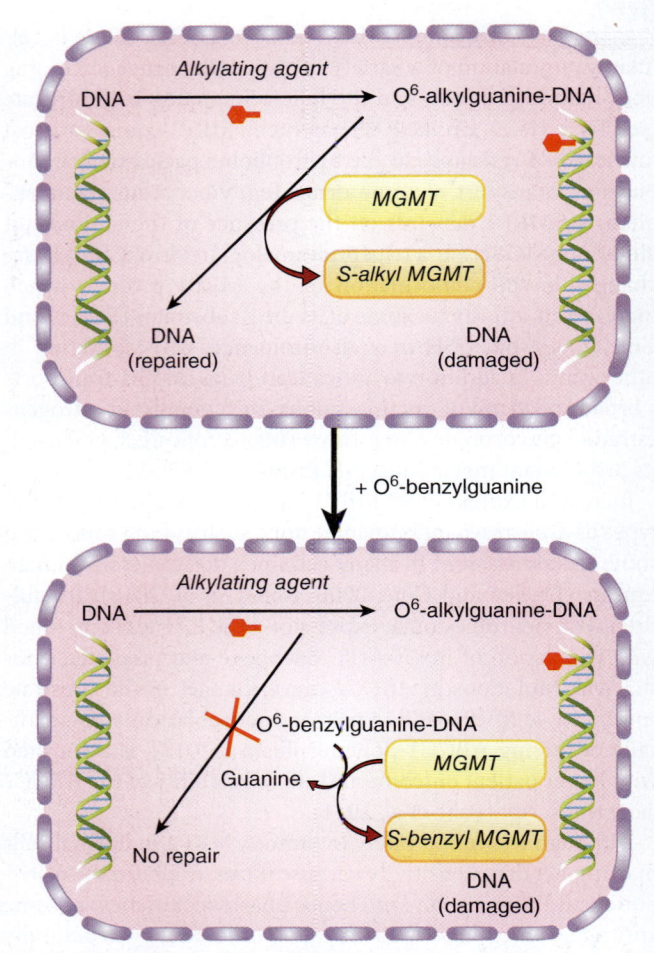

FIGURE 18–23 Resistance mediated by repair of an alkylated guanine base by MGMT and inhibition of this repair by O^6-benzylguanine. (*upper panel*) The DNA repair enzyme MGMT causes resistance by removing toxic adducts from the O^6 position of guanine in native DNA. It does this by transferring the alkyl group to a cysteine residue in the enzyme itself, resulting in auto-inactivation of enzyme. (*lower panel*) In the presence of exogenous O^6-benzylguanine, MGMT is no longer available to repair the DNA and resistance is circumvented.

the relative contribution of which depends on a variety of different factors (see Chap. 9, Sec. 9.3). Many human cancers probably have impairment in DNA repair pathways that contributes to their genomic instability, and such tumors are likely to be more sensitive to DNA-damaging agents. Regaining the capacity for certain types of DNA repair is a potential mechanism by which tumor cells can acquire resistance to DNA-targeting drugs. For example, exposure to platinum-containing drugs in *BRCA1* or *BRCA2* mutated ovarian cancer cells (which plays a crucial role in homologous recombination; see Chap. 9, Sec. 9.3.4) can select for drug-resistant cells in which additional mutations in *BRCA1* or *BRCA2* can result in partial restoration of protein function and thus drug resistance (Sakai et al, 2008; Christie et al, 2017).

Cells may survive if there is a defect in a single DNA repair gene because of redundancy in repair pathways, but may die if an alternative pathway is inhibited, a concept known as synthetic lethality (McLornan et al, 2014; see Chap. 19, Sec. 19.6.2). The concept of genetic synthetic lethality was first explored in model organisms such as *Drosophila melanogaster* and *Saccharomyces cerevisiae*. Genome-wide screening technologies have enabled the ability to map genes that interact synthetically, and to identify chemicals whose inhibition of one genetic network are synthetic lethal with mutations in a second genetic network (called chemo-genetic synthetic lethality; reviewed in Kaelin, 2005). This property can be exploited clinically, for example, by using an inhibitor of poly-(adenosine phosphate ribose) polymerase (PARP) to treat tumors with an existing mutation leading to a deficit in another DNA repair pathway; normal cells without a defect in a DNA repair pathway are spared (Chalmers et al., 2010; Mateo et al, 2015).

18.4.6 Apoptosis and Autophagy

Differences in the sensitivity of tumor cells to anticancer drugs can occur because of changes in the pathways that mediate cell death and survival. Types of cell death that have been observed following treatment with anticancer drugs include apoptosis, necrosis, mitotic catastrophe, and senescence, whereas autophagy may act (paradoxically) to enhance either death or survival of the cell. Apoptosis is initiated by the mitochondrial cytochrome c/Apaf-1/caspase-9 pathway (see Chap. 8, Sec. 8.4) while signaling through the death receptor pathway by drug-induced FasL upregulation seems less important, except possibly for 5-FU-induced cytotoxicity. The proapoptotic and antiapoptotic members of the bcl-2 family, the kinases and phosphatases that regulate their activity and subcellular localization, the initiator and effector caspases, the various inhibitors of apoptosis proteins (IAPs), as well as the presence of wild-type or mutant p53, are all examples of proteins that might influence the sensitivity of tumor cells to apoptotic cell death (Brown and Attardi, 2005; Mohammad et al, 2015).

Markers of apoptosis are observed commonly after treatment of malignant cells (or solid tumors) with anticancer drugs, but the effect of stimulating apoptotic pathways on sensitivity of anticancer drugs is variable. Some laboratory studies have shown that modulating these pathways can affect drug response, but several investigators have found little or no effect on drug sensitivity of solid tumors from modulating pathways of apoptosis (eg, Brown and Attardi, 2005). Proapoptotic inhibition of the MDM2-p53 pathway indicates that sensitivity of anticancer drugs can be increased in preclinical experiments and may be a promising strategy. A key determinant of whether the process of apoptosis might be modified to influence drug sensitivity is whether it is primary in causing lethal damage to cells, or simply represents a pathway whereby cells that have already sustained lethal and nonrepairable damage undergo cellular lysis. It appears likely that this depends on both the drugs used and the cell type that is treated.

Autophagy is a lysosomal degradation pathway for intracellular digestion of cellular macromolecules that maintains cellular metabolism in times of stress such as exposure to hypoxia or to cytotoxic drugs (see Chap. 8, Sec. 8.4.6 and Chap. 12, Sec. 12.3.6). When autophagy is activated, intracellular membrane vesicles form and engulf proteins, cytoplasm, organelles, and protein aggregates, and these vesicles are then delivered to lysosomes where they and their contents are degraded. Autophagy-associated pathways can promote cell survival by recycling breakdown products of macromolecules, especially under adverse conditions such as hypoxia (see Chap. 12, Sec. 12.3.6; White and DiPaola, 2009). Upregulation of autophagy has been observed in cells treated with anticancer drugs, and may lead to resistance to drugs and radiation (Tan et al, 2017). The development of inhibitors of autophagy is being investigated as a mechanism for overcoming resistance.

18.4.7 Drug Resistance and the Solid Tumor Environment

Sensitivity to drugs depends not only on the intrinsic sensitivity of the constituent tumor cells but also on the microenvironment and on contact between the tumor cells. Tumors have a complex extracellular matrix (see Chap. 10, Sec. 10.2 and Chap. 12, Sec. 12.2.2), and cells in common epithelial-derived tumors have close cellular contact. Solid tumors have a poorly formed vasculature, which leads to regions of hypoxia and extracellular acidity (see Chap. 11, Sec. 11.5, and Chap. 12, Sec. 12.2.3), and a requirement that anticancer drugs penetrate over relatively long intercapillary distances (as compared to those in normal tissues) to reach the target tumor cells (Minchinton and Tannock, 2006; Fig. 18–24). Variable concentration of nutrient metabolites in the extracellular environment, and other factors, lead to variable rates of cell proliferation before treatment, and of repopulation of surviving tumor cells after treatment, both of which influence drug sensitivity of experimental and clinical tumors.

Drug-resistance mechanisms that depend on the microenvironment may be explored by using model systems that maintain cellular interactions with other cells and with the extracellular matrix, thereby better reflecting how tumors in vivo are exposed to drugs. One model is provided by spheroids, in which malignant cells grow in contact with each other and with an extracellular matrix to form nodules in tissue culture (Durand, 1989; Ong et al, 2018; Fig. 18–25A). Alternatively, tumor cells can be grown on collagen-coated semiporous Teflon membranes to form multilayered cell cultures (MCCs) of relatively constant thickness to provide a useful model for studying drug penetration through tumor tissue (Hicks et al, 1997; Tannock et al, 2002; Fig. 18–25B). Drug can then be added on one side of the MCC and its time-dependent concentration measured on the other (Fig. 18–25C) to quantify the penetration of drugs through the MCC as compared to that through the semipermeable membrane alone (Fig. 18–25D).

18.4.7.1 Influence of Cell-Cell Contact and the Extracellular Matrix
Repeated drug treatment of solid tissue, either in the form of spheroids or tumor-bearing mice, may lead to drug resistance that is expressed only when the cells are grown in contact with one another. The tumor cells do not display drug resistance when grown without cell-cell

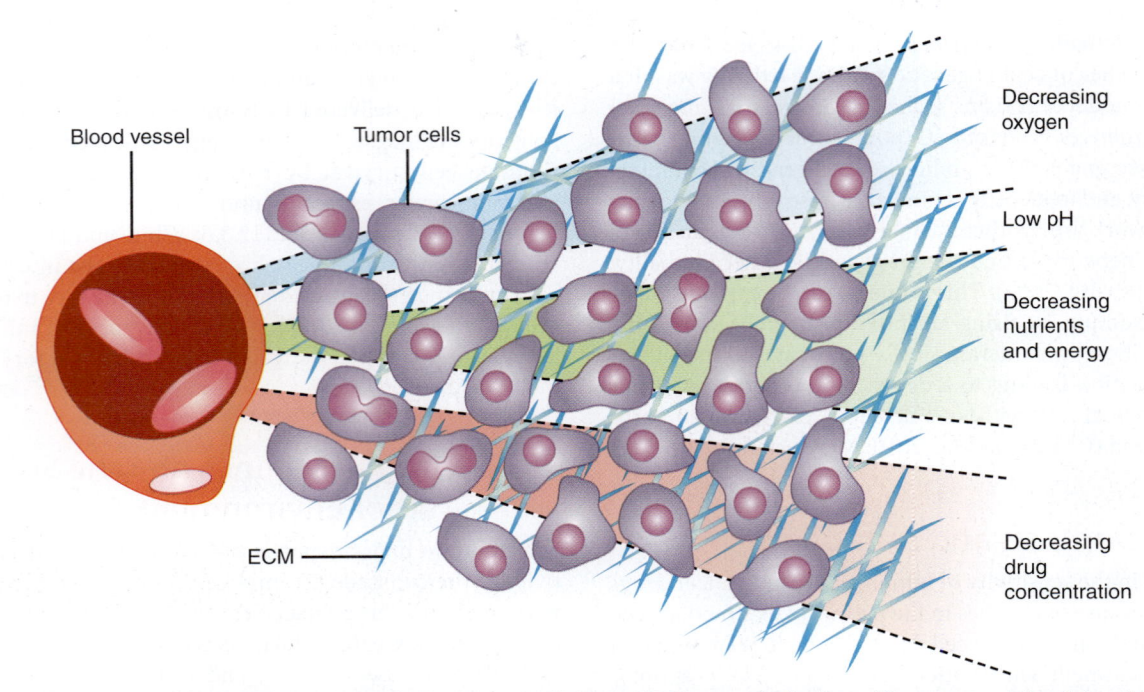

FIGURE 18–24 Representation of gradients of oxygen and other metabolites, and of cell proliferation and death in relation to blood vessels in solid tumors. *ECM*, extracellular matrix. (Reproduced with permission from Minchinton AI, Tannock IF. Drug penetration in solid tumours. *Nat Rev Cancer* 2006 Aug;6(8):583-592.)

contact as in dilute cell culture (Teicher et al, 1990). Further work suggests that drug resistance is dependent on integrin-mediated cell adhesion, and may be reversed by silencing of the gene encoding focal adhesion kinase, or by agents that inhibit adhesion between the cells (Zutter, 2007; Chen et al, 2010; see Chap. 10, Sec. 10.2). Integrin-mediated cell adhesion may influence multiple cellular properties, including cell proliferation, through regulation of cell-cycle checkpoints and upregulation of cell-cycle–inhibitory CDKs (Zutter, 2007). Hence these effects may be mediated in part by a reduction in the rate of cell proliferation in the solid tissue environment, with consequent resistance to cycle-active drugs.

The extracellular matrix (ECM) can provide tumor cells with protection against cell death mediated by anticancer drugs, described as cell adhesion–mediated drug resistance (CAMDR; Dickreuter and Cordes, 2017). CAMDR has been most studied in multiple myeloma, where myeloma cells interact with stroma in the bone marrow, leading to initiation of survival signals that are absent when the same cells are in suspension (Li and Dalton, 2006). Several strategies to circumvent this type of resistance have been proposed that target molecules in tumor cells and/or in the ECM that are required for cell adhesion. The activity of the proteasome inhibitor bortezomib, which has led to improved prognosis in patients with multiple myeloma, appears to depend on its ability to inhibit CAMDR (Noborio-Hatano et al, 2009).

18.4.7.2 Drug Resistance in Hypoxic Environments

Tumor vasculature is characterized by irregular blood flow and stasis, and by relatively large intercapillary distances in comparison to those in normal tissues (see Chap. 11, Sec. 11.5). Hence, tumor regions that are not in close proximity to the vasculature may be hypoxic, with low extracellular pH because of the production of lactic acid and poor clearance of this and other acidic products of metabolism (see Fig. 18–24). Hypoxia is widely recognized as a major factor leading to resistance of tumor cells to radiotherapy (see Chap. 16, Sec. 16.4), but the following mechanisms may also cause cells in hypoxic regions to be resistant to anticancer drugs.

Cells in nutrient-deprived regions of tumors tend to have a low rate of proliferation in comparison to cells situated close to functional blood vessels. Most anticancer drugs are more toxic to proliferating than to nonproliferating cells (see Chap. 17, Sec. 17.5). Thus, even if the drugs achieve potentially cytotoxic concentrations in these regions, the level of cell death may be limited. Surviving cells that were previously hypoxic may begin to proliferate following loss of killed cells closer to blood vessels, leading to an improvement in the distribution of oxygen and nutrient metabolites, and therefore may allow regrowth of the tumor (Saggar and Tannock, 2015).

Hypoxia and extracellular acidity have direct effects on the activity and/or uptake of some anticancer drugs, independent of proliferative status. As for ionizing radiation, the toxicity of some drugs is dependent on the production of free radicals, and this process depends on availability of oxygen. Drugs that require active transport into cells are dependent on ATP, and anaerobic metabolism is much less efficient than oxidative phosphorylation in producing ATP (see Chap. 12, Sec. 12.3). Drugs that are weak bases, such as doxorubicin, have a greater proportion of charged molecules under acidic conditions, which decreases their ability to cross the plasma membrane and be taken up into the cell, leading to decreased activity. In contrast, extracellular acidity may enhance the uptake of drugs that are weak acids, such as chlorambucil or melphalan.

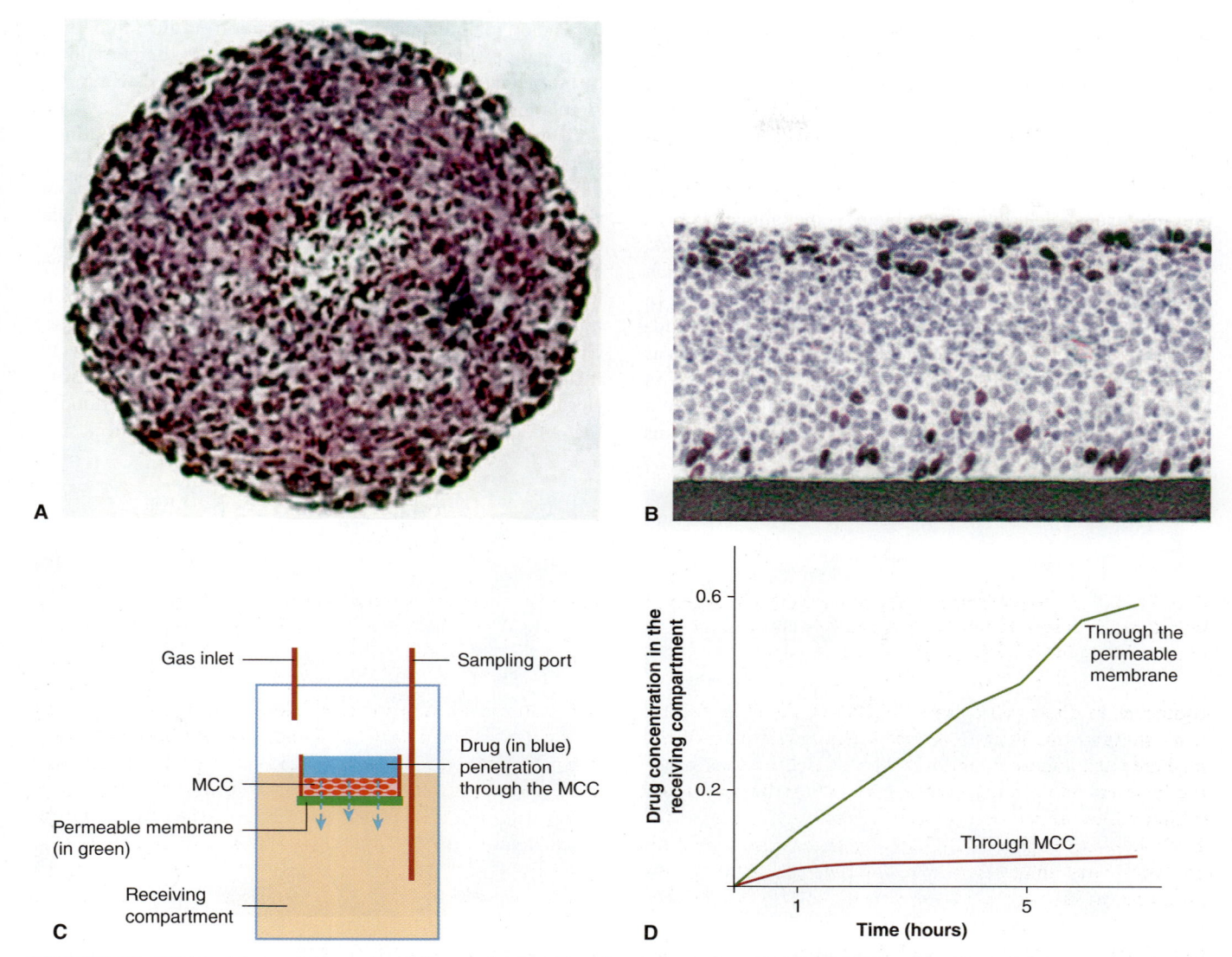

FIGURE 18–25 Models used for study of drug resistance that depends on the microenvironment found in solid tumors. **A)** Multicellular tumor spheroid. The distribution of fluorescent compounds may be imaged directly. **B)** Multilayered cell culture (MCC) grown on a collagen-coated Teflon membrane. **C)** The MCC is floated on medium in a larger vessel and drug can be added to the upper compartment in dilute agar and sampled as a function of time in the stirred lower compartment, on the other side of the MCC, to evaluate. **D)** The time-dependent transport of drug through the MCC as compared to that through the semiporous membrane alone. (Reproduced with permission from Trédan O, Galmarini CM, Patel K, et al: Drug resistance and the solid tumor microenvironment. *J Natl Cancer Inst* 2007 Oct 3;99(19):1441-1454.)

In general, however, the direct effects of hypoxia and acidity on drug sensitivity are smaller than those on radiation sensitivity.

Drugs are being developed that are selective for killing of hypoxic cells, and which might complement both radiotherapy and conventional chemotherapy (see Chap. 12, Sec. 12.4.4). Hypoxia-activated prodrugs are inactive in their native form but are activated by reduction under hypoxic conditions such as may occur in solid tumors, and may then kill tumor cells. The first agent to be tested clinically, tirapazamine, did not improve the activity of cisplatin and radiotherapy in randomized controlled trials, probably because it has poor diffusion characteristics into hypoxic regions. Newer agents, such as evofosfamide, have more favorable properties but thus far have failed to improve survival when combined with conventional chemotherapy in clinical trials (eg, Tap et al., 2017), although these trials had suboptimal design in that they did not select participants on the basis of tumor hypoxia. Low levels of hypoxia are observed in some normal tissues, including bone marrow, and may lead to some normal-tissue toxicity.

18.4.7.3 Drug Access and Tumor Cell Resistance

Effective treatment of solid tumors requires both that the constituent cells be sensitive to the drug(s) that are used and that the drugs achieve a sufficient concentration to exert lethal toxicity for all of the viable cells in the tumor. Thus, successful treatment depends on the efficient delivery of drugs through the vascular system of the tumor, and penetration of the drugs from tumor capillaries to reach tumor cells that are distant from them. Such cells will be in nutritionally deprived environments, as oxygen and other nutrients must gain access to the tumor by the same route, and may be relatively resistant to drugs for reasons described in the previous section (see Fig. 18–24).

The distribution of fluorescent or radiolabeled drugs in spheroids, and studies of their penetration through MCCs (see Fig. 18–25), indicate rather poor tissue penetration of multiple drugs, including doxorubicin, gemcitabine, taxanes, and methotrexate (Durand, 1989; Minchinton and Tannock, 2006). Smaller molecules distribute largely by diffusion, which depends on size, shape, charge, and solubility of the drug in the extracellular matrix, and "consumption" because of binding or metabolism by proximal cells. Larger molecules, such as therapeutic monoclonal antibodies, probably depend more on convection, which is inhibited by high levels of interstitial fluid pressure (Minchinton and Tannock, 2006). Both mechanisms depend on maintenance of a concentration gradient into tissue from tumor blood vessels, and distribution is therefore likely to be better for drugs with a prolonged lifetime within the circulation.

Drug distribution in relation to blood vessels in solid tumors can be quantified by using immunohistochemistry or autoradiography applied to tumor sections (Fig. 18–26). The blood vessels can be recognized by an antibody to an endothelial cell marker (eg, CD31), and patent vessels by an injected fluorescent marker, such as the carbocyanine dye DiOC7; hypoxic regions of tumors can be recognized by antibodies to injected markers of hypoxia such as pimonidazole or EF5 (see Chap. 12, Sec. 12.4.1). Drugs that can be recognized directly if they are fluorescent, such as doxorubicin or mitoxantrone (Fig. 18–26A, B and D), or by fluorescence-labeled antibodies that recognize pharmacodynamic markers of drug effect, such

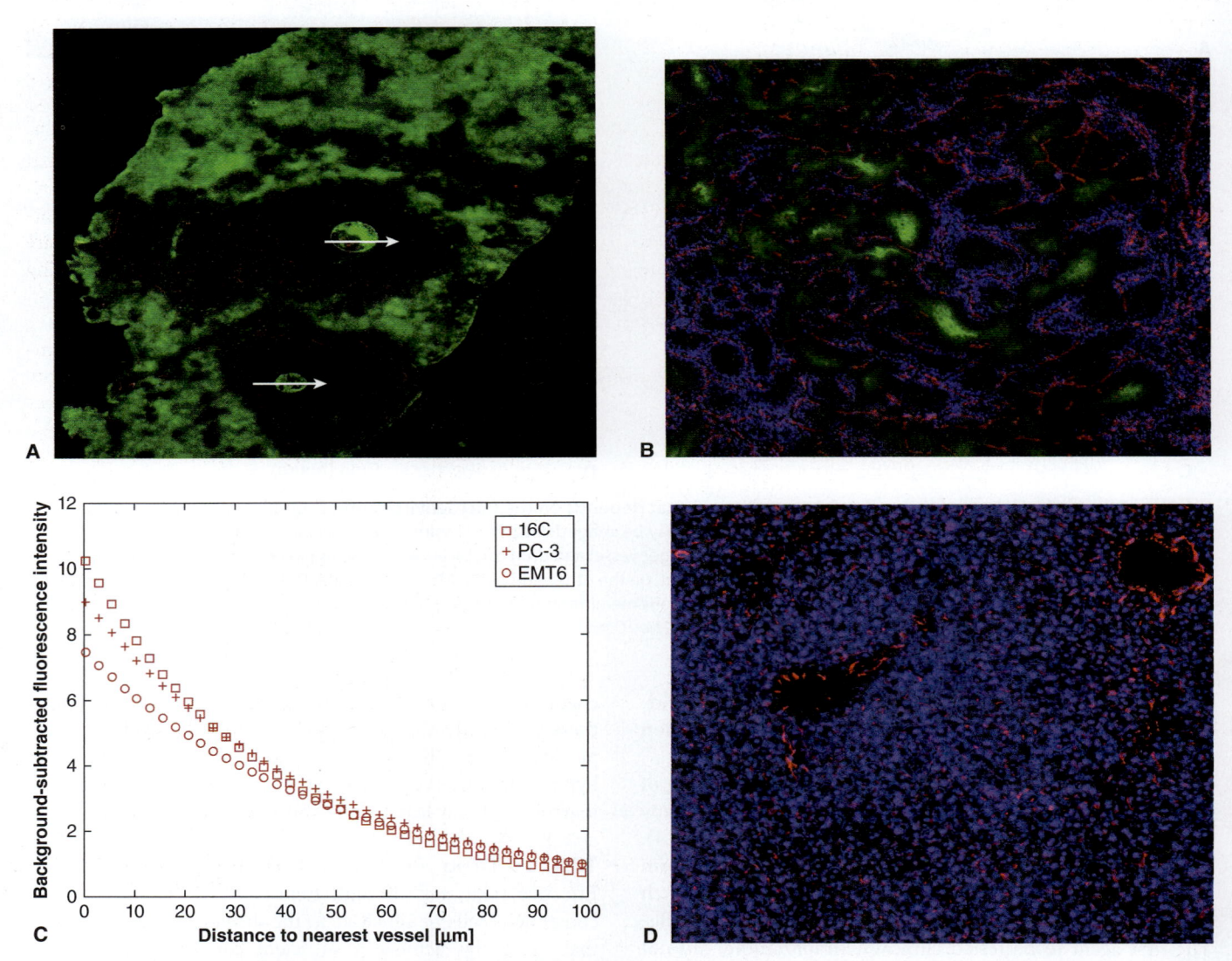

FIGURE 18–26 Drug distribution in tumor and normal tissue. **A)** Photomicrographs showing poor distribution of fluorescent mitoxantrone (green) into metastases (arrows) of a human breast carcinoma in the liver of a nude mice, as compared to normal liver. **B)** Distribution of doxorubicin (blue) in relation to blood vessels (red) and regions of hypoxia (green) in an experimental tumor. Note the perivascular distribution. **C)** Concentration of doxorubicin in relation to distance from blood vessels in 3 experimental tumors. **D)** Distribution of doxorubicin (blue) in relation to blood vessels (red) in normal mouse liver. (Part B: Reproduced with permission from Primeau AJ, Rendon A, Hedley D, et al: The distribution of the anticancer drug Doxorubicin in relation to blood vessels in solid tumors. *Clin Cancer Res* 2005 Dec 15;11(24 Pt 1):8782-8788.)

as changes in apoptosis (eg, activated caspase-3), cell proliferation (eg, Ki67), or DNA damage (eg, γH2AX). Computerized image analysis programs can relate drug concentration (eg, as measured by fluorescence of doxorubicin), or a marker of drug effect, with distance from the nearest blood vessel or nearest region of hypoxia over the whole area of a tumor section.

Studies using the above techniques show that there is a sharply decreasing gradient of many drugs from functional blood vessels of tumors (including human breast cancers) such that cells distal from blood vessels have minimal exposure after a single injection (see Fig. 18–26A–C; Lankelma et al, 1999; Primeau et al, 2005; Saggar et al, 2013). This gradient-type distribution contrasts with more uniform distribution of drugs in most normal tissues, which have an orderly and functional vascular system (see Fig. 18–26D), although the presence of P-glycoprotein, MRP4, and other membrane transporters in the blood–brain barrier leads to uniformly low drug concentrations in brain. Failure of drugs to penetrate tumor tissue in sufficient concentrations to kill cells distal from functional blood vessels is likely to be a major cause of poor clinical response.

Strategies have been proposed to modify or complement the distribution of anticancer drugs in solid tumors to improve therapeutic efficacy (Minchinton and Tannock, 2006). Agents that modify the stromal cells or ECM have been shown to improve drug distribution in experimental tumors (Olive et al, 2009; Provenzano et al, 2012), whereas hypoxia-activated prodrugs provide a potential method for complementing the action of conventional anticancer drugs that have limited penetration from tumor blood vessels. (see Chap. 12, Sec. 12.4.4)

18.4.8 Repopulation

Proliferation of surviving tumor cells between daily doses of fractionated radiotherapy is an important cause of failure to achieve local tumor control (see Chap. 16, Sec. 16.6.2). Presumably, this impediment is a result of improving nutrition in the environment of surviving tumor cells as a result of killing of other cells in the tumor and better availability of nutrient metabolites and oxygen. For chemotherapy, repopulation is likely to be more important because treatment courses are given typically at 3-week intervals, and in experimental studies, a higher rate of proliferation (ie, of repopulation) has been reported after treatment of tumors by chemotherapy than in untreated control tumors (reviewed in Kim and Tannock, 2005). This process of tumor "recovery" is analogous to repopulation of the bone marrow from stem cells that are stimulated to divide as a result of treatment.

Repopulation following chemotherapy has been modeled (Figure 18–27; Kim and Tannock, 2005). If there is no change in the rate of repopulation, a human tumor may show net growth because of this process, even if each course of chemotherapy leads to killing of 70% of the viable tumor cells (Fig. 18–27A). A changing rate of repopulation can cause regrowth following initial tumor shrinkage (Fig. 18–27B), even if there is a delay in onset of repopulation after drug treatment caused by the immediate cytostatic effects of drugs on surviving cells (Fig. 18–27C). Studies of experimental tumors have shown that quiescent hypoxic cells may reoxygenate and proliferate following chemotherapy; paradoxically, these originally nutrient-deprived cells may have died in an untreated tumor but are "rescued" by chemotherapy as a result of killing of proliferating cells close to blood vessels, and improvement in nutrition in their microenvironment (Saggar and Tannock, 2017).

Tumor shrinkage followed by regrowth is observed commonly when chemotherapy is used to treat human tumors. The above modeling indicates that this recovery can occur simply as a consequence of changes in the rate of repopulation of surviving cells after successive treatments and in the

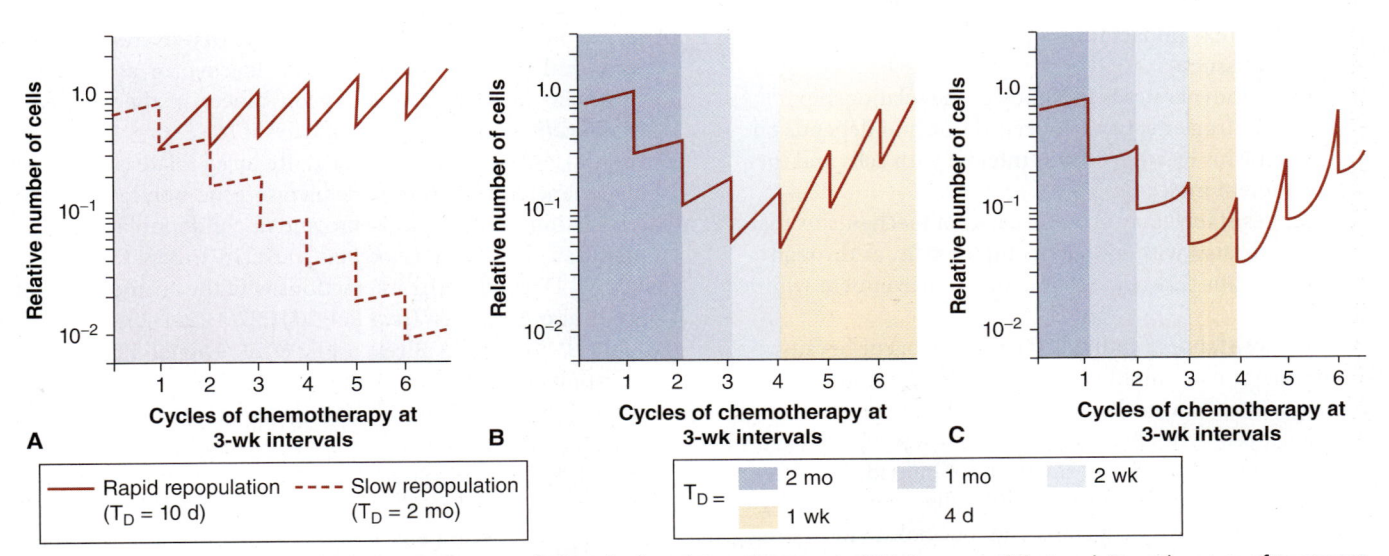

FIGURE 18–27 Models of cell killing and repopulation during chemotherapy. In (A) it is assumed that each 3-week course of treatment kills 70% of the tumor cells, and repopulation is shown with a doubling time of 10 days (solid line) or 2 months (dashed line). In (B) the rate of repopulation increases between successive cycles of chemotherapy so that doubling time decreases from 2 months to 4 days. In (C) the model allows for initial cytostatic effects on surviving tumor cells after each dose of chemotherapy. *Note that shrinkage and regrowth of tumors, observed commonly in the clinic, may occur as a result of accelerating repopulation and without any selection of drug-resistant cells.*

absence of any change in the intrinsic drug sensitivity of the constituent cells. As for radiotherapy, there are strategies that might be used to inhibit repopulation between courses of chemotherapy, and thereby avoid the effective drug resistance that is observed. One method is to change the "fractionation" and to give lower doses of drugs more frequently or continuously. However, this strategy is unlikely to be tumor specific and may also lead to inhibition of cell proliferation in critical normal tissues such as bone marrow. Other approaches include inhibition of growth factor receptors and prostaglandin E2 that may selectively stimulate tumor cell proliferation (Kurtova et al, 2015). Such agents will need to be short acting and discontinued just before the next cycle of chemotherapy, as anticancer drugs are likely to be more effective in killing cycling tumor cells.

SUMMARY

- Anticancer drugs are designated as chemotherapy (where cell killing is relatively nonspecific and usually maximum against proliferating cells) and targeted agents that inhibit one or more known molecular targets (reviewed in Chap. 19)
- Chemotherapy drugs are grouped broadly according to their mechanisms of action. Major families include alkylating agents and platins (that interact directly with DNA), antimetabolites, topoisomerase inhibitors, and agents that interact with microtubules.
- The efficacy of anticancer drugs depends on their pharmacokinetics: how the concentration of a drug and its metabolites changes with time after administration in different tissues; thus, efficacy depends on absorption, metabolism, distribution, and excretion. Understanding of pharmacokinetics provides insight into how dose and schedule may impact tumor response and toxicity to normal tissues.
- Pharmacodynamics is the study of the relationship between drug effect and concentration and depends on mechanisms by which drugs interact with cells and their constituent molecules.
- Drug resistance may occur because of mechanisms that are associated with individual tumor cells, or through mechanisms that relate to the microenvironment within tumors.
- Drug resistance of individual cells may occur because of mutation or amplification of genes, or because of epigenetic changes that lead to transient expression of cellular properties that are associated with drug resistance.
- Mechanisms that lead to resistance of individual cells include impaired drug uptake into cells, enhanced drug efflux from cells, changes in drug metabolism or in drug targets, repair of drug-induced damage (usually to DNA).
- Several ABC proteins are expressed on the surface of cells and can mediate enhanced efflux of multiple chemically unrelated drugs. Important members of this family that are expressed in human tumors include P-glycoprotein, MRP1, and ABCG2 (formerly known as BCRP). These proteins are also expressed in a polarized manner on cells in several normal tissues and influence the distribution of substrate drugs in the body.
- Drug resistance may occur when cells are in contact as a result of interactions with other cells or with the extracellular matrix, even though the same cells are drug sensitive when separated in tissue culture.
- Drug distribution is often poor in solid tumors, such that cells distant from functional blood vessels are exposed to only a low concentration of drug. Such cells are often slowly proliferating and hence more resistant to cycle active drugs. Agents that are activated under hypoxic conditions may have potential for overcoming this type of drug resistance.
- Repopulation of surviving tumor cells occurs between drug treatments, similar to repopulation of normal cells in bone marrow and other proliferating tissues. Accelerating repopulation during sequential courses of treatment may lead to tumor regrowth after an initial response, even if there is no selection of intrinsically drug-resistant cells.

REFERENCES

Allen TM, Cullis PR. Liposomal drug delivery systems: from concept to clinical applications. *Adv Drug Deliv Rev* 2013;65(1):36-48.

Allocati N, Masulli M, Di Ilio C, Federici L. Glutathione transferases: substrates, inhibitors and pro-drugs in cancer and neurodegenerative diseases. *Oncogenesis* 2018;7(1):8

An Q, Robins P, Lindahl T, Barnes DE. 5-Fluorouracil incorporated into DNA is excised by the Smug1 DNA glycosylase to reduce drug cytotoxicity. *Cancer Res* 2007;67:940-945.

André T, Boni C, Navarro M, et al. Improved overall survival with oxaliplatin, fluorouracil, and leucovorin as adjuvant treatment in stage II or III colon cancer in the MOSAIC trial. *J Clin Oncol* 2009;27(19):3109-3116.

Ashton LJ, Giffor AJ, Kwan E, et al. Reduced folate carrier and methylenetetrahydrofolate reductase gene polymorphisms: associations with clinical outcome in childhood acute lymphoblastic leukemia. *Leukemia* 2009;23(7):1348-1351.

Baker AF, Dorr RT. Drug interactions with the taxanes: clinical implications. *Cancer Treat Rev* 2001;27(4):221-233.

Barault L, Amatu A, Bleeker FE, et al. Digital PCR quantification of MGMT methylation refines prediction of clinical benefit from alkylating agents in glioblastoma and metastatic colorectal cancer. *Ann Oncol* 2015;26:1994-1999.

Brown JM, Attardi LD. The role of apoptosis in cancer development and treatment response. *Nat Rev Cancer* 2005;5(3):231-237.

Calvert AH, Newell DR, Gumbrell LA, et al. Carboplatin dosage: prospective evaluation of a simple formula based on renal function. *J Clin Oncol* 1989;7(11):1748-1756.

Chalmers AJ, Lakshman M, Chan N, Bristow RG. Poly(ADP-ribose) polymerase inhibition as a model for synthetic lethality in developing radiation oncology targets. *Semin Radiat Oncol* 2010;20(4):274-2781.

Chen Y, Wang Z, Chang P, et al. The effect of focal adhesion kinase gene silencing on 5-fluorouracil chemosensitivity involves an Akt/NF-kappaB signaling pathway in colorectal carcinomas. *Int J Cancer* 2010;127:195-206.

Christie EL, Fereday S, Doig K, Pattnaik S, Dawson SJ, Bowtell DDL. Reversion of BRCA1/2 germline mutations detected in circulating tumor DNA from patients with high-grade serous ovarian cancer. *J Clin Oncol* 2017;35(12):1274-1280.

Cole SPC, Bhardwaj G, Gerlach JH, et al. Overexpression of a transporter gene in a multidrug-resistant human lung cancer cell line. *Science* 1992;258:1650-1654.

David KA, Picus J. Evaluating risk factors for the development of ifosfamide encephalopathy. *Am J Clin Oncol* 2005;28(3):277-280.

Deeley RG, Cole SP. Substrate recognition and transport by multidrug resistance protein 1 (ABCC1). *FEBS Lett* 2006;580(4):1103-1111.

DeGorter MK, Conseil G, Deeley RG, Campbell RL, Cole SP. Molecular modeling of the human multidrug resistance protein 1 (MRP1/ABCC1). *Biochem Biophys Res Commun* 2008;365:29-34.

Dickreuter E, Cordes N. The cancer cell adhesion resistome: mechanisms, targeting and translational approaches. *Biol Chem* 2017;398(7):721-735.

Doyle LA, Yang W, Abruzzo LV, et al. A multidrug resistance transporter from human MCF-7 breast cancer cells. *Proc Natl Acad Sci USA* 1998;95(26):15665-15670.

Durand RE. Distribution and activity of antineoplastic drugs in a tumor model. *J Natl Cancer Inst* 1989;81(2):146-152.

Friboulet L, Olaussen KA, Pignon JP, et al. ERCC1 isoform expression and DNA repair in non-small-cell lung cancer. *N Engl J Med* 2013;368(12):1101-1110.

Gewirtz DA. A critical evaluation of the mechanisms of action proposed for the antitumor effects of the anthracycline antibiotics Adriamycin and daunorubicin. *Biochem Pharmacol* 1999;57(7):727-741.

Gordon AN, Fleagle JT, Guthrie D, Parkin DE, Gore ME, Lacave AJ. Recurrent epithelial ovarian carcinoma: a randomized phase III study of pegylated liposomal doxorubicin versus topotecan. *J Clin Oncol* 2001;19(14):3312-3322.

Henricks LM, Lunenburg CATC, Meulendijks D, et al. Translating DPYD genotype into DPD phenotype: using the DPYD gene activity score. *Pharmacogenomics* 2015;16(11):1277-1286.

Hicks KO, Ohms SJ, van Zijl PL, et al. An experimental and mathematical model for the extravascular transport of a DNA intercalator in tumours. *Br J Cancer* 1997;76(7):894-903.

Hollenstein K, Dawson RJ, Locher KP. Structure and mechanism of ABC transporter proteins. *Curr Opin Struct Biol* 2007;17:412-418.

Issa ME, Takhsha FS, Chirumamilla CS, et al. Epigenetic strategies to reverse drug resistance in heterogeneous multiple myeloma. *Clin Epigenetics* 2017;9:17.

Juliano RL, Ling V. A surface glycoprotein modulating drug permeability in Chinese hamster ovary cell mutants. *Biochim Biophys Acta* 1976;455(1):152-162.

Kaelin WG Jr. The concept of synthetic lethality in the context of anticancer therapy. *Nat Rev Cancer* 2005;5(9):689-698.

Kelland L. The resurgence of platinum-based cancer chemotherapy. *Nat Rev Cancer* 2007;7(8):573-584.

Kim JJ, Tannock IF. Repopulation of cancer cells during therapy: an important cause of treatment failure. *Nat Rev Cancer* 2005;5(7):516-525.

Kurtova AV, Xiao J, Mo Q, et al. Blocking PGE2-induced tumour repopulation abrogates bladder cancer chemoresistance. *Nature* 2015;517(7533):209-213.

Lankelma J, Dekker H, Luque FR, et al. Doxorubicin gradients in human breast cancer. *Clin Cancer Res* 1999;5(7):1703-1707.

Lenz H-J, Stintzing S, Loupakis F. TAS-102, a novel antitumor agent; a review of the mechanism of action. *Cancer Treat Rev* 2015;41(9):777-783.

Leslie EM, Deeley RG, Cole SPC. Multidrug resistance proteins in toxicology: role of P-glycoprotein, MRP1, MRP2 and BCRP (ABCG2) in tissue defense. *Toxicol Appl Pharmacol* 2005;204(3):216-237.

Li ZW, Dalton WS. Tumor microenvironment and drug resistance in hematologic malignancies. *Blood Rev* 2006;20(6):333-342.

Liu JJ, Lu J, McKeage MJ. Membrane transporters as determinants of the pharmacology of platinum anticancer drugs. *Curr Cancer Drug Targets* 2012;12(8):962-986.

Luria SE, Delbrück M. Mutations of bacteria from virus sensitivity to virus resistance. *Genetics* 1943;28(6):491-511.

Marchesi F, Turriziani M, Tortorelli G, Avvisati G, Torino F, De Vecchis L. Triazene compounds: mechanism of action and related DNA repair systems. *Pharmacol Res* 2007;56(4):275-287.

Marty M, Espie M, Llombart A, Monnier A, Rapoport BL, Stahalova V. Multicenter randomized phase III study of the cardioprotective effect of dexrazoxane (Cardioxane) in advanced/metastatic breast cancer patients treated with anthracycline-based chemotherapy. *Ann Oncol* 2006;17(4):614-622.

Mateo J, Carreira S, Sandhu S, et al. DNA-repair defects and olaparib in metastatic prostate cancer. *N Engl J Med* 2015;373(18):1697-1708.

Mathijssen RH, Marsh S, Karlsson MO, et al. Irinotecan pathway genotype analysis to predict pharmacokinetics. *Clin Cancer Res* 2003;9(9):3246-3253.

Matsson P, Pedersen JM, Norinder U, et al. Identification of novel specific and general inhibitors of the three major human ATP-binding cassette transporters P-gp, BCRP and MRP2 among registered drugs. *Pharm Res* 2009;26(8):1816-1831.

McLornan DP, List A, Mufti GJ. Applying synthetic lethality for the selective targeting of cancer. *N Engl J Med* 2014;371(18):1725-1735.

Minchinton AI, Tannock IF. Drug penetration in solid tumours. *Nat Rev Cancer* 2006;6(8):583-592.

Miwa M, Ura M, Nishida M, et al. Design of a novel oral fluoropyrimidine carbamate, capecitabine, which generates 5-fluorouracil selectively in tumours by enzymes concentrated in human liver and cancer tissue. *Eur J Cancer* 1998;34(8):1274-1281.

Mohammad RM, Muqbil I, Lowe L, et al. Broad targeting of resistance to apoptosis in cancer. *Semin Cancer Biol* 2015; 35(Suppl):S78-S103.

Mukhtar E, Adhami VM, Mukhtar H: Targeting microtubules by natural agents for cancer therapy. *Molec Cancer Ther* 2014;13(2):275-284.

Nies AT, Keppler D. The apical conjugate efflux pump ABCC2 (MRP2). *Pflugers Arch* 2007;453(5):643-659.

Noborio-Hatano K, Kikuchi J, Takatoku M, et al. Bortezomib overcomes cell-adhesion-mediated drug resistance through downregulation of VLA-4 expression in multiple myeloma. *Oncogene* 2009;28(2):231-242.

Olive KP, Jacobetz MA, Davidson CJ, et al. Inhibition of Hedgehog signaling enhances delivery of chemotherapy in a mouse model of pancreatic cancer. *Science* 2009;324(5933): 1457-1461.

Ong CS, Zhou X, Han J, et al. In vivo therapeutic applications of cell spheroids. *Biotechnol Adv* 2018;36(2):494-505.

Pajic M, Murray J, Marshall GM, et al. ABCC1/G2012T single nucleotide polymorphism is associated with patient outcome in primary neuroblastoma and altered stability of the ABCC1 gene transcript. *Pharmacogenet Genomics* 2011;21(5):270-279.

Primeau AJ, Rendon A, Hedley D, et al. The distribution of the anticancer drug doxorubicin in relation to blood vessels in solid tumors. *Clin Cancer Res* 2005;11(24 Pt 1):8782-8788.

Provenzano PP, Cuevas C, Chang AE, Goel VK, Von Hoff DD, Hingorani SR. Enzymatic targeting of the stroma ablates physical barriers to treatment of pancreatic ductal adenocarcinoma. *Cancer Cell* 2012;21(3):418-429.

Quaranta S, Thomas F. Pharmacogenetics of anti-cancer drugs: State of the art and implementation-recommendation of the French National Network of Pharmacogenetics. *Therapie* 2017;72(2):205-215.

Ramirez M, Rajaram S, Steininger RJ, et al. Diverse drug-resistance mechanisms can emerge from drug-tolerant cancer persister cells. *Nat Commun* 2016;7:10690.

Ratain MJ. Body-surface area as a basis for dosing of anti-cancer agents: science, myth, or habit? *J Clin Oncol* 1998; 16(7):2297-2298.

Relling MV, Evans WE. Pharmacogenomics in the clinic. *Nature* 2016;526(7573):343-350.

Riechelmann RP, Zimmermann C, Chin SN, et al. Potential drug interactions in cancer patients receiving supportive care exclusively. *J Pain Symptom Manage* 2008;35(5):535-543.

Robey RW, Pluchino KM, Hall MD, Fojo AT, Bates SE, Gottesman MM. Revisiting the role of ABC transporters in multidrug-resistant cancer. *Nat Rev Cancer* 2018;18(7):452-464.

Ronnekleiv-Kelly SM, Sharma A, Ahuja N. Epigenetic therapy and chemosensitization in solid malignancy. *Cancer Treat Rev* 2017;55:200-208.

Rothenberg ML, Meropol NJ, Poplin EA, Van Cutsem E, Wadler S. Mortality associated with irinotecan plus bolus fluorouracil/leucovorin: summary findings of an independent panel. *J Clin Oncol* 2001;19(18):3801-3807.

Saggar JK, Fung AS, Patel KJ, Tannock IF. Use of molecular biomarkers to quantify the spatial distribution of effects of anticancer drugs in solid tumors. *Mol Cancer Ther* 2013; 12(4):542-552.

Saggar JK, Tannock IF. Chemotherapy rescues hypoxic tumor cells and induces their reoxygenation and repopulation—an effect that is inhibited by the hypoxia-activated prodrug TH-302. *Clin Cancer Res* 2015;21(9):2107-2114.

Sakai W, Swisher EM, Karlan BY, et al. Secondary mutations as a mechanism of cisplatin resistance in BRCA2-mutated cancer. *Nature* 2008;451(7182):1116-1120.

Sau A, Pillizzari Tregno F, Valentino F, et al. Glutathione transferases and development of new principles to overcome drug resistance. *Arch Biochem Biophys* 2010;500(2):116-122.

Schroth W, Goetz MP, Hamann U, et al. Association between CYP2D6 polymorphisms and outcomes among women with early stage breast cancer treated with tamoxifen. *JAMA* 2009;302(13):1429-1436.

Sharma SV, Lee DY, Li B, et al. A chromatin-mediated reversible drug-tolerant state in cancer cell subpopulations. *Cell* 2010;141(1):69-80.

Sprauten M, Darrah TH, Peterson DR, et al. Impact of long-term serum platinum concentrations on neuro- and ototoxicity in cisplatin-treated survivors of testicular cancer. *J Clin Oncol* 2012;30(3):300-307.

Tan Q, Joshua AM, Wang M, et al. Up-regulation of autophagy is a mechanism of resistance to chemotherapy and can be inhibited by pantoprazole to increase drug sensitivity. *Cancer Chemother Pharmacol* 2017;79(5):959-969.

Tannock IF, Lee CM, Tunggal JK, et al. Limited penetration of anticancer drugs through tumor tissue: a potential cause of resistance of solid tumors to chemotherapy. *Clin Cancer Res* 2002;8(3):874-884.

Tap WD, Papai Z, Van Tine BA, et al. Doxorubicin plus evofosfamide versus doxorubicin alone in locally advanced, unresectable or metastatic soft-tissue sarcoma (TH CR-406/SARC021): an international, multicentre, open-label, randomised phase 3 trial. *Lancet Oncol* 2017;18(8):1089-1103.

Teicher BA, Herman TS, Holden SA, et al. Tumor resistance to alkylating agents conferred by mechanisms operative only in vivo. *Science* 1990;247(4949 Pt 1):1457-1461.

Tekade RK, Tekade M, Kesharwani P, D'Emanuele A. RNAi-combined nano-chemotherapeutics to tackle resistant tumors. *Drug Discov Today* 2016;21(11):1761-1774.

Trédan O, Galmarini CM, Patel K, Tannock IF. Drug resistance and the solid tumor microenvironment. *J Natl Cancer Inst* 2007;99:1441-1454.

White E, DiPaola RS. The double-edged sword of autophagy modulation in cancer. *Clin Cancer Res* 2009;15(17): 5308-5316.

Yu M, Ocana A, Tannock IF. Reversal of ATP-binding-cassette drug transporter activity to modulate chemoresistance: why has it failed to provide clinical benefit? *Cancer Metastasis Rev* 2013;32(1-2):211-227.

Zutter MM. Integrin-mediated adhesion: tipping the balance between chemosensitivity and chemoresistance. *Adv Exp Med Biol* 2007;608:87-100.

Molecular Targeted Therapies

Zachary Veitch and Philippe L. Bedard

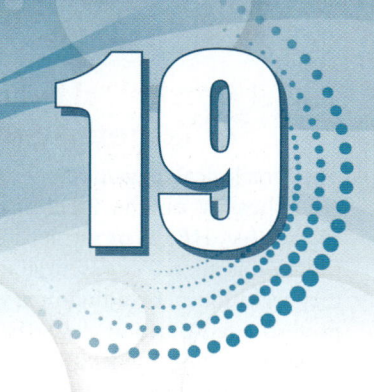

Chapter Outline

- **19.1 Introduction**
  - 19.1.1 Preclinical Development of Targeted Agents
  - 19.1.2 Pharmacokinetics and Pharmacodynamics
  - 19.1.3 Mechanisms of Action
  - 19.1.4 Mechanisms of Resistance
- **19.2 Biomarkers**
- **19.3 Antiangiogenic Receptor Tyrosine Kinase Inhibitors**
  - 19.3.1 Antiangiogenic Monoclonal Antibodies
  - 19.3.2 Antiangiogenic Small Molecule Tyrosine Kinase Inhibitors (TKIs)
  - 19.3.3 RET Inhibition
  - 19.3.4 c-KIT Inhibition
  - 19.3.5 FLT-3 Inhibition
  - 19.3.6 FGFR Inhibition
- **19.4 Inhibitors of the Epidermal Growth Factor Receptor Family**
  - 19.4.1 Inhibitors of EGFR
  - 19.4.2 Inhibitors of HER2
- **19.5 Inhibitors of Intracellular Receptor Tyrosine Kinase Pathways**
  - 19.5.1 Inhibitors of Phosphatidyl Inositol 3-Kinase (PI3K)
  - 19.5.2 Mammalian Target of Rapamycin Inhibitors (mTOR)
  - 19.5.3 Mitogen-Activated Protein Kinase Pathway Inhibitors (RAF/MEK)
- **19.6 Inhibitors of Cell Cycle, DNA Repair, Epigenetics, and Fusion Proteins**
  - 19.6.1 Cyclin-Dependent Kinase Inhibitors
  - 19.6.2 DNA Repair Inhibitors
  - 19.6.3 Epigenetic Inhibitors
  - 19.6.4 Fusion Protein Inhibitors
- **19.7 Other Targeted Therapies**
  - 19.7.1 Proteasome Inhibitors
  - 19.7.2 B-Cell Receptor (BCR) Pathway Inhibitors
  - 19.7.3 BH3 Inhibitors
  - 19.7.4 Hedgehog/SMO/Patch Pathway Inhibitors
  - 19.7.5 Selective Inhibitors of Nuclear Export
- **19.8 Future Development of Targeted Therapies**
- **Summary**
- **References**

19.1 INTRODUCTION

Advances in molecular biology have provided a better understanding of the complex cellular pathways that are critical to tumor formation and growth. Laboratory-based assays that can detect biologically relevant molecular alterations in tumor samples, including immunohistochemistry, in situ hybridization, DNA sequencing, gene expression, and epigenetic profiling, have informed the development of new classes of anticancer drugs that target aberrantly expressed molecular pathways. Compared with conventional cytotoxic chemotherapy, molecular targeted agents may offer greater tumor selectivity and different patterns of toxicity as the alterations they target are more common in, or in some cases exclusive to, tumors compared with normal tissues (see Chap. 17, Sec. 17.2). Biomarkers are increasingly used to aid in the selection of patients likely to respond to a particular class of molecular targeted agent and in some cases to identify mechanisms of resistance upon disease progression. Identifying patients likely to benefit is paramount, as targeted therapies comprise a rapidly expanding proportion of health care expenditures with new drugs routinely priced at more than $100,000 per year. Decisions to integrate these agents into routine cancer care must often weigh factors such as clinical benefit, toxicity, quality of life, and treatment cost for their practical application (Schnipper et al, 2016). This chapter will focus on the preclinical development and clinical application of molecular targeted agents and highlight the biologic basis of these therapies.

19.1.1 Preclinical Development of Targeted Agents

The preclinical development of targeted anticancer agents relies heavily on the identification and modulation of cell surface (eg, HER2) or intracellular (eg, PI3K) proteins whose function is altered or essential in malignancy. Various laboratory techniques including next generation sequencing (NGS), protein identification (eg, IHC), and functional genomic screens (eg, RNAi, CRISPR), are used to identify and characterize putative therapeutic targets.

Preclinical testing evaluates initially the biologic activity of novel agents in vitro using human (or sometimes animal) 2-dimensional (eg, cancer cell monolayers) or 3-dimensional (eg, organoids) cell cultures (Dhandapani and Goldman, 2017). The model systems used are selected typically based on their expression of a drug target(s) or tissue of interest, as well as ease of growth or manipulation. Although these models can validate pharmacologic and anticancer (eg, cytotoxic or antiproliferative) effects, as well as provide insights into predictors of drug sensitivity, in vitro systems are limited in their ability to model antitumor activity.

Animal models of human disease represent the de facto standard for preclinical evaluation of anticancer compounds before human testing, yielding important information on tumor response, pharmacokinetics, toxicity, and therapeutic indices. Mouse models of cancer are widely used to evaluate the in vivo efficacy of anticancer drugs. Murine and human cancer xenograft models are described further in Chapter 17, Section 17.4.2. These in vivo systems can recapitulate tumor biology, physiology, and microenvironmental effects to varying degrees but still have limitations as a result of cross-species differences. Interspecies incompatibilities such as ligand-receptor variability, lack of immune tumor response in immunodeficient mice, variable tumor microenvironments, and many others impact the extrapolation of experimental and nonclinical data to the clinical setting (Rubin and Gilliland, 2012).

Development of targeted agents using modern approaches has expanded and accelerated efforts to produce new cancer therapies. However, the preclinical activity of targeted compounds translates infrequently to benefit in humans, with only 5% of oncology drugs entering phase I clinical trials achieving regulatory (ie, US Food and Drug Administration) approval (Mullard, 2016).

19.1.2 Pharmacokinetics and Pharmacodynamics

Pharmacokinetics evaluates the absorption, distribution, metabolism, and excretion of drugs in a biological system; this is described commonly as what the "body does to the drug." Conversely, pharmacodynamics evaluates the relationship between a drug's concentration at the target site and its resulting effect; this is described as what the "drug does to the body." These concepts are discussed in Chap. 18, Sec. 18.2.

The therapeutic concentration required to produce a desired effect in animals can often exceed that which can be reached in humans. In addition, evaluation of drug combinations in murine models may not reflect the pharmacokinetic or pharmacodynamic effects seen in clinical testing. Such factors must be considered before testing a potential anticancer compound in people.

Knowledge of pharmacokinetics as well as probable toxicities based on testing in animals is necessary to identify a safe starting dose and to define expected dose-limiting toxicities for human testing. A thorough understanding of pharmacodynamic effects permits characterization of these in tumors or other tissues in early clinical testing, in order to confirm that the agent is exerting the intended biologic effect in patients. These correlative studies can define pharmacokinetic/pharmacodynamic relationships and inform determination of recommended doses for later stages of clinical development. Studies performed in early clinical testing must be interpreted in the context of preclinical data and may be key considerations for go/no go decision making (eg, if a drug has undesirable pharmacokinetic properties or fails to inhibit the intended biochemical target).

19.1.3 Mechanisms of Action

Targeted compounds differ from conventional chemotherapeutics by disrupting specific mutated or abnormally regulated cellular proteins that are involved in cancer proliferation and survival. A first step in the rational development of targeted agents is target identification: the identification of cellular proteins or pathways that are essential for cancer growth and may be amendable to selective disruption. Although some molecular targeted agents have direct cytotoxic effects on their cellular targets, many are cytostatic and act to arrest tumor growth by exploiting dependencies that are specific to cancer, relative to healthy cells. By comparison, the targets of standard chemotherapeutic agents are generally present in both healthy and cancerous tissues, and their action and therapeutic index is mediated by cytotoxic effects against all rapidly dividing cells (see Chap. 17, Sec. 17.5, and Chap. 18, Sec. 18.3). This toxicity results in both acute and cumulative side effects, often making prolonged administration difficult. Targeted therapies exhibit different side effect profiles from chemotherapy, which may allow their continuous or prolonged dosing. Toxicities of these agents can be drug-, target- or pathway-dependent and are linked generally to target expression in healthy tissues, the selectivity of the compound for its intended target, the diversity of receptors inhibited, and their specific role(s) in cellular functioning (Liu and Kurzrock, 2014).

Most targeted cancer therapies currently in the clinic have been developed against intrinsic cellular targets but others are designed to interact with components of the tumor microenvironment, including stromal and immune cells. Direct cancer cell targeting is accomplished primarily through the use of monoclonal antibodies (eg, trastuzumab) or small molecule inhibitors (eg, vemurafenib) (Fig. 19–1).

Intravenously administered chimeric or recombinant humanized monoclonal antibodies (predominantly IgG class)

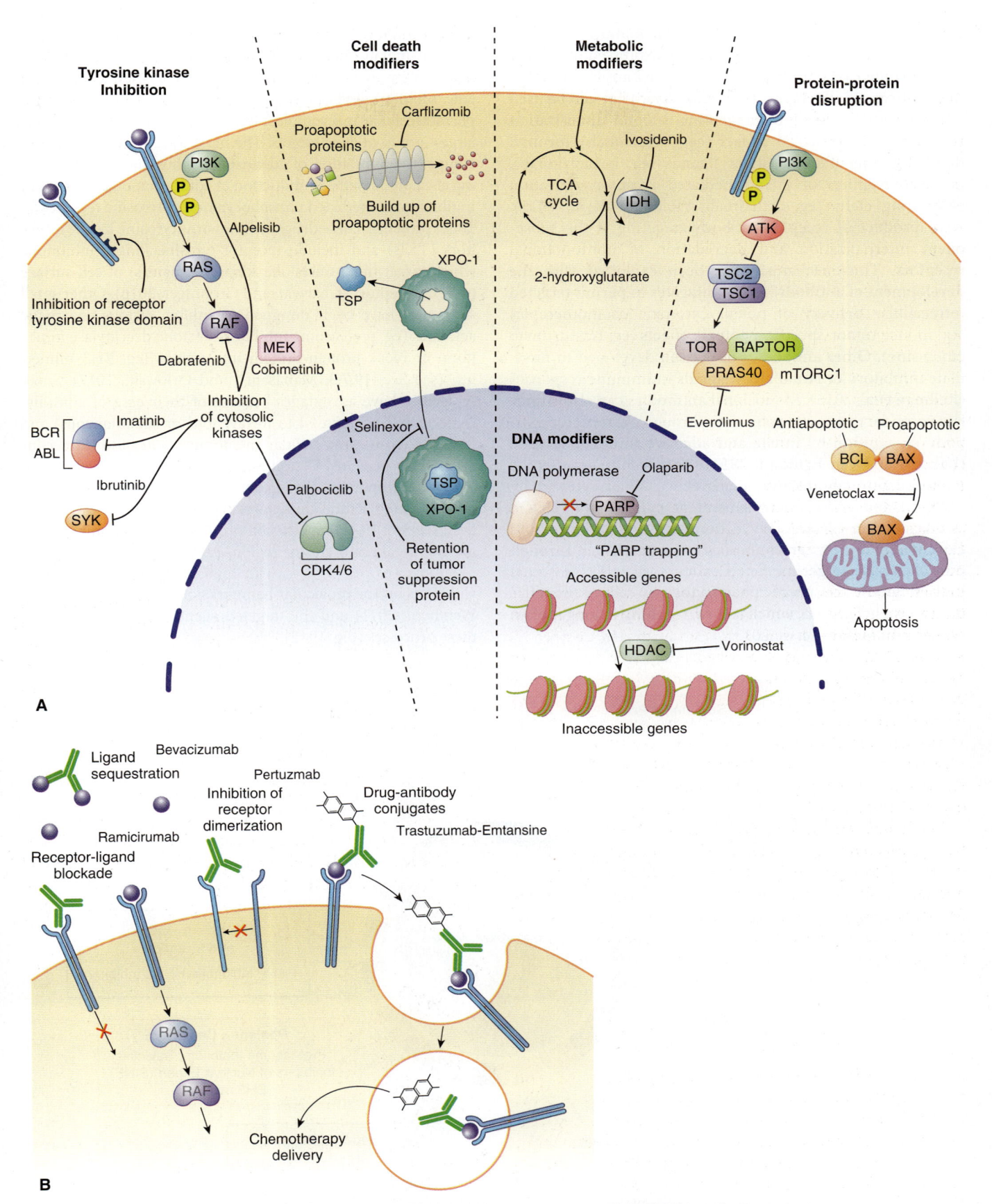

FIGURE 19-1 Mechanisms of action of antibody and small molecule molecular targeted therapies.

are designed to recognize specific external membrane–bound receptor epitopes that are preferentially expressed on cancer and, in some cases, immune cells. Targeted antibodies exert their anticancer effects in a variety of ways. They can be used to inhibit cell signaling by preventing receptor dimerization and activation at the cell surface (eg, pertuzumab), through direct binding of extracellular ligands (eg, bevacizumab), or by prevention of ligand-mediated receptor activation at binding clefts (eg, cetuximab) (Redman et al, 2015). A by-product of receptor-antibody targeting is the subsequent internalization and degradation of nonfunctional receptors. This mechanism has been exploited with the development of antibody-drug conjugates to permit targeted intracellular delivery of potent cytotoxic chemotherapies and induce tumor-specific cytotoxic effects (eg, trastuzumab emtansine). Other antibodies have been developed to modulate inhibitory or stimulatory signals in immune responses (Redman et al, 2015). Monoclonal antibodies can also stimulate secondary immune activation through Fc-receptor antibody recognition by innate and adaptive immune systems (Bakema and van Egmond, 2014). This secondary effect is mediated through antibody-dependent cellular cytotoxicity (ADCC) and complement-dependent cytotoxicity (CDC), as discussed in Chapter 21, Section 21.5.2. Metabolism and clearance of anticancer antibodies is accomplished through 2 mechanisms: target-mediated endocytosis with lysosomal degradation or nonspecific phagocytosis by cells of the reticuloendothelial system, which is slow, resulting in long molecular half-lives (Foltz et al, 2013).

Small molecule inhibitors are generally administered orally and are metabolized by CYP3A4 hepatic enzymes and to a lesser extent by other cytochrome P450 enzymes. Small molecule inhibitors are designed to bind and disrupt single or multiple intracellular macromolecules, with kinases representing the largest group of drug targets. The most common mechanism is competitive inhibition of adenosine triphosphate (ATP) binding at catalytic clefts, or induction of conformational changes to inhibit kinase mediated phosphorylation of tyrosine residues on target proteins. These drugs are known as tyrosine kinase inhibitors (TKIs) and include receptor-tyrosine kinase inhibitors, which target the intracellular kinase domain(s) of cell surface protein receptors (Gharwan and Groninger, 2016). Other small molecules have been designed to inhibit various enzymatic activities (eg, proteasome inhibitors, histone deacetylase inhibitors) or block protein-protein interactions (eg, BH3 mimetics) (see Sec. 19.7.3; Manasanch and Orlowski, 2017). Small molecules have advantages because of their ease of administration (oral as opposed to intravenous or subcutaneous) and their ability to cross cellular membranes and bind intracellular effector proteins. Drug design has facilitated development of novel compounds that target complex driver or resistance mutations (eg, osimertinib, targeting the EGFR T790M mutation; see Sec. 19.4.1) and fusion proteins (eg, ponatinib, targeting the breakpoint cluster region–Abelson [BCR-ABL] T315I mutation; see Sec. 19.6.4) with high selectivity. This chapter will focus on the molecular hallmarks of cancer (Hanahan and Weinberg, 2011) and the targeted agents designed to disrupt these processes (Fig. 19–2).

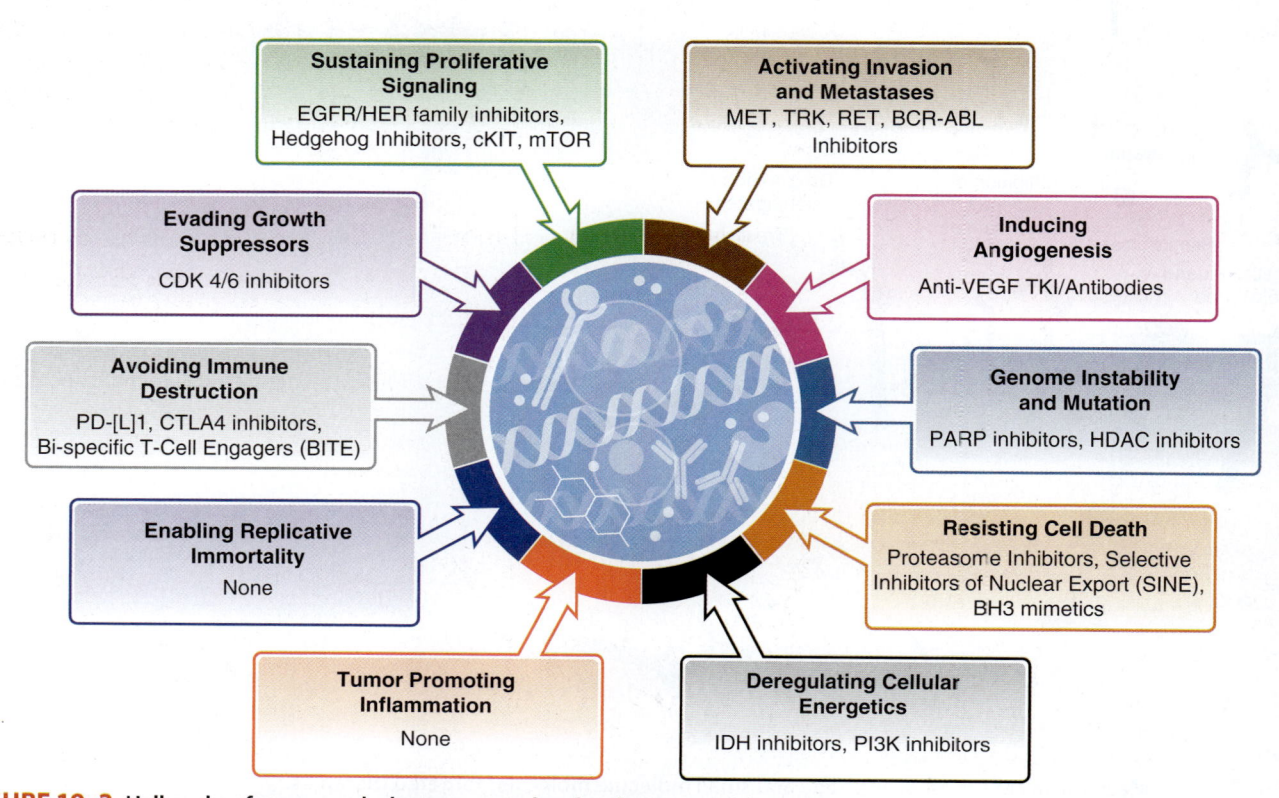

FIGURE 19–2 Hallmarks of cancer and where approved molecular targeted therapies act.

19.1.4 Mechanisms of Resistance

Resistance to targeted anticancer agents is a major challenge in oncology. Two forms of resistance are recognized: (1) intrinsic (primary, or de novo) resistance or (2) acquired (secondary, adaptive) resistance. Intrinsic or primary resistance may develop from an alteration (eg, mutation), presence of alternative pathways, or absence of a drug target from the onset of disease (Groenendijk and Bernards, 2014). Acquired or secondary resistance evolves from the selection of resistant clones following prolonged or repetitive anticancer treatments (Greaves and Maley, 2012). For example, cancer cells acquiring resistance to prolonged TKI therapy can gain mutations in their kinase domain that confer a survival advantage to a subset of clones, which proliferate to form the dominant cell population. Kinase mutations can occur in amino acids that regulate the selectivity of ligands (eg, TKIs) entering the ATP-binding cleft, known as "gatekeeper" mutations (Lovly and Shaw, 2014). Alternatively, alterations can arise in key amino acids that affect the steric hindrance or electrostatic potential of ATP-binding sites, thereby preventing ligands from entering the ATP-binding pocket; these are also known as "solvent-front" mutations.

Resistance mechanisms to targeted therapies are often drug class or target specific and consist of 3 general classifications, including (1) alteration of the drug target, (2) bypass activation of signaling pathways (in parallel or downstream), and (3) stimulation of alternate prosurvival pathways (Fig. 19–3; Lovly and Shaw, 2014). Alterations in drug targets include the aforementioned gatekeeper or solvent-front mutations (eg, ABL T315I in chronic myelogenous leukemia [CML]), target protein amplifications (eg, ALK and MET in lung cancer), decreased drug target expression (eg, ER-α in breast cancer), and splice variant alterations (eg, B-RAF^{V600E} in melanoma). Bypass activation of exogenously inhibited cell signaling pathways can occur in parallel through other receptor tyrosine kinases (eg, HER2 in lung), or through downstream activation of intracellular kinases that circumvent upstream inhibition (eg, KRAS in colorectal cancer). Increased stimulation of cell survival pathways (ie, YAP pathway in lung cancer) often acts to shift the balance in favor of prosurvival over proapoptotic signaling. Additional mechanisms of drug resistance including histologic change to a more aggressive pathology, alteration of the tumor microenvironment, epigenetic modifications (see Chap. 3, Sec. 3.4), expression of drug efflux transporters (see Chap. 18, Sec. 18.4.3), and epithelial-to-mesenchymal transition (see Chap. 13, Sec. 13.3.1).

19.2 BIOMARKERS

Cancers are heterogeneous in their behavior—even cancers with the same tissue of origin and histologic appearance under light microscopy can have very different rates of growth, treatment response, and patterns of metastatic dissemination. These features can in part be attributed to different underlying genetic or epigenetic changes that are responsible for tumor development and malignant behavior. A *biomarker* is defined as a characteristic that is objectively measured and evaluated as an indicator of normal biologic processes, pathogenic processes, or pharmacologic responses to a therapeutic intervention (Biomarkers Definitions Working Group, 2001). Another definition of a *biomarker* specific to cancer is a molecular, cellular, tissue, or process-based alteration that provides an indication of current, or more importantly, future behavior of a cancer (Hayes et al, 1996). Biomarkers may inform clinical decisions about drug treatment, either by identifying those who have an excellent prognosis and do not require drug treatment following surgery or radiotherapy or by discriminating

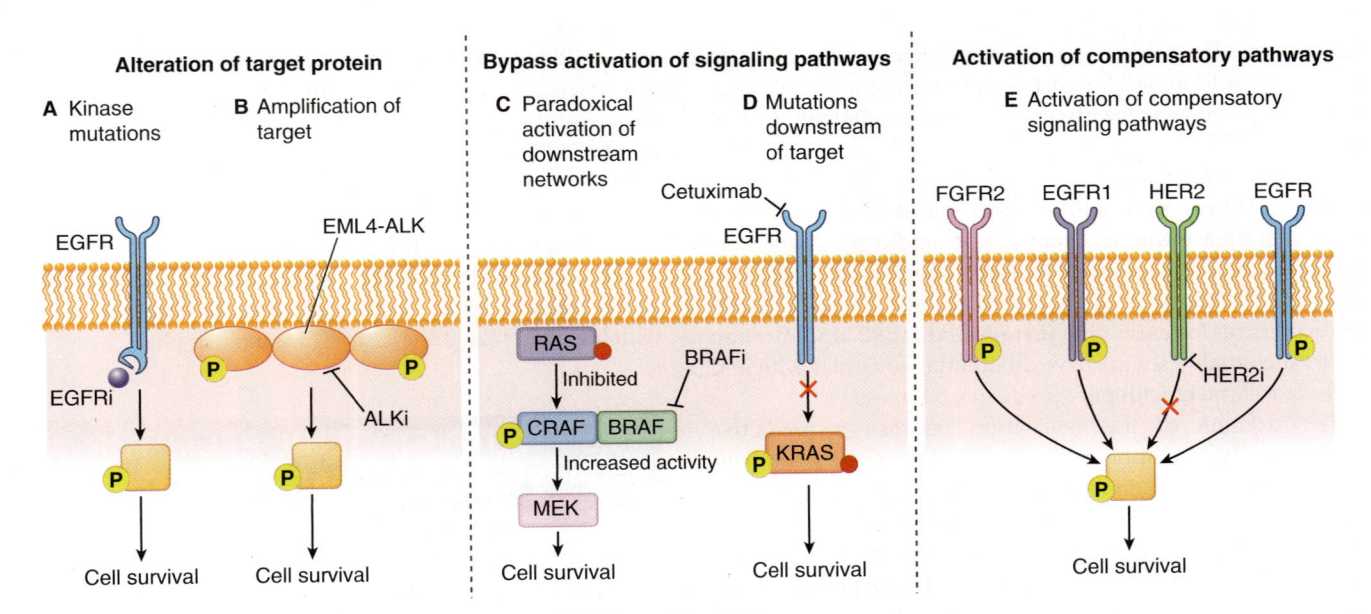

FIGURE 19–3 Mechanisms of resistance to molecular targeted therapies.

likelihood of response to a given treatment. Tailoring therapy for individual patients based on the results of biomarker testing can be used to reduce overtreatment, avoid toxicities, help control medical costs with less expensive anticancer drugs, and reduce attrition in early drug development by enriching studies with patients predicted to benefit. Although biomarkers can be used to guide all kinds of cancer interventions, including but not limited to screening, diagnosis, and the application of standard chemotherapies, the development of new molecular targeted therapies is linked increasingly to 1 or more biomarkers designed to identify distinct populations of patients who may benefit from such treatment.

Biomarkers can also be classified according to their potential application (see Table 19–1; FDA/CDER, 2018).

A *diagnostic biomarker* is measured to determine the presence of the disease and its specific subtype. Because of the cost and impact of screening large populations of individuals, diagnostic biomarkers used as screening tools must have high sensitivity and specificity if they are to have clinical utility for population health (see Chap. 22, Sec. 22.4). Currently, no diagnostic (blood-based) biomarkers are endorsed by clinical guidelines for population-level cancer screening. At the individual level, diagnostic biomarkers are used to confirm, stage, and monitor some human malignancies (eg, hepatocellular carcinoma: alpha-fetoprotein; prostate cancer: prostate-specific antigen) (Shaw et al, 2015).

A *prognostic biomarker* is measured before treatment to indicate outcome for patients untreated or receiving standard treatment. Prognostic biomarkers may identify patients with an expected favorable outcome who do not require intensive treatment, or they may indicate disease with poor prognosis that requires aggressive treatment. Examples of prognostic biomarkers used in early-stage breast cancer to determine adjuvant drug treatment include tumor size, nodal involvement, histologic grade, estrogen and progesterone receptor expression, *HER2* gene amplification, and multigene expression assays (Kwa et al, 2017). Patients have the same differential outcome for pure prognostic biomarkers with or without treatment, but biomarkers that are prognostic in the absence of treatment may also be predictive of the benefit from certain treatments or interventions (Fig. 19–4).

A *predictive biomarker* is measured before or over the course of the treatment to identify patients most likely to benefit from a given treatment. Examples of predictive biomarkers measured before treatment in early-stage breast cancer to determine adjuvant drug treatment include estrogen receptor expression for endocrine therapy and *HER2* amplification for trastuzumab. Patients have differential outcomes with and without treatment with pure predictive biomarkers.

The strength of the association between a predictive marker and the treatment effect is known as the *treatment-by-biomarker interaction* (Ballman, 2015). In a randomized clinical trial that evaluates a time-to-event endpoint such as disease-free, progression-free, or overall survival (OS) for experimental vs standard treatment, an *interaction effect* can be defined as the ratio of the hazard ratio (HR; see Chap. 22, Sec. 22.5.3) for the marker-positive subgroup divided by the hazard ratio for the marker-negative subgroup. For a *quantitative interaction effect*, the magnitude of the treatment effect varies for the marker positive and marker negative subgroups but is in the same direction. For a *qualitative interaction effect*, the direction of the treatment effect varies for the marker-positive and marker-negative subgroups (positive/negative or vice versa). An example of a *qualitative interaction* was observed in a randomized phase III trial that compared the EGFR tyrosine kinase inhibitor gefitinib vs standard chemotherapy with carboplatin and paclitaxel in advanced first-line non–small cell lung adenocarcinoma (Mok et al, 2009). In the subgroup of patients with EGFR-activating mutations, progression-free survival (PFS) was significantly longer among those who received gefitinib than among those who received carboplatin-paclitaxel, whereas in the subgroup of 176 patients who were negative for *EGFR* mutations, PFS was significantly longer among those who received carboplatin-paclitaxel.

Many biomarkers have been identified initially from subsets of patients enrolled in large clinical trials or in retrospective cohorts for whom tissue is available. In these settings, where patients are enrolled and treated without molecular preselection, putative biomarkers may be examined simultaneously to identify hypothesis-generating associations that can be validated in independent patient cohorts. There are several criteria that should be fulfilled before a biomarker can be used to inform treatment decisions in clinical practice. First, it should be biologically plausible that the biomarker identifies differences between subgroups of patients that may be clinically meaningful. Second, there should be sufficient in vitro and/or in vivo preclinical evidence available to support the biological association for the role of the biomarker in the pathogenesis of the disease. Third, the *analytical validity* of a biomarker should be established: the assay that is used to measure the biomarker should be accurate, reproducible, and reliable. Biomarkers used to inform clinical decisions should be evaluated in a clinical testing laboratory, with the appropriate certification and proficiency testing standards, with pre-defined cut-offs as identified through receiver operating characteristic curves (see Chap. 22, Sec. 22.4) that differentiate biomarker-positive from biomarker-negative groups. Fourth, a biomarker should be proven to have *clinical utility*—the result of measuring a biomarker leading to a clinical decision that has been shown with high level of evidence to improve clinical care. Although many biomarkers reported in the literature correlate with important clinical endpoints, they are only useful if their application leads to better patient outcomes, or similar outcomes with less cost, than if the assay(s) were not applied.

19.3 ANTIANGIOGENIC RECEPTOR TYROSINE KINASE INHIBITORS

Angiogenesis is the process through which new blood vessels are formed from the release of multiple proangiogenic factors in response to tumor hypoxia through hypoxia-inducible factor 1α (HIF-1α) signaling, or to other tumor properties and

TABLE 19-1 Indications for FDA-approved targeted anticancer therapies and their respective biomarkers.

Target	Drug Class	Drug	Indication	Biomarker
ALK	Small molecule	Alectinib	Non–small cell lung cancer	ALK translocation
	Small molecule	Brigatinib	Non–small cell lung cancer	ALK translocation
	Small molecule	Ceritinib	Non–small cell lung cancer	ALK translocation
	Small molecule	Crizotinib	Non–small cell lung cancer	ALK translocation
	Small molecule	Lorlatinib	Non–small cell lung cancer	ALK translocation
BCR-ABL1	Small molecule	Bosutinib	Acute/chronic myelogenous leukemia	BCR-ABL1 fusion
	Small molecule	Dasatinib	Acute lymphoblastic leukemia, chronic myelogenous leukemia	BCR-ABL1 fusion
	Small molecule	Imatinib	Acute lymphoblastic leukemia, chronic myelogenous leukemia	BCR-ABL1 fusion
	Small molecule	Nilotinib	Chronic myelogenous leukemia	BCR-ABL1 fusion
	Small molecule	Ponatinib	Chronic myelogenous leukemia	BCR-ABL1 fusion, T315I mutation
TRK	Small molecule	Larotrectinib	Solid tumors	TRK fusion
ROS1	Small molecule	Crizotinib	Non–small cell lung cancer	ROS1 translocation
PDFRA	Small molecule	Imatinib	Hypereosinophilic syndrome	FIP1L1-PDGFRA fusion
			Chronic eosinophilic leukemia	FIP1L1-PDGFRA fusion
			MDS/MPD	PDGFRA gene rearrangement
PIK3CA	Small molecule	Alpelisib	Breast cancer	PIK3CA mutation
BRAF	Small molecule	Dabrafenib*	Melanoma	BRAF V600E/K mutation
			Anaplastic thyroid cancer	BRAF V600E/K mutation
	Small molecule	Vemurafenib†	Melanoma	BRAF V600E/K mutation
	Small molecule	Encorafenib‡	Melanoma	BRAF V600E/K mutation
MEK	Small molecule	Cobimetinib	Melanoma	BRAF V600E/K mutation
	Small molecule	Trametinib	Melanoma	BRAF V600E/K mutation
			Anaplastic thyroid cancer	BRAF V600E/K mutation
	Small molecule	Binimetinib	Melanoma	BRAF V600E/K mutation
PARP	Small molecule	Niraparib	Ovarian cancer	germline BRCA1/2 mutation
	Small molecule	Olaparib	Ovarian cancer	germline BRCA1/2 mutation
			Breast cancer	germline BRCA1/2 mutation
	Small molecule	Rucaparib	Ovarian cancer	germline BRCA1/2 mutation
	Small molecule	Talazoparib	Breast cancer	germline BRCA1/2 mutation
BCL2	Small molecule	Venetoclax	Chronic lymphocytic leukemia	Chromosome 17p deletion
FGFR	Small molecule	Erdafitinib	Bladder cancer	FGFR2 or FGFR3 mutation
EGFR	Small molecule	Erlotinib	Non–small cell lung cancer	EGFR exon 19 deletion, exon 21 L858R mutation
	Small molecule	Afatinib	Non–small cell lung cancer	EGFR exon 19 deletion, exon 21 L858R mutation
	Small molecule	Gefitinib	Non–small cell lung cancer	EGFR exon 19 deletion, exon 21 L858R mutation
	Small molecule	Osimertinib	Non–small cell lung cancer	EGFR exon 19 deletion, exon 21 L858R mutation, T790M mutation
	Small molecule	Dacomitinib	Non–small cell lung cancer	EGFR exon 19 deletion, exon 21 L858R mutation
	Antibody	Cetuximab	Colorectal cancer	KRAS wild type
	Antibody	Panitumumab	Colorectal cancer	KRAS wild type, NRAS wild type
HER2	Antibody-drug conjugate	Ado-trastuzumab emtansine	Breast cancer	ERBB2 amplifcation and/or overexpresion
	Small molecule	Lapatinib	Breast cancer	ERBB2 amplifcation and/or overexpresion
	Small molecule	Neratinib	Breast cancer	ERBB2 amplifcation and/or overexpresion
	Antibody	Pertuzumab	Breast cancer	ERBB2 amplifcation and/or overexpresion
	Antibody	Trastuzumab	Breast cancer	ERBB2 amplifcation and/or overexpresion

(Continued)

TABLE 19–1 Indications for FDA-approved targeted anticancer therapies and their respective biomarkers. *(Continued)*

Target	Drug Class	Drug	Indication	Biomarker
FLT3	Small molecule	Midostaurin	Acute myeloid leukemia	FLT3 mutation
	Small molecule	Gilteritinib	Acute myeloid leukemia	FLT3 mutation
IDH1	Small molecule	Ivosidenib	Acute myeloid leukemia	IDH1 mutation
IDH2	Small molecule	Enasidenib	Acute myeloid leukemia	IDH2 mutation
KIT	Small molecule	Imatinib	Aggressive systemic mastocytosis	KIT D816V mutation
			Gastrointestinal stromal tumors	KIT (CD117) expression positive (Exon 9, Exon 11 mutation)

*Combination with trametinib.
†Combination with cobimetinib.
‡Combination with binimetinib.
Antihormone and immunotherapies have been omitted.
Data from Table of Pharmacogenomic Biomarkers in Drug Labeling. Food and Drug Administration. Updated 2/5/2020 https://www.fda.gov/drugs/science-research-drugs/table-pharmacogenomic-biomarkers-drug-labeling.

pathways. Vascular endothelial growth factor (VEGF) is a prominent signaling ligand in this process, with five VEGF isoforms (A, B, C, D, E) that bind to 3 main subtypes of VEGF receptors (VEGFR-1, -2, and -3; see Chap. 11, Sec. 11.4). Three approaches have been used to inhibit the VEGF signaling pathway, including (1) antibodies or other recombinant proteins that bind to circulating VEGF or (2) to its receptor (VEGFR) to prevent ligand-receptor interaction and (3) small molecules that inhibit intracellular tyrosine kinase activity. No predictive biomarkers for antiangiogenic therapy, beyond tumor histology, have been validated for clinical application. Resistance to antiangiogenic therapies is multifactorial and discussed further in Chapter 11.

19.3.1 Antiangiogenic Monoclonal Antibodies

Bevacizumab is a recombinant humanized monoclonal antibody against circulating VEGF-A ligand that prevents its interaction with VEGFR-1 and -2 on endothelial cells. It has limited anticancer effects when administered alone, but exhibits meaningful clinical activity when given together with cytotoxic chemotherapies for advanced colorectal (Keating, 2014), cervical (Tewari et al, 2017), ovarian, mesothelioma (Zalcman et al, 2016), non–small cell lung cancer (NSCLC), and renal cell carcinoma (in combination with interferon); although its use has declined in the management of NSCLC and renal cell carcinoma (RCC) as a result of more effective treatment options. Similar to bevacizumab, **ramucirumab** is a fully humanized monoclonal antibody inhibiting the VEGFR-2 receptor, the target of VEGF-A, -C, and -D ligands. Ramucirumab has been shown to delay progression of disease for previously treated NSCLC (Garon et al, 2012), hepatocellular carcinoma (HCC) (Zhu et al, 2019), and advanced gastric cancer, and in people with colorectal cancer who have progressive disease after receiving bevacizumab (Sanchez-Gastaldo et al, 2016). Typical of therapeutic monoclonal antibodies, which have long half-lives, ramucirumab and bevacizumab are administered intravenously at 2- to 3-week intervals. Side effects associated with both bevacizumab and ramucirumab include high

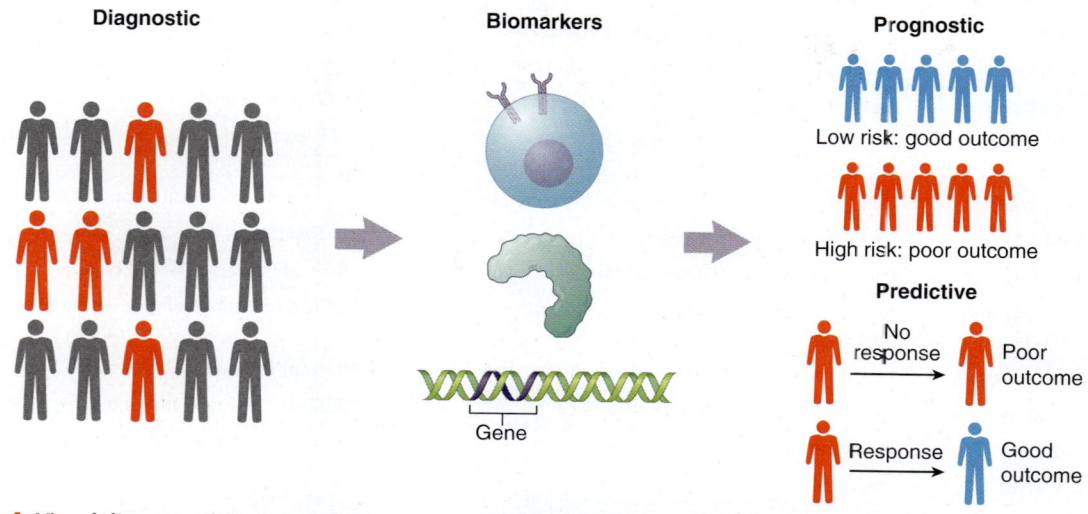

FIGURE 19–4 Visual diagram of diagnostic, prognostic, and predictive biomarkers in patient populations.

blood pressure, bleeding, proteinuria (high urine protein levels), development of clots, risk of gastrointestinal tract rupture (perforation), and impaired wound healing—effects that can be long lasting given the long biologic half-life of the antibody drugs.

Multiple costimulatory RTKs are also involved in angiogenesis, one of which is platelet-derived growth factor (PDGF) and its receptor (PDGFR). The PDGFR family of receptors (see Chap. 11, Sec. 11.4.2) have complementary functions to stimulate vascular growth through modulation of stromal cells and cancer-associated fibroblasts in the tumor microenvironment. Stimulation of proangiogenic PDGF/PDGFR pathways leads to epithelial mesenchymal transition, cell growth, and remodeling of the extracellular matrix, all of which may contribute to tumor growth or spread. **Olaratumab** is a recombinant human monoclonal antibody that inhibits PDGFRα signaling in tumor and stromal cells. Olaratumab demonstrated survival benefit in early-phase clinical trials for soft tissue sarcomas (Tap et al, 2016); however, a confirmatory phase III trial failed to confirm this benefit, highlighting the potential for initial signals from small, underpowered studies to be misleading. Side effects are more frequent when olaratumab is combined with doxorubicin chemotherapy and include higher rates of low white blood cells, hair loss, mouth sores, nausea, high blood glucose levels, and muscle pain.

19.3.2 Antiangiogenic Small Molecule Tyrosine Kinase Inhibitors (TKIs)

Small molecule TKIs have been developed to target a number of signaling enzymes in the angiogenesis pathway (see Chap. 11, Sec. 11.4). Most antiangiogenic TKIs are relatively nonselective and act by inhibiting multiple receptors (ie, VEGFR, PDGFR, FGFR, c-KIT, MET, RET, AXL, FLT-3, CSF1R) and/or intracellular targets (ie, RAF) (see Fig. 19–5). These off-target effects are often used to exploit specific receptor amplifications or mutations in certain tumor types and will be discussed in later sections (eg, c-KIT in gastrointestinal stromal tumors [GISTs]). Most TKIs that block VEGFR signaling are associated with class-effect toxicities including high blood pressure, proteinuria, rash, fatigue, diarrhea, mouth sores, nausea, and elevation of liver enzymes.

Sunitinib is a multitargeted TKI that inhibits VEGFR (1, 2, 3), PDGFR (α/β), c-KIT (CD117), the FMS-like tyrosine kinase 3 (FLT3), and other membrane-bound RTKs (ie, FGFR, RET, CSF1R). Approved treatment indications for sunitinib include favorable risk metastatic clear cell RCC (Sánchez-Gastaldo et al, 2017), GISTs (von Mehren and Joensuu, 2018), and pancreatic neuroendocrine tumors (Raymond et al, 2011). Dosing strategies for sunitinib vary by indication but often require dose reduction or modification of schedule to manage side effects. In addition to common TKI side effects, sunitinib carries an additional risk of thyroid dysfunction and painful hands and feet referred to as hand-foot syndrome (Segaert et al, 2009). **Pazopanib** and **axitinib** inhibit many of the same RTKs as sunitinib (Fig. 19–5) and are also used for treatment of metastatic RCC. Axitinib has also shown improved survival in combination with immunotherapy in RCC (Rini et al, 2019), and activity in alveolar soft part sarcoma, a rare sarcoma subtype (Wilky et al, 2019). Pazopanib is reported to have an improved side effect profile relative to sunitinib, although rates of liver enzyme elevation are more frequent.

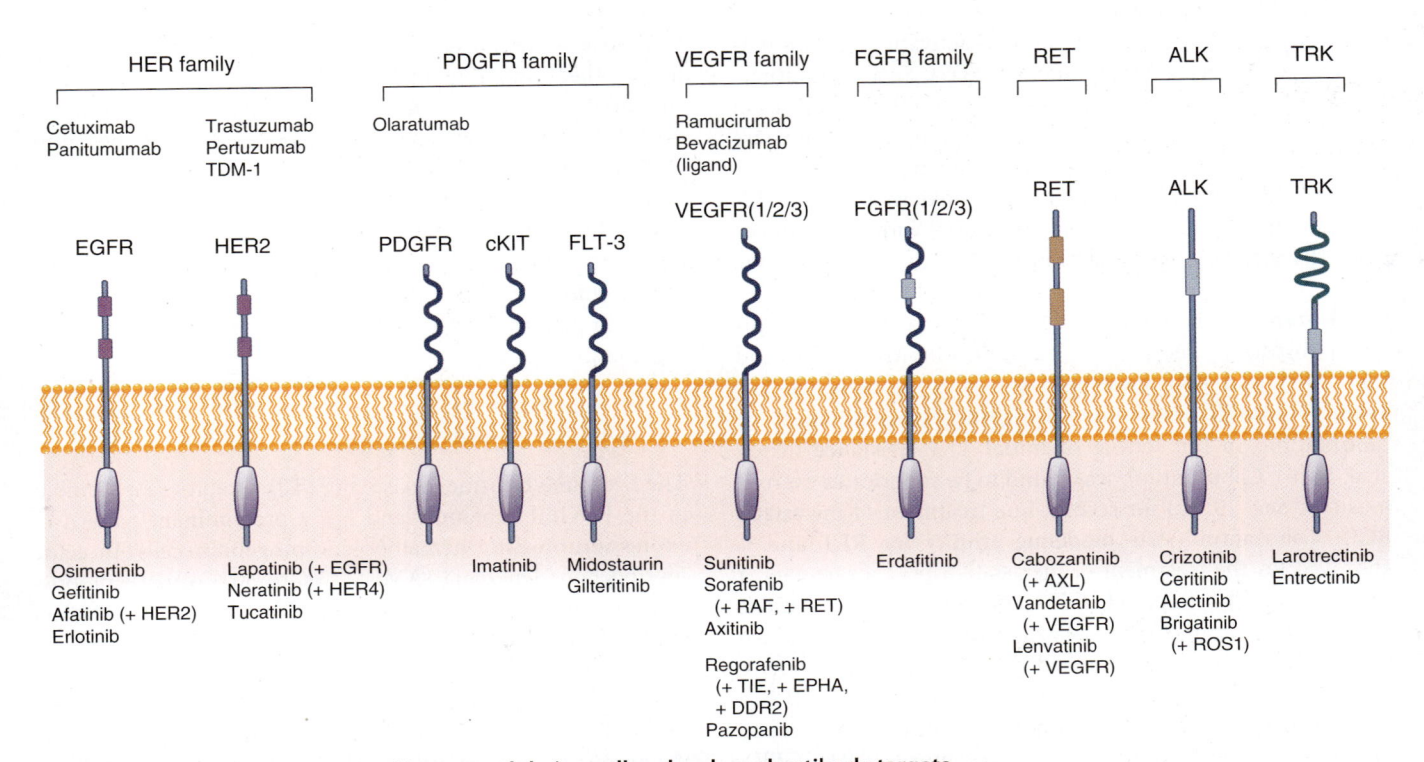

FIGURE 19–5 Receptor tyrosine kinases and their small molecule and antibody targets.

Sorafenib exhibits a similar spectrum of kinase inhibition to sunitinib and pazopanib but was identified preclinically as an inhibitor of the mitogen-activated protein kinase (MAPK) signaling pathway through cytosolic RAF kinase (ie, BRAF) inhibition (Wan et al, 2004) (see Fig. 19–5). Sorafenib also inhibits the RET receptor and is indicated for the management of advanced-stage unresectable HCC (Forner et al, 2018) and desmoid tumors (Gounder et al, 2018), metastatic differentiated thyroid cancer that is refractory to radioactive iodine (Brose et al, 2014), and to a lesser degree in metastatic RCC. Adverse events related to sorafenib are similar to those seen with other TKIs.

The multikinase inhibitor **regorafenib** also inhibits RAF and traditional angiogenic receptors but has an expanded spectrum of angiogenesis receptor inhibition including TIE2, DDR2, and Eph2A (Fig. 19–5). Regorafenib has been shown to delay progression in chemotherapy-refractory metastatic colorectal cancer (Grothey et al, 2013), metastatic GIST following imatinib and sunitinib failure, and in HCC for patients who have progressed after sorafenib treatment. Given its expanded spectrum of receptor inhibition, regorafenib is associated with more adverse events including greater risk of liver toxicity, diarrhea, high blood pressure, and hand-foot skin reaction, in addition to other common TKI side effects.

19.3.3 RET Inhibition

The rearranged during transfection (*RET*) proto-oncogene is a transmembrane glycoprotein involved in embryonic kidney and enteric nervous system development. Oncogenic activation of RET occurs predominantly through intrachromosomal rearrangements or fusion events (ie, RET-KIF5B in NSCLC; RET-CCDC6 in papillary thyroid cancer) with a variety of gene partners, or alternatively through activating point mutations in medullary thyroid cancer (MTC). Several multitargeted TKIs inhibit RET, which has prompted their application in RET-activated cancers, described below. RET inhibitors are in early clinical development and have shown promise for cancers with RET mutation with favorable toxicity profiles. This activity supports the notion that for cancers with strong oncogenic drivers, selective inhibition may maximize therapeutic index.

Cabozantinib is a multitargeted TKI that inhibits traditional angiogenic receptors in addition to c-MET, AXL, and RET. MET and AXL have been shown to be activated following sunitinib treatment, raising the potential utility of cabozantinib in the setting of initial TKI resistance (Zhou et al, 2016). Cabozantinib was found to be superior to everolimus (see Sec. 19.5.2) for second-line treatment of metastatic RCC. Cabozantinib has moderate affinity for RET and is approved for the treatment of metastatic MTC, a rare cancer characterized by frequent *RET*-activating point mutations (Schlumberger et al, 2017). Cabozantinib has also been shown to delay progression of advanced HCC in patients who have progressed after sorafenib treatment (Abou-Alfa et al, 2018).

Vandetanib inhibits RET in addition to VEGFR-2/3 and the human epidermal growth factor receptor (HER1/EGFR). This drug has been shown to delay progression compared to placebo in patients with advanced MTC with higher response rates for tumors harboring somatic *RET* M918T mutations (Wells et al, 2012). Cardiac conduction abnormalities are a side effect of vandetanib.

Lenvatinib is a multitargeted TKI that also inhibits RET, fibroblast growth factor receptor (FGFR), and VEGFR 1-3 receptors. Lenvatinib is noninferior to sorafenib and has been shown to delay progression as first-line treatment for HCC that is not amenable to surgery (Kudo et al, 2018). It is also approved as second-line treatment of metastatic RCC in combination with everolimus, or as first- or second-line therapy for iodine-refractory differentiated thyroid cancer (Schlumberger et al, 2015). Common side effects are similar to those of other TKIs with severe hypertension as a hallmark.

19.3.4 c-KIT Inhibition

The receptors c-KIT (CD117) and PDGFR are expressed on >90% of GISTs, with the majority harboring c-KIT-activating mutations in exon 11 (90%) or 9 (8%), and approximately 10% to 20% having mutations in PDGFRα (von Mehren and Joensuu, 2018). **Imatinib** was the first approved small molecule TKI in humans for the treatment of CML based on its ability to inhibit BCR-ABL fusion proteins (see Sec. 19.6.4). Secondary kinase targets of imatinib include c-KIT and PDGFR. Imatinib is indicated as neoadjuvant (treatment before surgery) and maintenance therapy (after surgery) for GISTs, and as first-line treatment for metastatic disease. Mutations in the c-KIT receptor at exon 11 have shown increased sensitivity to imatinib treatment for GISTs, whereas mutations in exon 9 have demonstrated relative resistance (Heinrich et al, 2003). The PDGFR D842V mutant isoform is an infrequent (5%) primary resistance mutation to imatinib therapy, whereas the majority of other mutations in PDGFR are sensitive to the drug. Acquired resistance to imatinib occurs through mutations in exon 13 and 17, for which second-generation c-KIT inhibitors have shown considerable promise. Fluid retention (limbs, face) is a known side effect of imatinib, with additional TKI side effects discussed in Section 19.6.4.1. Because of their off-target effects including c-KIT inhibition, sunitinib (second-line) and regorafenib (third-line) are also indicated in the treatment of GISTs in patients whose tumors have progressed after receiving imatinib.

19.3.5 FLT-3 Inhibition

The FMS-like tyrosine kinase-3 (FLT3) receptor is a member of the PDGFR subfamily and has a predominant pattern of expression on early hematopoietic progenitor cells. In acute myelogenous leukemia (AML), 25% to 30% of patients possess mutations in FLT3 such as an internal tandem duplication (FLT3-ITD) mutation or point mutations in codon D835 of the tyrosine kinase domain (FLT3-TKD) leading to constitutive activation and MAPK signaling. The more common FLT3-ITD is associated with an unfavorable prognosis, while the prognostic impact of FLT3-TKD is less well characterized.

Midostaurin is an oral multitargeted TKI with activity against FLT3 mutations. In a randomized phase III trial, the survival of patients with newly diagnosed FLT3-mutated AML was improved with midostaurin maintenance treatment administered following standard induction and consolidation chemotherapy (Stone et al, 2017).

Gilteritinib, a selective FLT3 inhibitor, was reported to improve overall survival and rates of complete remission in patients with relapsed or refractory FLT3-mutated AML compared with standard chemotherapy. Patients who had received prior midostaurin in this clinical trial had a poor response to gilteritinib, consistent with the presence of resistance to FLT3 inhibition. Midostaurin and gilteritinib are associated with high-grade anemia, and gilteritinib also carries a risk of low neutrophil counts with fever, and low platelets.

19.3.6 FGFR Inhibition

FGFRs are a group of single-pass, transmembrane RTKs with 4 family members (FGFR1 to FGFR4) that possess kinase domains (FGFR5 lacks a kinase domain). Overall, there are 18 fibroblast growth factor ligands that bind to FGFRs, which play a role in cell proliferation, growth, differentiation, migration, and survival. Alterations in FGFR, including somatic mutations, amplifications, and translocations, are found in a number of tumor types including bladder (20%-30%), breast (10%-18%), endometrial (13%), lung (squamous; 13%), and ovarian cancer (~9%) (Helsten et al, 2016). Despite frequent mutations in up to 7% of solid tumors, the role of FGFR is largely unknown and the response to FGFR inhibitors is poor in mixed-histology, targeted trials.

Erdafitinib is a first-generation FGFR-TKI that targets FGFR subtypes 1 to 4. In a pivotal phase II study evaluating erdafitinib in patients with advanced urothelial carcinoma with FGFR3 mutations or FGFR2/3 fusions who had progressed on prior therapy, high (40%) response rates and delayed cancer progression were observed (Loriot et al, 2019). Side effects of erdafitinib include low blood sodium, mouth sores, and fatigue. Serious side effects included retinal detachment and hand-foot syndrome. Mechanisms of clinical resistance to erdafitinib are yet to be described.

19.4 INHIBITORS OF THE EPIDERMAL GROWTH FACTOR RECEPTOR FAMILY

The human epidermal growth factor receptor (HER) family is composed of 4 transmembrane RTKs (HER1 [or EGFR]/HER2/HER3/HER4) that bind 11 related ligands leading to homo- or heterodimerization and prosurvival cell signaling through the MAPK and PI3K-AKT pathways (Fig. 19–5; see also Chap. 6, Sec. 6.2). Unlike conventional RTKs, HER2 lacks the ability to bind extracellular ligands, and HER3 possesses an inactive intracellular tyrosine kinase signaling domain requiring dimerization with other HER family members for signal propagation (Baselga and Swain, 2009). HER1/EGFR and HER2 are the best characterized HER family members with genomic alterations (mutations [EGFR] and amplifications [HER2]) representing both prognostic and predictive biomarkers of tumor behavior and response to targeted therapies.

19.4.1 Inhibitors of EGFR

Selective targeting of HER1/EGFR with small molecule TKIs is beneficial in the treatment of patients with activating mutations in EGFR. These mutations occur predominantly in lung cancers of adenocarcinoma histology (>90%) and to a lesser degree in other tumor types (eg, head and neck cancers). The frequency of EGFR mutations in NSCLC varies with smoking status (higher in nonsmokers), gender (female), and Asian (higher) vs non-Asian ancestry. More than 90% of oncogenic EGFR mutations include deletion of exon 19 or point mutation of L858R in exon 21 (Shi et al, 2014). EGFR-activating mutations are associated with more favorable prognosis in NSCLC and are highly responsive to targeted therapy. However, development of resistance (eg, T790M, a gatekeeper mutation) to early generation EGFR TKIs is common. Bypass resistance mechanisms to EGFR-TKIs also occur, including MET receptor amplification and exon 14 skipping (Awad et al, 2016).

In advanced colorectal cancer, antibody-based targeting of HER1/EGFR has an established clinical role. However, in contrast to the application of EGFR TKIs in NSCLC, the mutational status of EGFR is not used to guide the delivery of this therapy. Instead, the presence or absence of activating mutations in the downstream RAS oncogene is the relevant clinical biomarker, with treatment restricted to those with wild-type (nonmutated) RAS. Approximately 40% of colorectal patients possess mutated downstream *RAS* isoforms (*KRAS* or *NRAS*), which cause intrinsic resistance to anti-EGFR antibodies (Bertotti et al, 2015).

Cetuximab is a chimeric monoclonal antibody against extracellular EGFR, whereas **panitumumab** is a fully humanized monoclonal antibody against EGFR. Cetuximab was found to delay tumor progression in patients with non-RAS mutated metastatic colorectal cancer when used as first-line treatment in combination with chemotherapy. The identification of *KRAS* mutation as a predictive biomarker of EGFR targeting was achieved retrospectively, as initial studies enrolled all patients regardless of mutational status. In a secondary analysis of a phase III clinical trial using expanded *RAS* mutation testing (exon 3 and 4 in addition to exon 2) in patients receiving chemotherapy plus cetuximab, patients with *RAS* wild-type compared with *RAS*-mutated tumors demonstrated improvements in overall survival (Van Cutsem et al, 2015). Panitumumab has also been approved for non–*RAS*-mutated, metastatic colorectal cancer as first-line treatment in combination with chemotherapy. Similar results have been seen for wild-type vs mutated *RAS* and *BRAF* genes (Douillard et al, 2013). Large, randomized trials have also confirmed a survival advantage for single agent cetuximab and panitumumab in patients with chemotherapy refractory advanced colorectal cancer compared to best supportive care (Price et al, 2014). Cetuximab is also used for the treatment of locally advanced, human papillomavirus–negative, squamous cell cancers of the head and neck in combination with concurrent radiotherapy (Mehanna et al, 2019), or in the metastatic setting with platinum and fluorouracil–based chemotherapies (Vermorken et al, 2008). Mutational testing for *EGFR* (<3%) and *RAS* (4%-5%) is not performed commonly in head and neck cancers because of the low prevalence of mutations in this tumor type, and lower use of cetuximab compared with platinum chemotherapy for most patients with this disease (Suh et al, 2014).

Gefitinib and **erlotinib** are orally administered, first-generation small molecule TKIs of the intracellular portion of EGFR-associated tyrosine kinases (see Fig. 19-5 and Chap. 6, Sec. 6.2). Gefitinib was shown initially to prolong survival compared with standard carboplatin-paclitaxel chemotherapy when administered as the initial treatment for advanced NSCLC among nonsmokers or former light smokers in east Asia (Mok et al, 2009). In a preplanned subgroup analysis by *EGFR* mutational status (ie, exon 19 deletion, exon 21 L858R, exon 20 T790M), the presence of an *EGFR* gene mutation was a strong predictor of better outcome with gefitinib, whereas patients without these mutations had better outcome with chemotherapy (ie, EGFR mutation is a qualitative predictive biomarker) (Recondo et al, 2018). Gefitinib has also been shown to increase time to disease recurrence compared with cisplatin-vinorelbine in the adjuvant setting for patients with resected early-stage *EGFR* mutation–positive NSCLC, although overall survival data are not yet mature (Zhong et al, 2018). **Erlotinib** is indicated for patients with advanced NSCLC after progression on platinum or docetaxel chemotherapies regardless of EGFR status, based on a trial performed before the use of EGFR mutations as routine biomarkers (Shepherd et al, 2005). This study demonstrated a small improvement in overall survival, highlighting the utility of biomarker preselection for EGFR-TKIs. Erlotinib has also been studied in other EGFR wild-type settings, including in metastatic pancreatic cancer in combination with gemcitabine as first-line chemotherapy, where a statistically significant, but clinically negligible, improvement in survival was observed in an unselected population (Moore et al, 2007).

A limitation of first-generation EGFR-TKIs is the occurrence of intrinsic or acquired resistance mutations that render tumor cells insensitive to the inhibitory effects of these agents. **Afatinib** is an oral, second-generation irreversible pan-HER TKI, which has been evaluated in 2 first-line phase III studies of patients with metastatic EGFR-TKI–naïve lung adenocarcinoma with EGFR-activating mutation(s). Afatinib demonstrated extended time to progression over cisplatin-pemetrexed chemotherapy in one study, but relative equivalence compared to gefitinib in a second comparative trial. This general equivalence of afatinib (second-generation) compared to gefitinib (first-generation) is important, as it demonstrates that resistance mechanisms can often be multifactorial. Afatinib is also approved for the treatment of patients with metastatic or locally advanced squamous cell lung cancer after progression on platinum-based chemotherapy independent of EGFR status (Recondo et al, 2018). Many patients require dose interruption and/or reduction for common toxicities including rash, diarrhea, mouth sores, nail changes, and nausea and vomiting, again highlighting the important role of EGFR family proteins in normal tissue function.

Osimertinib is an oral, third-generation, irreversible EGFR-TKI that inhibits selectively both EGFR-TKI–sensitizing mutations and overcomes a key resistance mutation, EGFR T790M. The T790M mutation of EGFR leads to a substitution of the amino acid threonine with methionine at position 790 of exon 20 affecting ATP binding at the EGFR kinase domain. This gatekeeper mutation confers resistance to first- and second-generation EGFR-TKIs. T790M mutations can be detected through DNA sequencing of tumor samples or in blood samples containing cell-free, circulating tumor DNA (ctDNA) in approximately 50% of patients after progression on first- or second-generation EGFR-TKIs. Osimertinib approval was based on results of a phase III trial comparing osimertinib to platinum-based chemotherapy in patients with EGFR T790M mutant NSCLC progressing after prior EGFR-TKI therapy, where it delayed tumor progression by almost 6 months. Another randomized phase III trial of osimertinib vs gefitinib or erlotinib as initial treatment for untreated metastatic EGFR-mutant (ie, exon 19 del or exon 21 L858R) NSCLC also demonstrated superior time to disease progression (Recondo et al, 2018). Commonly acquired resistance mechanisms to front-line osimertinib are C797 and L792 EGFR mutations (25%), in addition to MET amplification (15%), which has led to the development of a combination of osimertinib with MET inhibition (savolitinib). Side effects of osimertinib are typically mild and include standard EGFR-TKI toxicities. More severe side effects include inflammatory lung disease, and potential for cardiac toxicity.

Inhibition of EGFR, which is expressed in gut and skin tissues, commonly causes diarrhea and skin toxicities. Skin toxicities manifest as an acne-like skin rash involving the face and upper trunk, which progresses over time to dry skin, fissures, and infection around nail beds. Development of a moderate to severe anti-EGFR–mediated rash has been correlated with improved survival and tumor response in patients with metastatic colon cancer receiving cetuximab or panitumumab (Petrelli et al, 2013). This correlation may reflect high endogenous EGFR expression in patient keratinocytes (skin cells), which are likely reflective of those on the tumor cell surface. Prophylactic measures, such as skin moisturizers, sunscreen, topical steroids, and oral antibiotics (doxycycline/minocycline) can reduce the severity of skin toxicities without affecting treatment efficacy. Hypomagnesemia is another common side effect of EGFR inhibition.

19.4.2 Inhibitors of HER2

HER2 amplification is a strong adverse prognostic marker in breast cancer in the absence of effective treatments targeting this pathway. Agents targeting these receptors represent some of the earliest effective biomarker-directed therapies for the treatment of solid tumors, although acquired resistance is common. Amplification of *HER2* and overexpression of its protein product occurs predominantly in patients with breast cancer (15%-20%), and to a lesser extent in patients with gastric (10%-20%), and metastatic colorectal (2%-6%) cancer. Amplification/overexpression of *HER2* at the tumor cell surface is a strong predictor of therapeutic response to HER2-targeted agents.

Trastuzumab is a fully humanized monoclonal antibody against HER2 and has improved survival when used in combination with chemotherapy for the treatment of women with HER2-overexpressing breast cancer in the neoadjuvant (before surgery), adjuvant, and metastatic setting (Baselga et al, 2017). Trastuzumab has also shown improved survival when used in combination with platinum and fluorouracil–based chemotherapy for treatment of advanced gastric or gastroesophageal junction cancers that overexpress HER2 (Bang et al, 2010). Symptomatic toxicities to trastuzumab are minimal, with serious side effects related to effects on cardiac myocytes including reduced heart contractility (as measured by ejection fraction) and, less commonly, symptomatic heart failure. Patients with pre-existing heart disease, prior chest wall radiation, and concomitant administration or previous exposure to cardiotoxic drugs (including anthracyclines) are at an increased risk of heart failure with trastuzumab therapy. Management of trastuzumab-related cardiotoxicity typically necessitates dose delay and, less often, discontinuation of therapy.

Pertuzumab is a monoclonal antibody directed against a different epitope of the extracellular domain of the HER2 receptor, and inhibits its homo- and/or heterodimerization with HER3 receptors. Women with advanced HER2-positive breast cancer treated with pertuzumab, trastuzumab, and docetaxel compared to trastuzumab and docetaxel alone had significantly improved overall survival (Singh et al, 2014). For patients with early-stage HER2-positive breast cancer, the addition of pertuzumab to standard chemotherapy with trastuzumab in the adjuvant setting produces only a small absolute improvement in invasive disease-free survival (von Minckwitz et al, 2017). In the neoadjuvant setting, pertuzumab improves pathologic complete response rates in women with breast cancer when used in combination with trastuzumab plus chemotherapy, but this combination has not shown improvements in long-term outcomes. Pertuzumab in combination with trastuzumab has also demonstrated improved objective response rates (32%) in patients with HER2-amplified, treatment-refractory metastatic colorectal cancer (Meric-Bernstam et al, 2019). Pertuzumab does not significantly increase the risk of trastuzumab-associated cardiotoxicity, although it is associated with an increased risk of diarrhea.

Trastuzumab emtansine (T-DM1) is an antibody-drug conjugate in which the potent cytotoxic antimicrotubule agent emtansine is conjugated to the trastuzumab antibody through a thioether linker. In a phase III trial, adjuvant T-DM1 was shown to significantly reduce recurrence rates compared with trastuzumab for patients with residual disease after neoadjuvant chemotherapy (von Minckwitz et al, 2019). T-DM1 is also approved as a single agent for treatment of patients with advanced HER2-positive breast cancer who have received prior taxane and trastuzumab (with or without pertuzumab) based therapies. A randomized phase III trial demonstrated longer time to progression and survival compared to capecitabine chemotherapy in combination with lapatinib, an EGFR/HER2 TKI (see below) (Singh et al, 2014). The most common side effects of T-DM1 include thrombocytopenia, liver enzyme elevation, and anemia.

Overexpression of HER2 on tumor cells is also the primary target of small molecule anti-HER2 therapies. **Lapatinib** and **neratinib** are orally administered, small-molecule TKIs of HER2 and HER1/EGFR tyrosine kinase receptors, and neratinib possesses additional activity against HER4 (note that HER3 does not have an active kinase domain). **Lapatinib** is used in combination with capecitabine for treatment of women with HER-2–overexpressing advanced breast cancer whose tumors have progressed on trastuzumab, but its efficacy has been surpassed by trastuzumab emtansine. Although lapatinib increases tumor response when given in the preoperative setting in combination with trastuzumab, this strategy did not improve survival when given as adjuvant therapy (Goss et al, 2013). Evaluation of adjuvant **neratinib** for 12 months compared with placebo in a randomized clinical trial demonstrated a small improvement in invasive disease–free survival at 5 years, which appeared to be limited to hormone receptor–positive, HER2-positive breast cancers. Substantial side effects (including diarrhea), high cost, and lack of mature data showing an improvement in overall survival limit its application (Martin et al, 2017). Like trastuzumab, lapatinib and neratinib can cause cardiac toxicity, although the incidence is low in appropriately selected patients. Lapatinib also causes toxicities not observed with trastuzumab, such as diarrhea, skin rash, and elevated liver enzymes and bilirubin related to its dual EGFR and HER2 targeting. Both drugs exhibit improved bioavailability with high-fat meals, possibly allowing dosing with food to reduce their high cost (Ratain and Cohen, 2007).

19.5 INHIBITORS OF INTRACELLULAR RECEPTOR TYROSINE KINASE PATHWAYS

19.5.1 Inhibitors of Phosphatidyl Inositol 3-Kinase (PI3K)

Phosphatidyl-inositol 3-kinase (PI3K) is a cytosolic lipid kinase composed of a catalytic (p110 $\alpha/\beta/\delta/\gamma$) and regulatory (p85/p55) subunit heterodimer that interacts directly with the intracellular portion of tyrosine kinase receptors and/or RAS proteins at the cell membrane. PI3K stimulates antiapoptotic and proliferative cell signaling via the AKT/mTOR pathway (Liu et al, 2009) (see Fig. 19–6 and Chap. 6, Sec. 6.2). The expression of catalytic subunit isoforms and the frequency of activating mutations are variable in solid and hematologic malignancies. In solid tumors, *PIK3CA*, encoding p110α, is one of the most commonly mutated oncogenes, with several

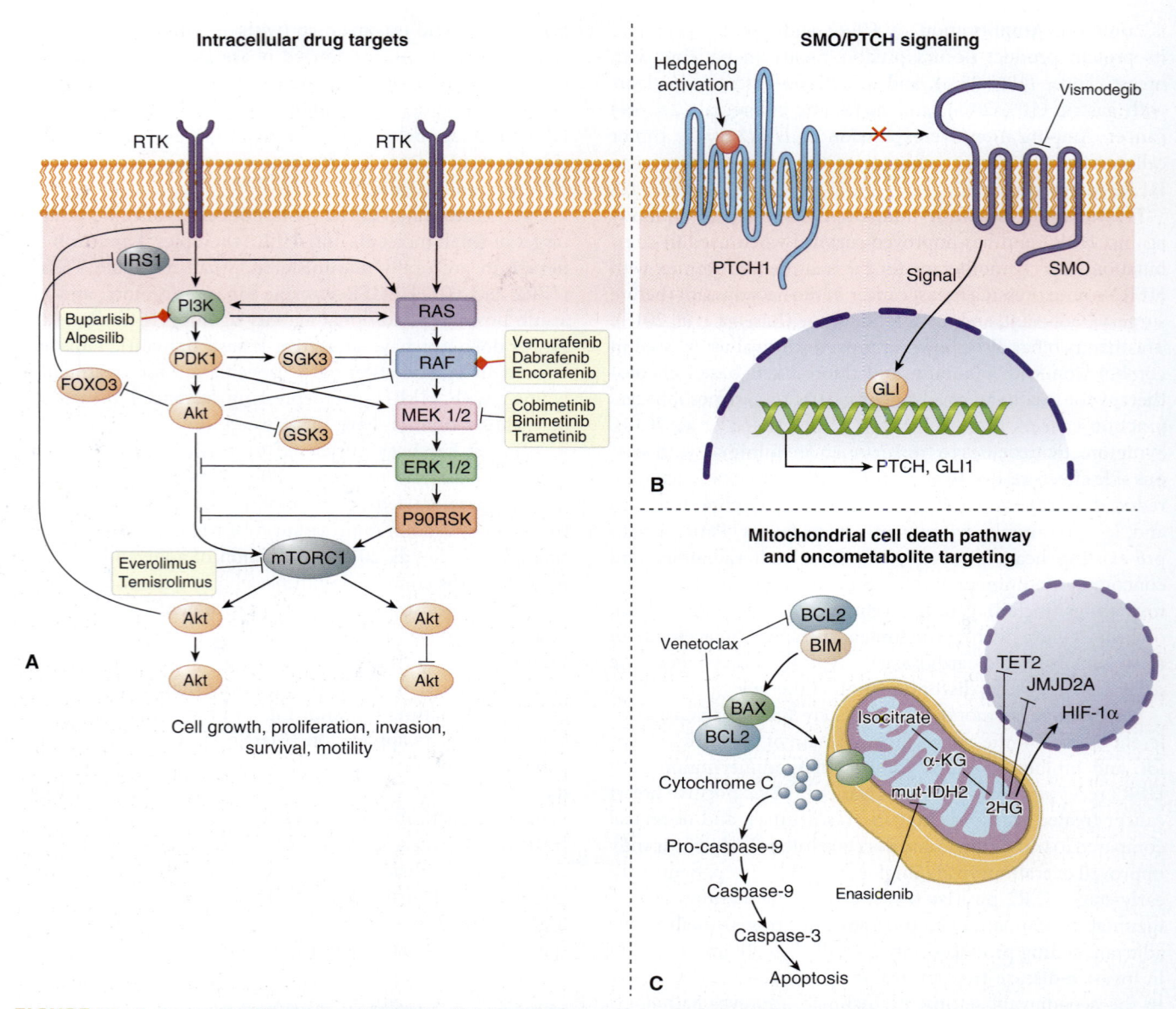

FIGURE 19–6 Conceptual figure showing intracellular pathway inhibition (PI3K, RAF/MEK, mTOR) and novel targeted therapies (BH3, SMO/PTCH). (Part A Modified with permission from Jahangiri A, Weiss WA. It takes two to tango: Dual inhibition of PI3K and MAPK in rhabdomyosarcoma. *Clin Cancer Res* 2013 Nov 1;19(21):5811-5813.)

recurrent activating hotspot mutations. Somatic mutations in the *PIK3CA* gene occur in up to 50% of endometrial cancers, 10% to 40% of breast cancers depending on subtype, and >10% of tumors across several histologies. In contrast, the PIK3-δ isoform is preferentially expressed (but not mutated) in lymphoid cells, where it is required for B-cell receptor signaling (Okkenhaug and Vanhaesebroeck, 2003). These mutations and tissue-specific isoform expressions have allowed for biomarker-(ie, PIK3CA) and histology-(ie, PIK3-delta expression in CLL) oriented development of PI3K inhibitors.

Several large randomized trials adding nonselective PI3K inhibitors to standard endocrine therapy have been conducted in hormone receptor–positive, HER2-negative breast cancer, where rates of activating mutations are ~30% to 40%. Although these trials have shown consistent small improvements in response rate or delayed progression, particularly among patients with *PIK3CA*-mutated cancers, their substantial toxicities and modest effectiveness have led to isoform-specific development. For example, subgroup analysis of 2 phase III clinical trials using the pan-PI3K inhibitor **buparlisib** (Awada et al, 2017) demonstrated a slight improvement in outcome, particularly in a *PIK3CA*-mutated breast cancer subset. Inhibitors selective for the α isoform have shown more encouraging results and a better side-effect profile, with toxicities reflecting the role of this pathway in normal cells. **Alpelisib** was recently shown to delay progression when added to fulvestrant in patients with ER-positive/HER2-negative PIK3CA-mutated breast cancer (André et al, 2018). The most commonly encountered toxicities with PIK3CA inhibitors are hyperglycemia, rash, nausea, and decreased appetite.

Development of PI3K-δ inhibitors in lymphoid malignancies has been more successful, given the tissue-specific role of this isoform. **Idelalisib** is a selective, oral small molecule inhibitor of the PI3K-δ catalytic domain. Idelalisib is used as monotherapy for the treatment of patients with indolent, non-Hodgkin lymphoma (NHL) after at least 2 prior systemic therapies, and for disease that is refractory to both rituximab and chemotherapy (Gopal et al, 2014). It is also approved for the treatment of relapsed chronic lymphocytic leukemia (CLL) for patients with significant coexisting medical conditions such as decreased kidney function or myelosuppression related to prior therapies. Improved outcomes in this population with substantial comorbidities were observed in a phase III trial (Furman et al, 2014). Side effects of idelalisib include low neutrophils, fever, diarrhea, bowel inflammation (colitis), and rash. Idelalisib can cause fatal or serious liver toxicity or colitis in approximately 15% to 20% of treated patients, as well as lung inflammation.

19.5.2 Mammalian Target of Rapamycin Inhibitors (mTOR)

The mammalian target of rapamycin (mTOR) is located downstream in the PI3K-AKT pathway. A primary function of mTOR is regulation of hypoxia-induced cell signaling by HIF-1α, which is implicated in angiogenesis and many other pathways (Fig. 19-6; see Chap. 12, Sec. 12.2.3). mTOR also interacts with estrogen receptor cell signaling and has been implicated in resistance of breast cancer to hormonal therapy (Yamnik and Holz, 2010; see Chap. 20, Sec. 20.4). **Everolimus** and **temsirolimus** are rapalogs (related to rapamycin): small molecule inhibitors of the mTOR Complex 1 (mTORC1). These agents act to inhibit this complex through allosteric disruption of protein binding, not via direct ATP-competitive inhibition of the mTOR catalytic site. These agents differ in their mode of administration (oral, continuous for everolimus vs intravenous, intermittent for temsirolimus), and in the settings in which they have been studied and approved for clinical use. Everolimus is approved in the treatment of metastatic renal cell carcinoma following anti-VEGFR TKI therapy with sorafenib or sunitinib, or in combination with lenvatinib (Sánchez-Gastaldo et al, 2017). In metastatic hormone receptor–positive, HER2-negative breast cancer, everolimus has been approved in combination with the aromatase inhibitor exemestane based on results of a phase III trial, which showed an improvement in PFS, but not overall survival, at the expense of added toxicity. Everolimus also delayed progression compared with best-supportive care in a phase III trial for patients with advanced, well-differentiated (or moderately differentiated in pancreas) neuroendocrine tumors of the pancreas, lung, or gastrointestinal tract (Yao et al, 2016). Temsirolimus leads to small improvements in survival of patients with poor-prognosis metastatic renal cell cancer, but its use has declined because of development of more effective therapies.

Inhibitors of mTOR have substantial toxicities, including metabolic disorders (high blood sugar, cholesterol, and lipids), hematologic toxicities (anemia and low lymphocytes), and gastrointestinal toxicities, such as mouth sores, nausea, and diarrhea. Less common but potentially life-threatening toxicities include allergic reactions and lung inflammation.

19.5.3 Mitogen-Activated Protein Kinase Pathway Inhibitors (RAF/MEK)

The classical RAS-MAPK pathway is an intracellular signaling mechanism involved in multiple prosurvival cellular functions (see Chap. 6, Sec. 6.2.4). In addition to the RAS proteins described previously (see Sec. 19.3), the cytosolic kinases RAF, MEK, and ERK provide downstream signal transduction and regulation of gene transcription. BRAF is a member of the RAF family of serine/threonine protein kinases. Mutations in the *BRAF* gene are seen in ~50% of melanomas (Davies et al, 2002) and in 20% to 50% of anaplastic thyroid cancers, and at a lower frequency in other tumor types such as NSCLC (1%-3%). Although multiple activating BRAF mutations have been recognized, the most common of these is the valine to glutamate substitution at amino acid 600 (V600E). These mutations result in constitutive activation of the BRAF protein and phosphorylation of its downstream substrates MEK1 and MEK2 (Sharma et al, 2006).

Dabrafenib and **vemurafenib** are orally administered small molecule inhibitors of mutant BRAF V600E/K. They undergo primary metabolism by CYP isoforms 3A4, 2C8 (dabrafenib), and 2D6 (vemurafenib) and were initially shown to be effective when used alone to treat patients with advanced melanomas. The combination of BRAF with the MEK inhibitors **cobimetinib** and **trametinib** for the treatment of *BRAF* mutation positive metastatic melanoma has improved treatment efficacy, based on inhibition of bypass activation (by MEK) of the MAPK pathway downstream of BRAF (Pelster and Amaria, 2019) (Figs. 19-3 and 19-6). Other BRAF/MEK inhibitors (**binimetinib** and **encorafenib**) have also shown efficacy in BRAF-mutated advanced melanoma (Dummer et al, 2018). In the adjuvant setting, the combination of dabrafenib plus trametinib for BRAF V600 mutation–positive stage III melanoma led to improvements in relapse-free survival compared with placebo, although early analyses have not shown an improvement in overall survival. Combination BRAF/MEK inhibition (eg, dabrafenib plus trametinib) has also shown activity in difficult-to-treat V600E mutation–positive anaplastic thyroid cancer (Subbiah et al, 2018), and for untreated BRAF V600E–mutant metastatic NSCLC (Planchard et al, 2017).

Single-agent BRAF inhibitor therapy is associated with a paradoxical overactivation of MAPK pathways and development of keratoacanthomas (typically benign skin tumors) and squamous cell carcinomas of the skin (Gibney et al, 2013). This side effect appears to be mitigated with the addition of downstream MEK inhibitors. Vemurafenib is associated with increased sensitivity to light (photosensitivity) compared with dabrafenib, and high–sun protection factor (SPF) sunscreens in addition to avoidance of direct sunlight are recommended while on BRAF inhibitor therapy. MEK inhibitors are generally associated with rash, nausea, diarrhea, fatigue, increased liver enzymes, venous thromboembolism (blood clots), and limb swelling. Risk of cardiac toxicity is amplified with combination therapy.

19.6 INHIBITORS OF CELL CYCLE, DNA REPAIR, EPIGENETICS, AND FUSION PROTEINS

19.6.1 Cyclin-Dependent Kinase Inhibitors

The cyclin-dependent kinase (CDK) family of proteins are critical regulators of the cell cycle. Efforts to target these proteins as anticancer therapy have only recently proven successful with the development of selective inhibitors of CDK4 and CDK6. CDK4/6 regulate the transition between the G1/S phases of the cell cycle and mediate progression through the restriction point, which is governed by the retinoblastoma (RB) transcriptional regulator (see Chap. 8, Sec. 8.2). Selective CDK4/6 inhibitors act by inhibiting the phosphorylation of RB in G1, leading to cell cycle arrest when RB function is intact. The development of several CDK4/6 inhibitors as adjuncts to endocrine therapy for hormone receptor–positive, HER2-negative breast cancer was inspired by the observation that cancer cell lines with this phenotype exhibited preferential sensitivity to one of these agents (palbociclib) in vitro (Finn et al, 2009). Three agents have been shown to improve outcomes in the first- or second-line setting when added to standard endocrine therapy. Although these agents are generally well tolerated, they add toxicity to endocrine therapy, most notably low neutrophil counts, anemia, and fatigue.

Palbociclib is an oral selective CDK4/6 inhibitor that is administered daily for 21 days of a 28-day cycle in combination with endocrine therapy. In a phase III trial, the addition of palbociclib to the aromatase inhibitor letrozole as initial systemic therapy for advanced hormone receptor (HR)–positive, HER2-negative breast cancer in postmenopausal women significantly delayed cancer progression (Eggersmann et al, 2019). A second trial combining palbociclib with the selective estrogen receptor degrader (SERD) fulvestrant in patients whose disease had recurred or progressed on an aromatase inhibitor resulted in a doubling of median PFS compared with fulvestrant alone, and a significant improvement in overall survival in patients who had sensitivity to prior endocrine therapy (Turner et al, 2018). **Ribociclib** and **abemaciclib** are CDK4/6 inhibitors that have undergone similar development to palbociclib, and are also approved for use with antihormonal agents for the treatment of hormone receptor–positive advanced breast cancer. Abemaciclib is the only CDK4/6 inhibitor that is approved as monotherapy after prior failure of endocrine and chemotherapy, based on a phase II trial (Dickler et al, 2017).

No predictive or prognostic molecular biomarkers (beyond ER) have been validated to guide therapy with CDK4/6 inhibitors. Correlative analyses of completed clinical trials have identified some predictors of benefit, including the baseline expression of cyclin E, and early changes in detectable ctDNA following treatment initiation (O'Leary et al, 2018). These findings, which reflect the potential power of so-called liquid biopsies to detect molecular changes and guide treatment, are encouraging but will need to be validated in additional studies before application in the clinical setting.

A key determinant of clinical resistance to CDK4/6 inhibition is loss of RB tumor suppressor function, which relieves dependence on CDKs at the G1 checkpoint. Although RB loss of function is a rare event (<3%) in untreated ER-positive breast cancer, this alteration is enriched in patients progressing on CDK4/6 inhibitors. Preclinical models have identified additional mechanisms of resistance, including amplification of cyclin E or CDK6, but their relevance in the clinical setting is less clear (Knudsen and Witkiewicz, 2017; see Chap. 8, Sec. 8.2.6).

Although the effects of each of the 3 CDK4/6 inhibitors on response rate and PFS have been remarkably consistent, the individual agents exhibit differences in their toxicity profiles, likely related to drug target selectivity. Palbociclib and ribociclib are associated with a higher incidence of neutropenia and mouth sores than abemaciclib whereas ribociclib is associated with elevation of liver enzymes and cardiac conduction disturbances. Although abemaciclib causes less myelosuppression, it is associated with substantial rates of diarrhea.

19.6.2 DNA Repair Inhibitors

Inhibition of the DNA repair enzyme poly(ADP-ribose) polymerase (PARP) represents a therapeutic approach based on the concept of synthetic lethality (see Chap. 9, Sec. 9.3.4 and Chap. 17, Sec. 17.2). Cancers in patients with *BRCA1* and *BRCA2* mutations develop from cells that undergo loss of heterozygosity at these sites that are functionally homologous recombination deficient (HRD) in the repair of DNA double-strand breaks. When this conservative mechanism of DNA double-strand break repair is lost, other mechanisms that are more error prone (eg, nonhomologous end joining [NHEJ]) predominate. Although the initial mechanism of PARP inhibitor action was thought to be inhibition of signaling processes required to repair single-stranded breaks, the development of clinical PARP inhibitors has revealed the role of "PARP trapping," whereby PARP inhibitors trap PARP1 on DNA, thereby impairing the progression of replication forks (Ashworth and Lord, 2018). Thus, in the presence of HRD, repair and resumption of replication is impeded, conferring a selective sensitivity in the context of BRCA1/2 deficiency. Tumors may also exhibit "BRCA-ness," a term defining a group of tumors that lack germline or somatic mutations in BRCA but share similar genomic features of HRD. Tumors with features of BRCA-ness may possess defects in genes intricately related to DNA repair such as *PALB2*, *ATR*, *RAD51*, or Fanconi anemia genes. Although *ATM* mutations are often considered in this context, the degree to which *ATM*-mutated cancers exhibit features of BRCA-ness is less clear and may depend on the tissue origin of the tumor.

BRCA deficiency is most commonly observed in serous ovarian cancers (11%-25%), resulting from an inherited germline deficiency followed by a somatic loss of heterozygosity (germline plus somatic gene loss), or arise from a somatic loss of both copies of BRCA within the tumor, without a predisposing germline deletion (somatic biallelic event). **Olaparib, rucaparib, and niraparib** are oral, selective PARP inhibitors that are approved as maintenance treatment for women with platinum-sensitive, relapsed BRCA-mutated high-grade serous epithelial, fallopian tube, or primary peritoneal cancer, who responded to prior platinum-based chemotherapy. Maintenance therapy with olaparib in patients with newly diagnosed advanced BRCA-mutated ovarian cancer who had a partial or complete response to platinum chemotherapy leads to a large (~70%) reduction in the probability of relapse at 3 years and is now standard-of-care (Moore et al, 2018).

PARP inhibitors have also been studied in breast cancer, initially in unselected patients, but more recently focused on germline BRCA carriers. Somatic loss of BRCA in nongermline carriers is observed less commonly in breast cancer (~5%) than in ovarian cancer (15%). Olaparib and **talazoparib** have been approved for the treatment of germline BRCA-mutated metastatic HER2-negative breast cancer, based on the results of phase III trials in which they were compared with non-platinum chemotherapy of investigators' choice (Robson et al, 2017). In these studies, improvements in PFS and response rates were observed. The design of these trials precludes the direct comparison of PARP inhibitors with platinum chemotherapy, which is active and a standard of care in BRCA1/2-related breast cancer. Both the mechanisms of action and available clinical data suggest that cross-resistance to platinum chemotherapy and PARP inhibitors may be common. BRCA mutations also occur in prostate and pancreatic cancers, and clinical trials are ongoing to define the role of PARP inhibitors in these populations.

Resistance to PARP inhibitors can occur through mechanisms such as reversion mutations in BRCA1 or BRCA2 resulting in a restoration of protein function, through drug-efflux transporters (eg, ABCB1 [P-gp], see Chap. 18, Sec. 18.4.3), acquisition of PARP functional mutations (with loss of PARP-DNA trapping), and loss of additional DNA repair genes involved in NHEJ (eg, P53BP1) (Lord and Ashworth, 2013). Common side effects of PARP inhibitors include nausea, vomiting, diarrhea, loss of appetite, fatigue, and low blood counts including anemia that require transfusion.

19.6.3 Epigenetic Inhibitors

19.6.3.1 Histone Deacetylase (HDAC) Inhibitors

Acetylation of histones by histone acetyltransferases (HATs) influences gene regulation by inducing a closed chromatin structure that limits accessibility of DNA/RNA transcriptional machinery (see Chap. 3, Sec. 3.2.2). Histone deacetylase (HDAC) catalyzes the removal of acetyl groups from lysine residues of nucleosomal histones, facilitating an open chromatin conformation and availability of gene transcription. Aberrant HDAC activity has been associated with the development of some human malignancies through selective regulation of proliferative and antiapoptotic genes (Ceccacci and Minucci, 2016). HDAC inhibitors have been developed that bind zinc ions at the active site of HDAC, thereby inhibiting its enzymatic function (Slingerland et al, 2014).

Vorinostat and **romidepsin** are approved HDAC inhibitors indicated in the management of relapsed and refractory cutaneous (CTCL) or peripheral T-cell lymphoma (PTCL) respectively. Two additional HDAC inhibitors, **belinostat** and **panobinostat** (in combination with dexamethasone and bortezomib) are approved for the treatment of relapsed or refractory PTCL and multiple myeloma, respectively. **Chidamide (tucidinostat)** is an oral HDAC inhibitor that has shown improved PFS in combination with exemestane compared to exemestane alone in hormone refractory metastatic breast cancer in a phase III trial (Jiang et al, 2019). As oral (vorinostat, panobinostat, chidamide) or intravenous (belinostat, romidepsin) monotherapy, side effects include diarrhea, nausea/vomiting, fatigue, infections and fever, bone marrow suppression, cardiac conduction abnormalities, loss of appetite, and liver dysfunction.

19.6.3.2 Isocitrate Dehydrogenase (IDH) Inhibitors

Isocitrate dehydrogenase 1 and 2 (IDH1/2) are metabolic enzymes involved in the tricarboxylic acid (TCA) or Krebs cycle and act by catalyzing the conversion of isocitrate to α-ketoglutarate (see Chap. 12, Sec. 12.3.1). Mutations in IDH 1 or 2 result in a change of enzymatic function leading to an accumulation of the oncometabolite D-2-hydroxyglutarate, a potent inhibitor of multiple α-ketoglutarate dependent enzymes involved in epigenetic regulation of DNA and histones (ie, TET1/2/3 family) (Fig. 19–6). This disruption of DNA regulation leads to modulation of gene expression through hypermethylation, perpetuating a prosurvival phenotype and attenuating cellular differentiation (Waitkus et al, 2018). IDH mutations (eg, IDH1 at R132) occur frequently in brain malignancies (astrocytomas, oligodendromas, and secondary glioblastomas), in ~10% to 30% of acute myeloid leukemias (AMLs), and in other tumor types including cholangiocarcinoma and chondrosarcomas (Molenaar et al, 2018). The association between IDH1/2 mutational status and survival in AML patients may vary with the specific mutation observed, although circulating levels of the D-2-hydroxyglutarate have been correlated with survival outcomes (DiNardo et al, 2013). Conversely, in malignant gliomas IDH-mutated tumors have an improved prognosis compared to those that are IDH wild-type.

Enasidenib is an oral, selective inhibitor of mutated IDH2 enzymes. In an early-phase clinical trial of relapsed or refractory IDH2-mutated AML patients, enasidenib demonstrated an overall response rate of approximately 40%, with median survival of about 9 months and prolonged survival in those achieving a complete response, leading to its regulatory approval (Stein et al, 2017). **Ivosidenib** is an orally administered, selective inhibitor of mutated IDH1 enzymes and conferred a similar degree of benefit in IDH1-mutated AML, resulting in its approval for relapsed/refractory IDH1 mutated

AML. A study of ivosidenib in IDH mutant cholangiocarcinoma has also reported that the drug has promising activity.

Common side effects of enasidenib and ivosidenib include nausea, vomiting, diarrhea, elevated bilirubin, electrolyte disturbances, cardiac conduction abnormalities, and myelosuppression. IDH differentiation syndrome is an on-target biological effect of these agents that occurs in patients with AML, resulting in multiorgan dysfunction that occurs in 4% to 7% of patients and can be life-threatening.

19.6.4 Fusion Protein Inhibitors

Oncogenic gene rearrangements occur in some malignancies, creating cytosolic or receptor tyrosine kinase fusion proteins that drive tumor cell growth. As described below, oncogenic fusions can be almost universal in certain diseases (eg, BCR-ABL in CML), or occur at low frequency, such as TRK fusions in solid tumors (~1%). The identification of fusion proteins has led to effective biomarker-directed therapies. The identification of rare but actionable fusion proteins (eg, TRK) adds complexity to the conduct of clinical trials and the use of agents targeting them in routine practice, where many patients must have tumor testing to identify whether they constitute the small proportion eligible for treatment.

19.6.4.1 BCR-ABL The breakpoint cluster region–Abelson (BCR-ABL) fusion protein is a constitutively active cytosolic kinase arising from reciprocal translocation of chromosome 9 and 22, known as the Philadelphia (Ph) chromosome (see Chap. 7, Sec. 7.5.1). BCR-ABL is present in >90% of patients with CML, and in approximately 25% of patients with acute lymphoblastic leukemias (ALLs) depending on age.

Imatinib is an orally administered small molecule TKI of ABL kinase and the BCR-ABL fusion protein. It was approved based on the phase III IRIS trial, demonstrating complete cytogenetic response (no detection of BCR-ABL–positive cells) of 76% at 18 months compared with interferon-alpha plus low-dose cytarabine chemotherapy (14% at the same time point), leading to a markedly prolonged survival (O'Brien et al, 2003). Resistance to imatinib in CML results from mutations that alter amino acids at the imatinib-binding site on ABL (ie, E255K, T135I) or prevent BCR-ABL from achieving the inactive conformation required for imatinib binding (Shah et al, 2002). Imatinib is also effective for treatment of BCR-ABL–positive AML and of GISTs based on its adjunct c-KIT inhibition, as well as other rare malignancies that have PDGFR rearrangements (see Sec. 19.3.4).

Second-generation BCR-ABL TKIs have been developed to overcome resistance and improve the speed, depth, and duration of response to TKI therapy. **Dasatinib** inhibits BCR-ABL and other targets. In a phase III trial, dasatinib was compared to imatinib as first-line treatment for chronic phase CML, demonstrating faster and higher rates of major molecular response (Rosti et al, 2017). In addition to the side effects seen with imatinib, dasatinib carries a serious risk of delayed heart toxicity, and high blood pressure in the lungs. **Nilotinib** is another inhibitor of BCR-ABL fusion proteins and other cytosolic kinases that was designed to bind with higher affinity than imatinib even in the presence of multiple resistance mutations. It also proved superior to imatinib in a phase III trial, but should be avoided in patients with cardiac conduction abnormalities.

Ponatinib is a third-generation BCR-ABL inhibitor designed to overcome the T315I mutation that confers resistance in up to 20% of first- and second-generation BCR-ABL TKIs. In a single-arm phase II trial, ponatinib led to high rates of complete cytogenetic response in BCR-ABL mutation–positive CML or ALL in patients who experienced resistance or unacceptable side effects to dasatinib or nilotinib, or with the imatinib-resistant T315I mutation. However, ponatinib carries a substantial risk of arterial or venous blood clots in about 25% of patients, in addition to heart and liver function abnormalities.

19.6.4.2 ALK and ROS-1 The anaplastic lymphoma kinase (ALK) gene undergoes somatic rearrangement in 4% to 5% of NSCLCs and to varying degrees in other malignancies. In lung cancer, the ALK gene most commonly undergoes fusion with the echinoderm microtubule-associated protein-like 4 (EML4) gene, giving rise to the constitutively active ALK-EML4 kinase. ROS-1 also undergoes gene rearrangement in 1% to 2% of non–small cell lung cancers. It is most commonly attached to the CD47 receptor gene yielding the CD74-ROS1 fusion kinase, although other ROS1 fusion genes have been identified. Similar to mutations in EGFR, gene rearrangements in ALK and ROS1 are associated with younger age, light/never smokers, and adenocarcinoma histology (Cancer Genome Atlas Research Network, 2014).

Crizotinib is a first-in-class, orally administered small molecule TKI targeting ALK, MET, and ROS-1 alterations. Crizotinib has demonstrated improvements in median PFS and response rates in platinum-pretreated or treatment-naïve ALK-rearranged NSCLC (Solomon et al, 2014). Because of the low rates of *ROS1* gene rearrangements, evaluation of this group in large prospective clinical trials is difficult, but small studies have demonstrated high response rates to crizotinib (Recondo et al, 2018). Side effects of crizotinib include visual disturbances, nausea, bowel disturbances, low neutrophils and liver dysfunction, and rare instances of lung inflammation. Resistance to crizotinib develops invariably within the first year or two of TKI therapy, with progression commonly occurring in the brain. Multiple resistance mechanisms can occur, including ALK tyrosine kinase domain point mutations (ie, L1196M), ALK amplification, and stimulation of other receptors that promote tumor cell survival (eg, c-KIT, EGFR).

The second-generation ALK small molecule TKIs **ceritinib, alectinib,** and **brigatinib** have been developed to overcome resistance mechanisms and to more effectively penetrate the blood-brain barrier to prevent and treat central nervous system (CNS) metastases. **Ceritinib** has 20-fold greater potency than crizotinib and also inhibits MET and ROS1 kinases in addition to penetrating the CNS and demonstrating activity against brain metastases. It has undergone similar development to crizotinib and has similar side effects in addition to cardiac conduction abnormalities. **Alectinib** has demonstrated significantly improved PFS and tumor response rates compared with platinum-based chemotherapy both in patients with untreated NSCLC and after progression on crizotinib. The phase III ALEX trial comparing alectinib to crizotinib for untreated ALK-positive NSCLC demonstrated superior PFS and enhanced prevention of CNS metastasis. Alectinib is associated with increased muscle pain but is generally better tolerated than crizotinib. Resistance mutations to second-generation ALK inhibitors include the G1202R point mutation (21%-43%), and ALK double mutants D1203N plus E1210K or D1203N plus F1174C (Recondo et al, 2018). Third-generation ALK inhibitors (eg, **lorlatinib**) for the treatment of mutation-positive NSCLC after progression on ceritinib and alectinib are showing promising results in early-phase clinical trials (Solomon et al, 2018).

19.6.4.3 TRK The neurotrophin family of receptor tyrosine kinases includes 3 transmembrane proteins (TrkA, TrkB, and TrkC) encoded by the *NTRK1*, *NTRK2*, and *NTRK3* genes, respectively (Chao, 2003). Involved in nervous system development and in neural maintenance in adults, NTRK receptor gene rearrangements (eg, *TPM3-NTRK1*) are uncommon, having been identified in only 1% or fewer adult malignancies. **Larotrectinib** is an oral selective TRK kinase inhibitor that achieved a response rate of 75% in patients with predominantly *NTRK*1- and *NTRK*3-fusion cancers across 17 tumor types in an early-phase clinical trial (Drilon et al, 2018). Larotrectinib was generally well tolerated, with mild liver enzyme elevation, nausea, and dizziness as the most common side effects. Resistance mutations developed primarily at the NTRK1 (G595R) and NTRK3 (G623R) solvent front positions, as well as NTRK1 F589L (a gatekeeper mutation).

19.7 OTHER TARGETED THERAPIES

19.7.1 Proteasome Inhibitors

The ubiquitin proteasome pathway is central in the maintenance of cellular homeostasis acting to degrade both functional and nonfunctional proteins that balance cell survival (eg, Bcl-2) vs death (eg, p53), and growth (eg, nuclear factor-κB [NF-κB]) vs senescence (eg, cyclin-dependent kinase inhibitor B1). Cancers have been shown to preferentially alter this balance through selective proteasomal degradation to favor a prosurvival phenotype (Manasanch and Orlowski, 2017). Targeted disruption of the proteasome catalytic domain (20S) is thought to increase cellular stress through simulation of the unfolded protein response, resulting in proapoptotic signaling and cancer cell death (see Chap. 8, Sec. 8.4). Proteasome inhibitors have also been shown to block prosurvival signals via NF-κB translocation to the nucleus and are antiangiogenic. Proteasome inhibitors are used routinely in the treatment of multiple myeloma and resistance to these agents is incompletely understood.

Bortezomib is a first-in-class reversible inhibitor of the β5-subunit catalytic site of the 20S proteasome. It is administered subcutaneous or intravenously and has a variable half-life and dosing schedule (once- or twice-weekly). It has been established as a backbone therapy in combination with various drug combinations for the treatment of transplant-ineligible, transplant-eligible, and relapsed or refractory multiple myeloma, and is one of the drugs that has led to marked improvement in survival for people with this disease (Hideshima et al, 2011). It is also used in the maintenance of 17p-deleted multiple myeloma posttransplant and for the treatment of mantle cell lymphoma. Side effects of bortezomib include neuropathy (nerve damage), which is worse with IV infusion, low platelets, nausea, diarrhea, fatigue, and risk for Varicella zoster virus reactivation. Prophylaxis with antivirals is recommended for all patients.

Carflizomib is a selective irreversible proteasome inhibitor that also binds the 20S catalytic subunit. It is indicated in the treatment of relapsed or refractory multiple myeloma either in combination with lenalidomide and dexamethasone or with dexamethasone alone. Treatment with carflizomib led to longer median PFS when compared with bortezomib (both with dexamethasone) in a phase III trial for patients with relapsed or refractory multiple myeloma, albeit with slightly more serious adverse events. Carflizomib carries a risk of kidney impairment and cardiovascular side effects, including high blood pressure and heart failure but causes less neuropathy than bortezomib.

Ixazomib is another proteasome inhibitor with a longer proteasome dissociation half-life (9.5 days) than bortezomib, but with the added advantage of oral dosing. Treatment with ixazomib led to improved PFS in a phase III trial when added to lenalidomide and dexamethasone, regardless of high-risk cytogenetic (ie, 17p deletion) abnormalities. Ixazomib is associated with delayed onset of low platelets and a higher incidence of rash.

19.7.2 B-Cell Receptor (BCR) Pathway Inhibitors

The B-cell receptor (BCR) is a transmembrane receptor located on the surface of B-lymphocytes and is activated in response to extracellular antigen recognition (see Chap. 21, Sec. 21.3). BCR signaling occurs through heterodimerization with transmembrane signal transduction subunits CD79A/B with downstream signaling through spleen tyrosine kinase (SYK), and Bruton's tyrosine kinase (BTK). These cytosolic kinases activate MAPK, PI3K-AKT, and NF-κB signaling leading to cell growth, survival, and DNA repair (Burger and Wiestner, 2018). Abnormal BCR signaling has been shown in a number of B-cell hematologic malignancies including chronic lymphocytic leukemia (CLL). Management of CLL is rapidly changing because of the significant efficacy and decreased toxicity of targeted therapies relative to historical standard of care chemotherapies. Specific subgroups of CLL patients possess high-risk cytogenetic abnormalities such as chromosome

17p13.1 deletion, *TP53* gene mutation, and unmutated immunoglobulin heavy-chain variable region (IGHV) genes that show relative resistance to chemotherapy and have poor prognosis (Parikh, 2018).

Ibrutinib is an oral, small molecule inhibitor that binds covalently to the ATP-binding cleft of BTK to abrogate downstream BCR signaling. It also has off-target inhibition effects on the chemokine receptors CXCL-12, CXCL-13, and CCL-19 involved in signaling, adhesion, and migration of malignant B cells (de Rooij et al, 2012). Ibrutinib is approved as first-line treatment of CLL regardless of 17p, *TP53*, or IGHV mutational status and is also indicated for the treatment of relapsed or refractory CLL as a single agent or in combination with bendamustine-rituximab. In a pivotal randomized phase III trial, ibrutinib plus rituximab compared to standard-of-care chemotherapy (FCR, fludarabine, cyclophosphamide, rituximab) resulted in significantly improved toxicity, PFS, and overall survival regardless of age, performance status, or high-risk cytogenetics with the exception of IGHV mutated status (Shanafelt et al, 2018). Ibrutinib has also shown efficacy in phase II trials in combination with the BH3 inhibitor venetoclax (see below) as initial treatment or in relapsed or refractory CLL (Jain et al, 2019). Adverse events associated with ibrutinib include higher rates of infection, tumor lysis syndrome, cardiac arrhythmias (atrial fibrillation), bleeding, myelosuppression, diarrhea, and kidney toxicity.

The second-generation, highly selective BTK inhibitor **acalabrutinib** (ACP-19) has an improved toxicity profile relative to ibrutinib with lower rates of atrial fibrillation, infection, and bleeding. Acalabrutinib is approved for the treatment of relapsed or refractory mantle cell lymphoma and has also shown benefit in the treatment of CLL (Byrd et al, 2016).

Genomic mechanisms of resistance to ibrutinib are thought to arise from mutations in BTK (eg, C481S) or from a loss in the autoinhibitory SH2 domain of downstream phospholipase C gamma 2 (PLCG2), leading to a constitutively active protein that is independent of BTK signaling (Mertens and Stilgenbauer, 2017). Histologically driven mechanisms of resistance to BTK inhibitors include transformation to a more aggressive form of lymphoma (ie, diffuse large B-cell lymphoma), also known as a Richter transformation.

19.7.3 BH3 Inhibitors

Programmed cell death or apoptosis is regulated by 2 mechanisms—the intrinsic (mitochondrial) and extrinsic (FAS ligand, death receptor) cell death pathway(s) (see Chap. 8, Sec. 8.4). The intrinsic cell death, or mitochondrial pathway, occurs in response to cellular damage and is mediated by the B-cell lymphoma 2 (BCL-2) family of proteins. This group of mitochondria-associated proteins maintains balance between proapoptotic (ie, BAX, BAK, BID) and antiapoptotic (ie, BCL-2, BCL-xL, BCL-W) cell signaling, with increased proapoptotic protein expression resulting in mitochondrial outer membrane permeabilization and programmed cell death. Inhibition of mitochondrial apoptosis is accomplished through sequestration of proapoptotic proteins by antiapoptotic proteins via the BCL-2 homology domain 3 (BH3), or other homology domains (BH1, BH2) (Fig. 19–1; Montero and Letai, 2018). One mechanism by which cancer cells avoid apoptosis is through the upregulation of antiapoptotic proteins or downregulation of proapoptotic proteins to favor cell survival (Cory and Adams, 2002).

Venetoclax is an oral, selective small-molecule BH3 mimetic that binds the antiapoptotic BCL-2 protein, displacing it from proapoptotic proteins and consequently stimulating the intrinsic apoptotic pathway (Fig. 19–6). Venetoclax is indicated in the management of 17p-deleted, relapsed, or refractory CLL as monotherapy, and in combination with low-dose cytarabine for the management of AML in treatment-naïve patients ≥65 years old. Venetoclax has also demonstrated benefit in a phase III trial comparing rituximab in combination with bendamustine or venetoclax as first-line therapy for relapsed or refractory CLL regardless of *IGHV* or *TP53* (17p) mutational status. Benefit was seen in all patient subgroups, although venetoclax was associated with an increased risk of low neutrophils (but without a corresponding increased risk of infection). As discussed previously, venetoclax has also shown considerable efficacy in combination with ibrutinib. Venetoclax is associated with electrolyte abnormalities, risk of tumor lysis syndrome, and diarrhea. Acquired resistance to venetoclax has been associated with a G101V mutation that reduces affinity of the BCL2 drug target by ~180-fold (Blombery et al, 2019).

19.7.4 Hedgehog/SMO/Patch Pathway Inhibitors

The hedgehog (HH) pathway is an important regulator of embryogenesis. Activation of the HH pathway involves binding of HH ligands (ie, Sonic) to the upstream Patched (PTCH1) transmembrane protein, leading to its degradation and release of Smoothened (SMO) protein into the primary cilia. This event prompts dissociation of the Suppressor of Fuse (SUFU) protein from glioma-associated oncology-gene homolog (GLI) transcriptional regulators leading to cell growth. Loss-of-function mutations in the HH pathway (PTCH1) are seen in familial (Gorlin syndrome) and sporadic basal cell carcinoma (BCC) in addition to medulloblastoma (see Chap. 6, Sec. 6.4.3; Briscoe and Thérond, 2013). Although most BCCs are indolent and readily removed by surgical resection, some progress to an advanced stage where surgery or radiotherapy may no longer be possible.

Vismodegib is an oral, first-in-class, small molecule inhibitor of SMO (Fig. 19–6). In an international, nonrandomized 2-cohort study, patients with metastatic or locally advanced BCC (unresectable based on specific surgical criteria) treated with vismodegib demonstrated overall response rates of about 30%, with approximately 20% of patients with locally advanced disease achieving a complete response (Sekulic et al, 2012). Side effects of vismodegib include muscle spasms, weight loss, fatigue, changed taste, and alopecia. Primary and secondary resistance rates to vismodegib are low (<10%), and most commonly occur from point mutations that impair drug target binding (ie, W535L) (Frampton and Basset-Séguin, 2018).

19.7.5 Selective Inhibitors of Nuclear Export

The nuclear pore complex is a transport channel that mediates the import and export of proteins and RNA from the nucleus to the cytoplasm (Fig. 19–1). CRM1 or exportin-1 (XPO1) is a nuclear export protein involved in drug resistance and is overexpressed in both solid tumors and hematologic malignancies (Sun et al, 2016). **Selinexor** is an oral, first-in-class, selective inhibitor of nuclear export (SINE) that blocks CRM1/XPO1, resulting in accumulation and activation of tumor suppressor proteins within the nucleus, resulting in growth inhibition and apoptosis. In a multicenter phase II trial, patients with relapsed or refractory multiple myeloma, who had already received at least 4 standard therapies, were treated with selinexor in combination with dexamethasone (Chari et al, 2018). Response rates for this heavily pretreated group was moderate (~20%) with manageable side effects, including low platelets, fatigue, nausea, diarrhea, and vomiting.

19.8 FUTURE DEVELOPMENT OF TARGETED THERAPIES

As described throughout this chapter, targeted therapies are a rapidly expanding and evolving group of anticancer agents. With the increased availability of clinical molecular profiling using next-generation sequencing and a greater understanding of cancer and its interaction with the immune system, the identification of actionable tumor alterations and therapies that exploit these strategies will drive drug development and the concept of personalized medicine (see Chap. 22, Sec. 22.2.3). The increasing complexity of clinical trials that evaluate common genomic alterations in multiple tumor types (basket trials) or evaluate multiple biomarkers in a specific tumor histology (umbrella trials) will refine the utility of targeted therapies as they pertain to individual patients (Cescon and Siu, 2017). The prospective collection and banking of patient biospecimens (ie, urine, stool, saliva, blood, tissue) on clinical trials will provide a unique opportunity to understand the interplay of the human microbiome with evolving tumor dynamics in the clinical setting (Deng and Nakamura, 2017). Emerging real-time profiling technologies, such as the evaluation of ctDNA in the blood, also offer the potential to detect actionable alterations in a minimally invasive manner and provide valuable information about tumor heterogeneity, molecular response to ongoing treatment, and the emergence of resistant clones (Cescon et al, 2020). The ability of single or combinations of targeted agents to improve outcomes and reduce treatment toxicities, though remaining affordable, will be at the forefront of future advances in systemic cancer treatment.

SUMMARY

► Targeted anticancer therapies aim to provide greater tumor selectivity by exploiting vulnerabilities in aberrantly expressed molecular pathways.
► Small molecule tyrosine kinase inhibitors (TKIs) and antibodies directed against cell surface receptors comprise the majority of molecular targeted agents.
► The identification and development of predictive and prognostic biomarkers can improve the clinical development and delivery of targeted therapies to patients most likely to benefit.
► Side effects from molecular targeted therapies are different than conventional chemotherapy and reflect the diversity of receptors that are inhibited in normal tissues.
► Intrinsic and acquired resistance to molecular targeted therapies are common, leading to disease progression.
► Development of new agents or combination therapies that inhibit the mutated protein targets or bypass mechanisms that confer acquired resistance is a rational path to improve cancer outcomes.

REFERENCES

Abou-Alfa GK, Meyer T, Cheng AL, et al. Cabozantinib in patients with advanced and progressing hepatocellular carcinoma. *N Engl J Med* 2018;379(1):54-63.

Amaya ML, Pollyea DA. Targeting the IDH2 pathway in acute myeloid leukemia. *Clin Cancer Res* 2018;24(20):4931-4936.

André F, Ciruelos EM, Rubovszky G, et al. LBA3_PRAlpelisib (ALP) + fulvestrant (FUL) for advanced breast cancer (ABC): results of the phase III SOLAR-1 trial. *Ann Oncol* 2018;29(suppl 8).

Antony J, Huang RYJ. AXL-driven EMT state as a targetable conduit in cancer. *Cancer Res* 2017;77(14):3725-3732.

Ashworth A, Lord CJ. Synthetic lethal therapies for cancer: what's next after PARP inhibitors? *Nat Rev Clin Oncol* 2018;15(9):564-576.

Atkinson AJ, Colburn WA, DeGruttola VG, et al. Biomarkers and surrogate endpoints: preferred definitions and conceptual framework. *Clin Pharmacol Ther* 2001;69(3):89-95.

Awad MM, Oxnard GR, Jackman DM, et al. MET exon 14 mutations in non–small-cell lung cancer are associated with advanced age and stage-dependent MET genomic amplification and c-met overexpression. *J Clin Oncol* 2016;34(7):721-730.

Awada A, Jagiełło-Gruszfeld A, Baselga J, et al. Buparlisib plus fulvestrant versus placebo plus fulvestrant in postmenopausal, hormone receptor-positive, HER2-negative, advanced breast cancer (BELLE-2): a randomised, double-blind, placebo-controlled, phase 3 trial. *Lancet Oncol* 2017;18(7):904-916.

Bakema JE, van Egmond M. Fc receptor-dependent mechanisms of monoclonal antibody therapy of cancer.

In: Clarke A, Compans RW, Cooper M, eds. *Current Topics in Microbiology and Immunology*. vol. 382. Berlin: Springer; 2014: 373-392.

Ballman KV. Biomarker: predictive or prognostic? *J Clin Oncol* 2015;33(33):3968-3971.

Bang YJ, Van Cutsem E, Feyereislova A, et al. Trastuzumab in combination with chemotherapy versus chemotherapy alone for treatment of HER2-positive advanced gastric or gastro-oesophageal junction cancer (ToGA): a phase 3, open-label, randomised controlled trial. *Lancet* 2010;376(9742):687-697.

Baselga J, Coleman RE, Cortés J, Janni W. Advances in the management of HER2-positive early breast cancer. *Crit Rev Oncol/Hematol* 2017;119:113-122.

Baselga J, Swain SM. Novel anticancer targets: revisiting ERBB2 and discovering ERBB3. *Nat Rev Cancer* 2009;9(7):463-475.

Bertotti A, Papp E, Jones S, et al. The genomic landscape of response to EGFR blockade in colorectal cancer. *Nature* 2015;526(7572):263-267.

Blombery P, Anderson MA, Gong J, et al. Acquisition of the recurrent Gly101Val mutation in BCL2 confers resistance to venetoclax in patients with progressive chronic lymphocytic leukemia. *Cancer Discov* 9(3):342-353.

Briscoe J, Thérond PP. The mechanisms of Hedgehog signalling and its roles in development and disease. *Nat Rev Mol Cell Biol* 2013;14(7):416-429.

Brose MS, Nutting CM, Jarzab B, et al. Sorafenib in radioactive iodine-refractory, locally advanced or metastatic differentiated thyroid cancer: a randomised, double-blind, phase 3 trial. *Lancet* 2014;384(9940):319-328.

Burger JA, Wiestner A. Targeting B cell receptor signalling in cancer: preclinical and clinical advances. *Nat Rev Cancer* 2018;18(3):148-167.

Byrd JC, Harrington B, O'Brien S, et al. Acalabrutinib (ACP-196) in relapsed chronic lymphocytic leukemia. *N Engl J Med* 2016;374(4):323-332.

Cancer Genome Atlas Research Network. Comprehensive molecular profiling of lung adenocarcinoma. *Nature* 2014 July 31;511(7511):543-550.

Ceccacci E, Minucci S. Inhibition of histone deacetylases in cancer therapy: lessons from leukaemia. *Br J Cancer* 2016;114(6):605-611.

Cescon DW, Bratman S, Chan SM, et al. Circulating tumor DNA and liquid biopsy in oncology. *Nat Cancer* 2020;1:276-290.

Cescon D, Siu LL. Cancer clinical trials: the rear-view mirror and the crystal ball. *Cell* 2017;168(4):575-578.

Chari A, Vogl DT, Dimopoulos MA, et al. Results of the Pivotal STORM Study (Part 2) in Penta-Refractory Multiple Myeloma (MM): deep and durable responses with oral selinexor plus low dose dexamethasone in patients with penta-refractory MM. *Blood* 2018;132(suppl 1):598 LP-598.

Chao M. Neurotrophins and their receptors: A convergence point for many signalling pathways. *Nat Rev Neurosci* 2003;4:299-309.

Collisson EA, Campbell JD, Brooks AN, et al. Comprehensive molecular profiling of lung adenocarcinoma. *Nature* 2014;511(7511):543-550.

Cory S, Adams JM. The Bcl2 family: regulators of the cellular life-or-death switch. *Nat Rev Cancer* 2002;2(9):647-656.

Davies H, Bignell GR, Cox C, et al. Mutations of the BRAF gene in human cancer. *Nature* 2002;417(6892):949-954.

de Rooij MFM, Kuil A, Geest CR, et al. The clinically active BTK inhibitor PCI-32765 targets B-cell receptor- and chemokine-controlled adhesion and migration in chronic lymphocytic leukemia. *Blood* 2012;119(11):2590-2594.

Deng X, Nakamura Y. Cancer precision medicine: from cancer screening to drug selection and personalized immunotherapy. *Trends Pharmacol Sci* 2017;38(1):15-24.

Dhandapani M, Goldman A. Preclinical cancer models and biomarkers for drug development: new technologies and emerging tools. *J Mol Biomark Diagn* 2017;8(5):356.

Dickler MN, Tolaney SM, Rugo HS, et al. MONARCH 1, a phase II study of abemaciclib, a CDK4 and CDK6 inhibitor, as a single agent, in patients with refractory HR+/HER2- metastatic breast cancer. *Clin Cancer Res* 2017;23(17):5218-5224.

DiNardo CD, Propert KJ, Loren AW, et al. Serum 2-hydroxyglutarate levels predict isocitrate dehydrogenase mutations and clinical outcome in acute myeloid leukemia. *Blood* 2013;121(24):4917-4924.

Dlugosz A, Agrawal S, Kirkpatrick P. Vismodegib. *Nat Rev Drug Discov* 2012;11(6):437-438.

Douillard J-Y, Oliner KS, Siena S, et al. Panitumumab-FOLFOX4 treatment and RAS mutations in colorectal cancer. *N Engl J Med* 2013;369(11):1023-1034.

Drilon A, Laetsch TW, Kummar S, et al. Efficacy of larotrectinib in TRK fusion–positive cancers in adults and children. *N Engl J Med* 2018;378(8):731-739.

Dummer R, Ascierto PA, Gogas HJ, et al. Overall survival in patients with BRAF-mutant melanoma receiving encorafenib plus binimetinib versus vemurafenib or encorafenib (COLUMBUS): a multicentre, open-label, randomised, phase 3 trial. *Lancet Oncol* 2018;19(10):1315-1327.

Eggersmann TK, Degenhardt T, Gluz O, Wuerstlein R, Harbeck N. CDK4/6 inhibitors expand the therapeutic options in breast cancer: palbociclib, ribociclib and abemaciclib. *BioDrugs* 2019;33(2):125-135.

FDA/CDER. Table of pharmacogenomic biomarkers in drug labeling. https://www.fda.gov/drugs/scienceresearch/ucm572698.htm. Published 2018. Accessed August 5, 2019.

Finn RS, Dering J, Conklin D, et al. PD 0332991, a selective cyclin D kinase 4/6 inhibitor, preferentially inhibits proliferation of luminal estrogen receptor-positive human breast cancer cell lines in vitro. *Breast Cancer Res* 2009;11(5):R77.

Foltz IN, Karow M, Wasserman SM. Evolution and emergence of therapeutic monoclonal antibodies. *Circulation* 2013;127(22):2222-2230.

Forner A, Reig M, Bruix J. Hepatocellular carcinoma. *Lancet* 2018;391(10127):1301-1314.

Frampton JE, Basset-Séguin N. Vismodegib: a review in advanced basal cell carcinoma. *Drugs* 2018;78(11):1145-1156.

Furman RR, Sharman JP, Coutre SE, et al. Idelalisib and rituximab in relapsed chronic lymphocytic leukemia. *N Engl J Med* 2014;370(11):997-1007.

Garon EB, Cao D, Alexandris E, John WJ, Yurasov S, Perol M. A randomized, double-blind, phase III Study of Docetaxel and Ramucirumab Versus Docetaxel and Placebo in the Treatment of Stage IV Non–Small-Cell Lung Cancer After Disease Progression After 1 Previous Platinum-Based Therapy (REVEL): treatment rationale and study design. *Clin Lung Cancer* 2012;13(6):505-509.

Gharwan H, Groninger H. Kinase inhibitors and monoclonal antibodies in oncology: clinical implications. *Nat Rev Clin Oncol* 2016;13(4):209-227.

Gibney GT, Messina JL, Fedorenko IV, Sondak VK, Smalley KSM. Paradoxical oncogenesis—the long-term effects of BRAF inhibition in melanoma. *Nat Rev Clin Oncol* 2013;10(7):390-399.

Gopal AK, Kahl BS, de Vos S, et al. PI3Kδ inhibition by idelalisib in patients with relapsed indolent lymphoma. *N Engl J Med* 2014;370(11):1008-1018.

Goss PE, Smith IE, O'Shaughnessy J, et al. Adjuvant lapatinib for women with early-stage HER2-positive breast cancer: a randomised, controlled, phase 3 trial. *Lancet Oncol* 2013;14(1):88-96.

Gounder MM, Mahoney MR, Van Tine BA, et al. Sorafenib for advanced and refractory desmoid tumors. *N Engl J Med* 2018;379(25):2417-2428.

Greaves M, Maley CC. Clonal evolution in cancer. *Nature* 2012;481(7381):306-313.

Groenendijk FH, Bernards R. Drug resistance to targeted therapies: Déjà vu all over again. *Mole Oncol* 2014;8(6):1067-1083.

Grothey A, Cutsem EV, Sobrero A, et al. Regorafenib monotherapy for previously treated metastatic colorectal cancer (CORRECT): an international, multicentre, randomised, placebo-controlled, phase 3 trial. *Lancet* 2013;381(9863):303-312.

Hanahan D, Weinberg RA. Hallmarks of cancer: the next generation. *Cell* 2011;144(5):646-674.

Harrison PT, Huang PH. Exploiting vulnerabilities in cancer signalling networks to combat targeted therapy resistance. *Essay Biochem* 2018;62(4):583-593.

Hayes DF, Bast RC, Desch CE, et al. Tumor marker utility grading system: a framework to evaluate clinical utility of tumor markers. *J Natl Cancer Inst* 1996;88(20):1456-1466.

Heinrich MC, Corless CL, Demetri GD, et al. Kinase mutations and imatinib response in patients with metastatic gastrointestinal stromal tumor. *J Clin Oncol* 2003;21(23):4342-4349.

Helsten T, Elkin S, Arthur E, Tomson BN, Carter J, Kurzrock R. The FGFR landscape in cancer: analysis of 4,853 tumors by next-generation sequencing. *Clin Cancer Res* 2016;22(1):259-267.

Hideshima T, Richardson PG, Anderson KC. Mechanism of action of proteasome inhibitors and deacetylase inhibitors and the biological basis of synergy in multiple myeloma. *Mol Cancer Ther* 2011;10(11):2034-2042.

Jahangiri A, Weiss WA. It takes two to tango: dual inhibition of PI3K and MAPK in rhabdomyosarcoma. *Clin Cancer Res* 2013;19(21):5811-5813.

Jain N, Keating M, Thompson P, et al. Ibrutinib and venetoclax for first-line treatment of CLL. *N Engl J Med* 2019;380(22):2095-2103.

Jiang Z, Li W, Hu X, et al. 283O_PRPhase III trial of chidamide, a subtype-selective histone deacetylase (HDAC) inhibitor, in combination with exemestane in patients with hormone receptor-positive advanced breast cancer. *Ann Oncol* 2018. https://doi.org/10.1093/annonc/mdy424.011.

Keating GM. Bevacizumab: a review of its use in advanced cancer. *Drugs* 2014;74(16):1891-1925.

Knudsen ES, Witkiewicz AK. The strange case of CDK4/6 inhibitors: mechanisms, resistance, and combination strategies. *Trends Cancer* 2017;3(1):39-55.

Kudo M, Finn RS, Qin S, et al. Lenvatinib versus sorafenib in first-line treatment of patients with unresectable hepatocellular carcinoma: a randomised phase 3 non-inferiority trial. *Lancet* 2018;391(10126):1163-1173.

Kwa M, Makris A, Esteva FJ. Clinical utility of gene-expression signatures in early stage breast cancer. *Nat Rev Clin Oncol* 2017;14(10):595-610.

Lim SY, Lee JH, Diefenbach RJ, Kefford RF, Rizos H. Liquid biomarkers in melanoma: detection and discovery. *Mole Cancer* 2018;17(1):8.

Liu P, Cheng H, Roberts TM, Zhao JJ. Targeting the phosphoinositide 3-kinase pathway in cancer. *Nat Rev Drug Discov* 2019;8(8):627-644.

Liu S, Kurzrock R. Toxicity of targeted therapy: implications for response and impact of genetic polymorphisms. *Cancer Treat Rev* 2014;40(7):883-891.

Lord CJ, Ashworth A. Mechanisms of resistance to therapies targeting BRCA-mutant cancers. *Nat Med* 2013;19(11):1381-1388.

Loriot Y, Necchi A, Park SH, et al; BLC2001 Study Group. Erdafitinib in locally advanced or metastatic urothelial carcinoma. *N Engl J Med* 2019;381(4):338-348.

Lovly CM, Shaw AT. Molecular pathways: resistance to kinase inhibitors and implications for therapeutic strategies. *Clin Cancer Res* 2014;20(9):2249-2256.

Manasanch EE, Orlowski RZ. Proteasome inhibitors in cancer therapy. *Nat Rev Clin Oncol* 2017;14(7):417-433.

Martin M, Holmes FA, Ejlertsen B, et al. Neratinib after trastuzumab-based adjuvant therapy in HER2-positive breast cancer (ExteNET): 5-year analysis of a randomised, double-blind, placebo-controlled, phase 3 trial. *Lancet Oncol* 2017;18(12):1688-1700.

Mehanna H, Robinson M, Hartley A, et al. Radiotherapy plus cisplatin or cetuximab in low-risk human papillomavirus-positive oropharyngeal cancer (De-ESCALaTE HPV): an open-label randomised controlled phase 3 trial. *Lancet* 2019;393(10166):51-60.

Meric-Bernstam F, Hurwitz H, Raghav KPS, et al. Pertuzumab plus trastuzumab for HER2-amplified metastatic colorectal cancer (MyPathway): an updated report from a multicentre, open-label, phase 2a, multiple basket study. *Lancet Oncol* 2019;20(4):518-530.

Mertens D, Stilgenbauer S. Ibrutinib-resistant CLL: unwanted and unwonted! *Blood* 2017;129(11):1407-1409.

Mok TS, Wu Y-L, Thongprasert S, et al. Gefitinib or carboplatin–paclitaxel in pulmonary adenocarcinoma. *N Engl J Med* 2009;361(10):947-957.

Molenaar RJ, Maciejewski JP, Wilmink JW, van Noorden CJF. Wild-type and mutated IDH1/2 enzymes and therapy responses. *Oncogene* 2018;37(15):1949-1960.

Montero J, Letai A. Why do BCL-2 inhibitors work and where should we use them in the clinic? *Cell Death Differentiation* 2018;25(1):56-64.

Moore K, Colombo N, Scambia G, et al. Maintenance olaparib in patients with newly diagnosed advanced ovarian cancer. *N Engl J Med* 2018;379(26):2495-2505.

Moore MJ, Goldstein D, Hamm J, et al. Erlotinib plus gemcitabine compared with gemcitabine alone in patients with advanced pancreatic cancer: a phase III trial of the National Cancer Institute of Canada Clinical Trials Group. *J Clin Oncol* 2007;25(15):1960-1966.

Mullard A. Parsing clinical success rates. *Nat Rev Drug Discov* 2016;15(7):447-447.

O'Brien SG, Guilhot F, Larson RA, et al. Imatinib compared with interferon and low-dose cytarabine for newly diagnosed chronic-phase chronic myeloid leukemia. *N Engl J Med* 2003;348(11):994-1004.

O'Leary B, Hrebien S, Morden JP, et al. Early circulating tumor DNA dynamics and clonal selection with palbociclib and fulvestrant for breast cancer. *Nat Commun* 2018;9(1):896.

Okkenhaug K, Vanhaesebroeck B. PI3K in lymphocyte development, differentiation and activation. *Nat Rev Immunol* 2003;3(4):317-330.

Parikh SA. Chronic lymphocytic leukemia treatment algorithm 2018. *Blood Cancer J* 2018;8(10):93.

Pelster MS, Amaria RN. Combined targeted therapy and immunotherapy in melanoma: a review of the impact on the tumor microenvironment and outcomes of early clinical trials. *Ther Adv Med Oncol* 2019;11:175883591983082.

Petrelli F, Borgonovo K, Barni S. The predictive role of skin rash with cetuximab and panitumumab in colorectal cancer patients: a systematic review and meta-analysis of published trials. *Targeted Oncol* 2013;8(3):173-181.

Planchard D, Smit EF, Groen HJM, et al. Dabrafenib plus trametinib in patients with previously untreated BRAFV600E-mutant metastatic non-small-cell lung cancer: an open-label, phase 2 trial. *Lancet Oncol* 2017;18(10): 1307-1316.

Price TJ, Peeters M, Kim TW, et al. Panitumumab versus cetuximab in patients with chemotherapy-refractory wild-type KRAS exon 2 metastatic colorectal cancer (ASPECCT): a randomised, multicentre, open-label, non-inferiority phase 3 study. *Lancet Oncol* 2014;15(6):569-579.

Ratain MJ, Cohen EE. The value meal: how to save $1,700 per month or more on lapatinib. *J Clin Oncol* 2007; 25(23):3397-3398.

Raymond E, Dahan L, Raoul J-L, et al. Sunitinib malate for the treatment of pancreatic neuroendocrine tumors. *N Engl J Med* 2011;364(6):501-513.

Recondo G, Facchinetti F, Olaussen KA, Besse B, Friboulet L. Making the first move in EGFR-driven or ALK-driven NSCLC: first-generation or next-generation TKI? *Nat Rev Clin Oncol* 2018;15(11):694-708.

Redman JM, Hill EM, AlDeghaither D, Weiner LM. Mechanisms of action of therapeutic antibodies for cancer. *Mol Immunol* 2015;67(2):28-45.

Rini BI, Plimack ER, Stus V, et al. Pembrolizumab plus axitinib versus sunitinib for advanced renal-cell carcinoma. *N Engl J Med* 2019;380(12):1116-1127.

Robson M, Im SA, Senkus E, et al. Olaparib for metastatic breast cancer in patients with a germline BRCA mutation. *N Engl J Med* 2017;377(6):523-533.

Rosti G, Castagnetti F, Gugliotta G, Baccarani M. Tyrosine kinase inhibitors in chronic myeloid leukaemia: which, when, for whom? *Nat Rev Clin Oncol* 2017;14(3):141-154.

Rubin EH, Gilliland DG. Drug development and clinical trials—the path to an approved cancer drug. *Nat Rev Clin Oncol* 2012;9(4):215-222.

Sanchez-Gastaldo A, Gonzalez-Exposito R, Garcia-Carbonero R. Ramucirumab clinical development: an emerging role in gastrointestinal tumors. *Targeted Oncol* 2016;11(4):479-487.

Sánchez-Gastaldo A, Kempf E, González del Alba A, Duran I. Systemic treatment of renal cell cancer: a comprehensive review. *Cancer Treat Rev* 2017;60:77-89.

Schlumberger M, Elisei R, Müller S, et al. Overall survival analysis of EXAM, a phase III trial of cabozantinib in patients with radiographically progressive medullary thyroid carcinoma. *Ann Oncol* 2017;28(11):2813-2819.

Schlumberger M, Tahara M, Wirth LJ, et al. Lenvatinib versus placebo in radioiodine-refractory thyroid cancer. *N Engl J Med* 2015;372(7):621-630.

Schnipper LE, Davidson NE, Wollins DS, et al. Updating the American Society of Clinical Oncology Value Framework: revisions and reflections in response to comments received. *J Clin Oncol* 2016;34(24):2925-2934.

Segaert S, Chiritescu G, Lemmens L, Dumon K, Van Cutsem E, Tejpar S. Skin toxicities of targeted therapies. *Eur J Cancer* 2009;45:295-308.

Sekulic A, Migden MR, Oro AE, et al. Efficacy and safety of vismodegib in advanced basal-cell carcinoma. *N Engl J Med* 2012;366(23):2171-2179.

Shah NP, Nicoll JM, Nagar B, et al. Multiple BCR-ABL kinase domain mutations confer polyclonal resistance to the tyrosine kinase inhibitor imatinib (STI571) in chronic phase and blast crisis chronic myeloid leukemia. *Cancer Cell* 2002; 2(2):117-125.

Shanafelt TD, Wang V, Kay NE, et al. A randomized phase III study of ibrutinib (PCI-32765)-based therapy vs. standard fludarabine, cyclophosphamide, and rituximab (FCR) chemoimmunotherapy in untreated younger patients with chronic lymphocytic leukemia (CLL): a trial of the ECOG-ACRIN cancer. *Blood* 2018;132(suppl 1):LBA-4.

Sharma A, Tran MA, Liang S, et al. Targeting mitogen-activated protein kinase/extracellular signal–regulated kinase kinase in the mutant (V600E) B-raf signaling cascade effectively inhibits melanoma lung metastases. *Cancer Res* 2006; 66(16):8200-8209.

Shaw A, Bradley MD, Elyan S, Kurian KM. Tumour biomarkers: diagnostic, prognostic, and predictive. *BMJ* 2015;351:h3449.

Shepherd FA, Rodrigues Pereira J, Ciuleanu T, et al. Erlotinib in previously treated non–small-cell lung cancer. *N Engl J Med* 2005;353(2):123-132.

Shi Y, Au JSK, Thongprasert S, et al. A prospective, molecular epidemiology study of EGFR mutations in Asian Patients with Advanced Non–Small-Cell Lung Cancer of Adenocarcinoma Histology (PIONEER). *J Thorac Oncol* 2014;9(2): 154-162.

Singh JC, Jhaveri K, Esteva FJ. HER2-positive advanced breast cancer: optimizing patient outcomes and opportunities for drug development. *Br J Cancer* 2014;111(10):1888-1898.

Slingerland M, Guchelaar HJ, Gelderblom H. Histone deacetylase inhibitors. *Anti-Cancer Drugs* 2014;25(2):140-149.

Solomon BJ, Besse B, Bauer TM, et al. Lorlatinib in patients with ALK-positive non-small-cell lung cancer: results from a global phase 2 study. *Lancet Oncol* 2018;19(12): 1654-1667.

Solomon BJ, Mok T, Kim DW, et al. First-line crizotinib versus chemotherapy in ALK-positive lung cancer. *N Engl J Med* 2014;371(23):2167-2177.

Stein EM, DiNardo CD, Pollyea DA, et al. Enasidenib in mutant IDH2 relapsed or refractory acute myeloid leukemia. *Blood* 2017;130(6):722-731.

Stone RM, Mandrekar SJ, Sanford BL, et al. Midostaurin plus chemotherapy for acute myeloid leukemia with a FLT3 mutation. *N Engl J Med* 2017;377(5):454-464.

Subbiah V, Kreitman RJ, Wainberg ZA, et al. Dabrafenib and trametinib treatment in patients with locally advanced or metastatic BRAF V600–mutant anaplastic thyroid cancer. *J Clin Oncol* 2018;36(1):7-13.

Suh Y, Amelio I, Guerrero Urbano T, Tavassoli M. Clinical update on cancer: molecular oncology of head and neck cancer. *Cell Death Dis* 2014;5(1):e1018-e1018.

Sun Q, Chen X, Zhou Q, Burstein E, Yang S, Jia D. Inhibiting cancer cell hallmark features through nuclear export inhibition. *Signal Transduct Targeted Ther* 2016;1:16010.

Tap WD, Jones RL, Van Tine BA, et al. Olaratumab and doxorubicin versus doxorubicin alone for treatment of soft-tissue sarcoma: an open-label phase 1b and randomised phase 2 trial. *Lancet* 2016;388(10043):488-497.

Tewari KS, Sill MW, Penson RT, et al. Bevacizumab for advanced cervical cancer: final overall survival and adverse event analysis of a randomised, controlled, open-label, phase 3 trial (Gynecologic Oncology Group 240). *Lancet* 2017;390(10103):1654-1663.

Turner NC, Slamon DJ, Ro J, et al. Overall survival with palbociclib and fulvestrant in advanced breast cancer. *N Engl J Med* 2018;379(20):1926-1936.

Van Cutsem E, Lenz HJ, Köhne CH, et al. Fluorouracil, leucovorin, and irinotecan plus cetuximab treatment and RAS mutations in colorectal cancer. *J Clin Oncol* 2015; 33(7):692-700.

Vermorken JB, Mesia R, Rivera F, et al. Platinum-based chemotherapy plus cetuximab in head and neck cancer. *N Engl J Med* 2008;359(11):1116-1127.

von Mehren M, Joensuu H. Gastrointestinal stromal tumors. *J Clin Oncol* 2018;36(2):136-143.

von Minckwitz G, Huang CS, Mano MS, et al. Trastuzumab emtansine for residual invasive HER2-positive breast cancer. *N Engl J Med* 2019;380(7):617-628.

von Minckwitz G, Procter M, de Azambuja E, et al. Adjuvant pertuzumab and trastuzumab in early HER2-positive breast cancer. *N Engl J Med* 2017;377(2):122-131.

Waitkus MS, Diplas BH, Yan H. Biological role and therapeutic potential of IDH mutations in cancer. *Cancer Cell* 2018;34(2):186-195.

Wan PTC, Garnett MJ, Roe SM, et al. Mechanism of activation of the RAF-ERK signaling pathway by oncogenic mutations of B-RAF. *Cell* 2004;116(6):855-867.

Wells SA, Robinson BG, Gagel RF, et al. Vandetanib in patients with locally advanced or metastatic medullary thyroid cancer: a randomized, double-blind phase III trial. *J Clin Oncol* 2012;30(2):134-141.

Wilky BA, Trucco MM, Subhawong TK, et al. Axitinib plus pembrolizumab in patients with advanced sarcomas including alveolar soft-part sarcoma: a single-centre, single-arm, phase 2 trial. *Lancet Oncol* 2019;20(6):837-848.

Yamnik RL, Holz MK. mTOR/S6K1 and MAPK/RSK signaling pathways coordinately regulate estrogen receptor alpha serine 167 phosphorylation. *FEBS Lett* 2010 Jan 4; 584(1):124-128.

Yao JC, Fazio N, Singh S, et al. Everolimus for the treatment of advanced, non-functional neuroendocrine tumours of the lung or gastrointestinal tract (RADIANT-4): a randomised, placebo-controlled, phase 3 study. *Lancet* 2016; 387(10022):968-977.

Zalcman G, Mazieres J, Margery J, et al. Bevacizumab for newly diagnosed pleural mesothelioma in the Mesothelioma Avastin Cisplatin Pemetrexed Study (MAPS): a randomised, controlled, open-label, phase 3 trial. *Lancet* 2016; 387(10026):1405-1414.

Zhong WZ, Wang Q, Mao WM, et al. Gefitinib versus vinorelbine plus cisplatin as adjuvant treatment for stage II–IIIA (N1–N2) EGFR-mutant NSCLC (ADJUVANT/ CTONG1104): a randomised, open-label, phase 3 study. *Lancet Oncol* 2018;19(1):139-148.

Zhou L, Liu XD, Sun M, et al. Targeting MET and AXL overcomes resistance to sunitinib therapy in renal cell carcinoma. *Oncogene* 2016;35(21):2687-2697.

Zhu AX, Kang YK, Yen CJ, et al. REACH-2 Study Investigators. Ramucirumab after sorafenib in patients with advanced hepatocellular carcinoma and increased α-fetoprotein concentrations (REACH-2): a randomised, double-blind, placebo-controlled, phase 3 trial. *Lancet Oncol* 2019; 20(2):282-296.

Hormones and Cancer

Nathan Lack and Etienne Leygue

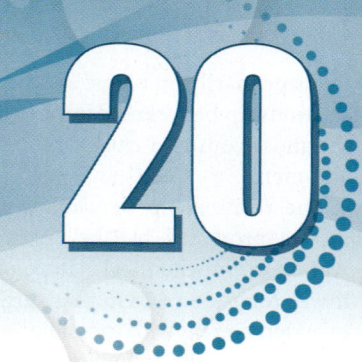

Chapter Outline

20.1 Introduction
20.2 Basic Mechanisms of Steroid Hormone Action
    20.2.1 Synthesis and Metabolism of Steroid Hormones
    20.2.2 Transport of Steroid Hormones in the Bloodstream
    20.2.3 Steroid Receptors
    20.2.4 Classical Mechanism of Steroid Receptor Action
    20.2.5 Nonclassical Mechanisms of Steroid Receptor Action
    20.2.6 Quantification of Steroid Hormone Receptor
20.3 Natural History of Breast and Prostate Cancer
    20.3.1 Risk Factors for Breast and Prostate Cancer
    20.3.2 Development and Progression of Breast and Prostate Cancers
20.4 Breast Cancer: Hormonal Therapies and Resistance
    20.4.1 Hormonal Therapy
    20.4.2 Hormonal Therapy for Different Stages of Breast Cancer
    20.4.3 Resistance to Hormone Therapy
    20.4.4 New Approaches to Hormonal Treatment of Breast Cancer
20.5 Prostate Cancer: Hormone Therapy and Resistance
    20.5.1 Hormonal Therapy
    20.5.2 Intermittent Hormonal Therapy for Prostate Cancer
    20.5.3 Hormone and Chemoprevention Strategies for Prostate Cancer
    20.5.4 Mechanisms of Resistance to Hormonal Therapies for Prostate Cancer
    20.5.5 Novel Androgen Deprivation Therapy for Prostate Cancer
20.6 Paraneoplastic Endocrine Syndromes
    20.6.1 Hypercalcemia
    20.6.2 Cushing Syndrome
    20.6.3 Syndrome of Inappropriate Antidiuretic Hormone Secretion (SIADH)
    20.6.4 Paraneoplastic Hypoglycaemia
Summary
References

20.1 INTRODUCTION

The word *hormone* was first used in Modern Medicine by the English physician Ernest Henry Starling (1866-1927), when he described the chemical messengers that travel through the body from the cells of production to a target organ. This word comes directly from the Greek verb ὁρμῶ (ormo), that means "to lunge" or "rush forward" as these messengers "rush" from the cells of origin toward the target organ. Today, the term *hormone* refers to those chemical messengers that travel through the bloodstream between cellular sites and regulate physiology and behavior. Hormones belong to 3 major classes: eicosanoids, steroids, and peptidic products. Even though isolated cells from organs such as the heart or the intestines secrete hormones and hence can be considered endocrine cells, endocrine glands are typically defined as those specific regions of the body where endocrine cells are concentrated. These regions include the hypothalamus, pituitary, thyroid, parathyroids, thymus, pancreas, pineal, adrenals, ovaries, and testes. As hormones are the only way outside of the nervous system for our organs to communicate, they are involved in almost all physiological processes including digestion, respiration, lactation, reproduction, response to stress, movement, growth, and many others. Given their ubiquitous roles in cellular physiology, it is not surprising they are also critical to both tumorigenesis and tumor progression. Many common cancer types are driven by inappropriate hormone signaling, including prostate, breast, endometrium, ovary, thyroid, testes, and bone cancers (Henderson et al, 1982). In this chapter, we will focus primarily on breast and prostate cancers to illustrate the relationship between hormones and cancer as they are among the most common causes of cancer-related death in women and men.

The relationship between prostate enlargement and hormones produced by the testes has long been recognized. Although the chemical nature of androgens was not known, it was reported in 1895 that surgical castration (orchiectomy) of elderly men with prostate enlargement, presumably due to benign prostatic hyperplasia, resulted in rapid atrophy of prostatic tissue. Following the isolation of "testosterone" as the most potent androgenic compound in the testes in 1935, Huggins and Hodges later demonstrated the efficacy of surgical orchiectomy for the treatment of metastatic prostate cancer, for which Huggins received the Nobel Prize in Physiology or Medicine in 1966. Similarly, a link between estrogen and breast cancer growth was established at the end of the 19th century, when Beatson demonstrated that removal of ovaries (oophorectomy) helped in the treatment of metastatic breast cancer in some premenopausal women. However, a molecular basis for this observation was not forthcoming until the 1960s with the discovery of the estrogen receptor, followed by the demonstrated expression of estrogen receptors in some human breast tumors by Elwood Jensen.

Evidence for a direct link between sex steroids and the carcinogenic process leading to breast and prostate tumors, was first provided by Robert Noble. He reported that prolonged exposure to estrogen, androgen, or combinations of the two, caused breast and prostate cancers in rats. More recently, the successful use of the antiestrogen tamoxifen to reduce the incidence of breast cancer in high-risk women supports a direct link between estrogen action and breast tumor formation. Similar to breast cancer, the development of prostate cancer requires the presence of androgen. Eunuchs, who cannot produce significant levels of androgens, rarely, if ever, develop prostate cancer. Therefore, these hormones not only contribute to the development of normal mammary and prostate glands, but also to the dysplastic and neoplastic processes that occur in these tissues.

This chapter will describe primarily how hormones affect cancers. We will explore the intrinsic connections existing between steroid hormones and cancers of the breast and prostate in the context of basic mechanisms of hormone action, natural history of the two diseases, and their treatment with hormonally based therapies. We will conclude with a succinct description of paraneoplastic endocrine syndromes that result from the production of hormones by various types of tumors.

20.2 BASIC MECHANISMS OF STEROID HORMONE ACTION

Breast and prostate cancer are dependent primarily on two steroid hormones for their growth and proliferation: estrogen and androgen. The bioavailability of these compounds at the site of action depends on several factors, including synthesis, transport, and expression of specific receptors within the target cell.

20.2.1 Synthesis and Metabolism of Steroid Hormones

All steroids are synthesized from the common precursor cholesterol, through a cascade of reactions involving specific enzymes (Fig. 20–1). The synthesis of a particular steroid in an endocrine gland relies on the presence of those enzymes responsible for the transition of one compound to another.

The primary site of synthesis of estrogens in premenopausal women is the para-follicular region of the ovary. Synthesis follows the menstrual cycle and is regulated via the gonad-hypothalamus-pituitary feedback axis, as indicated in Figure 20–2. In postmenopausal women, however, estrogens originate mainly in adipose tissue and skin, where androgens are converted to estradiol-17β by aromatase cytochrome P450 and 17β-hydroxysteroid dehydrogenases (Miettinen et al, 2000; Simpson, 2000).

In men, the vast majority of androgen (90%) is synthesized in Leydig cells of the testes with the remaining ~10% being made primarily in the adrenal cortex. As illustrated in Figure 20–2, most testosterone is secreted by the testes whereas the major adrenal androgens are dehydroepiandrosterone (DHEA) and its sulfate derivative. Although these adrenal hormones are weak androgens, they can be converted in other tissues to testosterone. As with estrogen synthesis in the ovary, testosterone production in the testis is regulated by a negative feedback loop involving luteinizing hormone (LH) and luteinizing hormone-releasing hormone (LHRH) via the gonad-hypothalamus-pituitary feedback axis (see Fig. 20–2). Although there are diurnal fluctuations in the secretion of androgens, their production, unlike estrogen production, does not follow a regular cyclical pattern. Also, even though there is no clear equivalent to the menopause in men, there is a progressive decrease in testosterone levels with age, which is accompanied by some degree of testicular failure.

20.2.2 Transport of Steroid Hormones in the Bloodstream

As hydrophobic molecules in an aqueous environment, most steroid hormones are transported in the blood bound to proteins, predominantly sex hormone–binding globulin (SHBG) and albumin. Only approximately 2% of total steroid hormones are in an unbound form, ultimately providing the biologically active fraction. SHBG also plays a role in permitting certain steroid hormones to act without entering the cell: estrogens and androgens bind with high affinity to SHBG, which, in turn, interacts with a specific, high-affinity receptor (SHBG-R) on cell membranes that induce a signal via a G-protein/cAMP (Kahn et al, 2002). The steroid/SHBG-R/SHBG complex generates messages that have effects on the transcriptional activity of intracellular receptors for steroid hormones.

Hormones and Cancer **489**

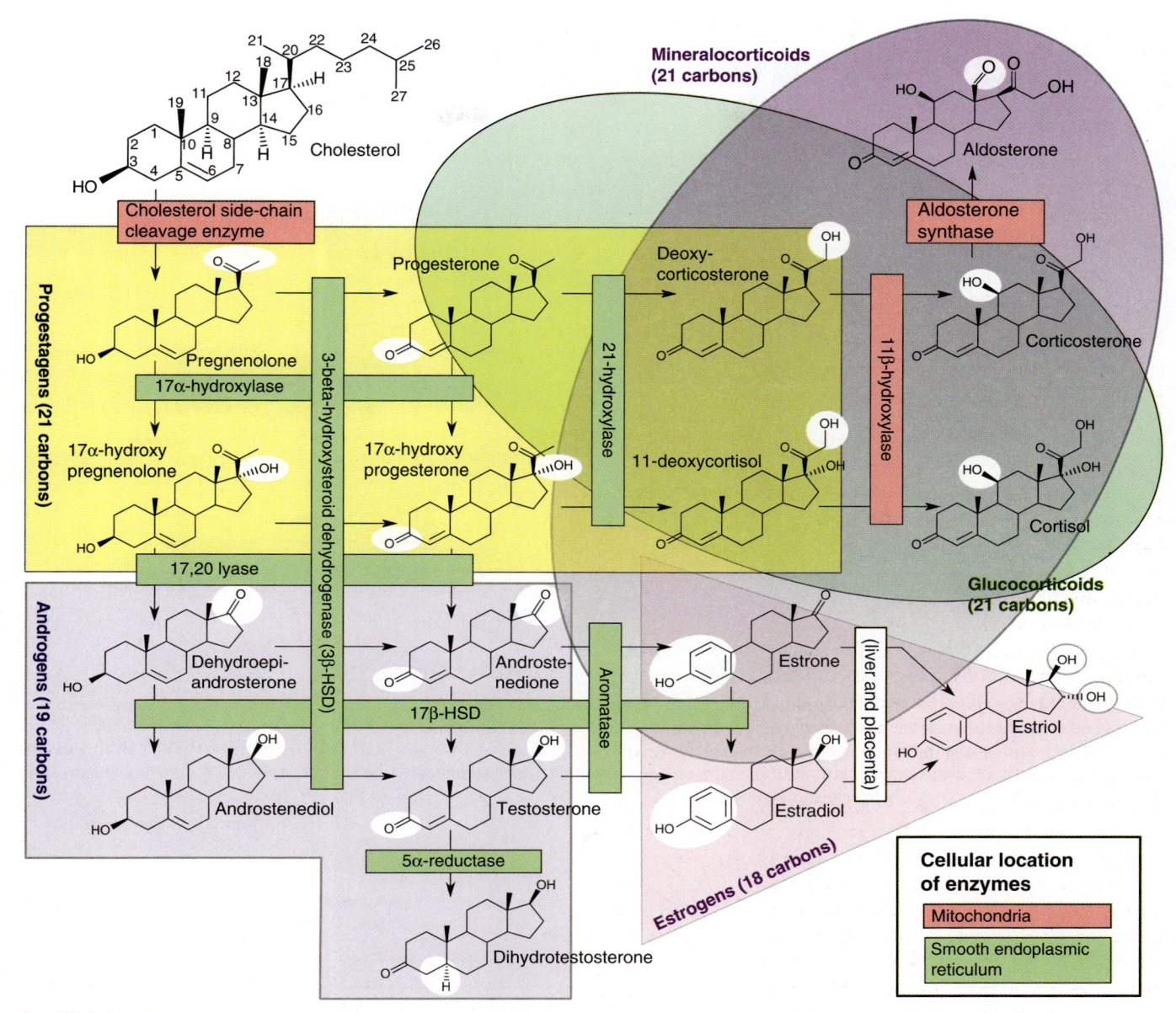

FIGURE 20–1 Steroidogenesis. Changes in molecular structure from a precursor are highlighted in white. (Reproduced with permission from Häggström M, Richfield D: Diagram of the pathways of human steroidogenesis. *WikiJournal of Medicine* 2014;1(1) https://en.wikipedia.org/wiki/File:Steroidogenesis.svg.)

Hence, SHBG not only modulates the amount of ligand available to bind to these steroid receptors but may also alter their activity through interaction with the cell membrane. Factors that influence the levels of SHBG and albumin will affect the bioactivity of steroid hormones. For example, SHBG production is stimulated by both estrogens and by the antiestrogen tamoxifen, whereas androgens and progestins have been shown to suppress it. In addition, SHBG can be expressed inside the cytoplasm of prostate cells from de novo synthesis which, through binding to steroids such as dihydrotestosterone (DHT), can affect the intracellular concentration of free androgens (Kahn et al, 2002). Once they reach their target cells, unbound steroids such as estrogens and androgens diffuse passively into the cell and act through their respective specialized steroid receptors.

20.2.3 Steroid Receptors

Steroid receptors belong to the nuclear receptor superfamily, which contains 48 members in humans. Members of this superfamily act mostly as ligand-regulated transcription factors and they share similarities with respect to their structural homology and functional properties. As shown in Figure 20–3, each member of the steroid receptor family possesses a modular structure composed of the following:

1. an N-terminal region containing ligand-independent transcriptional activating functions (collectively referred to as activating function-1 or AF1);

2. a centrally located DNA-binding domain of approximately 65 amino acids having two zinc fingers (see Chap. 6, Sec. 6.2.6);

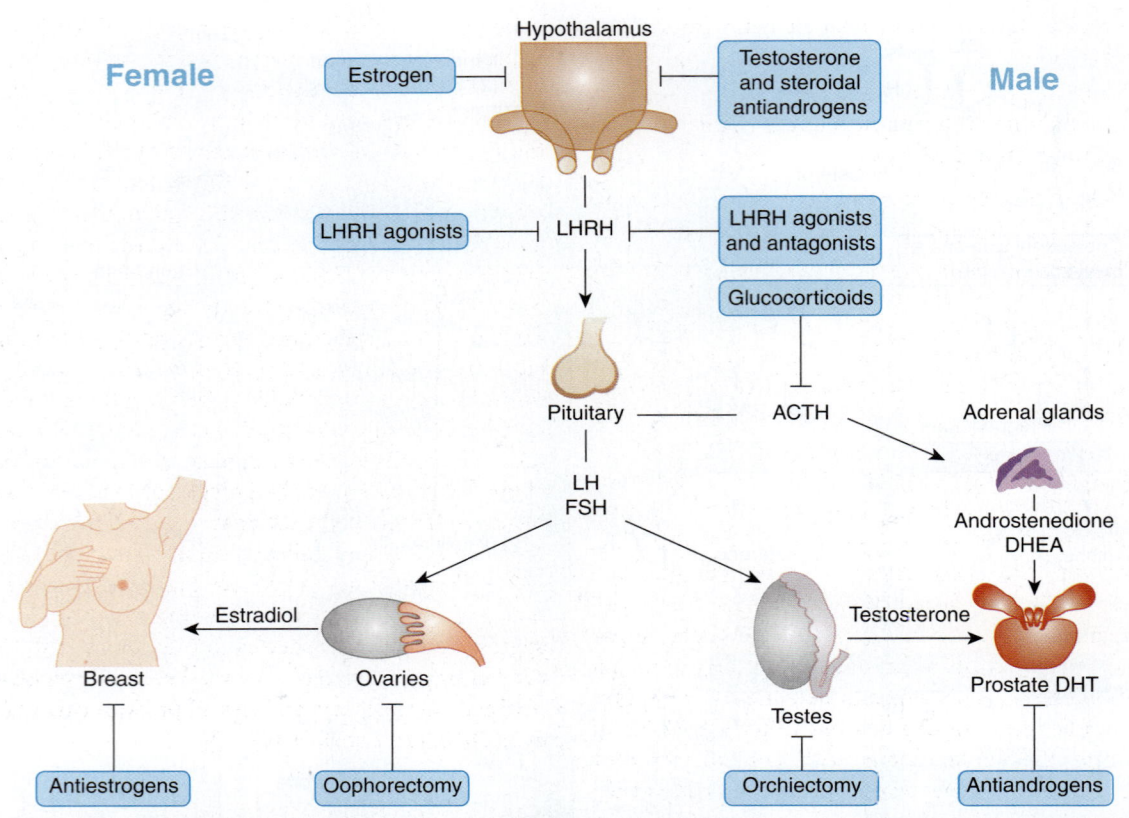

FIGURE 20–2 **The gonadal–hypothalamic–pituitary axis.** The pathways and feedback loops that regulate the production of estrogens in females and androgens in males and their target tissues are shown. The procedures and agents used for blocking the synthesis and activity of androgens and estrogens at the various steps in the pathway are highlighted. Note that luteinizing hormone–releasing hormone (LHRH) agonists initially stimulate release of luteinizing hormone (LH) followed by its inhibition. *ACTH,* adrenocorticotropic hormone; *DHEA,* dehydroepiandrosterone; *DHT,* dihydrotestosterone; *FSH,* follicle-stimulating hormone.

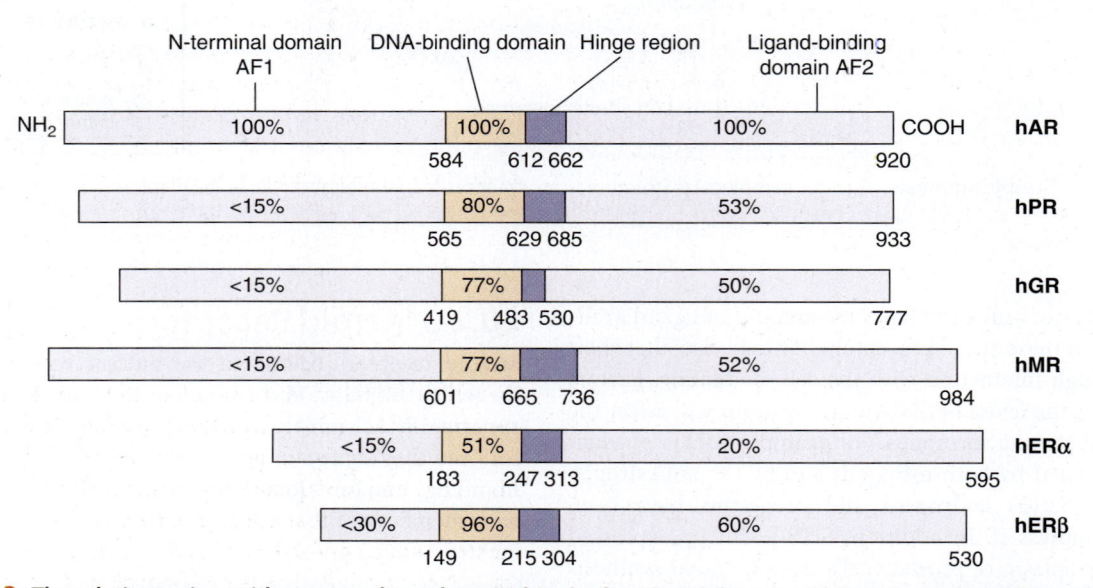

FIGURE 20–3 **The relative amino acid sequence homology within the functional domains of the principal members of the family of human (h) steroid hormone receptors.** The relative amino acid sequence homology (represented by the percentages indicated in boxes) for hERβ is in reference to hERα, whereas all the other receptors are relative to hAR. The numbers correspond to the amino acid positions from the N-terminus (NH$_2$), AF1 and AF2 refer to the transcriptional *a*ctivation *f*unction 1 and 2 that reside in the N-terminal and ligand-binding domains, respectively. *AR,* Androgen receptor; *ER,* estrogen receptor; *GR,* glucocorticoid receptor; *MR,* mineralocorticoid receptor; *PR,* progestin receptor.

3. a hinge region that contains signal elements for nuclear localization; and
4. a ligand-binding domain in the C-terminal region of the protein containing a ligand-dependent transcriptional activating function (called AF2).

AF1 and AF2, through interactions with coregulators (coactivators or corepressors), function independently or synergistically, depending on the gene promoter and/or cell context (Aranda and Pascual, 2001; Lonard and O'Malley, 2007). Between members of the family of steroid receptors, the N-terminal region has the highest degree of amino acid sequence variability, whereas the DNA-binding domain has the most shared homology.

20.2.3.1 Estrogen Receptors
There are 2 estrogen receptors (ERs), ERα and ERβ, that are encoded by 2 separate genes (see Fig. 20-3). Several variant isoforms of each ER, generated by alternative RNA splicing, may also be expressed (Murphy et al, 1998). Even though the centrally located DNA-binding domains of ERα and ERβ (see Fig. 20-3) are highly homologous (>95% identity), their ligand-binding domains are only 60% identical. This suggests that these 2 receptors likely bind similar genomic regions but differ substantially with respect to their interactions with coregulators and hence their effects on gene transcription. As with other steroid receptors, the ligand-binding domain contains a ligand-dependent dimerization function, and a ligand-dependent transactivation function, AF2. Similarly, a ligand-independent transactivation function, AF1, is present in the N-terminal domain. This latter domain is also different in ERα and ERβ. ERs are subject to multiple post-translational modifications such as phosphorylation, which can regulate receptor activity, transcriptional activity, DNA binding, protein turnover, and ligand sensitivity (Ward and Weigel, 2009). Besides these 2 classical nuclear estrogen receptors, membrane receptors recognized by estrogens have also been described. These nonclassical receptors, which correspond to either variant forms of ERα or to a G protein-coupled receptor (GPR30), are suspected to be involved in the rapid nongenomic roles played by estrogen (see Sec. 20.2.5; Arnal et al, 2017; Molina et al, 2017).

20.2.3.2 Androgen Receptor
Androgens act primarily through the androgen receptor (AR). This receptor is encoded by sequences on the X chromosome. As it is encoded by a single allele in males, it is susceptible to genetic defects that can cause phenotypes ranging from minor undervirilization to a complete female phenotype known as *androgen insensitivity syndrome*. The normal, wild-type AR has a molecular weight of approximately 110 kDa, but truncated variants have been observed in a variety of prostate cancers. These variants lack the ligand-binding domain of the AR but are still functional, even in the absence of androgen (Hu et al, 2009). In this chapter, AR refers only to the wild-type, 110-kDa form.

Relative to other steroid receptors, the AR has one of the largest N-terminal domains, which make up >50% of the 920 amino acid sequence (see Fig. 20-3). A unique feature of the AR relative to other members of this family is the occurrence of several stretches of the same amino acids (termed *homopolymeric*) in the N-terminal domain. These tracts include 17 to 29 repeating glutamine residues, starting approximately at amino acid 59, 9 proline residues at amino acid 372, and a 24-residue glycine stretch beginning at amino acid 449. These repeating tracts have been shown to modulate the folding and structural integrity of the N-terminal domain (Davies et al, 2008), and there is evidence of an inverse relationship between variations in their lengths and the transcription levels of mRNAs (Robins et al, 2008). Not surprisingly, these variations result in biological effects: for example, an abnormal extension of the polyglutamine tract to 40 or more residues is associated with neurodegenerative diseases such as X-linked spinal and bulbar muscular atrophy (La Spada et al, 1991). Older studies suggested that a decreased size of these homopolymers was associated with an increased risk or more aggressive form of prostate cancer (Stanford et al, 1997). However, in larger more-recent work, there has been no association between CAG repeats and risk of prostate cancer (Lindström et al, 2010; Price et al, 2010).

20.2.4 Classical Mechanism of Steroid Receptor Action

An overview of how steroid hormones regulate growth and differentiation of their target cells is shown in Figure 20-4. Most of the steroid hormone that enters the cell is derived from the small unbound fraction entering by passive diffusion. On entry into the cell, the steroid or its active metabolic derivative (eg, DHT) binds directly to a predominantly cytoplasmic (androgen receptor) or nuclear (estrogen receptor) steroid receptor protein. The steroid-receptor complex then undergoes an activation step involving a conformational change and shedding of heat shock (including HSP70, HSP90, and HSP40) and other chaperone proteins, which are necessary to maintain the receptor in a competent ligand-binding state (Aranda and Pascual, 2001). Activation of the androgen receptor causes an intracellular looping between the NTD and LBD that exposes a nuclear localization signal which drives the translocation of the activated nuclear receptor. Once in the nucleus, the activated androgen receptor and estrogen receptor dimerize and then bind to specific DNA motifs called hormone-responsive elements (HREs) found in the promoters/enhancer regions of hormone-regulated genes (Aranda and Pascual, 2001). The receptor-DNA complexes, in turn, associate dynamically with coactivators that create a favorable chromatin environment allowing basal transcriptional components to initiate the transcription of genes, whose messenger RNAs (mRNAs) are translated into proteins that elicit specific biological responses.

20.2.4.1 Binding of Steroid Receptors to DNA
As transcription factors, steroid receptors modulate gene

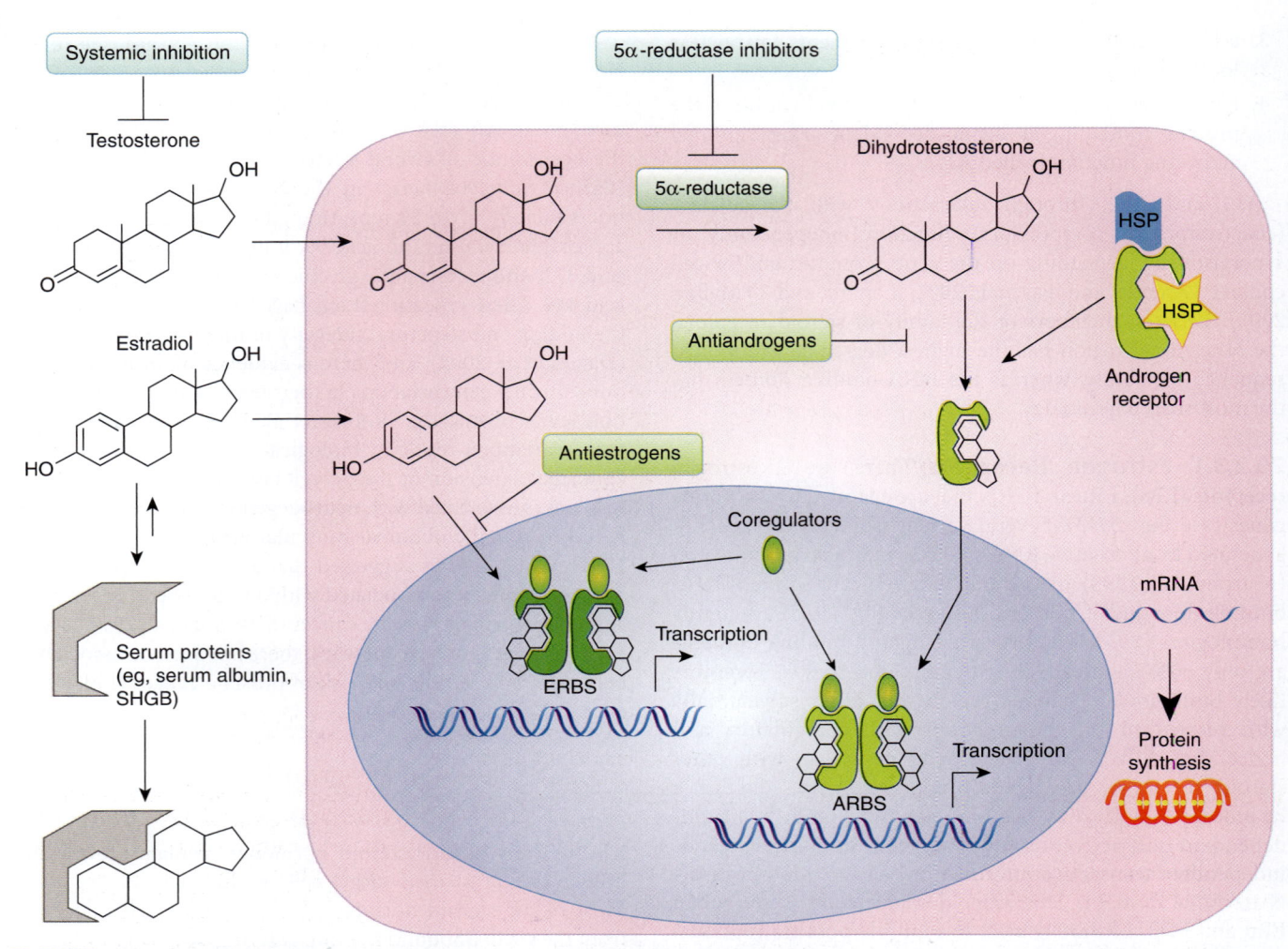

FIGURE 20–4 Schematic pathways for the classical mechanism of action of testosterone and estradiol in hormone target cells. A relatively simplistic overview of the key events in steroid hormone action with the sites at which the hormone signal can be inhibited is indicated. Although the dynamics of estrogen and androgen action are similar, testosterone is generally converted to the potent dihydrotestosterone, which binds to a cytoplasmic form of the androgen receptor and is translocated into the nucleus, whereas estradiol binds directly to its receptor in the cell nucleus. *ARE*, androgen-responsive element; *ERE*, estrogen-responsive element; *HSP*, heat shock protein; *SHBG*, sex hormone-binding globulin.

expression by first binding to specific DNA sequences in the promoter/enhancer regions of hormone-regulated genes (see Fig. 20–5). Most of hormone receptor binding sites are located in enhancers rather than promoters. The α-helix structure of the first zinc finger of the DNA-binding domain of a receptor is the primary discriminator for binding to different DNA sequence motifs of HREs (Aranda and Pascual, 2001). Members of the nuclear receptor family typically bind as dimers to pairs of a similar DNA sequence motif, AGNNCA (N = any nucleotide), which comprises the HRE found in the promoters of steroid regulated genes (Glass, 1994). Steroid receptors can also bind as homodimers or associated complexes to multiple enhancers that are often hundreds of kilobase pairs distal to target genes. These bound sites induce gene transcription by chromosomal looping to the proximal promoter and subsequent activation of RNA polymerase II through the mediator complex (Fullwood et al, 2009). Nuclear receptors can be further subdivided based on the primary sequence of their DNA-binding motif; AGGTCA for the ER and thyroid receptor subfamily, and AGAACA for the AR, glucocorticoid receptor (GR), or progestin receptor (PR). In general, 2 or more sets of interacting HREs in a regulatory element are required to elicit a steroid-mediated response (Rennie et al, 1993; Klinge, 1999).

The very high sequence homology of HREs has raised the question as to how steroid receptors govern hormone-specific responses. Although there is no definitive answer, the interaction with unique combinations of coregulators, pioneer factors, epigenetic modifications, and other binding proteins that are cell-specific likely alters steroid-receptor specific gene regulation. Other parameters may also be important, such as the availability of receptor and ligand, the activity of proximal transcription factors, the cooperative binding of receptors to 2 or more DNA-binding sites, and altered DNA target motif recognition.

20.2.4.2 Interaction of Steroid Receptors with Coregulator Proteins
Nuclear receptors regulate gene

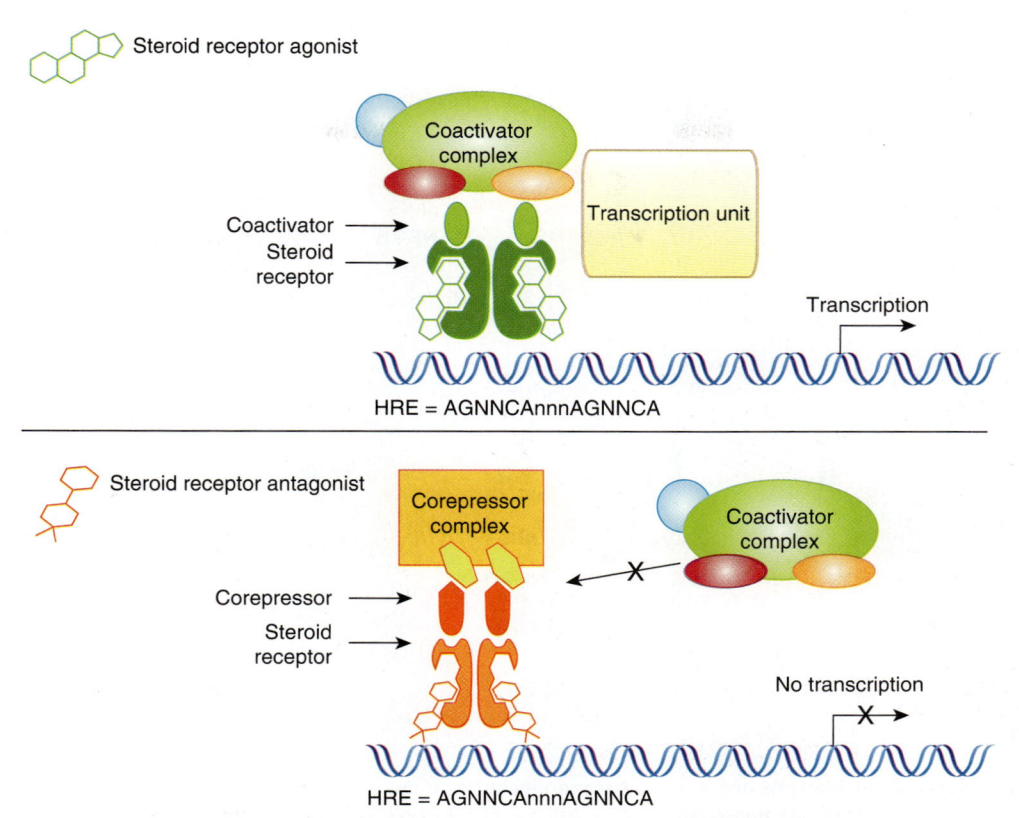

FIGURE 20–5 **Illustration of the role of coactivators and corepressor in regulation of steroid receptor action.** In the presence of agonistic ligands (eg, estradiol for estrogen receptor [ER] and DHT for androgen receptor [AR]), the steroid receptor-DNA complexes associate dynamically with coactivators, which, in turn, recruit other proteins, forming a large coactivator complex. This complex can have multiple chromatin remodeling activities. Some coregulators have histone acetyl-transferase (HAT) activity, which results in dynamic nucleosomal histone acetylation and increased access of basal transcription complexes (that include RNA polymerase II) to the promoters of target genes. In the presence of antagonistic ligands (eg, tamoxifen for ER and bicalutamide for AR), the receptors are in a different conformational state) and the receptor-DNA complexes dynamically associate with corepressors (Co-R) with histone deacetyl-transferase (HDAC) activities, which condense chromatin and destabilize basal transcription units. This results in reduced transcription of target genes. *HRE*, hormone-responsive element.

transcription mainly through the recruitment of coregulator protein complexes to the enhancer regions of target genes (Stashi et al, 2014; see Fig. 20–5). Coregulators fall into 2 main classes, coactivators and corepressors, which enhance or repress transcription, respectively.

Although the auxiliary molecular components involved and the exact dynamics of their interactions remain to be identified, a general pattern has emerged. The coactivators and corepressors mediate both AF1 and AF2 activities of steroid receptors. Their mechanism of transcriptional activation is thought to involve 2 stages (Perissi and Rosenfeld, 2005; Rosenfeld et al, 2006). First, when recruited to the receptor by direct protein-protein binding, coregulators promote the local remodeling of chromatin structure directly through acetyltransferase or deacetylase activity and through their ability to recruit other proteins with chromatin remodeling activity. Second, cofactor complexes recruit and/or stabilize the basal transcription machinery by protein-protein interactions so as to enable efficient transcription of the target gene by RNA polymerase II (Perissi and Rosenfeld, 2005). Overall, it is suspected that receptors that are not bound to their ligands, or those bound to antagonists (Fig. 20–5), form complexes with corepressors that inversely inhibit the transcription of specific genes.

It is uncertain which coactivators are necessary or sufficient for transcriptional activation. In MCF-7 breast cancer cells ERα and a number of coactivators associate rapidly with target promoters in an extremely dynamic, cyclic fashion and the SRC/NCOA/p160 class of coactivators is sufficient for gene activation (Shang et al, 2000; Metivier et al, 2003). It is likely that the relative availability of coregulators will vary in different tissues and may even be restricted to specific tissues. Also, although the occurrence of receptor-specific coregulators has not been confirmed, many coregulators bind preferentially to certain receptors. For example, a repressor of ER transcriptional activity, called *r*epressor of *e*strogen receptor *a*ctivity (REA) is active on ERα or ERβ but not other steroid receptors (Montano et al, 1999). Its mechanism of action involves a competition with coactivators such as SRC-1 (Wang et al, 2016) for binding to the ligand-binding domain of ER. Furthermore, a member of the SRC/NCOA family, SRC-3/NCOA3 or *a*mplified *i*n *b*reast *c*ancer 1 (AIB1) may have a role in breast cancer as it is amplified and overexpressed in some

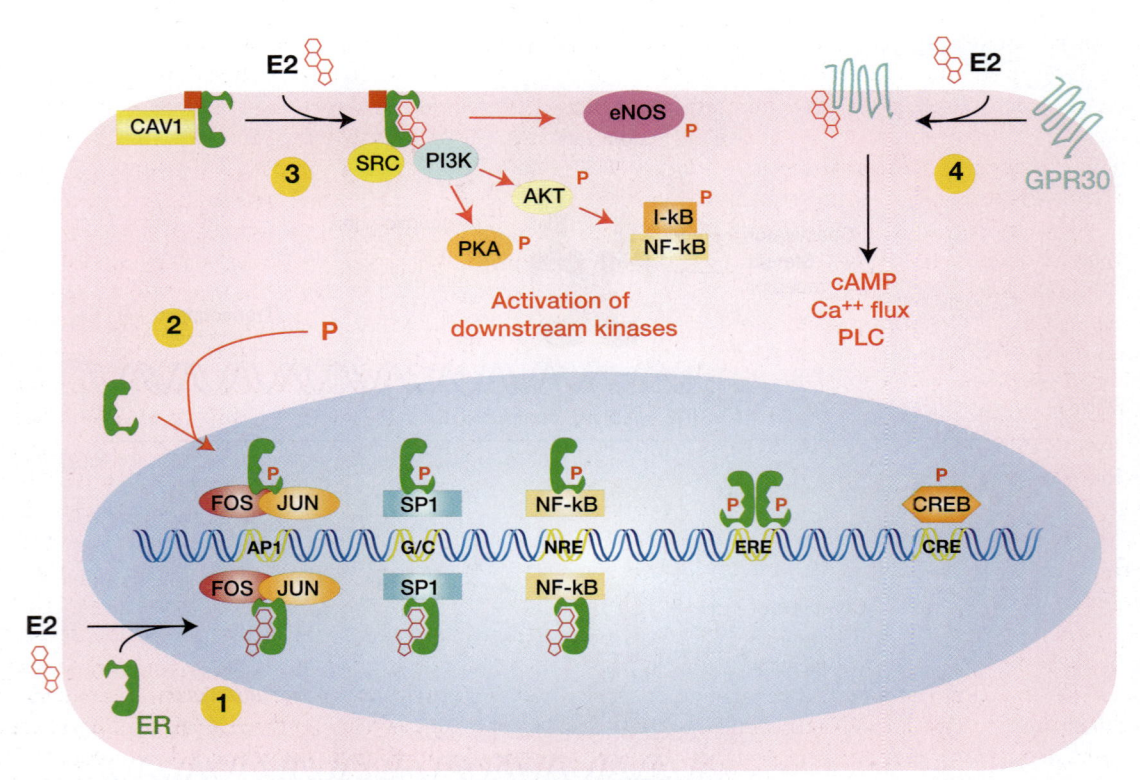

FIGURE 20–6 Non classical mechanisms of action of estrogen receptor. 1- Once activated upon binding of estrogen (E2), the estrogen receptor (green ER) can be recruited by other transcription factors (such as FOS-JUN, SP1 or NF-kB) on their respective DNA response elements (AP1: 5'-ATGAGTCAT-3', G/C box: 5'-G/T-GGGCGG-G/A-G/A-C/T-3', NRE: 5'-GGG-A/G-NN-T/C-T/C-CC-3') to control the transcription of genes devoid of Estrogen responsive element. **2-** Alternatively, Phosphorylation specific events (red arrows, red P) are sufficient to activate the estrogen receptor in the absence of ligand. **3-** Nongenomic pathways or rapid effect, have also been described, which can involve a small pool of ER, palmitoylated (red square) on Cys 447 and interacting with caveolin-1 (CAV1). Upon E2 activation and interactions with protein kinases (SRC and PI3K), a cascade of rapid phosphorylations is started which involves kinases (AKT, PKA), transcription factors (I-kB, NF-kB, CREB) and the endothelial NO synthase (eNOS). **4-** Interestingly, a G-Protein-coupled receptor (GPR30), activated upon binding of estrogen and inducing Calcium and cAMP releases as well as Phospholipase C activation, has also been involved in the rapid non genomic effect of Estrogens. CRE: cAMP-response element: 5'-TGACGTCA-3'.

breast tumors and such overexpression has been correlated with tamoxifen resistance (Xu et al, 2009).

20.2.5 Nonclassical Mechanisms of Steroid Receptor Action

In addition to the classical mechanism of action described above, which involves the induced transcription of target genes following the ligand-dependent recruitment of receptor homodimers on regulatory DNA sequence, steroid receptors have been found to act through other mechanisms (Fig. 20–6).

First, ligand-activated steroid receptors can induce transcription of target genes without contacting the DNA directly, through protein-protein interactions with other transcription factors that are themselves in direct contact with DNA via their own specific response elements (Ratman et al, 2013; Arnal et al, 2017). Thus, steroid receptors can tether other transcription factors to modulate positively or negatively their activity. For example, ERα can interact with SP1 or AP-1 (FOS-JUN) transcription factors and activate the transcription of genes such as RARα, insulin-like growth factor-binding protein–4 or transforming growth factor α (see Chap. 6, Sec. 6.2.6). This mechanism appears to be very common, as the majority of the DNA sites where AR/ER bind do not contain a classical HRE sequence. Intriguingly, recent studies have demonstrated that AR binding can induce expression of enhancer RNAs that act as transregulatory elements able to alter gene expression at different chromosomal locations (Hsieh et al, 2014).

ER and AR can also be activated without ligand through crosstalk with a variety of growth factor networks (Levin and Hammes, 2016). Growth factors such as epidermal growth factor (EGF) and/or insulin-like growth factor (IGF)–1 bind to their respective tyrosine kinase receptors located in the plasma membrane of target cells and activate signal transduction pathways involving activation of other kinases; these events can lead to phosphorylation of steroid receptors. For example, mitogen-activated protein kinase (MAPK) that is activated by growth factor signaling (see Chap. 6, Sec. 6.2.4) can directly phosphorylate both ERs and the AR. Similarly, interleukin-6 and protein kinase A can activate the AR and ERα directly in the absence of the appropriate steroid ligand. Interleukin-6 may also bind to and influence AR activity without inducing phosphorylation of the AR. In addition, growth factor/phosphorylation pathways have the ability to influence steroid hormone receptor signaling via their ability to modulate coactivators by phosphorylation (Han et al, 2009). As discussed later, these alternative pathways for regulation of ER and AR activity could have a profound influence on the emergence of hormone independence in tumors that have not lost their hormone receptors.

There is further evidence that not all effects of steroid hormones are mediated via the regulation of genomic or transcriptional events. Transcription-independent effects of estrogen occur rapidly in target cells, within seconds to a few minutes. For estrogen, examples of nongenomic effects include modulation of calcium ion flux, effects on membrane channels in the central nervous system and peripheral excitable cells, membrane-associated interactions with growth factor receptors, and interactions with survival/apoptosis pathways. There is evidence that membrane-associated ERs coupled to G proteins or nitric oxide–generating systems mediate some of these actions. Other steroid hormones such as progesterone and testosterone may also influence cells via related mechanisms.

The overall importance of nontranscriptional actions of estrogen and androgen in cancer remains unknown. There are multiple levels of estrogen interaction with growth factor receptor kinases and the signal transduction pathways that they regulate. Therefore, nongenomic and genomic actions of estrogen are likely to be integrated with and complementary to each other. Unraveling this molecular complexity has important implications with respect to new therapeutic combinations and approaches (Arpino et al, 2008). High-throughput experiments, which combine the power of chromatin immunoprecipitation, global run on and deep sequencing are starting to shed light on the highly complex relationship between steroid receptors and gene transcription (Hah and Kraus, 2014; Pomerantz et al, 2015). Understanding the molecular events triggered by hormones in cancer cells is critical to identifying new pharmacologic targets to fight these diseases.

20.2.6 Quantification of Steroid Hormone Receptor

ERα and PR are biomarkers in breast cancer and can help predict the likelihood of response to endocrine therapy. In a population of breast cancer patients with advanced disease, 30% to 40% will respond to endocrine therapy. If the primary breast tumor is both ERα and PR positive, 70% to 80% of women will respond positively. Yet if the cancer is both ERα and PR negative, only <10% will respond to endocrine therapy. In prostate cancer, the AR status does not provide a similar predictive power, as almost all tumors are sensitive to endocrine therapy (~90%). Assessing AR expression therefore does not provide any prognostic or diagnostic value in primary cancer because nearly all tumors possess a functioning AR and will be affected by androgen withdrawal. AR expression is, however, important when diagnosing neuroendocrine prostate cancer (see Sec. 20.5.3).

ERα and PR are measured routinely in breast cancer biopsies by immunohistochemistry (IHC) using well-characterized, specific monoclonal antibodies, as outlined in Figure 20–7A. IHC methods (Fitzgibbons et al, 2010; Hammond et al, 2010) can both determine the receptor expression as well as assess its heterogeneity in tumor tissue. An example of ER heterogeneity within a breast tumor is shown in Figure 20–7B. Heterogeneity refers to the observation that both ER-positive and ER-negative breast cancer cells can be present to varying degrees within any breast cancer biopsy sample, in addition to the presence of other types of cells (vascular cells, infiltrating cells of the immune system, normal stromal fibroblasts, normal breast adipocytes, and normal breast epithelial cells). Semiquantitative methods are used to evaluate ER and PR by IHC, with positive results generally reported when more than 1% of tumor nuclei stain positively (Hammond et al, 2010). There is a correlation between benefit and increasing ER level, which can be assessed by combining the level of staining intensity (1 low, 2 medium, 3 high) with the percentage (1%-100%) of tumor cells positively stained to give H-scores or Allred scores (Brouckaert et al, 2013). Results can vary, however, among laboratories, especially in the low to middle range of the receptor spectrum. In order to homogenize results across centers, guidelines for standard operating procedures for tissue collection, assay validation, quality control, and interpretation have been published (Fitzgibbons et al, 2010; Hammond et al, 2010; Duffy et al, 2017). Ultimately, assessment of hormone receptor status relies on the critical "reading/interpretation" of stained tumor tissues by a trained pathologist. This remains time consuming and still subject to individual variations. Intense research remains underway, which aims at automatizing the whole process, from staining to interpretation of results (Zarrella et al, 2016; Ahern et al, 2017).

ER and PR can also be assayed at their mRNA levels, usually as a part of a multiple genes signature assessment of the tumor. This is now routinely assessed as part of a 21-gene (Oncotype DX) or 70-gene (Mammaprint) expression analysis using reverse transcription and quantitative polymerase chain reaction technology (see Chap. 2, Sec. 2.2.5). These assays are critical, as they help predict the benefit of adding or not chemotherapy to hormonal therapy in women with ERα breast cancer (Sparano et al, 2015; Cardoso et al, 2016). The use of such tests has been associated with a decreased use of adjuvant chemotherapy (Bhutiani et al, 2018).

20.3 NATURAL HISTORY OF BREAST AND PROSTATE CANCER

20.3.1 Risk Factors for Breast and Prostate Cancer

20.3.1.1 Risk Factors for Breast Cancer Female gender and increasing age are the major risk factors for human breast cancer. However, all factors that increase the cumulative exposure to estrogen have been established as positive risk factors. These include not only early menarche and late menopause but also obesity in postmenopausal women as adipose tissue is the main source of estrogen in postmenopausal women. Factors that reduce the cumulative exposure to estrogens, such as early first pregnancy, multiple full-term pregnancies, oophorectomy in premenopausal

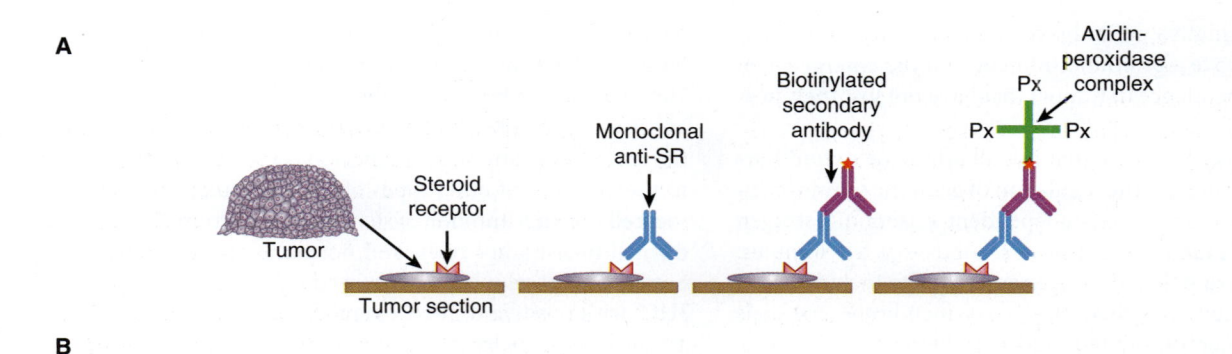

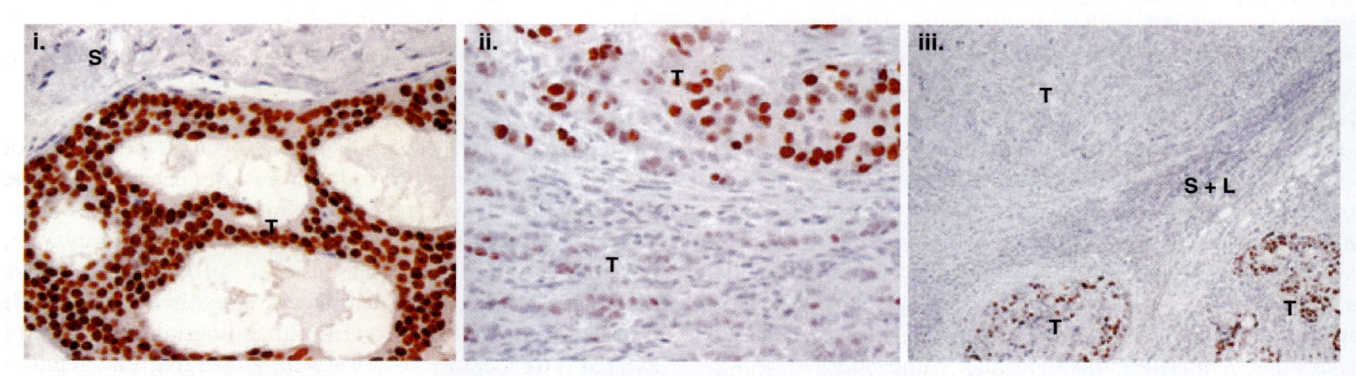

FIGURE 20–7 Immunohistochemical–avidin-biotin complex method. **A)** Determination of hormone receptors in tumor tissue. Thin sections of tumor are cut from formalin-fixed, paraffin-embedded biopsy specimens. The section is next exposed to a monoclonal antibody specific for the steroid receptor (SR) being assessed. The section is then exposed to a second biotinylated antibody specific for the first antibody. Finally, avidin-peroxidase complex is added, followed by a chromogen, and color appears where the SR is located. **B)** Immunohistograms illustrating heterogeneity of human breast cancer biopsy samples. Brown staining represents ERα positivity. *T*, invasive breast cancer; *S*, stromal and connective tissue elements; *L*, lymphocytes. **(i)** Homogenous expression of ERα within an invasive breast cancer, with negative adjacent vessels and stroma. **(ii)** Moderate heterogeneity of expression of ERα within an invasive breast cancer, with strong expression within solid nests of tumor cells in the upper field and weak or negative expression within less-cohesive clusters of tumor cells in the lower field. Stromal and lymphocytic elements are negative for ERα. **(iii)** Marked heterogeneity of expression of ERα within an invasive tumor metastatic to an axillary lymph node. In the upper part of the section one metastatic component is homogenously ERα –ve and in the lower part of the section, the other component is moderate to highly ERα +ve. These 2 different elements are separated in this field of view by a band of fibrous stroma and infiltrating lymphocytes.

women, and physical activity, are associated with a reduced risk of breast cancer. Consistent with these observations, increased serum levels of estrogens are associated with postmenopausal breast cancer. Use of hormone replacement therapies in menopausal women, particularly those that combine estrogen and progestin, also increases the risk of breast cancer (Banks et al, 2008).

Breast cancer is influenced by genetic factors as women with a family history of breast cancer are at increased risk of the disease. Women that carry a germline mutation within genes that encode the DNA repair proteins *BRCA1* and *BRCA2* present with an inherited predisposition to breast cancer (see Chap. 9, Sec. 9.5). However, only 5% of all breast cancers can be attributed to inherited mutations in these genes and less than 10% overall can be attributed to an inherited predisposition. Therefore, environmental factors are very important for the development of breast cancer. This is highlighted by the observation that Asian women who have migrated to Western countries have an increased rate of breast cancer in a few generations (Ziegler et al, 1993). Most breast cancers are sporadic, although polymorphisms in genes associated with the biosynthesis of estrogens (Thompson and Ambrosone, 2000) and factors that regulate ER activity such as the AR (Giguere et al, 2001) may influence breast cancer development.

The major role of estrogen in breast cancer is thought to result from its proliferative effect on breast epithelium. However, a complex interplay of steroid hormones, growth factors, extracellular matrix, and their respective receptors is likely involved. Genotoxic effects of steroids cannot be excluded, although the relative roles of the different mechanisms remain unclear (Lin et al, 2009; Pauklin et al, 2009).

20.3.1.2 Risk Factors for Prostate Cancer

Carcinogenesis of the prostate involves genetic and environmental influences, but no obvious etiologic agent has been identified. Risk factors include family history, age, and race (Hsing and Chokkalingam, 2006). First-degree male relatives of prostate cancer patients diagnosed younger than 60 years have an approximately 4-fold increase in risk, and those men with relatives who have breast cancer have a higher risk of prostate cancer. Men carrying germline mutations of genes involved in DNA repair, especially *BRCA2*, have an increased risk of developing more aggressive prostate cancer compared to noncarriers (Pritchard et al, 2016). Hereditary factors affect most commonly men with early-onset disease and are responsible for relatively few cases (<10%). Diet may also be important in prostate cancer development as, similar to breast cancer, the high consumption of red meat in a North American diet is associated with an increased risk of prostate cancer (Denis et al, 1999). The association of obesity with numerous hormonal changes that influence endocrine pathways may also contribute to prostate cancer development and progression (Calle and Kaaks, 2004).

Prostate cancer is a disease of the elderly, with more than 75% of cancers diagnosed in men older than 65 years. However, microfoci of high-grade prostatic intraepithelial neoplasia (PIN), the presumed precursor of the disease, can be found in men in their third and fourth decade of life. Most of the early tumors are microscopic, generally well to moderately differentiated, and tend to be multifocal. The frequency with which these neoplastic lesions are seen in autopsy material is similar among African Americans, European Americans, and Japanese men, but the incidence of clinical disease is higher in African American men and lower in Japanese men. However, in Japanese immigrants, the incidence of prostate cancer rises to levels near those of European Americans within 2 generations, suggesting the involvement of diet or environmental factors. Collectively, these observations suggest that the critical event in the natural history of prostate cancer is tumor promotion rather than tumor initiation, and that promotion and progression of this cancer are strongly influenced by epigenetic or hormonal signaling.

20.3.2 Development and Progression of Breast and Prostate Cancers

20.3.2.1 Development and Progression of Breast Cancer
Cellular events associated with the natural history of breast cancer are depicted in Figure 20–8A. Most invasive breast cancers arise from the epithelial cells of the terminal duct lobular unit (TDLU). Histopathological studies have identified a series of premalignant breast lesions referred to as hyperplasia without atypia, usual ductal hyperplasia (UDH), atypical hyperplasia (AH), and ductal carcinoma in situ (DCIS). Each of these lesions is associated with an increased risk of developing invasive breast cancer. For example, AH is associated with a 5-fold increased risk, and DCIS is associated with a 10-fold increased risk (Page et al, 2000).

Normal development of the mammary gland is dependent on the presence of ERα. Mice lacking the gene encoding ERα (*Esr1*) form only a small rudimentary ductal remnant (Korach, 1994). However, only 7% to 17% of normal human breast epithelial cells express ERα by immunochemistry (Clarke et al, 1997). In contrast, more than 70% of human breast tumors are ER-alpha positive (ERα+). Most hyperplastic lesions, with or without atypia, show increased expression of ERα and increased frequency of ER+ cells compared to normal epithelium. Similarly, more than 70% of DCIS are ERα+, similar to invasive breast cancer (Allred and Mohsin, 2000). In normal breast epithelial cells, ERα and Ki67, a marker of cell proliferation, are rarely, if ever, coexpressed (Anderson et al, 1998); this finding suggests that either ERα-expressing cells are incapable of proliferating or that ERα must be downregulated before

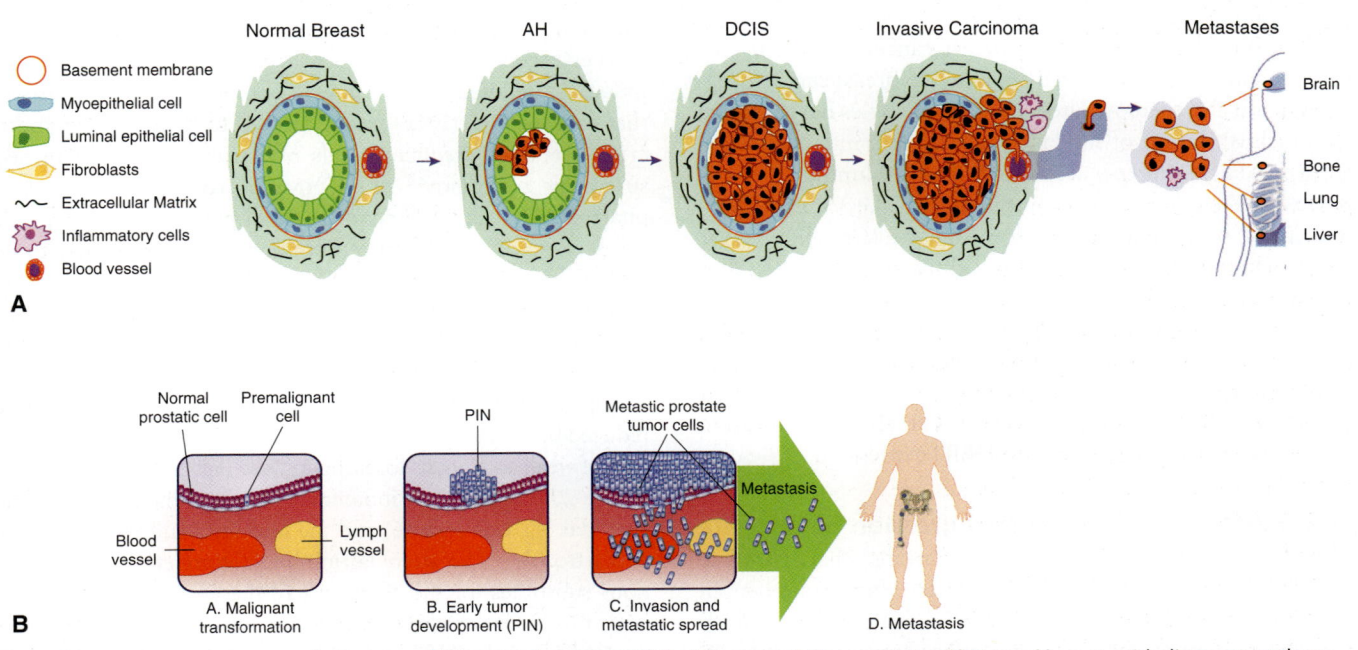

FIGURE 20–8 An overview of the natural history of cancers of the breast and the prostate. **A)** Normal breast epithelium can undergo a stepwise transition from a series of premalignant breast lesions referred to as atypical hyperplasia (AH), and ductal carcinoma in situ (DCIS) leading to invasive carcinoma and metastasis. **B)** A normal prostate epithelial cell can develop into a premalignant tumor cell that can give rise to prostatic intraepithelial neoplasia (PIN), and then become an invasive carcinoma.

normal breast epithelial cells can proliferate. This inverse relationship between growth and ERα expression is maintained in UDH, but is lost in AH, DCIS, and ERα+ invasive breast cancer cells (Shoker et al, 1999). Thus, an alteration in estrogen responsiveness and/or mechanism of estrogen action occurs during the development of breast cancer.

ERβ, which is also expressed in both normal and neoplastic human breast tissues (Leygue et al, 1998; Roger et al, 2001), does not seem to play a pivotal role in the development of the mammary gland. Indeed, mice disrupted for the gene encoding ERβ (*Esr2*) develop a fully functional duct system (Couse and Korach, 1999). Expression of ERβ, which is higher than that of ERα in the normal human breast, tends to generally decline during breast cancer development (Leygue et al, 1998; Roger et al, 2001).

Until recently, the standard molecular classifiers of breast cancers employed to select patients for specific treatments were the presence or absence of ERα, the progesterone receptor (PR), and HER2/ErbB2. In the presence of ERα, the tumor still depends on estrogen for its growth, and these cancers are more likely to respond to estrogen withdrawal therapies. The presence of the PR, a target gene of ER, implies that ER signaling is functional in these tumors. Similarly, an overexpressed/amplified HER2 reflects a dependence on this growth factor receptor for proliferation. HER2/ErbB2 is amplified and/or overexpressed in up to 20% of all breast tumors, and these tumors are aggressive and traditionally had a poor outcome. The development of humanized antibodies (eg, trastuzumab) targeting HER2 has improved the outcome for these patients (Di Cosimo and Baselga, 2010). Unfortunately, not all ERα+ tumors respond to hormone therapy and not all HER2/ErbB2 amplified lesions decrease on trastuzumab treatment. Molecular profiling technologies are being used to find additional markers for classifying human breast cancer to provide the basis of a more individualized approach to breast cancer prognostication and therapy. These new technologies have resulted in the classification of human breast tumors into 6 different subtypes. These subtypes are called luminal A, luminal B, HER2 overexpressing, basal-like, normal breast-like (Sorlie, 2004) and, most recently, a claudin-low subtype (Creighton et al, 2010). These different subtypes are clinically relevant as they are associated with different clinical outcomes. ERα and PR are expressed in the luminal A and B subtypes, although about half of the HER2-overexpressing subtype also can express ERα. However, these molecular classifications remain research tools and are not yet used routinely in clinical practice, in contrast to the determination of ER, PR, and HER2 expression.

20.3.2.2 Development and Progression of Prostate Cancer

The two pathological conditions that correlate frequently with latent and clinical prostate cancer are benign prostatic hyperplasia (BPH) and PIN. BPH shares many biologic properties with prostate cancer, including androgen regulation of growth and increasing prevalence with advancing age. However, BPH is not a premalignant lesion and does not increase the risk of cancer. A more likely source that leads to initiation of prostate cancer is PIN. This is characterized by cytologic atypia of proliferating luminal epithelium within preexisting acini and ducts with no penetration of the basement membrane (see Fig. 20–8*B*). A wide spectrum of molecular/genetic abnormalities is common to both high-grade PIN and prostate cancer including expression of the AR in the luminal epithelium (Sakr and Partin, 2001; Vukovic et al, 2007). In addition to being a precursor for prostate cancer, it is likely that PIN predates invasive cancer by at least a decade and thus may serve as a predictive marker for the disease.

Although questions still remain about the hypothesis, there is increasing evidence that prostate and other cancers may arise as a consequence of genetic alterations in a stem cell population (Lawson and Witte, 2007; see Chap. 13, Sec. 13.3.2). The longevity of stem cells makes them more likely to develop genetic alterations over time that may eventually culminate in cancer. Moreover, unlike mature prostate cells, primitive stem cells can thrive under androgen depletion as these cells are not believed to express AR (Wang et al, 2009; Packer and Maitland 2016). This therefore introduces an intriguing model whereby cancer stem cells can repopulate the tumor following hormone therapy. These findings may be of critical importance to identify novel therapeutic approaches for future clinical management.

20.4 BREAST CANCER: HORMONAL THERAPIES AND RESISTANCE

20.4.1 Hormonal Therapy

Endocrine therapies for patients with ER+ breast cancer are aimed at inhibiting the proliferative effect of estrogen on breast cancer cells. As outlined in Figure 20–2, this aim can be achieved in 2 ways: decreasing the level of circulating and/or local estrogen, or blocking the action of estrogen on the target tissue. As detailed in Section 20.2.6, only those breast tumors that express ERα (ERα+) are expected to benefit from endocrine therapies. Reduced levels of estrogen can be achieved surgically, by removal of the ovaries (oophorectomy), and pharmacologically. Premenopausal women can either opt for surgical or radiation-induced oophorectomy, or choose to be treated with LHRH agonists, which initially stimulate and then block the LHRH receptor in the pituitary gland; this leads to a reduction in levels of gonadotrophins, which stimulate the ovary to synthesize estrogens.

In postmenopausal women, residual levels of estrogen can be reduced by selective aromatase inhibitors that inhibit the conversion of weak androgens to estrogens (see Fig. 20–1). As shown in Figure 20–9, aromatase inhibitors fall into 2 main classes—the steroidal (eg, exemestane) and the nonsteroidal (eg, anastrozole and letrozole). The steroidal inhibitors compete with endogenous substrates for the active site of the enzyme, and are processed to intermediates that bind irreversibly to the active site, causing inhibition. The nonsteroidal inhibitors also compete with the endogenous substrates for the active site, but form a strong, although reversible, coordinate bond with the heme iron atom, excluding endogenous substrates and oxygen from the enzyme. Removal of the nonsteroidal inhibitor results in reversal

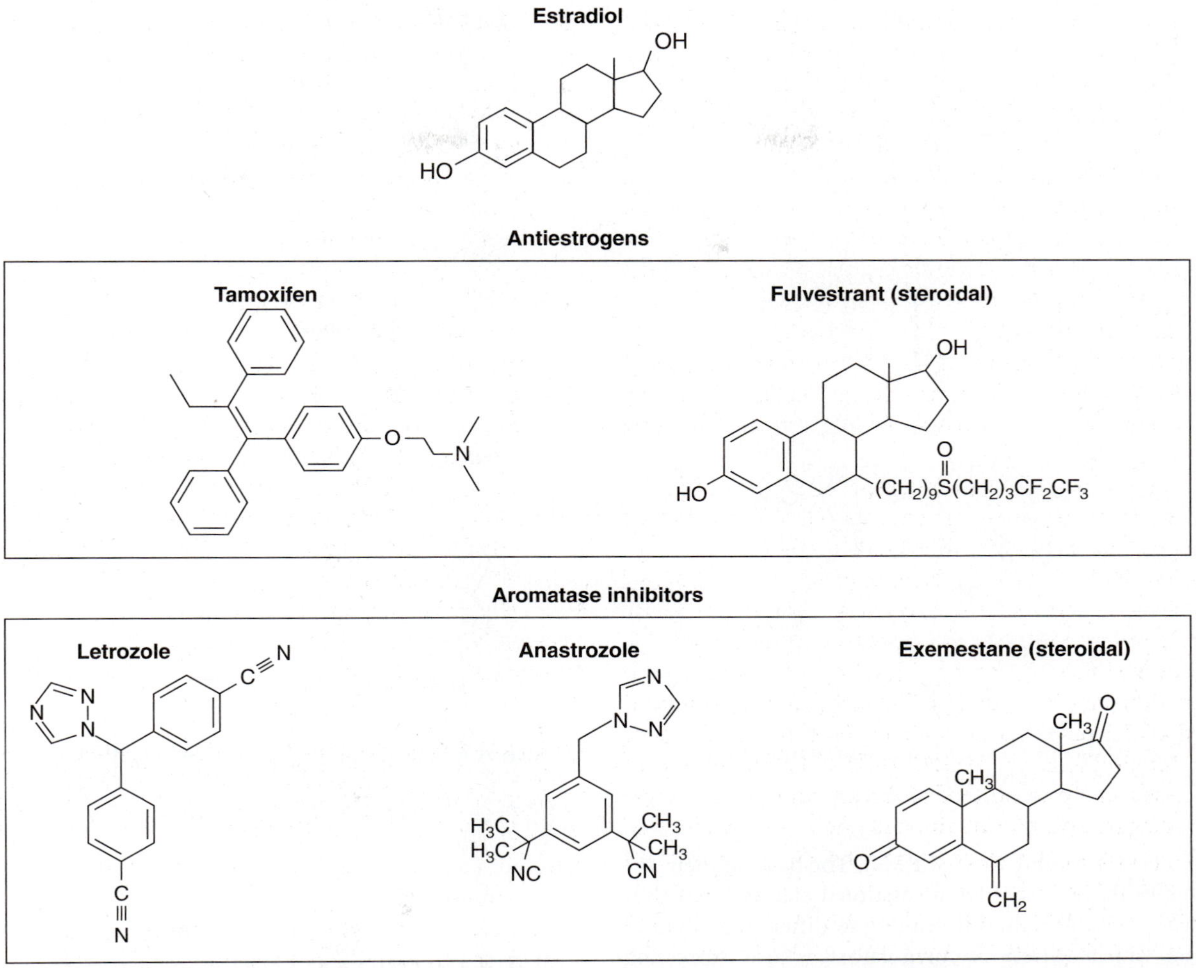

FIGURE 20–9 Structures of antiestrogens and aromatase inhibitors. The antiestrogens block estrogen binding to its receptor, and the steroidal forms also increase turnover of the receptor protein. The aromatase inhibitors block the formation of estrogens from androgen precursors.

of enzyme inhibition. These agents are preferred alternatives to tamoxifen (see below) as first-line treatment of postmenopausal women. Aromatase inhibitors are not effective alone in premenopausal women with ERα+ breast cancer: the aromatase inhibitor-induced reduction in plasma estrogen decreases the negative feed-back loop and ultimately increases follicle-stimulating hormone (FSH), which increases estrogen secretion by the ovary.

The nonsteroidal antiestrogen tamoxifen has been for decades the agent of choice for first-line endocrine therapy for the treatment of ER+ breast cancer (see Fig. 20–9). Tamoxifen leads to improved survival when used as adjuvant therapy for women of all ages with ERα+ breast cancer, and also decreases the incidence of breast cancer in women at high risk for the disease. Tamoxifen and its more active metabolites, 4-hydroxytamoxifen and N-Desmethyl-4-hydroxy-tamoxifen (endoxifen), inhibit competitively the binding of estradiol to the ligand-binding site of the ER in a dose-dependent manner. Because tamoxifen requires metabolism to more active metabolites, alterations in the activity of the enzymes responsible for its metabolism (Fig. 20–10) may affect an individual's responsiveness to tamoxifen. As discussed below, alterations in this metabolism can be involved in resistance to endocrine therapy.

When tamoxifen or similar compounds bind to the ER, they cause conformational changes that allow the inactive receptor to bind to DNA but not to activate transcription (see Fig. 20–11). X-ray crystallography studies of the ER ligand domain bound to either estradiol or 4-hydroxytamoxifen show that estradiol binding causes formation of a hydrophobic cleft on the surface of this domain that serves as a docking site for coactivators. In contrast, antiestrogens displace this part of the receptor, thereby blocking coactivator access (Shiau et al, 1998). Compounds like tamoxifen have both estrogenic and antiestrogenic properties, depending on the cell type or the promoter of any particular target gene. Because tamoxifen neutralizes the ligand-dependent AF-2 activation domain but not the DNA binding of the estrogen receptor, it is believed that estrogenic effects result from participation of the AF-1 ligand-independent activation domain. Tamoxifen has estrogenic effects in bone and in cardiovascular tissue (which are desirable to prevent osteoporosis and cardiac disease) and in the uterus (which is undesirable, as it may stimulate proliferation and lead to a small increase in the incidence of uterine cancer). Compounds with different selectivity in their estrogenic and antiestrogenic properties are referred to as selective

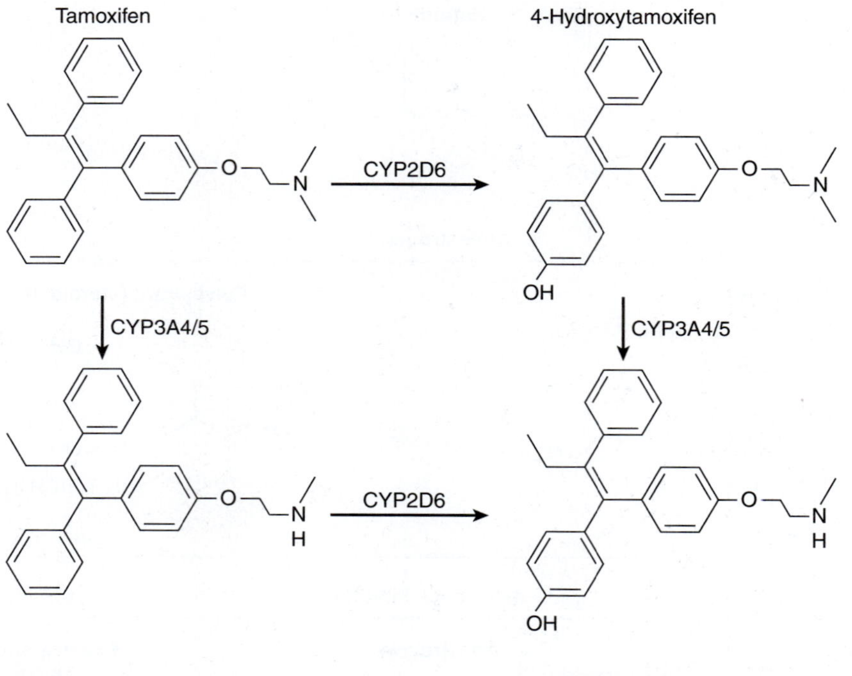

FIGURE 20-10 Metabolism of tamoxifen to more active metabolites such as 4-hydroxytamoxifen and N-desmethyl-4-hydroxytamoxifen (endoxifen).

estrogen receptor modulators (SERMs). The basis of their differences is in the different conformational changes that they induce when bound to the ER, leading to differential abilities to interact with a variety of coregulators, whose expression and/or activation will vary between cell types and tissues, as illustrated in Figure 20-10. As breast tumors often develop resistance to tamoxifen without loss of ER expression, and because tamoxifen has undesirable estrogenic properties in the uterus, other SERMs have been investigated for their usefulness in breast cancer treatment and prevention. For example, raloxifene is a SERM that has estrogenic effects in bone and the cardiovascular system, but is antiestrogenic in the breast and uterus (O'Regan and Jordan, 2001). A clinical trial (Study of Tamoxifen and Raloxifene [STAR]) found raloxifene to have comparable efficacy to tamoxifen in breast cancer prevention in high-risk women, without increasing the risk of endometrial cancer (Vogel et al, 2006).

Steroidal antiestrogens, such as fulvestrant (see Fig. 20-11), show little if any estrogenic activity (in particular in the uterus) but remain active to treat some women whose breast cancers have acquired resistance to tamoxifen. The mechanism of action of these "pure" antiestrogens is distinct from the partial antiestrogens such as tamoxifen, in that they downregulate ER expression by increasing its degradation, and inactivate the ER complex (O'Regan and Jordan, 2001). Such compounds have been named selective estrogen receptor downregulators (SERDs). Because of its steroidal nature, fulvestrant is not suitable for oral administration and is administered by intramuscular injection. High-dose progestin treatment that is used (now rarely) as a third-line endocrine treatment may also act partially by downregulating expression of the ER in breast tumors.

20.4.2 Hormonal Therapy for Different Stages of Breast Cancer

Systemic adjuvant therapy given after surgical removal of the primary tumor is aimed at eliminating subclinical, micrometastatic cancer cell deposits that may have spread from the original tumor site. Adjuvant hormonal therapies, such as tamoxifen or ovarian ablation in premenopausal women and tamoxifen or aromatase inhibitors (given for 5 years) in postmenopausal women, have been shown to increase both relapse-free and overall survival of women with ER+ early breast cancer, when used either alone, or following adjuvant chemotherapy (Early Breast Cancer Trialists' Collaborative Group, 2005). Hormonal therapies can also prolong survival and maximize the quality of life of women with metastatic breast cancer. Hormonal treatments are often used in sequence, and women who respond to initial endocrine treatment have approximately a 50% chance of responding to a second agent, whereas other hormonal agents, including fulvestrant and megestrol acetate, may lead to further responses when used as third-line treatment. Despite the responsiveness of advanced ER+ breast cancer to initial endocrine therapy, tumors eventually develop resistance to all forms of endocrine therapy.

Neoadjuvant (preoperative) endocrine therapy (with or without chemotherapy) is used in some women to reduce the size of their primary breast cancer, thereby allowing assessment of response to treatment and increasing the possibility of breast-conserving surgery.

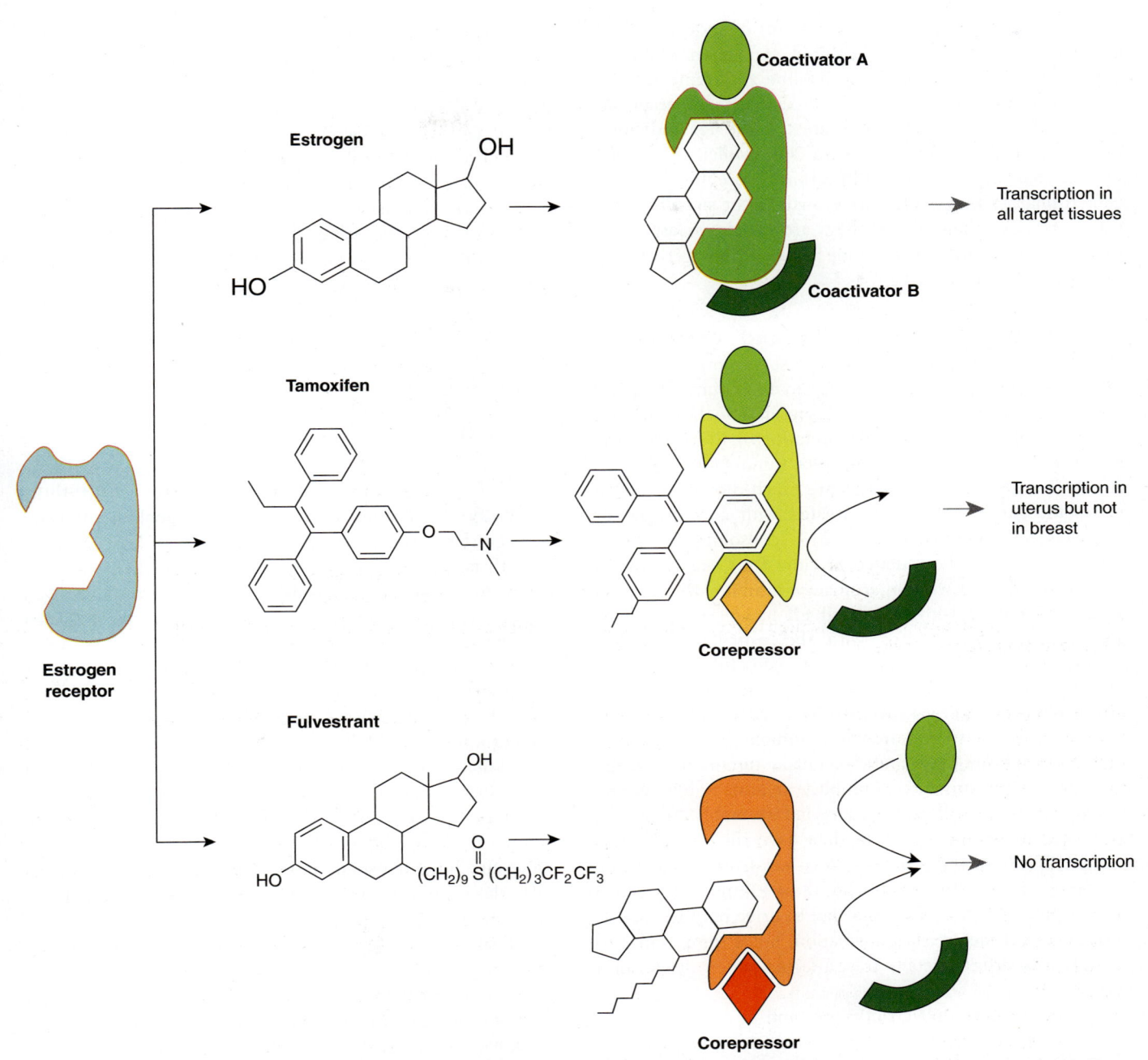

FIGURE 20–11 Schematic of conformational changes induced by different SERMs (estrogen, tamoxifen, and fulvestrant) resulting in differential recruitment of coregulators and differential activity. Estrogen binds to the estrogen receptor (ER), causing a conformational change that leads to docking of appropriate coactivators (hypothetical coactivator A and coactivator B) with ER in all target tissues and resulting in enhanced transcription of target genes. Tamoxifen binds to ER giving rise to a different conformation such that it docks coactivator A and a hypothetical corepressor that in one tissue (breast) inhibits estrogen action but in another tissue partially activates estrogen action (uterus). Another SERM called *fulvestrant* binds to ER, resulting in a different conformation such that it only docks the corepressor and inhibits estrogen action in both target tissues.

20.4.3 Resistance to Hormone Therapy

Although most ERα+ cancers respond initially to hormone therapy, many eventually acquire the ability to grow despite treatment because of "acquired resistance." Other cancers have "intrinsic" or de novo resistance to hormonal therapy. Resistance of cancer cells to anticancer drugs results from multiple mechanisms (Cree and Charlton, 2017; see Chap. 18, Sec. 18.4).

Six hallmarks of anticancer drug resistance have been identified: (1) alteration of drug targets; (2) expression of drug efflux pumps; (3) expression of detoxification mechanisms; (4) reduced susceptibility to apoptosis and cell death; (5) increased ability to repair DNA damage; (6) altered proliferation. These mechanisms can lead to de novo and acquired resistance to tamoxifen, although the mechanisms may differ, because de novo tamoxifen-resistant ER+ breast tumors are also generally resistant to other forms of endocrine therapy whereas tumors with acquired tamoxifen resistance may respond to second- and third-line endocrine therapy. Some mechanisms of resistance to endocrine therapy are general, but other mechanisms are specific for individual therapies (Musgrove and Sutherland, 2009; Miller, 2010). Multiple mechanisms, such as modification of receptor/cofactors, altered pharmacology, alternate growth factor signaling activation, and/or enhanced autophagy are used by breast cancer cells to escape control by hormone therapy (Clarke et al, 2015; Murphy and Dickler, 2016).

20.4.3.1 Modification of ERs and Cofactors.
A substantial proportion of ER+ breast tumors are either resistant de novo to endocrine therapy or acquire resistance after treatment with endocrine therapies despite the continued expression of ER. The presence of mutations in ERα is relatively rare in naïve nontreated primary ER+ tumors (Koboldt et al, 2012). However, such mutations are much more frequent in metastatic cancers of women treated with antiestrogen or aromatase inhibitors (Toy et al, 2013; Jeselsohn et al, 2014): ERα was found to be mutated in almost 40% of tumors of women pre-treated with an aromatase inhibitor (Fribbens et al, 2016). Women with a mutated ER had poorer outcome when subsequently treated with the aromatase inhibitor exemestane than with the antiestrogen fulvestrant (see Fig. 20–9) whereas those with a wild-type ERα had the same progression-free survival (Fribbens et al, 2016). This suggests not only that exposure to aromatase inhibitors increases ERα mutations but that these mutations make tumors more likely to resist further aromatase inhibitor treatment but do not interfere with their ability to respond favorably to further antiestrogen treatment. Recent data have shown that these mutant ERs have transcriptomes distinct from those of the wild-type ER. Investigating further these ER mutant-selective transcriptomes, which are suspected to drive both endocrine resistance and metastastase formation, holds the promise to identify new drug targets to treat affected patients (Jeselsohn et al, 2018).

The ability to recruit coactivators and/or corepressors to a promoter plays an important role in transcriptional regulation by a steroid hormone (see Figs. 20–5 and 20–11). Experimental alteration of the relative expression and/or activity of coactivator and corepressor causes target cells to interpret tamoxifen either as an antiestrogen or an estrogen. Alterations of specific coactivators, such as the nuclear coactivators (NCOA)-2 and -3, both amplified in about 8% of primary tumors (Koboldt, 2012), have been described in human breast tumors (Groner and Brown, 2017), and correlations with resistance to tamoxifen have been reported (Musgrove and Sutherland, 2009; Osborne and Schiff, 2011). Because coregulators are essential to ER signaling, altered expression and/or activity could affect sensitivity of tumors to aromatase inhibitors as a result of estrogen independence of growth and survival pathways. Growth factor/phosphorylation pathways can also influence steroid hormone receptor pathways via their ability to modulate coactivators by phosphorylation (Han et al, 2009) and may influence the emergence of hormone independence.

20.4.3.2 Altered Pharmacology
A potential mechanism behind tamoxifen resistance involves altered uptake and/or metabolism of this drug by the tumor: reduced intratumoral drug concentrations might be insufficient to control cell proliferation. Because CYP2D6 is the major enzyme responsible for the generation of endoxifen, the active metabolite of tamoxifen (see Fig. 20–10), it has been proposed that individuals with CYP2D6 gene polymorphisms that reduce enzymatic activity may benefit less from tamoxifen (Hoskins et al, 2009; Kiyotani et al, 2010). However, large studies show minimal differences in outcome when high and low metabolizers are treated (Regan et al, 2012), and CYP2D6 is only one factor modulating resistance to tamoxifen (Province et al, 2014).

20.4.3.3 Alternate Growth Factor Signaling Pathways
Activation of growth factor signaling pathways can interfere with hormone therapy in at least 2 ways. Growth factors such as IGF-I, heregulin, and EGF have the ability to activate ER signaling in the absence of estrogen through phosphorylation of coregulators or of the ER itself (see Fig. 20–6). This activation involves mainly PI3K/AKT/mTOR and RAF/MEK/ERK (see Chap. 6, Sec. 6.2). Similar phosphorylations occur for the ligand-independent activation of ER by protein kinase A, protein kinase C, pp90rsk1, and protein kinase B. The expression and/or activity of many of these kinases are often increased in breast tumors compared with normal breast tissue, and specific phosphatases that deactivate these kinases are expressed at higher levels in some breast cancer cell lines with altered responses to estrogen. Thus, an altered phosphorylation profile of the ER and/or its coregulators may underlie progression to hormone resistance (Xu et al, 2009; Skliris et al, 2010).

Activation of growth factor pathways also stimulates survival and proliferation thereby directly interfering with the expected negative impact of hormone therapy on cell growth (Clarke et al, 2015; Murphy and Dickler, 2016). For example, sustained activation of the PI3K/AKT/mTOR pathway can protect breast cancer cells against tamoxifen-induced apoptosis through upregulation of the antiapoptotic protein BCL-2 (Campbell et al, 2001; see Chap. 8, Sec. 8.4).

Multiple levels of crosstalk that exist between ER and other transcription factors and coregulator proteins play a critical role in progression to hormone independence. For example, the crosstalk between ER and HER2/Neu causes tamoxifen to act as an estrogen agonist in breast cancer cells that express high levels of AIB1 and HER2, resulting directly in de novo resistance (Shou et al, 2004). Interestingly, the drug gefitinib, an inhibitor of EGFR, blocks this crosstalk and restores the antiproliferative effect of tamoxifen. The interactions between ER and many other signaling pathways provide a rationale for treatments that combine antiestrogens or aromatase inhibitors together with drugs that inhibit specific molecular pathways. For example, abemaciclib, a cyclin-dependent kinase 4 and 6 (CDK4/6) inhibitor, was found to increase both progression-free and overall survival of patients treated with fulvestrant (Sledge et al, 2017). Supported by the results of other clinical trials, CDK4/6 inhibitors such as palbociclib, ribociclib or abemaciclib are now used routinely with hormonal agents as second or third line therapy for ER+ breast cancer (see Chap. 19, Sec. 19.6.1).

20.4.3.4 Enhanced Autophagy
Autophagy is a process used by cells to recycle their defective components, such as proteins or organelles (Kaur and Debnath, 2015; see Chap. 8, Sec. 8.4.6 and Chap. 12, Sec. 12.3.6). These cellular components are first stored in autophagosomes, which then fuse with lysosomes to allow their decomposition and followed by recycling of essential elements. Cancer cells use autophagy to survive stress, such as that induced by hypoxia or drug effects. Autophagy may also contribute to tumor dormancy and to resistance to hormone therapy (Jain et al, 2013): inhibiting autophagy in tamoxifen-resistant MCF-7 breast cancer cells restored their sensitivity to the drug (Qadir et al, 2008; Clarke et al, 2015).

The inherent ability of cancer cells to combine resistance mechanisms to overcome therapy in many different ways is one of the critical challenges faced by clinicians (Fig. 20–12).

20.4.4 New Approaches to Hormonal Treatment of Breast Cancer

Several clinical trials (https://www.breastcancertrials.org/bct_nation/home.seam) of combinations of endocrine therapies with targeted biological agents are ongoing, based on different therapeutic strategies (Murphy and Dickler, 2016; Liu et al, 2017). These include but are not limited to

A- **Switching endocrine agents:** for example aromatase inhibitors (steroidal or not) before or after various antiestrogens (SERDs).

B- **Cotreatments with endocrine agents targeting a specific pathway:** For example, mTOR inhibitor (evolerimus) alone or combined with exemestane; antiestrogen fulvestrant plus or minus a PIK3 inhibitor (pictilisib); exemestane plus or minus HDAC inhibitor (entinostat); fulvestrant plus an antibody targeting the programmed cell death receptor PD-1 (pembrolizumab). Comibining Cyclin-dependent kinase 4/6 inhibitors (CDKIs such as palbociclib or ribociclib) with either aromatase inhibitors or fulvestrant has been found to significantly benefit patients with ER positive-Her2-negative metastic breast cancer (Gao et al.,2019).

Better understanding of the mechanisms responsible for resistance to endocrine therapies could lead to changes in sequencing and scheduling of treatment. For example, the development of resistance to aromatase inhibitors through upregulation of growth factor and survival pathways might be reversed by periods of time off treatment. In addition, the use of pharmaco-genetics to identify patients more likely to have adverse side effects or less likely to benefit from a particular treatment is another important focus in cancer therapy (see Chap. 18, Sec. 18.2.3).

20.5 PROSTATE CANCER: HORMONE THERAPY AND RESISTANCE

20.5.1 Hormonal Therapy

When organ confined, prostate cancer is potentially curable by prostatectomy or radiation therapy. However, in men with locally advanced or metastatic disease, treatment with androgen deprivation therapy (ADT) is the first-line treatment. By inhibiting the critical androgen-dependent signaling pathway, the prostate cancer cells will activate apoptosis and inhibit their proliferation (see Fig. 20–4). Approximately 90% of patients with metastatic prostate cancer will respond to ADT, as indicated by a fall in the serum marker of the disease, prostate-specific antigen (PSA), and by an improvement in symptoms (most often pain caused by metastases in bone). However, although the cancer initially responds to this treatment, it always develops resistance. Treatment is associated with a median progression-free survival of 1-2 years and overall survival of 2-4 years. However, even after chemical or surgical castration, most tumors that grow remain dependent on androgens; hence, those cancers are termed "castration-resistant" prostate cancer (CRPC).

Androgen deprivation therapy works by either interfering with the synthesis of androgens or the ability of androgens to interact with the AR. Bilateral orchiectomy (castration) is the most direct way to block androgen stimulation of the prostate and has the advantages of low morbidity, low cost, and high compliance. However, the associated psychological problems have decreased its practice in favor of chemical castration using LHRH agonists. LHRH agonists include goserelin, leuprolide, and buserelin, which can be administered as long-acting (3-6 months) formulations to block the secretion of LH by desensitizing the pituitary gland and thereby inhibiting the synthesis of testosterone by the testis (see Fig. 20–2). Initially, LHRH agonists cause a rise in both LH and testosterone that increase AR signaling and cause a "flare" with tumor proliferation. This can be diminished by temporary coadministration of an antiandrogen to inhibit AR signaling in the tumor cells. Alternatively, the use of the LHRH antagonists degarelix or relugolix avoids this flare and does not require coadministration of antiandrogens.

Antiandrogens bind directly to the AR within the prostate cell and antagonize the action of both testicular and adrenal androgens (see Fig. 20–4). Apart from transient use to prevent the flare associated with LHRH agonists, they are usually added as second-line hormonal therapy at the time of progression. Early antiandrogens, including cyproterone acetate, were steroidal homologs that, although clinically effective, had progestational activity that reduced LH and plasma testosterone. These agents were largely replaced by early nonsteroidal antiandrogens, such as flutamide and bicalutamide (Fig. 20–13), that are moderately effective androgen antagonists but have no

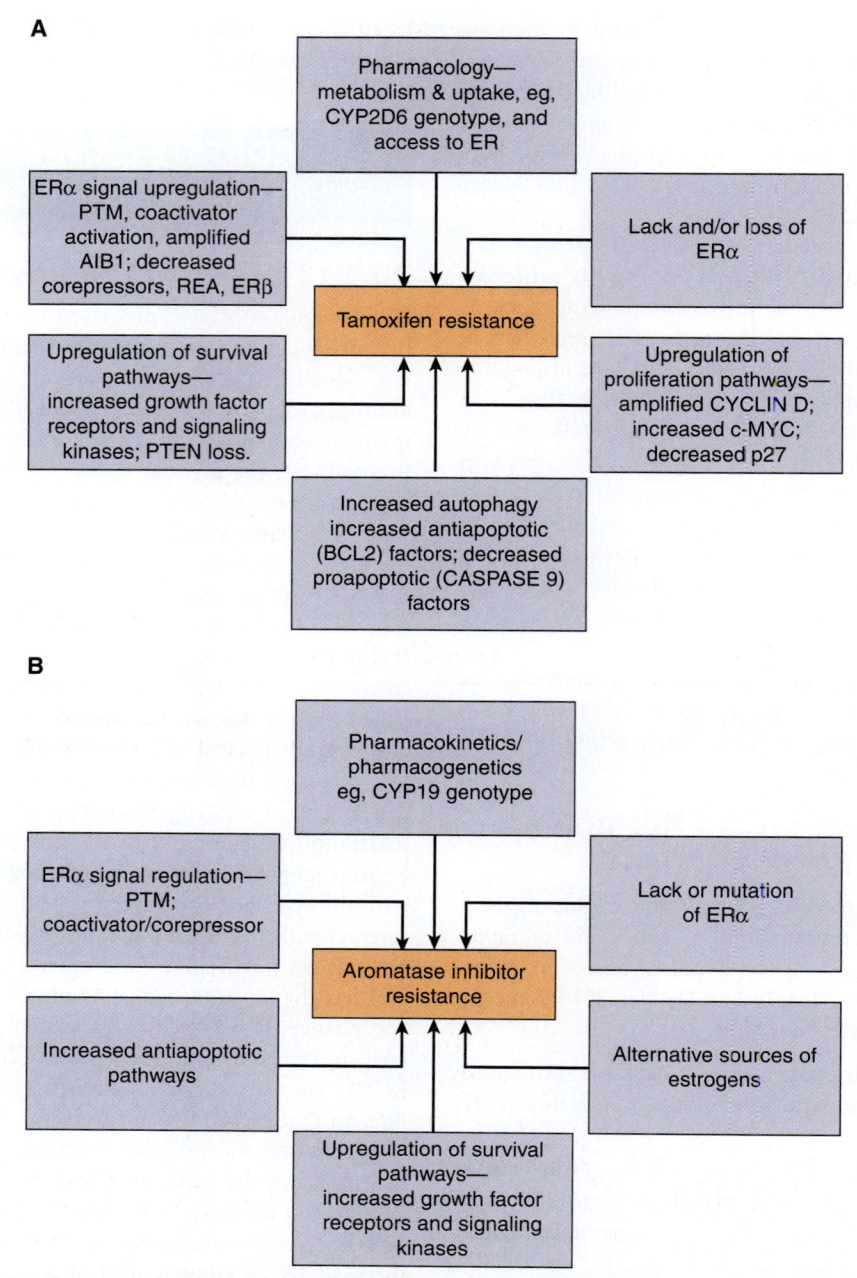

FIGURE 20-12 Summary of the multiple mechanisms of resistance to (A) tamoxifen and (B) aromatase inhibitors in human breast cancer. *REA*, repressor of ER activity; *PTM*, post-translational modifications.

gonadotropic or hypothalamic feedback activity. Building on the clinical success of these first nonsteroidal antiandrogens, the structurally related but more potent drug enzalutamide (MDV3100) was developed (Tran et al, 2009). Enzalutamide binds the AR with greater affinity than bicalutamide, impairs its nuclear translocation, and may have negative effects on the binding of AR to androgen response elements and the recruitment of coactivators. Randomized phase III trials have shown that enzalutamide improves the survival of men with CRPC, whose disease has progressed after receiving chemotherapy (Scher et al, 2012), and delays emergence of hormone resistance and improves survival of men with CRPC when given prior to chemotherapy (Beer et al, 2014).

De novo steroidogenesis can also be inhibited by abiraterone acetate, a specific and potent inhibitor of cytochrome p450 17A1 (Figs. 20–1 and 20–13; see also Sec. 20.5.3). CYP17A1 is a critical enzyme in both gonadal and nongonadal androgen biosynthesis. By inhibiting this enzyme, both the conversion of pregnenolone and progesterone to their 17α-hydroxy derivatives as well as the subsequent formation of dehydroepiandrosterone and androstenedione are blocked. The metabolite Δ(4)-abiraterone is also itself a potent antiandrogen that directly antagonizes the AR (Li et al, 2015). Because of concurrent inhibition of glucocorticoid synthesis and compensatory increase in adrenocorticotropic hormone (ACTH), abiraterone is given with low-dose steroids such as prednisone to

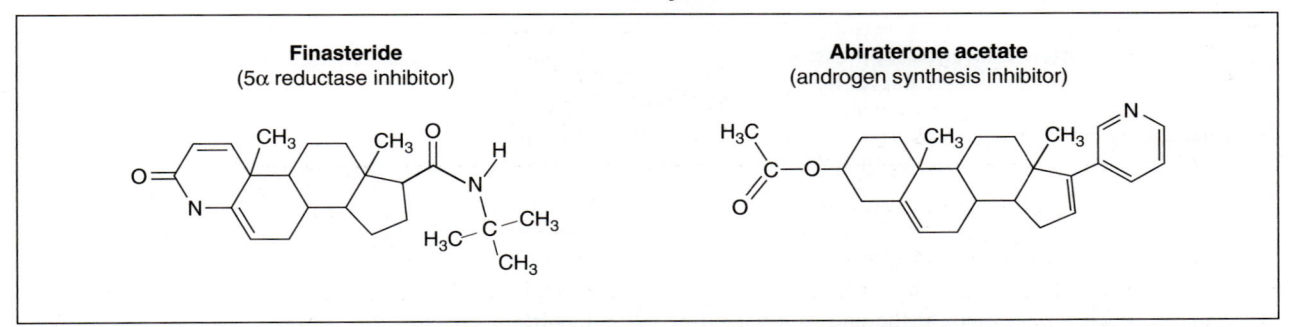

FIGURE 20–13 Structures of antiandrogens and antienzymes that block androgen metabolism. The antiandrogens block androgen binding to its receptor. The antienzymes inhibit the conversion of testosterone to the more active form dihydrotestosterone (5α reductase inhibitors) or block androgen synthesis (abiraterone acetate).

reduce the severity and incidence of mineralocorticoid activity–related adverse events. Glucocorticoids inhibit production of ACTH, which decreases production of weak androgens by the adrenal gland that can also lead to tertiary responses (see Fig. 20-2). Abiraterone acetate has shown a substantial improvement in time to disease progression for men with metastatic castration-resistant prostate cancer, and like enzalutamide, has improved survival when used to treat metastatic prostate cancer, both in men after and before they have received chemotherapy (de Bono et al, 2011; Ryan et al, 2013; 2015). Abiraterone acetate has also been shown in two concordant randomized clinical trials to lead to substantial improvement in survival of men with aggressive prostate cancer when given concurrently with classical ADT, and it has become the new standard of care (Fizazi et al, 2017; James et al, 2017). Trials with enzalutamide or the related drug apalutamide in combination with classical ADT have shown similar efficacy to abiraterone.

Irrespective of the type of ADT, the side effects can include hot flushes, loss of libido and sexual potency, gynecomastia, lethargy, depression, loss of bone and muscle mass, and metabolic syndrome with increased diabetes. Although a meta-analysis found no link between ADT and cardiovascular death, there may be increased cardiac morbidity in those patients with pre-existing health problems (D'Amico et al, 2015). One unexpected side effect of antiandrogens is that about 20% of patients who respond and then progress to CRPC have a further clinical response following discontinuation of treatment. The underlying molecular mechanism responsible for the "antiandrogen withdrawal syndrome" is not fully understood, but may relate to altered AR ligand specificity and inadvertent activation of the AR by antiandrogen.

20.5.2 Intermittent Hormonal Therapy for Prostate Cancer

In addition to acting as mitogens to induce DNA synthesis and cell proliferation, androgens are potent differentiating agents. In studies with castrated rodents, administration of small amounts of androgen was shown to induce markers of differentiation in the prostate without stimulating rounds of cell proliferation. This conditioning effect of androgens on surviving

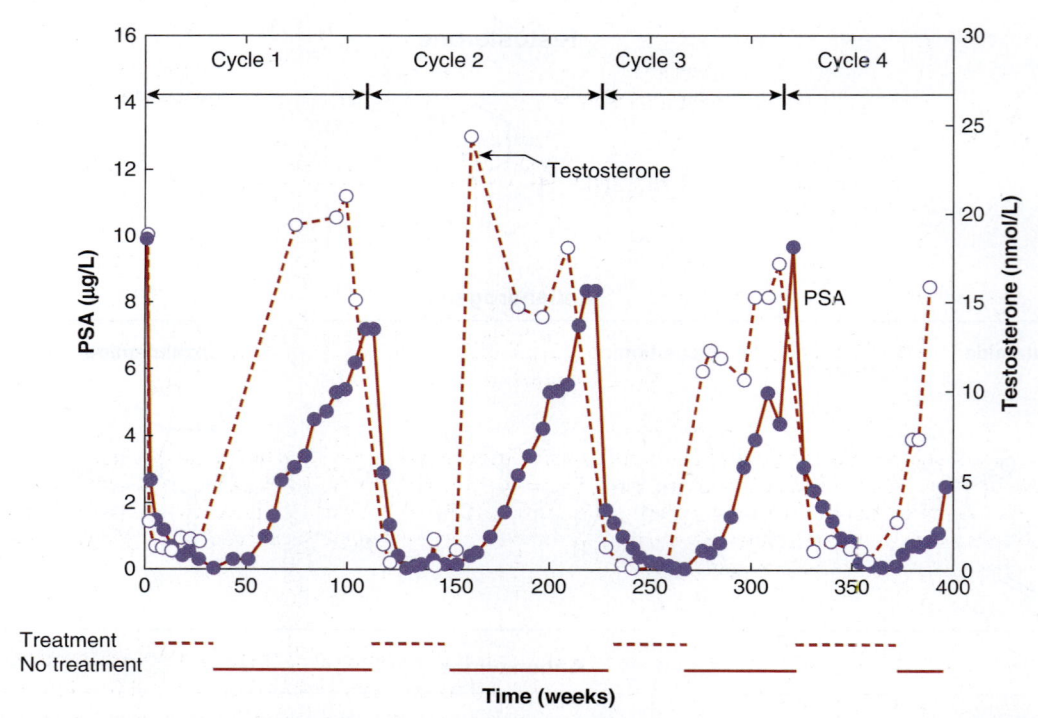

FIGURE 20–14 Intermittent androgen suppression. Approximately 8 years after radical prostatectomy and radiation treatment for positive surgical resection margins, the patient was started on a regimen of intermittent androgen suppression when his serum PSA had increased from a nadir of 0.6 to 10.4 µg/L. He was treated with a combination of antiandrogen (cyproterone acetate) and LHRH agonist (leuprolide acetate). The patient has undergone 4 cycles of androgen withdrawal and replacement over a period of more than 7 years. Open circles indicate serum testosterone values (nmol/L) and closed circles are serum levels of PSA (µg/L). (Used with permission from Dr N. Bruchovsky.)

cells allowed them to retain desirable, hormone-regulated traits, and the capacity to undergo apoptosis following ADT. The effect of androgen replacement at the end of a period of ADT-induced regression of the androgen-dependent Shionogi mouse mammary carcinoma was first tested by transplantation into noncastrated males. This cycle of transplantation and castration-induced apoptosis was repeated and relative to one-time castration, intermittent androgen suppression approximately tripled the time to androgen independence (Akakura et al, 1993). Other experimental models of hormone-dependent prostate cancer have confirmed these effects. Figure 20–14 shows a representation of how intermittent hormone suppression might regulate tumor growth.

Prospective clinical trials have evaluated intermittent hormonal therapy and have found that intermittent treatment is as effective, but not more effective, than continuous androgen suppression, while reducing treatment-related toxicity, drug costs, and improved quality of life, including recovery of sexual potency (Magnan et al, 2015).

In addition to intermittent treatment, ADT has also been investigated before or after primary treatments for localized prostate cancer, such as prostatectomy or radiation therapy, or concurrent with radiation therapy. Neoadjuvant hormone treatment can lead to a reduction in tumor size, but such therapy has not been shown to improve survival following radical surgery. However, the combination of radiation and hormonal therapy for locally advanced prostate cancer does prolong survival (Warde et al, 2011). The concurrent administration of ADT and the cytotoxic chemotherapeutic agent docetaxel also results in improved survival in men with untreated metastatic prostate cancer (Sweeney et al, 2015; James et al, 2016).

20.5.3 Hormone and Chemoprevention Strategies for Prostate Cancer

Epidemiologic studies of prostate cancer suggest that diet and lifestyle likely contribute more to prostate carcinogenesis than racial or familial factors (see Sec. 20.3.1.2). The observation that premalignant prostatic lesions (e.g. PIN) occur with almost equal frequency in different racial populations with both high and low risk of prostate cancer implies that the limiting step is progression from subclinical to locally invasive carcinoma. The evidence that androgen stimulation over a long period of time is a necessary prerequisite for prostate cancer makes it an obvious target for chemoprevention. The potential preventive role of finasteride (see Fig. 20–13), which blocks the intracellular metabolism of testosterone to the more potent DHT, was tested to see if it would decrease the risk of prostate cancer. In a phase III trial of 18,000 men older than 50 years, treatment with finasteride for 7 years was shown to cause a cumulative reduction of 25% in early-stage, organ-confined, low-grade prostate cancer (Thompson et al, 2003). However, neither this nor other 5α-reductase inhibitors decreased the prevalence of higher-grade potentially lethal prostate cancer.

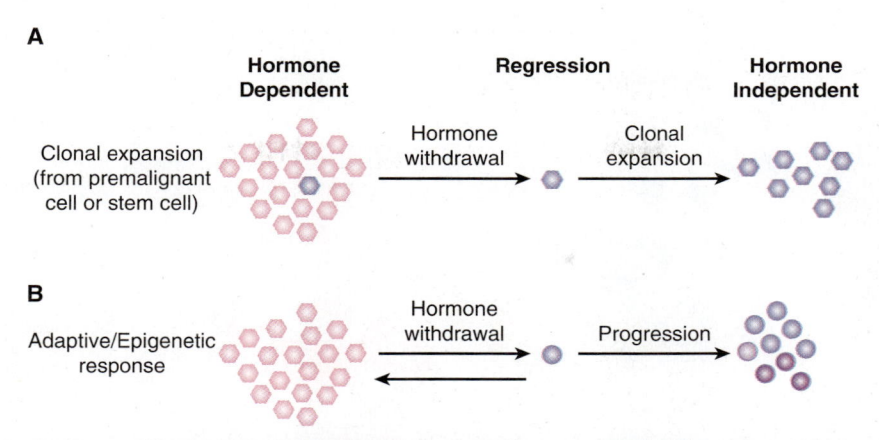

FIGURE 20–15 Clonal selection and epigenetic/adaptive mechanisms for emergence of hormone independence in tumors. **A)** On hormone withdrawal, hormone-dependent cells are killed, leaving behind preexisting hormone-independent clones that repopulate the tumor. **B)** On hormone withdrawal, most cells are killed except for those expressing critical cell-survival genes. When reexposed to hormone, the pattern of gene expression reverts and the tumor regrows in response to hormone. However, through further adaptive changes in gene expression patterns, the cells no longer require hormone to sustain their growth.

20.5.4 Mechanisms of Resistance to Hormonal Therapies for Prostate Cancer

Although hormonal therapy is initially effective in most men, the cancer almost always develops resistance. This can occur via somatic mutations that provide a growth or survival advantage. This mechanism suggests that many different genetically related clones are present and that hormonal therapy kills all but the resistant population of cells, which subsequently becomes the dominant phenotype of the tumor (Fig. 20–15). Supporting this model, there is a shared genetic lineage between early- and late-stage cancers (Beltran, 2016). Resistance can also occur by epigenetic modifications that alter the cellular differentiation. By changing the cellular state, the dependencies of the cancer may change and introduce drug resistance. Environmental stress, including ADT, or paracrine signaling can induce cellular plasticity, which allows differentiation (see Chap. 13, Sec. 13.3.2). Overall, these genetic and epigenetic modifications, either individually or in combination can induce resistance through several mechanisms, including androgen receptor amplification, androgen receptor alterations, coactivator overexpression, and intratumoral androgen production (Fig. 20–16). The relative importance of each mechanism is dependent on both the patient's cancer and the type of treatment.

20.5.4.1 Androgen Receptor Amplification

Approximately 60% of prostate tumors have amplification of wild-type *AR* after progression on ADT (Robinson et al, 2015). This occurs typically by copy number amplification of either the AR gene or the regulatory elements that control AR expression (Quigley et al, 2018; Takeda et al, 2018). In *AR* gene-amplified tumors, PSA immunostaining appears to be about twice as dense as in tumors with no amplification, indicating that *AR* gene amplification leads to upregulation of the PSA gene (and possibly other androgen-regulated genes). Thus patients with *AR* gene amplification may have elevated serum PSA concentrations without a clear correlation with tumor burden (Koivisto and Helin, 1999).

20.5.4.2 Androgen Receptor Alterations

Estimates of the incidence of somatic point mutations in the *AR* gene range from 0% to 30% of patients with CRPC, with a tendency for *AR* mutations to occur more frequently in advanced, metastatic disease. Also, men treated with antiandrogens are more likely to have *AR* mutations as compared to men treated solely by surgical castration or LHRH agonists (Taplin et al, 1999). Almost all of the mutations associated with resistance occur in the ligand-binding domain (LBD) of the AR. These *AR* mutations show a range of effects from partial or complete loss of function to diverse transactivational activity (Shi et al, 2002). The well-characterized threonine-to-alanine (T878A) mutation in the AR-LBD of the LNCaP human prostate cancer cell line has been shown to alter androgen-binding specificity, such that it can be activated by high concentrations of virtually any steroid or antiandrogen (Duff and McEwan, 2005). Similar types of mutations have been observed in some men who manifest with antiandrogen withdrawal syndrome, suggesting that these AR mutations cause antiandrogens to act as AR agonists. In those patients treated with enzalutamide, AR mutations have been observed in circulating cell-free DNA (Lallous et al, 2016) though they are rarely observed (Robinson et al, 2015).

Truncated forms of the AR that lack a ligand-binding site have been proposed to be involved in ADT resistance and CRPC progression (Hu et al, 2009). Numerous AR variants have been identified but they share a common structural feature of truncation or exon skipping of the AR-LBD (Ware et al, 2014). Although these variants are unable to bind androgens, they are constitutively active and therefore intrinsically resistant to all currently approved antiandrogens.

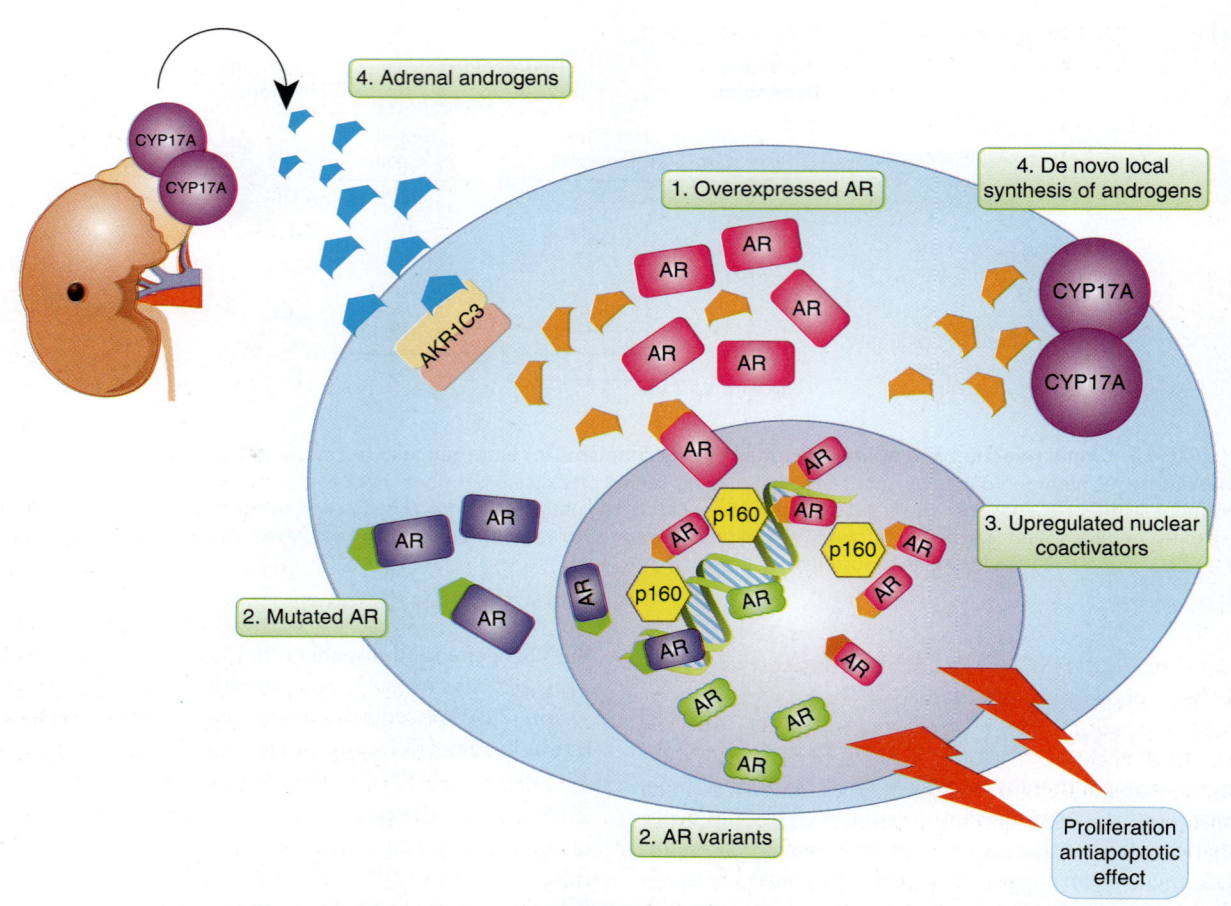

FIGURE 20–16 Summary of the multiple mechanisms of castration-resistant prostate cancer. Key regulatory proteins are the androgen receptor (AR), cytochrome P450 17A1 (CYP17A), p160 family members including SRC-1 and TIF2/SRC-2 (P160)s.

These variants can be detected at low levels in normal prostate tissue and untreated primary prostate cancer but their expression increases in CRPC. Recent clinical work demonstrated a clear correlation between expression of the AR-V7 variant and resistance to abiraterone and enzalutamide (Antonarakis et al, 2014). However, the presence of AR variants cannot predict consistently the response to ADT (Bernemann et al, 2017).

Immunohistochemical analysis of biopsies from all stages and grades of prostate cancer shows that the AR is generally retained (Crnalic et al, 2010). However, with the growing clinical use of the more potent hormonal agents abiraterone and enzalutamide, there has been an increase in prostate cancers with reduced or absent AR expression (Alanee et al, 2015). These cancers upregulate neuroendocrine markers such as chromogranin A, synaptophysin, CD56, and NSE. Such neuroendocrine prostate cancers (NEPC) often have histologic features similar to small-cell carcinomas; as they do not express AR they are intrinsically resistant to ADT. Although NEPCs occur rarely de novo (<5%), treatment with second-generation hormone therapy has been proposed to push the cancer into this AR-independent state. NEPCs generally have mutations in RB1, PTEN, and TP53 with amplification of MYCN and aurora kinase A (Beltran et al, 2011). However, such mutations are not exclusive to NEPC and have also been found in CRPC with histologic properties of an adenocarcinoma.

20.5.4.3 Overexpression of Coactivators

Overexpression of coactivators can lower the ligand threshold of the AR such that physiological concentrations of adrenal androgens are adequate to drive androgen-regulated transcription (Chmelar et al, 2007). Immunohistochemical evaluation of human prostate cancer samples demonstrated overexpression of the coactivator SRC-1 in approximately half of nontreated prostate cancers, as well as high levels of both SRC-1 and SRC-2 in the majority of castration-resistant tumors (Gregory et al, 2001). Other coactivators that are involved in prostate cancer progression and in the development of a castration-resistant state include members of the mediator complex (MED1), which is involved in AR-mediated transcription and AR chaperones such as heat shock protein Hsp 27 and cell division cycle Cdc 37. The *MED1* gene is overexpressed in both AR-positive and AR-negative prostate cancer cell lines, as well as in clinically localized prostate cancers, suggesting that MED1 hyperactivity might promote prostate tumor formation (Vijayvargia et al, 2007).

20.5.4.4 Intratumoral Androgen Production

There is extensive clinical evidence that the tumor itself can synthesize androgen to evade ADT (Fig. 20–16). Expression of genes that mediate androgen synthesis (eg, AKR1C2 and AKR1C1 involved in the production of 3α-androstanediol and 3β-androstanediol from 5α-DHT), are elevated or modified in CRPC but not primary tumors (Knudsen and Penning, 2010). In support of this model, intracellular testosterone levels in many CRPC cells have been shown to be adequate for activation of androgen-dependent genes (Locke et al, 2008). This mechanism of resistance may explain partially the clinical success of abiraterone acetate, which can not only inhibit adrenal and testicular androgen synthesis but also that of testosterone in prostatic tissue.

20.5.5 Novel Androgen Deprivation Therapy for Prostate Cancer

As the progression to CRPC occurs despite a continued dependence on AR signaling, inhibition of the AR with novel therapeutics still remains one of the most promising pharmacologic targets. This has lead to the approval of the structurally related antiandrogens apalutamide and darolutamide. These compounds have improved potency and/or pharmacokinetics as compared to enzalutamide, but the clinical efficacy is comparable. Other agents are being developed to target different sites on the AR including the N-terminal domain (Andersen et al, 2010) and the DNA-binding domain (Dalal et al, 2014): they offer potential efficacy against all isoforms of AR including the constitutively active variants. There has also been some research, although not yet clinically successful, with compounds that induce AR degradation (Omlin et al, 2015). Further research is ongoing to develop effective AR inhibitors that inhibit this critical signaling pathway through novel mechanisms.

20.6 PARANEOPLASTIC ENDOCRINE SYNDROMES

Paraneoplastic endocrine syndromes are defined as systemic manifestations of malignancy caused by hormones released by cancer cells (Dimitriadis et al, 2017). The term "paraneoplastic" was first introduced in 1949 by Guichard and Vignon to describe the neurologic symptoms observed in a patient bearing a uterine tumor. Because the effects observed could not be attributed to the local presence of cancer cells in the nervous system, the word was used to describe phenomena resulting from the existence of cancer cells in distant regions. It is now recognized that cancer cells of both endocrine and nonendocrine lineage can secrete hormones or cytokines that can lead to metabolic changes and to specific clinical syndromes. Some of these syndromes can manifest themselves before a cancer is diagnosed and can then lead to earlier detection of the disease (Pelosof and Gerber, 2010). The most common paraneoplastic endocrine syndromes are hypercalcemia, Cushing syndrome, syndrome of inappropriate antidiuretic hormone secretion (SIADH), and hypoglycemia.

20.6.1 Hypercalcemia

Hypercalcemia is observed in more than 10% of all advanced cancer patients and is associated with an extremely poor prognosis. It occurs primarily by ectopic production of parathyroid hormone in squamous cell tumors and small cell lung cancer, but has been also described in other malignancies including colorectal (Galindo et al, 2016) and neuroendocrine cancers (Kaltsas et al, 2010). Hypercalcemia can also occur rarely from the release of vitamin D by some lymphomas. Hypercalcemia is not always paraneoplastic; it can result from the direct release of calcium by the osteolytic activity of metastases in bone from breast, lung, kidney, and other cancers.

20.6.2 Cushing Syndrome

This syndrome is caused by prolonged overexposure to cortisol, and approximately 10% of cases are paraneoplastic (Pelosof and Gerber, 2010). In half of these instances, the syndrome is caused by secretion of ACTH by either small cell lung cancer or bronchial carcinoid. It can also be attributable to the synthesis of this hormone by neuroendocrine cells from the thymus, the pancreas, ovary, or prostate. Ectopic ACTH production can be linked directly to demethylation of the regulatory regions of the proopiomelanocortin gene, which acts as the hormone precursor (Newell-Price, 2003).

20.6.3 Syndrome of Inappropriate Antidiuretic Hormone Secretion (SIADH)

This syndrome affects 2% of all cancer patients, with the majority associated with small cell lung cancers. It is caused by high concentrations of the antidiuretic hormone that increases retention of solute-free water by the kidney leading to low levels of sodium in the blood. Antidiuretic hormone is secreted normally by the hypothalamus and stored in the posterior hypophysis, but it can be produced ectopically by small lung cancer cells, and less frequently by prostate and breast cancer cells (Thajudeen and Salahudeen, 2016).

20.6.4 Paraneoplastic Hypoglycaemia

Although relatively rare compared to the syndromes described above, paraneoplastic hypoglycaemia can result from the production of insulin-like factors such as insulin-like growth factor 1, insulin-like growth factor 2, or glucagon-like peptide 1 by nonpancreatic tumor cells. Some mesenchymal, kidney, and ovary tumors have been found to secrete these factors.

SUMMARY

▶ Breast and prostate cancer share many common epidemiologic and biological features. Many factors contribute to their etiology, but a Western-type diet appears to be a major factor associated with high incidence.

- Both breast and prostate cancer require long-term exposure to sex-steroid hormones to develop. A direct causal link to overstimulation with estrogens and androgens respectively has been demonstrated in animal tumor models; conversely, a protective effect has been observed from treatments that block the action of these hormones (eg, prepubertal castration or administration of antihormonal drugs).
- Estrogens and androgens share many features in their mechanism of action: both are synthesized from common precursors (ie, cholesterol); both are carried mainly by the same protein in the blood (ie, SHGB [sex hormone–binding globulin]); and both bind to structurally related intracellular receptors. Both types of hormone-receptor complexes, in turn, bind to comparable regulatory DNA sequences at promoters/enhancers of genes and interact with similar sets of coregulator proteins to activate or repress gene expression.
- Approximately 70% of breast carcinomas are ER+, and approximately 50% of these will respond to endocrine therapy. By comparison, most prostate cancers are AR+ and most (~90%) respond to hormonal therapy. Therefore, ER assays are performed routinely in women with breast cancer, and only ER+ tumors are hormonally treated, whereas no receptor-based selection process is applied to prostate tumors.
- Treatment modalities used to kill hormone-dependent breast or prostate tumor cells are based on the same principles: either blocking the synthesis of the steroid hormone or blocking the steroid receptor. Unfortunately, endocrine therapy for locally advanced or metastatic disease is not curative as the tumors progress from hormone dependence to hormone independence.
- Potential mechanisms leading to hormone independence include ascendancy of alternative signal transduction pathways; receptor gene mutations or amplifications; ligand-independent receptor crosstalk with growth factors or kinases; autocrine synthesis of androgens; and upregulation of cell-survival genes.
- Combining and alternating treatments targeting steroid hormone action and other signaling pathways critical for cell growth holds the promise to strongly benefit cancer patients.

REFERENCES

Ahern TP, Beck AH, Rosner BA, et al. Continuous measurement of breast tumor hormone receptor expression: a comparison of two computational pathology platforms. *J Clin Pathol* 2017;70(5):428-434.

Akakura K, Bruchovsky N, Goldenberg SL, et al. Effects of intermittent androgen suppression on androgen-dependent tumors. Apoptosis and serum prostate-specific antigen. *Cancer* 1993;71(9):2782-2790.

Alanee S, Moore A, Nutt M, et al. Contemporary incidence and mortality rates of neuroendocrine prostate cancer. *Anticancer Res* 2015;35(7):4145-4150.

Allred DC, Mohsin SK. Biological features of premalignant disease in the human breast. *J Mammary Gland Biol Neoplasia* 2000;5(4):351-364.

Anderson E, Clarke RB, Howell A. Estrogen responsiveness and control of normal human breast proliferation. *J Mammary Gland Biol Neoplasia* 1998;3(1):23-35.

Andersen RJ, Mawji NR, Wang J, et al. Regression of castrate-recurrent prostate cancer by a small-molecule inhibitor of the amino-terminus domain of the androgen receptor. *Cancer Cell* 2010;17(6):535-546.

Antonarakis ES, Lu C, Wang H, et al. AR-V7 and resistance to enzalutamide and abiraterone in prostate cancer. *N Engl J Med* 2014;371(11):1028-1038.

Aranda A, Pascual A. Nuclear hormone receptors and gene expression. *Physiol Rev* 2001;81(3):1269-1304.

Arnal JF, Lenfant F, Metivier R, et al. Membrane and nuclear estrogen receptor alpha actions: from tissue specificity to medical implications. *Physiol Rev* 2017;97(3):1045-1087.

Arpino G, Wiechmann L, Osborne CK, Schiff R. Crosstalk between the estrogen receptor and the HER tyrosine kinase receptor family: molecular mechanism and clinical implications for endocrine therapy resistance. *Endocr Rev* 2008;29(2):217-233.

Banks E, Canfell K, Reeves G. HRT and breast cancer: recent findings in the context of the evidence to date. *Womens Health (Lond Engl)* 2008;4(5):427-431.

Beer TM, Armstrong AJ, Rathkopf DE, et al. Enzalutamide in metastatic prostate cancer before chemotherapy. *N Engl J Med* 2014;371(5):424-33.

Beltran H, Rickman DS, Park K, et al. Molecular characterization of neuroendocrine prostate cancer and identification of new drug targets. *Cancer Discov* 2011;1(6):487-95.

Bernemann C, Schnoeller TJ, Luedeke M, et al. Expression of AR-V7 in circulating tumour cells does not preclude response to next generation androgen deprivation therapy in patients with castration resistant prostate cancer. *Eur Urol* 2017;71(1):1-3.

Brouckaert O, Paridaens R, Floris G, et al. A critical review why assessment of steroid hormone receptors in breast cancer should be quantitative. *Annals Oncol* 2013;24(1):46-53.

Bhutiani N, Egger ME, Ajkay N, et al. Multigene signature panels and breast cancer therapy: patterns of use and impact on clinical decision making. *J Am Coll Surg* 2018;226(4):406-412.

Calle EE, Kaaks R. Overweight, obesity and cancer: epidemiological evidence and proposed mechanisms. *Nat Rev Cancer* 2004;4(8):579-591.

Campbell RA, Bhat-Nakshatri P, Patel NM, et al. Phosphatidylinositol 3-kinase/AKT-mediated activation of estrogen receptor alpha: a new model for anti-estrogen resistance. *J Biol Chem* 2001;276(13):9817-9824.

Cardoso F, van't Veer LJ, Bogaerts J, et al. 70-gene signature as an aid to treatment decisions in the early-stage breast cancer. *N Eng J Med* 2016;375(8):717-729.

Chmelar R, Buchanan G, Need EF, et al. Androgen receptor co-regulators and their involvement in the development and progression of prostate cancer. *Int J Cancer* 2007;120(4): 719-733.

Clarke RB, Howell A, Potten CS, Anderson E. Dissociation between steroid receptor expression and cell proliferation in the human breast. *Cancer Res* 1997;57(22):4987-4991.

Clarke R, Tyson JJ, Dixon JM. Endocrine resistance in breast cancer—an overview and update. *Mol Cell Endocrinol* 2015;418:220-234.

Couse JF, Korach KS. Estrogen receptor null mice: what have we learned and where will they lead us? *Endocr Rev* 1999;20(3):358-417.

Cree IA, Charlton P. Molecular chess? Hallmarks of anti-cancer drug resistance. *BMC Cancer* 2017;17(1):10.

Creighton CJ, Chang JC, Rosen JM. Epithelial-mesenchymal transition (EMT) in tumor-initiating cells and its clinical implications in breast cancer. *J Mammary Gland Biol Neoplasia* 2010;15(2):253-260.

Crnalic S, Hörnberg E, Wikström P, et al. Nuclear androgen receptor staining in bone metastases is related to a poor outcome in prostate cancer patients. *Endocr Relat Cancer* 2010;17(4):885-895.

Dalal K, Roshan-Moniri M, Sharma A, et al. Selectively targeting the DNA-binding domain of the androgen receptor as a prospective therapy for prostate cancer. *J Biol Chem* 2014;289(38):26417-26429.

D'Amico AV, Chen MH, Renshaw A, et al. Long-term follow-up of a randomized trial of radiation with or without androgen. *JAMA* 2015;314(12):1291-1293.

Davies P, Watt K, Kelly SM, et al. Consequences of polyglutamine repeat length for the conformation and folding of the androgen receptor amino-terminal domain. *J Mol Endocrinol* 2008;41(5):301-314.

de Bono JS, Logothetis CJ, Molina A, et al. Abiraterone and increased survival in metastatic prostate cancer. *N Engl J Med* 2011;364(21):1995-2005.

Denis L, Morton MS, Griffiths K. Diet and its preventive role in prostatic disease. *Eur Urol* 1999;35(5-6):377-387.

Di Cosimo S, Baselga J. Management of breast cancer with targeted agents: importance of heterogenicity. *Nat Rev Clin Oncol* 2010;7(3):139-147.

Dimitriadis GK, Angelousi A, Weickert MO, et al. Paraneoplastic endocrine syndromes. *Endocr Relat Cancer* 2017;24(6):173-190.

Duff J, McEwan IJ. Mutation of histidine 874 in the androgen receptor ligand-binding domain leads to promiscuous ligand activation and altered p160 co-activator interactions. *Mol Endocrinol* 2005;19(12):2943-2954.

Duffy MJ, Harbeck N, Nap M, et al. Clinical use of biomarkers in breast cancer: updated guidelines from the european group on tumor markers (EGTM). *Eur J Canc* 2017;75: 284-298.

Early Breast Cancer Trialists' Collaborative Group. Effects of chemotherapy and hormonal therapy for early breast cancer on recurrence and 15-year survival: an overview of the randomised trials. *Lancet* 2005;365:1687-1717.

Fitzgibbons PL, Murphy DA, Hammond ME, et al. Recommendations for validating estrogen and progesterone receptor immunohistochemistry assays. *Arch Pathol Lab Med* 2010;134(6):930-935.

Fizazi K, Tran N, Fein L, et al. Abiraterone plus prednisone in metastatic, castration-sensitive prostate cancer. *N Engl J Med* 2017;377(4):352-360.

Fribbens C, O'Leary B, Kilburn L, et al. Plasma ESR1 mutations and the treatment of estrogen receptor–positive advanced breast cancer. *J Clin Oncol* 2016;34(25):2961-2968.

Fullwood MJ, Liu MH, Pan YF, et al. An oestrogen-receptor-alpha-bound human chromatin interactome. *Nature* 2009;462(7269):58-64.

Galindo RJ, Romao I, Valsamis A, et al. Hypercalcemia of malignancy and colorectal cancer. *World J Oncol* 2016;7(1):5-12.

Gao JF, Cheng J, Bloomquist E, et al. CDK4/6 inhibitor treatment for patients with hormone receptor-positive, Her2-negative, advanced or metastatic breast cancer: a US food and drug administration pooled analysis. *Lancet* 2020;21:250-260.

Giguere Y, Dewailly E, Brisson J, et al. Short polyglutamine tracts in the androgen receptor are protective against breast cancer in the general population. *Cancer Res* 2001; 61(15):5869-5874.

Glass CK. Differential recognition of target genes by nuclear receptor monomers, dimers, and heterodimers. *Endocr Rev* 1994;15(3):391-407.

Gregory CW, He B, Johnson RT, et al. A mechanism for androgen receptor-mediated prostate cancer recurrence after androgen deprivation therapy. *Cancer Res* 2001;61(11):4315-4319.

Groner AC, Brown M. Role of steroid receptor and coregulator mutations in hormone-dependent cancers. *J Clin Invest* 2017;127(4):1126-1135.

Hah N, Kraus WL. Hormone-regulated transcriptomes: lessons learned from estrogen signaling pathways in breast cancer cells. *Mol Cell Endocrinol* 2014;382(1):652-664.

Hammond ME, Hayes DF, Dowsett M, A, et al. American Society of Clinical Oncology/College of American Pathologists guideline recommendations for immunohistochemical testing of estrogen and progesterone receptors in breast cancer. *Arch Pathol Lab Med* 2010;134:907-922.

Han SJ, Lonard DM, O'Malley BW. Multi-modulation of nuclear receptor co-activators through posttranslational modifications. *Trends Endocrinol Metab* 2009;20(1):8-15.

Henderson BE, Ross RK, Pike MC, Casagrande JT. Endogenous hormones as a major factor in human cancer. *Cancer Res* 1982;42(8):3232-3239.

Hoskins JM, Carey LA, McLeod HL. CYP2D6 and tamoxifen: DNA matters in breast cancer. *Nat Rev Cancer* 2009; 9(8):576-586.

Hsieh CL, Fei T, Chen Y, et al. Enhancer RNAs participate in androgen receptor-driven looping that selectively enhances gene activation. *Proc Natl Acad Sci* 2014;111(20):7319-7324.

Hsing AW, Chokkalingam AP. Prostate cancer epidemiology. *Front Biosci* 2006;11:1388-1413.

Hu R, Dunn TA, Wei S, et al. Ligand-independent androgen receptor variants derived from splicing of cryptic exons signify hormone-refractory prostate cancer. *Cancer Res* 2009;69(1):16-22.

Jain K, Paranandi KS, Sridharan S, et al. Autophagy in breast cancer and its implications for therapy. *Am J Cancer Res* 2013;3(3):251-265.

James ND, Sydes MR, Clarke NW, et al. Addition of docetaxel, zoledronic acid, or both to first-line long-term hormone therapy in prostate cancer (STAMPEDE): survival results from an adaptive, multiarm, multistage, platform randomised controlled trial. *Lancet* 2016;387(10024):1163-1177.

James ND, de Bono JS, Spears MR, et al. Abiraterone for prostate cancer not previously treated with hormone therapy. *N Engl J Med* 2017;377(4):338-351.

Jeselsohn R, Yelensky R, Buchwalter G, et al. Emergence of constitutively active estrogen receptor-α mutations in pretreated advanced estrogen receptor-positive breast cancer. *Clin Cancer Res* 2014;20(7):1757-1767.

Jeselsohn R, Bergholz JS, Pun M, et al. Allele-specific chromatin recruitment and therapeutic vulnerabilities of ESR1 activating mutations. *Cancer Cell* 2018;33(2):173-186.

Kahn SM, Hryb DJ, Nakhla AM, et al. Sex hormone-binding globulin is synthesized in target cells. *J Endocrinol* 2002;175(1):113-120.

Kaltsas G, Androulakis II, de Herder WW, et al. Paraneoplastic syndromes secondary to neuroendocrine tumours. *Endocr Relat Cancer* 2010;17(3):173-193.

Kaur J, Debnath J. Autophagy at the crossroads of catabolism and anabolism. *Nat Rev Mol Cell Biol* 2015;16(8):461-472.

Kiyotani K, Mushiroda T, Imamura CK, et al. Significant effect of polymorphisms in CYP2D6 and ABCC2 on clinical outcomes of adjuvant tamoxifen therapy for breast cancer patients. *J Clin Oncol* 2010;28(8):1287-1293.

Klinge CM. Estrogen receptor binding to estrogen response elements slows ligand dissociation and synergistically activates reporter gene expression. *Mol Cell Endocrinol* 1999;150(1-2):99-111.

Knudsen KE, Penning TM. Partners in crime: deregulation of AR activity and androgen synthesis in prostate cancer. *Trends Endocrinol Metab* 2010;21(5):315-324.

Koboldt DC, Fulton RS, McLellan MD, et al. Comprehensive molecular portraits of human breast tumours. *Nature* 2012;490(7418):61-70.

Koivisto PA, Helin HJ. Androgen receptor gene amplification increases tissue PSA protein expression in hormone-refractory prostate carcinoma. *J Pathol* 1999;189(2):219-223.

Korach KS. Insights from the study of animals lacking functional estrogen receptor. *Science* 1994;266:1524-1527.

Lallous N, Volik SV, Awrey S, et al. Functional analysis of androgen receptor mutations that confer anti-androgen resistance identified in circulating cell-free DNA from prostate cancer patients. *Genome Biol* 2016;17:10.

La Spada AR, Wilson EM, Lubahn DB, et al. Androgen receptor gene mutations in X-linked spinal and bulbar muscular atrophy. *Nature* 1991;352(6330):77-79.

Lawson DA, Witte ON. Stem cells in prostate cancer initiation and progression. *J Clin Invest* 2007;117(8):2044-2050.

Leygue E, Dotzlaw H, Watson PH, Murphy LC. Altered estrogen receptor alpha and beta messenger RNA expression during human breast tumorigenesis. *Cancer Res* 1998;58(15):3197-3201.

Levin ER, Hammes SR. Nuclear receptors outside the nucleus: extranuclear signalling by steroid receptors. *Nat Rev Mol Cell Biol* 2016;17(12):783-797.

Li Z, Bishop AC, Alyamani M, et al. Conversion of abiraterone to D4A drives anti-tumour activity in prostate cancer. *Nature* 2015;523(7560):347-51.

Lin C, Yang L, Tanasa B, et al. Nuclear receptor-induced chromosomal proximity and DNA breaks underlie specific translocations in cancer. *Cell* 2009;139(6):1069-1083.

Lindström S, Ma J, Altshuler D, et al. A large study of androgen receptor germline variants and their relation to sex hormone levels and prostate cancer risk. Results from the National Cancer Institute Breast and Prostate Cancer Cohort Consortium. *J Clin Endocrinol Metab* 2010;95(9):E121-E127.

Liu CY, Wu CY, Petrossian K, et al. Treatment for the endocrine resistant breast cancer: Current options and future perspectives. *J Steroid Biochem Mol Biol* 2017;172:166-175.

Locke JA, Guns ES, Lubik AA, et al. Androgen levels increase by intratumoral de novo steroidogenesis during progression of castration-resistant prostate cancer. *Cancer Res* 2008;68(15):6407-6415.

Lonard DM, O'Malley BW. Nuclear receptor coregulators: judges, juries, and executioners of cellular regulation. *Mol Cell* 2007;27(5):691-700.

Magnan S, Zarychankxi R, Pilote L, et al. Intermittent vs continuous androgen deprivation therapy for prostate cancer: a system review and meta-analysis. *JAMA Oncol* 2015;1(9):1261-1269.

Metivier R, Penot G, Hübner MR, et al. Estrogen receptor-alpha directs ordered, cyclical, and combinatorial recruitment of cofactors on a natural target promoter. *Cell* 2003;115(6):751-763.

Miettinen M, Isomaa V, Peltoketo H, et al. Estrogen metabolism as a regulator of estrogen action in the mammary gland. *J Mammary Gland Biol Neoplasia* 2000;5(3):259-270.

Miller WR. Aromatase inhibitors: prediction of response and nature of resistance. *Expert Opin Pharmacother* 2010;11(11):1873-1887.

Molina L, Figueroa CD, Bhoola KD, et al. GPER-1/GPR30 a novel estrogen receptor sited in the cell membrane: therapeutic coupling to breast cancer. *Expert Opin Ther Targets* 2017;21(8):755-766.

Montano MM, Ekena K, Delage-Mourroux R, et al. An estrogen receptor-selective co-regulator that potentiates the effectiveness of antiestrogens and represses the activity of estrogens. *Proc Natl Acad Sci U S A* 1999;96(12):6947-6952.

Murphy CG, Dickler MN2. Endocrine resistance in hormone-responsive breast cancer: mechanisms and therapeutic strategies. *Endocr Relat Cancer* 2016;23(8):337-52.

Murphy LC, Dotzlaw H, Leygue E, et al. The pathophysiological role of estrogen receptor variants in human breast cancer. *J Steroid Biochem Mol Biol* 1998;65(1-6):175-180.

Musgrove EA, Sutherland RL. Biological determinants of endocrine resistance in breast cancer. *Nat Rev Cancer* 2009;9(9):631-643.

Newell-Price J. Proopiomelanocortin gene expression and DNA methylation: implications for Cushing's syndrome and beyond. *J Endocrinol* 2003;177(3):365-372.

O'Regan RM, Jordan VC. Tamoxifen to raloxifene and beyond. *Semin Oncol* 2001;28(3):260-273.

Osborne CK, Schiff R. Mechanisms of endocrine resistance in breast cancer. *Annu Rev Med* 2011;62:233-247.

Packer JR, Maitland NJ. The molecular and cellular origin of human prostate cancer. *Biochim Biophys Acta* 2016;1863(6 Pt A):1238-1260.

Page DL, Jensen RA, Simpson JF, Dupont WD. Historical and epidemiologic background of human premalignant breast disease. *J Mammary Gland Biol Neoplasia* 2000;5(4):341-349.

Pauklin S, Sernandez IV, Bachmann G, et al. Estrogen directly activates AID transcription and function. *J Exp Med* 2009;206(1):99-111.

Pelosof LC, Gerber DE. Paraneoplastic syndromes: an approach to diagnosis and treatment. *Mayo Clin Proc* 2010;85(9):838-854.

Perissi V, Rosenfeld MG. Controlling nuclear receptors: the circular logic of cofactor cycles. *Nat Rev Mol Cell Biol* 2005;6(7):542-554.

Pomerantz MM, Li F, Takeda DY, et al. The androgen receptor cistrome is extensively reprogrammed in human prostate tumorigenesis. *Nat Genet* 2015;47(11):1346-1351.

Price DK, Chau CH, Till C, et al. Androgen receptor CAG repeat length and association with prostate cancer risk: results from the prostate cancer prevention trial. *J Urol* 2010;184(6):2297-2302.

Pritchard CC, Mateo J, Walsh MF, et al. Inherited DNA-repair gene mutations in men with metastatic prostate cancer. *N Engl J Med* 2016;375:443-453.

Province MA, Altman RB, Klein TE. Interpreting the CYP2D6 results from the International Tamoxifen Pharmacogenetics Consortium. *Clin Pharmacol Ther* 2014;96(2):144-146.

Qadir MA, Kwok B, Dragowska WH, et al. Macroautophagy inhibition sensitizes tamoxifen-resistant breast cancer cells and enhances mitochondrial depolarization. *Breast Cancer Res Treat* 2008;112(3):389-403.

Quigley DA, Dang HX, Zhao SG, et al. Genomic hallmarks and structural variation in metastatic prostate cancer. *Cell* 2018;174:758-769.

Ratman D, Vanden Berghe W, Dejager L, et al. How glucocorticoid receptors modulate the activity of other transcription factors: a scope beyond tethering. *Mol Cell Endocrinol* 2013;380(1-2):41-54.

Regan MM, Leyland-Jones B, Bouzyk M, et al. CYP2D6 genotype and tamoxifen response in postmenopausal women with endocrine-responsive breast cancer: the Breast International Group 1-98 Trial. *J Natl Cancer Inst.* 2012;104(6):441-451.

Rennie PS, Bruchovsky N, Leco KJ, et al. Characterization of two cis-acting DNA elements involved in the androgen regulation of the probasin gene. *Mol Endocrinol* 1993;7(1):23-36.

Robins DM, Albertelli MA, O'Mahony OA. Androgen receptor variants and prostate cancer in humanized AR mice. *J Steroid Biochem Mol Biol* 2008;108(3-5):230-236.

Robinson D, Van Allen EM, Wu YM, et al. Integrative clinical genomics of advanced prostate cancer. *Cell* 2015;161(5):1215-1228.

Roger P, Sahla ME, Makela S. Decreased expression of estrogen receptor beta protein in proliferative preinvasive mammary tumors. *Cancer Res* 2001;61(6):2537-2541.

Rosenfeld MG, Lunyak VV, Glass CK. Sensors and signals: a coactivator/corepressor/epigenetic code for integrating signal-dependent programs of transcriptional response. *Genes Dev* 2006;20(11):1405-1428.

Ryan CJ, Smith MR, De Bono JS, et al. Abiraterone in metastatic prostate cancer without previous chemotherapy. *N Engl J Med* 2013;368:138-148.

Ryan CJ, Smith MR, Fizazi K, et al. Abiraterone acetate plus prednisone versus placebo plus prednisone in chemotherapy-naive men with metastatic castration-resistant prostate cancer (COU-AA-302): final overall survival analysis of a randomised, double-blind, placebo-controlled phase 3 study. *Lancet Oncol* 2015;16(2):152-160.

Saad F, Fizazi K, Jinga V, et al. Orteronel plus prednisone in patients with chemotherapy-naive metastatic castration-resistant prostate cancer (ELM-PC 4): a double-blind, multicentre, phase 3, randomised, placebo-controlled trial. *Lancet Oncol* 2015;16(3):338-348.

Sakr WA, Partin AW. Histological markers of risk and the role of high-grade prostatic intraepithelial neoplasia. *Urology* 2001;57(4 Suppl 1):115-120.

Scher HI, Fizazi K, Saad F, et al. Increased survival with enzalutamide in prostate cancer after chemotherapy. *N Engl J Med* 2012;367(13):1187-1197.

Shang Y, Hu X, DiRenzo J, et al. Cofactor dynamics and sufficiency in estrogen receptor-regulated transcription. *Cell* 2000;103(6):843-852.

Shi XB, Ma AH, Xia L, et al. Functional analysis of 44 mutant androgen receptors from human prostate cancer. *Cancer Res* 2002;62(5):1496-1502.

Shiau AK, Barstad D, Loria PM, et al. The structural basis of estrogen receptor/co-activator recognition and the antagonism of this interaction by tamoxifen. *Cell* 1998;95(7):927-937.

Shoker BS, Jarvis C, Sibson DR, et al. Oestrogen receptor expression in the normal and pre-cancerous breast. *J Pathol* 1999;188(3):237-244.

Shou J, Massarweh S, Osborne CK, et al. Mechanisms of tamoxifen resistance: increased estrogen receptor-HER2/neu cross-talk in ER/HER2-positive breast cancer. *J Natl Cancer Inst* 2004;96(12):926-935.

Simpson ER. Biology of aromatase in the mammary gland. *J Mammary Gland Biol Neoplasia* 2000;5(3):251-258.

Skliris GP, Nugent ZJ, Rowan BG, et al. A phosphorylation code for oestrogen receptor-alpha predicts clinical outcome to endocrine therapy in breast cancer. *Endocr Relat Cancer* 2010;17(3):589-597.

Sledge GW, Toi M, Neven P, et al. Monarch 2: Abemaciclib in combination with fulvestrant in women with HR+/HER– advanced breast cancer who had progressed while receiving endocrine therapy. *J Clin Oncol* 2017;35(25):2875-2884.

Sorlie T. Molecular portraits of breast cancer: tumour subtypes as distinct disease entities. *Eur J Cancer* 2004;40(18):2667-2675.

Sparano JA, Gray RJ, Makower DF, et al. Prospective validation of a 21-gene expression assay in breast cancer. *N Eng J Med* 2016;373(21):2005-2014.

Stanford JL, Just JJ, Gibbs M, et al. Polymorphic repeats in the androgen receptor gene: molecular markers of prostate cancer risk. *Cancer Res* 1997;15:1194-1198.

Stashi E, York B, O'Malley BW. Steroid receptor coactivators: servants and masters for control of systems metabolism. *Trends Endocrinol Metab* 2014;25(7):337-347.

Sweeney CJ, Chen YH, Carducci M, et al. Chemohormonal therapy in metastatic hormone-sensitive prostate cancer. *N Engl J Med* 2015;373(8):737-746.

Takeda DY, Spisak S, Seo J-H, et al. A somatically acquired enhancer is a noncoding driver in advanced prostate cancer. *Cell* 2018;174:422-432.

Taplin ME, Bubley GJ, Ko YJ, et al. Selection for androgen receptor mutations in prostate cancers treated with androgen antagonist. *Cancer Res* 1999;59(11):2511-2515.

Thajudeen B, Salahudeen AK. Role of tolvaptan in the management of hyponatremia in patients with lung and other cancers: current data and future perspectives. *Cancer Manag Res* 2016;8:105-114.

Thompson IM, Goodman PJ, Tangen CM, et al. The influence of finasteride on the development of prostate cancer. *N Engl J Med* 2003;349(3):215-224.

Thompson PA, Ambrosone C. Molecular epidemiology of genetic polymorphisms in estrogen metabolizing enzymes in human breast cancer. *J Natl Cancer Inst Monogr* 2000;27:125-134.

Toy W, Shen Y, Won H, et al. ESR1 ligand-binding domain mutations in hormone-resistant breast cancer. *Nat Genet* 2013;45(12):1439-1445.

Tran C, Ouk S, Clegg NJ, et al. Development of a second-generation antiandrogen for treatment of advanced prostate cancer. *Science* 2009;324(5928):787-790.

Vijayvargia R, May MS, Fondell JD. A coregulatory role for the mediator complex in prostate cancer cell proliferation and gene expression. *Cancer Res* 2007;67(9):4034-4041.

Vogel VG, Costantino JP, Wickerham DL, et al. Effects of tamoxifen vs raloxifene on the risk of developing invasive breast cancer and other disease outcomes: the NSABP Study of Tamoxifen and Raloxifene (STAR) P-2 trial. *JAMA* 2006;295(23):2727-2741.

Vukovic B, Beheshti B, Park P, et al. Correlating breakage-fusion-bridge events with the overall chromosomal instability and in vitro karyotype evolution in prostate cancer. *Cytogenet Genome Res* 2007;116(1-2):1-11.

Wang L, Lonard DM, O'Malley BW. The role of steroid receptor coactivators in hormone dependent cancers and their potential as therapeutic targets. *Horm Canc* 2016;7(4):229-235.

Wang X, Kruithof-de Julio M, Economides KD, et al. A luminal epithelial stem cell that is a cell of origin for prostate cancer. *Nature* 2009;461(7263):495-500.

Ward RD, Weigel NL. Steroid receptor phosphorylation: assigning function to site-specific phosphorylation. *Biofactors* 2009;35(6):528-536.

Warde P, Mason M, Ding K, et al. Combined androgen deprivation therapy and radiation therapy for locally advanced prostate cancer: a randomised phase III trial. *Lancet* 2011;378(9809):2104-2111.

Ware KE, Garcia-Blanco MA, Armstrong AJ, et al. Biologic and clinical significance of androgen receptor variants in castration resistant prostate cancer. *Endocr Relat Cancer* 2014;21(4):87-103.

Xu J, Wu RC, O'Malley BW. Normal and cancer-related functions of the p160 steroid receptor co-activator (SRC) family. *Nat Rev Cancer* 2009;9(9):615-630.

Zarrella ER, Coulter M, Welsh AW, et al. Automated measurement of estrogen receptor in breast cancer: a comparison of fluorescent and chromogenic methods of measurement. *Lab Invest* 2016;96(9):1016-1025.

Ziegler RG, Hoover RN, Pike MC, et al. Migration patterns and breast cancer risk in Asian-American women. *J Natl Cancer Inst* 1993;85(22):1819-1827.

The Immune System and Immunotherapy

21

Samuel D. Saibil, Ben X. Wang, and Marcus O. Butler

Chapter Outline

- 21.1 Introduction to the Immune System
- 21.2 Innate Immunity
  - 21.2.1 Antigen Presentation
  - 21.2.2 Maturation of Dendritic Cells
  - 21.2.3 Innate Lymphoid Cells
- 21.3 Adaptive Immunity
  - 21.3.1 Generation of Lymphocyte Diversity
  - 21.3.2 T-Cell Activation
  - 21.3.3 T-Cell Memory
  - 21.3.4 T-Cell Subsets
  - 21.3.5 Modulation of T-Cell Activation
  - 21.3.6 T-Cell Tolerance
- 21.4 Tumor Immunology
  - 21.4.1 Tumor-Associated Antigens
  - 21.4.2 Tumor-Associated Antigen–Specific T Cells in Humans
  - 21.4.3 Immune Surveillance
  - 21.4.4 T-Cell Infiltration and Disease Prognosis
  - 21.4.5 Barriers to Antitumor Immunity
- 21.5 Immunotherapy
  - 21.5.1 Introduction
  - 21.5.2 Monoclonal Antibodies for Cancer Therapy
  - 21.5.3 In Vivo Immunomodulation
  - 21.5.4 Immune Checkpoint Inhibitors
  - 21.5.5 Adoptive T-Cell Therapy
- Summary
- References

21.1 INTRODUCTION TO THE IMMUNE SYSTEM

One feature that is common to all organisms is the ability to defend themselves against challenges in the environment in which they live. Mammals have a complex phalanx of defenses against bacteria, viruses, and parasites, which comprise the immune system. The immune system can be characterized broadly as having 2 major arms: *innate immunity* and *adaptive immunity*. The innate immune system is the "first line of defense" against pathogens and includes macrophages and dendritic cells that function in part to present antigens to the cells in the adaptive immune system. The adaptive arm of the immune system is mediated by lymphocytes and responds with higher specificity to pathogens. Key cells of the adaptive immune system are helper T cells (T_H) that express a marker known as CD4, cytotoxic T lymphocytes (CTL) that are distinguished by the CD8 marker, and B cells that produce antibodies. The molecular components of pathogens that are recognized by T and B cells are referred to broadly as antigens.

The adaptive immune system has evolved to respond to an initial encounter with a variety of foreign pathogens as well as a potential secondary encounter with the same pathogen. These challenges have shaped the development of the immune system to have the properties of diversity, specificity, and memory. Diversity enables an individual to respond to a broad array of possible pathogens, while at the same time generating exquisite specificity to elements of specific pathogens, ensuring a focused response to a given pathogen while minimizing collateral damage to the host tissues. Memory is the ability of the immune system to respond rapidly to a pathogen that has been encountered previously thus quickly clearing the offending organism.

Another feature of the immune system is that it generally does not attack the host's own tissues. This recognition of "self" vs "non-self" and the ability to avoid attacking self-tissues is referred to as *self-tolerance*. Although these mechanisms of tolerance are critical to avoid autoimmunity, they are impediments that need to be overcome in antitumor immunity.

21.2 INNATE IMMUNITY

21.2.1 Antigen Presentation

One of the main functions of the innate immune system is to present antigens to the adaptive immune system to orchestrate a functional immune response. Dendritic cells (DCs) are highly specialized and efficient antigen-presenting cells

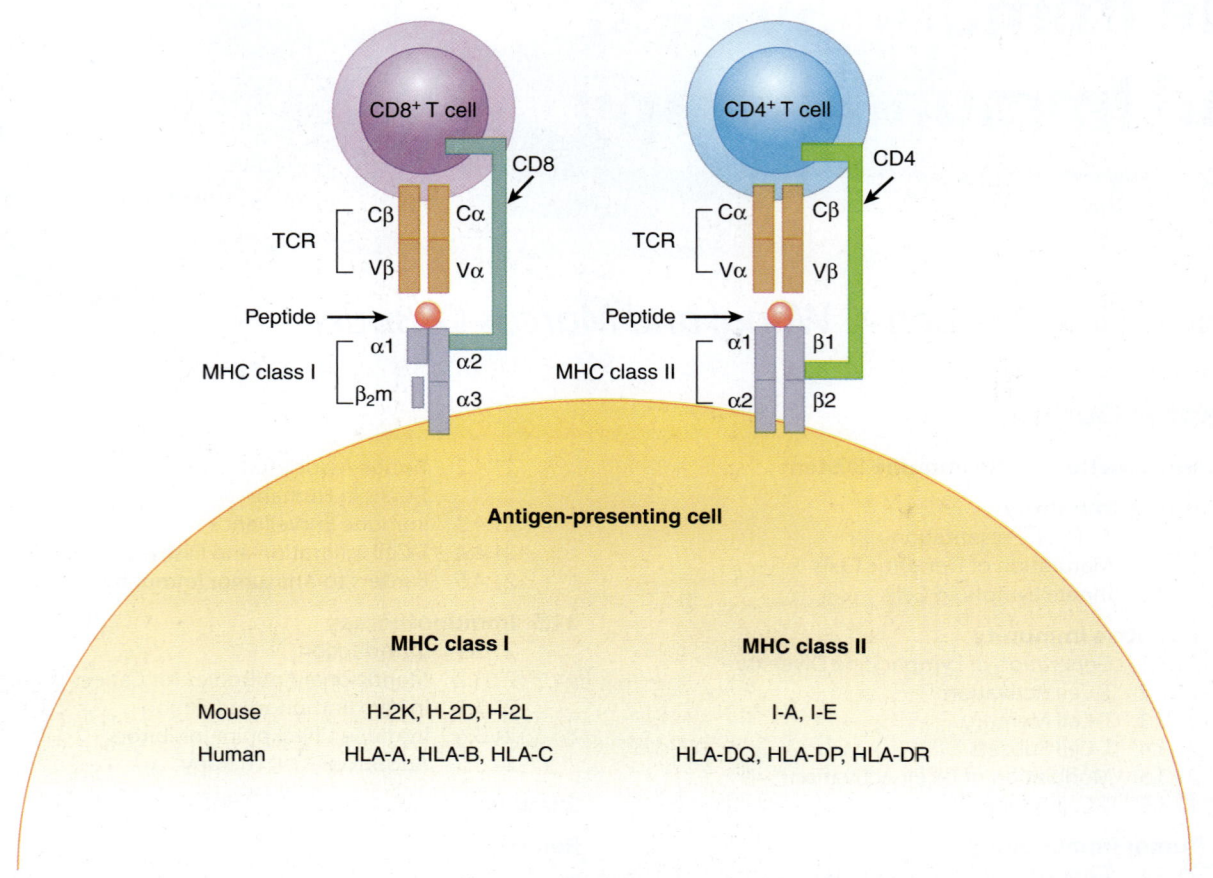

FIGURE 21–1 T-cell recognition of antigens in the context of MHC molecules. The α/β dimer of the T-cell receptor (TCR) recognizes peptide fragments on the surface of antigen-presenting cells (APCs). The TCR on CD4+ T cells binds MHC class II molecules bearing an antigenic peptide. This interaction is stabilized by the CD4 coreceptor from the surface of the CD4+ T-cell binding to the MHC class II molecule. The TCR on CD8+ T cells binds MHC class I molecules bearing an antigenic peptide. This interaction is stabilized by the CD8 coreceptor. The nomenclature of MHC alleles in human and mouse is listed at the bottom of the figure. $β_2m$, $β_2$-microglobulin.

(APCs). One key function that differentiates DCs from other "professional" APCs, such as macrophages and B cells, is their ability to activate naïve T cells. Antigens are presented to T cells by major histocompatibility complex (MHC) molecules. The MHC consists of a series of proteins encoded by highly polymorphic codominantly expressed genes. As a result, each individual expresses a particular combination of MHC alleles that is different between individuals, and a huge diversity exists in populations. There are 2 main types of MHC molecules. MHC class I molecules are expressed on almost all cells. MHC class II molecules are expressed primarily on APCs such as macrophages, DCs and B cells, or their expression can be induced on cells by inflammation. The mouse MHC class I molecules are referred to as H-2K, H-2D, and H-2L; the mouse MHC class II molecules are I-A and I-E. The human MHC is composed of 3 class I molecules, HLA-A, HLA-B, and HLA-C, and 3 class II molecules, HLA-DQ, HLA-DP, and HLA-DR. Class I heterodimers comprise a transmembrane α-chain noncovalently bound to the nonpolymorphic $β_2$-microglobulin protein ($β_2m$). The class II MHC molecule is expressed on the cell surface as an α and β heterodimer. A schematic of MHC class I and II molecules is depicted in Figure 21–1.

The functions of MHC class I and II molecules are to bind and display peptide fragments for T-cell recognition. These peptides may be derived from self-proteins or foreign proteins. The peptide-binding cleft of MHC molecules contains the regions of highest polymorphism within the molecule and has an impact on the array of peptides that may be bound. Class I and class II differ in the size of peptides that can bind the cleft. MHC class I binds smaller peptide fragments (8-11 amino acids), whereas class II binds larger fragments of proteins (15-18 amino acids).

The 3 major pathways by which peptides can be processed and loaded into the binding cleft of MHC molecules are referred to as the exogenous, endogenous, and cross-presentation pathways. These pathways are depicted in Figure 21–2. The exogenous pathway is the predominant pathway for class II loading, whereas the proteins processed through the endogenous and cross-presentation pathways result in class I loading. The endogenous pathway occurs in most cells, whereas the other 2 pathways (exogenous and cross-presentation) occur primarily in APCs.

The exogenous pathway of protein processing begins when an APC acquires material from outside the cell by phagocytosis

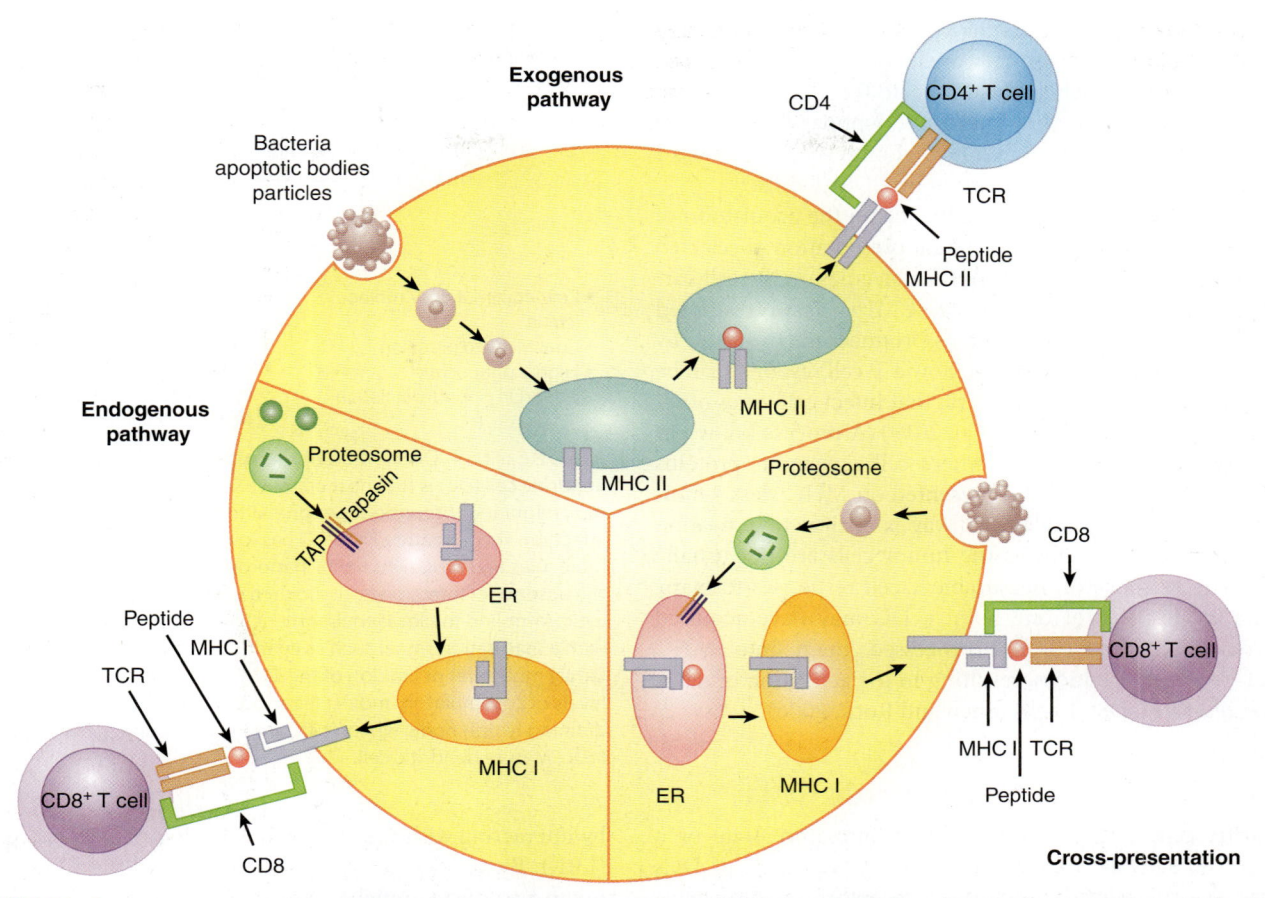

FIGURE 21–2 Antigen-processing pathways in the antigen-processing cell (APC). There are 3 pathways of antigen processing by the APC: exogenous, endogenous, and cross-presentation. The exogenous pathway processes proteins produced outside the APC and places their peptides on MHC class II for recognition by CD4+ T cells (upper right). Proteins derived from apoptotic bodies, bacteria, and particulate antigens are processed into peptides by the exogenous pathway. The exogenous pathway occurs in phagocytic cells, including B cells, macrophages, and dendritic cells. The endogenous pathway places cell-produced peptides into the peptide-binding groove of MHC class I for recognition by CD8+ T cells (lower left). The endogenous pathway is responsible for immune recognition of viral peptides or self-peptides. Peptides are cleaved from proteins in the cytosol by the proteasome. The peptides enter the endoplasmic reticulum (ER) in a process dependent on the transporter associated with antigen processing (TAP) and are loaded onto MHC class I, with the help of a cofactor, tapasin. MHC class I is then shuttled to the cell surface. This pathway occurs in most cells, not just APCs, allowing sensing of viral infection in all cell types. The cross-presentation pathway (lower right) also loads peptides onto MHC class I for recognition by CD8+ T cells, but the proteins that are processed are not cell-intrinsic and are instead taken up from the surrounding environment. This pathway is important for detecting viruses that infect cells other than APCs and tumor antigens taken up in the form of tumor apoptotic bodies. The cross-presentation pathway is most efficient in dendritic cells.

or receptor-mediated endocytosis. This exogenous material is processed initially in an acidified early endosome by pH-sensitive proteases. The endosome containing the fragmented protein finally fuses with a vesicle containing newly formed MHC class II molecules where the peptides then bind in the cleft of the MHC molecule. MHC class II is produced in the endoplasmic reticulum. When the protein is produced, a chaperone protein known as the invariant chain initially occupies the peptide-binding groove. As the MHC-invariant complex leaves the Golgi apparatus, the invariant chain targets the complex to enter the endosomal pathway where proteases known as cathepsins digest the invariant chain until only a small fragment known as CLIP (class II-associated invariant chain-derived peptide) remains in the binding cleft. The MHC II–CLIP complex next associates with proteins that aid in the release of CLIP, freeing the peptide-binding groove for occupancy by the extrinsically obtained peptides. After this peptide exchange, the complex is shuttled to the cell membrane, where it is available to be recognized by CD4+ T cells (Bryant and Ploegh, 2004; Trombetta and Mellman, 2005).

The endogenous pathway is responsible for loading cell-intrinsic proteins in the binding cleft of MHC class I molecules. Proteins are digested by a large macromolecular complex known as the proteosome. The proteosome normally processes self-proteins and when a cell is exposed to inflammatory cytokines, such as interferon-γ (IFN-γ) or tumor necrosis factor–α (TNF-α), the structure of the proteosome is altered into a structure known as the *immunoproteasome*, which is more efficient at processing peptides with high binding efficiency to the MHC class I peptide-binding cleft. Self-proteins are cleaved into short fragments by the proteosome in the cytoplasm and are then shuttled into the endoplasmic reticulum by the TAP protein complex. As the peptides are guided into the ER by the TAP transporter, they are loaded onto empty MHC class I molecules, which are held close to the TAP complex by the protein Tapasin. In viral infections, peptides derived from the virus will be processed and loaded onto the MHC class I molecule resulting in viral detection by CD8+ T cells.

Efficient activation of T cells depends on the acquisition of antigens by APCs and the subsequent presentation of selected peptides in combination with MHC molecules on the cell surface for recognition by T cells. Because MHC class I–restricted peptides are derived from proteins produced intrinsically by the cell, a conundrum arises as to how a T-cell response can be initiated against viruses or bacteria that infect cell types other than APCs (Sanchez-Paulete et al, 2019). A process known as cross-presentation can occur where cell-exogenous proteins can be taken up by DCs and presented on MHC class I molecules (see Fig. 21–2). This pathway is critical to activation of tumor-specific T cells, as the tumor cells are not usually APCs. The presence of measurable T-cell responses to many tumors implies that at one point a DC may have acquired tumor-derived proteins and processed them into MHC class I–restricted peptides, resulting in the activation of naïve tumor-reactive CD8+ T cells (Shen and Rock, 2006).

21.2.2 Maturation of Dendritic Cells

Dendritic cells (DCs) can exist in an immature state or a mature (ie, activated) state (Fig. 21–3). Maturation of DCs occurs via specialized cell-surface receptors or intracellular receptors that recognize pathogen-associated molecular patterns. These receptor classes include Toll-like receptors (TLRs), nucleotide-binding domain and leucine-rich repeat receptors (NLRs), the retinoic acid–inducible gene-like receptors (RLRs), and c-type lectins (Iwasaki and Medzhitov, 2010). The best-studied receptors are the TLR family of proteins (Kawasaki and Kawai, 2014). The ligands for TLRs include viral/bacterial DNA and RNA, bacterial lipids, and endogenously derived molecules, such as heat shock proteins and uric acid crystals that alert the immune system to tissue damage. There are at least 13 identified TLRs in mammals, 9 of which are conserved between human and mouse (TLR1 to TLR9). TLR4 is one of the best-characterized TLRs; the pathogen-associated ligand for TLR4 is lipopolysaccharide (LPS), a molecule found on the outer membrane of gram-negative bacteria. TLR9 recognizes unmethylated CpG (cytosine phosphate guanine) DNA structures (Hemmi et al, 2000), which are plentiful in bacterial DNA but rare in mammals. Activation of TLR9 by CpG DNA results in production of the cytokines interleukin (IL)-12 and TNF-α, which contribute to the induction of cell-mediated immunity and have shown antitumor effects in animal models. TLR agonists are under clinical investigation alone and in combination with immune checkpoint inhibitors (Sec. 21.5.3.2; Wang et al, 2018).

The NOD-like and RIG-I-like families of proteins (NLRs and RLRs) detect the presence of bacteria and viruses, respectively. NLR proteins sense bacterial products in the cytoplasm

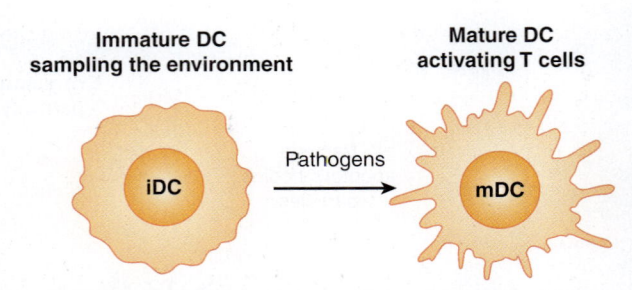

FIGURE 21–3 Dendritic cell maturation and migration. The dendritic cell (DC) is the most effective sentinel for the immune system, migrating throughout peripheral tissues seeking damage or infection. The immature DC (iDC) has low expression of costimulatory molecules and MHC. This limits inappropriate activation of T cells in the absence of infection or tissue damage. The iDC is highly phagocytic, sampling the local environment for antigens. On encounter with a maturation signal such as ligands for the Toll-like receptor (TLR) family molecules or ligation of the CD40 molecule, the iDC increases levels of costimulatory molecules and MHC and migrates to the local draining lymph node, where it can interact with and activate T cells. mDC, Mature dendritic cell.

by interacting with the C-terminal leucine-rich repeat regions (LRR). Bacterially derived products bind to the LRR, resulting in a conformational change in intracellular NOD proteins. This change activates the NOD proteins resulting in recruitment of signaling kinases and activation of caspase-1 (CASP)-1 through binding to caspase recruitment domains (CARDs). This activation results in both de novo cytokine transcription via activation of the nuclear factor-kappa B (NF-κB) and AP1 transcription factors (see Chap. 6, Sec. 6.2.6) and activation of IL-1 through CASP-1 activity (Franchi et al, 2009). RLRs are also localized in the cytoplasm but bind viral-derived RNA sequences. The RLR family contains several members, such as RIG-I, MDA-5, and LGP2. These proteins bind modifications found in the 5′ end of virally produced RNAs that are not found in mammalian RNA. Detection of viral RNA in the cytoplasm results in activation of NF-κB and IRF3 (interferon regulatory factor 3), thereby inducing inflammatory cytokine and type-1 interferon production by the infected cell (Kawai and Akira, 2008).

After the detection of pathogens via these different receptor families, the APC becomes mature and upregulates expression of MHC class II and other costimulatory molecules that contribute to the activation of T cells (see Fig. 21–3). In addition, mature APCs are induced to secrete cytokines and chemokines that promote immune function in a variety of ways. Signaling through TLRs also induces a change in migration of the APC. DCs will change their responsiveness to chemokine signals and migrate out of the peripheral tissues and localize ("home") to lymph nodes, thus increasing their chances of encountering a T cell with specificity to the pathogen that activated the DC. Monocytes and macrophages will migrate in the opposite pattern, entering the infected or damaged tissue where they take part in pathogen clearance or tissue repair, at the same time acting as local APCs to maintain activation of T cells at the site of infection.

21.2.3 Innate Lymphoid Cells

Innate lymphoid cells (ILCs) are a group of cells that, like T and B cells of the adaptive immune system, are derived from a common lymphoid progenitor cell. Unlike T and B cells, these cells lack adaptive antigen receptors generated via recombination of genetic elements. Instead, ILCs express multiple different receptors that are encoded in the germline and recognize pre-specified target molecules on host or foreign cells. Initially, natural killer (NK) cells were the only identified group of ILCs, but there are now three major recognized subgroups, labeled Group 1, 2 and 3 ILCs. Each group is defined by the requirement for specific transcription factors to induce their development and by the production of similar effector cytokines (Vivier et al, 2018). Each group of ILCs can be further subdivided into multiple subsets of cells with different properties and function. The importance of ILC biology in the immune response is just beginning to be appreciated.

In the context of tumor immunology, the role of Group 1 ILCs has been the best defined. Group 1 ILCs, which require the transcription factor T-bet for their development, include highly cytotoxic NK cells as well as ILC1 cells, which display lower expression of the cytolytic molecule perforin. NK cells have an important role in controlling tumors as they can be activated to lyse cells that have decreased levels of class I MHC expression (Lanier, 2005). Whereas T cells may recognize tumors due to novel antigens that arise by mutation, so called "altered self", NK cells can recognize loss of antigen presentation, so called "missing self". Thus, NK cells may be able to control tumors that have lost class I MHC expression and are thereby able to evade CD8+ T cells. Accordingly, there is interest in utilizing NK cells as cellular therapies for cancer (Franks et al, 2020). However, a subset of NK cells, dubbed NKregs, has been identified with ability to inhibit the expansion of tumor infiltrating lymphocytes in tissue culture (Crome et al, 2017). Thus, like ILCs, different subsets of NK cells can display a wide range of function. Some NK cells suppress tumors via direct lysis of tumor cells whilst others might promote tumor growth by regulating cells of the adaptive immune system. Further work to decipher the complexity of NK and ILC1 biology is required to help optimize therapeutic approaches utilizing NK cells.

21.3 ADAPTIVE IMMUNITY

21.3.1 Generation of Lymphocyte Diversity

B and T cells express highly specific receptors that recognize antigen. The B-cell receptor (BCR) and T-cell receptor (TCR) are generated uniquely in each cell as the consequence of genomic DNA rearrangements. The BCR is a membrane-bound form of the soluble immunoglobulin (antibody) that will be produced by that cell on activation, as a consequence of the ability to bind a specific antigen. BCRs can bind to antigens in their native form, so that the B cell can detect unprocessed antigens. In contrast, the TCR is not secreted, and stimulation via the TCR may lead to the activation of the T-cell response. Antigen recognition by T cells is also different from antigen recognition by B cells. T cells do not react to antigen in its unprocessed form, but rather recognize peptide fragments bound in the MHC of APCs (as described above; see also Fig. 21–2). These differences allow B and T cells to defend the host in 2 different ways: by directly recognizing the pathogen and by recognizing cells infected by the pathogen.

The TCR is composed of 2 protein chains joined together by disulfide bonds (Fig. 21–4A). This dimer can be composed of either α and β chains or γ and δ chains. The αβ TCR is present on the majority of mature T cells found in the blood and lymphoid organs whereas γδ TCR-bearing T cells are found primarily in the skin and intestine. The TCR is expressed at the cell surface in a molecular complex that includes proteins that have intracellular signaling domains (immunoreceptor tyrosine activation motifs [ITAMs]): CD3δε, CD3γε, and TCRζζ. Once the TCR is bound by specific peptide-MHC complexes, the ITAMs in the CD3 and TCR molecules aggregate together and initiate an intracellular signaling cascade (Brownlie and Zamoyska, 2013).

The TCR chains are not encoded as single transcripts; rather, they are the result of genomic DNA rearrangements that bring together different gene segments and splice them into a combined exon (see Fig. 21–4B). This genomic splicing is dependent on an enzyme known as *recombination activation gene recombinase* (*RAG* recombinase) that is expressed exclusively in developing T and B cells (Krangel, 2009). The TCRα chain is composed of 2 separate rearranged gene segments brought together during recombination. Variable (V) gene segments undergo rearrangement with joining (J) gene segments and are expressed together with constant (C) regions, forming the α chain of the TCR. The β chain has 3 rearranged gene segments: variable, diversity (D), and joining regions that undergo rearrangement and are expressed with the constant region of the β locus. The large number of possible combinations of VJ in the α chain and VDJ in the β chain results in enormous diversity among T-cell populations, especially as each mature T cell will rearrange its own TCR independently (Krangel, 2009; see Fig. 21–4B). In addition, a strategy called "N region diversity" occurs that generates additional nucleotides during the rearrangement process, which increases the repertoire of antigens that can be recognized by each TCR. The specificity of the TCR for a defined peptide bound in the groove of an MHC molecule is determined by regions of the TCR called complementarity determining regions (CDRs). Interactions of the CDR with the peptide-MHC complex are a result of the combination of the V chains expressed, as well as the diversity generated by pairing of the VJ and VDJ gene segments.

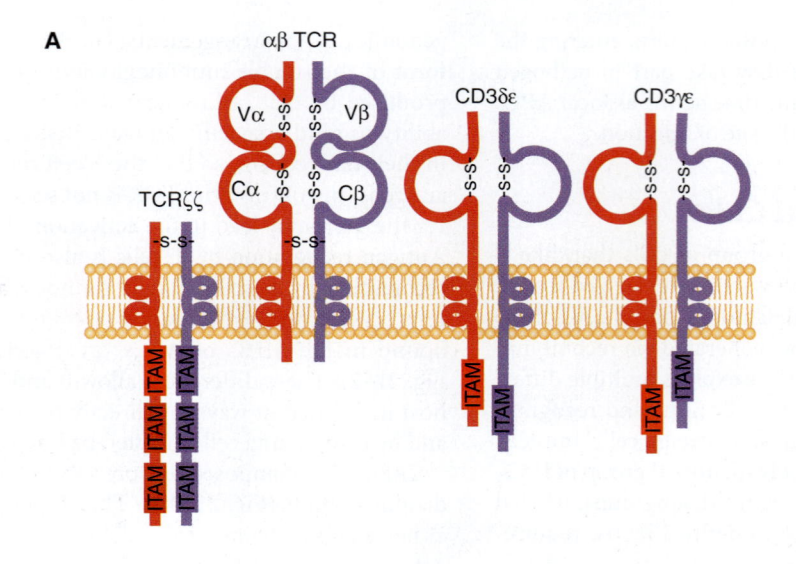

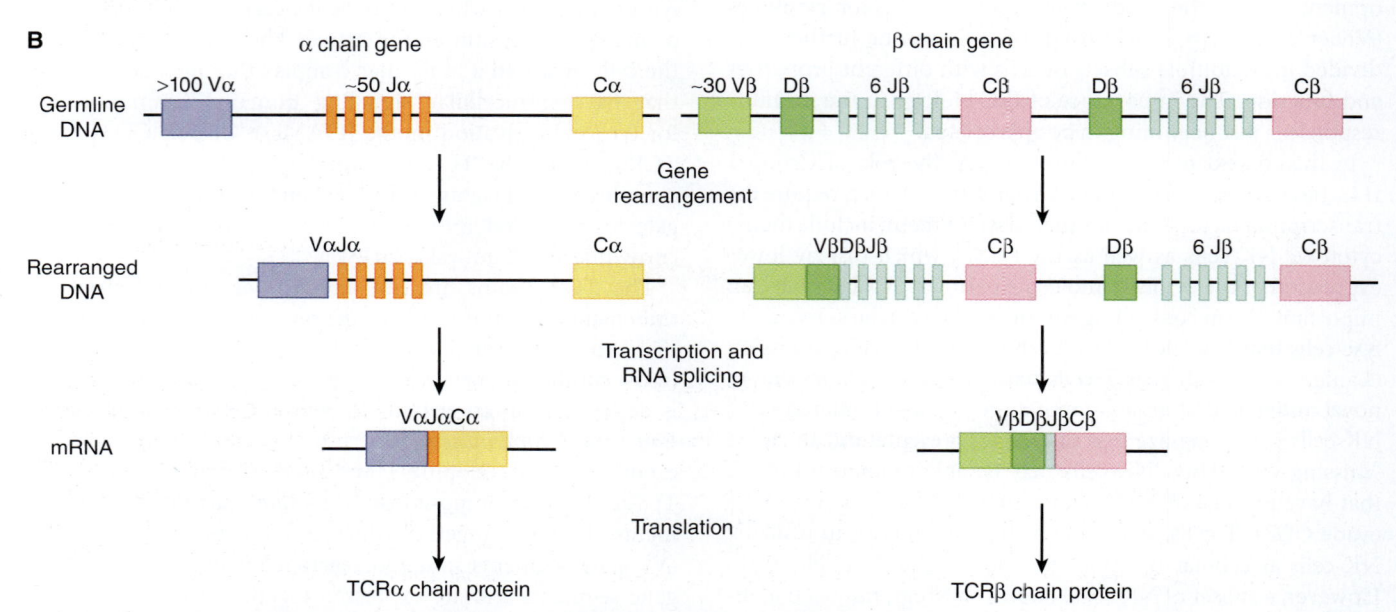

FIGURE 21–4 The αβ T-cell receptor (αβ TCR). A) The TCR is composed of 2 chains, α and β, each containing 2 immunoglobulin domains formed by an intrachain disulfide bond. The αβ TCR is associated with the dimeric proteins CD3δε, CD3γε, and TCRζζ, and together, they comprise the TCR complex. *ITAM*, Immunoreceptor tyrosine-based activation motifs. **B)** The variable (V), diversity (D), joining (J), and constant (C) domains are encoded by corresponding gene segments that undergo somatic rearrangement to generate the αβ TCR heterodimer. Following V(D)J gene rearrangement and transcription, the RNA is spliced to the C gene segment. The resulting messenger RNA (mRNA) encodes the TCR chains that dimerize to form the complete TCR protein. A small pool of effector CD8+ T cells become memory T cells: T effector memory (TEM) and T central memory (TCM) cells. These memory subsets can be defined by their localization, surface molecule expression, and function. *4-1BB*, tumor necrosis factor receptor superfamily member 9; *OX40*, tumor necrosis factor receptor superfamily member 4; *PD-1*, programmed cell death protein 1; *TIGIT*, T cell immunoreceptor with immunoglobulin (Ig) and immunoreceptor tyrosine-based inhibition motif (ITIM) domain.

21.3.2 T-Cell Activation

The functional status of a mature T cell depends on whether it expresses a receptor that can bind to a peptide-MHC molecule expressed by a mature APC. T cells can exist in a *naïve* or resting state, or they can be *effector* T cells, which means that they have engaged a mature DC bearing their cognate antigen and have differentiated subsequently into functional T cells. Alternatively, they can be *memory* T cells, which are previously activated antigen-specific cells that persist after the pathogen has been eliminated. These 3 states (naïve, effector, and memory) impart different phenotypic and functional properties (Fig. 21–5). These stages of development have been studied most extensively in the CD8+ MHC class I–restricted lineage of T cells, and thus much of the following information will refer to CD8+ T cells; however, they also broadly apply to CD4+ T cells.

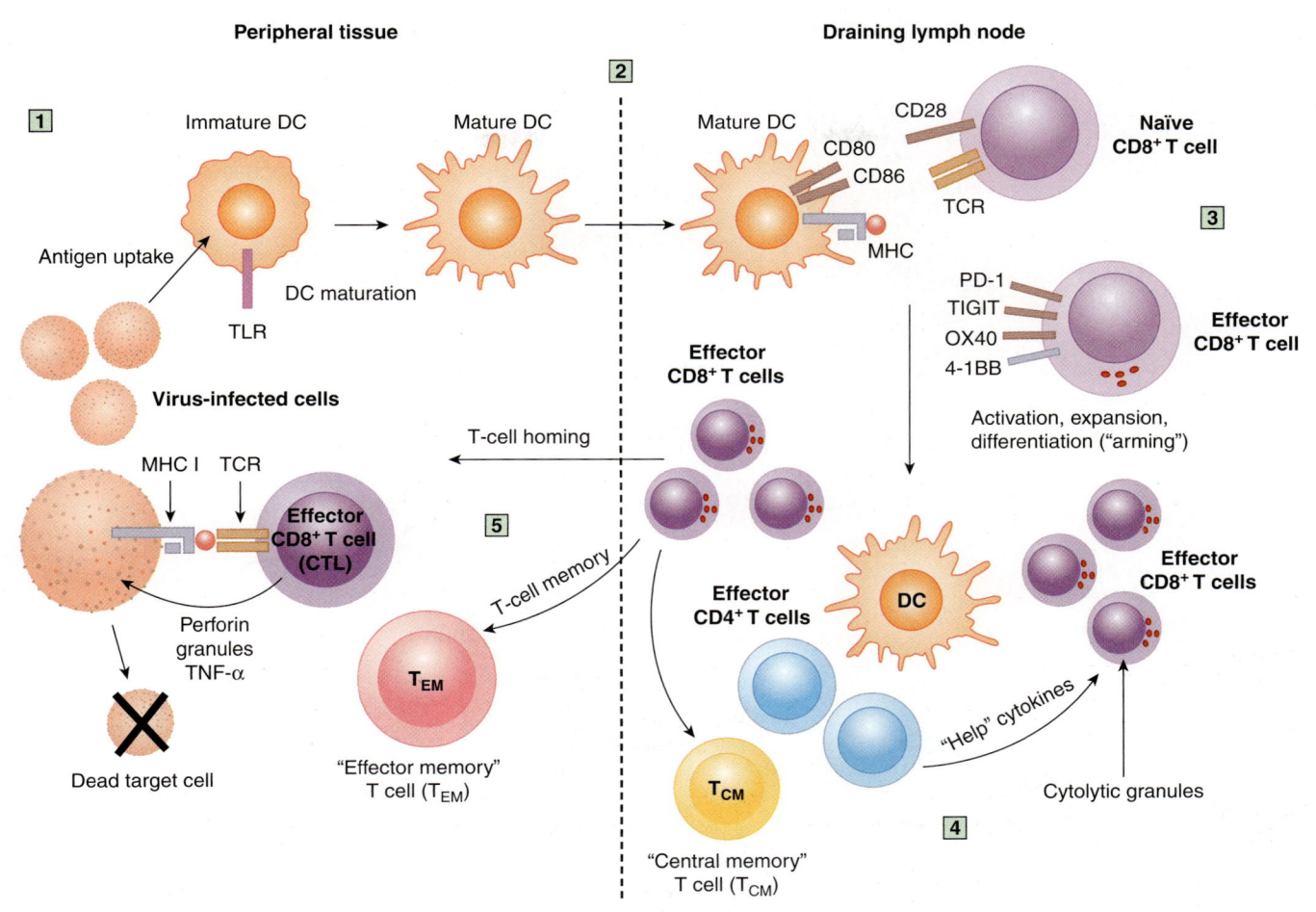

FIGURE 21-5 The stages of a cytotoxic T-cell response. 1) CD8+ T-cell immune responses begin when a DC is activated by a pathogen or inflammatory signal in the periphery. Antigens are picked up by the DC and processed into peptides and placed onto MHC class I molecules via the cross-presentation pathway. **2)** Mature DCs migrate to T-cell areas in the lymph nodes, where they interact with naïve T cells. **3)** The T cell recognizes its cognate peptide bound to MHC class I on the DC, resulting in activation of the T cell and the expression of activation markers such as 4-1BB, OX40, PD-1 and TIGIT. If the TCR signal is followed by costimulation by CD28 on the T cell interacting with CD80 and CD86 on the DC, the T cell will begin to proliferate, expanding the clone of the T cell that has specificity to the antigen. **4)** The CD8+ T cell will become armed by exposure to 'help' cytokines released by effector CD4+ T helper cells, resulting in cytolytic granule formation. **5)** The T cell then exits the lymph node and traffics to sites of inflammation to engage and kill cells that present the cognate antigenic peptide on their MHC class I molecules.

Most T-cell responses can be subdivided into 3 phases: activation (also known as priming), expansion, and contraction (Fig. 21–6). A naïve T cell has a high threshold for activation, which means that when a mature T cell encounters its cognate antigen–MHC complex for the first time, it is slow to respond and requires several signals to initiate proliferation and acquisition of effector function. The DC is the main cell responsible for T-cell activation. During priming, a DC acquires antigen and matures at the site of infection and travels to the draining lymph node where it enters the T-cell area and interacts with the T cells resident there. An "integrin" receptor–ligand interaction occurs between leukocyte function–associated antigen (LFA)-1 and LFA-2 on the T cell and intercellular adhesion molecule (ICAM) expressed on the DC. These interactions initially slow migration of the DC past the naïve T cell and then help bring their cell membranes into close proximity, allowing MHC-TCR interactions (Dustin and Cooper, 2000; Fig. 21–6). If a mature DC presents a peptide on its MHC molecules that is recognized by the specific TCR on the T cell, a signal will be sent into the T cell. This antigen-specific recognition, together with other receptor ligand interactions, promotes a functional T-cell response. One of the well-studied molecules that leads to optimal T-cell activation is CD28. The ligands of CD28 are CD80 (B7-1) and CD86 (B7-2), which are upregulated on the surface of mature DCs. This CD28 costimulatory signal results in the production of IL-2, a cytokine critical for T-cell proliferation and survival (Fig. 21–6). T-cell activation also results in the increased expression of several other molecules, including CD40L, which is the ligand for the TNF family member CD40 that is present on the surface of the DC. The binding of CD40 on the DC results in the upregulation of costimulatory molecules, cytokines, and increased DC survival, allowing for prolonged antigen presentation (Quezada et al, 2004). The positive feedback loop between T cells and the DC results in expansion of antigen-specific T-cell clones. These expanded T cells are now functional effector T cells that change their

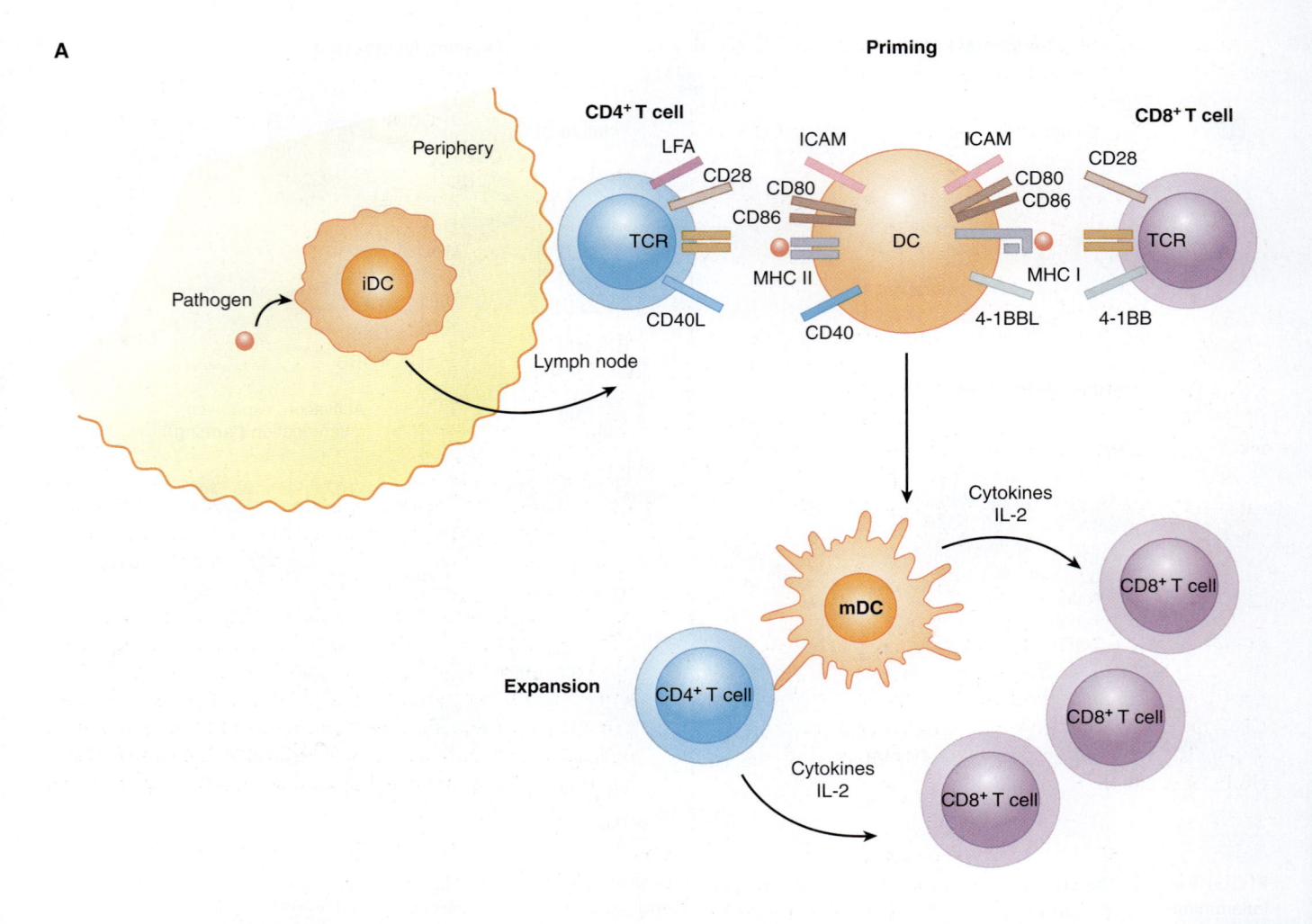

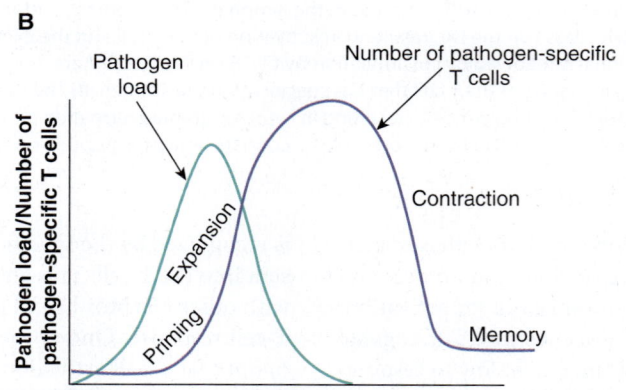

FIGURE 21–6 T-cell activation: priming, expansion, and contraction. A) After sensing tissue damage or infection in a peripheral tissue, the DC bearing antigen migrates to the T-cell area of a draining lymph node. DCs and T cells mingle in the lymph node, adhering to one another through interactions between LFA (lymphocyte function-associated antigen) on the T cell and ICAM (intercellular adhesion molecule) on the DC. T cells with a TCR that is specific for the antigen obtained at the site of infection will interact with the DC and signal through the antigen-specific TCR. At the same time, CD28 on the T cell will bind to CD80 and CD86 on the DC. This signal is referred to as *costimulation*. CD4+ T cells will express CD40 ligand (CD40L) that binds to CD40 on the DC, promoting the antigen-bearing DC's survival and increasing cytokine production. 4-1BB expressed by activated antigen-specific CD8+ T cells binds 4-1BBL expressed by DCs to promote T cell survival. Antigen-specific CD8+ and CD4+ T cells that receive these signals will then begin to divide. These expanded antigen-specific T cells then travel to the peripheral tissues to clear the infection. **B)** The T-cell immune response can be divided into several phases. Priming occurs when an antigen is first presented to naïve T cells and they are induced to expand for the first time. As the levels of antigen wane because of clearance by the immune system, contraction of the antigen-specific T-cell clones occurs. After contraction, a greater number of specific T cells remain than before the infection. These cells are referred to as memory T cells and have properties that allow them to react rapidly to reinfection with the same pathogen. *4-1BB*, tumor necrosis factor receptor superfamily member 9; *4-1BBL*, tumor necrosis factor receptor superfamily member 9 ligand; *IL*, interleukin.

chemokine and integrin expression patterns; they leave the lymph nodes and home to sites of inflammation.

21.3.3 T-Cell Memory

After the pathogen that initiated a T-cell response has been cleared, the effector T cells that responded to that pathogen disappear, leaving only a small pool of specialized T cells behind, known as *memory T cells*. These cells respond rapidly on a reencounter with the appropriate antigen and thus offer protection from subsequent infections with the same pathogen. Memory T cells are CD8+ and can be subdivided into 2 categories: T effector memory (T_{EM}) and T central memory (T_{CM}) cells (Fig. 21–5). These subsets can be defined by their localization, surface molecule expression, and function. The T_{CM} cells are found in secondary lymphoid tissues. These cells express the chemokine receptor CCR7, express high levels of CD62L, and do not have preformed lytic granules. T_{CM} cells most likely represent a pool of antigen-specific CD8+ T cells that are ready to expand again on a second encounter with their cognate antigen. The T_{EM} cells are found in nonlymphoid tissues: these cells have preformed cytolytic granules and are ready to act immediately at the sites of pathogen entry. T_{EM} cells are identified by virtue of the profile CD8+, CD62 low, and CCR7−. The maintenance of memory CD8+ T cells is dependent in part on 2 cytokines, IL-7 and IL-15 (Kalia et al, 2006).

21.3.4 T-Cell Subsets

Cytotoxic T lymphocytes (CTLs) are CD8+ T cells that possess the ability to kill target cells directly if the TCR is specific for peptides presented by MHC class I molecules expressed by the target cell. Differentiation of the CD8+ T cell from a resting naïve T cell into a mature CTL includes the formation of cytolytic granules (see Fig. 21–5). The cytolytic granules contain the molecule perforin and proteases of the granzyme family. After TCR engagement on the CTL, the cytolytic granules fuse quickly with the cell membrane, releasing perforin and granzymes. Perforin forms pores in the target cell membrane allowing the granzyme proteases to enter. Granzymes initiate cleavage of proteins inside the target cell, and the result is apoptosis. (see Chap. 8, Sec. 8.4)

T-helper (T_H) cells express the CD4 coreceptor and recognize peptides presented by MHC class II molecules. T_H cells can be divided into several subgroups that are defined by their functional properties and/or their ability to produce a defined cytokine profile (Fig. 21–7). The first identified T_H cell subsets were termed T_H1 and T_H2 and represented 2 discrete pathways of CD4+ mature T-cell differentiation. T_H1 cells express the transcription factor T-BET (Magombedze et al, 2013); they produce high levels of the cytokines IL-2, TNF-α, and IFN-γ, and induce IL-12 production by APCs. A T_H1 cell augments primarily a CD8+ CTL-type response focused on elimination of intracellular pathogens, such as viruses and intracellular bacteria. T_H2 cells mediate humoral (antibody) responses that

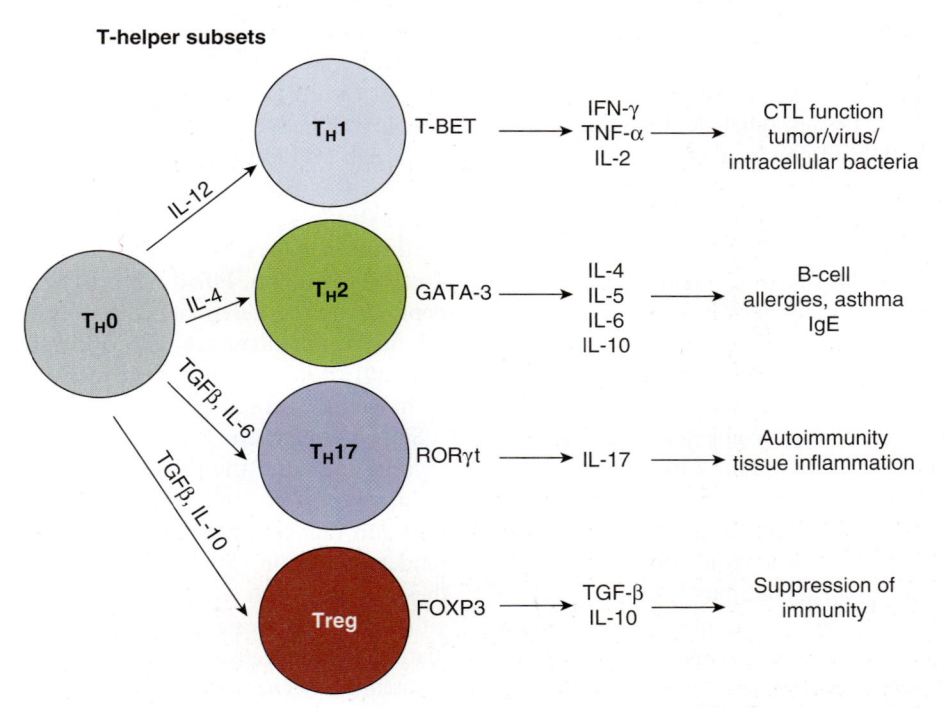

FIGURE 21–7 T-helper cell subsets. T-helper (T_H) cells express the CD4 coreceptor and recognize peptides presented on MHC class II molecules of APCs. After activation through TCR engagement, the T cell goes down 1 of 4 differentiation pathways, resulting in different effector functions. These pathways begin when a naïve CD4+ T cell (T_H0) is activated in the presence of different cytokine and signaling conditions. The differentiation pathways rely on transcriptional patterns enforced by specific transcription factors. After differentiation, the subsets produce signature sets of cytokines that characterize their final effector function. *CTL*, cytotoxic T lymphocyte; *FOXP3*, forkhead box P3; *GATA3*, GATA binding protein 3; *IL*, interleukin; *IFN*, interferon; *IgE*, immunoglobulin E; *RORγT*, RAR-related orphan receptor gamma, isoform 2; *T-BET*, T-box transcription factor 21; *TGF-β*, transforming growth factor beta; *TNF-α*, tumor necrosis factor alpha.

are directed generally against extracellular pathogens and parasites. The T_H2 T cell produces IL-4 among other cytokines: binding of IL-4 to its receptor on CD4⁺ T cells results in signal transducers and activators of transcription 6 (STAT6) activation and transcription of GATA3, which is the master transcription factor (see Chap. 6, Sec. 6.2.6) required for T_H2 cell function (Zhu et al, 2004).

The T_H17 subset is named for the ability to produce the cytokine IL-17, which is believed to act on local tissues to promote inflammation (McGeachy and Cua, 2008). These cells are involved in many types of autoimmune diseases (Gutcher and Becher, 2007) and have a possible role in antitumor responses (Ji and Zhang, 2010).

Regulatory T cells (Tregs) represent another CD4⁺ T-cell population that has the ability to inhibit immune responses. This subset is key for preventing autoimmune diseases. In the mouse, they have been shown to express the markers CD25 and FoxP3, and their presence is dependent on the transcription factor FoxP3. There are 2 major sources of Tregs. One subset develops during thymic selection and is called natural Treg (nTreg). The second group of Tregs originates from mature peripheral CD4⁺ T cells that are converted into regulatory cells through signals in their environment; they are referred to as induced Tregs (iTregs) (Jonuleit and Schmitt, 2003; Josefowicz et al, 2012).

21.3.5 Modulation of T-Cell Activation

A major advance in anticancer immunotherapy has been the introduction of agents, which modulate immune activation. Activation of T cells is required and desirable to resolve many infections, but uncontrolled T-cell activation may result in damage to the surrounding tissues. A balance between costimulatory activators and inhibitory molecules enables inhibition of a T-cell response when appropriate. Two of these inhibitory molecules are cytotoxic T-lymphocyte antigen (CTLA)-4 and programmed death (PD)-1, which are the targets of several approved immunotherapy drugs belonging to the class of immune checkpoint inhibitors (see Sec. 21.5.4).

Ipilimumab, the first approved checkpoint inhibitor (Sec. 21.5.4.1), targets CTLA-4, which is upregulated on the T-cell surface early after TCR engagement, although it is constitutively found on Tregs. CTLA-4 competes with CD28 for binding with CD80 and CD86 and CTLA-4 has a higher affinity than CD28 for CD80 and CD86. Clustering of CD80/86 on the surface of APCs sends a signal to the APC to activate an enzyme called indoleamine 2,3-deoxygenase (IDO), which, in turn, metabolizes tryptophan and inhibits T-cell proliferation (Sec. 21.5.4.3). Signaling through CTLA-4 into the T-cell recruits the Src homology domain-containing phosphatase (SHP)-1 and interrupts the TCR signal. The critical role of CTLA-4 in inhibiting T-cell responses is evident in mice that have been genetically manipulated to lack the CTLA-4 protein (CTLA-4 "knockout" mice), as these mice develop severe autoimmunity and unregulated lymphoproliferation (Fife and Bluestone, 2008).

PD-1, like CTLA-4, is expressed on activated CD4⁺ and CD8⁺ T cells but has a unique mechanism of action. Engagement of PD-1 results in interference with TCR-mediated signaling and blocks the function and survival of effector T cells. (Greenwald et al, 2005). There are 2 known ligands for PD-1. PD-L1 (B7-H1) exhibits broad expression; it is found on many nonhematopoietic cells, as well as immune cells, including APCs. The expression of PD-L2 is restricted mainly to APCs. Expression of PD-L1 has been found on many tumor cells and correlates with poor prognosis. Expression of PD-L1 on tumor cells as well as other cell populations is increased by IFN-γ, which is produced by activated T cells (Gibbons Johnson and Dong, 2017). Tregs have been shown to express both PD-1 and PD-L1 (Fife and Bluestone, 2008). Agents targeting PD-1 and PD-L1 are now in routine use for treatment of several types of cancer (see Sec. 21.5.4.2).

21.3.6 T-Cell Tolerance

Because the rearrangements of the TCR are random, inevitably combinations will arise that are specific for self-antigens. One of the main roles of the thymus is the production of functional, but not autoreactive, T cells. This process can be broken down into 2 major events (Klein et al, 2014). First, a T cell must express a TCR that is able to interact with self-MHC molecules. This process is known as *positive selection* and is important for selecting only those T cells that express receptors that recognize self-MHC, as all foreign peptides are presented by self MHC. As a consequence of positive selection, each T cell in the repertoire is selected for recognition of the different MHC molecules in a given host; selection is based on weak interactions between the TCR and MHC presenting self-peptide. Cells that cannot bind to self-MHC do not receive any signal through their TCR and undergo apoptosis ("no selection"). In contrast, T cells that have TCRs with high avidity to self-peptides presented by the MHC are deleted; this process is referred to as "negative selection." Alternatively, some high-avidity, self-reactive thymocytes are rendered tolerant by a process called *anergy*, which results in T-cell inactivation. Finally, T cells with high avidity to self-peptides may differentiate into Tregs, which play a critical role in the maintenance of peripheral tolerance (Josefowicz et al, 2012). A schematic of the model of thymocyte selection is shown in Figure 21–8.

Some autoreactive T cells escape negative selection in the thymus and enter the periphery. It is likely that this process occurs when some self-antigens are not expressed in the thymus and therefore potentially self-reactive T cells cannot be rendered tolerant. The mechanisms involved in preventing these T cells with self-specificity from becoming activated either can be intrinsic to the T cell or a result of immune regulation by other cells.

Intrinsic mechanisms of peripheral tolerance include *deletion* and *anergy*, which are similar to the self-tolerance mechanisms that occur in the thymus. DCs have the ability to imprint the "fate" of deletion or anergy of mature self-reactive T cells. DCs can display self-antigen that has been acquired from tissues and, if the DC is in a resting state, it renders T cells tolerant to these self-antigens. However, as described in Section 21.2.2,

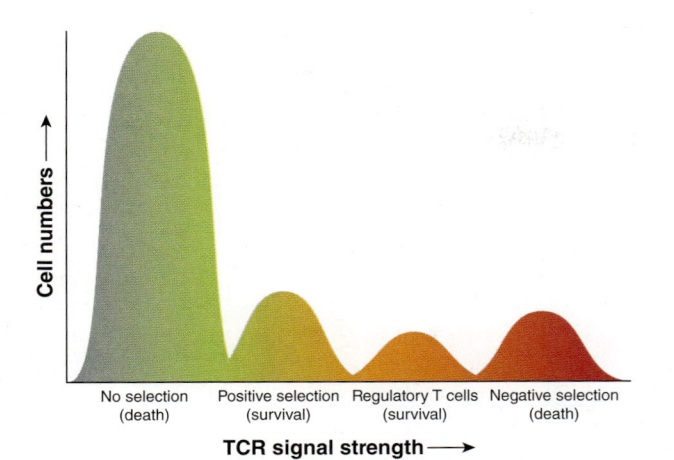

FIGURE 21-8 Thresholds of T-cell selection. T cells are selected during development in the thymus for their ability to bind peptides in the context of self-MHC molecules but will not be activated by self-peptides to become effector cells. Random genomic rearrangements of the TCR genes result in receptors with various affinities for self-peptides bound by MHC. T cells that cannot bind to self-MHC do not receive any signal through their TCR and undergo apoptosis ("no selection"). Cells that bind self-MHC, but do not react strongly to self-peptides, finish development and enter the periphery as naïve T cells ("positive selection"). T cells with intermediate affinity to self-peptides will differentiate into regulatory T cells (Tregs). Finally, T cells that develop high-affinity TCRs, which would result in strong affinity to "self," are deleted ("negative selection").

DCs also have the ability to activate the immune system. The distinction that permits the induction of T-cell tolerance or T-cell immunity is the "functional status" of the DC: resting or steady-state DCs present peptide-MHC complexes that can lead to induction of tolerance, whereas mature or activated DCs induce immunity (Steinman et al, 2003).

There are certain thresholds or concentrations of self-antigen–MHC complexes that are required to induce tolerance (Naeher et al, 2007). If tissue-specific antigens are not presented at an immunologically detectable level, T-cell ignorance is the result. In this situation, self-reactive T cells exist in the T-cell repertoire in a naïve or ignorant state. However, if these cells encounter antigen in an immune-stimulatory setting, these cells can be activated to destroy self-tissues. This scenario has been demonstrated experimentally in many models, including a mouse model of multiple sclerosis where myelin fragments are injected with a powerful immune stimulator (complete Freund adjuvant [CFA]). These myelin antigens are presented to naïve self-reactive T cells in the context of local inflammation induced by the CFA. The myelin-specific T cells then become activated and attack the myelin sheaths in the nervous system (Constatinescu et al, 2011).

Tregs are critical for the maintenance of peripheral immune tolerance in both mouse and man. Mice lacking Treg expression because of a mutation in the *foxp3* gene (the transcription factor that is required for Tregs) succumb to severe multi-organ autoimmune disease. In humans, mutations impairing Treg development or function are correlated with the fatal autoimmune disease known as immune dysregulation, polyendocrinopathy, enteropathy, X-linked (IPEX; Wildin and Freitas, 2005). Current models propose that Tregs are antigen specific but suppress T-cell responses in a nonspecific manner. Tregs encounter antigen and then subsequently suppress the function of T cells with various other antigen specificities in the local vicinity through "bystander suppression." Tregs function to mediate this phenomenon through both cell contact- and soluble factor-mediated mechanisms. Activated Tregs possess the ability to kill directly both T cells and APCs in their local environment by producing granzyme B that can enter surrounding cells and induce apoptosis (Gondek et al, 2005). This targeted elimination can reduce the quantity of activated T cells in an inflammatory site and terminate antigen presentation. Tregs have also been shown to inhibit killing by CTLs by impairing granule exocytosis (Mempel et al, 2006). The high levels of CTLA-4 present on Tregs bind to CD80 and CD86 on APCs, resulting in increased intracellular levels of the tryptophan-metabolizing enzyme IDO (Orabona et al, 2004). These high IDO levels then cause depletion of tryptophan from the local environment, thereby inhibiting T-cell proliferation (Munn and Mellor, 2016). Tregs also express high levels of the IL-2 receptor CD25, and as a consequence, Tregs bind IL-2 more rapidly than other T cells in the local area. Thus, Tregs may function in part by limiting the amount of this T-cell growth factor available to effector cells nearby. Activated Tregs have been shown to secrete the anti-inflammatory cytokines IL-10 and transforming growth factor (TGF)-β (Sakaguchi et al, 2009); TGF-β also has antiproliferative functions and may contribute to limiting immune responses.

21.4 TUMOR IMMUNOLOGY

The immune system is equipped to recognize and eliminate foreign threats such as bacteria and viruses. However, the immune system is also capable of recognizing tumors and mounting an immune response against them, even though they are derived from the host's own cells. Several strategies that activate or enhance the immune response to tumors have been devised over the last few decades as therapies for cancer.

21.4.1 Tumor-Associated Antigens

One fundamental aspect that was critical to move the field of tumor immune therapy forward was the identification of tumor-associated antigens (TAAs). TAAs are intracellular or extracellular proteins that are expressed preferentially by tumor cells, but often can be expressed by normal cells. These proteins are processed and presented on MHC class I and II molecules in a similar manner to proteins of nontumor origin (eg, self-proteins, or viral or bacterial proteins), as described above. Therefore, specific T cells can recognize TAAs through their TCRs. The identification of TAAs was important for tumor immunology and immunotherapy as it allowed for the detection and characterization of T cells that can recognize specific TAAs. It also allows for the design of immunotherapy that focuses on activation of TAA-specific T.

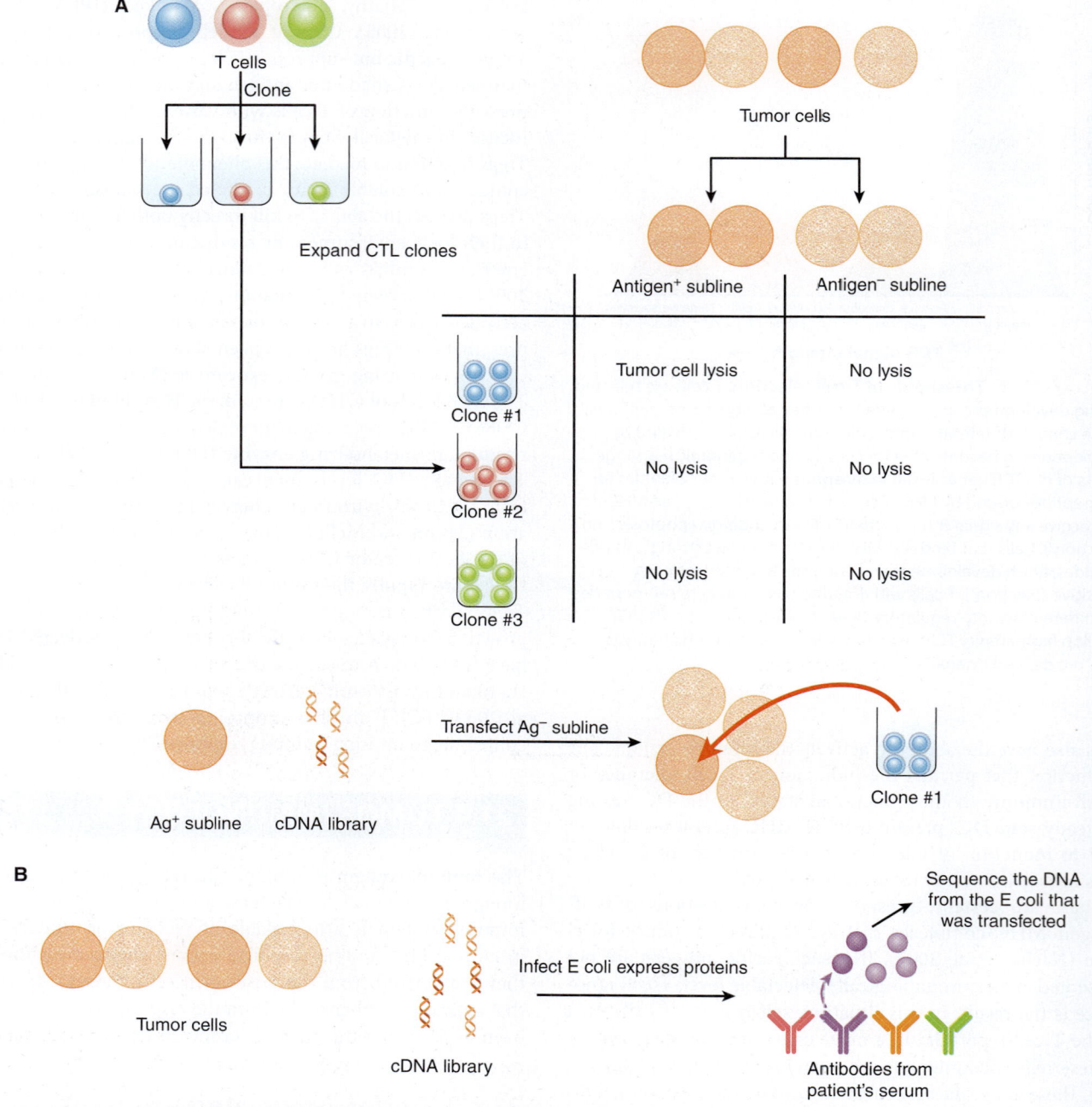

FIGURE 21–9 Approaches for identifying TAAs. A) CTLs from a cancer patient are cloned by plating them at 1 cell per well and expanding each clone. Autologous tumor cells are cultured in vitro and various sublines are obtained, some of which are "antigen-loss" variants. The CTL clones are tested for their ability to lyse the tumor cell sublines. If a clone is able to lyse one subline, but not another, the antigen expressed by the former is identified by transfecting antigen-negative target cells with cDNA libraries derived from the antigen-positive tumor cells. The DNA encoding the target antigen (the TAA) is isolated based on the ability of the CTL clone to lyse the target cell that was transfected with the TAA. **B)** In the SEREX approach, expression libraries composed of cDNAs isolated from autologous tumor cells are cloned into phage expression vectors which are used to infect *Escherichia coli* (E.coli). Serum samples from cancer patients (which should contain antibodies that recognize TAAs) are used to screen these libraries. Clones that are bound by antibodies are then isolated and sequenced.

21.4.1.1 Identification of Tumor-Associated Antigens

The first TAA was identified by Boon and colleagues (van der Bruggen et al, 1991). Using a panel of CTL clones isolated from a patient with metastatic melanoma in combination with various sublines of melanoma tumor cells derived from the same patient, the authors identified a gene whose product was targeted by a particular CTL clone. This gene was not expressed in normal tissues. Furthermore, T cells from the original patient could recognize melanoma cell lines established from other human leukocyte antigen (HLA)-A–matched patients that also expressed the same TAA. Through this approach, the MAGE, BAGE, and GAGE families of TAAs were identified (see below).

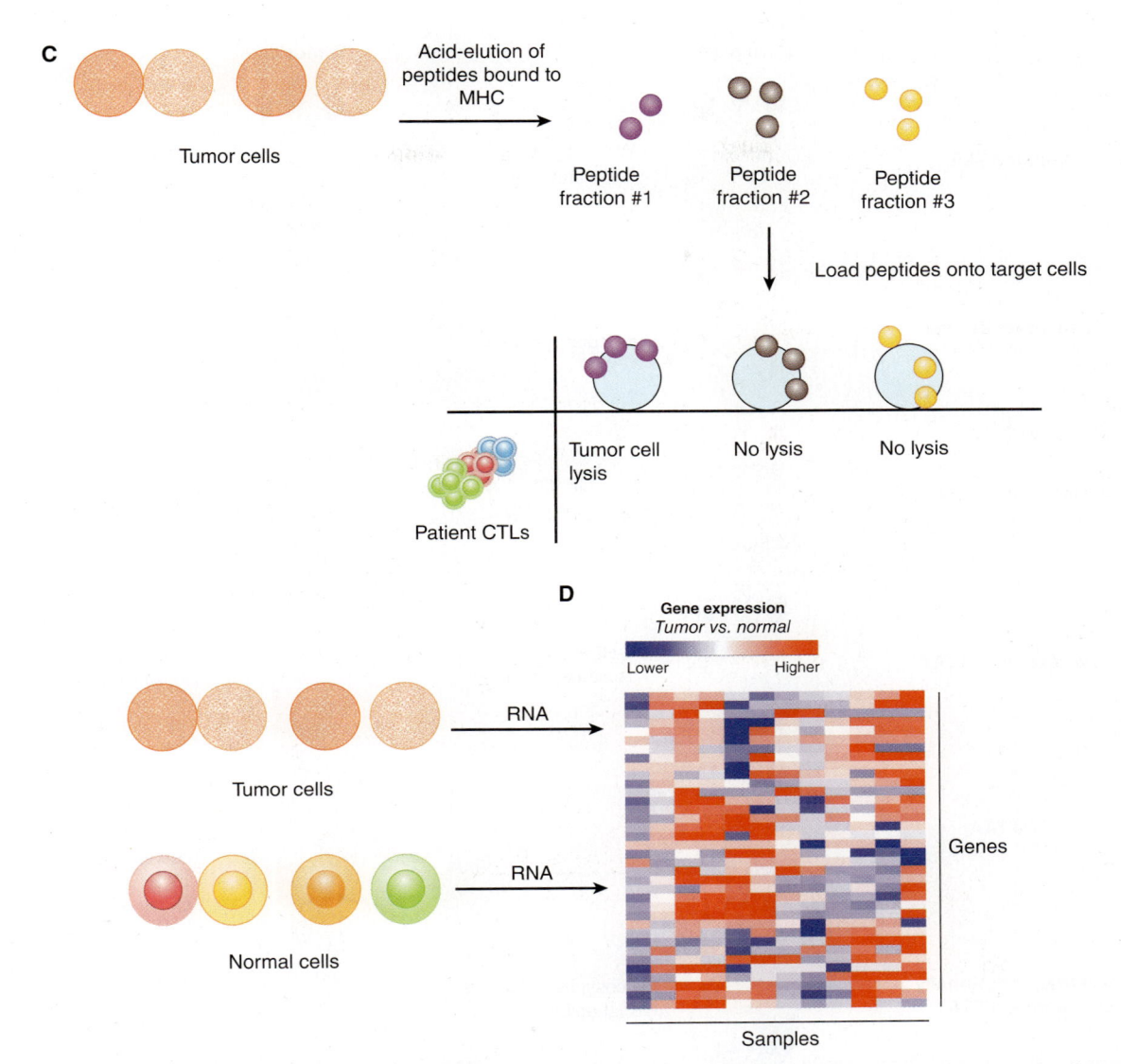

FIGURE 21-9 (*Continued*) Other methods to identify TAAs include (**C**) the acid-elution of MHC-bound peptides from tumor cells and subsequent screening of peptide fractions for recognition by T cells from cancer patients, and (**D**) gene expression microarray analysis for upregulated RNA transcripts in tumor cells compared with normal cells.

Other approaches have successfully identified many TAAs. One method is referred to as SEREX (*se*rological analysis of *r*ecombinant cDNA *ex*pression libraries; Sahin et al, 1995). Serum samples taken from cancer patients were postulated to contain antibodies that recognize TAAs. Expression libraries composed of complementary DNAs (cDNAs) isolated from autologous tumor cells were cloned into phage expression vectors and used to infect Escherichia coli (E.coli). These libraries were screened using patient serum and the clones that were bound by antibodies were isolated and sequenced. The TAA recognized by the antibody was then identified based on the DNA sequence. Confirmation of the identified protein as a TAA was established in various ways, including evaluating protein expression in normal and malignant tissues. Clinically relevant TAAs, such NY-ESO-1, were thus identified using the SEREX approach. Other methods to identify TAAs include the acid-elution of MHC-bound peptides from tumor cells and subsequent screening of peptide fractions for recognition by T cells from cancer patients and, more recently, gene expression microarray analyses (see Chap. 2, Sec. 2.2.12) of tumor cells compared with normal cells. These approaches are depicted in Figure 21–9.

Once a TAA has been identified, it is important to identify the peptide sequences in that protein that can be recognized by various TCRs. One approach has been to identify peptides that can be presented by HLA-A*0201 molecules and recognized by human T cells (Kawashima et al, 1998). HLA-A*0201 is prevalent in Caucasians and is often the focus of studies involving unique peptides that bind this HLA molecule. First, peptides that contained amino acid motifs that would be predicted to bind the HLA-A*0201 molecule were identified. The ability to bind HLA-A*0201 was verified using MHC-binding assays. These peptides were then tested for their ability to expand peptide-specific T cells from the peripheral blood T-cell population of HLA-A*0201–positive donors. These expansions were achieved by stimulating T cells with autologous DCs that had

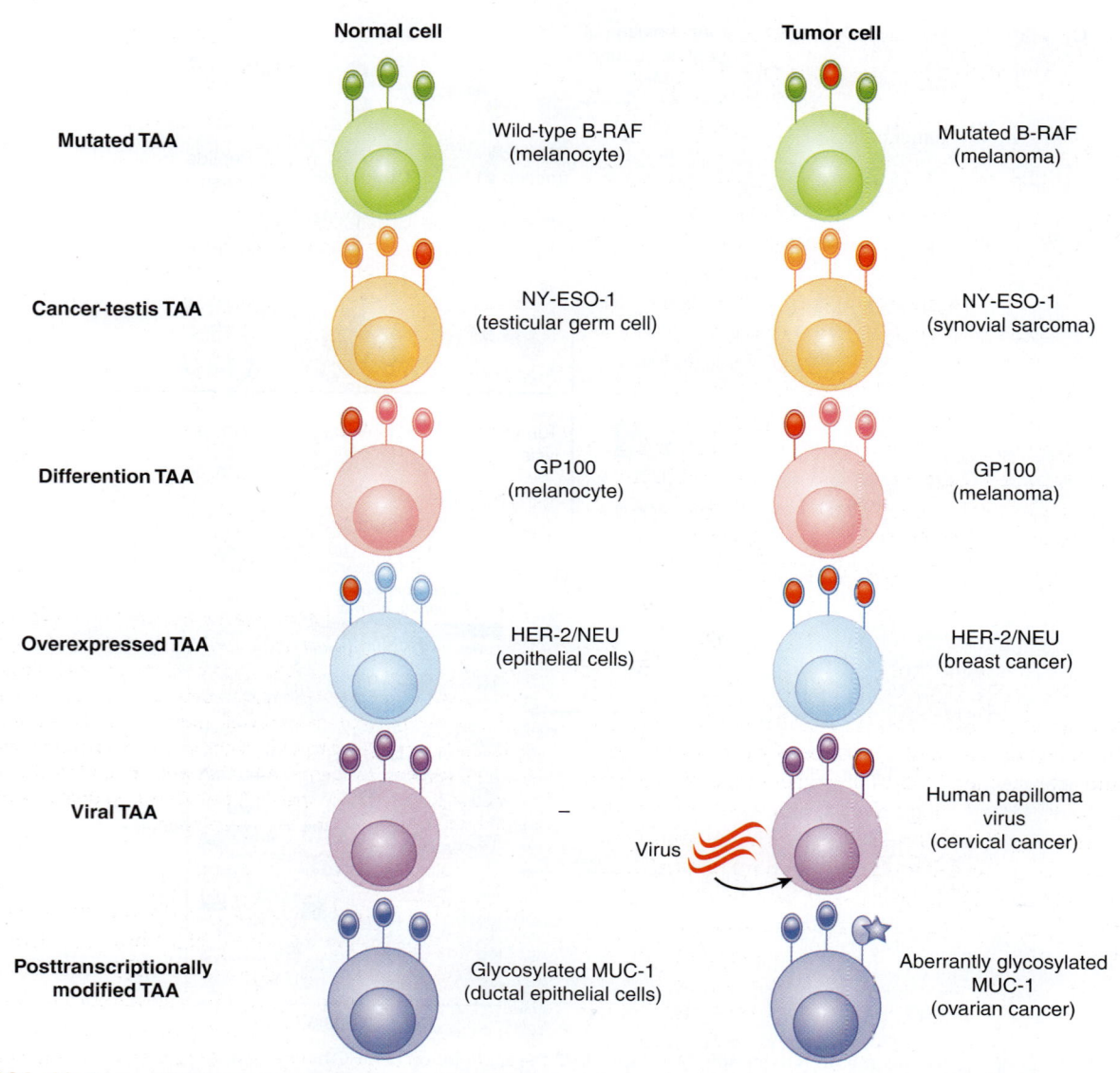

FIGURE 21–10 Types of tumor-associated antigens (TAAs). Various classes of TAAs are depicted and an example of each type of TAA is given. Expression on a normal cell and a tumor cell is shown. TAAs are depicted in red.

been exposed to the peptide of interest. After multiple rounds of peptide stimulation, the expanded T cells were tested for their ability to lyse peptide-coated target cells. Using this approach, multiple immunogenic peptides of the MAGE-A2, MAGE-A3, carcinoembryonic antigen (CEA), and human epidermal growth receptor (HER)-2/neu proteins were identified.

21.4.1.2 Types of Tumor-Associated Antigens
TAAs can be classified into several broad categories: (a) mutation antigens, (b) cancer-testis antigens, (c) differentiation antigens, (d) overexpressed antigens, (e) viral antigens, and (f) antigens with unique posttranslational modifications (Fig. 21–10).

Mutation antigens are generally proteins that harbor mutations that are unique to an individual tumor, although some mutations such as the BRAF V600E mutation in melanoma are common to a subset of patients. Both driver and passenger mutations alter the amino acid coding sequences resulting in the expression of mutated proteins that are processed and presented on the cell surface in the context of MHC. As these sequences are unique "neoantigens," they can be recognized as foreign by a T-cell response resulting in antitumor immunity (Gubin et al, 2015; Yarchoan et al, 2017).

The expression of cancer-testis antigens is restricted to tumor cells and normal placental trophoblasts and testicular germ cells, and therefore represent appealing targets for immunotherapy. Cancer-testis antigens include the MAGE, BAGE, and GAGE proteins, as well as the commonly expressed NY-ESO-1.

Differentiation antigens are proteins that are expressed on both normal tissues and tumors derived from a particular tissue. For example, gp100, Melan-A/MART-1, and tyrosinase are expressed on normal melanocytes as well as malignant melanoma. Other differentiation antigens include the B-cell antigens CD19 and CD20 (B cell–derived malignancies) and prostate-specific antigen (PSA-prostate cancer). Differentiation antigens also include oncofetal antigens, such as α-fetoprotein and CEA, which are expressed in various tissues during fetal development and are re-expressed on tumors.

TAAs are expressed on various normal tissues, but with higher expression on tumor cells. For example, Wilms tumor-1 (WT-1) is expressed in a proportion of breast cancers, lung cancers, and other tumor cells. Mesothelin is expressed on pancreatic cancer, mesothelioma, and ovarian cancer.

Viral TAAs are expressed by tumors that are induced by viral transformation. This includes Epstein-Barr virus (EBV)–induced tumors such as some lymphomas and nasopharyngeal carcinoma, human papilloma virus (HPV)–induced cervical neoplasias, and Merkel cell carcinoma–associated polyoma virus.

Another class of TAAs consists of proteins where posttranslational modification occurs differently in normal cells compared with tumor cells. T cells are able to distinguish between the same peptide with different posttranslational modifications, such as differential glycosylation levels. For example, mucin-1 (MUC-1) proteins are generally hypoglycosylated in tumor cells compared with normal cells (Schietinger et al, 2008).

21.4.2 Tumor-Associated Antigen–Specific T Cells in Humans

The development of MHC-peptide multimer reagents has enabled the direct detection of T cells specific for various TAAs (Bakker and Schumacher, 2005). This reagent generally consists of soluble MHC class I molecules (eg, HLA-A*0201) folded together with a peptide of interest (eg, a peptide derived from a tumor-associated protein that is known to bind that particular HLA allele) (Fig. 21–11). In the classical "tetramer," each MHC molecule is tagged covalently with a molecule of biotin. Multiple MHC-peptide complexes are then aggregated together using streptavidin, which possesses 4 biotin-binding sites. The multimeric nature of the reagent allows for higher-avidity binding of specific TCRs, and any bound cells can be detected by flow cytometric analysis of the fluorochrome-conjugated streptavidin moiety. Although MHC-peptide multimers have also been constructed using MHC class II molecules and class II-binding peptides, they are generally not as robust as MHC class I–derived multimers (Vollers and Stern, 2008).

Early studies using HLA-A*0201 MHC-peptide multimers were able to identify the presence of peripheral T cells that could recognize melanoma-associated antigens such as Melan-A/MART-1 and tyrosinase. These tumor-specific T cells could be detected by ex vivo staining of tumor-infiltrated lymph nodes, without the need for in vitro stimulation or expansion using specific peptides (Romero et al, 1998). The presence and function of tumor-specific T cells have also been demonstrated for other cancers. Numerous studies have demonstrated that some women with breast cancer have pre-existing immunity against breast TAAs. In one study, 7 of 13 breast cancer patients had detectable tumor-specific T-cell responses at the time of diagnosis (Rentzsch et al, 2003). This response was demonstrated by evaluating the induction of IFN-γ RNA transcripts in response to stimulation with peptides derived from several common antigens expressed by breast cancers: MUC-1, HER-2/NEU, CEA, NY-ESO-1, and SSX-2. HER-2/NEU is expressed by a variety of cancers and preexisting immunity to HER-2/NEU has been demonstrated in patients whose cancers expressed HER-2/NEU (breast, ovarian, lung, colorectal, prostate) (Sotiropoulou et al, 2003). After a brief restimulation of peripheral blood T cells ex vivo with HER-2/NEU peptide-exposed DCs, effector function of the restimulated T cells was evaluated by enzyme-linked immunospot (ELISPOT) assay (production of IFN-γ on a per-cell basis) and CTL assay (ability to kill target cells). Hence, immune tolerance against tumors is incomplete, as TAA-specific T cells can be detected in cancer patients. However, it was not until the development of immune modulating therapies that result in blockade of immune checkpoints that therapeutic efficacy has been observed (see Sec. 21.5.4).

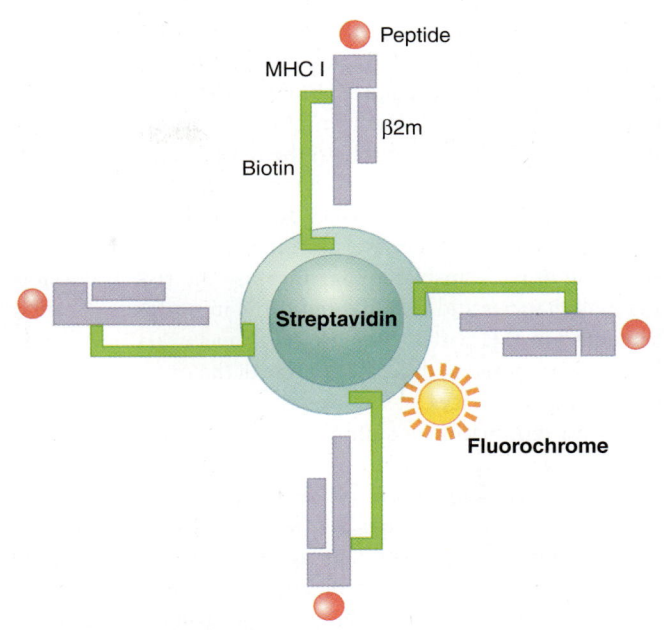

FIGURE 21–11 Structure of an MHC-peptide multimer. An MHC-peptide tetramer is depicted, where 4 MHC class I–peptide complexes are complexed together. Each MHC class I molecule is biotinylated; each biotinylated MHC class I–peptide complex is bound via the biotin molecule to a streptavidin molecule, and the streptavidin molecule is conjugated to a fluorochrome. These peptides can be tumor-associated antigens (TAAs) that when bound to MHC class I can be recognized by tumor-specific T cells. These reagents are helpful for monitoring tumor-specific T-cell responses.

21.4.3 Immune Surveillance

Numerous studies provide evidence in support of cancer immune surveillance (Swann and Smyth, 2007). That the immune system eliminates tumor cells was shown using various immunodeficient mice: (a) mice deficient in the Rag protein and therefore lacking all T and B cells, (b) mice deficient in the receptor for the immunostimulatory cytokine interferon-γ (IFN-γ receptor 1 knockout mice), and (c) mice deficient in the key intracellular signaling molecule downstream of IFN-γ receptor signaling (*Stat1* knockout mice). These immunodeficient mice developed MCA-induced and spontaneous tumors at a higher frequency and with faster kinetics compared with immunocompetent mice (Kaplan et al, 1998; Shankaran et al, 2001). Patients with acquired immunodeficiency syndrome (AIDS) as a result of human immunodeficiency virus (HIV) infection are more susceptible to the development of Kaposi's sarcoma, non-Hodgkin's B-cell lymphoma, and cervical cancer – these are also called AIDS-defining cancers (Yarchoan and Uldrick, 2018). Likewise, immunosuppression of patients receiving organ transplants may increase the risk of developing malignancies and also highlights the importance of cancer screening in this patient population (Engels, 2017). A model has been proposed to describe the role of the immune response during various stages of tumor progression, which includes 3 phases: elimination, equilibrium, and escape (Swann and Smyth, 2007) (Fig. 21–12).

During the elimination phase of immune surveillance, the immune system recognizes tumor cells and mounts a response against the tumor. During the equilibrium phase, the immune system and the tumor are in dynamic equilibrium, where the combination of the genomic instability of tumor cells and selective pressure exerted by the antitumor immune response results in editing, or "sculpting" of the tumor cell population. The elimination of certain tumor cells by the immune system results in the selection of less immunogenic tumors. During the escape phase, enough tumor cell variants arise that the tumor can escape elimination by the immune system. Escape may be partly a result of reduced immunogenicity of tumor cells, such as reduced expression of TAAs, or downregulation of MHC class I, but there are many mechanisms whereby the tumor can evade the immune system. These mechanisms include negative regulatory immune cell types, immunosuppressive factors produced by tumor cells, and surface receptors that dampen the T-cell response.

21.4.4 T-Cell Infiltration and Disease Prognosis

The importance of T-cell immunity in reducing clinical tumor burden in humans is highlighted in part by studies evaluating tumor tissues for infiltration by immune cells. In many studies where immunohistochemical or gene expression analyses of tumor tissue are performed, the data show an association between immune cell (especially T-cell) infiltration and better prognosis (eg, Tuthill et al, 2002; Zhang et al, 2003; Galon et al, 2006). In an example of this type of study, genomic analysis for RNA expression was performed for 75 colorectal tumors (Galon et al, 2006). Expression levels of a cluster of T_H1-related genes showed a statistically significant inverse correlation with

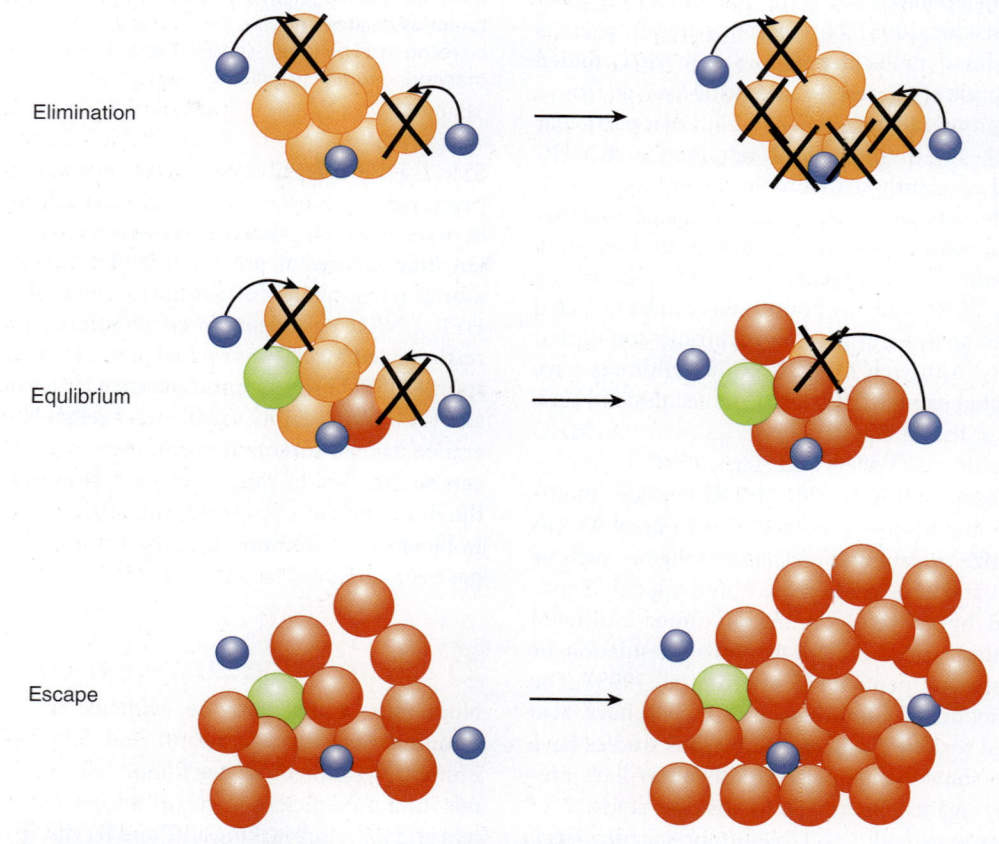

FIGURE 21–12 **The 3 Es of cancer immune-editing.** In this model, immunoediting is composed of 3 main phases. During the *elimination phase*, the immune system recognizes tumor cells and mediates their elimination. During the *equilibrium phase*, the immune system and the tumor are in dynamic equilibrium, where the combination of genomic instability of tumor cells and selective pressure exerted by the antitumor immune response results in editing, or "sculpting" of the tumor cell population. The elimination of certain tumor cells by the immune system results in the selection of less immunogenic tumors. During the *escape phase*, enough tumor cell variants arise that the tumor can escape elimination by the immune system. *Blue*, immune cell; *orange/green/red*, tumor cells.

tumor recurrence, thus implicating the T_H1 response in dampening progression of human tumors. In the same study, immunohistochemistry for immune cell infiltration in paraffin-embedded tissue microarrays constructed from 415 colorectal tumors was also performed. High densities of CD3+ T cells, CD8+ T cells, granzyme B (a cytotoxic granule produced by lytic T cells), and CD45RO (a T-cell activation marker) were found in patients without recurrence compared to patients with recurrence. In a multivariate analysis, the density of CD3+ cells in tumors was shown to be an independent prognostic factor, and these T-cell markers proved to be a better predictor of patient survival than standard histopathologically based staging methods. Interestingly, a CD8+ T-cell infiltration of the tumor microenvironment and an IFNγ expression profile have been associated with clinical response to immunotherapy with immune checkpoint blockade (Tumeh et al, 2014; Ayers et al, 2017).

21.4.5 Barriers to Antitumor Immunity

Despite the evidence that the immune system can respond to tumor cells, it is difficult to estimate the relative importance of antitumor immunity in tumor progression. It is clear that when tumors do develop, the immune response is unable to control tumor growth. Various mechanisms can lead to failure of immune-mediated tumor control; many of them are the same mechanisms that prevent autoimmunity and thereby suppress immune responses against self-tissues. Various mechanisms of peripheral T-cell tolerance are discussed above (see Sec. 21.3.6): T-cell deletion, T-cell anergy, and the function of negative regulatory cells and molecules have all been demonstrated to possess a negative impact on the immune response to tumors in various models. It is the recognition of immune checkpoint molecules and their blockade that has resulted in the successful immunotherapeutic treatment of some types of cancer (see Sec. 21.5.4).

21.5 IMMUNOTHERAPY

21.5.1 Introduction

Our improved understanding of tumor immunology has led to a growing list of immunotherapeutic agents being approved for use against cancers. One broad category of agents consists of monoclonal antibodies (mAbs). Although the mechanisms of action of various mAbs are not always related to the antitumor T-cell response that is discussed above—many function in a manner completely independent of T cells—they are important players in cancer therapy.

Immunotherapy that is aimed at augmenting antitumor T-cell immunity can be broadly categorized into (a) in vivo immune modulators that use either general/nonspecific or specific approaches and (b) adoptive cell therapy. Each category encompasses many different strategies—some investigational and some approved for therapy. Those strategies selected for discussion in this chapter are listed in Table 21-1.

General immunomodulation refers to strategies that augment general T-cell responses, in a "nonspecific" or "polyclonal"

TABLE 21-1 Selected approaches to cancer immunotherapy.

Monoclonal Antibody Therapies	(See Table 21-2)
Immune modulation (immune-activating agents)	Bacillus of Calmette and Guérin (BCG)*
	Interferon-α*
	Interleukin-2*
	Imiquimod*
Immune modulation (immune checkpoint blockade)	Anti-CTLA-4 blockade (ipilimumab)*
	Anti-PD-1*
	Anti-PD-L1*
	Combination anti-PD-1 and anti-CTLA-4*
Immune modulation (specific approaches)	Vaccination with:
	Tumor-associated proteins
	Tumor-associated peptides
	Irradiated tumor cells
	Talimogene Laherparepvec
Adoptive cell therapies	Dendritic cells
	Sipuleucel-T*
	Antigen-specific T-cell clones/lines
	Tumor-infiltrating lymphocytes
	TCR (T cell receptor) T cells
	CAR (chimeric antigen receptor) T cells*

*Currently FDA approved.

manner. This type of immunotherapy includes the use of cytokines (eg, INF-α, IL-2), immunologic adjuvants (TLR agonists), and agents that target immunomodulatory molecules such as CTLA-4, PD-1, and PD-L1, known as checkpoint inhibitors. Specific immunotherapy focuses on the activation and enhancement of the number of T cells that can recognize TAAs by using vaccine strategies. Although vaccination often refers to a prophylactic strategy to prevent disease, vaccination may also refer to therapy aimed at eliciting antitumor immune responses to eliminate established cancers. Vaccine approaches include the use of TAAs or peptides derived from TAAs. Other approaches are based on vaccination using whole tumor cells (autologous or allogeneic) that have been irradiated to prevent their proliferation following infusion. In adoptive cell therapy, immune cells (autologous or allogeneic) such as DCs and T cells are manipulated ex vivo and then reinfused.

21.5.2 Monoclonal Antibodies for Cancer Therapy

Monoclonal antibodies (mAbs) bind specifically to their target protein and can block the target protein's function, trigger signaling downstream of the target protein, or deliver conjugated toxins to cells expressing the target protein. Current Food and Drug Administration (FDA)–approved mAbs include those that target antigens expressed by tumor cells (eg, CD20 on non-Hodgkin lymphoma and chronic lymphocytic leukemia), molecules that promote tumor growth (eg, epidermal growth factor receptor and HER-2), or angiogenic molecules

TABLE 21-2 Monoclonal antibodies approved for cancer therapy as of 2020.

Monoclonal Antibody	Cancer Targeted	Target Molecule	Type of mAb
Alemtuzumab	CLL	CD52	Humanized IgG$_1$
Bevacizumab	Colorectal, lung cancer	VEGF	Humanized IgG$_1$
Blinatumomab	ALL	CD19	Mouse
Cetuximab	Colorectal cancer	EGFR	Chimeric IgG$_1$
Daratumumab	Multiple myeloma	CD38	Human IgG$_1$
Elotuzumab	Multiple myeloma	SLAM7	Humanized IgG$_1$
Gemtuzumab	AML	CD33	Humanized IgG$_4$
Ibritumomab tiuxetan	NHL	CD20	Mouse
Ofatumumab	CLL	CD20	Human IgG$_1$
Panitumumab	Colorectal cancer	EGFR	Human IgG$_2$
Pertuzumab	Breast cancer	Her-2/neu	Humanized IgG$_1$
Ramucirumab	Gastric cancer	VEGFR2	Human IgG$_1$
Rituximab	NHL, CLL	CD20	Chimeric IgG$_1$
Tositumomab	NHL	CD20	Mouse
Trastuzumab	Breast cancer	HER-2/neu	Humanized IgG$_1$

Abbreviations: ADCC, Antibody-dependent cell-mediated cytotoxicity; *ALL*, Acute lymphocytic leukemia; *AML*, acute myelogenous leukemia; *CLL*, chronic lymphocytic leukemia; *EGFR*, epidermal growth factor receptor; *IgG*, immunoglobulin G; *NHL*, non-Hodgkin lymphoma; *VEGF*, vascular endothelial growth factor.

(eg, vascular endothelial growth factor). Table 21–2 lists examples of antibodies approved for cancer therapy as of 2020.

21.5.2.1 Production of Monoclonal Antibodies

An mAb that recognizes a given protein target is derived from an antibody molecule that was produced by a single B cell. Originally, mAbs were produced by fusing B cells from the spleen of an animal that had been immunized with the target protein, with a myeloma cell line that was selected for the inability to produce immunoglobulin (Fig. 21–13A). Clones of these fused cells (called *hybridomas*) that secreted antibodies with the desired specificity were isolated and used to produce large amounts of the monoclonal antibody of interest. In recent years, this approach has been superseded by recombinant technologies (Fig. 21–13B).

21.5.2.2 Types of Therapeutic Antibodies

Initially, therapeutic antibodies that recognize human proteins were generated by immunization of animals (eg, mice) with human proteins. However, mouse antibodies have limited therapeutic value for several reasons. Mouse Fc domains (the "constant" domains of an antibody that are conserved among all antibodies of a particular class) are not recognized as efficiently as human Fc domains by human immune cells, and such recognition is required for some of the mechanisms of action of antibody therapy. Also, mouse antibodies are recognized as foreign proteins by the human immune system, preventing repetitive antibody administration. One solution has been the generation of *chimeric antibodies*, which are engineered to contain the variable (Fv) region from a mouse antibody and the human constant (Fc) regions. Another approach is to generate *humanized antibodies* where the hypervariable region of the variable antigen-binding domain (Fv) is derived from a mouse antibody and the rest of the Fv and the entire Fc region is derived from human sequences. To completely circumvent neutralizing antibodies with xenogeneic sequences, many current therapeutic antibodies are fully human. These antibodies can be isolated from mice that have been engineered to express only human antibodies, or they can be isolated by a phage display approach, where libraries of random recombinations of human antibody genes are expressed in bacteriophage. The antibody-expressing phage are then screened for the ability to bind the target protein. Figure 21–13C illustrates these types of antibodies.

21.5.2.3 Mechanisms of Action of Antibodies

Antibodies that bind to receptors on the cell surface can block receptor signaling (by steric blockade of ligand binding) or can trigger receptor signaling (by aggregation of multiple receptors). Antibodies can also lead to lysis of cells that express the molecule targeted by the antibody. Target-cell lysis can occur by activation of the complement protein cascade or by initiation of antibody-dependent cell-mediated cytotoxicity (ADCC) (Fig. 21–14). The complement cascade is initiated by binding of the Fc domain of immunoglobulin (Ig)G to a complement protein, which then leads to a cascade of cleavage of various complement system proteins. The end result of this cascade is the formation of a protein complex called the membrane attack complex (MAC) on the target cell (in this case, the tumor cell) that leads to pore formation and lysis of the target cell. Other proteins activated by the complement cascade are able to mediate chemoattraction of various immune cells to the site of tumor. ADCC, in contrast, is initiated on binding of the Fc region of antibodies by Fc receptors (FcRs). FcRs are expressed on various innate immune cell types, and the activation of FcRs leads to activation of cytotoxic activity against target cells. For example, FcγRIIIA is expressed by natural killer (NK) cells, and binding of this receptor by

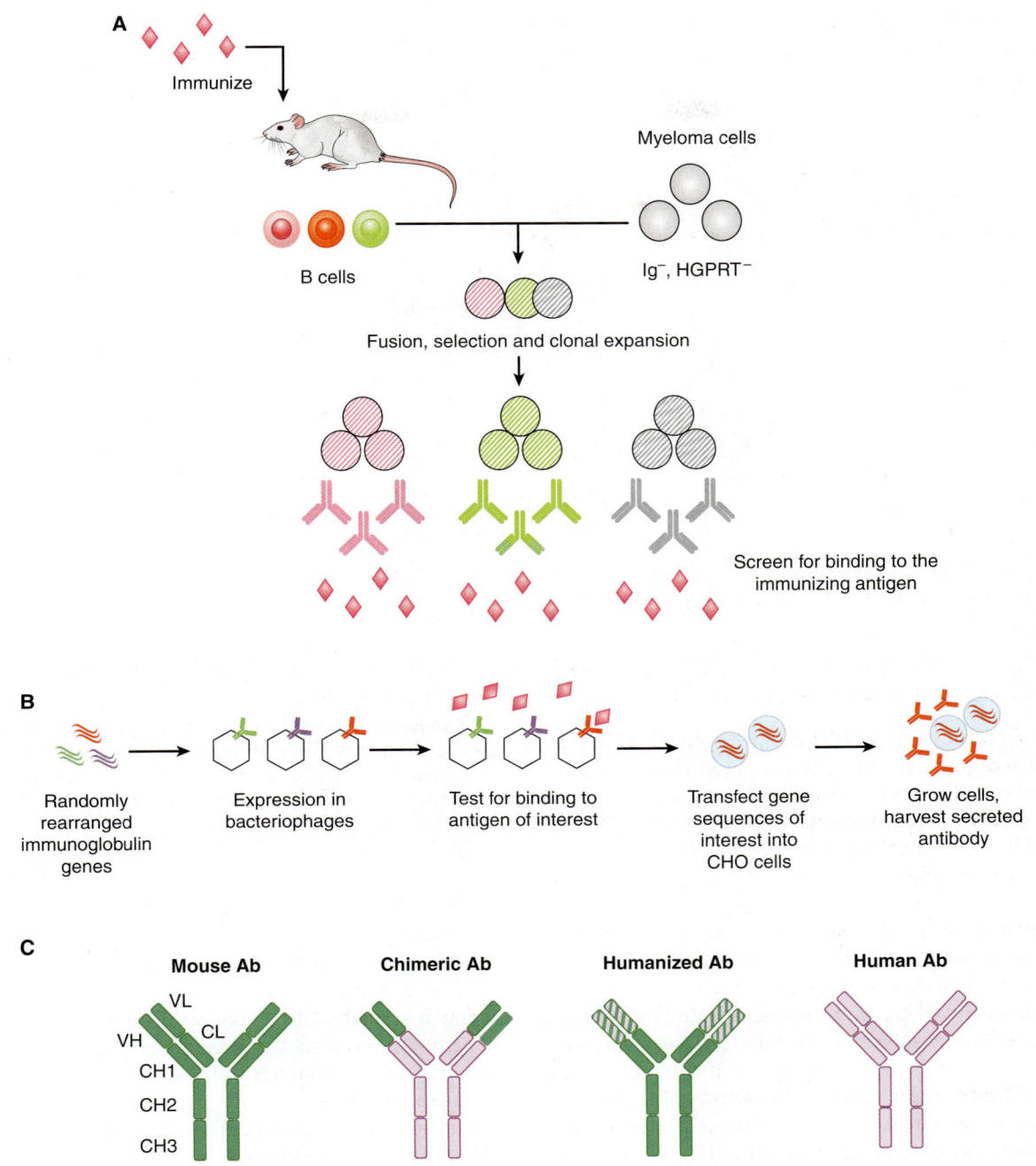

FIGURE 21-13 Methods of monoclonal antibody production. **A)** mAbs were initially produced by the fusion of B cells with a specialized myeloma cell line. Fused cells were cloned and then the clone that produced the antibody of interest was selected for antibody production. **B)** Other methods are based on recombinant technologies, where the desired antibody genes are transfected into cells such as Chinese hamster ovary (CHO) cells and antibodies are harvested from culture supernatants. In this example, the antibody genes of interest are identified by screening bacteriophages for binding to the antigen of interest. The bacteriophages have been engineered to express antibodies that are the product of random rearrangement of immunoglobulin genes. **C)** Antibodies are modified to produce chimeric, humanized, and completely human forms to avoid recognition and rejection when used as therapy. *Ig*, immunoglobulin. *HGPRT*, hypoxanthine-guanine phosphoribosyltransferase.

the Fc region of an IgG molecule activates NK cell–mediated lysis of the target cell (see Sec. 21.2.3). Trastuzumab and pertuzumab, which inhibit signaling through the HER-2/neu growth receptor (see Chap. 19, Sec. 19.4.2), have been shown to mediate antitumor activity via ADCC (Scheuer et al, 2009). Because ADCC is a potentially important mechanism mediating the action of therapeutic antibodies, the most effective antibodies should be engineered or selected to bind well to activating FcRs and to bind poorly to the inhibitory FcγIIB (Nimmerjahn and Ravetch, 2008).

21.5.2.4 Modified Antibodies
Antibodies can be modified in various ways in order to alter their therapeutic function. For example, bispecific T cell–engager molecules

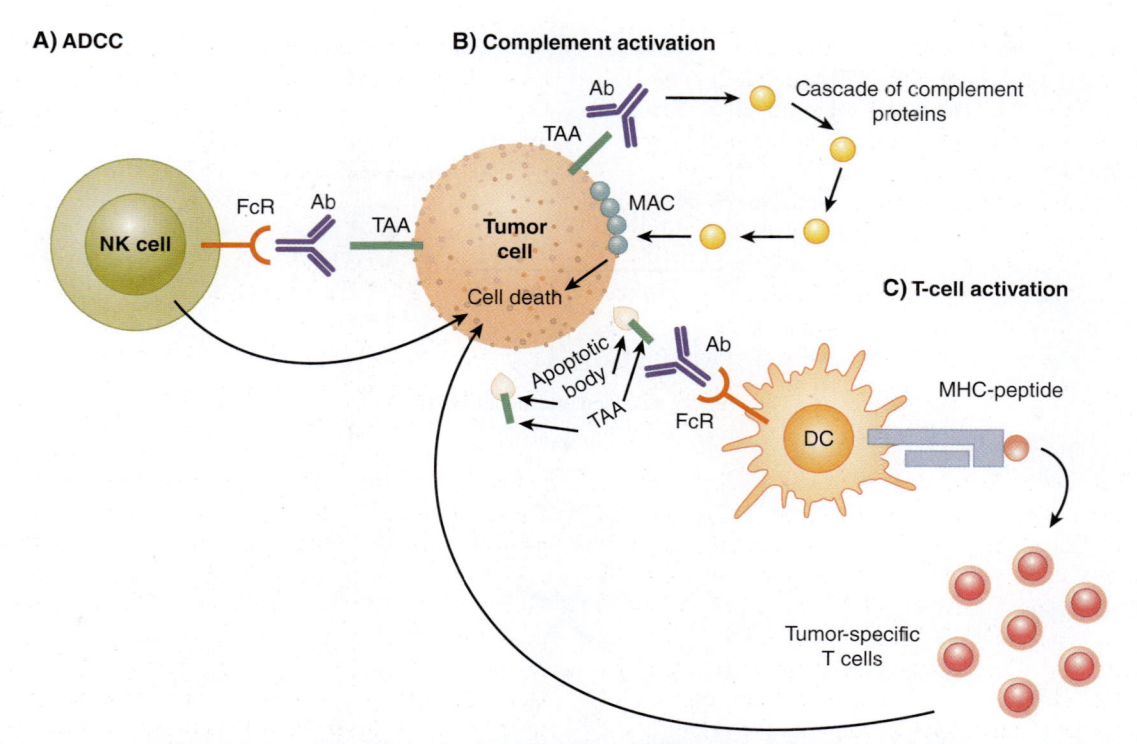

FIGURE 21–14 Tumor-specific antibodies can promote tumor regression by multiple mechanisms. In addition to either blocking or triggering cell-surface receptors, antibodies can lead to immune-mediated elimination of tumor cells. **A)** ADCC is induced when antibodies (Abs) bound to tumor-associated antigens (TAAs) on the surface of tumor cells are then bound by Fc receptors (FcR) expressed by natural killer (NK) cells. Triggering of the Fc receptors activates the cytolytic activity of NK cells. **B)** Complement activation is induced by binding of complement proteins to the Fc domain of antibody/antigen complexes. One of the end results of the complement cascade is the formation of the membrane attack complex (MAC) in the cell membrane of target cells, leading to cell death. **C)** Antibodies can also bind to tumor antigens present on apoptotic bodies formed when tumor cells undergo apoptosis during the normal cycle of proliferation and cell death. By this route, tumor antigens are taken up by DCs via Fc receptors. Tumor antigens can be processed by the DCs and presented as peptide-MHC complexes to T cells. Tumor-specific T cells can then be activated and mediate antitumor activities including cytotoxic activity against tumor cells.

(BiTE) consist of 2 Fv fragments, each with different specificities, linked together with a flexible linker (Wolf et al, 2005). Blinatumomab, a BiTE that is specific for CD3 and CD19 and is approved for the treatment of acute lymphoblastic leukemia, has been shown to mediate regression of non–Hodgkin B-cell lymphomas (Bargou et al, 2008). This agent is specific for CD19 (expressed on B cell–related malignancies) and CD3 (to recruit T cells to tumor cells). TCR-based bispecific biologics link the specificity of a TCR with anti-CD3 and are being investigated for the treatment of melanoma expressing GP100 (Boudousquie et al, 2017).

Several FDA-approved antibodies for cancer have been modified to deliver toxic or radioactive molecules to tumor cells. For example, gemtuzumab is fused to the toxin ozogamicin, ibritumomab tiuxetan is conjugated to yttrium-90, trastuzumab is fused with the chemotherapeutic agent emtansine, and tositumomab is conjugated to iodine-131.

21.5.3 In Vivo Immunomodulation

21.5.3.1 Immunomodulatory Agents and Cytokines

These were the first successful immunotherapy agents, which resulted in immune activation for clinical benefit. For several decades, Bacillus Calmette-Guérin (BCG), a live-attenuated strain of *Mycobacterium bovis*, has been used in preventing the recurrence of superficial bladder carcinoma. BCG is administered intravesically, and its mechanism of action is related to its immunostimulatory activity resulting in promotion of antineoplastic cytokines IL-2, TNF-α, and IFN-γ and infiltration of T cells into the bladder wall (Patard et al, 1998).

Since the 1980s, cytokines have been used in the treatment of cancer. IFN-α is produced by many cell types, including cells of the immune system such as T cells, B cells, NK cells, DCs, and macrophages, and has direct antitumor effects, as well as a role in immunomodulation (Dunn et al, 2006). IFN-α can directly inhibit proliferation of tumor cells, downregulate expression of oncogenes, and induce tumor-suppressor genes. It also possesses antiangiogenic activity.

IFN-α therapy induces responses in more than 90% of patients with hairy cell leukemia and has been used in other hematologic cancers, such as chronic myelogenous leukemia, myeloma, and low-grade non-Hodgkin lymphoma. Although approved for patients with melanoma and renal cell carcinoma, the overall clinical response rate is relatively low, and high-dose IFN-α therapy is associated with severe toxicities, including hypotension, vomiting, fever, and diarrhea; its use has been superseded by checkpoint inhibitors.

Interleukin-2 (IL-2) is a cytokine that acts primarily to stimulate proliferation of T cells and NK cells. High-dose IL-2 therapy is an approved treatment for renal cell carcinoma and melanoma, but the clinical response rate is low and therapy is associated with substantial toxicity. Although IL-2 promotes effector T-cell responses and can function to reverse anergy of effector T cells, IL-2 is not an ideal agent to promote immunity because it also promotes the expansion of Tregs, which can act to suppress anticancer immune responses. Novel versions and mimics of cytokines such as IL-2 and IL-15 are under investigation. These agents hold the promise of inducing anticancer effects while obviating toxicity (Charych et al, 2016; Silva et al, 2019).

21.5.3.2 Toll-Like Receptor Agonists
TLRs are a family of molecules that are stimulated by conserved molecular motifs that are present on various microorganisms (Akira et al, 2006; see also Sec. 21.2.2). The TLRs are expressed by many cell types, including cells of the innate immune system such as macrophages and DCs. Interactions between TLRs and corresponding ligands lead to activation of innate immune cells, which promote elimination of the microorganism through various mechanisms, including production of interferons and proinflammatory cytokines.

Because TLRs activate APCs such as DCs, they can enhance the ability of DCs to stimulate antitumor T-cell responses.

Imiquimod is a synthetic Toll-like receptor 7 (TLR7) agonist that is approved for treatment of superficial basal cell carcinoma, genital warts, and actinic keratosis. Treatment is generally effective for superficial basal cell carcinoma, with complete clearance rates of approximately 75% or higher (compared to a few percent in placebo-treated groups). Various TLR ligands are under investigation in animal models and early clinical trials for cancer immunotherapy either alone or in combination with other agents (Smith et al, 2018).

21.5.3.3 Therapeutic Cancer Vaccines
In order to focus the antitumor immune response, one strategy has been to enhance a specific immune response against tumor-associated antigens (see Sec. 21.4.2). Mature DCs are highly efficient antigen-presenting cells and therefore are central players in the induction of T-cell responses; administration of DCs that present TAAs to induce antitumor T cells in vivo has been performed (Tacken et al, 2007). In general, these DCs are obtained by in vitro differentiation of bone marrow progenitor cells (for mice) or peripheral blood monocytes (for humans) (Fig. 21–15). Granulocyte-macrophage colony-stimulating factor (GM-CSF) and IL-4 are used commonly to stimulate differentiation. Some of the methods for loading DCs with TAAs include loading peptides derived from TAAs onto surface MHC molecules, incubating DCs with whole TAA proteins, and transfecting or transducing DCs with DNA encoding

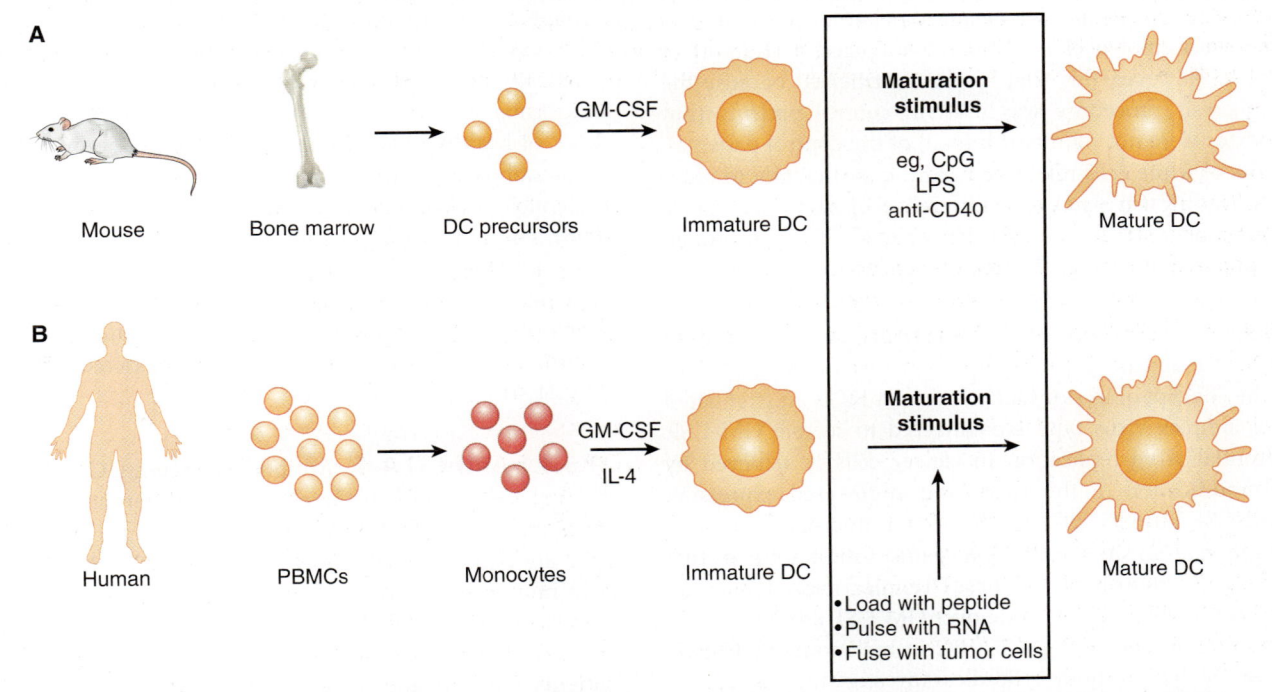

FIGURE 21–15 Generating DCs for therapy. Common methods for generating DCs for vaccination are shown. A) For mouse studies, DC precursors are obtained from bone marrow cells and differentiated into immature DCs in vitro using GM-CSF. (B) For human studies, monocytes are obtained from peripheral blood mononuclear cells by a variety of methods, including elutriation, plastic adherence, or isolation of CD14+ cells. Monocytes are then differentiated into immature DCs in vitro using GM-CSF and IL-4. For both mouse and human studies, immature DCs are manipulated to present tumor-associated antigens. This can be done by a variety of approaches, including exposing them to peptides or RNA, or fusing the DCs with tumor cells. DC maturation is induced by stimuli such as TLR ligands (eg, LPS or CpG oligodeoxynucleotides) or agonistic anti-CD40 antibody. Mature DCs presenting TAAs are then ready for infusion. *GM-CSF*, granulocyte-macrophage colony-stimulating factor. *LPS*, lipopolysaccharides. *PBMCs*, peripheral blood mononuclear cells.

TAAs. TAA-loaded DCs may also be exposed to a variety of maturation stimuli in order to enhance their immunogenicity. These stimuli include agonistic anti-CD40 antibody, various TLR ligands (eg, CpG oligodeoxynucleotides, poly I:C, LPS), and cytokine cocktails (eg, a cocktail of IL-1β, IL-6, tumor necrosis factor (TNF), and prostaglandin E2) (Fig. 21–15).

Clinical trials based on DC vaccination have demonstrated that this approach is associated with minimal toxicity, and there is some evidence for clinical effectiveness (Palucka and Bancherau, 2012, 2014). However, with the success of immune checkpoint blockade, vaccines have remained the subject of investigation either as monotherapy or in combination with immunomodulators.

21.5.3.4 Sipuleucel-T
Sipuleucel-T was the first autologous cellular therapy for cancer to receive FDA approval. The therapeutic product is produced by leukapheresis from a patient to be treated for prostatic cancer. The leukapheresis product is transported to a central facility where the cells are processed and incubated with a fusion protein of a prostate TAA (prostatic acid phosphatase [PAP]) and the cytokine GM-CSF (Small et al, 2000). The cellular product is then reinfused into the same patient. The premise of this therapy is that APCs, such as DCs, will take up the fusion protein. The PAP will be processed and presented by MHC molecules on the surface of APCs and will thus be able to stimulate PAP-specific T cells to mediate antitumor activity. The functions of GM-CSF include promoting the differentiation of DCs. A phase III trial showed a survival benefit for advanced prostate cancer patients treated with sipuleucel-T compared to placebo (Kantoff et al, 2010). However, this trial has been criticized because the leukapheresis procedure was used in control patients (but leukocytes were not reinfused into all of the control patients), and loss of white cells might be harmful, particularly to older adults, leading (in part) to a difference in survival because of poorer outcome in controls (Huber et al, 2012). Although conceptually interesting, this treatment is no longer used.

21.5.3.5 Talimogene Laherparepvec (T-Vec)
Immunotherapy using genetically engineered oncolytic viruses uses the concept of in situ vaccination. TVEC is an attenuated herpes simplex virus type 1 engineered to secrete GM-CSF. Preferential virus replication in cancer cells is achieved by gene-modification of the virus, and engineered expression of GM-CSF attracts DCs to the tumor microenvironment, resulting in an in situ vaccination against tumor antigens that are released during oncolysis. Phase III clinical trials showing an increased durable response rate over GM-CSF administration has resulted in approval for T-VEC in melanoma metastatic to skin or lymph nodes. Studies investigating its use in combination with other immune modulators and in other cancers are ongoing (Conry et al, 2018).

21.5.4 Immune Checkpoint Inhibitors

Despite the glimmer of activity seen with previous types of immunotherapy, it was not regarded as a meaningful treatment modality for cancer. This has changed over the past decade, and immunotherapy is now an important treatment modality alongside surgery, radiation, and chemotherapeutics. This paradigm shift has occurred primarily because of the development of immune checkpoint inhibitors that target cytotoxic T lymphocyte–associated protein 4 (CTLA-4) or programmed cell death protein 1 (PD-1) pathways and has resulted in improved survival rates in multiple tumor types. Despite the success of immune checkpoint inhibitors, many questions remain about their mechanisms of action and their optimal utilization in the clinic.

The breakthrough in immunotherapy occurred following the basic laboratory insights of James Allison and Tasaku Honjo who were awarded the 2018 Nobel Prize for Physiology or Medicine. They demonstrated, through a series of studies beginning in the 1990s, the importance of these pathways in providing an immunologic "brake" or checkpoint on the immune response (Fig. 21–16; Ishida et al, 1992; Krummel and Allison, 1995; Chambers et al, 1997; Nishimura et al, 1999). Previous immunotherapy treatments may have failed in part due to failure to address counterregulatory processes, which are employed by the immune system to prevent autoimmunity and runaway immune responses. Drs. Allison and Honjo and others showed that overcoming these immune checkpoints could unleash meaningful anticancer effects.

Initially there was confusion regarding the function of CTLA-4, which is structurally similar to CD28 and was thought to be a positive regulator of T cells. A key breakthrough occurred when Allison and others defined the negative regulatory role of CTLA-4 through experiments with genetically modified mice. CTLA-4 was shown to be critical for normal immune function, preventing the inappropriate attack of healthy tissue. In animal models, targeting CTLA-4 with antibodies could prevent the development of tumors and enable the elimination of established tumors (Leach et al, 1996). The group led by Honjo originally cloned PD-1 in 1992, which provides another important checkpoint of T cells. Subsequent work identified and characterized the ligands PD-L1, which is broadly expressed in the tissues and tumor microenvironment, and PD-L2, which has more restricted expression (Fig. 21–16).

21.5.4.1 Anti-CTLA-4.
Antibodies targeting CTLA-4 were the first to be tested in the clinic. Two different therapeutic antibodies were developed, one being a fully humanized IgG2 antibody (tremelimumab; Ribas, 2008) and the other a fully humanized IgG1 antibody (ipilimumab; Weber 2009). Tremelimumab failed to demonstrate benefit in clinical trials but ipilimumab increased overall survival significantly in patients with advanced melanoma compared to treatment with chemotherapy (Hodi et al. 2010). Moreover, among the approximately 15% to 20% of patients who responded to ipilimumab, many of the responses were durable and some lasted many years (Schadendorf et al, 2015).

Despite the negative regulatory role of CTLA-4 signaling being well established, the mechanism(s) whereby anti-CTLA-4 blockade induces antitumor immunity and results

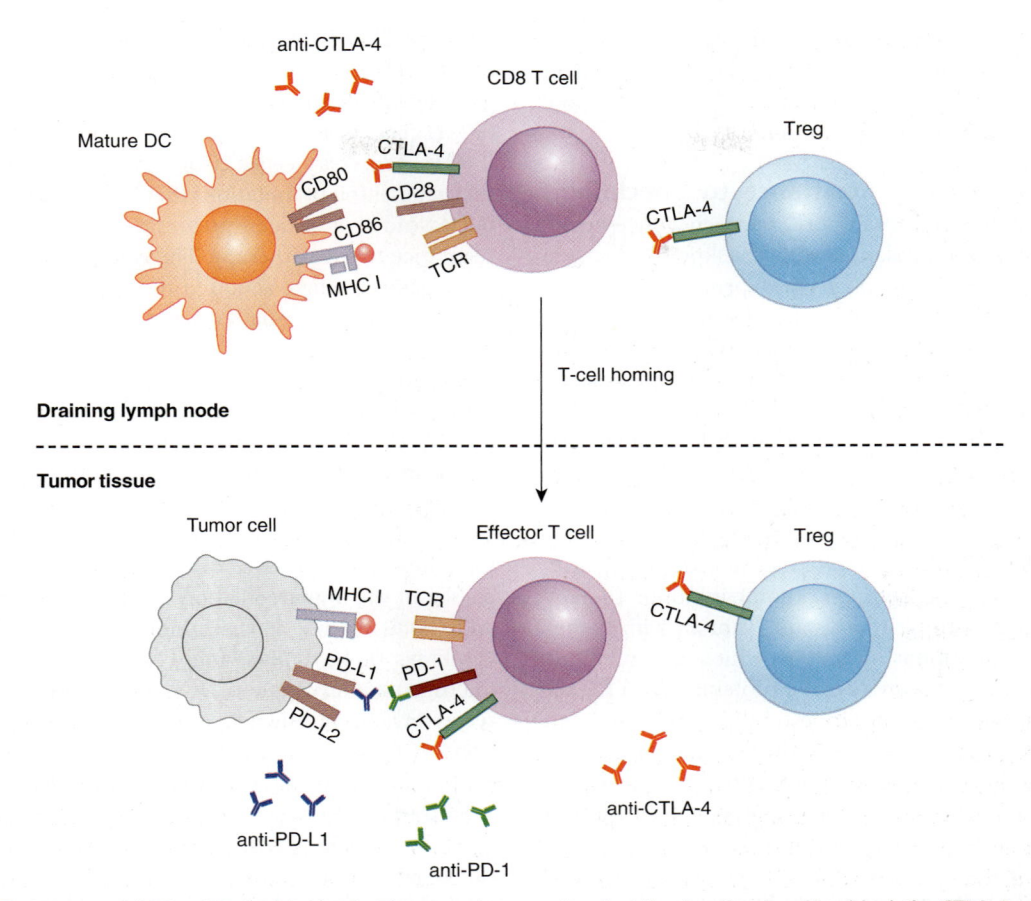

FIGURE 21–16 CTLA-4 and PD-1/PD-L1 blockade. Therapeutic monoclonal antibodies developed to block the CTLA-4 and PD-1/L1 immune checkpoint pathways have been approved for the treatment of cancers. CTLA-4 blockade prevents the downregulatory interaction between CD80 and CD86 with CTLA-4 and allows stimulation via CD28, which occurs primarily in lymph node structures during priming. CTLA-4 blocking mAbs may also bind to T regulatory (Treg) cells, which highly express CTLA-4. Blocking antibodies that bind to PD-1 or PD-L1 prevent suppressive signaling through PD-1, which is expressed on activated antigen-experienced cells. This blockade unleashes antitumor T-cell activity by T cells in the tumor microenvironment.

in durable disease control is still under investigation. There remains some debate whether the predominant target of anti–CTLA-4 blockade is to "release the brakes" on effector T cells or to inhibit the suppressive activity of Tregs. CTLA-4 blockade is thought to enhance effector T cells by the following mechanisms: Anti–CTLA-4 antibodies may prevent the interaction of CD80 and CD86 with CTLA-4, thereby allowing for prolonged interaction of CD80 and CD86 with the positive costimulatory receptor CD28 (see Fig. 21–16). In addition, CTLA-4 blockade may inhibit the CTLA-4–mediated negative intracellular signals that shut down effector T cells. There is also strong evidence that CTLA-4 suppresses effector T cells in a non–cell-autonomous fashion, that is, by inhibiting the suppressive activity of Tregs (Bachmann et al, 1999; Read et al, 2000). More recently, it has been suggested that ipilimumab depletes Treg cells in the tumor via ADCC that is dependent on the presence of macrophages that express the Fc gamma receptor IIIA (FcγRIIIA) (Romano et al, 2015). A potential reason for the lack of clinical activity of tremelimumab is due to an inability to deplete Tregs via ADCC, because tremelimumab is not the optimal IgG isotype to engage the FcγRIIIA. However, other studies have suggested that anti-CTLA-4 results in clinical benefit via mechanisms that do not result in Treg depletion (Sharma et al, 2019).

21.5.4.2 Anti-PD-1/PD-L1

There are several different antibodies that target either PD-1 or PD-L1 and are approved for use in the clinic. These antibodies block the interaction of PD-1 with its major ligand PD-L1, as well as with PD-L2 in the case of anti-PD-1 antibodies (Fig. 21–16). As with anti-CTLA-4, uncertainty exists regarding the cellular and molecular mechanisms that underpin the clinical activity of these agents. Although blocking inhibitory PD-1 signals to T cells in the tumor microenvironment contributes to the mechanism of action of these agents, the therapeutic significance of blocking PD-1/PD-L1 signals on other cell types present in the microenvironment, such as macrophages and NK cells, is being investigated (Hartley et al, 2018; Hsu et al, 2018). Despite these mechanistic uncertainties, PD-1 blockade is now part of the standard of care for renal cell cancer, bladder cancer, non–small cell lung cancer, head and neck cancer, as well as melanoma. Unfortunately, even though anti-PD-1/L1 agents have demonstrated activity against multiple different tumor types, the majority of cancer patients still will not benefit from treatment with an agent targeting the PD-1 axis. A major focus of research is to better understand the cellular and molecular mechanisms of resistance to these agents, as well as other checkpoint inhibitors.

21.5.4.3 Mechanisms of Resistance to Checkpoint Inhibitors.
A useful framework to approach conceptually resistance to immune modulation with checkpoint blockade is to consider 3 major overlapping types: primary resistance, adaptive resistance and acquired resistance (Sharma et al, 2017). Tumors that display primary resistance to checkpoint blockade are referred to as immunologically "cold" or "immune deserts" that are not infiltrated by T cells and do not appear to elicit an adaptive immune response. Tumors with low mutational burdens do not have a sufficient number of novel antigens that allow them to be recognized by the immune system and thus display primary resistance. Efforts are ongoing to utilize tumor mutational burden (TMB) as a biomarker in order to identify patients who will benefit from checkpoint inhibitor therapy vs those who will be primarily resistant. Tumors with higher numbers of nonsynonymous mutations, which are mutations that alter the amino acid sequence of a protein, have a higher response rate to immune checkpoint inhibitors (Yarchoan et al, 2017). This is most likely due to the fact that an increase in mutational burden increases that number of novel peptides from which "neo-antigens" can be generated and recognized by the immune system.

Tumors that display adaptive resistance elicit an antitumor response, but this response is quickly blunted by immunosuppressive factors (Kim et al, 2018). It is termed "adaptive resistance" because many of these immunosuppressive factors, including the expression of PD-L1, are induced by the presence of antitumor T cells expressing inflammatory cytokines (Spranger et al, 2013). These induced immunosuppressive factors include the upregulation of other coinhibitory molecules and their ligands, such as LAG3 and TIGIT, as well as the recruitment of suppressive cells that include Tregs, myeloid-derived suppressor cells (MDSCs), and anti-inflammatory M2 macrophages. Other mechanisms of adaptive resistance include the production of suppressive cytokines, such as IL-10 and TGF-beta, as well as the expression of enzymes such as indoleamine 2,3-dioxygenase (IDO) and arginase-1 (ARG1). IDO and ARG1 deplete key amino acids, tryptophan and arginine, respectively, from the tumor microenvironment that are required for an effective antitumor T-cell response (Mondanelli et al, 2017). In addition to these mechanisms, there are likely multiple other complex regulatory networks that can suppress the reinvigorated antitumor response induced by treatment with checkpoint inhibitors and result in adaptive tolerance.

Acquired resistance is similar to adaptive resistance but applies to patients who respond to immunotherapy for months or even years before their tumors become resistant and progress. Serial analysis of the tumors from 4 melanoma patients who had been treated with anti-PD-1 therapy for months before progressing led to the identification of mutations associated with the acquired resistance phenotype. Mutations had developed in either Janus kinase (JAK) 1 or JAK2 (see Chap. 6, Sec. 6.3.1), essential kinases for signaling downstream of the gamma interferon receptor, or in the beta-2-microglobulin (β2M) gene, which is essential for antigen presentation by class I MHC (Zaretsky et al, 2016). These findings demonstrated that acquisition of mutations that inhibit inflammatory signaling cascades or antigen presentation to CD8$^+$ T cells lead to resistance to PD-1 therapy. The extent to which mutations in these genes mediate acquired resistance to anti-PD-1 therapy in larger numbers of patients and in tumors of differing histology is being investigated.

Factors produced by tumor cells, or by other cells in the tumor microenvironment, are also known to suppress antitumor T-cell responses. Two examples of tumor-related immunosuppressive factors are TGF-β and IDO. TGF-β is produced by tumor-associated macrophages, tumor cells, and Tregs and exerts immunosuppressive effects on multiple cell types, including DCs and effector T cells. TGF-β signaling in DCs results in the downregulation of MHC class II, CD40, CD80, and CD86, as well as the inhibition of the proinflammatory cytokines IL-12, IFN-α, and TNF-α. Thus, TGF-β induces a tolerogenic phenotype in DCs. These tolerogenic DCs themselves have been shown to secrete TGF-β leading to the induction of Tregs in mouse and human models. The immune suppressive effect of TGF-β on T cells is also well established. TGF-β signaling results in suppression of granzyme A, granzyme B, and FAS ligand in CTLs. In addition, induced Tregs can be generated by TGF-β (see Sec. 21.3.4).

Clinical trials for various agents aimed at blocking the effect of TGF-β have been conducted (Flavell et al, 2010). Blocking strategies include small molecule inhibitors, delivery of antisense molecules, and the use of blocking antibodies. Clinical responses have been limited, but further investigation into the immunologic effect of these strategies and combination of TGF-β blockade with other immunotherapeutic strategies might lead to improved responses.

IDO is an important immunosuppressive mediator (Munn and Mellor, 2016). IDO is an enzyme involved in oxidative catabolism of tryptophan, and because tryptophan is important for T-cell proliferation and activation, depletion of tryptophan by IDO inhibits T-cell responses. IDO-secreting tumor cells and DCs have been found in patients with various cancers, including melanoma, breast cancer, and colon cancer. IDO-secreting DCs have also been found in tumor-draining lymph nodes and, furthermore, these IDO-secreting DCs can induce anergy of tumor-specific T cells in vivo. Immunohistologic detection of IDO in tumor-draining lymph nodes of melanoma patients revealed that IDO expression correlated with poor prognosis (Munn et al, 2004; Lee et al, 2005).

Understanding the mechanisms by which tumor-specific T cells fail to control tumor growth may form the basis for designing therapeutic strategies. For example, unresponsive tumor-specific T cells may need to be rescued ex vivo and then reinfused; negative regulatory molecules may need to be blocked; or deleted tumor-specific T cells may need to be replenished. Immunosuppressive molecules present in the tumor microenvironment may also need to be inhibited. It is likely that a combination of these approaches will lead to the most effective approaches to immunotherapy.

21.5.4.4 Combination Immune Checkpoint Blockade

Overcoming resistance to checkpoint inhibitors is a major area of investigation, and combining agents with different targets, such as anti-PD-1 and anti-CTLA-4 agents is one strategy that has increased the rates of clinical response in tumors, including melanoma, renal cell cancer, and a subset of patients with NSCLC (Postow et al, 2015; Hellmann et al, 2018; Motzer et al, 2018). However, the increased efficacy of combining anti-PD-1 and anti-CTLA-4 regimen is accompanied by markedly increased toxicity. Other novel combinations, such as those targeting LAG3 or TIGIT combined with anti-PD-1/-L1, or combinations of a checkpoint inhibitor with an antibody targeting costimulatory molecules such as OX40 or 4-1BB are also being tested. A lack of understanding of many aspects of the biology of these molecules has prevented the rational design of novel combination regimens as well the selection of the optimal target patient populations, and many combinations have failed to provide benefit in early trials (Iafolla et al, 2018). Checkpoint blockade is also being tested in combination with different treatment modalities, including chemotherapy, targeted therapy, radiation therapy, as well as vaccines and cellular therapies. Positive effects have been observed, particularly with some combinations of chemotherapy and anti-PD-1 treatment (Paz-Ares et al, 2018; Schmid et al, 2018). Future combination regimens are exploring advances in personalized medicine to develop "bespoke" immunotherapy treatments using checkpoint inhibitors in tandem with therapies targeting patient-specific tumor antigens or by selecting the combination treatment regimen based on the expression of an investigational biomarker (Sathyanarayanan and Neelapu, 2015).

21.5.5 Adoptive T-Cell Therapy

Infusion of T cells that can recognize and destroy tumor cells is a major area of interest for immunotherapy. That transferred T cells can mediate potent antitumor effects has been demonstrated by donor lymphocyte infusions, which are the standard treatment for patients with relapsed leukemia following allogeneic bone marrow transplantation. Lymphocytes from allogeneic bone marrow transplantation donors are stored and infused if the leukemia patient relapses following bone marrow transplantation. These lymphocytes mediate regression of the relapsed leukemia primarily via an allogeneic response (a so-named graft-vs-leukemia effect). For patients with relapsed chronic myelogenous leukemia, about 70% of patients treated with donor lymphocyte infusion experience complete remission (Kolb et al, 2004).

Adoptive T-cell therapy based on a tumor antigen–specific response is based on ex vivo expansion and manipulation of patient-derived T cells followed by reinfusion in an autologous manner. General approaches to generate T cells for adoptive cell therapy are depicted in Figure 21–17 and described below.

21.5.5.1 Adoptive Cell Therapy with Tumor-Infiltrating Lymphocytes

Under normal circumstances, T cells do not infiltrate tissues, and the presence of tumor-infiltrating lymphocytes (TILs) suggested to investigators that TILs could represent a source of tumor-specific T cells for therapy. TILs can be obtained following dissociation of tumor tissue, and expansion of TILs can be undertaken ex vivo in the presence of various T-cell growth factors such as IL-2. Adoptive transfer of bulk populations of TILs has been performed in trials for various cancers, including melanoma, ovarian cancer, renal cell carcinoma, and non–small cell lung cancer. Collectively, these trials demonstrate that adoptive transfer of TILs is clinically active (Rohaan et al, 2019).

High clinical response rates have been reported when patients with metastatic melanoma were treated with TIL-based protocols in a series of trials. In these protocols, patients were given nonmyeloablative lymphodepleting chemotherapy (cyclophosphamide and fludarabine) immediately prior to infusion of TILs (10^{10} to 10^{11} cells) and high-dose IL-2 therapy. The clinical utility of this approach now that checkpoint inhibitors are available is uncertain but under investigation in clinical studies for immunotherapy-resistant disease or in combination.

21.5.5.2 Adoptive Cell Therapy with Tumor-Specific T Cells

One source of T cells for adoptive cell therapy is expanded antigen-specific T cells from the peripheral blood of cancer patients as either T cell clones or lines enriched for antigen specificity. This approach is advantageous in that the peptide specificity of the transferred T cells is well defined, and peripheral blood T cells have not been subjected to immunosuppressive factors present within the tumor microenvironment. Potential drawbacks for this approach include the possibility that these T cells may not home to the tumor site. It is also possible that tumor cells do not express the peptide recognized by the T-cell clones and will escape detection by the T cells.

The general approach to generating nonengineered tumor-specific T cells for therapy involves stimulation of bulk peripheral blood T cells with peptides derived from TAAs of interest. The most well studied TAA-derived peptides are those that bind the HLA-A*0201 MHC molecule, and therefore these trials have been generally limited to HLA-A*0201–positive patients. Peptide-stimulated T cells are then cultured under limiting dilution conditions in order to expand a population of T cells derived from a single clone. All T cells expanded from a single T cell will express identical TCRs and therefore can be considered clones. Alternatively, antigen-specific T cells can be sorted by various techniques, expanded, and then infused as T-cell lines with enriched specificity. CD8+ T-cell and CD4+ T-cell lines and clones have been used in early-phase clinical trials, which have demonstrated that this approach is associated with low toxicity (Ott et al, 2019).

21.5.5.3 Chimeric Antigen Receptor T Cells

A major challenge of immunotherapy is that many TAAs are derived from self and are subject to regulatory mechanisms to prevent

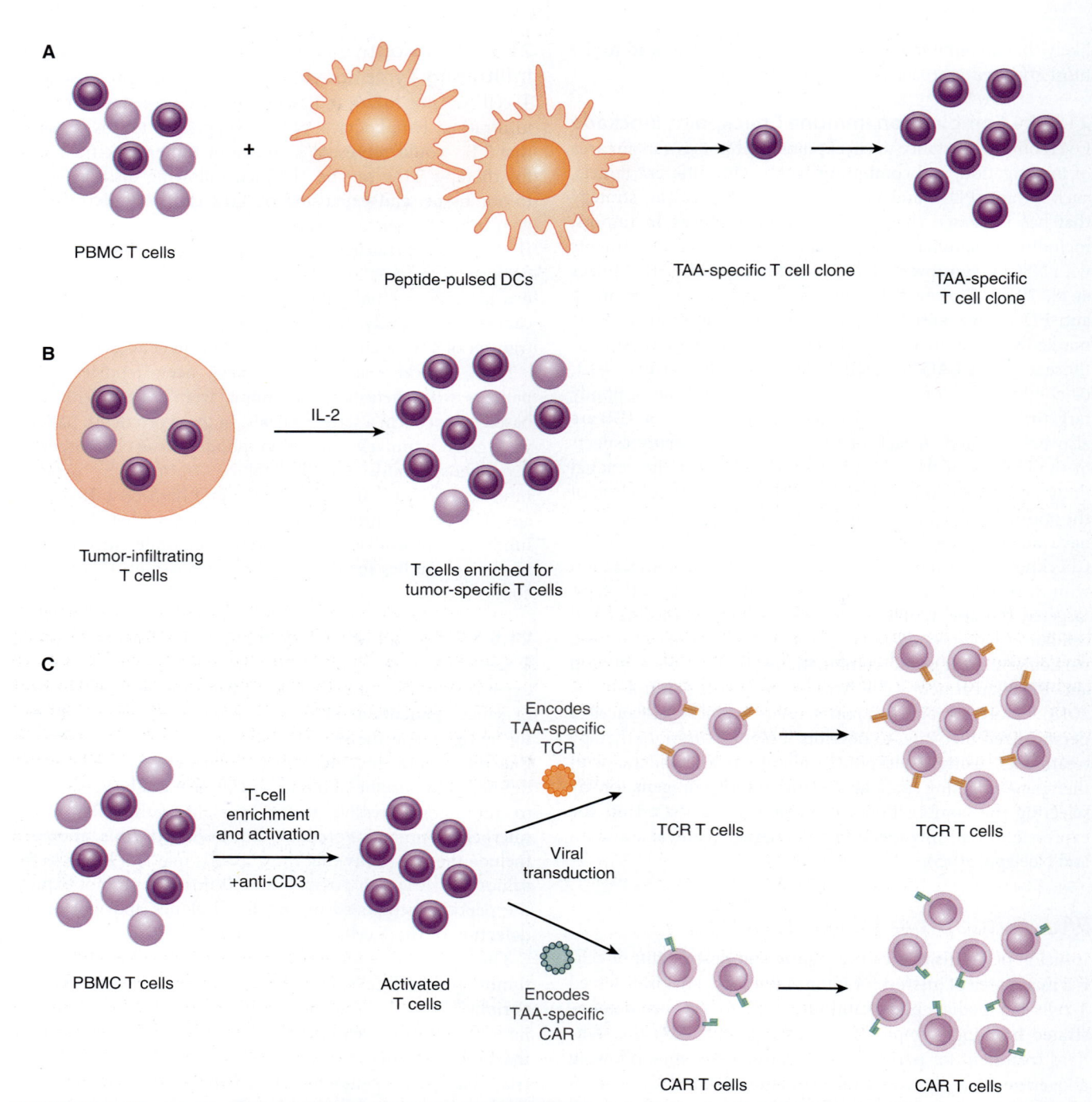

FIGURE 21-17 In vitro approaches to adoptive T-cell therapy. Adoptive T-cell therapy consists of 3 main types of therapy: **A)** Endogenous T cells can be expanded in an antigen-specific manner to large numbers for adoptive transfer. To generate tumor-specific T-cell clones or lines, peripheral blood mononuclear cells (PBMCs) are isolated and the bulk T-cell population is stimulated with antigen-presenting cells such as DCs that have been exposed to peptides derived from tumor-associated antigens (TAAs). Through successive rounds of stimulation and expansion, tumor-specific T cells are selectively expanded. **B)** Tumor-infiltrating lymphocyte (TIL) therapy involves the surgical excision of a tumor sample, which is processed in the laboratory. To generate TILs, tumor tissue is dissociated and the bulk population of TILs is expanded in vitro using a T-cell growth factor (eg, IL-2). In theory, the resulting T-cell population is enriched for tumor-specific T cells. TIL samples are expanded in a rapid expansion protocol to large numbers (10^{10}-10^{11}) and infused after lymphodepleting chemotherapy. TIL are further supported in vivo by administration of IL-2 post infusion. **C)** To generate gene-engineered T cells, peripheral blood lymphocytes are stimulated in vitro with anti-CD3 engagement and then exposed to a retroviral or lentiviral vector with the expression of an engineered receptor (TCR or CAR). The exogenous receptor redirects the lymphocyte to eliminate the tumor cell target.

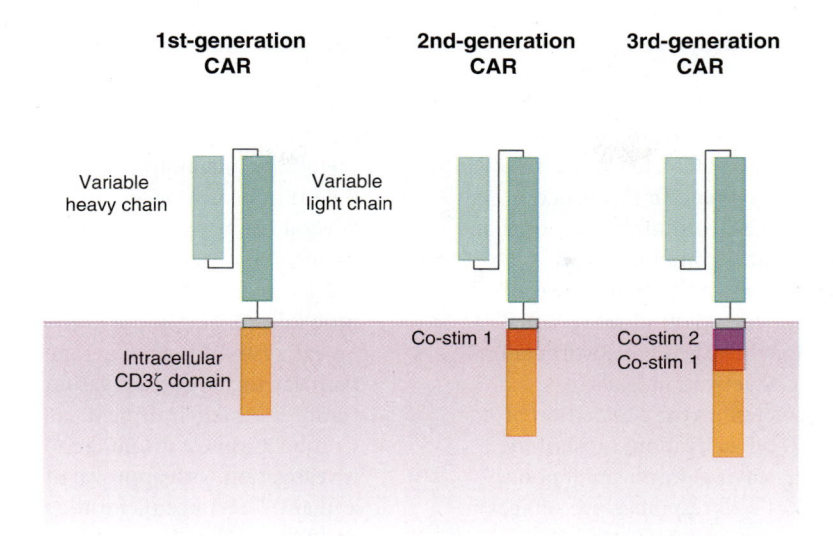

FIGURE 21–18 Production and use of chimeric antigen receptor (CAR) T cells. First-generation CARs are composed of an extracellular antigen-binding domain, a transmembrane domain, and intracellular CD3ζ domain containing ITAM motifs for T-cell activation. Second- and third-generation CARs have 1 or 2 additional intracellular costimulatory domains (CD28, 4-1BB, OX40, CD27). *ITAM*, Immunoreceptor tyrosine-based activation motifs.

autoreactivity. Consequently, T-cell responses expanded from tumors or from the periphery must overcome these hurdles. One strategy is the redirection of T cells through synthetic engineering to endow these cells with antitumor activity. With the development of gene-transfer techniques, it has become possible to exogenously express receptors in T cells that endow them with tumor specificity (Sadelain et al, 2017). This is accomplished through the use of retroviral or lentiviral vectors that encode for chimeric antigen receptors (CARs), which combine an extracellular antigen-binding domain with an intracellular T-cell activating signaling domain, or the alpha and beta chains of a tumor antigen–specific T-cell receptor (TCR) (June et al, 2018). The CAR T-cell approach involves a synthetic receptor that consists of an extracellular domain that can specifically bind a target molecule on the cancer cell, a transmembrane domain, and an intracellular domain that provides a positive signal when the receptor binds target. Although this strategy was first proposed in the 1990s, a breakthrough occurred when second-generation constructs, which incorporated costimulatory domains were used in the clinic to target CD19-expressing tumors (Fig. 21–18). Remarkable success with CD19-targeting CAR T cells has been achieved in the treatment of B-cell leukemias and lymphomas using second-generation dual-signaling CARs (Locke et al, 2019; Schuster et al, 2019).

Success with gene-engineered T-cell approaches has been linked to the ability of adoptively transferred T cells to engraft and persist, which can be enhanced in most cases by preinfusion lymphodepletion. Rapid in vivo expansion of transferred cells can result in unique acute toxicities associated with the release of cytokines (cytokine release syndrome), which may be fatal and require treatment with anti-IL6/IL6R agents or corticosteroids (Neelapu et al, 2018). Mechanisms of resistance include the emergence of tumor cells, which have downregulated the target antigen. Additionally, extension of the CAR T-cell approach to solid tumors has been challenging because of a lack of targets restricted to the tumor. However as proof of concept for a gene-engineered T-cell approach in solid tumors, T cells engineered to encode a TCR that recognizes the cancer-testes antigen, NY-ESO-1, have been successful in targeting NY-ESO-1–expressing tumors, most notably synovial sarcoma (Robbins et al, 2011; D'Angelo et al, 2018).

SUMMARY

The Immune System

▶ The 2 arms of the immune system are innate immunity and adaptive immunity. One of the functions of the innate immune system is to detect the presence of pathogens and present antigens to cells of the adaptive immune system. Dendritic cells (DCs) are efficient antigen-presenting cells (APCs). When DCs encounter pathogens, they differentiate from an immature to a mature state. Mature DCs have the ability to efficiently activate T cells.

▶ Antigens are presented to T cells by major histocompatibility complex (MHC) molecules. The antigens presented by MHC molecules are peptide fragments that can be derived from self or foreign proteins. There are 2 main types of MHC molecules: MHC class I and MHC class II, which present antigen to $CD8^+$ and $CD4^+$ T cells, respectively.

▶ B cells recognize antigens in their native form via a B-cell receptor (BCR). The BCR is a membrane-bound form of the soluble immunoglobulin (antibody) that will be produced by that B cell on activation. T cells

- recognize antigens as peptide fragments that are presented by MHC molecules via the T-cell receptor (TCR). The TCR is expressed on the surface of T cells and is not secreted. The diversity of BCR and TCR specificities is partly a result of a DNA rearrangement process called V(D)J rearrangement. In this process, selected gene segments from a large number of possible gene segments are spliced into a combined exon.
- A T-cell response is induced when TCRs are engaged by their cognate peptide-MHC ligand. Productive T-cell activation also requires signaling through costimulatory molecules (eg, CD28). T-cell activation leads to proliferation of the T cell as well as the acquisition of effector functions. After T-cell activation, most of the activated T cells disappear, leaving only a small pool of memory T cells behind. T-cell responses are subject to suppression by various mechanisms, including downregulation via molecules such as cytotoxic T-lymphocyte antigen (CTLA)-4 and programmed death (PD)-1.
- There are various types of T cells. Cytotoxic T lymphocytes (CTLs) can kill target cells and generally express the CD8 coreceptor. T helper cells (T_H cells) express the CD4 coreceptor and secrete various cytokines depending on their particular T_H cell subtype (T_H1, T_H2, T_H17, etc).
- Various mechanisms help to establish T-cell tolerance to self-antigens. For example, during T-cell development in the thymus, T cells that strongly recognize self-antigens are eliminated. Self-reactive T cells that escape thymic development can be suppressed by various peripheral tolerance mechanisms, including regulatory T cells (Tregs).
- Tumor-associated antigens (TAAs) are proteins that are expressed preferentially (or uniquely) by tumor cells. Types of TAAs include mutated self-proteins, cancer-testis antigens, proteins normally expressed during differentiation, overexpressed self-proteins, and viral antigens.
- The immune system can survey the body for tumor cells and eliminate them, a concept termed "cancer immune surveillance."
- Monoclonal antibodies (mAbs) bind specifically to their target protein. Monoclonal Ab therapy has various possible mechanisms of action: blockade of receptor signaling, triggering of receptor signaling, activation of the complement cascade leading to target cell lysis, or target cell lysis via antibody-dependent cell-mediated cytotoxicity. In addition, mAb therapy may enhance T-cell priming as a result of enhanced uptake and presentation of antigens.
- Barriers that inhibit the T-cell response against tumors include signaling through immune checkpoints where activated T cells are downregulated. Approved drugs that mediate immune checkpoint blockade include mAbs that target CTLA-4 and PD-1/PD-L1 pathways. These agents are immune modulators that augment antitumor immune responses in a general/nonspecific manner and can result in long-term disease control.
- The first immune checkpoint-blocking drug is ipilimumab, which blocks CTLA-4 and is approved for metastatic melanoma. CTLA-4 is upregulated early in the immune response.
- Several mAbs have been approved that block the PD-1 pathway and target either PD-1 or its counterreceptor PD-L1. PD-1 expression on activated T cells is upregulated later in the immune response and is present on exhausted T cells. Therapeutic action of blocking this pathway includes reactivation of resident T cells in the tumor microenvironment.
- Combinations of immune modulators are under investigation with approval of combined anti-CTLA-4 and anti-PD-1 agents for the treatment of melanoma and renal cell cancer.
- Adoptive cell therapy involves the culture and expansion of immune cells in the laboratory and then reinfusion of these cells as an antitumor agent. Approved cell products for anticancer therapy include cells engineered with a chimeric antigen receptor (CAR), which targets the B-cell antigen CD19 that is expressed on some leukemias and lymphomas.

REFERENCES

Akira S, Uematsu S, Takeuchi O. Pathogen recognition and innate immunity. *Cell* 2006;124(4):783-801.

Ayers M, Lunceford J, Nebozhyn M, et al. IFN-γ-related mRNA profile predicts clinical response to PD-1 blockade. *J Clinl Invest* 2017;127(8):2930–2940.

Bachmann MF, Kohler G, Ecabert B, et al. Cutting edge: lymphoproliferative disease in the absence of CTLA-4 is not T cell autonomous. *J Immunol* 1999;163(3):1128-1131.

Bakker AH, Schumacher TN. MHC multimer technology: current status and future prospects. *Curr Opin Immunol* 2005;17(4):428-433.

Bargou R, Leo E, Zugmaier G, et al. Tumor regression in cancer patients by very low doses of a T cell-engaging antibody. *Science* 2008;321(5891):974-977.

Boudousquie C, Bossi G, Hurst J, Rygiel KA, Jakobsen BK, Hassan NJ. Polyfunctional response by ImmTAC (IMCgp100) redirected CD8+ and CD4+ T cells. *Immunology* 2017;152(3):425–438.

Brownlie RJ, Zamoyska R. T cell receptor signalling networks: branched, diversified and bounded. *Nat Rev Immunol* 2013;13(4):257-269.

Bryant P, Ploegh H. Class II MHC peptide loading by the professionals. *Curr Opin Immunol* 2004;16(1):96-102.

Chambers CA, Sullivan TJ, Allison JP. Lymphoproliferation in CTLA-4-deficient mice is mediated by costimulation-dependent activation of CD4+ T cells. *Immunity* 1997;7(6):885-895.

Charych DH, Hoch U, Langowski JL, et al. NKTR-214, an engineered cytokine with biased il2 receptor binding, increased tumor exposure, and marked efficacy in mouse tumor models. *Clin Cancer Res* 2016;22(3):680–690.

Conry RM, Westbrook B, McKee S, Norwood TG. Talimogene laherparepvec: First in class oncolytic virotherapy. *Hum Vaccin Immunother* 2018;14(4):839–846.

Constantinescu CS, Farooqi N, O'Brien K, Gran B. Experimental autoimmune encephalomyelitis (EAE) as a model for multiple sclerosis (MS). *Br J Pharmacol* 2011;164(4):1079–1106.

Crome SQ, Nguyen LT, Lopez-Verges S, et al. A distinct innate lymphoid cell population regulates tumor-associated T cells. *Nat Med* 2017;23:368–375.

D'Angelo SP, Melchiori L, Merchant MS, et al. Antitumor activity associated with prolonged persistence of adoptively transferred NY-ESO-1 c259T cells in synovial sarcoma. *Cancer Discov* 2018;8(8):944–957.

Dunn GP, Koebel CM, Schreiber RD. Interferons, immunity and cancer immunoediting. *Nat Rev Immunol* 2006;6(7): 836-848.

Dustin ML, Cooper JA. The immunological synapse and the actin cytoskeleton: molecular hardware for T cell signaling. *Nat Immunol* 2000;1(1):23-29.

Engels EA. Cancer in Solid Organ Transplant Recipients: There Is Still Much to Learn and Do. *Am J Transplant* 2017;17(8):1967-1969.

Fife BT, Bluestone JA. Control of peripheral T-cell tolerance and autoimmunity via the CTLA-4 and PD-1 pathways. *Immunol Rev* 2008;224:166-182.

Flavell RA, Sanjabi S, Wrzesinski SH, et al. The polarization of immune cells in the tumour environment by TGFbeta. *Nat Rev Immunol* 2010;10(8):554-567.

Franchi L, Warner N, Viani K, et al. Function of Nod-like receptors in microbial recognition and host defense. *Immunol Rev* 2009;227(1):106-128.

Franks SE, Wolfson B, Hodge JW. Natural born killers: NK cells in cancer therapy. *Cancers (Basel)* 2020;12:2131.

Galon J, Costes A, Sanchez-Cabo F, et al. Type, density, and location of immune cells within human colorectal tumors predict clinical outcome. *Science* 2006;313(5795):1960-1964.

Gibbons Johnson RM, Dong H. Functional expression of programmed death-ligand 1 (B7-H1) by immune cells and tumor cells. *Front Immunol* 2017;8:961.

Gondek DC, Lu LF, Quezada SA, et al. Cutting edge: contact-mediated suppression by CD4⁺CD25⁺ regulatory cells involves a granzyme B-dependent, perforin-independent mechanism. *J Immunol* 2005;174(4):1783-1786.

Greenwald RJ, Freeman GJ, Sharpe AH. The B7 family revisited. *Ann Rev Immunol* 2005;23:515–548.

Gubin MM, Artyomov MN, Mardis ER, Schreiber RD. Tumor neoantigens: building a framework for personalized cancer immunotherapy. *J Clin Invest* 2015;125(9): 3413–3421.

Gutcher I, Becher B. APC-derived cytokines and T cell polarization in autoimmune inflammation. *J Clin Invest* 2007; 117(5):1119-1127.

Hartley GP, Chow L, Ammons DT, Wheat WH, Dow SW. Programmed cell death ligand 1 (PD-L1) signaling regulates macrophage proliferation and activation. *Cancer Immunol Res* 2018;6(10):1260-1273.

Hellmann MD, Ciuleanu TE, Pluzanski A, et al. Nivolumab plus Ipilimumab in Lung Cancer with a High Tumor Mutational Burden. *N Engl J Med* 2018;378(22):2093-2104.

Hemmi H, Takeuchi O, Kawai T, et al. A Toll-like receptor recognizes bacterial DNA. *Nature* 2000;408(6813):740-745.

Hodi FS, O'Day SJ, McDermott DF, et al. Improved survival with ipilimumab in patients with metastatic melanoma. *N Engl J Med* 2010;363(8):711-723.

Hsu J, Hodgins JJ, Marathe M, et al. Contribution of NK cells to immunotherapy mediated by PD-1/PD-L1 blockade. *J Clin Invest* 2018;128(10):4654-4668.

Huber ML, Haynes L, Parker C, Iversen P. Interdisciplinary critique of sipuleucel-T as immunotherapy in castration-resistant prostate cancer. *J Natl Cancer Inst* 2012;104(4):1-7.

Iafolla MAJ, Selby H, Warner K, Ohashi PS, Haibe-Kains B, Siu LL. Rational design and identification of immuno-oncology drug combinations. *Eur J Cancer* 2018;95:38-51.

Ishida Y, Agata Y, Shibahara K, et al. Induced expression of PD-1, a novel member of the immunoglobulin gene superfamily, upon programmed cell death. *EMBO J* 1992;11(11):3887-3895.

Iwasaki A, Medzhitov R. Regulation of adaptive immunity by the innate immune system. *Science* 2010;327(5963):291-295.

Ji Y, Zhang W. Th17 cells: positive or negative role in tumor? *Cancer Immunol Immunother* 2010;59:979-987.

Jonuleit H, Schmitt E. The regulatory T cell family: distinct subsets and their interrelations. *J Immunol* 2003;171(12): 6323-6327.

Josefowicz SZ, Lu LF, Rudensky AY. Regulatory T cells: mechanisms of differentiation and function. *Annu Rev Immunol* 2012;30:531-564.

June CH, Sadelain M. Chimeric antigen receptor therapy. *N Engl J Med* 2018;379(1):64–73.

Kalia V, Sarkar S, Gourley TS, et al. Differentiation of memory B and T cells. *Curr Opin Immunol* 2006;18(3):255-264.

Kantoff PW, Higano CS, Shore ND, et al. Sipuleucel-T immunotherapy for castration-resistant prostate cancer. *N Engl J Med* 2010;363(5):411-422.

Kaplan DH, Shankaran V, Dighe AS, et al. Demonstration of an interferon gamma-dependent tumor surveillance system in immunocompetent mice. *Proc Natl Acad Sci U S A* 1998;95(13):7556-7561.

Kawai T, Akira S. Toll-like receptor and RIG-I-like receptor signaling. *Ann N Y Acad Sci* 2008;1143:1-20.

Kawasaki T, Kawai T. Toll-like receptor signaling pathways. *Front Immunol* 2014;5:461.

Kawashima I, Hudson SJ, Tsai V, et al. The multi-epitope approach for immunotherapy for cancer: identification of several CTL epitopes from various tumor-associated antigens expressed on solid epithelial tumors. *Hum Immunol* 1998;59(1):1-14.

Kim TK, Herbst RS, Chen L. Defining and understanding adaptive resistance in cancer immunotherapy. *Trends Immunol* 2018;39(8):624-631.

Klein L, Kyewski B, Allen PM, et al. Positive and negative selection of the T cell repertoire: what thymocytes see (and don't see). *Nat Rev Immunol* 2014;14(6):377-391.

Kolb HJ, Schmid C, Barrett AJ, et al. Graft-versus-leukemia reactions in allogeneic chimeras. *Blood* 2004;103(3):767-776.

Krangel MS. Mechanics of T cell receptor gene rearrangement. *Curr Opin Immunol* 2009;21(2):133-139.

Krummel MF, Allison JP. CD28 and CTLA-4 have opposing effects on the response of T cells to stimulation. *J Exp Med* 1995;182(2):459-465.

Lanier LL. NK cell recognition. *Annu Rev Immunol* 2005;23:225-274.

Leach DR, Krummel MF, Allison JP. Enhancement of antitumor immunity by CTLA-4 blockade. *Science* 1996;271(5256):1734-1736.

Lee JH, Torisu-Itakara H, Cochran AJ, et al. Quantitative analysis of melanoma-induced cytokine-mediated immunosuppression in melanoma sentinel nodes. *Clin Cancer Res* 2005;11(1):107-112.

Locke FL, Ghobadi A, Jacobson CA, et al. Long-term safety and activity of axicabtagene ciloleucel in refractory large B-cell lymphoma (ZUMA-1): a single-arm, multicentre, phase 1-2 trial. *Lancet Oncol* 2019;20(1):31-42.

Magombedze G, Reddy PB, Eda S, Ganusov VV. Cellular and population plasticity of helper CD4(+) T cell responses. *Front Physiol* 2013;4:206.

McGeachy MJ, Cua DJ. Th17 cell differentiation: the long and winding road. *Immunity* 2008;28(4):445-453.

Mempel TR, Pittet MJ, Khazaie K, et al. Regulatory T cells reversibly suppress cytotoxic T cell function independent of effector differentiation. *Immunity* 2006;25(1):129-141.

Mondanelli GS, Ugel U, Grohmann Bronte V. The immune regulation in cancer by the amino acid metabolizing enzymes ARG and IDO. *Curr Opin Pharmacol* 2017;35:30-39.

Motzer RJ, Tannir DF, McDermott O, et al. Nivolumab plus ipilimumab versus sunitinib in advanced renal-cell carcinoma. *N Engl J Med* 2018;378:1277-1290.

Munn DH, Sharma MD, Hou D, et al. Expression of indoleamine 2,3-dioxygenase by plasmacytoid dendritic cells in tumor-draining lymph nodes. *J Clin Invest* 2004;114(2):280-290.

Munn DH, Mellor AL. IDO in the tumor microenvironment: inflammation, counter-regulation, and tolerance. *Trends Immunol* 2016;37(3):193-207.

Naeher D, Daniels MA, Hausmann B, et al. A constant affinity threshold for T cell tolerance. *J Exp Med* 2007;204(11):2553-2559.

Neelapu SS, Tummala S, Kebriaei P, et al. Chimeric antigen receptor T-cell therapy—assessment and management of toxicities. *Nat Rev Clin Oncol* 2018;15(1):47-62.

Nimmerjahn F, Ravetch JV. Fcgamma receptors as regulators of immune responses. *Nat Rev Immunol* 2008;8(1):34-47.

Nishimura H, Nose M, Hiai H, et al. Development of lupus-like autoimmune diseases by disruption of the PD-1 gene encoding an ITIM motif-carrying immunoreceptor. *Immunity* 1999;11(2):141-151.

Orabona C, Grohmann U, Belladonna ML, et al. CD28 induces immunostimulatory signals in dendritic cells via CD80 and CD86. *Nat Immunol* 2004;5(11):1134-1142.

Ott PA, Dotti G, Yee C, Goff SL. An Update on Adoptive T-Cell Therapy and Neoantigen Vaccines. *Am Soc Clin Oncol Educ Book* 2019;39:e70-e78.

Palucka K, Banchereau J. Cancer immunotherapy via dendritic cells. *Nat Rev Cancer* 2012;12(4):265-277.

Palucka K, Banchereau J. SnapShot: cancer vaccines. *Cell* 2014;157(2):516-516e1.

Patard JJ, Saint F, Velotti F, et al. Immune response following intravesical bacillus Calmette-Guerin instillations in superficial bladder cancer: a review. *Urol Res* 1998;26(3):155-159.

Paz-Ares L, Luft A, Vicente D, et al. Pembrolizumab plus chemotherapy for squamous non-small-cell lung cancer. *N Engl J Med* 2018;379(21):2040-2051.

Postow MA, Chesney J, Pavlick AC, C. et al. Nivolumab and ipilimumab versus ipilimumab in untreated melanoma. *N Engl J Med* 2015;372(21):2006-2017.

Quezada SA, Jarvinen LZ, Lind EF, et al. CD40/CD154 interactions at the interface of tolerance and immunity. *Annu Rev Immunol* 2004;22:307-328.

Read S, Malmstrom V, Powrie F. Cytotoxic T lymphocyte-associated antigen 4 plays an essential role in the function of CD25(+)CD4(+) regulatory cells that control intestinal inflammation. *J Exp Med* 2000;192(2):295-302.

Rentzsch C, Kayser S, Stumm S, et al. Evaluation of pre-existent immunity in patients with primary breast cancer: molecular and cellular assays to quantify antigen-specific T lymphocytes in peripheral blood mononuclear cells. *Clin Cancer Res* 2003;9(12):4376-4386.

Ribas A. Overcoming immunologic tolerance to melanoma: targeting CTLA-4 with tremelimumab (CP-675,206). *Oncologist* 2008;13(suppl 4):10-15.

Robbins PF, Morgan RA, Feldman SA, et al. Tumor regression in patients with metastatic synovial cell sarcoma and melanoma using genetically engineered lymphocytes reactive with NY-ESO-1. *J Clin Oncol* 2011;29(7):917–924.

Rohaan MW, Wilgenhof S, Haanen JBAG. Adoptive cellular therapies: the current landscape. *Virchows Arch* 2019;474(4):449-461.

Romano E, Kusio-Kobialka M, Foukas PG, et al. Ipilimumab-dependent cell-mediated cytotoxicity of regulatory T cells ex vivo by nonclassical monocytes in melanoma patients. *Proc Natl Acad Sci U S A* 2015;112(19):6140-6145.

Romero P, Dunbar PR, Valmori D, et al. Ex vivo staining of metastatic lymph nodes by class I major histocompatibility complex tetramers reveals high numbers of antigen-experienced tumor-specific cytotoxic T lymphocytes. *J Exp Med* 1998;188(9):1641-1650.

Sadelain M, Riviere I, Riddell S. Therapeutic T cell engineering. *Nature* 2017;545(7655):423–431.

Sahin U, Tureci O, Schmitt H, et al. Human neoplasms elicit multiple specific immune responses in the autologous host. *Proc Natl Acad Sci U S A* 1995;92(25):11810-11813.

Sakaguchi S, Wing K, Onishi Y, et al. Regulatory T cells: how do they suppress immune responses? *Int Immunol* 2009;21(10):1105-1111.

Sanchez-Paulete AR, Teijeira A, Cueto FJ, et al. Antigen cross-presentation and T-cell cross-priming in cancer immunology and immunotherapy. *Ann Oncol* 2017;28(suppl 12):xii44-xii55.

Sathyanarayanan V, Neelapu SS. Cancer immunotherapy: strategies for personalization and combinatorial approaches. *Mol Oncol* 2015;9(10):2043-2053.

Schadendorf D, Hodi FS, Robert C, et al. Pooled analysis of long-term survival data from phase II and phase III trials of ipilimumab in unresectable or metastatic melanoma. *J Clin Oncol* 2015;33(17):1889-1894.

Scheuer W, Friess T, Burtscher H, et al. Strongly enhanced antitumor activity of trastuzumab and pertuzumab combination treatment on HER2-positive human xenograft tumor models. *Cancer Res* 2009;69(24):9330-9336.

Schietinger A, Philip M, Schreiber H. Specificity in cancer immunotherapy. *Sem Immunol* 2008;20(5):276-285.

Schmid P, Adams S, Rugo HS, et al. Atezolizumab and nab-paclitaxel in advanced triple-negative breast cancer. *N Engl J Med* 2018;379(22):2108-2121.

Schuster SJ, Bishop MR, Tam CS, et al. Tisagenlecleucel in adult relapsed or refractory diffuse large B-cell lymphoma. *N Engl J Med* 2019;380(1):45-56.

Shankaran V, Ikeda H, Bruce AT, et al. IFNgamma and lymphocytes prevent primary tumour development and shape tumour immunogenicity. *Nature* 2001;410(6832):1107-1111.

Sharma A, Subudhi SK, Blando J, et al. Anti-CTLA-4 immunotherapy does not deplete FOXP3+ regulatory T cells (Tregs) in human cancers. *Clin Cancer Res* 2019;25(4):1233-1238.

Sharma P, Hu-Lieskovan S, Wargo JA, Ribas A. Primary, adaptive, and acquired resistance to cancer immunotherapy. *Cell* 2017;168(4):707-723.

Shen L, Rock KL. Priming of T cells by exogenous antigen cross-presented on MHC class I molecules. *Curr Opin Immunol* 2006;18(1):85-91.

Silva D-A, Yu S, Ulge UY, et al. De novo design of potent and selective mimics of IL-2 and IL-15. *Nature* 2019;565(7738):186–191.

Small EJ, Fratesi P, Reese DM, et al. Immunotherapy of hormone-refractory prostate cancer with antigen-loaded dendritic cells. *J Clin Oncol* 2000;18(23):3894-3903.

Smith M, Garcia-Martinez E, Pitter MR, et al. Trial watch: toll-like receptor agonists in cancer immunotherapy. *Oncoimmunology* 2018;7(12):e1526250.

Sotiropoulou PA, Perez SA, Iliopoulou EG, et al. Cytotoxic T-cell precursor frequencies to HER-2 (369-377) in patients with HER-2/neu-positive epithelial tumours. *Br J Cancer* 2003;89(6):1055-1061.

Spranger S, Spaapen RM, Zha Y, et al. Up-regulation of PD-L1, IDO, and T(regs) in the melanoma tumor microenvironment is driven by CD8(+) T cells. *Sci Transl Med* 2013;5(200):200ra116.

Steinman RM, Hawiger D, Nussenzweig MC. Tolerogenic dendritic cells. *Annu Rev Immunol* 2003;21:685-711.

Swann JB, Smyth MJ. Immune surveillance of tumors. *J Clin Invest* 2007;117(5):1137-1146.

Tacken PJ, de Vries IJ, Torensma R, et al. Dendritic-cell immunotherapy: from ex vivo loading to in vivo targeting. *Nat Rev Immunol* 2007;7:790-802.

Trombetta ES, Mellman I. Cell biology of antigen processing in vitro and in vivo. *Annu Rev Immunol* 2005;23:975-1028.

Tumeh PC, Harview CL, Yearley JH, et al. PD-1 blockade induces responses by inhibiting adaptive immune resistance. *Nature* 2014;515(7528):568-571.

Tuthill RJ, Unger JM, Liu PY, et al. Risk assessment in localized primary cutaneous melanoma: a Southwest Oncology Group study evaluating nine factors and a test of the Clark logistic regression prediction model. *Am J Clin Pathol* 2002;118(4):504-511.

van der Bruggen P, Traversari C, Chomez P, et al. A gene encoding an antigen recognized by cytolytic T lymphocytes on a human melanoma. *Science* 1991;254(5038):1643-1647.

Vivier E, Artis D, Colonna M, et al. Innate lymphoid cells: 10 years on. *Cell* 2018;174:1054-1066.

Vollers SS, Stern LJ. Class II major histocompatibility complex tetramer staining: progress, problems, and prospects. *Immunology* 2008;123(3):305-313.

Wang D, Jiang W, Zhu F, Mao X, Agrawal S. Modulation of the tumor microenvironment by intratumoral administration of IMO-2125, a novel TLR9 agonist, for cancer immunotherapy. *Int J Oncol* 2018;53(3):1193-1203.

Weber J. Ipilimumab: controversies in its development, utility and autoimmune adverse events. *Cancer Immunol Immunother* 2009;58(5):823-830.

Wildin RS, Freitas A. IPEX and FOXP3: clinical and research perspectives. *J Autoimmun* 2005;25(suppl):56-62.

Wolf E, Hofmeister R, Kufer P, et al. BiTEs: bispecific antibody constructs with unique anti-tumor activity. *Drug Discov Today* 2005;10(18):1237-1244.

Yarchoan M, Johnson BA, Lutz ER, Laheru DA, Jaffee EM. Targeting neoantigens to augment antitumour immunity. *Nat Rev Cancer* 2017;17(4):209-222.

Yarchoan R, Uldrick TS. HIV-Associated Cancers and Related Diseases. *N Engl J Med* 2018;378(11):1029-1041.

Zaretsky JM, Garcia-Diaz A, Shin DS, et al. Mutations associated with acquired resistance to PD-1 blockade in melanoma. *N Engl J Med* 2016;375:819-829.

Zhang L, Conejo-Garcia JR, Katsaros D, et al. Intratumoral T cells, recurrence, and survival in epithelial ovarian cancer. *N Engl J Med* 2003;348(3):203-213.

Zhu J, Min B, Hu-Li J, et al. Conditional deletion of Gata3 shows its essential function in T(H)1-T(H)2 responses. *Nat Immunol* 2004;5(11):1157-1165.

Guide to Clinical Studies

Eitan Amir

Chapter Outline

- 22.1 Introduction
- 22.2 Cancer Genomics and Clinical Studies
- 22.3 Treatment
  - 22.3.1 Purpose of Clinical Trials
  - 22.3.2 Personalized Cancer Medicine and Its Evaluation
  - 22.3.3 Limitations of and Sources of Bias in Clinical Trials
  - 22.3.4 Importance of Randomization
  - 22.3.5 Choice and Assessment of Outcomes
  - 22.3.6 Survival Curves and their Comparison
  - 22.3.7 Statistical Issues
  - 22.3.8 Meta-analysis
  - 22.3.9 Patient-Reported Outcomes
  - 22.3.10 Health Outcomes Research
  - 22.3.11 Cost-Effectiveness
- 22.4 Diagnosis and Screening
  - 22.4.1 Diagnostic Tests
  - 22.4.2 Sources of Bias in Diagnostic Tests
  - 22.4.3 Tests for Screening of Disease
  - 22.4.4 Tests During Follow-up of Treated Tumors
  - 22.4.5 Bayes Theorem and Likelihood Ratios
- 22.5 Prognosis
  - 22.5.1 Identification of Prognostic Factors
  - 22.5.2 Evaluation of Prognostic Factor Studies
  - 22.5.3 Predictive Markers
- Summary
- References
- Bibliography

22.1 INTRODUCTION

To select the optimal treatment for patients, clinical oncologists need to be skilled at critically evaluating data from clinical studies and interpreting these appropriately. Clinicians should also be proficient in the application of diagnostic tests, assessment of risk, and the estimation of prognosis. Equally, scientists involved in translational research should be aware of the problems and pitfalls in undertaking clinical studies. The practice of oncology is increasingly incorporating genomic assessment both to provide information on prognosis and to allow optimal choice of therapy. This chapter provides a critical overview of methods used in clinical research.

22.2 CANCER GENOMICS AND CLINICAL STUDIES

The field of cancer genomics is growing rapidly as a result of advances in DNA sequencing technologies (see Chap. 2, Sec. 2.2.10). This information is having an impact on cancer treatment, including intensive research into personalized cancer medicine, whereby attempts are made to match treatment with a molecular targeted agent to a mutation predicted to render the tumor sensitive (see Section 22.3.2). Genomic information is also adding to classical prognostic factors to produce more refined estimates of prognosis, and of prediction of response to different types of treatment (see Section 22.5).

Two main methods are available to study the cancer genome:

1. Whole-genome sequencing (WGS) is the backbone technology that supports the in-depth sequencing of the entire human genome (Metzker, 2009).
2. Targeted genome sequencing refers to strategies that enrich for DNA regions that are believed to be involved in tumor biology. This includes the whole exome or panels of genes recurrently altered in cancer (Robison, 2010).

Genomic analysis can provide in-depth information about a number of mutations in cancer. Not all these mutations have clinical significance. Therefore, a classification of mutations has been suggested (Sukhai et al, 2016). This classification provides information as to whether the identified mutation has been shown to be prognostic or predictive in the tumor site tested (class 1) or a different tumor site (class 2), or whether its significance is uncertain (classes 3-5). The classification of somatic alterations will continue to evolve as clinical data accumulate and as new therapies are developed.

High-throughput genotyping platforms such as microarrays (see Chap. 2, Sec 2.2.12) have been used successfully for genotyping clinical samples (Thomas et al, 2007). Microarrays allow for testing of large amounts of biological material through high-throughput miniaturized, multiplexed, and parallel processing and detection methods. The development of DNA microarray technology holds promise for improvements in the diagnosis, prognosis, and tailoring of treatment. The technical aspects of creating gene expression profiles are described in Chapter 2, Sections 2.2.12 and 2.5.2.

The ability to investigate the transcription of thousands of genes concurrently by using DNA microarrays poses a variety of analytical challenges. Microarray data sets are commonly very large and can be affected by numerous variables. Challenges to microarray analysis include methods for taking into account the effects of background noise, removal of poor-quality and low-intensity data, and choice of a statistical test for determination of significant differences between tumor and control samples (see Chap. 2, Sec. 2.5.2).

Progress has also been made in using circulating tumor DNA, with this approach showing some promise in detecting minimal residual disease, or identifying mutations associated with a particular disease type (Newman et al, 2014). RNA is much less stable than DNA in circulating blood, and although RNA preserved in extracellular vesicles can provide information about tumor recurrence, RNA-based studies have been limited by poor reproducibility, and RNA assays are not yet ready for clinical use (SEQC/MAQC-III Consortium, 2014).

A variety of tests for the identification of statistically significant changes are used. These include a spectrum from simple tests such as the t test or analysis of variance, to nonparametric smoothing analyses or Bayesian methods. These methods should be tailored to the specific microarray data set and should take into account multiple comparisons. Use of a P-value cutoff of less than 0.05 applied to a single comparison means that the false-positive rate will be less than about 5%, but this level of false positivity is too high for microarray data because most analyses comprise multiple significance tests. Consequently, there has been a shift from the use of P values to the false-discovery rate (FDR; see Chap. 2, Sec. 2.6), which is defined as the expected proportion of false positives among the declared significant results.

The analysis of gene expression profiles is evolving rapidly, and several methodologic issues surrounding the use of microarrays in prognostic or other studies have been reported (see also Chap. 2, Sec 2.6). Concerns about standardization and reliability of genomic analyses as well as data suggesting that "false-positive" overexpression or "false-negative" underexpression of genes may occur if microarray experiments are not replicated (Ioannidis et al, 2009). To limit these types of error, central repositories for genomic data have been established such as the Cancer Genome Atlas (https://cancergenome.nih.gov), an international collaboration that has generated comprehensive maps of the key genomic changes in 33 types of cancer.

Genomic testing remains limited by a number of analytic factors. First, many identified mutations are of limited clinical significance. All cancers arise as a result of somatically acquired mutations either in the presence or absence of germline mutations. That does not mean, however, that all mutations in a cancer genome are of importance. Second, there is intratumor heterogeneity so that genomic testing will reveal different sequences in biopsies taken from different parts of most tumors and from their metastases (Gerlinger et al, 2012; Swanton, 2012; see also Chap 13, Sec 13.2.3). Additionally, genomic testing often uses archival tissue, which may not be representative of the status of the disease at the time of testing. Finally, genomic analysis does not take into account epigenetic effects or the influence of post-translation changes, which occur in many cancers (Chan et al, 2014).

22.3 TREATMENT

22.3.1 Purpose of Clinical Trials

Clinical trials are used to assess the effects of specific interventions on the health of individuals. Possible interventions include treatment with drugs, radiation, or surgery; modification of diet, behavior, or environment; and surveillance with physical examination, blood tests, or imaging tests. This section focuses on trials of treatment.

Clinical trials may be separated conceptually into *explanatory* trials, designed to evaluate the biological effects of treatment, and *pragmatic* trials, designed to evaluate the practical effects of treatment (Schwartz et al, 1980). This distinction is crucial, because treatments that have desirable biological effects (eg, the ability to kill cancer cells and cause tumor shrinkage) may not have desirable effects in practice (ie, may not lead to improvement in duration or quality of life). Table 22–1 lists the major differences between explanatory and pragmatic trials.

The evaluation of new cancer treatments usually involves progression through a series of clinical trials. Phase I trials are designed to evaluate the relationship between dose and toxicity and aim to establish a tolerable dose and schedule of administration. Phase II trials are designed to screen treatments for their antitumor effects in order to identify those worthy of further evaluation. Phase I and phase II trials are explanatory—they assess the biological effects of treatment on host and tumor in small numbers of subjects to guide decisions about further research. Randomized phase III trials are designed to determine the usefulness of new treatments in the management of patients and are therefore pragmatic. Randomization is the process of assigning participants to experimental and control (existing) therapy, with each participant having a prespecified (usually equal) chance of being assigned to any group.

Phase I Trials: Phase I trials are used commonly to define the recommended dose and schedule for future study, the so-called

TABLE 22–1 Classification of clinical trials.

Characteristic	Explanatory (Phase I and Phase II Trials)	Pragmatic (Phase III Trials)
Purpose	To guide further research and not to formulate treatment policy	To select future treatment policy
Treatment and dosing	To assist in selecting a schedule and to define the maximal tolerated dose (Phase I) and to seek evidence of biological activity (Phase II)	Choose treatment schedule and dose that is tolerated for the target population based on earlier trials
Assessment criteria	Criteria that give biological information (such as inhibition of intended target), tumor response, and dose-dependent toxicity	Should reflect benefit to patients, such as overall survival, quality of life, and toxic effects
Choice of patients	Patients most likely to demonstrate an effect	Patients representative of those to whom the treatment will be applied
Entry criteria	Idealized conditions: exclude patients with conditions that might decrease chance of showing an effect	Real-life conditions: include patients who are expected to receive treatment at end of trial

recommended phase II dose. Historically, the recommended dose for further study has been the maximum tolerable dose (MTD) of a new drug, with the phase I trial focusing on evaluating the relationship between dosage and toxicity, and on pharmacokinetics and pharmacodynamics (see Chap. 18, Sec. 18.2.1). Small numbers of patients are treated at successively higher doses until the maximum acceptable degree of toxicity is reached. However, with the development of drugs that have a known molecular target, there is sometimes little relationship between dose and toxicity, and the recommended phase II dose can be based on pharmacokinetic and/or pharmacodynamic parameters (ideally based on whether the drug inhibits its putative molecular target in tumor tissue, although that is rarely studied in practice).

Many variations have been used in the design of phase I trials; a typical design is to use a low initial dose, unlikely to cause severe side effects, based on tolerance in animals. A *modified Fibonacci sequence* is then used to determine dose escalations: Using this method, the second dose level is 100% higher than the first, the third is 67% higher than the second, the fourth is 50% higher than the third, the fifth is 40% higher than the fourth, and all subsequent levels are 33% higher than the preceding levels. Three patients are treated at each level until any potentially dose-limiting toxicity is observed. Six patients are treated at any dose where such dose-limiting toxicity is encountered. The MTD is defined as the maximum dose at which dose-limiting toxicity occurs in fewer than one-third of the patients tested.

This design is based on experience that few patients have life-threatening toxicity and on the assumption that the MTD is also the most effective anticancer dose. It has been criticized because most patients receive doses that are well below the MTD and are therefore participating in a study where they have little chance of therapeutic response. Adaptive trials using accelerated titration where fewer patients are treated at the lowest doses, and Bayesian dose-finding designs where the magnitude of dose increments is determined by toxicity observed at lower doses, have been suggested as methods to address this limitation (Simon et al, 1997; Yin et al, 2006). Furthermore, it has been suggested that for some molecular-targeted agents, use of MTD is less meaningful. First, MTD (which is defined typically in the first cycle of treatment) generally defines acute toxicity. The use of targeted agents is usually chronic and long-term tolerability is often different from acute tolerability. Second, early clinical trials of biological agents demonstrated that maximal beneficial effects could be seen at doses lower than the MTD. This led to the concept of the optimal biological dose, which is defined as the dose that produces the maximal beneficial effects with the fewest adverse events (Adjei, 2006). Despite difficulties in determination of the optimal biological dose (Parulekar and Eisenhauer, 2004), the use of nontoxicity endpoints to define the recommended phase II dose for targeted agents is increasing (Hansen et al, 2017).

Historically, phase I trials were performed in unselected patients with a variety of cancers. Recently, there have been attempts to enrich early-phase drug development with patients most likely to benefit from treatment such as inclusion of patients with specific tumor histologies or tumors harboring a particular genomic aberration irrespective of their underlying histology. Phase I trials often have dose *expansion cohorts* in which a larger number of patients are treated at the recommended phase II dose (Manji et al, 2013). The aim of these cohorts is to increase knowledge about both safety and potential efficacy of the experimental drug. These cohorts can improve the efficiency of the drug development process and allow for more patients to be treated at a potentially effective dose.

Phase II Trials: Phase II trials are designed to determine whether a new treatment has sufficient anticancer activity to justify further evaluation, although particularly when evaluating targeted agents, they should ideally provide information about target inhibition and, hence, mechanism of action. They usually include highly selected patients with a given type of cancer and may use a molecular biomarker to define patients most likely to respond (eg, expression of the estrogen receptor in women with breast cancer when evaluating a hormonal agent; see Chap. 20, Sec. 20.4). Phase II trials are suitable for guiding decisions about further research but are rarely suitable for making decisions about patient management. Phase II trials may be single-arm or randomized. Single-arm phase II trials are simple and require small sample sizes, but their results usually need to be compared to historical controls. Single-arm phase II studies usually exclude patients with "nonevaluable" disease, and use outcome measures such as the proportion of patients whose tumors shrink or disappear (response rate) as the primary measure of outcome. Their sample size is calculated to distinguish active from inactive therapies according to whether response rate is greater or less than some arbitrary or historical level. The resulting sample size is inadequate to provide a precise estimate of activity. Tumor response rate is a reasonable end point for assessing the anticancer activity of a cytotoxic drug; however, response rate is a suboptimal end point in trials evaluating targeted agents, which can modify time to tumor progression without causing major tumor shrinkage (El-Maraghi and Eisenhauer, 2008). Single-arm trials may be preferred for single agents with tumor response end points. They may also be preferable in less common tumor sites where accrual is challenging. However, the availability of an appropriate estimate of historical response rate is an important limitation—particularly for biomarker-driven studies, where the biomarker may have prognostic effects that are not well-defined.

Randomized phase II designs are more complex, require substantially more patients as compared with single-arm trials, but do provide more robust preliminary evidence of comparative efficacy. Typically, randomized phase II trials use endpoints such as progression-free survival (PFS) and may be more suitable for the study of targeted agents. Randomized designs may be favorable for trials of combination therapy and with time-to-event end points (Gan et al, 2010). The literature is confusing, however, because phase II trials, especially those with randomized designs, have sometimes been reported and interpreted as if they did provide definitive answers to questions about patient management.

Phase III Trials: Phase III trials are designed to answer questions about the usefulness of treatments in patient management. Questions about patient management are usually comparative, as they involve choices between alternatives—that is, an experimental vs the current standard of management. The current standard may include other anticancer treatments or may be "best supportive care" without specific anticancer therapy. The aim of a phase III trial is to estimate the difference in outcome associated with a difference in treatment, sometimes referred to as the *treatment effect*. Ideally, alternative treatments are compared by administering them to groups of patients that are equivalent in all other respects, that is, by randomization of suitable patients between the current standard and the new experimental treatment. Randomized controlled phase III trials are currently regarded as the best, and often only, reliable means of determining the usefulness of treatments in patient management. Phase III drug trials are often conducted in order to register drug treatment for particular indications, which requires approval by agencies such as the United States Food and Drug Administration (FDA) or the European Medicines Agency (EMA). Their end points should reflect patient benefit, such as duration and quality of survival. Most randomized phase III clinical studies are designed to show (or exclude) statistically significant improvements in overall survival, although many cancer trials use putative surrogate end points such as disease-free survival (DFS) or PFS as the primary end point. The use of a surrogate end point is only clinically meaningful if it has been validated as predicting for improvement in overall survival or quality of life (see below).

One criticism of the structure of clinical trials is that it takes a long time for drugs to go from initial (phase I) testing to regulatory approval (based on results of phase III trials). More adaptive designs have been introduced to try to speed up drug development. The multiarm, multistage trial design (Royston et al, 2003) is an approach for conducting randomized trials. It allows several agents or combinations of agents to be assessed simultaneously against a single control group in a randomized design. Recruitment to research arms that do not show sufficient promise in terms of an intermediate outcome measure may be discontinued at interim analyses. In contrast, recruitment to the control arm and to promising research arms continues until sufficient numbers of patients have been entered to assess the impact in terms of the definitive primary outcome measure. By assessing several treatments in one trial, this design allows the efficacy of drugs to be tested more quickly and with smaller numbers of patients compared with a program of separate phase II and phase III trials. The STAMPEDE trial for men with prostate cancer is an excellent example of this type of trial; it has provided practice-changing evidence to improve survival for men with metastatic disease, while simultaneously rejecting ineffective treatments (James et al, 2016, 2017).

Adaptive clinical trials may also accelerate drug development. In adaptive trials prespecified changes to eligibility criteria, sample size or outcome measures may change during the study depending on results observed after the trial has begun. Most commonly, adaptive decisions are based on Bayesian analysis.

A criticism of classical drug development is that in an era of molecular-targeted therapy, treatments are often provided on an empirical basis with few trials assessing novel methods for enriching participants for those most likely to benefit from the experimental therapy. Trials with biomarkers selecting patients likely to benefit have needed smaller sample size to detect similar levels of benefit to those not using biomarkers (Amir et al, 2011). Some agents (eg, imatinib for the treatment of patients with gastrointestinal stromal tumors [GISTs] and ceritinib for the treatment of anaplastic lymphoma kinase [ALK]–mutated non–small cell lung cancer) did not need randomized phase III trials to detect substantial benefits. There are 2 broad ways to select patients for targeted drugs based on biomarkers. In the enrichment approach, all patients are assessed prospectively for presence of the biomarker, and only those with the biomarker are included in the trial (eg, trastuzumab in human epidermal growth factor receptor 2 [HER2]–positive breast cancer). In the retrospective approach, the presence or absence of a biomarker is determined in all treated patients and related to the probability of response to a targeted agent (eg, panitumumab in colorectal cancer in relation to K-ras mutations). The enrichment approach leads to greater economic value across the drug development pathway and could reduce both the time and costs of the development process (Trusheim et al, 2011).

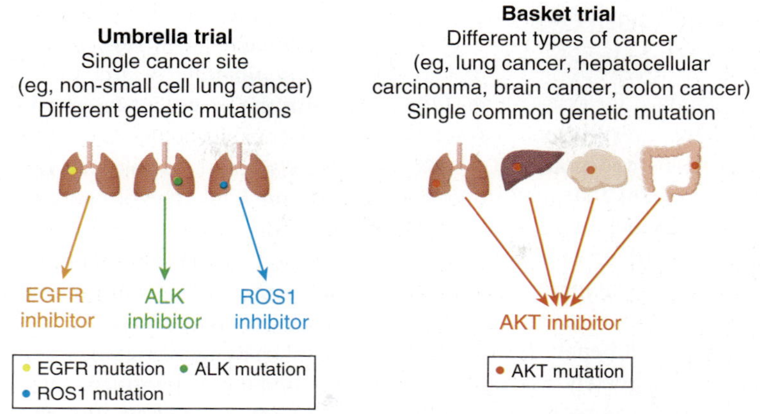

FIGURE 22–1 **Umbrella and Basket Studies.** The figure illustrates examples of umbrella and basket studies.

22.3.2 Personalized Cancer Medicine and Its Evaluation

Initial attempts at personalized cancer medicine relied on the observation of differential protein expression (such as the estrogen receptor in breast cancer) or major chromosomal abnormalities (such as the BCR/ABL translocation or Philadelphia chromosome in chronic myelogenous leukemia). With the increasing availability of genomic sequencing platforms, it has been possible to identify specific oncogenic mutations. Identification of recurrent somatic mutations has led to the successful development of targeted agents against the epidermal growth factor receptor (EGFR) and ALK in non–small cell lung cancer as well as BRAF in melanoma. Other genomic aberrations have been identified as conferring either de novo or acquired resistance to treatment (eg, KRAS mutations in the treatment of colon cancer with anti-EGFR therapy or the T790M mutation after anti-EGFR treatment for non-small cell lung cancer).

For targeted agents with a putative biomarker of benefit, early-phase trials aim to identify a recommended phase II dose, but also to provide some preliminary evidence of the utility of biomarker selection. For this, two common methods are basket and umbrella studies (see Fig. 22–1). *Basket trials* are based on the hypothesis that the presence of a molecular marker (determined typically by genomic analysis of an individual patient's cancer) predicts response to a therapy targeting that marker independent of tumor histology. *Umbrella studies* are designed to test the impact of different drugs targeting different pathways, each tied to one of the various molecular alterations that occur within a particular cancer.

There have been a number of attempts to provide large-scale sequencing of tumors in order to allow patients to enroll in basket or umbrella studies (Tannock and Hickman, 2016). However, despite up to half of patients having genomic aberrations compatible with therapeutic targeting, fewer than 1 in 7 patients receive treatment based on individual genomic analysis, and there does not appear to be a substantial beneficial effect from such a strategy. Possible reasons for this include that not all putative biomarkers provide utility for treatment selection and also that intratumoral heterogeneity results in limited benefit from treatments, which may only be effective against some clones (Bedard et al, 2013).

Personalized cancer medicine is reliant on the availability of robust predictive biomarkers. The most robust assessment of a biomarker entails randomized allocation to an experimental group where treatment is selected on the basis of the biomarker (biomarker positive patients receiving a drug targeting the involved pathway and biomarker negative patients receiving standard treatment) and a control group which receives standard treatment without biomarker assessment (see Le Tourneau et al, 2015, for an example). Any difference seen between the arms is explained by the utility of the biomarker in selecting the optimal treatment. However, this method is inefficient as invariably some patients in the experimental arm will be biomarker negative and will therefore receive the same treatment as the control group leading to dilution of effect of a targeted drug. Consequently, this design is seldom used. Instead, randomized trials collect biomarker status at baseline and then allocate patients to a targeted drug or standard treatment. A post hoc analysis is then performed to evaluate if treatment effect is different in biomarker-positive and biomarker-negative patients. If there is a statistical interaction between the treatment allocation and the biomarker status, this suggests that the biomarker predicts benefit for the treatment under investigation. An example of this is the identification that benefit from the anti-EGFR antibodies cetuximab and panitumumab was seen only in patients with KRAS wildtype colon cancer (Lièvre et al. 2006; Amado et al, 2008; Karapetis et al, 2008).

More recently, attention has focused on immunotherapy (see Chap. 21, Sec. 21.5). The concept of such treatment is to upregulate the host immune response thereby allowing self-selection of anticancer targets. This difference in mechanism of action is reflected in the methods for early clinical trials of targeted agents and immunotherapeutics. In contrast to agents targeting oncogenes or dysregulated oncogenic pathways, immunotherapy drugs typically have been developed empirically in a manner similar to cytotoxic chemotherapy as attempts at the identification of a reliable biomarker of benefit (eg, PDL-1 expression) have not shown promise.

22.3.3 Limitations of and Sources of Bias in Clinical Trials

Randomized trials are the gold standard for assessment of the efficacy and safety of new medical interventions. However, there remain a number of limitations and potential sources of bias (Tannock et al, 2016a). Problems that may influence the interpretation of randomized trials include study initiation based on inadequate preclinical and early clinical studies; use of narrow eligibility criteria such that participants in trials do not reflect patients treated in the community; the use of surrogate endpoints that do not reflect patient benefit (ie, duration or quality of survival); failure to adequately assess health-related quality of life or patient-reported outcomes, especially when the goals of treatment are palliative; reporting of statistically significant but clinically irrelevant results; underestimation of the toxicity; and biased reporting, both in the primary publication and by the media. Many of these are addressed in the section below.

Important characteristics of the patients enrolled in a clinical trial include demographic data (eg, age and gender), clinical characteristics (the stage and pathological type of disease), general well-being, and activities of daily life (performance status), as well as other prognostic factors. Phase III trials are most likely to have positive outcomes if they are applied to homogenous populations. Consequently, most clinical trials have multiple exclusion criteria, such that patients with selected comorbidities and use of some concomitant medications are often excluded. For this and other unknown reasons, patients enrolled in clinical trials often have better outcomes (even if receiving standard treatment) than patients who are seen in routine practice (Chua and Clarke, 2010). Eligibility criteria of phase III trials have become more restrictive with regard to certain comorbidities (eg, cardiovascular disease) and receipt of certain concurrent medications (Srikanthan et al, 2016). Consequently, many patients treated in routine practice would not meet the eligibility criteria of registration trials of therapies approved for their disease (Treweek et al, 2015).

Treatment outcomes for patients with cancer often depend as much on their initial prognostic characteristics as on their subsequent treatment, and imbalances in prognostic factors (which can include genomic features) can have profound effects on the results of a trial. The reports of most randomized clinical trials include a table of baseline prognostic characteristics for patients assigned to each arm. The *P* values often reported in these tables are misleading, as any differences between the groups, other than the treatment assigned, *are known* to have arisen by chance. The important question as to whether any such imbalances influence the estimate of treatment effect is best answered by an analysis that is adjusted for any imbalance in prognostic factors (see Sec. 22.5).

Adherence refers to the extent to which a treatment is delivered as intended. It depends on the willingness of physicians to prescribe treatment as specified in the protocol and the willingness of patients to take treatment as prescribed by the physician. Patient adherence with oral medication is variable and may be a major barrier to the delivery of efficacious treatments (Hershman et al, 2010).

Contamination occurs when people in one arm of a trial receive the treatment intended for those in another arm. This may occur if people allocated to placebo obtain active drugs from elsewhere, as has occurred in trials of treatments for HIV infection. This type of contamination is rare in trials of anticancer drugs but common in trials of dietary treatments, vitamin supplements, or other widely available agents. The effect of contamination is to blur distinctions between treatment arms.

Crossover is a related problem that influences the interpretation of trials assessing survival duration. It occurs when people allocated to one treatment subsequently receive the alternative treatment when their disease progresses. Although defensible from pragmatic and ethical viewpoints, crossover changes the nature of the question being asked about survival duration. In a 2-arm trial without crossover, the comparison is of treatment A vs treatment B, whereas with crossover, the comparison is of treatment A followed by treatment B vs treatment B followed by treatment A.

Cointervention occurs when treatments are administered that may influence outcome but are not specified in the trial protocol. Examples are blood products and antibiotics in drug trials for acute leukemia, or radiation therapy in trials of systemic adjuvant therapy for breast cancer. Because cointerventions are not allocated randomly, they may be distributed unequally between the groups being compared and can contribute to differences in outcome.

22.3.4 Importance of Randomization

Well-conducted randomized trials provide a high level of evidence about the value of a new treatment (Table 22–2). The ideal comparison of treatments comes from observing their effects in groups that are otherwise equivalent, and randomization is the only effective means of achieving this. Comparisons between historical controls, between concurrent but nonrandomized controls, or between groups that are allocated to different treatments

TABLE 22–2 Hierarchy of evidence.

Level	Study Methods
High	Systematic review/metaanalysis
	Randomized controlled trial
	Cohort study
	Case-control study
	Case series
	Case report
	Expert Opinion
Low	Laboratory data

Data from Guyatt GH, Haynes RB, Jaeschke RZ, et al. Users' Guides to the Medical Literature: XXV. Evidence-based medicine: principles for applying the Users' Guides to patient care. Evidence-Based Medicine Working Group. *JAMA* 2000 Sep 13;284(10):1290-1296.

by clinical judgment, are almost certain to generate groups that differ systematically in their baseline prognostic characteristics. Important factors that are measurable can be accounted for in the analysis; however, important factors that are poorly specified—such as comorbidity, a history of complications with other treatments, the ability to comply with treatment, or family history— cannot. Comparisons based on historical controls are particularly prone to bias because of changes over time in factors other than treatment, including altered referral patterns, different criteria for selection of patients, and improvements in supportive care. These changes over time are difficult to assess and difficult to adjust for in analysis. Such differences tend to favor the most recently treated group and to exaggerate the apparent benefits of new treatments.

Stage migration causes systematic variation (Fig. 22–2), and occurs when patients are assigned to different clinical stages because of differences in the precision of staging investigations rather than differences in the true extent of disease. This can occur if patients staged very thoroughly as part of a research protocol are compared with patients staged less thoroughly in the course of routine clinical practice, or if patients staged with newer more-accurate tests are compared with historical controls staged with older, less-accurate tests. Stage migration is important because the introduction of new and more sensitive diagnostic tests produces apparent improvements in outcome for each anatomically defined category of disease in the absence of any real improvement in outcome for the disease overall (Feinstein et al, 1985). This paradox arises because, in general, the patients with the worst prognosis in each category are reclassified as having more advanced disease. As illustrated in Figure 22–2, a portion of those patients initially classified as having localized disease (stage I) may be found to have regional spread if more sensitive imaging is used, and a portion of those initially classified as having only regional spread (stage II) will be found to have systemic spread (stage III). As a consequence, the prognosis of each category of disease improves in the absence of any real improvement in the prognosis of the disease overall.

The major benefit of randomization is the unbiased distribution of *unknown* and *unmeasured* prognostic factors between treatment groups. However, it is only ethical to allocate patients to treatments randomly when there is uncertainty about which treatment is best. The difficulty for clinicians is that this uncertainty, known as *equipoise*, usually resides among physicians collectively rather than within them individually.

Random allocation of treatment does not ensure that the treatment groups are equivalent, but it does ensure that any differences in baseline characteristics are a result of chance. Consequently, differences in outcome must be a result of either chance or treatment. Standard statistical tests estimate the probability (P value) that differences in outcome, as observed, might be a result of chance alone. The lower the P value, the less plausible is the *null hypothesis* that the observed difference is a result of chance, and the more plausible is the *alternate hypothesis* that the difference is a result of treatment.

Imbalances in known prognostic factors can be reduced or avoided by *stratifying* and *blocking* groups of patients with similar prognostic characteristics during the randomization procedure. For example, in a trial of adjuvant hormone therapy for breast cancer, patients might be stratified according to the presence or absence of lymph node involvement, hormone receptor expression, and menopausal status. *Blocking* ensures that treatment allocation is balanced for every few patients within each defined group (strata). This is practical only for a small number of strata. Randomization in multicenter trials is often blocked and stratified by treatment center to account for differences between centers; however, this carries the risk that when there is almost complete accrual within a block, the physicians may know the arm to which the next patient(s) will be assigned, creating the possibility of selection bias (see below). An alternative approach to adjust for imbalances in prognostic factors is to use multivariable statistical methods (see Sec. 22.5.1 and Chap. 4, Sec. 4.4).

For randomization to be successfully implemented and to reduce bias, the randomization sequence must be adequately

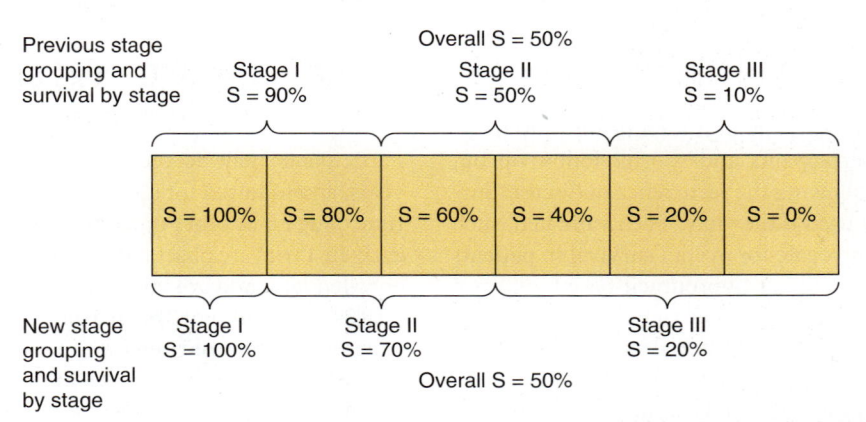

FIGURE 22–2 Stage migration. The diagram illustrates that a change in staging investigations may lead to the apparent improvement of results within each stage without changing the overall results. In the hypothetical example, patients are divided into 6 equal groups, each with the indicated survival. Introduction of more-sensitive staging investigations moves patients into higher-stage groups, as shown, but the overall survival of 50% remains unchanged.

concealed so that the investigators, involved health care providers, and participants are not aware of the upcoming assignment. The absence of adequate allocation concealment can lead to selection bias, one of the very problems that randomization is supposed to eliminate. Historically, allocation concealment was achieved by the use of opaque envelopes, but in multicenter studies, centralized internet-based allocation systems are now used.

If feasible, it is preferable that both physicians and patients be unaware of which treatment is being administered. This optimal double-blind design prevents bias. Evidence for bias in nonblinded randomized trials comes from the observation that they lead more often to apparent improvements in outcome from experimental treatment and increased drop-out from the control arm than blinded trials and that assignment sequences in randomized trials have sometimes been deciphered (Chalmers et al, 1983; Wood et al, 2008). Of note, even in blinded trials inadvertent unblinding can occur if one arm has a unique toxicity profile. In such scenarios, the effort of blinding may not be justified.

22.3.5 Choice and Assessment of Outcomes

The measures used to assess a treatment should reflect the goals of that treatment. Treatment for advanced cancer is often given with palliative intent—to prolong survival or reduce symptoms without realistic expectation of cure. Survival duration has the advantage of being an outcome that can be measured unambiguously, but if a major goal of treatment is improved quality of life, then appropriate methods should be used to measure quality of life (see Section 22.3.9). Anticancer treatments may prolong survival through toxic effects on the cancer or may shorten survival through toxic effects on the host. Similarly, anticancer treatments may improve quality of life by reducing cancer-related symptoms or may worsen quality of life by adding toxicity due to treatment. Patient benefit depends on the trade-off between these positive and negative effects.

Proposed surrogate or indirect measures of patient benefit, such as tumor shrinkage, DFS, or PFS, can sometimes provide an early indication of efficacy, but they are rarely substitutes for more direct measures of patient benefit. For example, the use of DFS rather than overall survival in studies of adjuvant treatment requires fewer participants and shorter follow-up but ignores what happens following the recurrence of disease. Surrogate measures can be used if they have been validated, such as the use of DFS as a surrogate for overall survival in patients with colorectal cancer receiving fluorouracil-based adjuvant treatment (Sargent et al, 2005). Higher tumor response rates or improvements in PFS or DFS do not always translate into longer overall survival or better quality of life (Ng et al, 2008). Changes in the concentration of tumor markers in serum, such as prostate-specific antigen (PSA) for prostate cancer or cancer antigen 125 (CA125) in ovarian cancer, have been used as outcome measures in certain types of cancer.

Levels of these markers may reflect tumor burden in general, but the relationship is quite variable; there are individuals with extensive disease who have low levels of a tumor marker in serum. The relationship between serum levels of a tumor marker and outcome is also variable. In men who have received local treatment for early-stage prostate cancer, the reappearance of PSA in the serum indicates disease recurrence. In men with advanced prostate cancer, however, baseline levels of serum PSA may not be associated with duration of survival, and changes in PSA following treatment are not consistently related to changes in symptoms. Newer biomarkers such as circulating tumor cells or circulating tumor DNA provide information on prognosis (Ocaña et al, 2016), but have not been shown to provide useful information for treatment planning and have therefore not been included in practice guidelines.

In cancer trials, patients are excluded sometimes from the analysis on the grounds that they are "not evaluable." Reasons for nonevaluability vary, but may include death soon after treatment was started or failure to receive the full course of treatment. It may be permissible to exclude patients from analysis in explanatory phase II trials that are seeking to describe the biological effects of treatment; these trials indicate the effect of treatment in those who were able to complete it. It is seldom appropriate to exclude patients in randomized trials, which should reflect the conditions under which the treatment will be applied in practice. Such trials test a policy of treatment, and the appropriate analysis for a pragmatic trial is by *intention to treat*: patients should be included in the arm to which they were allocated regardless of their subsequent course.

For some events (eg, death) there is no doubt as to whether the event has occurred, but assignment of a particular cause of death (eg, whether it was cancer related) may be subjective, as is the assessment of tumor response, recognition of tumor progression or recurrence, and therefore determination of PFS or DFS. The compared groups should be followed with similar types of evaluation so that they are equally susceptible to the detection of outcome events such as recurrence of disease. Whenever the assessment of an outcome is subjective, variation between observers should be examined. Variable criteria of tumor response and imprecise tumor measurement have been documented as causes of variability in clinical trials.

22.3.6 Survival Curves and Their Comparison

Participants may be recruited to clinical trials over several years, and followed for an additional period to determine their time of death or other outcome measure. Participants enrolled early in a trial are observed for a longer time than participants enrolled later and are more likely to have died by the time the trial is analyzed. For this reason, the distribution of survival times is the preferred outcome measure for assessing the influence of treatment on survival. Survival duration is defined as the interval from some convenient "zero time," usually the date of enrollment or randomization in a study, to the time of death of any cause. Participants who have died provide actual observations of survival duration. Participants who were alive at last follow-up provide *censored* (incomplete) observations of survival duration; their eventual survival duration will be at least

TABLE 22–3 Calculation of actuarial survival.

Follow-up Interval (A)	Number at Risk (B)	Number Dying (C)	Number Withdrawn Alive (D)	Probability of Dying During Interval (E)	Probability of Surviving During Interval (F)	Overall Probability of Survival (G)
0	100	—	—	—	—	1
1	100	8	2	0.080	0.920	0.920
2	90	3	2	0.033	0.967	0.890
3	85	1	0	0.012	0.988	0.879
4	84	3	1	0.036	0.964	0.847
5	80	7	3	0.088	0.912	0.773
6	70	6	4	0.086	0.914	0.706
7	60	5	5	0.083	0.917	0.648
8	50	1	4	0.020	0.980	0.635
9	45	1	2	0.022	0.978	0.621
10	42	1	1	0.024	0.976	0.606

Note: A. Follow-up intervals may be of any convenient size; usually days, weeks, or months. B. Number at risk means number of patients alive at the start of the interval. C. Number dying is number of patients dying during each interval. D. Number withdrawn alive refers to patients alive who have not been followed longer than the interval after randomization. E. Probability of dying during each interval is number of patients dying (C) divided by the number at risk (B). F. Probability of survival during each interval is the complement (1 − E) of the probability of dying. G. Overall probability of survival is the cumulative product of the probabilities in (F). The numbers in this column may be plotted against time as an actuarial survival curve.

as long as the time to their last follow-up. Most cancer trials are analyzed before all participants have died, so a method of analysis, which accounts for censored observations, is required.

Actuarial survival curves provide an estimate of the eventual distribution of survival duration (when everyone has died), based on the observed survival duration of those who have died and the censored observations of those still living. Actuarial survival curves are preferred to simple cross-sectional measures of survival because they incorporate and describe all of the available information. Table 22–3 illustrates the *life-table method* for construction of an actuarial survival curve. The period of follow-up after treatment is divided into convenient short intervals—for example, weeks or months. The probability of dying in a particular interval is estimated by dividing the number of people who died during that interval by the number of people who were known to be alive at its beginning ($E = C/B$ in Table 22–3). The probability of surviving a particular interval, having survived to its beginning, is the complement of the probability of dying in it ($F = 1 − E$). The actuarial estimate of the probability of surviving for a given time is calculated by cumulative multiplication of the probabilities of surviving each interval until that time (Fig. 22–3).

The *Kaplan-Meier method* of survival analysis, also known as the *product limit method*, is identical to the actuarial method

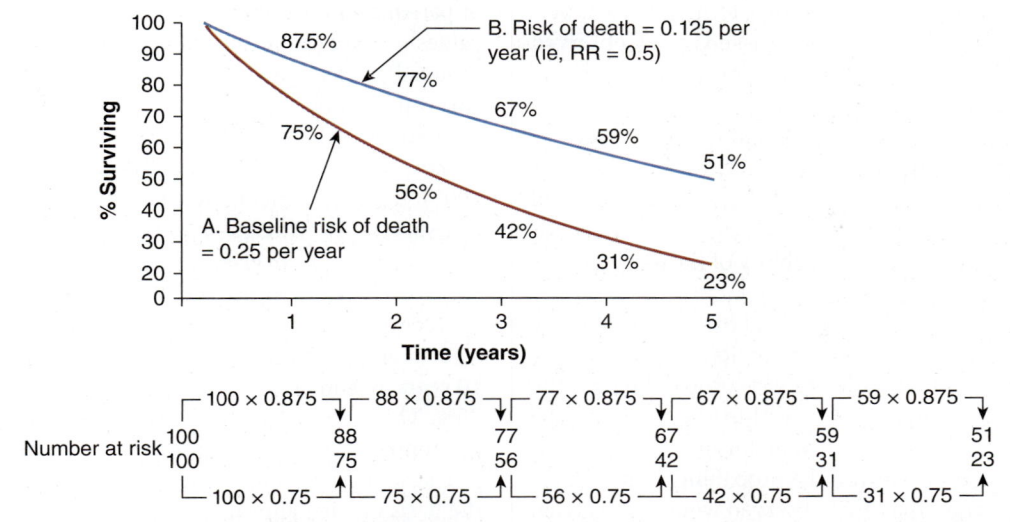

FIGURE 22–3 Hypothetical survival curves for 2 patient groups. In a 1-year interval, patients in group A have a 25% probability of dying, whereas those in group B have a 12.5% probability of dying (ie, relative risk [RR] = 0.5). At the end of 5 years, 77% of patients in group A have died (survival rate = 23%). Note that although the hazard rate of death in group B = 0.5, by the end of 5 years, the cumulative risk of death is 49%, not 0.5 × 77% (= 38.5%).

except that the calculations are performed at each death rather than at fixed intervals. The Kaplan-Meier survival curve is depicted graphically with the probability of survival on the y-axis and time on the x-axis: vertical drops occur at each death. The latter part of a survival curve is often the focus of most interest, as it estimates the probability of long-term survival; however, it is also the least-reliable part of the curve, because it is based on fewer observations and therefore more liable to error. The validity of all actuarial methods depends on the time of censoring being independent of the time of death; that is, those who have been followed for a short period of time or who are lost to follow-up are assumed to have similar probability of survival as those who have been followed longer. The most obvious violation of this assumption occurs if participants are lost to follow-up because they have died or are too sick to attend clinics. This situation is termed informative censoring. Informative censoring is often applied to patients who discontinue therapy without progressive disease or to patients who die of causes other than cancer. Particularly if the rate of informative censoring differs between the arms of a randomized trial, it can introduce a postrandomization bias and may ignore the potential detrimental effect of one of the treatments on noncancer outcomes (Templeton et al, 2020).

Overall survival curves do not take into account the cause of death, whereas cancer-specific survival curves are constructed by considering only death due to cancer; patients dying from other causes are treated as censored observations at the time of their death. However, there may be uncertainty about the influence of cancer or its treatment on death: deaths from cardiovascular causes, accidents, or suicides, for example, may all occur as an indirect consequence of cancer or its treatment.

The first step in comparing survival distributions is visual inspection of the survival curves. Ideally, there will be indications of both the number of censored observations and the number of people at risk at representative time points, often indicated beneath the curve (see Fig. 22–3). Curves that cross are difficult to interpret, because this means that short-term survival is better in one arm, whereas long-term survival is better in the other. Two questions must be asked of any observed difference in survival curves: (1) whether it is clinically important and (2) whether it is likely to have arisen by chance. The first is a value judgment that will be based on factors such as absolute magnitude of the observed effect, toxicity, baseline risk, and cost of the treatment (see Sec. 22.3.11). The second is a question of statistical significance, which, in turn, depends on the size of the difference, the variability of the data, and the sample size of the trial.

The precision of an estimate of survival (or anther outcome measure) is conveniently described by its *95% confidence interval*, which implies that there is a 95% probability that the true value of the measurement lies within the interval. The *statistical significance* of a difference in survival distributions is expressed by a P value, which is the probability that a difference as large as or larger than that observed would have arisen by chance alone. Several statistical tests are available for calculating the P value for differences in survival distributions. The *log-rank test* and the *Wilcoxon test* are used most commonly: both methods compare the difference between the observed number of deaths and the number expected if the curves were equivalent. Because the Wilcoxon test gives more weight to early follow-up times when the number of patients is greater, it is less sensitive than the log-rank test to differences between survival curves that occur later in follow-up.

Survival analyses can be adjusted, in principle, for any number of prognostic variables. For example, in a trial comparing the effects of 2 regimens of adjuvant chemotherapy on the survival of women with early-stage breast cancer, an unadjusted analysis would compare the survivals of the 2 treatment groups directly. The estimate of the treatment effect can be adjusted for imbalances in known prognostic factors such as spread to axillary lymph nodes and hormone-receptor expression by including them in a multivariable analysis using the *Cox proportional hazards model* (Tibshirani, 1982; see Sec. 22.5.1 and Chap. 4, Sec. 4.4.3). In large randomized trials, such adjustments rarely affect the conclusions, because the likelihood of major imbalances is small.

Differences in the distribution of survival times for 2 treatments compared in a randomized trial may be summarized in several ways:

1. The absolute difference in the median survival or in the proportion of patients who are expected to be alive at a specified time after treatment (eg, at 5 or 10 years).
2. The hazard ratio (HR): ie, the ratio of the probability of dying during any specific time interval between the 2 arms. (Note that there is an implicit assumption, termed proportional hazards, that this ratio is constant, an assumption that is frequently invalid.)
3. The number of patients who would need to be treated to prevent 1 death over a given period of time.

Differences in data presentation may create substantially different impressions of clinical benefit. For example, a substantial reduction in hazard ratio may correspond to only a small improvement in absolute survival and a large number of patients who would need to be treated to save 1 life. These values depend on the expected level of survival in the control group. For example, a 25% relative improvement in overall survival (ie, HR = 0.75) has been found for use of adjuvant combination chemotherapy in younger women with breast cancer (Early Breast Cancer Trialists Collaborative Group, 2005). If this treatment effect is applied to women with a control survival at 10 years of about 50%, it will lead to an absolute increase in survival of approximately 12%; between 8 and 9 women would need to be treated to save 1 life over that 10-year period. The same 25% reduction in hazard ratio would lead to an approximately 6% absolute increase in survival at 10 years in women where control survival at 10 years is around 75%. This corresponds to 1 life saved over 10 years for every 17 women treated. When presented with different summaries of trials, physicians may select the experimental treatment on the basis of what appears to be a substantial reduction in hazard or odds ratio, but reject treatment on the basis of a smaller increase in absolute survival or a large number of patients that need to be treated to save 1 life, even though these represent

TABLE 22-4 Number of patients required to detect or exclude an improvement in survival. Data assume $\alpha = 0.05$; power, $1 - \beta = 0.90$.

	\multicolumn{11}{c}{Expected Survival in Experimental Group}
		0	0.1	0.2	0.3	0.4	0.5	0.6	0.7	0.8	0.9	1.0
Expected survival in control group	0		150	75	50	35	30	25	20	15	15	10
	0.1			430	140	75	50	35	25	20	15	15
	0.2				625	185	90	55	40	30	20	15
	0.3					755	210	100	60	40	25	20
	0.4						815	215	100	55	35	25
	0.5							815	210	90	50	30
	0.6								755	185	75	35
	0.7									625	140	50
	0.8										430	75
	0.9											150
	1.0											

different expressions of the same effect (Chao et al, 2003). Note also that because the number of patients at risk changes with time, the absolute gain in survival does not equal the product of the hazard ratio and the cumulative risk of death in the control group (see Fig. 22–3).

22.3.7 Statistical Issues

The number of participants required for a randomized clinical trial where the primary endpoint is duration of survival depends on several factors:

1. The minimum difference in survival rates that is considered clinically important: the smaller the difference, the larger the number of participants required.
2. The number of deaths expected with the standard treatment used in the control arm: a smaller number of participants is required when the expected survival is either very high or very low (see Table 22–4).
3. The probability of (willingness to accept) a false-positive result (alpha, or type I error): the lower the probability, the larger the number of participants required.
4. The probability of (willingness to accept) a false-negative result (beta, or type II error): the lower the probability, the larger the number of participants required.

The minimum difference that is clinically important is the smallest difference that would lead to the adoption of a new treatment. This judgment will depend on the severity of the condition being treated and the feasibility, toxicity, and cost of the treatment(s). Based on such information, the required number of patients to be entered into a trial can be estimated from tables similar to Table 22–4. The acceptable values for the error probabilities are matters of judgment. Values of 0.05 for alpha (false-positive error) and 0.1 or 0.2 for beta (false-negative error) are well-entrenched. There are good arguments for using lower (more stringent) values, although perhaps even more important is that trials should be repeated by independent investigators before their results are used to change clinical practice. Conclusions about the outcome of a clinical trial should not be based on the P value alone. The American Statistical Association released guidance on the interpretation of statistical testing focusing on the fact that P values do not provide a measure of the size of the effect or the importance of the result nor can a P value be used to provide evidence regarding a hypothesis (Wasserstein and Lazar, 2016).

In a trial assessing survival duration, it is the number of deaths rather than the number of participants that determines the reliability of its conclusions. For example, a trial with 1000 participants and 200 deaths will be more reliable than a trial with 2000 participants and 150 deaths. From a statistical point of view, this means that it is more efficient to perform trials in participants who are at a high risk of death. It also explains the value of prolonged follow-up; longer follow-up means more deaths, which produce more reliable conclusions. In reports of randomized trials, evaluation of results is often based on a small absolute difference in the number of events between groups, such that a change of only a few events in one group could change the conclusions of the trial. The fragility index is a metric that can identify the number of events required to change statistically significant to nonsignificant results. Application of the fragility index has shown that results from randomized trials in high impact journals frequently hinge on 3 or fewer events (Walsh et al, 2014).

22.3.7.1 Power The power of a trial refers to its ability to detect a difference between treatments when in fact they do differ. The power of a trial is the complement of beta, the type II error (power = 1 – beta). Table 22–4 shows the relationship between the expected difference between treatments and the number of patients required. A randomized clinical trial that seeks to detect an absolute improvement in survival of 20%, compared with a control group receiving standard treatment whose expected survival is 40%, will require approximately

108 patients in each arm at α = 0.05 and a power of 0.9. This means that a clinical trial of this size has a 90% chance of detecting an improvement in survival of this magnitude. Detection of a smaller difference between treatments—for example, a 10% absolute increase in survival—would require approximately 410 patients in each arm. A substantial proportion of published clinical trials are too small to detect clinically important differences reliably. If an underpowered study finds "no statistically significant difference" associated with the use of a given treatment, the results may mask a clinically important therapeutic gain that the trial was unable to detect. In contrast, some trials have become so large that they can detect very small differences in survival, which are statistically significant but may not be clinically meaningful. For example, in the APHINITY trial exploring the addition of pertuzumab to chemotherapy and trastuzumab in early-stage breast cancer, investigators reported a statistically significant improvement in DFS (HR 0.81, P = .045), however, this translated to a 0.9% difference in 3-year DFS (von Minckwitz et al, 2017).

Concerns that advances in cancer therapy may provide limited meaningful benefit to patients has resulted in oncology societies attempting to provide a standardized approach to grading clinical benefit, thereby aiding the counseling of patients about the benefit of different drug options and providing structure for reimbursement decisions by payers. These include the European Society for Medical Oncology Magnitude of Clinical Benefit Scale (Cherny et al, 2015) and the American Society of Clinical Oncology Value Framework (Schnipper et al, 2016). These tools have differing grading systems and constructs of clinical benefit and there is only modest concordance between them (Del Paggio et al, 2017). As such, neither has been accepted universally.

22.3.8 Meta-analysis

Meta-analysis is a method by which data from individual randomized clinical trials that assess similar treatments (eg, adjuvant chemotherapy for breast cancer vs no chemotherapy) are combined to give an overall estimate of treatment effect. Meta-analysis can be useful because (1) the results of individual trials are subject to random error and may give misleading results, and (2) a small effect of a treatment (eg, approximately 5% improvement in absolute survival for node-negative breast cancer from use of adjuvant chemotherapy) may be difficult to detect in individual trials. Detection of such a small difference will require several thousand patients to be randomized, yet it may be sufficiently meaningful to recommend adoption of the new treatment as standard.

Meta-analysis requires the extraction and combination of data from trials addressing the question of interest. The preferred method involves collection of data on individual patients (date of randomization, date of death, or date last seen if alive) that were entered in individual trials, although literature-based approaches are also recognized. The trials will, in general, compare related strategies of treatment to standard management (eg, radiotherapy with or without chemotherapy for stage III non–small cell lung cancer) but may not be identical (eg, different types of chemotherapy might be used).

Meta-analysis is typically a 2-stage process. First, summary statistics (such as risk or hazard ratios) are calculated for each individual study. Then a summary (pooled) effect estimate is calculated as a weighted average of the effects of the intervention in the individual studies. All methods of meta-analysis should incorporate a test of heterogeneity—an assessment of whether the variation among the results of the separate studies is compatible with random variation, or whether it is large enough to indicate inconsistency in the effects of the intervention across studies (interaction).

Data are presented typically in forest plots as in Figure 22–4, which illustrates the comparison of a strategy (in this example, ovarian ablation as adjuvant therapy for breast cancer) used alone vs no such treatment (upper part of figure) and a related comparison where patients in both arms also receive chemotherapy (lower part of figure). Here, each trial included in the meta-analysis is represented by a symbol, proportional in area to the weighting applied to each trial, and by a horizontal line representing its confidence interval. A vertical line represents the null effect, and a diamond beneath the individual trials represents the overall treatment effect and confidence interval. If this diamond symbol does not intersect the vertical line representing the null effect, a significant result is declared.

The potential for bias and methodologic quality can be assessed in a meta-analysis. A funnel plot is a simple scatter plot in which a measure of each study's size or precision is plotted against a measure of the effect of the intervention. Symmetrical funnel plots suggest, but do not confirm absence of publication bias, but do not rule out limitations in methodologic quality.

Meta-analysis is an expensive and time-consuming procedure. Important considerations are as follows:

1. Attempts should be made to include the latest results of all trials; unpublished trials should be included to avoid publication bias.
2. Because of publication bias and other reasons, meta-analyses obtained from reviews of the literature tend to overestimate the effect of experimental treatment as compared with a meta-analysis based on data for individual patients obtained from the investigators (Stewart and Parmar, 1993).
3. Because meta-analysis may combine trials with related but different treatments (eg, less-effective and more-effective chemotherapy), the results may underestimate the effects of treatment that could be obtained under optimal conditions.

There is extensive debate in the literature about the merits and problems of meta-analyses and their advantages and disadvantages as compared with a single, large, well-designed trial (Parmar et al, 1996; Buyse et al, 2000; Noble, 2006). A well-performed meta-analysis uses all the available data, recognizes that false-negative and false-positive trials are likely to be common, and may limit the inappropriate influence of individual trials on practice.

Study name	Deaths/patients Allocated ablation	Allocated control	Obs −Exp	Var of O−E	Annual odds of death Ratio (and CIs), ablation: control	Reduction (% and SD)
(a) Ovarian ablation in the absence of chemotherapy						
Christie A	76/88	80/90	−7.3	33.7		
Norwegian RH	24/68	43/83	−9.1	15.9		
NSABP B-03*	75/129	2(35/55)	−2.3	21.2		
Saskatchewan CF	59/143	62/112	−11.6	28.2		
PMH Toronto*	133/216	143/204	−11.7	48.6		
Bradford RI (stratum 1)	5/22	7/20	−1.4	2.9		
(a) Subtotal*	372/666 (55.9%)	405/619 (65.4%)	−43.4	150.5		24% (P = .0006)
(a) Ovarian ablation in the presence of chemotherapy						
Bradford RI (stratum 2)	5/21	4/17	0.6	1.9		
Toronto–Edmonton	56/119	52/122	3.1	25.1		
BCCA Vancouver	21/57	21/54	−1.4	10.0		
IBCSG/Ludwig II	85/139	91/142	−5.9	39.8		
SWOG 7827 B	42/136	49/126	−5.0	21.7		
(b) Subtotal*	209/472 (44.3%)	217/461 (47.1%)	−8.6	98.5		8% (P > .1)
Total (a + b)	581/1138 (51.1%)	622/1080 (57.6%)	−52.0	249.0		18.4% (P = .001)

Treatment effect P = .001

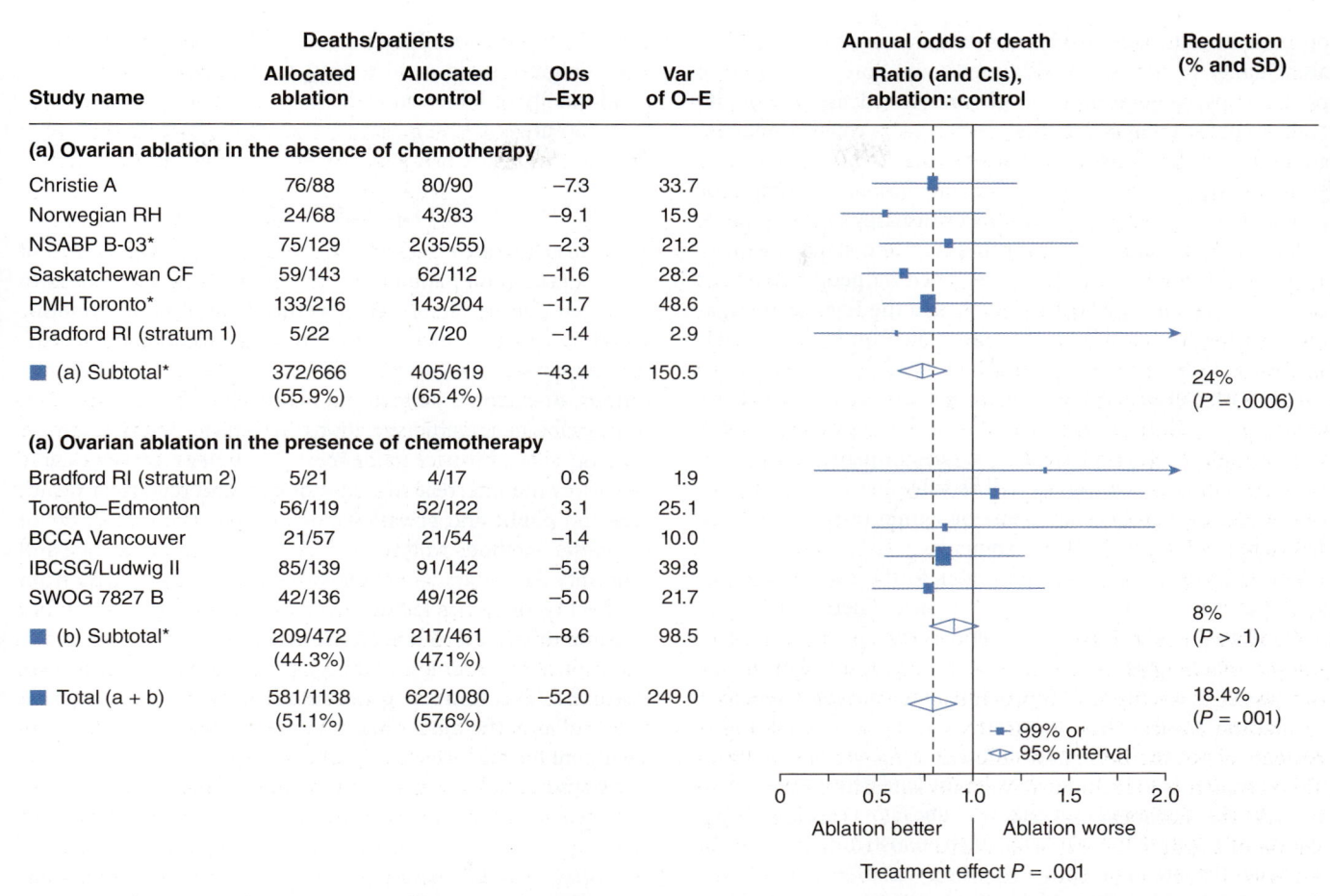

FIGURE 22–4 Presentation of results of a metaanalysis in a forest plot. Each trial is represented by a square symbol, whose area is proportional to the number of patients entered, and by a horizontal line. These represent the mean and 95% confidence interval for the ratio of annual odds of death in the experimental and standard arms. A vertical line drawn through odds ratio 1.0 represents no effect. The trials are separated into those asking a simple question (in this example, ovarian ablation vs no adjuvant treatment for early breast cancer) and a related but more complex question (ovarian ablation plus chemotherapy vs chemotherapy alone). Diamonds represent overall mean odds ratios and their 95% confidence intervals for the 2 subsets of trials and for overall effect. The vertical dashed line represents mean reduction in annual odds of death for all trials. (Reproduced with permission from Ovarian ablation in early breast cancer: overview of the randomised trials. Early Breast Cancer Trialists' Collaborative Group. *Lancet* 1996 Nov 2;348(9036):1189-1196.)

22.3.9 Patient-Reported Outcomes

Reporting of adverse events in clinical trials is crucial to ensure patients' safety and clinicians' understanding of the toxicity profiles of new anticancer drugs. The Common Terminology Criteria for Adverse Events (CTCAE), developed by the US National Cancer Institute (NCI) is a classification system for the severity of adverse events of anticancer drugs (https://ctep.cancer.gov/protocolDevelopment/electronic_applications/ctc.htm). The CTCAE was introduced in the 1980s when most anticancer drugs were cytotoxic chemotherapeutic agents, were given intermittently, and had transient, but acute, toxic effects. The use of CTCAE may be suboptimal for modern targeted agents, which are given continuously and can cause recurrent or chronic symptomatic toxicities (Seruga et al, 2016). More recently, the NCI helped develop a patient-reported outcomes version of the CTCAE (PRO-CTCAE), which integrates patient perspective into adverse event reporting in clinical trials (Basch et al, 2014). A recent study randomized patients with metastatic breast, lung, genitourinary, or gynecologic cancer to regular reporting of PRO-CTCAE vs usual practice where patients report concerns during visits to the outpatient clinic: This trial demonstrated better quality of life and duration of overall survival for those with more frequent monitoring of symptoms (Basch et al, 2017).

Physician-evaluated performance status and patient-reported outcomes such as quality of life are correlated, but are far from identical, and both can provide independent prognostic information in clinical trials (see Sec. 22.5.2). Patient-reported outcomes include symptom scales (eg, for pain or fatigue) and measures of quality of life. Physicians and other health professionals are quite poor in assessing the level of symptoms of their patients, and simple methods for grading symptoms by patients, such as the Functional Assessment of Cancer Therapy (FACT) Scale or the Edmonton Symptom Assessment Scale (Cella et al, 1993; Nekolaichuk et al, 1999) can give valuable information about palliative (or toxic) effects on patients with cancer who are participating in clinical trials. Quality of life is a multidimensional concept reflecting physical, psychological, spiritual, and social aspects of life and self-assessment is essential. *Instruments* (questionnaires) addressing differing aspects of health-related quality of life are available: they range from generic instruments designed for people with a variety of conditions or diseases to instruments designed for patients with a specific type and stage of cancer. The FACT-General (FACT-G), developed for people receiving cancer treatments (Cella et al, 1993); and the European Organization for Research and Treatment of Cancer Core Quality of Life Questionnaire (EORTC QLQ-C30), developed for people with cancer participating in international clinical trials (Aaronson et al, 1993) are used most often to evaluate people with cancer. Both combine a core questionnaire relevant to most patients with cancer, as well as subscales that allow subjects to evaluate additional disease or symptom-specific items. They are available in multiple languages.

The *validity* of an instrument refers to the extent to which it measures what it is supposed to measure. There is no objective, external gold standard for comparison, so indirect methods are used to gauge the validity of quality-of-life instruments (Aaronson et al, 1993). Examples include *convergent validity*, the degree of correlation between instruments or scales purporting to measure similar attributes, and *discriminant validity*, or the degree to which an instrument can detect differences between different aspects of quality of life. *Face validity* and *content validity* refer to the extent to which an instrument addresses the issues that are important. *Responsiveness* refers to the detection of changes in quality of life with time, such as those caused by effective treatment, whereas *predictive validity* refers to the prognostic information of a quality-of-life scale in predicting an outcome such as duration of survival. Validated quality-of-life scales are often strong predictors of survival (see Sec. 22.5.2).

Validity is *conditional*—it cannot be judged without specifying for what and for whom it is to be used. Good validity of a questionnaire in symptomatic men with advanced hormone-resistant prostate cancer does not guarantee good validity in men with earlier-stage prostate cancer, for whom pain might be less important and sexual function more important. Differences between interventions, such as toxicity profiles, might influence validity. For example, nausea and vomiting might be important in a trial of cisplatin-based chemotherapy, whereas sexual function might be more important in a trial of hormonal therapy. The context in which an instrument is to be used and the context(s) in which its validity was assessed must be reexamined for each application. Furthermore, it is important that an a priori hypothesis for palliative outcomes is defined and preferable that the proportion of patients with palliative response is reported (Joly et al, 2007).

There are methodologic challenges to using patient-reported outcomes. Attrition because of incomplete data collection remains a challenge and can confound quality-of-life analysis (patients with poor quality of life are less likely to complete questionnaires). Patient perceptions of their quality of life can change over time (eg, "good quality of life" may be quite different for a patient who has survived cancer as compared to someone without the disease; this is known as response-shift). Psychological defenses also tend to conserve perception of good quality of life even in the presence of worsening symptoms (Sprangers, 1996).

22.3.10 Health Outcomes Research

Outcomes research seeks to understand the *end results* of various factors on patients and populations. It can be used to assess prognostic factors, such as the effect of socioeconomic status on cancer survival (Booth et al, 2010), to compare different approaches to the management of specific medical conditions, to examine patients' and clinicians' decision making, to describe geographic variations in clinical practice, and to develop or test practice guidelines. Outcomes research usually addresses the interrelated issues of cost and quality of health care and public and private sector interest. The availability of computer methods to link large databases (eg, incidence and mortality data from cancer registries and treatment data from hospital records) has facilitated the ability of health outcomes research to address important clinical questions.

Various methodologic designs are used in outcomes research. These include cohort studies, case-control studies, and studies of the uptake and outcome of new evidence-based treatment for management (see also Chap. 4, Sec. 4.3). Most of these studies use a retrospective cohort design. End points in outcomes research are usually clinical, economic, or patient-centered. Clinical outcomes include mortality or medical events (eg, hospitalization) as a result of an intervention. Economic outcomes include direct and indirect health costs (see Sec. 22.3.11). A major difference between outcomes research and randomized trials is that outcomes research lacks randomized controls, but it provides a "real-world" assessment of an intervention without the restrictive eligibility criteria of randomized trials. Therefore, results of outcomes research are often more generalizable. Table 22–5 describes the strengths and weaknesses of data derived from randomized trials and health outcome studies. An example of the utility of outcomes research comes from the Prostate Cancer Outcomes Study. In this project, the Surveillance, Epidemiology, and End

TABLE 22–5 Strengths and Weaknesses of Randomized Trials and Population-based health outcome studies.

RCTs	Population-Based Studies
Precise measures of efficacy under ideal conditions	Difficulty in eliminating bias and confounders of effect
Poor measure of effectiveness under real-life conditions	Can estimate effectiveness in the general population
Limited information on toxicity	Assess toxicity under real-life conditions
Applicability to clinical practice can be limited	Evaluate uptake of treatment in general population

Data from Booth CM, Tannock IF. Randomised controlled trials and population-based observational research: partners in the evolution of medical evidence. *Br J Cancer* 2014 Feb 4;110(3):551-555.

Results (SEER) database of the United States National Cancer Institute was used to assess the outcomes of approximately 3500 men who had been diagnosed with primary invasive prostate cancer. Unlike many randomized trials, this study included a substantial number of men of different ethnic origins and socioeconomic groups, who had been treated in a variety of settings. This methodology enabled investigators to assess racial differences in stage at diagnosis and in treatment to help explain the significantly higher mortality rates from prostate cancer among black men in the United States (Hoffman et al, 2001).

The gold standard for assessing a medical intervention remains the randomized trial. However, randomized trials are not feasible in all settings, and such trials tend to be conducted in highly selected populations. Outcomes research aims to bridge the transition from evidence obtained in clinical trials to evaluate effectiveness of an intervention in usual clinical practice. Disadvantages to outcomes research include lack of randomized comparisons and the likelihood that causality may be attributed to several interventions, not only the one of interest. An example of this is the exploration of screening mammography for breast cancer. Outcomes data show improved outcomes after the introduction of screening in many populations. Unfortunately, it remains unclear whether the improved outcomes can be associated with mammography alone or a combination of mammography, improvements in treatment, and patient awareness and the establishment of multidisciplinary teams (Welch, 2010).

22.3.11 Cost-Effectiveness

Pharmacoeconomic evaluations play an integral role in the funding decisions for cancer drugs. The basic premise of the evaluation of cost-effectiveness is to compare the costs and consequences of alternative interventions, and to determine which treatment offers best value for limited resources. There are several methods available to evaluate economic efficiency, including cost minimization, cost benefit, and cost effectiveness analysis (Canadian Agency for Drugs and Technology in Health, 2006; Shih and Halpern, 2008). With respect to anticancer drugs, cost utility analysis (a type of cost-effectiveness analysis) is the preferred method because it considers differences in cost, survival, and quality of life between 2 competing interventions. In its most common form, a new strategy is compared to a reference standard to calculate the incremental cost-effectiveness ratio (ICER):

$$\text{ICER} = \frac{\text{Cost (new)} - \text{Cost (old)}}{\text{Effectiveness (new)} - \text{Effectiveness (old)}} \quad [\text{Eq. 22.1}]$$

In Equation 22.1, the ICER may be expressed as the increased cost per life-year gained, which can be estimated from differences in survival when the new treatment is compared with the standard treatment in a randomized controlled trial. The increase in survival can be adjusted for differences in quality of survival by multiplying the median survival with each treatment by the "utility" of the survival state, where "utility" is a factor between zero and 1 that is a measure of the relative quality of life of patients following each treatment (as compared to perfect health) (Shih and Halpern, 2008). The ICER is then expressed as the increased cost to gain one quality-adjusted life-year (QALY); in practice, utility is often difficult to estimate, and in the absence of major differences in toxicity between new and standard treatment, the simpler increase in cost-per-life-year gained is often used.

If the ICER falls below a predefined threshold, the new treatment is considered cost-effective, otherwise it is considered cost-ineffective. A major challenge in the use of pharmacoeconomic modeling for estimating drug cost is in establishing the threshold for value. The World Health Organization has proposed to use multiples of a country's per capita gross domestic product (GDP) to establish thresholds for economic value. Products less than or equal to the per capita GDP would be considered very cost effective, 1 to 3 times would be cost effective, and more than 3 times would be cost ineffective (Murray et al, 2000). However, individual jurisdictions have set different thresholds. For example, the National Institute for Clinical Excellence in the United Kingdom has established a threshold ICER of £30,000 (~US$50,000) per QALY gained (Devlin and Parkin, 2004), whereas the Canadian Agency for Drugs and Technologies in Health have set a threshold of CA$100,000 for cancer drugs. There remains no consensus as to what threshold is appropriate, but by convention, cutoffs of $100,000 to $150,000 per QALY are used often for public funding of new treatments in developed countries; much lower costs per QALY can be supported in the developing world (Sullivan et al, 2011).

In principle, the added costs per QALY gained can be used by public health systems to make choices between funding quite different health interventions. For example, a health jurisdiction might compare the cost-effectiveness ratio from extending the use of renal dialysis to that from introduction of a new anticancer drug, and select that which provides the lower cost for a given increase in QALYs or life-years.

22.4 DIAGNOSIS AND SCREENING

22.4.1 Diagnostic Tests

Diagnostic tests are used to screen for cancer in people who are symptom free, establish the existence or extent of disease in those suspected of having cancer, and follow changes in the extent and severity of the disease during therapy or follow-up. Diagnostic tests are used to distinguish between people with a particular cancer and those without it. Test results may be expressed quantitatively on a continuous scale or qualitatively on a categorical scale. The results of serum tumor marker tests, such as PSA, are usually expressed quantitatively as a concentration, whereas the results of imaging tests, such as a computed tomography (CT) scan, are usually expressed qualitatively as normal or abnormal. To assess how well a diagnostic test discriminates between those with and without disease, it is necessary to have an independent means of classifying those with

562 CHAPTER 22

	Disease status	
	Disease present (D+)	Disease absent (D−)
Test positive (T+)	True positive (TP) T+D+	False positive (FP) T+D−
Test negative (T+)	False negative (FN) T−D+	True negative (TN) T−D−

"Vertical properties" calculated from columns:
- Sensitivity = TP/(TP+FN)
- Specificity = TN/(TN+FP)
- False-negative rate = FN/(FN+TP)
- False-positive rate = FP/(FP+TN)

"Horizontal properties" calculated from rows:
- Positive predictive value = TP/(TP+FP)
- Negative predictive value = TN/(TN+FN)

FIGURE 22–5 Selection of a cutoff point for a diagnostic test defines 4 subpopulations as shown. Predictive values (but not sensitivity and specificity) depend on the prevalence of disease in the population tested.

High prevalence (50%)

	D+	D−		
T+	80	10	Sensitivity	80%
			Specificity	90%
T−	20	90	Predictive value (+)	89%

Intermediate prevalence (~9%)

	D+	D−		
T+	80	100	Sensitivity	80%
			Specificity	90%
T−	20	900	Predictive value (+)	44%

Low prevalence (~1%)

	D+	D−		
T+	80	1000	Sensitivity	80%
			Specificity	90%
T−	20	9000	Predictive value (+)	7.4%

FIGURE 22–6 Test properties and disease prevalence. Examples of application of a diagnostic test to populations in which disease has high, intermediate, or low prevalence. The predictive value of the test decreases when there is a low prevalence of disease.

and without disease—a "gold standard." This might be the findings of surgery, the results of a biopsy, or the clinical outcome of patients after prolonged follow-up. If direct confirmation of the presence of disease is not possible, the results of a range of different diagnostic tests may be the best standard available.

Simultaneously classifying the subjects into diseased (D+) and nondiseased (D−) according to the gold standard test and positive (T+) or negative (T−) according to the diagnostic test being assessed defines 4 subpopulations (Fig. 22–5). These are true-positives (TPs: people with the disease in whom the test is positive), true-negatives (TNs: people without the disease in whom the test is negative), false-positives (FPs: people without the disease in whom the test is positive), and false-negatives (FNs: people with the disease in whom the test is negative).

Test performance can be described by indices calculated from the 2 × 2 table shown in Figure 22–5. "Vertical" indices are calculated from the columns of the table and describe the frequency with which the test is positive or negative in people whose disease status is known. These indices include sensitivity (the proportion of people with disease who test positive) and specificity (the proportion of people without disease who test negative). These indices are characteristic of the particular test and do not depend on the prevalence of disease in the population being tested. The sensitivity and specificity of a test can be applied directly to populations with differing prevalence of disease.

"Horizontal" indices are calculated from the rows of the table and describe the frequency of disease in individuals whose test status is known. These indices indicate the predictive value of a test—for example, the probability that a person with a positive test has the disease (positive predictive value) or the probability that a person with a negative test does not have the disease (negative predictive value). These indices depend on characteristics of both the test (sensitivity and specificity) and the population being tested (prevalence of disease in the study population). The predictive value of a test cannot be applied directly to populations with differing prevalence of disease.

Figure 22–6 illustrates the influence of disease prevalence on the performance of a hypothetical test assessed in populations with high, intermediate, and low prevalence of disease. Sensitivity and specificity are constant, as they are independent of prevalence. As the prevalence of disease declines, the positive predictive value of the test declines. This occurs because although the *proportions* of TP results among diseased subjects and FP results among nondiseased subjects remain the same, the *absolute numbers* of TP and FP results differ. In Figure 22–6, for the high-prevalence population, the absolute number of false positives (10) is small in comparison with the absolute number of true positives (80): a positive result is 8 times more likely to come from a subject with disease than a subject without disease, and the positive predictive value of the test is relatively high. In the low-prevalence population, the absolute number of false positives (1000) is large in comparison with the absolute number of true positives (80): a positive result is 12.5 times more likely to come from a subject without disease, and the positive predictive value is relatively low. For this reason, diagnostic tests that may be useful in patients where there is already suspicion of disease (high-prevalence situation) may not be of value as screening tests in a less selected population (low-prevalence situation; see Sec. 22.4.3).

If a quantitative test is to be used to distinguish subjects with or without cancer, then a cutoff point must be selected that distinguishes positive results from negative results. Quantitative test results are often reported with a normal or reference range. This is the range of values obtained from some arbitrary proportion, usually 95%, of apparently healthy individuals; the corollary is that 5% of apparently healthy people will have values outside this range. Diagnostic test results are rarely conclusive about the presence or absence of diseases such as cancer; more often, they just raise or lower the likelihood that it is present.

Figure 22–7 shows the effects of choosing different cutoff points for a diagnostic test. A cutoff point at level *A* provides some separation of subjects with and without cancer, but

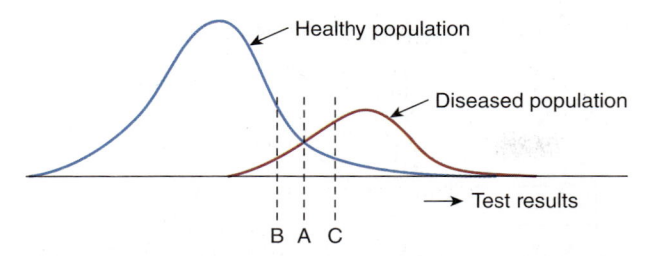

FIGURE 22-7 Interpretation of a diagnostic test (eg, PSA for prostate cancer) requires the selection of a cutoff point that separates negative from positive results. The position of the cutoff point (which might be set at A, B, or C) influences the proportion of patients who are incorrectly classified as being healthy or having disease.

because of overlap, there is always some misclassification. If the cutoff point is increased to level C, fewer subjects without cancer are wrongly classified (ie, the specificity increases) but more people with cancer fall below the cutoff and will be incorrectly classified (ie, the sensitivity decreases). A lower cutoff point at level B has the opposite effect: more subjects with cancer are correctly classified (sensitivity increases), but at the cost of incorrectly classifying larger numbers of people without cancer (specificity decreases). This trade-off between sensitivity and specificity is a feature of all diagnostic tests.

The 2 × 2 table and the indices derived from it (see Fig. 22–5) provide a simple and convenient method for describing test performance at a single cutoff point, but they give no indication of the effect of using different cutoff points. A receiver operating characteristic (ROC) curve provides a method for summarizing the effects of different cutoff points on sensitivity, specificity, and test performance. Figure 22–8 shows examples of ROC curves. The ROC curve plots the true-positive rate (TPR; which equals sensitivity) against the false-positive rate (FPR; which equals 1 − specificity) for different cutoff values. The "best" cutoff point is the one that offers the best compromise between TPR and FPR. This is represented by the point on the ROC curve closest to the upper left-hand corner. Statistically, ROC curves represent the balance between sensitivity and specificity with the area under the ROC curve (AUC; also known as the C-statistic) showing a model's discriminatory accuracy. An AUC of 0.5 is no better than a flip of a coin, whereas an AUC of 1.0 represents a perfect test. Realistically, an AUC of 0.7 or 0.8 is consistent with good discriminatory accuracy.

22.4.2 Sources of Bias in Diagnostic Tests

The performance of a diagnostic test is usually evaluated in a research study to estimate its usefulness in clinical practice. Differences between the conditions under which a test is evaluated, and the conditions under which it will be used, may produce misleading results. Important factors relating both to the people being tested and the methods being used are summarized in Table 22–6 (see also Jaeschke et al, 1994; Scales et al, 2008). If a test is to be used to identify patients with colon cancer, then the study sample should include people with both localized and advanced disease (a wide clinical spectrum). The sample should also include people with other clinical conditions that might be mistaken for colon cancer (eg, diverticular disease) in order to evaluate the ability of the test to distinguish between these conditions, or to detect colon cancer in its presence (comorbidity). If there are different histologic types of a cancer, then the test should be evaluated in a sample of patients who have these different histologic types.

The evaluation of diagnostic test performance requires subjects to be classified by both disease status (diseased or nondiseased) and test status (positive or negative). For the evaluation to be valid, the 2 acts of classification must be independent. If either the classification of disease status is influenced by the

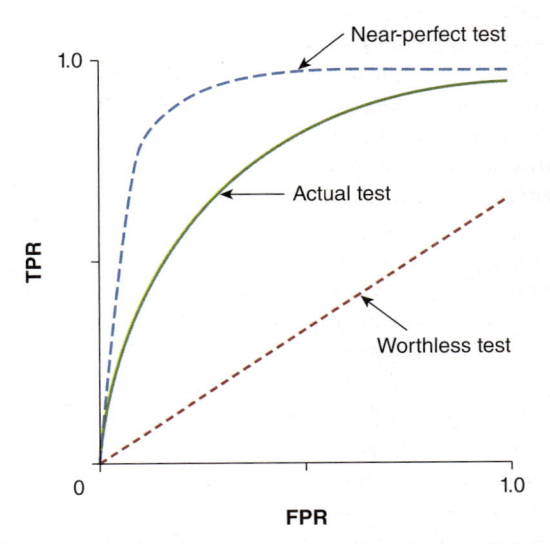

FIGURE 22-8 Curves showing receiver operating characteristics in which the true-positive rate (TPR) is plotted against the false-positive rate (FPR) of a diagnostic test as the cutoff point is varied. The performance of the test is indicated by the shape of the curve, as shown.

TABLE 22-6 Factors that may distort the estimated performance of a diagnostic test.

Spectrum of patients for evaluation of the test
Clinical spectrum: Should include patients with a wide range of features of the disease
Comorbid spectrum: Should include patients with a wide range of other diseases
Pathologic spectrum: Should include patients with a range of histological types of disease
Potential sources of bias in test evaluation
Exclusion of equivocal cases
Work-up bias: Results of the test influence the choice of subsequent tests that confirm or refute diagnosis
Test review bias: Results of the test influence the interpretation of subsequent tests to establish diagnosis
Diagnostic review bias: Knowledge of the disease influences the interpretation of the test
Incorporation bias: Test information is used as a criterion to establish diagnosis

test result or the interpretation of the test result is influenced by disease status, then there will be an inappropriate and optimistic estimate of test performance (see below and Table 22–6).

Workup bias arises if the results of the diagnostic test under evaluation influence the choice of other tests used to determine the subject's disease status. For example, suppose that the performance of a positron emission tomographic (PET) scan is to be evaluated as an indicator of spread of hitherto locoregional lung cancer by comparing it with the results of mediastinal lymph node biopsy. Workup bias will occur if only patients with abnormal PET scans are selected for mediastinoscopy, because regional spread in patients with normal PET scans will remain undetected. This leads to an exaggerated estimate of the predictive value of PET scanning.

Test-review bias occurs when the subjective interpretation of one test is influenced by knowledge of the result of another test. For example, a radiologist's interpretation of a PET scan might be influenced by knowledge of the results of a patient's CT scan. Using the CT scan to help interpret the results of an ambiguous PET scan may lead to a systematic overestimation of the ability of PET scan to identify active tumor. The most obvious violation of independence of the test and the method used to establish diagnosis arises when the test being evaluated is itself incorporated into the classification of disease status.

Diagnostic-review bias occurs when knowledge of an earlier test (e.g. a diagnostic core biopsy) affects or influences how the final diagnosis (e.g. final surgical pathology) is established (Schmidt and Factor, 2013).

22.4.3 Tests for Screening of Disease

Tests have been developed to screen an asymptomatic population to detect precancerous lesions or early cancers that are more amenable to treatment than cancers detected without screening. There are factors that influence the value of a screening program other than the sensitivity and specificity of the screening test. First, the cancer must pass through a preclinical phase that can be detected by the screening test. Slowly growing tumors, or those that arise from premalignant lesions, are more likely to meet this criterion. Second, treatment must be more effective (ie, more likely to achieve cure or more likely to prolong survival) for screen-detected patients than for those treated after symptoms develop: if the outcome of treatment is uniformly good or bad regardless of the time of detection, then screening will be of no benefit. Third, the prevalence of cancer in the population must be relatively high for a screening program to be effective. Finally, the screening test must be acceptable to the target population: painful and inconvenient tests are unlikely to be accepted as screening tools by asymptomatic individuals.

The primary goal of a screening program is to reduce *disease-specific mortality*, that is, the proportion of people in a population who die of a given cancer in a specified time. Other end points often reported in screening studies include stage of diagnosis and *case fatality rate* (the proportion of patients with the disease who die in a specified period). However, these intermediate end points are affected by several types of bias, particularly length-time bias and lead-time bias.

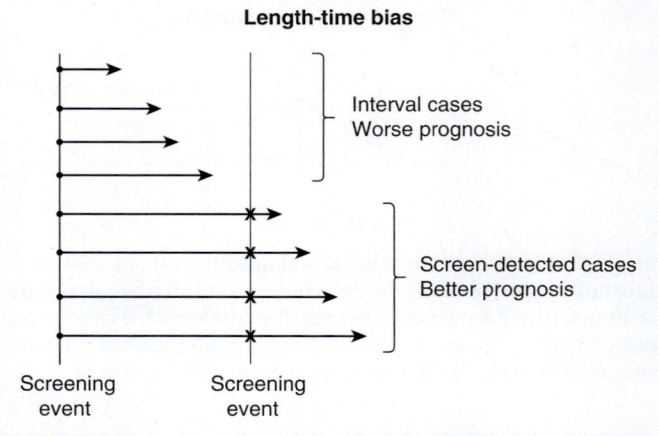

FIGURE 22–9 Illustration of length-time bias in a screening test. The test is more likely to detect disease that is present for a long time (ie, slowly growing disease). Horizontal lines represent the length of time that disease is present prior to clinical diagnosis.

Length-time bias is illustrated in Figure 22–9. The horizontal lines in the figure represent the length of time from inception of disease to the time it produces clinical signs or symptoms and would be diagnosed in the absence of screening. Long lines indicate slowly progressing disease, and short lines indicate rapidly progressing disease. A single examination, such as screening for breast cancer with mammography (represented in the figure by a vertical line), will intersect (detect) a larger number of long lines (people with more indolent disease) than short lines (people with aggressive disease). Thus, a screening examination will selectively identify those people with slowly progressing disease. An extreme result of length time bias is overdiagnosis, which describes a scenario in which a cancer identified by a screening test is so indolent that it would not cause any symptoms for the duration of that patient's lifetime. All screening tests are susceptible to overdiagnosis, but it can be difficult to quantify this effect as it requires all patients in a screening trial to be followed until death.

Lead-time bias is illustrated in Figure 22–10. Four critical time points in the clinical course of a person with cancer are indicated in Figure 22–10: the time of disease inception (0), the time at which the disease becomes incurable (1), the time of diagnosis (2), and the time of death (3). Many patients with common cancers are currently incurable by the time their disease is diagnosed, and the aim of a screening test is to advance the time of diagnosis to a point where the disease is curable. Even if the cancer is incurable despite the earlier time of diagnosis, survival will appear to be prolonged by early detection because of the additional time (the lead-time) that the disease is known to be present (Fig. 22–10). In screening for breast cancer with mammography, the lead-time is estimated to be approximately 2 years. Advancing the date of diagnosis may be beneficial if it increases the chance of cure. However, if it does not increase the chance of cure, then advancing the date of diagnosis may be detrimental, because patients spend a longer time with the knowledge that they have incurable disease.

The strongest study design for evaluating the impact of a screening test involves the randomization of people to have the

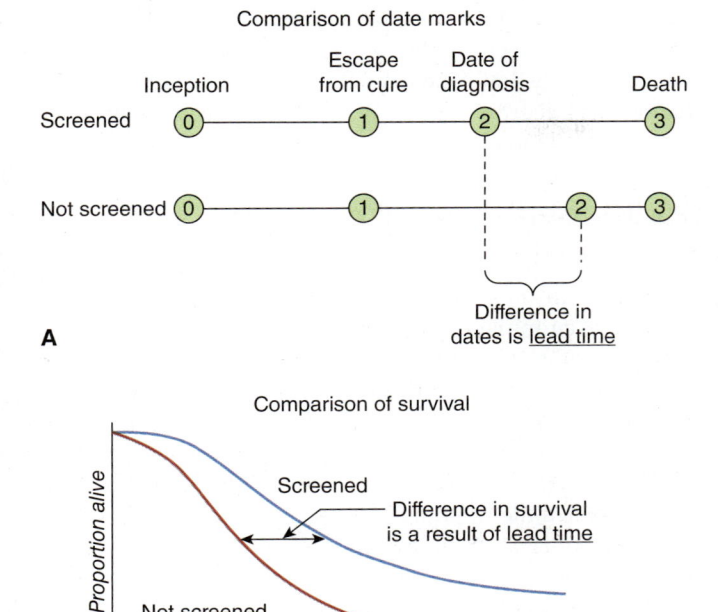

FIGURE 22–10 Illustration of lead-time bias. **A)** Application of a test may lead to earlier diagnosis without changing the course of disease. **B)** There is an improvement in survival when measured from time of diagnosis.

test or to be followed in the usual way without having the test. The most important outcome measures that are assessed in such a trial include overall survival, disease-specific survival, and quality of life. Both randomized trials and those using health outcomes methods have demonstrated reductions in mortality rates as a result of breast cancer associated with mammographic screening in postmenopausal women (Kalager et al, 2010), cervical cancer with exfoliative cytology-based (Laara et al, 1987) or acetic acid–based screening (Shastri et al, 2014) and colorectal carcinoma with fecal occult blood testing (Towler et al, 1998). However, an overview of the quality of trials of screening mammography has questioned whether there is a true reduction in mortality (Gøtzsche and Jørgensen, 2013). Also, there has been a decrease in disease-specific mortality, but an increase in death rate from all causes in some trials (Black et al, 2002). Some screening procedures might be harmful in that they lead to investigations with some associated morbidity and mortality. Randomized trials have demonstrated a small benefit associated with screening people at high risk for lung cancer using CT scans (National Lung Screening Trial, 2010), whereas trials evaluating the value of PSA screening for prostate cancer have either shown no benefit (Andriole et al, 2009) or a small decrease in disease-specific mortality (Schröder et al, 2009).

22.4.4 Tests During Follow-up of Treated Tumors

Among patients who have had a complete response to curative-intent treatment, most follow-up tests can be viewed as a form of screening for local or metastatic recurrence. Consequently, many of the requirements for an effective screening test described above also apply to follow-up tests. Because most clinically evident recurrent cancers are not curable (particularly metastatic recurrences), it is uncommon that early intervention to treat asymptomatic recurrence will produce a true improvement in mortality due to disease. Studies of follow-up tests that report improvement in case-fatality rates usually suffer from lead-time bias. As with screening studies, randomized trials provide the best methodology to compare the utility of alternative approaches to follow-up. Four randomized, controlled clinical trials involving 3055 women with breast cancer, found no difference in overall or disease-specific survival between patients observed with intensive radiologic and laboratory testing and those observed with clinical visits and mammography (Rojas et al, 2005). These findings demonstrate that for follow-up tests to improve survival, they must detect recurrences for which curative treatment is available; unfortunately, for most common tumors in adults, such treatment is rarely available.

22.4.5 Bayes Theorem and Likelihood Ratios

The results of diagnostic tests are rarely conclusive about the presence or absence of disease, and prognostic tests are rarely definitive about the course of disease. The utility of these tests is that they raise or lower the probability of observing a particular disease or prognosis (Jaeschke et al, 1994). This concept is embodied in *Bayes theorem*. This theorem allows an initial estimate of a probability to be adjusted to take account of new information from a diagnostic or prognostic test, thus producing a revised estimate of the probability. The initial estimate is referred to as the *prior* or *pretest probability*; the revised estimate is the *posterior* or *posttest probability*.

For example, the pretest probability of breast cancer in a 45-year-old American woman presenting for screening mammography is approximately 3 in 1000 (the prevalence of disease in women of this age). If her mammogram is reported as "suspicious for malignancy," then her post-test probability of having breast cancer rises to approximately 300 in 1000, whereas if the mammogram is reported as "normal," then her post-test probability of having breast cancer falls to approximately 0.4 in 1000 (Kerlikowske et al, 1996).

Bayes theorem describes the mathematical relationship between the new post-test probability, the former prior probability (ie, the prevalence of disease in the tested population), and the additional information provided by a test (or clinical trial). This relationship can be expressed with 2 formulae that look different but are logically equivalent. For a diagnostic test with the characteristics defined in Figure 22–5, *the probability form of Bayes theorem* can be expressed as

Post-test probability =

$$\frac{\text{sensitivity} \times \text{prevalence}}{(\text{sensitivity} \times \text{prevalence}) + (1 - \text{specificity})(1 - \text{prevalence})}$$

[Eq. 22.2]

The alternative form of the Bayes theorem is expressed in terms of a likelihood ratio and is much easier to use. The *likelihood ratio* is a useful concept that for any test result represents the ratio of the probability that disease is present to the probability that it is absent. For a positive diagnostic test, the likelihood ratio is the likelihood that the positive test represents a true positive rather than a false positive:

$$\text{Likelihood Ratio of a positive test result} = \frac{\text{sensitivity}}{1-\text{specificity}} = \frac{\text{true positive rate}}{\text{false positive rate}} \quad \text{[Eq. 22.3]}$$

For a negative diagnostic test, the likelihood ratio is the likelihood that the negative result represents a false negative rather than a true negative (ie, *false negative rate/true negative rate*). A good diagnostic test has a high likelihood ratio for a positive test (ideally >10) and a low likelihood ratio for a negative test (ideally <0.1).

22.5 PROGNOSIS

A prognosis is a forecast of expected course and outcome for a patient with a particular stage of disease. It may apply to the unique circumstances of an individual or to the general circumstances of a group of individuals. People with apparently similar types and stages of cancer live for different lengths of time, have different patterns of progression, and respond differently to the same treatments. Variables associated with the outcome of a disease that can account for some of this heterogeneity are known as *prognostic factors*, and they may relate to the tumor, the host, or the environment. An increasing number of tumor-related factors, including various gene signatures and somatic alterations (see Sec. 22.2; Chap. 2, Sec. 2.6), have been found to convey prognostic information.

Differences in prognostic characteristics often account for larger differences in outcome than do differences in treatment. For example, in women with primary breast cancer, differences in survival according to lymph node status are much greater than differences in survival according to treatment. Imbalances in the distribution of such important prognostic factors in clinical trials, which compare different treatments, may produce biased results by either obscuring true differences or creating spurious ones. Furthermore, the effects of treatment may be different in patients with differing prognostic characteristics. For example, the prognosis of hormone receptor–negative breast cancer is worse than that of hormone receptor–positive disease; however, the benefit from adjuvant chemotherapy for hormone receptor–negative patients is greater.

A *predictive test* evaluates the probability of outcome after some form of treatment. Prognostic factors (eg, for overall survival) may or may not predict the likelihood of benefit to a particular treatment. For example, the recurrence score of the 21-gene expression predictor, Oncotype DX for women with breast cancer provides both prognostic and predictive information. The predictive role of the Oncotype DX assay was assessed in patients with node-negative, estrogen receptor–positive tumors who were to receive standard hormonal therapy. Absolute benefit from chemotherapy was minimal when the recurrence score was low, whereas patients whose primary tumors had a high recurrence score derived additional benefit from adjuvant chemotherapy (Paik et al, 2006).

22.5.1 Identification of Prognostic Factors

Two stages are often used in the characterization of prognostic factors. In an initial exploratory analysis (sometimes called a "training set"), apparent patterns and relationships are examined and are used to generate hypotheses. In confirmatory analyses, the level of support for a prespecified hypothesis is examined critically using different "validation sets" of data; ideally different investigators in different institutions to those that generated the "training set" should undertake at least one of these confirmatory studies. Most studies evaluate a number of "candidate" prognostic factors with varying levels of prior support.

In univariable analysis, the strength of association between each candidate prognostic factor and the outcome is assessed separately. Univariable analyses are simple to perform, but they do not indicate whether different prognostic factors are providing the same or different information. For example, in women with breast cancer, lymph node status and hormone receptor status are both found to be associated with survival duration in univariable analysis; however, they are also found to be associated with one another. Univariable analysis will not provide a clear indication as to whether measuring both factors provides more prognostic information than measuring either factor alone. Multivariable analyses are more complex, but adjust for the simultaneous effects of several variables on the outcome of interest (see also Chap. 4, Sec. 4.4.3). Variables that are significant when included together in a multivariable model provide independent prognostic information.

Cox proportional hazards regression is a commonly used form of multivariable modeling of potential prognostic factors and can be used to model time-to-relapse or time-to-death in a cohort of patients who have been followed for different lengths of time. The method models the "hazard function" of the event, which is defined as the rate at which the event (eg, relapse) occurs. The effect of the presence (compared to absence) of a prognostic factor on the event rate, called the *hazard ratio*, represents the change in the rate of events caused by the presence or absence of the prognostic factor. For example, if the outcome of interest is tumor recurrence, a hazard ratio of 2 represents a 2-fold increase in the risk of recurrence (negative effect) as a result of the presence of the prognostic factor. A hazard ratio of 1 implies that the prognostic factor does not have an effect. The greater (or smaller) the value of the hazard ratio above or below 1 the larger the negative (or positive) effect of the prognostic factor.

The Cox proportional hazards method assumes that the relative effect of a given prognostic factor compared to the "baseline" is constant throughout the patient's follow-up period (ie, there is a constant "proportional hazard"). A Cox model may also assume that a given increase in the level of a factor has the same prognostic significance throughout the range of its measured values. Finally, variables may "interact" with each other biologically, and such interaction will not be accounted for in a Cox model unless a specific "interaction term" is included. For many factors of clinical interest, these assumptions may be incorrect, and the Cox model may then provide misleading estimates of prognostic value.

22.5.2 Evaluation of Prognostic Factor Studies

Methods of classifying cancer are based on factors known to influence prognosis, such as anatomic extent and histology of the tumor. The widely used TNM system for staging cancers is based on the extent of the primary tumor (T), the presence or absence of regional lymph node involvement (N), and the presence or absence of distant metastases (M). Other attributes of the tumor that have an influence on outcome, such as histologic grade or specific biomarkers such as estrogen receptor expression in breast cancer or EGFR mutation in non–small cell lung cancer, are also included as prognostic factors in the analysis and reporting of therapeutic trials. The identification of novel prognostic factors using the methods of molecular biology is an area of active investigation. Guidelines for selecting useful prognostic factors have been suggested by Altman (2001). The utility of a prognostic factor depends on the accuracy with which it can be measured. For example, the size and extent of the primary tumor are important prognostic factors in men with early prostate cancer, but there is substantial variability between observers in assessing these attributes: this variation contributes to the variability in outcome among patients assigned to the same prognostic category by different observers.

Several factors may diminish the validity of studies that report the discovery of a "significant" prognostic factor. Prognostic studies usually report outcomes for patients who are referred to academic centers and/or who participate in clinical studies. These patients may differ systematically from patients with similar malignancies in the community as they are selected for better performance status and fewer comorbidities, leading to *referral bias*. Also, patients who participate in clinical trials tend to have better outcomes than those who do not participate in clinical trials, even if they receive similar treatment (Peppercorn et al, 2004; Chua and Clarke, 2010). Thus population-based data—for example, data from cancer registries—may provide more pertinent information regarding overall prognosis than data from selected patients referred to academic centers or enrolled in clinical trials. However, the *relative* influence of a prognostic factor is less likely to be affected by referral bias than the *absolute* influence on prognosis for that disease. For example, if hormone receptor status influences survival of women with breast cancer irrespective of treatment administered, then it is likely to influence survival within each center, even if the absolute survival of patients may differ between centers. Ideally, a prognostic study should include all identified cases within a large, geographically defined area.

Objective criteria, independent of knowledge of the patients' initial prognostic characteristics, must be used to assess the relevant outcomes such as disease recurrence or cause of death in studies of prognosis. *Workup bias*, *test-review bias*, and *diagnostic-review bias*, discussed in Section 22.4.2, have their counterparts in studies of prognosis. For example, a follow-up bone scan in a patient with breast cancer that is equivocal may be more likely to be read as positive (ie, indicating recurrence of disease) if it is known that the patient initially had extensive lymph node involvement or that she subsequently developed proven bone metastases. To avoid these biases, all patients should be assessed with the same frequency, using the same tests, interpreted with the same explicit criteria and without knowledge of the patient's initial characteristics or subsequent course.

Several deficiencies in statistical analysis are common in prognostic factor studies. Typically, a large number of candidate prognostic factors are assessed in univariable analyses, and those factors exhibiting some degree of association, often defined by a P value less than .05, are included in a starting set of variables for the multivariable analysis. The final multivariable model usually contains only the subset of these variables that remain significant when simultaneously included in the same model. A multivariable model reported in a study that contains 10 prognostic variables may be the result of hundreds of different statistical comparisons, so that there is a high chance of detecting spurious associations. The large numbers of comparisons performed make the P values provided with most multivariable prognostic models invalid unless the model is prespecified before analysis begins. Alternatively, methods to adjust for multiple testing such as use of false-discovery rate (discussed in Section 22.2) can be considered. Similarly, for a factor that is measured on a continuous or ordinal scale, it is not valid to identify an "optimal" cut-point using the study cohort, and then demonstrate that the factor is associated with prognosis in the same cohort. Such results usually will not be applicable to other groups of patients. Cut points should be defined prior to analysis, and the prognostic model developed using a "training set" of patients must be tested in a separate "validation set."

Prognostic factor studies need to assess sufficient patients to allow detection of potentially significant effects. A rough but widely accepted guideline is that a minimum of 10 outcome events should have occurred for each prognostic factor assessed. Thus, in a study assessing prognostic factors for survival in 200 patients of whom 100 have died, no more than 10 candidate prognostic factors should be assessed.

Studies of new biological markers often demonstrate that they are associated with known prognostic factors (eg, tumor grade). Although this might provide insight into biology of the tumor, it does not indicate the prognostic value of the marker. Furthermore, even if a multivariable analysis adds the new marker preferentially into a prognostic model and excludes a recognized prognostic factor, this does not necessarily indicate the superior prognostic value of the marker in clinical practice. The analysis of models that are used to include and exclude variables that are associated with each other will depend on

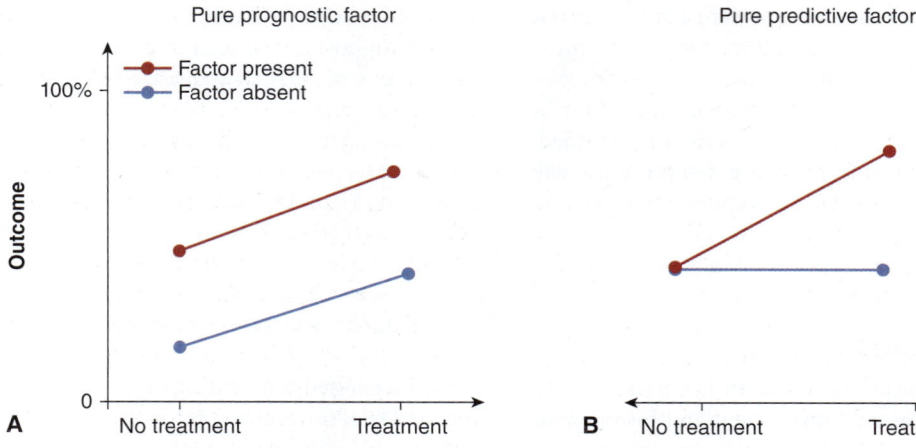

FIGURE 22-11 Differences between prognostic predictive tests.

the data set used: the results may not give the same preference between the 2 markers for different cohorts of patients with minor differences in outcome. Also, because conventional prognostic factors are generally easier to measure than novel biological markers, the practical question is whether the new marker provides clinically important *additional* prognostic information after controlling for known prognostic factors, rather than whether the new marker can replace an old one.

Prognostic classifications based solely on attributes of the tumor ignore patient-based factors known to affect prognosis such as performance status, quality of life, and the presence of other illnesses (comorbidity). Performance status, a measure of an individual's physical functional capacity, is one of the most powerful and consistent predictors of prognosis across the spectrum of malignant disease (Weeks, 1992). Studies in individual cancers, as well as a systematic review (Viganò et al, 2000), have consistently demonstrated strong, independent associations between simple measures of quality of life, obtained by patients completing validated questionnaires (see Sec. 22.3.9), and survival. Incorporation of these measures in clinical studies can reduce the heterogeneity that remains after accounting for attributes of the tumor.

22.5.3 Predictive Markers

Predictive markers are characteristics that are associated with treatment response. Statistically they are associated with an interaction effect with treatment. In contrast, prognostic tests are associated with improved outcomes independent of treatment (Fig. 22-11). Predictive tests for the selection of cancer drugs would ideally mirror the routine use of cultures of bacteria causing infections in testing for sensitivity to antibiotics. Assays to predict the clinical activity of anticancer drugs, in which tumor biopsies or cells derived from them are exposed to the drugs in tissue culture, followed by a test that evaluates killing of the tumor cells, have been described for several decades but none of them has proven reliable or useful.

Predictive assays that are in routine clinical use include analysis of estrogen (ER) and/or progesterone receptor (PgR) expression (see Chap. 20, Sec. 20.4): most oncologists would not consider endocrine therapy for women with breast cancer in the absence of a positive test for tumor cell expression of ER and/or PgR. Other established predictive tests include the analysis of HER2 overexpression or amplification in breast or gastric cancer for the use of HER2-targeted therapy, the presence of EGFR mutations in non–small cell lung cancer for EGFR inhibitors or the presence of BRAF mutations in melanoma for BRAF inhibitors. Despite their routine use, validation of these tests is suboptimal. The tests are prone to methodologic problems with interobserver and interlaboratory variation occurring in up to 20% of the patients.

Molecular techniques may lead to progress in the development of predictive tests. The antitumor activity of an increasing number of targeted therapeutics is based on the presence of specific biomarkers although the clinical utility of many biomarkers remains uncertain. This has created a need for real-time detection of genetic aberrations. Some cancer mutations occur at similar DNA bases in tumors from different patients (recurrent mutations). It is therefore possible to use assays that test for single bases (a process referred to as *mutation genotyping*) to detect these aberrations (Tran et al, 2012). There are only a few clinically validated recurrent mutations, but their repertoire is increasing, and they are being evaluated as predictive mutations for the numerous molecular targeted agents in development.

SUMMARY

▶ The evaluation of new treatments and technologies in clinical trials remains the backbone of clinical research in oncology.
▶ Data from genomic analyses are having an impact in cancer treatment as well as being the subject of intensive research into personalized cancer medicine.
▶ The promise of personalized cancer medicine is becoming a reality for a small subgroup of patients; however, for the majority the advances in genomic

technology has not resulted in improvement in treatment selection and cancer outcomes.
- Increasing use of health outcomes research, based on analysis of registries or other large databases will help in assessing the impact of health interventions at a societal level and provide a more generalizable assessment of the impact of new cancer treatments than may be observed from highly selected patients enrolled on clinical trials.
- Although tumor relapse and duration of survival are important outcomes and are easily measured in trials, they are often not the most relevant measures of treatment success. In many cases, treatment is offered to reduce symptoms, or there may be a choice between different treatments with apparently equivalent antitumor activity. In such trials, symptom control and quality of life is important.
- As diagnostic technologies and treatments continue to advance, oncologists must be able to conduct, evaluate, and interpret studies to define the best use of them. Although the methodologic principles that define valid, high-quality studies have been established, enthusiasm to adopt new technology often leads to studies that are subject to well-described biases and do not aid the rational use of the studied test.

REFERENCES

Aaronson NK, Ahmedzai S, Bergman B, et al. The European Organisation for Research and Treatment of Cancer QLQ-C30: a quality of life instrument for use in international clinical trials in oncology. *J Natl Cancer Inst* 1993;85(5): 365-376.

Adjei AA. What is the right dose? The elusive optimal biologic dose in phase I clinical trials. *J Clin Oncol* 2006;24(25): 4054-4055.

Altman DG. Systematic reviews of evaluations of prognostic variables. *BMJ* 2001;323(7306):224-228.

Amado RG, Wolf M, Peeters M, et al. Wildtype KRAS is required for panitumumab efficacy in patients with metastatic colorectal cancer. *J Clin Oncol* 2008;26(10):1626-1634.

Amir E, Seruga B, Martinez-Lopez J, et al. Oncogenic targets, magnitude of benefit, and market pricing of antineoplastic drugs. *J Clin Oncol* 2011;29(18):2543-2549.

Basch E, Reeve BB, Mitchell SA, et al. Development of the National Cancer Institute's patient-reported outcomes version of the Common Terminology Criteria For Adverse Events (PRO-CTCAE). *J Natl Cancer Inst* 2014; 106(9):dju244.

Basch E, Deal AM, Dueck AC, et al. Overall survival results of a trial assessing patient-reported outcomes for symptom monitoring during routine cancer treatment. *JAMA* 2017;318(2):197-198.

Bedard PL, Hansen AR, Ratain MJ, et al. Tumour heterogeneity in the clinic. *Nature* 2013;501(7467):355-364.

Black WC, Haggstrom DA, Welch HG. All-cause mortality in randomized trials of cancer screening. *J Natl Cancer Inst* 2002;94(3):369-375.

Booth CM, Li G, Zhang-Salomons J, Mackillop WJ. The impact of socioeconomic status on stage of cancer at diagnosis and survival: a population-based study in Ontario, Canada. *Cancer* 2010;116(17):4160-4167.

Booth CM, Tannock IF. Randomised controlled trials and population-based observational research: partners in the evolution of medical evidence. *Br J Cancer* 2014; 110(3):551-555.

Bush RS. Cancer of the ovary: natural history. In: Peckham MJ, Carter RL, eds. *Malignancies of the Ovary, Uterus and Cervix: The Management of Malignant Disease, Series #2.* London: Edward Arnold; 1979:26-37.

Buyse M, Piedbois P, Piedbois Y, Carlson RW. Meta-analysis: methods, strengths, and weaknesses. *Oncology (Williston Park)* 2000;14(3):437-443.

Canadian Agency for Drugs and Technology in Health. *Guidelines for the Economic Evaluation of Health Technologies.* 3rd ed. Ottawa, Canada; 2006. http://www.cadth.ca/media/pdf/186_EconomicGuidelines_e.pdf. Accessed November 8, 2010.

Cella DF, Tulsky DS, Gray G, et al. The functional assessment of cancer therapy scale: development and validation of the general measure. *J Clin Oncol* 1993;11(3):570-579.

Chalmers TC, Celano P, Sacks HS, Smith H Jr. Bias in treatment assignment in controlled clinical trials. *N Engl J Med* 1983;309(22):1358-1361.

Chan CH, Jo U, Kohrman A, et al. Posttranslational regulation of Akt in human cancer. *Cell Biosci* 2014;4(1):59.

Chao C, Studts JL, Abell T, et al. Adjuvant chemotherapy for breast cancer: how presentation of recurrence risk influences decision-making. *J Clin Oncol* 2003;21(23):4299-4305.

Cherny NI, Sullivan R, Dafni U, et al. A standardised, generic, validated approach to stratify the magnitude of clinical benefit that can be anticipated from anti-cancer therapies: the European Society for Medical Oncology Magnitude of Clinical Benefit Scale (ESMO-MCBS). *Ann Oncol* 2015;26(8):1547-1573.

Chua W, Clarke SJ. Clinical trial information as a measure of quality cancer care. *J Oncol Pract* 2010;6(3):170-171.

Del Paggio JC, Sullivan R, Schrag D, et al. Delivery of meaningful cancer care: a retrospective cohort study assessing cost and benefit with the ASCO and ESMO frameworks. *Lancet Oncol* 2017;18(7):887-894.

Devlin N, Parkin D. Does NICE have a cost-effectiveness threshold and what other factors influence its decisions? A binary choice analysis. *Health Econ* 2004;13(5):437-452.

Early Breast Cancer Trialists Collaborative Group (EBCTCG). Effects of chemotherapy and hormonal therapy for early breast cancer on recurrence and 15 years survival: an overview of the randomised trials. *Lancet* 2005;365:1687-1717.

Early Breast Cancer Trialists Collaborative Group. Ovarian ablation in early breast cancer: Overview of the randomised trials. *Lancet* 1996;348(9036):1189-1196.

El-Maraghi RH, Eisenhauer EA. Review of phase II trial designs used in studies of molecular targeted agents: outcomes and predictors of success in phase III. *J Clin Oncol* 2008;26(8):1346-1354.

Feinstein AR. Clinical *Epidemiology: The Architecture of Clinical Research*. Philadelphia, PA: Saunders; 1985.

Feinstein AR, Sosin DM, Wells CK. The Will Rogers phenomenon: stage migration and new diagnostic techniques as a source of misleading statistics for survival in cancer. *N Engl J Med* 1985;312:1604-1608.

Gan HK, Grothey A, Pond GR, Moore MJ, Siu LL, Sargent D. Randomized phase II trials: inevitable or inadvisable? *J Clin Oncol* 2010;28(15):2641-2647.

Gerlinger M, Rowan AJ, Horswell S, et al. Intratumor heterogeneity and branched evolution revealed by multiregion sequencing. *N Engl J Med* 2012;366(10):883-892.

Gøtzsche PC, Jørgensen KJ. Screening for breast cancer with mammography. *Cochrane Database Syst Rev* 2013; 6:CD001877.

Guyatt GH, Haynes RB, Jaeschke RZ, et al. Users' Guides to the Medical Literature: XXV. Evidence-based medicine: principles for applying the Users' Guides to patient care. Evidence-based medicine working group. *JAMA* 2000;284:1290-1296.

Hansen AR, Cook N, Amir E, et al. Determinants of the recommended phase 2 dose of molecular targeted agents. *Cancer* 2017;123(8):1409-1415.

Hayes DF, Trock B, Harris AL. Assessing the clinical impact of prognostic factors: when is "statistically significant" clinically useful? *Breast Cancer Res Treat* 1998;52(1-3): 305-319.

Hershman DL, Kushi LH, Shao T, et al. Early discontinuation and nonadherence to adjuvant hormonal therapy in a cohort of 8,769 early-stage breast cancer patients. *J Clin Oncol* 2010;28(27):4120-4128.

Hoffman RM, Gilliland FD, Eley JW, et al. Racial and ethnic differences in advanced-stage prostate cancer: the Prostate Cancer Outcomes Study. *J Natl Cancer Inst* 2001;93(5): 388-395.

Ioannidis JP, Allison DB, Ball CA, et al. Repeatability of published microarray gene expression analyses. *Nat Genet* 2009;41(2):149-155.

Jaeschke R, Guyatt GH, Sackett DL; for the Evidence-Based Medicine Working Group. Users' guides to the medical literature: III. How to use an article about a diagnostic test. *JAMA* 1994;271(9):389-391, 703-707.

James ND, Sydes MR, Clarke NW, et al. Addition of docetaxel, zoledronic acid, or both to first-line long-term hormone therapy in prostate cancer (STAMPEDE): survival results from an adaptive, multiarm, multistage, platform randomised controlled trial. *Lancet* 2016;387(10024):1163-1177.

James ND, de Bono JS, Spears MR, et al. Abiraterone for prostate cancer not previously treated with hormone therapy. *N Engl J Med* 2017;377(4):338-351.

Joly F, Vardy J, Pintilie M, Tannock IF. Quality of life and/or symptom control in randomized clinical trials for patients with advanced cancer. *Ann Oncol* 2007;18(12):1935-1942.

Kalager M, Zelen M, Langmark F, Adami HO. Effect of screening mammography on breast-cancer mortality in Norway. *N Engl J Med* 2010;363(13):1203-1210.

Karapetis CS, Khambata-Ford S, Jonker DJ, et al. K-ras mutations and benefit from cetuximab in advanced colorectal cancer. *N Engl J Med* 2008;359(17):1757-1765.

Kerlikowske K, Grady D, Barclay J, et al. Likelihood ratios for modern screening mammography: risk of breast cancer based on age and mammographic interpretation. *JAMA* 1996;276(1):39-43.

Laara E, Day NE, Hakama M. Trends in mortality from cervical cancer in the Nordic countries: association with organised screening programmes. *Lancet* 1987;1(8544): 1247-1249.

Le Tourneau C, Delord JP, Gonçalves A, et al. Molecularly targeted therapy based on tumour molecular profiling versus conventional therapy for advanced cancer (SHIVA): a multicentre, open-label, proof-of-concept, randomised, controlled phase 2 trial. *Lancet Oncol* 2015;16(13): 1324-1334.

Lièvre A, Bachet JB, Le Corre D, et al. KRAS mutation status is predictive of response to cetuximab in colorectal cancer. *Cancer Res* 2006;66(8):3992-3995.

Manji A, Brana I, Amir E, et al. Evolution of clinical trial design in early drug development: systematic review of expansion cohort use in single-agent phase I cancer trials. *J Clin Oncol* 2013;31(33):4260-4267.

Metzker ML. Sequencing technologies: the next generation. *Nat Rev Genet* 2009;11(1):31-46.

Murray CJ, Evans DB, Acharya A, et al. Development of WHO guidelines in generalized cost effectiveness analysis. *Health Econ* 2000;9(3):235-251.

National Lung Screening Trial. Press release: Lung cancer trial results show mortality benefit with low-dose CT. National Cancer Institute. http://www.cancer.gov/newscenter/press-releases/NLSTresultsRelease. Accessed November 1, 2010.

Nekolaichuk CL, Maguire TO, Suarez-Almazor M, et al. Assessing the reliability of patient, nurse, and family caregiver symptom ratings in hospitalized advanced cancer patients. *J Clin Oncol* 1999;17(11):3621-3630.

Newman AM, Bratman SV, To J, et al. An ultrasensitive method for quantitating circulating tumor DNA with broad patient coverage. *Nat Med* 2014;20(5):548-554.

Ng R, Pond GR, Tang PA, et al. Correlation of changes between 2-year disease-free survival and 5-year overall survival in adjuvant breast cancer trials from 1966 to 2006. *Ann Oncol* 2008;19(3):481-486.

Noble JH Jr. Meta-analysis: methods, strengths, weaknesses, and political uses. *J Lab Clin Med* 2006;147(1):7-20.

Ocaña A, Díez-González L, García-Olmo DC, et al. Circulating DNA and survival in solid tumors. *Cancer Epidemiol Biomarkers Prev* 2016;25(2):399-406.

Paik S, Shak S, Tang G, et al. A multigene assay to predict recurrence of tamoxifen-treated, node negative, estrogen receptor positive breast cancer. *J Clin Oncol* 2006;24: 3726-3734.

Parmar MKB, Stewart LA, Altman DG. Meta-analyses of randomised trials: when the whole is more than just the sum of the parts. *Br J Cancer* 1996;74:496-501.

Parulekar WR, Eisenhauer EA. Phase I trial design for solid tumor studies of targeted, non-toxic agents: theory and practice. *J Natl Cancer Inst* 2004;96(13):990-997.

Peppercorn JM, Weeks JC, Cook EF, et al. Comparison of outcomes in cancer patients treated within and outside clinical trials: conceptual framework and structured review. *Lancet* 2004;363(9405):263-270.

Robison K. Application of second-generation sequencing to cancer genomics. *Brief Bioinform* 2010;11(5):524-534.

Rojas MP, Telaro E, Russo A, et al. Follow-up strategies for women treated for early breast cancer. *Cochrane Database Syst Rev* 2005;(1):CD001768.

Royston P, Parmar MK, Qian W. Novel designs for multi-arm clinical trials with survival outcomes with an application in ovarian cancer. *Stat Med* 2003;22(14):2239-2256.

Sargent DJ, Wieand HS, Haller DG, et al. Disease-free survival versus overall survival as a primary end point for adjuvant colon cancer studies: individual patient data from 20,898 patients on 18 randomized trials. *J Clin Oncol* 2005;23(34):8664-8670.

Scales CD Jr, Dahm P, Sultan S, et al. How to use an article about a diagnostic test. *J Urol* 2008;180(2):469-476.

Schröder FH, Hugosson J, Roobol MJ, et al. Screening and prostate-cancer mortality in a randomized European study. *N Engl J Med* 2009;360(13):1320-1328.

Schwartz D, Flamant R, Lellouch J. *Clinical Trials*. London, UK: Academic Press; 1980.

Shih YC, Halpern MT. Economic evaluations of medical care interventions for cancer patients: how, why, and what does it mean? *CA Cancer J Clin* 2008;58(4):231-244.

SEQC/MAQC-III Consortium. A comprehensive assessment of RNA-seq accuracy, reproducibility and information content by the Sequencing Quality Control Consortium. *Nat Biotechnol* 2014;32:903-914.

Schmidt RL, Factor RE. Understanding sources of bias in diagnostic accuracy studies *Arch Pathol Lab Med* 2013;137:558-565.

Schnipper LE, Davidson NE, Wollins DS, et al. Updating the American Society of Clinical Oncology Value Framework: revisions and reflections in response to comments received. *J Clin Oncol* 2016;34(24):2925-2934.

Seruga B, Templeton AJ, Badillo FE, et al. Under-reporting of harm in clinical trials. *Lancet Oncol* 2016;17(5):e209-e219.

Shastri SS, Mittra I, Mishra GA, Gupta S, Dikshit R, Singh S, Badwe RA. Effect of VIA screening by primary health workers: randomized controlled study in Mumbai, India. *J Natl Cancer Inst* 2014;106(3):dju009.

Simon R, Freidlin B, Rubinstein L, Arbuck SG, Collins J, Christian MC. Accelerated titration designs for phase I clinical trials in oncology. *J Natl Cancer Inst* 1997;89(15):1138-1147.

Sprangers MAG. Response-shift bias: a challenge to the assessment of patients' quality of life in cancer clinical trials. *Cancer Treat Rev* 1996;22(Suppl A):55-62.

Srikanthan A, Vera-Badillo F, Ethier J, et al. Evolution in the eligibility criteria of randomized controlled trials for systemic cancer therapies. *Cancer Treat Rev* 2016;43: 67-73.

Stewart LA, Parmar MKB. Meta-analysis of the literature or of individual patient data: is there a difference? *Lancet* 1993;341:418-422.

Sukhai MA, Craddock KJ, Thomas M, et al. A classification system for clinical relevance of somatic variants identified in molecular profiling of cancer. *Genet Med* 2016;18(2):128-136.

Sullivan R, Peppercorn J, Sikora K, et al. Delivering affordable cancer care in high-income countries. *Lancet Oncol* 2011;12(10):933-980.

Swanton C. Intratumor heterogeneity: evolution through space and time. *Cancer Res* 2012;72:4875-4882.

Tannock IF, Hickman JA. Limits to personalized cancer medicine. *N Engl J Med* 2016;375(13):1289-1294.

Tannock IF, Amir E, Booth CM, et al. Relevance of randomised controlled trials in oncology. *Lancet Oncol* 2016a;17(12):e560-e567.

Templeton AJ, Ace O, Amir E, Tannock IF. Informative censoring – a neglected cause of bias in oncology trials. *Nat Rev Clin Oncol* 2020;17:327-328.

Thomas RK, Baker AC, Debiasi RM, et al. High-throughput oncogene mutation profiling in human cancer. *Nat Genet* 2007;39(3):347-351.

Tibshirani R. A plain man's guide to the proportional hazards model. *Clin Invest Med* 1982;5(1):63-68.

Towler B, Irwig L, Glasziou P, et al. A systemic review of the effects of screening for colorectal cancer using the faecal occult blood test, hemoccult. *BMJ* 1998;317(7158):559-565.

Tran B, Dancey JE, Kamel-Reid S, et al. Cancer genomics: technology, discovery, and translation. *J Clin Oncol* 2012;30(6):647-660.

Treweek S, Dryden R, McCowan C, et al. Do participants in adjuvant breast cancer trials reflect the breast cancer patient population? *Eur J Cancer* 2015;51(8):907-914.

Trusheim MR, Burgess B, Hu SX, et al. Quantifying factors for the success of stratified medicine. *Nat Rev Drug Discov* 2011;10(11):817-833.

Viganò A, Dorgan M, Buckingham J, et al. Survival prediction in terminal cancer patients: a systematic review of the medical literature. *Palliat Med* 2000;14(5):363-374.

von Minckwitz G, Procter M, de Azambuja E, et al. Adjuvant pertuzumab and trastuzumab in early HER2-positive breast cancer. *N Engl J Med* 2017;377(2):122-131.

Walsh M, Srinathan SK, McAuley DF, et al. The statistical significance of randomized controlled trial results is frequently fragile: a case for a Fragility Index. *J Clin Epidemiol* 2014;67(6):622-628.

Walter S. In defense of the arcsine approximation. *Statistician* 1979;28:219-222.

Wasserstein RL, Lazar NA. The ASA's statement on p-values: context, process, and purpose. *Am Stat* 2016;70:129-133.

Weeks J. Performance status upstaged? *J Clin Oncol* 1992;10(12):1827-1829.

Welch HG. Screening mammography—a long run for a short slide? *N Engl J Med* 2010;363(13):1276-1278.

West HJ. Novel precision medicine trial designs: umbrellas and baskets. *JAMA Oncol* 2017;3(3):423.

Wood L, Egger M, Gluud LL, et al. Empirical evidence of bias in treatment effect estimates in controlled trials with different interventions and outcomes: meta-epidemiological study. *BMJ* 2008;336(7644):601-605.

Yin G, Li Y, Ji Y. Bayesian dose-finding in phase I/II clinical trials using toxicity and efficacy odds ratios. *Biometrics* 2006;62:777-784.

BIBLIOGRAPHY

Crowley J. *Handbook of Statistics in Clinical Oncology*. New York, NY: Dekker; 2001.

Fletcher RH, Fletcher SW. *Clinical Epidemiology: The Essentials*. Baltimore, MD: Lippincott Williams & Wilkins; 2005.

Hulley SB. *Designing Clinical Research*. Philadelphia, PA: Lippincott Williams & Wilkins; 2007.

Sackett DL, Haynes RB, Guyatt GH, Tugwell P. *Clinical Epidemiology: A Basic Science for Clinical Medicine*. Boston, MA: Little, Brown; 1991.

Index

Note: Page numbers followed by *f* and *t* indicate figures and tables, respectively.

A

AAs. *See* Antiangiogenic agent(s) (AAs)
ABC. *See* ATP-binding cassette (ABC) transporters
ABCB5, in melanoma, 317
ABCB1 gene, 449, 450
ABCC1 gene, 449, 450, 451
ABCG2/BCRP, and multidrug resistance, 449, 449*f*, 449*t*, 451
Abemaciclib, 177, 476
  and fulvestrant, combined, 502–503
  with hormonal agents, for breast cancer, 503
Abiraterone acetate, 504–505, 505*f*
  mechanism of action of, 505*f*
  resistance, 509
  structure of, 505*f*
Abnormalization, 250*f*, 264, 264*f*
Abscission, 174–175
Abscopal effects, of radiation, 363, 375
ABT-510, 268
Acalabrutinib, indications for, 480
Accelerated repopulation, 423*f*
  of irradiated cells, 390–392, 391*f*
Acetaldehyde dehydrogenase(s) (ALDHs), 88, 91, 434
2-Acetylaminofluorene
  carcinogenicity, dose–response relationship and, 107, 107*f*
  potency as carcinogen, 107*t*
Acetyl-CoA, and epigenetics, 59, 59*f*
Acidity
  and cellular drug uptake, 299
  combined treatment and, 421–424, 422*t*
  in solid tumors, 453, 454*f*
    and drug resistance, 284, 454–455
  in tumor microenvironment, 230, 284
Acidosis, in tumor microenvironment, 284
ACIS. *See* Automated Cancer Information System (ACIS)
Acquired resistance, 446, 538
ACTH. *See* Adrenocorticotropic hormone (ACTH)
Actin. *See also* Smooth muscle actin
  integrins and, 124–125
Activating function-1 (AF1), 489–491, 490*f*, 493
Activating function-2 (AF2), 490*f*, 491, 493
Active transport, drug uptake by, 448–449
Actuarial survival curves, 555, 555*f*, 555*t*
Acute lymphoblastic (lymphocytic) leukemia (ALL)
  B-ALL
    chromosomal abnormalities in, 7*t*
    molecular lesions in, 7*t*
    relapse, treatment of, 409
  BCR-ABL in, 478
  chromosomal abnormalities in, 7*t*
  gene fusion in, 145, 147*t*, 150
  initiating cells, diverse clones in, 310
  MLL1 mutations in, 58
  molecular lesions in, 7*t*
  monoclonal antibody therapy for, 532*t*
  oncogenes in, 142*t*
  Philadelphia chromosome-negative, treatment of, 410
  Pre-B
    chromosomal abnormalities in, 7*t*
    molecular lesions in, 7*t*
  targeted therapy for, 467*t*
  T-cell (T-ALL), NOTCH signaling in, 128
  T-cell precursor, RAS-MAPK mutations in, 119
  tumor-suppressor genes in, 142*t*
Acute myelogenous (myeloid) leukemia (AML)
  cancer stem cells in, 314–315, 315*f*
  CBL-b mutations in, 134
  chromosomal abnormalities in, 7*t*
  DNA methyltransferase mutations in, 58, 58*f*
  epigenetic variants in, as biomarkers for precision cancer medicine, 63
  EZH2 mutations in, 58
  gene fusion in, 147*t*, 150
  with *IDH2* mutation, treatment of, 409
  IDH1/2 mutations in, 59–60, 63, 291, 477–478
  MLL1 mutations in, 58
  molecular lesions in, 7*t*
  monoclonal antibody therapy for, 532*t*
  oncogenes in, 142*t*
  PTPN11 mutations in, 123
  secondary
    alkylating agents and, 432
    directed drug delivery for, 410
  smoking and, 87*f*
  targeted therapy for, 467*t*, 468*t*
  TET2 mutations in, 58, 63
  therapy-related, chromosomal abnormalities in, 7*t*
  tumor-suppressor genes in, 142*t*
Acute promyelocytic leukemia (APML), differentiation therapy in, 321, 322*f*
ADAM, 127, 227, 259, 260*f*
  and cancer progression, 237–238, 237*t*
ADAM10
  and cancer progression, 237–238, 237*t*
  and metastasis, 231*f*, 232
ADAM12, and cancer progression, 237–238, 237*t*
ADAM17, and cancer progression, 237–238, 237*t*
ADAM inhibitors, 128
ADAM proteinase, in NOTCH signaling, 127
Adams-Oliver syndrome, 128
ADAMTS, 259, 260*f*
Adaptive immunity, 519–525
  cells of, 515
Adaptive resistance, 538
Adaptive therapy, 321, 322*f*
Adaptor proteins, 116, 117*f*
ADC. *See* Antibody drug conjugates (ADC); Apparent diffusion coefficient (ADC) imaging
ADCC. *See* Antibody-dependent cell-mediated cytotoxicity (ADCC)
Additivity, of combined drugs, 419–420, 420*f*
Adenoid cancer, NOTCH signaling in, 128
Adenomatous polyposis coli (APC), 125–126
Adenosine, 230
  analogs, 440
  structure of, 440*f*
Adenosine monophosphate-activated protein kinase (AMPK), and tumor metabolism, 286*f*, 288
Adenosine triphosphate (ATP)
  generation, by malignant cells, 284–287, 285*f*, 287*f*
  production
    in glutamine metabolism, 289, 289*f*
    in glycolysis, 284–287, 285, 286*f*
Adenoviruses, as vectors, 23
Adherence, definition of, 552
Adhesion molecules, 258–259, 259*f*
ADHs. *See* Alcohol dehydrogenase(s) (ADHs)
Adjuvant treatment, 243, 429
Adoptive (T-cell) cell therapies, 531, 531*t*, 539–541, 540*f*
  with tumor-infiltrating lymphocytes, 539, 540*f*
  with tumor-specific T cells, 539, 540*f*
Ado-trastuzumab emtansine, indications for, 467*t*
Adrenal cancer, tumor-suppressor genes in, 142*t*
Adrenocorticotropic hormone (ACTH)
  ectopic production of, 509
  in paraneoplastic Cushing syndrome, 509
Adriamycin. *See* Doxorubicin
ADT. *See* Androgen deprivation therapy (ADT)
AF1. *See* Activating function-1 (AF1)
AF2. *See* Activating function-2 (AF2)
Afatinib, 142*t*, 403, 469*f*
  adverse effects, 472
  indications for, 467*t*, 472
  mechanism of action of, 472
Affymetrix arrays, 18
Aflatoxin B_1, 74, 98
  carcinogenesis, *p53* mutation and, 102
  metabolic activation of, 100, 101*f*
  potency as carcinogen, 107, 107*t*
  structure of, 99*f*
  and viral infection, in hepatocellular carcinoma, 102
Aflibercept, 268*t*, 269–270
Age, and tumor angiogenesis, 266
Age distribution, and incidence rate, 70
Age-standardized rates, 70–71
  sex differences in, 72*f*, 73–74
Agilent, 18
AIB1 (amplified in breast cancer 1), 493–494
AIDS-defining cancers, 530
AIF. *See* Apoptosis-inducing factor (AIF)
AKT, 120–121, 120*f*, 149, 230
AKT1
  and oxidative stress, 290–291, 290*f*
  and tumor metabolism, 286*f*, 288
AKT gene, cancer-associated mutations in, 153–154, 153*f*
AKT kinase, 175
Alagille syndrome, 128
Alcohol
  and head and neck cancer, 87–88
    genomic risk study of, 88
  smoking and, and cancer risk, 85*f*, 88
Alcohol dehydrogenase(s) (ADHs), 88
Aldo-keto reductase, 100
Aldophosphamide, 433, 434*f*
Alectinib, 142*t*, 469*f*, 478–479
  indications for, 467*t*
Alemtuzumab, 409, 532*t*
ALK. *See* Anaplastic lymphoma kinase (ALK)
ALK gene, 142*t*
Alkylating agents, 432–436
  adverse effects of, 432
  bifunctional, 432
  mechanism of action of, 432, 452
  monofunctional, 432
  resistance to, 446*t*, 451
  and second malignancy, 418
  toxicity of, 432
O^6-Alkylguanine DNA alkyltransferase. *See* O^6-Methylguanine-DNA methyltransferase (MGMT)

573

ALL. *See* Acute lymphoblastic (lymphocytic) leukemia (ALL)
Allison, James, 3, 536
all-trans retinoic acid (ATRA), in APML treatment, 321, 322f
Alpelisib, 121, 474
　indications for, 467t
　mechanism of action of, 463f, 474f
Alpha-fetoprotein, 528
Alpha-ketoglutarate (α-KG), and epigenetic enzyme activity, 59, 59f
αSMA. *See* Smooth muscle actin, α-SMA
ALT. *See* Alternative lengthening of telomeres (ALT)
ALT-associated PML bodies (APBs), 215
Altered self, 519
Alternate hypothesis, 553
Alternative lengthening of telomeres (ALT), 212, 214, 215–216
American Society of Clinical Oncology, Value Framework, 558
Ames test, 105–106, 105f
Amifostine
　protective effects of, 421
　radioprotective effects of, 389
Amino acid(s), synthesis of, 287, 287f
80-Amino-acid motif. *See* Death domain (DD)
4-Aminobiphenyl, 107
　bioactivation, CYP enzymes in, 109
2-Amino-3-methylimidazo[4,5-f]quinoline (IQ), 99f, 100
Aminopeptidase(s), 259, 260f
AML. *See* Acute myelogenous (myeloid) leukemia (AML)
Amphiregulin, and cancer progression, 237–238, 237t
AMPK. *See* Adenosine monophosphate-activated protein kinase (AMPK)
Amplicons, 145
Amsterdam signature, 243
Anal cancer, human papillomavirus and, 85
Analysis of variance (ANOVA), 83, 548
Anaphase, 167, 170, 173f, 174
　early, 166f
　late, 166f
Anaphase promoting complex (APC), 208, 209f
Anaphase-promoting complex/cyclosome (APC/C), 167, 168f, 169–170, 169f, 170f, 172–174, 173f, 178–180
Anaplastic lymphoma kinase (ALK), targeted therapy and, 467t, 469f, 478–479
Anastrozole, 498, 499f
　structure of, 499f
Anchoring filaments, 250f
Androgen(s)
　adrenal, 488
　intratumoral production of, in prostate cancer, 508–509, 508f
　nontranscriptional actions of, 494f, 495
　and prostate cancer, 488, 508–509, 508f
　synthesis of, 488, 489f, 490f
　transport in blood, 488–489
Androgen deprivation therapy (ADT)
　adverse effects, 505
　intermittent, 505–506
　for prostate cancer, 503–505
　　resistance to, 507–508, 508f
Androgen insensitivity syndrome, 491
Androgen receptor(s), 490f, 491
　activation of, 491–494, 492f
　alterations, in prostate cancer, 507–508, 508f
　alternative regulatory pathways for, 494–495, 494f
　amplification, in prostate cancer, 507, 508f
　crosstalk with growth factor networks, 494–495
　DNA binding by, 492, 492f
　homopolymers in, 491
　inhibitors, advances in, 509
　mutations, in prostate cancer, 507–508, 508f
Androgen suppression, intermittent, 505–506, 506f
Anemia. *See also* Fanconi anemia
　aplastic, 215
　prognostic significance of, 382
　and radiotherapy, 299
　treatment of, 279
Anergy, 524
Aneuploidy, 179–180, 277
　and prognosis, 280
Angiogenesis, 2, 143, 233, 283, 466–468
　cell populations involved in, 249–251, 251f
　definition of, 248
　developmental, 251, 252f
　hypoxia and, 263–265, 264f, 295f, 296f, 297, 297f
　inhibitors of, 259–260, 261f
　intussusceptive, 252, 261f, 262
　mechanisms of, 252–255, 253f
　molecular regulators of, 253f, 256–262, 256f, 257t, 259f–262f
　MYC and, 151f
　nonproductive, 255
　pathologic, stimulators involved in, 257t
　protease regulation of, 259, 260f
　sprouting, 252–254, 253f, 261f
　stimulators of, 259–260, 261f
　targetable, molecular spectrum of, 272
　tumor, 262–266, 283
　　coagulation system and, 260
　　comorbidity and, 266
　　genetic background and, 266
　　modifiers of, 266–267
　　molecular regulators of, 256, 257t
　　onset of, 263
　　platelets and, 260
　　progression of, 263
　　unique characteristics of, 266–267
　　vascular aging and, 266
　in tumor progression, 260, 262f
　vascular splitting in, 252, 262f
Angiogenesis enhancement therapy, 272
Angiogenesis inhibitors, endogenous, 257t
Angiogenic effectors, 257t
Angiogenic hot spots, 264f
Angiogenic sprouts, 253f, 254
Angiogenic switch, 260, 262f, 263, 297
Angiogenin, 257t
Angiopoietin, 258, 265
　ANG1, 257t, 258
　　in angiogenesis, 254, 254f
　　hypoxia and, 297f
　　and lymphangiogenesis, 254f, 255
　　and vascular maturation, 255
　ANG2, 257t, 258, 270
　　in angiogenesis, 254, 254f
　　and lymphangiogenesis, 254f, 255
　ANG4, 258
　and TIE2, 254f, 258
Angiostatin, 257t, 260, 268
ANGPT4, and metastasis, 231f, 233
Animal(s). *See also* Mice
　bioassays in
　　for carcinogens, 106–107
　　dose–response relationship and, 106–107, 107f
　imaging of, 338–340, 339f, 340f
　organ specificity of metastasis in, 235, 235f
　safety pharmacology studies of anticancer drugs in, 418–419
　studies of molecular signatures of exposure and risk in, 109
　studies of targeted agents in, 462
Ankyrin, 127, 127f, 229, 229f
Anoikis, 181, 226
ANOVA. *See* Analysis of variance (ANOVA)
Antagonism, of combined drugs, 419–420, 421f
Anthracenediones, 442–443
Anthracycline(s), 442–443
　adverse effects of, pharmacogenetic studies of, 89, 89t
　dosage and administration of, 443
　resistance to, 446t, 449t, 450
Antiandrogens, 490f
　advances in (novel approaches), 509
　adverse effects, 505
　nonsteroidal, 503–504
　in prostate cancer treatment, 503–505
　structure of, 505f
Antiandrogen withdrawal syndrome, 505
Antiangiogenesis, 248, 263
　aging and, 266
Antiangiogenic agent(s) (AAs), 267–270, 268t, 269f
　adverse effects, 271
　ANG/TIE2 inhibitors as, 270
　based on activity of endogenous angiogenesis inhibitors, 268
　combinations of, 270
　first-generation exogenous, 268
　indirectly acting, designed to block oncogenic pathways, 268t
　molecularly targeted, 268–269, 268t
　originally developed for non-antiangiogenic indications, 268t
　resistance to, 270
　targeting angiogenic cells, 268t, 269f
　targeting growth factors, 268–270, 268t, 269f
　targeting oncogenic pathways, 268t, 269f, 271
　therapeutic response to, biomarkers of, 271
　toxicity of, 271
　tumor specificity of, 271
　VEGF/VEGFR inhibitors as, 268–270, 268t
Antiangiogenic therapies, 267–270, 268t, 269f
　challenges of, 271–272
　opportunities associated with, 271–272
Antibiotic resistance gene(s), in gene transfer methods, 23–24
Antibody-based anticancer therapy, 409. *See also* Monoclonal antibody(ies) (mAb); *specific agent*
　indications for, 467t
　mechanism of action of, 462–464, 463f
Antibody-dependent cell-mediated cytotoxicity (ADCC), 464, 532–533, 534f, 537
Antibody drug conjugates (ADC), 409
Anticancer drug(s). *See also specific drug*
　active, identification of, 406–407
　active metabolites of, 430
　activity, modifiers of, 421
　alkylating agents as, 432–436
　antimetabolites as, 436–440

antimicrotubular agents as, 443–445
as carcinogens, 417–418
cell death caused by, types of, 453
and cognitive dysfunction, 417
combinations
 additive effects of, 419–420, 420f, 421f
 antagonism of, 419–420, 421f
 dose-response relationships and, 419–420, 420f, 421f
 effects on therapeutic index, 419
 subadditive effects of, 420, 421f
 supra-additive effects of, 420, 421f
 synergy of, 419–420, 420f, 421f
 therapeutic benefit of, mechanisms of, 419
 toxicity of, 419
cost utility analysis for, 561
development of, 177. See also Clinical trials
 accelerated, 550
 functional genomic screens and, 405–406
 high throughput DNA sequencing and, 404
 rational drug design in, 407, 407f
 RNA sequencing and, 404, 405f
 strategies for, 404–407
diarrhea caused by, 417
diffusion in tissue, 280, 280f
directed delivery of, 410
dose
 and antitumor effect, 414, 414f
 and normal tissue toxicity, 414, 414f
dose–response curves for, 414–415, 414f
dosing, in individual patients, 431
drug interactions with, 430
effective dose-50 (ED-50), 414, 414f
fatigue caused by, 417
first-in-human phase I trial, 411f
 preclinical data needed for, 418–419
hair loss caused by, 417
and hand-foot syndrome, 417, 439
human studies of, 462
infertility caused by, 417
liposomal, 445–446
mechanism of action of, determination of, 412
myelosuppressive, 415–416, 416f
 dosage and administration of, 415–416
nanoparticle formulations of, 446
nausea and vomiting caused by, 417
new strategies using, 407–410
normal tissue toxicity of, 414–415, 414f
 determinants of, 418
pharmacodynamic/pharmacokinetic relationships of, 462
potential targets for, identification of, 404
preclinical evaluation of, 410–414, 411f
 in vitro, 410–412, 411f
 in vivo, 411f, 412–414, 413f
and proliferating tissues, 278
and radiation, combined, 421–424, 422f, 422t, 423f
with radiation therapy, effects on therapeutic index, 419, 421–424, 422t, 423f, 424f
and radiation toxicity, 424
resistance to. See also Drug resistance
 molecular mechanisms of, 446–448, 446t, 447f
safety pharmacology studies of, 418–419
screening for
 chemical libraries in, 406
 in libraries of known drugs, 407
 natural product libraries in, 406–407
side effects of, 415, 417

starting dose, for first-in-human phase I trial, 419
targeted. See Molecular targeted therapies; Targeted agents
targets, determination of, 412
therapeutic index of, 414–415, 414f, 431
 combination therapy and, 419
 modifiers and, 421
topoisomerase inhibitors as, 440–443
toxic dose-05 (TD-05), 414, 414f
toxic dose-50 (TD-50), 414f
toxicity of, 414–419
 in bone marrow, and treatment scheduling, 415–416
 genetic polymorphisms leading to, 431–432
 modifiers of, 421
 in mucosa, 416–417
Anti-CRISPR, 30
Antiestrogens
 in breast cancer treatment, 490f, 498–499
 mechanism of action of, 500
 structure of, 499f
Antifolates, 436–437
Antigen(s), 515. See also Tumor-associated antigens (TAAs)
 cross-presentation of, 517f, 518
 T-cell recognition of, 516–518, 516f, 517f
Antigen presentation, 515–518
Antigen-presenting cell(s) (APCs), 515–516, 516f
 Tregs and, 525
Antigen-processing pathways, 516–518, 517f
Anti-inflammatory agents, radioprotective effects of, 389
Antimetabolites, 436–440. See also specific agent
 cell-cycle specificity of, 436
 dosage and administration of, 436
 resistance to, 446, 446t
Antimicrotubular agents, 443–445. See also specific agent
Antioxidants
 and cellular effects of radiation, 351–352
 dietary, and cancer chemoprevention, 110
 radioprotective effects of, 389
 and reactive oxygen species accumulation, 290, 290f
Antisense oligonucleotides, in anticancer therapy, 409–410
Antitumor immunity
 barriers to, 531
 and tumor progression, 529–530, 530f
Antivascular agents, 268t
Aortic valve, bicuspid, 128
AP1, 518
Apalutamide, 505, 509
APBs. See ALT-associated PML bodies (APBs)
APC. See Adenomatous polyposis coli (APC); Anaphase promoting complex (APC)
APC/C. See Anaphase-promoting complex/cyclosome (APC/C)
APC gene, 142t
APCs. See Antigen-presenting cell(s) (APCs)
APHINITY trial, 558
Aplastic anemia, 215
APL or APML. See Acute promyelocytic leukemia (APML)
Apoptosis, 97, 167, 181, 224, 226, 523, 524, 534f
 BCL-2 family in, 182, 182f, 184f
 in Caenorhabditis elegans, 182, 182f
 caspases in, 182–183
 death receptor pathway, 183f, 184–185

deregulation
 and developmental defects, 185–186
 and disease, 185–186
drug sensitivity and, 446t, 453
drugs promoting, 407
hypoxia and, 296, 296f, 297f
inhibition, by tumor promoters, 102
in mammalian cells, 182, 182f, 183f
mechanisms of, 181–182, 182f
mitochondrial pathway, 183f, 184, 474f, 480
modifications, in cancer, 188
morphologic changes during, 181, 181f
MYC and, 150, 151f
and necroptosis, 187f
quantification of, 410
radiation-induced, 353, 353f, 356, 363, 386
regulation of, 480
resistance to, 143, 149
sphingomyelin/ceramide-mediated, in irradiated cells, 363
suppression, in cancer cells, 122
in treatment response, 446t, 453
Apoptosis-inducing factor (AIF), 182
Apoptotic index, 410
Apparent diffusion coefficient (ADC) imaging, 334, 335f
Aprepitant, for nausea and vomiting, 417
ara-C. See Cytosine arabinoside
Area under the curve (AUC), 430–431, 431t
Arginase-1 (ARG1), 538
Arginine-glycine-aspartic acid (RGD) peptides, integrin-blocking, 125
Argonaute proteins, 24
ARNT. See Aryl hydrocarbon receptor nuclear translocator (ARNT)
Aromatase inhibitors, 3. See also specific agent
 adverse effects of, pharmacogenetic studies of, 89, 89t
 in breast cancer treatment, 498–499
 nonsteroidal, 498–499, 499f
 resistance, 503
  in breast cancer, 501–503, 504f
 steroidal, 498, 499f
 structure of, 499f
Aromatic amines
 as carcinogens, 99f
 metabolic activation of, 100, 101f
Arresten, 260
Arsenic trioxide, in APML treatment, 321
Artemis, 203, 203f
 and radiosensitivity, 362f
Arteriogenesis, 251–252, 252f, 261f, 264
Arteriole(s), 250f
Arylamine N-acetyltransferases (NATs), 100
 activity, genetic variations in, and cancer risk, 108
Aryl hydrocarbon receptor nuclear translocator (ARNT), 295, 295f
ASA 404. See Vadimezan
Asbestos, and lung cancer, 1, 104
Ascertainment bias, 80t
ASF1, and alternative lengthening of telomeres, 215
Aspirin, and methotrexate, interactions of, 437
Association, tests for, 83
Astrocytoma, IDH1/2 mutations in, 477
Ataxia-telangiectasia (AT), 200t, 210
 and anticancer drug toxicity, 418
 and radiosensitivity, 359, 360f, 361, 389
Ataxia-telangiectasia and Rad3 related (ATR). See ATR (ATM- and Rad3-related)

Ataxia telangiectasia mutated (ATM)
        protein, 203, 203f, 210
    cell-cycle checkpoint activation
            downstream of, 207–208, 208f
    and cell-cycle checkpoints, 205–208, 206f, 357
    mutations, and radiosensitivity, 378
    and radiosensitivity, 360f, 362, 362f
    and risk from carcinogen exposure, 108
ATG genes, 291
ATLD. See AT-like disorder (ATLD)
AT-like disorder (ATLD), 200t, 204, 210
ATM. See Ataxia telangiectasia
        mutated (ATM) protein
ATM gene, 180, 210
    defects, and BRCA-ness, 476
ATP. See Adenosine triphosphate (ATP)
ATP-binding cassette (ABC) transporters.
        See also specific transporter
    drug resistance mediated by, reversal of, 451
    and multidrug resistance, 449, 449t
    physiologic roles of, 449, 449f, 452
    structure of, 450, 450f
ATR (ATM- and Rad3-related), 205
    cell-cycle checkpoint activation
            downstream of, 207–208, 208f
    and cell-cycle checkpoints, 205–208, 357
ATRA. See all-trans retinoic acid (ATRA)
ATR gene, 180
    defects, and BRCA-ness, 476
ATRX, and alternative lengthening
        of telomeres, 215
AUC. See Area under the curve (AUC)
AURKA, 166f
Aurora kinase (AUR)
    AUR A, 172–174, 173f
    AUR B, 172–174, 173f, 179
    inhibitors, 3, 178, 180
Autofluorescence imaging, 338, 338f
Automated Cancer Information System (ACIS), 74
Autophagosome, 291, 292f
Autophagy, 133, 181, 186–187, 284, 291–292, 453
    cellular functions in cancer, 291–292
    enhanced
        and resistance to hormonal
            therapy, 503, 504f
        and tumor dormancy, 503
    hypoxia and, 292, 292f, 296, 296f, 297f
    inhibition, 292
    morphologic changes during, 181, 181f
    process of, 291, 292f
    and tamoxifen resistance in breast
            cancer, 503, 504f
Autoradiography, 276
Avian leukosis virus (AVL), 150
AVL. See Avian leukosis virus (AVL)
Axitinib, 268t, 270, 469, 469f
Azacitidine, 60–61, 148t
5'-Aza-deoxycytidine, 195
Azo dyes, as carcinogens, 98, 104

B

Bacille Calmette-Guérin (BCG), 534
Bacteriophage, 106
BAGE, 528
BAK, 184, 184f
Bannayan-Riley-Ruvalcaba syndrome, 156
B[a]P. See Benzo[a]pyrene
BARD1 protein, 158
Basal cell carcinoma (BCC), 196
    hedgehog inhibitors for, 129
    hedgehog signaling in, 129

Base excision repair (BER), 198–200, 199f
    defects, cancer-prone human syndromes
            associated with, 200t
    long-patch, 199
    short-patch, 199
Basement membrane, 226
    of vasculature, 250f
Base pair(s), 6–7, 8f
Basic zipper proteins, 122
Basket trials, 481, 551, 551f
BAX, 182, 184, 184f
Bayesian methods, 548
Bayes theorem, 565–566
BCC. See Basal cell carcinoma (BCC)
B-cell receptor (BCR), 519
B-cell receptor (BCR) pathway
        inhibitors, 479–480
B cells (B lymphocytes), 515, 516
    antigen recognition by, 519
BCG. See Bacille Calmette-Guérin (BCG)
Bcl-2, 149
    and apoptosis, 453
    small molecule inhibitors of, 407
    targeted therapy and, 409
BCL-2, and apoptosis, 188
BCL2 gene, 24, 145, 196
BCL-2 homology domain 3. See BH3
BCL-2 homology (BH) regions, 182,
        184f. See also BH3
BCL-2 proteins, 480
    anti-apoptotic, 184f
    in apoptosis, 143, 182, 182f, 184f
    deregulation or deficiency, and
            disease, 185–186
    pro-apoptotic, 184, 184f
    and tamoxifen resistance, 502
    targeted therapy and, 467t
    ubiquitination of, 184
BCR. See B-cell receptor (BCR)
BCR-ABL, targeted therapy and, 478
BCR-ABL1, targeted therapy and, 467t
BCR-ABL fusion gene, 142t, 144,
        147t, 150, 404, 408
BCR-ABL inhibitors, 464, 464f
BCR-ABL protein kinase, 2, 148f, 150
Beclin 1, 187f
Belinostat, 61, 477
Bendamustine, 433
    indications for, 434
    structure of, 432, 433f
Benign prostatic hyperplasia (BPH), 488, 498
Benzidine, 104
    potency as carcinogen, 107t
Benzo[a]pyrene
    as carcinogen, 98, 99f
    CYP1A1-activated, and DNA adduct
            formation in lung cancer, 108, 108f
    metabolic activation of, 100, 100f
BER. See Base excision repair (BER)
Berkson's bias, 75, 80t
BETi. See Bromodomain inhibitors (BETi)
Bevacizumab, 268–269, 268t, 269f,
        403–404, 468–469, 469f, 532t
    mechanism of action of, 463f, 464
B16F10 cells, 235, 235f
BH3, 182, 184f
    pro-apoptotic proteins and, 182, 184f
BH3 inhibitors, 480
BH3 mimetics, 188, 464, 464f, 480
Bias
    ascertainment, 80t

assessment, in meta-analysis, 558
    in cancer screening, 80–81, 80t
    in case-control studies, 75–76
    in clinical trials, 552, 554
    confounding and, 78–79, 79f
    in cross-sectional study, 77–78
    detection, 80t
    diagnostic-review, 564, 567
    in diagnostic tests, sources of, 563–564, 563t
    in epidemiologic studies, 75–78, 80t
    experimenter's, 80t
    in familial studies, 78
    information, 79–80, 80t
    interviewer, 80t
    lead-time, 80–81, 80t, 564–565, 565f
    length-time, 80, 564, 564f
    overdiagnosis, 80, 80t
    prevalence, 77
    publication, 92, 558
    recall, 76, 79, 80t
    referral, 567
    sampling, 79–80, 80t
    selection, 79–80, 80t, 554
    self-selection, 80t
    survival, 78, 80t
    test-review, 564, 567
    workup, 564, 567
Bicalutamide, 503–504
    structure of, 505f
BID, 184, 184f, 185
BIK, 184, 184f
Bile duct carcinoma, tumor-suppressor
        genes in, 142t
BIM, 184, 184f, 188
Binimetinib, 475–476
    indications for, 467t
    mechanism of action of, 474f
Bioavailability
    absolute, 430
    factors affecting, 430
    P-glycoprotein inhibition and, 450
    relative, 430
BioGRID, 44
BioID, 30
Bioinformatics, 41
    machine learning and, 342
Bioluminescence, in imaging of animal
        models, 340, 340f
Biomarker(s), 465–466, 550. See
        also Tumor markers
    analytical validity of, 466
    and cancer risk, evaluation of, 91
    for carcinogen exposure, 107–108, 108f
    classification of, by potential appplication in
            anticancer therapy, 466, 467t–468t
    clinical use of, 465–466
    path to, 90, 91f
    clinical utility of, demonstration of, 466
    development of, steps in, 90, 91f
    diagnostic, 466, 468f
    discovery of, 90, 91f
        with proteomics, challenges for,
            36–37, 36f
    of genetic instability, 195
    for hypoxia, 294
    identification of, 109, 466
    and personalized medicine, 551
    pharmacogenomic evaluation of, 88
    predictive, 466, 468f
    prognostic, 466, 468f
    as prognostic indicators, 554

prognostic significance of, 567–568
of therapeutic response to
antiangiogenic agents, 271
Biorientation, 209
Biotin, in fluorescence in situ hybridization, 11
Biotin, in proteomics, 30
Biotin ligase(s), 30
Bispecific T cell–engagers (BiTEs), 409, 533–534
Bisphosphonates, adjuvant treatment with, in breast cancer, 243
Bisulfite sequencing, 307
single-cell genome-wide, 307
BiTEs. See Bispecific T cell–engagers (BiTEs)
Bladder cancer
Bacille Calmette-Guérin for, 534
carcinogens and, 104
gene fusion in, 147t
oncogenes in, 142t
radiotherapy for, with concomitant nicotinamide and carbogen, 383
risk, genetic variations in, 108
schistosomal infection and, 85, 103
secondary, cyclophosphamide and, 432
smoking and, 87, 87f
targeted therapy for, 467t
treatment of, hypoxia and, 298t
tumor-suppressor genes in, 142t
Bleomycin, 415
adverse effects, 445
indications for, 445
mechanism of action of, 445
mucosal damage caused by, 417
pharmacokinetics of, 445
pulmonary fibrosis caused by, 445
Bleomycin hydrolase, 445
Blinatumomab, 403–404, 409, 532t, 533–534
Blocking, of groups of patients, 553
Blood-brain barrier, 249
Blood cancer. See also Hematologic malignancies
hedgehog inhibitors for, 129
Blood supply. See also Angiogenesis; Vasculogenesis
and cell proliferation in tumors, 280, 280f
Blood transfusion(s), 299
and radiotherapy, 382
Blood vessels
anticancer therapy targeted to, 267–272, 268t, 269f
adverse effects, 271
alternative approaches, 271–272
therapeutic response to, biomarkers for, 271
tumor specificity of, 271
differentiated vs. undifferentiated, prognostic significance of, 309
invasion by cancer, 261f
permeabilization of, 261f
tumor-initiating, 267
Bloom syndrome, 200t
Blotting technique(s), 9–10, 10f. See also Northern blotting; Southern blotting; Western blotting
BMDCs. See Bone marrow–derived regulatory and progenitor cells (BMDCs)
BMI1 signaling, 313, 314t
BMP. See Bone morphogenetic protein(s) (BMP)
BMS-777607, 134
BMS-906024, 128
BMT. See Bone marrow transplantation (BMT)
BNCT. See Boron neutron capture therapy (BNCT)

Body surface area (BSA), and drug dosing, 431
Body weight. See also Obesity
and cancer prevention, 110
BOK, 184f
Bombina variegata-secreted protein 8 (Bv8), 257t, 258
Bone cancer. See also Multiple myeloma (MM)
gene fusion in, 147t
Bone marrow
anticancer drug toxicity in, and treatment scheduling, 415–416
cell proliferation in, 278–279, 278t
precursor cells in, proliferation and maturation of, 415, 416f
Bone marrow–derived regulatory and progenitor cells (BMDCs), 249, 251f, 252, 265
Bone marrow transplantation (BMT), lymphocyte infusions after, 539
Bone morphogenetic protein(s) (BMP)
and metastasis, 233, 234f
and tumor dormancy, 236
Bone scan, SPECT for, 335
Bonferroni correction, 43, 92
Borealin, 209
Boron neutron capture therapy (BNCT), 374
Bortezomib, 133, 271, 408
adverse effects, 479
indications for, 479
mechanism of action of, 454, 479
Bosutinib, 142t
indications for, 467t
Boveri, Theodore, 140, 143f
BPH. See Benign prostatic hyperplasia (BPH)
Brachytherapy, 350, 372–373
computer-controlled, 372
high-dose-rate, 370, 371f, 372
low-dose-rate, 370, 372
pulsed-dose, 372
BRAF
targeted therapy and, 467t, 475–476
V600 mutants, 404, 528
B-RAF gene, 142t
V600 mutants, 154–155, 404
BRAF inhibitors, 119–120
and keratoacanthomas, 475
for melanoma, 321
and secondary squamous cell carcinoma, 418
and secondary squamous cell carcinoma, 418
BRAF kinase, 2
mutations, in cancer, 119
BRAF/MEK inhibitors, 475–476
BRAF mutations, 2
activating, cancer associated with, 154–155, 154f
in melanoma, 119–120, 154, 154f, 196, 306–307, 307f, 320, 528, 528f, 568
and targeted therapy, 158–159, 404
and treatment, 321
targeted therapy for, 155, 158–159, 404, 475–476
BRAF-SND1 fusion gene, 147t
Bragg peak, 351, 351f, 374
Brain-derived neurotrophic factor (BDNF), receptor, 114f
Brain metastases, 233
branched evolution of, 320
private mutations in, 320
Brain tumors
cancer stem cells in, 315–316
radiomics studies of, 342–343, 344f

BRCA1, 202–203
BRCT domain, 158
and oxidative stress, 290
RING domain, 157–158
structure of, 157–158
BRCA2, 202–203
structure of, 158
BRCA1 and BRCA2 genes, 1, 142t, 180, 202–203, 211
automated sequencing of, 15f
and cancer-prone syndromes, 200t
mutations of, 157, 405–406, 476–477
and drug resistance, 452, 477
and risk from carcinogen exposure, 108
BRCA-ness, 476
Breakage-fusion-bridge cycle, 213
Breakpoint cluster region–Abelson. See BCR-ABL
Breast(s)
atypical hyperplasia (AH), 497–498, 497f
ductal carcinoma in situ (DCIS), 497–498, 497f
usual ductal hyperplasia (UDH), 497–498
Breast cancer
adjuvant therapy for
and cognitive dysfunction, 417
decision-making about, recurrence risk presentation and, 556–557
and second malignancies, 418
age-standardized incidence and mortality rates for, 72, 72f
alcohol and, 87–88
biomarkers in
predictive, 466
prognostic, 466
bone metastases, 235
formation of, 233, 234f
BRCA1/2 and, 157, 496
BRCA-deficient, treatment of, 3
BRCA1- or BRCA2-mutant, treatment of, 158
BRCA1/2-related, platinum chemotherapy for, 477
cancer stem cells in, 316–317, 319
and chemoresistance, 320
case fatality rate for, 71
CBL-b expression in, 134
CDK4/6 inhibitor therapy, 177
cellular radiosensitivity in, 378t
clonal and subclonal evolution of, 310
copy-number variations in, 17
Cowden syndrome and, 156
development and progression of, 497–498, 497f
driver mutations in, and treatment, 310
ERBB2(HER-2) in, 152
ERBB1 mutations in, 151
ER-positive, 3, 497–498
chemoprevention of, 110
gene enhancer methylation in, 56
resistance to hormonal therapy, 500–503, 504f
treatment of, 498–500
estrogen and, 495–496
estrogen/progesterone receptor status, 568
prognostic significance of, 495
and treatment outcomes, 89, 498
estrogen receptor coregulators in, 493–494
estrogen receptor heterogeneity in, 495, 496f
estrogen-responsive, 3
familial. See Familial breast and ovarian cancer
gene enhancer methylation in, 56
gene expression classifiers for, 3
gene expression profiling, 495
and survival prediction, 43

Breast cancer (*Cont.*)
  70-gene signature in, 43
  genetic and epigenetic heterogeneity of, interdependence of, 319
  genetic factors and, 496
  germline BRCA-mutated, 496
    treatment of, 477
  growth rate of, 276*f*
  HER2/ErbB2 in, 498, 568
  HER2 in, and targeted therapy, 158–159, 472–473
  HER2-negative
    hormone receptor-positive, 474, 476
    treatment of, 158, 474, 475, 476, 477
  Her2/neu status, and treatment outcomes, 89
  HER-2-overexpressing, treatment of, 409, 472–473
  HER2 status of, 3
    FISH of, 12
  heterogeneity of
    and chemoresistance, 320
    clinical significance of, 320
    and radioresistance, 320
  histopathology of, and imaging, integration of, 341, 342*f*
  hormonal therapy for, 498–500
    adjuvant, 500
    combined with targeted therapy, 503
    neoadjuvant (preoperative), 500
    new approaches to, 503
    resistance to, 500–503, 504*f*
    by stage, 500
    and switching of endocrine agents, 503
  hormone-sensitive, cell line derived from, 23
  imaging, and histopathology, integration of, 341, 342*f*
  and immunity against breast TAAs, 529
  incidence of, time trends in, 72*f*, 74
  invasiveness gene signature in, 319
  magnetic resonance imaging of, 341, 342*f*
  metastases and relapse
    genomic evolution of, 311, 320
    principal sites of, 234*t*
    treatment to prevent, 243
  microRNAs in, 147
  molecular profiling of, 3, 498
  monoclonal antibody therapy for, 532*t*
  MRI in, 334–335
  natural history of, 497*f*
  NOTCH signaling in, 128
  oncogenes in, 142*t*
  outcomes with, factors affecting, 561
  P-glycoprotein increase in, prognostic significance of, 450
  photoacoustic imaging of, 341, 342*f*
  PIK3CA-mutated, 474
  PI3-kinase signaling alterations in, 153, 153*f*
  PTEN promoter methylation in, 157, 157*f*
  risk factors for, 495–496
  screening
    and outcomes, 561
    and overdiagnosis, 72
  second malignancy after, 418
  sex steroids and, 488
  SIADH with, 509
  smoking and, 87*f*
  subtypes, 498
  targeted therapy for, 467*t*
  treatment, 2, 3
    multigene signatures and, 243, 495, 566

  triple-negative, 157
    anti-PD-1 mAb efficacy in mice, 134
    tumor-suppressor genes in, 142*t*
    variant enhancer loci in, 57
    WNT pathway inhibitors for, 127
    WNT signaling in, 126
Breast Cancer Association Consortium, 92
Breast cancer resistance protein (BCRP). *See* ABCG2/BCRP
Bremsstrahlung radiation, 350
Brigatinib, 142*t*, 469*f*, 478–479
  indications for, 467*t*
5-Bromodeoxyuridine, 277, 277*f*
Bromodomain inhibitors (BETi), 60*f*, 61–62
Bromodomain proteins, 61
Bronchial carcinoid, Cushing syndrome with, 509
Bronticuzumab, 128
Bruton tyrosine kinase (BTK), 479
Bruton tyrosine kinase (BTK) inhibitor, 479–480
  resistance to, 480
BSA. *See* Body surface area (BSA)
BUB1, and mitotic spindle checkpoint, 208–209, 209*f*
BUB1, 180
BUB3, and mitotic spindle checkpoint, 208–209, 209*f*
BUBR1 protein, 195
  and mitotic spindle checkpoint, 208–209, 209*f*
  MYC and, 151*f*
BUBR1 gene, 180
Buparlisib, 474
  mechanism of action of, 474*f*
Burkitt lymphoma (BL)
  chromosomal abnormalities in, 7*t*, 148*f*
  EBV and, 86, 149
  gene fusion in, 147*t*
  molecular lesions in, 7*t*
  MYC upregulation in, 150
Burrows-Wheeler transform, 15
Buserelin, in prostate cancer treatment, 503
Busulfan
  adverse effects, 434
  indications for, 434
  mechanism of action of, 434
Bv8. *See* Bombina variegata-secreted protein 8 (Bv8)
Bystander effect, 299, 363, 363*f*
Bystander suppression, 525

C
Cabazitaxel, 444
Cabozantinib, 268*t*, 469*f*, 470
CADASIL, 128
Cadherins, 228–230, 229*f*, 284
  and metastasis, 232
  vascular endothelial, 258–259, 259*f*
  and vascular maturation, 255
Caenorhabditis elegans, apoptosis in, 182, 182*f*
CAFs. *See* Cancer-associated fibroblasts (CAFs)
CAK. *See* CDK-activating kinase (CAK)
Calpains, 226*t*, 228
CAMDR. *See* Cell adhesion–mediated drug resistance (CAMDR)
Camptothecin
  mechanism of action of, 440
  pharmacology of, 440–441
  structure of, 441*f*
Camptothecin derivatives, resistance to, 449*t*
CAMs. *See* Cell adhesion molecules (CAMs)
Cancer-associated fibroblasts (CAFs), 238, 239*f*, 265, 281–283, 309, 309*f*
  molecular markers for, 282, 282*t*

Cancer biology, historical perspective on, 1–2
Cancer cell lines, 23
Cancer discoveries, timeline of, 139–141, 143*f*
Cancer Genome Atlas, 176, 548
Cancer incidence, 72
Cancer-initiating cells, 314
Cancer prevalence, 72
Cancers of unknown primary (CUP), epigenetic identity and, 63, 64*f*
Cancer stem cell (CSC)–derived endothelium, 261*f*
Cancer stem cells (CSCs), 2, 306, 313–317
  in brain tumors, 315–316
  in breast cancer, 316–317, 319
  in colorectal cancer, 315, 317
  functional classification of, 314
  in hematologic malignancies, 314–315, 315*f*
  hypoxia and, 297, 297*f*
  and integrin signaling, 228
  markers for, 314
  in melanoma, 316*f*, 317
  in metastasis, 236
  number of, in tumor, and dose response in radiotherapy, 375–377, 377*f*
  origin of, 314
  prognostic significance of, 319–320
  in prostate cancer, 315, 498
  radioresistance in, 362, 377
  radiosensitivity of, 378
    and dose response in radiotherapy, 375
    factors affecting, 377
  in recurrence, 236
  repopulation by, after hormone therapy, 498
  signaling pathways in, 313, 314*t*
  in solid tumors, 315–317, 316*f*
  and tumor angiogenesis, 267
  and xenograft formation, 313–314
Cancer stem cells (CSCs) hypothesis, 313, 314*f*
  criticism of, 317, 318*f*
Cancer treatment
  cancer heterogeneity and, 320–323, 322*f*
  future directions for, 3–4
  image guidance in, 341–342
  recent advances in, 2–3
  response to, clonal dynamics in, 311
Capecitabine
  enzymatic activation of, 439, 439*f*
  and hand-foot syndrome, 417, 439
  indications for, 439
  metabolism of, 439
  pharmacology of, 439
  structure of, 438*f*
  toxicity of, 439
Capillaries, 249, 250*f*
Carbogen breathing, with concomitant nicotinamide, in radiotherapy, 383
Carbonic anhydrase-9 (CA-9), hypoxia and, 294
Carbon ions, in radiotherapy, 374
Carbon tetrachloride, potency as carcinogen, 107*f*
Carboplatin
  dosage and administration of, 431, 435
  indications for, 435–436
  mechanism of action of, 435
  pharmacokinetics of, 435
  pharmacology of, 435
  structure of, 435, 435*f*
  toxicity of, 435–436
Carboxyaminotriazole, 268
Carcinoembryonic antigen, 527, 528
Carcinogen(s), 1, 97
  animal bioassays for, 106–107

anticancer drugs as, 417–418
assays for, 103, 104t
  cellular transformation, 106
  long-term, 104t
  short-term, 104–106, 104t
chemical, 98–103
  assessment of, 103–107, 104f
    features that cause difficulty in, 104, 105t
  EPA classification of, 103
  exogenous vs. endogenous, 102
  potency, range of, 107, 107t
DNA-adducted, identification of, 105
exposure
  biomarkers for, 107–108, 108f
  risk from, genetic variation in, 108
genotoxic, 97–98, 98–100, 99f
  direct-acting, 99, 99f
nongenotoxic, 97–98
population epidemiology of, 104
Carcinogen-adduct formation, 101
  as biomarker for cancer risk, 108, 108f
  studies of, 70, 98
Carcinogenesis, 97–110. See also Malignant transformation
  alkylating agents and, 432
  DNA methylation in, 20, 54–57, 55f, 56f
  epigenetic changes associated with, 54–57, 55f, 56f, 225, 225f
  genetic changes associated with, 225, 225f
  microRNAs in, 24
  models of, 97–98
  molecular epidemiology of, 107–109
  molecular signatures of exposure and risk in, 108–109
  secondary, 356
  stages of, 98–97
Carcinogenic risk, assessment of, 103–107, 104f
Carcinoid, bronchial, Cushing syndrome with, 509
CARDs. See Caspase recruitment domains (CARDs)
Carfilzomib, 133, 408
  adverse effects, 479
  indications for, 479
  mechanism of action of, 463f, 479
CAR-T cells, and WNT-related disease, 127
Case-cohort study design, 75–76
Case-control studies, 75–76, 75f
  bias in, 80t
  nested, 75–76
  population-based, 75
Case fatality rate/ratio, 71, 564
Case series, 76
Caspase(s)
  in apoptosis, 182–183
  CASP1, 518
  CASP8, modifications, and cancer, 188
  and death receptor apoptotic pathway, 185
  "executioner," 182
  "initiator," 182
  mammalian, 182, 185f
  proinflammatory, 183
  substrates for, 183
  ubiquitination of, 184
Caspase recruitment domains (CARDs), 518
Castration-resistant prostate cancer (CRPC)
  definition of, 503
  intratumoral androgen production in, 508–509, 508f
  mechanisms of, 507–509, 507f, 508f

Catalase, 290
β-Catenin, 229–230, 229f
  in WNT signaling, 125–126, 126f, 229
Cathepsin inhibitors, 228
Cathepsins, 226t, 227–228, 259, 260f
  and metastasis, 231f, 232
  in tumor microenvironment, 284
CBL-b, 132
  genetic alterations of, 134
c-CBL, 132
CCDC6-RET fusion gene, 147t
CD3, 519, 520f
  monoclonal antibody against, 533–534
CD4, 515, 516f
CD8, 515, 516f
CD19, 528
  monoclonal antibody against, 532t, 533–534
CD20, 528
  monoclonal antibody against, 532t
  radiolabeled antibodies against, 374
  rituximab and, 409
CD24, in breast cancer, 316f, 317, 319
CD25, 524, 525
CD28, 521, 522f, 537
CD33, monoclonal antibody against, 532t
CD34, 249, 278
CD38, monoclonal antibody against, 532t
CD40, 149, 521, 522f
CD44, 229–230, 229f, 284
  in breast cancer, 316f, 317, 319
  in colorectal cancer, 317
CD52
  alemtuzumab and, 409
  monoclonal antibody against, 532t
CD80, 521, 521f, 522f, 537
CD82, and metastasis, 232
CD86, 521, 521f, 522f, 537
CD133
  in brain tumors, 315–316, 316f
  in colorectal cancer, 317
    prognostic significance of, 319
  in glioblastoma, 318
    and chemoresistance, 320
    prognostic significance of, 319
  in melanoma, 317
2CdA. See Cladribine (2CdA)
CDC. See Complement-dependent cytotoxicity (CDC)
CDC20, 168f, 170, 173f
CDC25, 168f, 169, 172
  MYC and, 150, 151f
CDC25A, and cell-cycle checkpoints, 357
CDC25C, and cell-cycle checkpoints, 357
CDH1, 168f, 170, 170f
CDK-activating kinase (CAK), 168f
CDK inhibitor proteins (CKIs), 164f, 168f, 169
  with hormonal agents, for breast cancer, 503
CDKIs. See Cyclin-dependent kinase inhibitor(s) (CDKIs)
CDKN2A, 176
  and angiogenesis, 265
CDKs. See Cyclin-dependent kinase(s) (CDKs)
CD40L, 521, 522f
cDNA. See Complementary DNA (cDNA)
CD74-ROS1 fusion gene, 147t
CDRs. See Complementarity-determining regions (CDRs)
CDT1, 165f, 170 172, 172f
CEA. See Carcinoembryonic antigen
Cell(s). See also Stem cell(s); Tumor cells
  cancer, isolation of, 307

drug-resistant, selection of, 448
drug-tolerant persister, 448
irradiated. See also Cell survival
  dose-sparing effect, 359
  repair of damage in vivo, 359, 360f
  repair of potentially lethal damage in, 359–360
  repair of sublethal damage, 358–359
  repopulation, 359
  sublethal damage to, 358, 359f
  survival curves, 355, 355f
  surviving fraction, 355
isolation
  from hematologic malignancies, 38
  from solid tumors, 38, 307
molecular analysis in, 38–41
pluripotent, 318
radiation damage in, 351–353
senescent, in tumors, 143
single
  molecular analysis of, 307
  phenotypic analysis of, 307
stromal. See also Stroma/Stromal cells
  isolation of, 307
super state, 318
totipotent, 318
Cell adhesion
  integrin-mediated, in solid tumors, and drug resistance, 454
  reduced, and metastasis, 231–232, 231f
Cell adhesion–mediated drug resistance (CAMDR), 454
Cell adhesion molecules (CAMs), 226, 228–230, 229f, 284
  in angiogenesis, 259
  epithelial (EpCAM), in detection of circulating tumor cells, 233
Cell–cell contact, in solid tumors, and drug resistance, 453–454
Cell culture, 1, 23
  and cancer heterogeneity, 308
  malignant transformation in, assays for, 106
  multilayered. See Multilayered cell cultures (MCCs)
  preclinical evaluation of anticancer drugs in, 410–412, 411f
Cell cycle, 163–167
  in cancer cells, 122
  CDK inhibitors and, 476
  and cell growth, 175–176, 176f
  checkpoints, 164f, 167, 172, 177f, 178
    and genome stability, 205–210
    inactivation, 209–210
    modification in cancer, 180
    radiation-induced, 356–357, 358f
    silencing, by adaptation, 209–210
    as therapeutic target, 180–181
  control, molecular mechanisms of, 167–170, 168f
  DNA damage response and, 177f, 178
  dysregulation, in cancer, 177
  G_0 phase, 164, 164f, 167, 171, 171f, 276
  G_1 phase, 163–165, 164f, 165f, 166f, 167, 170–171, 170f, 276–277, 277f
  and radiosensitivity, 358f
  G_2 phase, 163–165, 164f–166f, 167, 172, 172f, 276–277, 277f
  radiation-induced checkpoints and, 356–357, 358f
  and radiosensitivity, 358f
  growth factors and, 122
  G_1/S transition, 170, 170f, 171, 171f, 178

Cell cycle (Cont.)
  in cancer, 176–177, 177f
    radiation-induced checkpoints and, 356–357, 358f
    G_2/M transition, 170, 170f, 173f, 178, 277f
    checkpoints and, 178, 357
    metaphase-anaphase transition, 170
    M phase, 163–164, 164f, 167, 172, 172f, 276–277
    and radiosensitivity, 358f
  phases of, 163–164, 164f
    chemotherapy and, 411
    and radiation-induced damage, 356–357, 357f, 358f
    progression through, molecular mechanisms regulating, 170–175
    and radiosensitivity, redistribution in, 359
    regulators, degradation of, 169–170
    S phase, 163–165, 164f, 165f, 166f, 167, 170, 172, 172f, 276–277, 277f
      radiation-induced checkpoints and, 356–357, 358f
      and radiosensitivity, 358f
    telophase/G_1, 172f
    therapeutic targeting of, in cancer, 177–178, 177f
Cell-cycle analysis, 276–278, 277f, 278f
Cell cycle–targeting agents, 177
Cell death, 163, 181–188. See also Apoptosis; Necrosis; Senescence
  accidental, 181
  autophagic, 186–187. See also Autophagy
  chemotherapy and, 457–458, 457f
  control of, modifications, in cancer, 188
  drug-induced, assays, 410
  immunogenic, 187–188
  mitotic catastrophe and, 353f, 354, 356, 364
  modification by tumor promoters, 102
  modifiers, mechanism of action of, 463f
  morphologic changes during, 181, 181f
  pathways, radiation and, 353–354, 353f
  post-mitotic, 353f
  pre-mitotic, 353f
  radiation-induced, in normal tissue, 386
  radiation-related, 352, 353–356, 353t
  regulated, 181
  in tumors, 279
Cell growth, 175–176, 176f
  therapeutic targeting of, in cancer, 177–178, 177f
Cell lines
  derived from cancers, 23
  human, gene essentiality in, online resource on, 28
  online resource on, 23
Cell of origin, 109
Cell proliferation, 2, 163
  aneuploidy and, 179
  in bone marrow, 278–279, 278t
  in cancer, 176–177, 179
    telomere maintenance and, 215–216
    combined radiation and drug treatment and, 422–423
  combined treatment and, 421–424, 422t
  hypoxia and, 296, 296f, 297f
  in intestine, 278t, 279, 279f
  Ki67 as marker of, 277–278, 278f, 279
  modification by tumor promoters, 102
  molecular control of, 163–176
  MYC and, 151f
  in normal tissues, 278–279, 278t
  therapeutic targeting of, in cancer, 177–178
  in tumors, 279–280
    blood supply and, 280, 280f
    and prognosis, 280–281
Cell repopulation
  chemotherapy and, 457–458, 457f
  and tumor control after radiotherapy, 390–392, 391f, 422–423, 422t, 423f
  chemotherapy and, 422–423, 422t, 423f
CellSearch, 233, 320
Cell survival
  after radiation, 353f, 354, 354f
    assays for, 354–356, 354f, 355f
    as stochastic process, 355
    target-theory model of, 356, 367–368, 367f
  hypoxia and, 296, 296f, 297f
Cell survival curves. See also Survival curves
  for irradiated cells, 355, 355f
  in preclinical evaluation of anticancer drugs, 410–412, 412f
Cell transformation assays, 106
Cellular crisis, 214
Cellular energetics, deregulation, MYC and, 151f
Cellular FLICE-like inhibitory protein (cFLIP), 185
Cellular signaling, 113–134
  cytoplasmic tyrosine kinase in, 123–125
  developmental, 125–131
  dysregulation of, 113
  growth factors in, 113–123
  intracellular, after radiation, 363
  normal functions of, 113
  transcriptional response to, 121–122, 121f
  and tumor response to radiotherapy, 377
  ubiquitin-mediated proteolysis in, 131–134
Censored observations, 554–556
Centriole(s), 164, 164f, 166f, 179
Centromere(s), 164f, 167
Centrosome cycle, 164–165, 166f
Centrosomes, 164, 164f, 173f
  extra, 179
Cerebellar tumors, pediatric, fetal transcriptional programs in, 19
Cerebro-oculo-facio-skeletal syndrome (COFS), 200t
Ceritinib, 142t, 469f, 478–479, 550
  indications for, 467t
Cervical cancer
  cellular radiosensitivity in, and tumor response prediction, 378, 379f
  gene fusion in, 147t
  in HIV-infected (AIDS) patients, 529
  human papillomavirus and, 73, 85–86, 103, 149
  hypoxic
    prognostic significance of, 381, 382f
    radiotherapy for, and prognosis, 381–382, 382f
    surgical treatment, and prognosis, 381
  imaging of, 337f
  magnetic resonance imaging of, 330f
  oncogenes in, 142t
  PI3-kinase signaling alterations in, 153, 153f
  radiotherapy for, blood transfusion and, 382
  smoking and, 87
  staining of, 330f
  treatment of, hypoxia and, 298t
  tumor-suppressor genes in, 142t
  WNT signaling in, 126
Cetuximab, 115, 142t, 268t, 271, 403, 408, 465f, 469f, 471–472, 532t, 551
  indications for, 467t
  mechanism of action of, 464
  with radiation therapy, 375, 376f
CFI-400945, 181, 187
cFLIP. See Cellular FLICE-like inhibitory protein (cFLIP)
c-FOS, 119, 119f
cGAS, in intercellular response to radiation, 363–364
CGH. See Comparative genomic hybridization (CGH)
Charged particles, linear energy transfer of, 351, 351f, 351t
Checkpoint kinase 1 (CHK1), 121, 158, 357
Checkpoint kinase 2 (CHK2), 357
Chemical carcinogens, 98–103
Chemical libraries, 406
  with DNA barcoding and sequencing, 406
Chemical shift imaging (CSI), 334. See also Magnetic resonance spectroscopy imaging (MRSI)
Chemo-genetic interaction, 199–200, 453
Chemokine receptor(s) (CCR), 523
  and metastasis, 233
Chemokines
  and cancer progression, 237–238, 237t
  and metastasis, 231f
  production of, by antigen-presenting cells, 518, 518f
  in tumor microenvironment, 283
Chemoprevention, 109–110
  of prostate cancer, 110, 506
Chemoreceptors, in nausea and vomiting, 417
Chemotherapy, 177, 403, 429. See also Anticancer drug(s); Drug therapy; specific drug
  alkylating agents for, 432–436
  antimetabolites for, 436–440
  antimicrotubular agents for, 443–445
  and anti-PD-1 treatment, combined, 539
  cell-cycle dependent, 278
  cell killing during, 457–458, 457f
  cell repopulation during, 457–458, 457f
  curative, 431
  dosage and administration of, 415–416
  dosing, in individual patients, 431
  liposomal drugs for, 445–446
  metronomic, antiangiogenic effects of, 268t, 271
  miscellaneous agents for, 445
  palliative, 429
    dosage and administration of, 431
  resistance to, cancer heterogeneity and, 320, 321
  response to, cell proliferation and, 280–281
  second malignancy after, 418
  side effects of, 462
    and proliferating tissues, 278
  and targeted agents, combined, and therapeutic index, 419
  topoisomerase inhibitors for, 440–443
  toxicity, 462
Chest radiography, spatial resolution in, 331
Chidamide, 477
Childhood cancer
  global trends in, 74
  risk factors for, 74
ChIP. See Chromatin immunoprecipitation (ChIP)
Chi-squared test, 83
Chlorambucil
  dosage and administration of, 433
  indications for, 433

pharmacology of, 433
structure of, 432, 433f
toxicity of, 433
uptake
  extracellular acidity and, 454–455
  pH and, 299
Chloride intracellular ion channels (CLIC) proteins, 255
Chondrotin sulfate, 226
Chromatid(s), radiation-induced damage to, cell-cycle phase and, 356–357, 357f
Chromatin, 52, 52f
  accessible, 52, 52f, 53, 54f. See also Euchromatin
  bivalent, 53
  compacted, 52, 52f, 53, 54f. See also Heterochromatin
  posttranslational modifications, 195
  and reversible drug tolerance in cancer cells, 448
Chromatin accessibility profile, of cancers of unknown primary, 63
Chromatin factor(s)
  as drug targets in cancer treatment, 60–62
  genetic variants in, as biomarkers for precision cancer medicine, 62–63
  mutations, in cancer, 57–58, 58f
Chromatin immunoprecipitation (ChIP), 20
  ChIP-on-chip, 22
  ChIP-Seq, 22
Chromatin interactions, anchors of, 57, 57f
  epigenetic variants at, 57, 58f
Chromatin-modifying protein(s)
  erasers, 53. See also Epigenetic enzyme(s), erasers
  readers, 53. See also Epigenetic enzyme(s), readers
  writers, 53. See also Epigenetic enzyme(s), writers
Chromatin states, 51, 52, 53
Chromatogram, 14
Chromoplexy, 311
Chromosomal abnormalities, 179–180
  after irradiation, 356
  carcinogen-related, detection of, 105
  FISH detection of, 12–13
  in lymphoid malignancies, 6, 7t
  in myeloid malignancies, 6, 7t
  nomenclature for, 6, 7t
Chromosomal analysis, 6
Chromosomal instability (CIN), 178, 179–180
  radiation-related, 356
Chromosomal passenger complex (CPC), 209
Chromosome(s), 167
  banding, 6
  in cell cycle, 164–165, 164f
  instability, 195
  metaphase, 6
  missegregation of, 179
  painting, 13, 13f
  radiation-induced damage to, cell-cycle phase and, 356–357, 357f
Chromothripsis, 14, 179–180, 311
Chronic eosinophilic leukemia, targeted therapy for, 467t
Chronic lymphocytic leukemia (CLL)
  B-cell
    ATM gene and, 210
    chromosomal abnormalities in, 7t
    molecular lesions in, 7t

BCR signaling in, 479–480
drug treatment of, 407
high-risk subgroups, 479–480
microRNAs in, 24, 147
monoclonal antibody therapy for, 532t
NOTCH signaling in, 128
relapsed, treatment of, 475
targeted therapy for, 467t, 479–480
treatment of, 409
tumor-suppressor genes in, 142t
WNT pathway inhibitors for, 127
Chronic myeloid (myelogenous) leukemia (CML), 140
  BCR-ABL in, 478
    FISH detection of, 12f, 13
    and targeted therapy, 158–159
  blast crisis, 150
    chromosomal abnormalities in, 7t
    molecular lesions in, 7t
  chromosomal abnormalities in, 7t
  endothelial transdifferentiation in, 255
  gene fusion in, 145, 147t, 150, 404
  imatinib resistance in, 408
  karyotyping in, 6f
  molecular lesions in, 7t
  oncogenes in, 142t
  Philadelphia chromosome in, 148f, 150
  relapse, after bone marrow transplantation, 539
  targeted therapy for, 150, 467t
  treatment of, 2, 408
  tumor-suppressor genes in, 142t
CID. See Collision-induced fragmentation (CID)
Cilengitide, 125, 268t, 270
  plus verapamil, 125
CIMP. See CpG island methylator phenotype (CIMP)
CIN. See Chromosomal instability (CIN)
CIP/KIP, 169
circRNA. See RNA (ribonucleic acid), closed circular (circRNA)
Circulating tumor cells (CTCs), 232–233
  clinical significance of, 63–64, 320
  detection of, 233
  gene expression, prognostic significance of, 233
  and metastasis, 232
  as prognostic indicators, 554
  whole-genome sequencing of, 320
Circulating tumor DNA (ctDNA), 3, 320, 481, 548
  epigenetic profiling of, 63–65, 64f
  methylation, profiling of, 64–65, 64f
  as prognostic indicator, 554
Cisplatin
  adverse effects of, pharmacogenetic studies of, 89, 89t
  cellular uptake of, 447f, 449
  indications for, 435
  mechanism of action of, 435, 452
  nephrotoxicity of, 430
  neurotoxicity of, 435
  ototoxicity of, 435
  pharmacokinetics of, 435
  with radiation therapy, 375, 376f
  resistance to, 435, 446, 446f, 447f
  structure of, 435, 435f
  time-concentration curve for, 430
  toxicity of, 435
CKIs. See CDK inhibitor proteins (CKIs)
c-KIT
  inhibition of, 470
  targeted therapy and, 469, 469f

C-KIT, imatinib and, 408
Cladribine (2CdA), 440
  cellular uptake of, 448–449
  structure of, 440f
Class II-associated invariant chain-derived peptide (CLIP), 517
Clearance, of drug, 430–431, 431t
CLIC. See Chloride intracellular ion channels (CLIC) proteins
Clinical benefit, grading of, 558
Clinical target volume (CTV), for radiotherapy, 372, 372f, 373f
Clinical trials
  adaptive, 550
  bias in, 552
  biomarkers and, 550
  blinded, 554
  cointervention and, 552
  contamination of, 552
  criticisms of, 550
  crossover in, 552
  double-blind, 554
  exclusion criteria, 552
  explanatory, 548, 549t
  limitations of, 552
  of molecular targeted therapies, 549, 550
  multiarm multistage design, 550
  non-evaluable subjects and, 554
  outcome assessment in, 554
  outcome selection in, 554
  phase I, 411f, 548–549, 549t
    design of, 549
    dose expansion cohorts in, 549
    preclinical data needed for, 418–419
    starting dose for, 419
  phase II, 548, 549–550, 549t
    randomized, 549–550
    single-arm, 549–550
  phase III, 548, 549t, 550
    eligibility criteria, 552
    randomized controlled, 548, 550
  power of, 557–558
  pragmatic, 548, 549t
  purpose of, 548–550
  randomized, 552
    required number of patients for, 557, 557t
  statistical issues in, 557
  results, factors affecting, 552
  of targeted therapy, 481
CLIP. See Class II-associated invariant chain-derived peptide (CLIP)
CLL. See Chronic lymphocytic leukemia (CLL)
Clonogenic survival, after radiation, 353f, 356
CLPTM1L gene, 88
Clustering methods, 43
CML. See Chronic myeloid (myelogenous) leukemia (CML)
CMMRD. See Constitutional mismatch repair deficiency (CMMRD) syndrome
c-MYC, 184
  hypoxia and, 296
CNVs. See Copy-number variations (CNVs)
Coagulation factors
  and metastasis, 231f
  targeted therapy against, 271
  VIIa, 259
Coagulation system, and tumor angiogenesis, 260
Cobimetinib, 463f, 467t, 468t, 475
  indications for, 467t
  mechanism of action of, 474f
Cockayne syndrome (CS), 200, 210, 362, 362f

COFS. *See* Cerebro-oculo-facio-skeletal syndrome (COFS)
Cognitive dysfunction, anticancer drug-related, 417
Cohesin, 172, 173f, 174
 and chromatin interactions, 57, 57f
Cohesinopathies, 200t
Cohort(s)
 definition of, 76
 disease-specific, 76
 prospective, 76
 retrospective, 76
Cohort study, 75f, 76–77
 bias in, 80t
 confounders in, 77
 observational, 76
 outcome in, 77
 prospective, 76–77
 retrospective, 76
Cointervention, and clinical trials, 552
Colcemid, 6
Collagen, 226, 228, 229f
Collision-induced fragmentation (CID), 32, 32f
Colon, high-grade dysplasia/early cancer, 338f
Colony-forming assays, 354–356, 354f, 410–411
Colorectal cancer
 age-standardized incidence and mortality rates for, 72, 72f
 alcohol and, 87–88
 B-RAF mutations in, 154, 154f
 cancer stem cells in, 315, 317
  and chemoresistance, 320
 cellular radiosensitivity in, 378t
 clonal subpopulations in, 310
 colitis and, 102–103
 copy-number variations in, 17
 CpG island methylator phenotype (CIMP) in, 57
 development
  epigenetic changes associated with, 225, 225f
  genetic alterations during, 225, 225f, 310
  simultaneous parallel evolution in, 310
 DNMT inhibitors and viral mimicry response in, 62
 epigenetic modifications at promoters and, 56
 gene enhancer methylation in, 56
 gene fusion in, 147t
 genetic heterogeneity of, 309–310
 hedgehog signaling in, 129
 and hypercalcemia, 509
 incidence of, time trends in, 72f, 74
 KRAS in, 551
 KRAS mutations in, 154, 154f
  and treatment outcomes, 89
 metastases, origins of, 311
 metastasis, principal sites of, 234t
 microRNAs in, 147
 microsatellite instability in, 309–310
 monoclonal antibody therapy for, 532t
 mutations in, 310
 oncogenes in, 142t
 PI3-kinase signaling alterations in, 153, 153f
 PTEN promoter methylation in, 157, 157f
 RAS-MAPK mutations in, 119
 screening
  ctDNA-targeted sequencing assay in, 65
  liquid biopsy ctDNA test for, 64–65
  and prevalence, 72
 SEPT9 (*Septin9*) promoter methylation in, 65
 smoking and, 87f
 targeted therapy for, 467t

TGF-β signaling in, 130
 tumor-suppressor genes in, 142t
 variant enhancer loci in, 56–57, 56f
 WNT signaling in, 125, 126
Combretastatin A 4-phosphate (CA4p), 268t, 271
Comet assay, 105, 211, 212t
Common Terminology Criteria for Adverse Events (CTCAE), 559
 patient-reported outcomes version (PRO-CTCAE), 559
 scale for, 384
Comobidity(ies), and tumor angiogenesis, 266
Comparative genomic hybridization (CGH), 13
Complement activation, 532, 534f
Complementarity
Complementarity-determining regions (CDRs), 519
Complementary DNA (cDNA), 8–9, 9f
 in polymerase chain reaction, 11
Complement-dependent cytotoxicity (CDC), 464
Compton effect, 350
Computed tomography (CT), 3, 329, 330f, 331–332, 332f, 333f, 337f
 agents for, 332f
 of animal models, 339
 contrast-enhanced, 329
 dynamic, 332
 dynamic contrast-enhanced, 332
 functional, 332
 in lung cancer screening, 332
 machine learning and, 342
 perfusion, 332
 radiomics and, 342–343
 radiotherapy guidance, 341
 screening, for lung cancer, 565
 in screening for cancer, 332
 test phantoms in, 341
Confidence interval, 78
 95%, 82–83, 82f, 556
Confounders, 70
 in case-control studies, 75
 in cohort study, 77
 definition of, 78–79, 79f
Confounding, 85
 bias and, 78–79, 79f
 controlling for, 79. *See also* Regression analysis
 in epidemiologic studies, 78–79, 79f
 vs. interaction, 85
Consortia, 92
Constitutional mismatch repair deficiency (CMMRD) syndrome, 200t
Contamination, of clinical trial, 552
Content validity, 560
Continuous Hyperfractionated Accelerated Radiotherapy (CHART), 395
Convergent validity, 560
Copanlisib, 175
Copy-number variations (CNVs), 15–17, 18f
 in cancer, 17
 heritable germline, 17
 pan-cancer patterns of, 17
Cornelia de Lange syndrome, 200t
Cost-effectiveness, 561
Costimulation, 522f
Cowden syndrome, 156
COX-2. *See* Cyclooxygenase 2 (COX-2)
Cox proportional hazards model, 42, 84, 84t, 556, 566–567

CPC. *See* Chromosomal passenger complex (CPC)
CPDs. *See* Cyclobutane pyrimidine dimers (CPDs)
CpG dinucleotides, 20, 21f, 52, 53f, 146
 methylation of, 52–53
CpG island methylator phenotype (CIMP), 57, 58f
CpG islands, 52, 146, 149, 195, 448
 in promoters, methylation at, 52
CPT-11. *See* Irinotecan
CRC. *See* Colorectal cancer
Creatinine clearance, 430
CREB-binding protein (CBP), 126
cre-loxP system, 27, 28f
Cremophor EL, 445
CRISPR
 off-switch (protein inhibitors) for, 30
 off-target effects of, 30
CRISPR-Cas, 28–30, 29f, 70, 212
 functional genomic screens, for identification of potential drug targets, 405–406
Crizotinib, 142t, 469f, 478–479
 indications for, 467t
CRM1, 481
Crohn's disease, TGF-β signaling in, 130
Crosslinking mass spectrometry, 30
Crossover, in clinical trials, 552
Cross-presentation, of antigens, 517f, 518
Cross-sectional studies, 77–78, 77t
 bias in, 80t
CRPC. *See* Castration-resistant prostate cancer (CRPC)
Cryo-electron microscopy (cryo-EM), 30, 38
Cryo-electron tomography (cryo-ET), 38
Crystallography, 37
CS. *See* Cockayne syndrome (CS)
CSCs. *See* Cancer stem cells (CSCs)
CSI. *See* Chemical shift imaging (CSI)
CSL transcription factors, in NOTCH signaling, 127–128, 127f
C_{ss}. *See* Steady-state plasma drug concentration
CST, 214f, 215
CT. *See* Computed tomography (CT)
CTCAE. *See* Common Terminology Criteria for Adverse Events (CTCAE)
CTCF, and chromatin interactions, 57, 57f, 58f
CTCFL/BORIS, promoter, demethylation at, 55
CTCs. *See* Circulating tumor cells (CTCs)
ctDNA. *See* Circulating tumor DNA (ctDNA)
CtIP, 202, 202f, 203, 203f
CTLs. *See* Cytotoxic T lymphocytes (CTLs)
CTV. *See* Clinical target volume (CTV)
c-type lectin-like receptor 2 (CLEC2), 255
CULLIN-3, 185
Cullin-RING ligases (CRLs), 132
Cumulative incidence sampling, 75
CUP. *See* Cancers of unknown primary (CUP)
Cushing syndrome, paraneoplastic, 509
Cutaneous T-cell lymphoma, treatment of, 408, 477
CXCL8, in cancer progression, 237t, 238
CXCL10, 188
CXCL12, and cancer-associated fibroblasts, 282
CXCR4, and metastasis, 235
Cyclin(s), 164f, 167–169, 168f, 169f
 A-type, 167–169, 169f, 170–171, 170f, 171, 171f, 174
 B-type, 167–169, 169f, 170–171, 172, 173f, 174, 178

CDK binding, 167–169, 169f
and cell-cycle checkpoints, 357
D1, MYC and, 150, 151f
D-type, 169, 169f, 171, 171f
  growth factor signaling and, 122
E-type, 169, 169f, 171, 171f, 476
prognostic significance of, 280–281
CYCLIN D1, 176
Cyclin-dependent kinase(s) (CDKs)
  CDK1, 164f, 166f, 167, 169, 169f, 170–174, 172, 173f
    and cell-cycle checkpoints, 357
  CDK2, 164f, 167–169, 169f, 170–171, 170f
    and cell-cycle checkpoints, 357
  CDK4, 169, 169f
    inhibitors, 476
    MYC and, 150, 151f
  CDK4/6, 164f
    inhibitors, 177, 177f, 502–503
  CDK6, 169, 169f
    inhibitors, 476
  CYCLIN-bound, 164f, 167–169, 168f
  prognostic significance of, 280–281
  regulation of, 167–169
Cyclin-dependent kinase inhibitor(s) (CDKIs), 476. *See also specific agent*
  and hormonal therapy, combined, for breast cancer, 503
  prognostic significance of, 280–281
  resistance to, 476
  toxicity of, 476
Cyclobutane pyrimidine dimers (CPDs), 350, 362
Cyclooxygenase 2 (COX-2), and metastasis, 225f, 231f, 233
Cyclophosphamide, 415, 433
  bladder cancer caused by, 432
  bladder irritation caused by, 432, 434
  dosage and administration of, 433
  indications for, 433
  metabolism of, 433, 434f
  pharmacology of, 433
  structure of, 432, 433f
  toxicity of, 433–434
Cyclosporine, 451
CYP. *See* Cytochrome P450 (CYP)
Cyproterone acetate, 503, 506f
Cystatins, 228
Cysteine proteases, 226t, 227–228
Cytarabine, cellular uptake of, 448–449
Cytarabine and daunorubicin, liposomal, for AML, 410
Cytidine analogs, 439–440
Cytochrome P450 (CYP), 430
  activity, classification of, 432
  carcinogen bioactivation by, 99–100, 100f, 101f
  chemoprevention strategies targeted to, 109
  CYP1A1
    and B[a]P DNA adducts as biomarkers for lung cancer risk, 108, 108f
    genetic variations in, and lung cancer risk, 108
  CYP1A2, activity, oncogenic vs. protective effects of, 109
  CYP17A1, inhibitor of, 504, 505f
  CYP2D6, and tamoxifen therapy for breast cancer, 500f, 502, 504f
  polymorphisms, and tamoxifen treatment, 432
  and small molecule inhibitors, 464
CyTOF, 41, 307
Cytogenetics, 5–6
  nomenclature for, 6, 7t

Cytokines, 113, 230
  antiangiogenic, 268
  and cancer-associated fibroblasts, 282, 282t
  in cancer-related extracellular vesicles, 262
  immunomodulatory agents and, 534–535
  in irradiated tissue, 385–386
  and late radiation damage in lung, 387, 388f
  production of
    by antigen-presenting cells, 518, 518f
    by innate lymphoid cells, 519
  proinflammatory, and metastasis, 231f
  receptors for, 123–124, 124f
  signaling, 123–124, 124f
  in tumor microenvironment, 283
Cytokinesis, 167, 173f, 174–175
Cytoplasmic proteins, and cancer-associated fibroblasts, 282, 282t
Cytosine analogs, as DNMT inhibitors, 60
Cytosine arabinoside
  adverse effects, 440
  dosage and administration of, 440
  indications for, 440
  mechanism of action of, 439–440
  mucosal damage caused by, 417
  pharmacokinetics of, 440
  resistance, 439–440, 446t
  structure of, 439, 439f
Cytosine phosphate guanine (CpG). *See* CpG
Cytoskeletal components, and cancer-associated fibroblasts, 282, 282t
Cytoskeletal remodeling, and metastasis, 231f
Cytotoxic T-lymphocyte antigen (CTLA), CTLA-4, 524
  functions of, 536
  immune checkpoint inhibitor targeting, 536–537, 537f
Cytotoxic T lymphocytes (CTLs), 515, 523, 525
  hypoxia and, 298
  in tumors, 283

D

Dabrafenib, 119–120, 142t, 475–476
  indications for, 467t
  mechanism of action of, 463f, 474f
Dacarbazine (DTIC)
  mechanism of action of, 434
  metabolism of, 434
DACH. *See* Diaminocyclohexane (DACH)
Dacomitinib, indications for, 467t
DAG. *See* Directed acyclic graphs (DAG)
Damage-associated molecular pattern molecules (DAMPs), 103, 187–188
DAMPs. *See* Damage-associated molecular pattern molecules (DAMPs)
DAPT, 321
Daratumumab, 532t
DARC. *See* Duffy antigen receptor for chemokine (DARC)
Darolutamide, 509
Dasatinib, 142t
  indications for, 467t
  mechanism of action of, 478
  side effects of, 478
Data-independent mass spectrometry (DIA), 37
Data set(s), -omic
  gene signatures, 43
  statistical analysis of, 42–43
  unsupervised clustering of, 43
Daunorubicin, 442–443

resistance to, 449t
structure of, 443f
DBF4-dependent kinase (DDK), 171
D-boxes, 168f
DCE-CT. *See* Dynamic contrast-enhanced computed tomography (DCE-CT)
DCE-MR. *See* Dynamic contrast-enhanced magnetic resonance (DCE-MR)
DCIS. *See* Ductal carcinoma in situ (DCIS)
3D-CRT. *See* Radiotherapy, 3-dimensional (3D) conformal
DCs. *See* Dendritic cells
ddNTPs. *See* Dideoxynucleotides (ddNTPs)
DDR. *See* DNA damage response (DDR)
DDR2, targeted therapy and, 469f, 470
2-DE. *See* Two-dimensional gel electrophoresis (2-DE)
Death domain (DD), 184
Death effector domain (DED), 185, 185f
Death-inducing signaling complex (DISC), 185
Death receptor(s)
  DR3, 184–185
  DR4 (TRAILR1), 184–185
  DR5 (TRAILR2), 184–185
  DR6, 184
  modifications, and cancer, 188
Death receptor apoptotic pathway, 183f, 184–185
Decitabine, 60–61
DED. *See* Death effector domain (DED)
Degarelix, in prostate cancer treatment, 503
Degrons, 131f, 132, 168f
Dehydroepiandrosterone (DHEA), 488, 489f, 490f
Delayed response genes, 122
Deletion(s), 144–146, 145f, 146f
DELTA-LIKE, 127, 127f
Delta-like ligand 1 (DLL1), 258
Delta-like ligand 3 (DLL3), 258
Delta-like ligand 4 (DLL4), 258
  in angiogenesis, 254–255, 254f, 257t
  antiangiogenic therapy targeted to, 272
Delta-Like Ligand 4 receptor (DLL-4), monoclonal antibodies against, 128
Demcizumab, 128
DEN. *See* Diethylnitrosamine (DEN)
Dendritic cells, 515–516
  and angiogenesis, 251
  generation of, for cancer vaccines, 535–536, 535f
  hypoxia and, 297f, 298
  maturation of, 518–519, 518f
  migration of, 518–519, 518f
  and T-cell activation, 521, 521f, 522f
  and T-cell immunity, 524–525
  and T-cell tolerance, 524–525
Denosumab, 233
Deoxycytidine, structure of, 439f
Deoxyuridine monophosphate (dUMP), 436, 437f, 438
DER. *See* Dose-enhancement ratio (DER)
Desert hedgehog (*DHH*), 128
N-Desmethyl-4-hydroxy-tamoxifen. *See* Endoxifen
Desmin, 282, 282t
Detection bias, 80t
Deubiquitinating enzymes (DUBs), 131, 131f, 132–133, 168f, 169–170
Developmental signaling, 125–131
Dexrazoxane, cardioprotective effects of, 421, 443
DFS. *See* Disease-free survival (DFS)
DGCR8. *See* DiGeorge syndrome critical region gene 8 (DGCR8)

DHEA. *See* Dehydroepiandrosterone (DHEA)
DHFR. *See* Dihydrofolate reductase (DHFR)
DIA. *See* Data-independent mass spectrometry (DIA)
Diagnostic-review bias, 564, 567
Diagnostic tests, 561–563
　bias in, sources of, 563–564, 563t
　cutoff point for, 562–563, 562f, 563f
　likelihood ratio and, 566
　negative predictive value of, 562, 562f
　performance of
　　disease prevalence and, 562, 562f
　　factors affecting, 563, 563t
　positive predictive value of, 562, 562f
　quantitative, 562
　sensitivity of, 562–563, 562f
　specificity of, 562–563, 562f
Diaminocyclohexane (DACH), 435
Diarrhea, 279
　antiangiogenic therapy and, 271
　anti-EGFR-mediated, 472
　drug-induced, 417
　irinotecan and, 417, 432, 442
Dibenz[a,h]anthracene, as carcinogen, 98
Dibromochloropropane, potency as carcinogen, 107t
Dicer, 24, 25f, 406f
Dideoxynucleotides (ddNTPs), in DNA sequencing, 14
Diet
　and cancer chemoprevention, 109, 110
　and prostate cancer risk, 497
Dietary exposure(s), and cancer risk, evaluation of, 90–91
Diethylnitrosamine (DEN), 99f, 103, 107
　metabolic activation of, 100, 101f
Difference gel electrophoresis (DIGE), 34
Differentiation therapy, 321
Diffusion
　facilitated, drug uptake by, 448
　passive, drug uptake by, 448
Diffusion-weighted imaging (DWI), 334, 335f
DIGE. *See* Difference gel electrophoresis (DIGE)
DiGeorge syndrome critical region gene 8 (DGCR8), 24, 25f
Digoxigenin, 11, 13
Dihydrofolate reductase (DHFR), 436–437, 437f, 447f
Dihydropyrimidine dehydrogenase (DPD), 438, 438f
　deficiency, and 5-fluorouracil toxicity, 88–89, 418, 432, 438
Dihydrotestosterone, 110, 489, 490f, 491, 492f
Dimethylcarbamoyl chloride, 99f
Dimethylnitrosamine, potency as carcinogen, 107f
Dinaciclib, 177
Dipeptidyl peptidases, 259, 260f
Directed acyclic graphs (DAG), 84
DISC. *See* Death-inducing signaling complex (DISC)
Discriminant validity, 560
Disease-free survival (DFS), 382f, 473, 550, 554
Disease-specific mortality, 564
Disheveled (DSH, DVL in mammals), 126, 126f
Distribution(s), 82, 82f
DJ1
　and oxidative stress, 290–291, 290f
　in Parkinson disease, 290–291
DLL4. *See* Delta-like ligand 4 (DLL4)
DNA (deoxyribonucleic acid). *See also* Nucleic acid(s)

alkylation, chemical carcinogens and, 101f
amplification of
　CGH detection of, 13
　in polymerase chain reaction, 10–11, 11f
　SNP arrays for, 14
analysis, Southern blotting technique for, 9–10, 9f, 10f
aralkylation, chemical carcinogens and, 100f
arylamination, chemical carcinogens and, 101f
in cancer-related extracellular vesicles, 262
cloned, as probe, 9, 9f
cloning of, 8–9, 9f
damage, 194–195, 194f
　alkylating agents and, 432
　assays, 211–212, 212t
　and carcinogenesis, 97–98, 224–225
　carcinogens causing, 99–100, 99f–101f
　checkpoints, 177f, 178
　chemoprevention targeted to, 109
　consequences of, 101–102
　drug-mediated, 446, 446t, 447f, 452–453, 452f
　endogenous ("background" levels of), 102
　by hydroxyl radicals, and radiotherapy, 379, 380f
　oxidative, 101
　　short-term assays for, 105
　patterns of, 101
　radiation-related, 352, 352f, 353t, 356
　short-term assays for, 105
　and tumor initiation, 97–98
deletions
　CGH detection of, 13
　FISH detection of, 12–13
demethylation, 53f
　at gene promoters, in carcinogenesis, 55
distribution of, fluorescent indicators of, 277, 277f
double-strand breaks
　assays for, 211–212, 212t
　cell response to, 177f, 178
　and homologous recombination, 178, 201–203, 202f, 358f, 361–362, 452, 476–477
　and nonhomologous end joining, 178, 202, 203–204, 203f, 358f, 361–362, 452
　and radiosensitivity, 359–360, 360f
　repair of, 54, 201–204, 358f, 360–362, 452
　　defects, cancer-prone human syndromes associated with, 200t, 210–212
　signaling pathways induced by, 206–208, 206f
　and drug resistance, 448
hybridization of, 7
hydroxymethylcytosine, 21, 53
hypermethylation, 57, 188
　and drug resistance, 448
hypomethylation, 60–61
in intercellular response to ionizing radiation, 363–364
interstrand crosslinks, repair, 204–205, 205f
local multiply damaged sites, radiation-related, 352, 352f
methylation, 52–53, 53f, 195. *See also* Methylated DNA
　at anchors of chromatin interactions, 57
　in cancer screening, 64–65
　in cancers of unknown primary, 63, 64f
　and carcinogenesis, 20, 54–57, 55f, 56f, 146–147
　and cellular reprogramming, 52
　of circulating tumor DNA (ctDNA), 64–65, 64f

de novo, in development, 53, 53f
　and drug resistance, 448
　and epigenetic changes, 20, 20f, 54–57, 55f, 56f
　epigenetics and, 59, 59f
　at gene enhancers, and carcinogenesis, 56–57, 56f
　and genomic stability, 52
　maintenance, 53, 53f
　methods for analyzing, 20–22, 21t
　in pan-cancer screening test, 65
　substrate for, 59, 59f
modifiers, mechanism of action of, 463f
overreplication, block to, 171–172, 172f
phosphate-deoxyribose backbone, 8f
recognition sequences cut by restriction enzymes, 7–9, 9f
repair, 54, 101–102, 102, 105–106, 350
　assays, 211–212
　BRCA1 in, 158, 452
　BRCA2 in, 158, 452
　and carcinogenesis, 224–225
　cell cycle-related radiosensitivity and, 358f
　combined treatment and, 422t
　defects
　　and anticancer drug toxicity, 418
　　and cancer-prone human syndromes, 200t, 210–212
　　and DNA-targeting drug efficacy, 452
　　and radiosensitivity, 362
　and drug resistance, 446, 446t, 447f, 452–453, 452f
　genetic variations in, and cancer risk, 108
　hypoxia and, 298, 299
　inhibition, and tumor response to radiotherapy, 378–379
　inhibitors, 476–477
　mutations associated with, and radiosensitivity, 378–379
　pathways, 197–205
　and radiosensitivity, 358f, 359–360
　by reversal of DNA damage, 197
replication, 6, 8f, 163–164, 164f, 165f
　damage repair, defects, cancer-prone human syndromes associated with, 200t
　error-prone, 102
　initiation, 171–172, 172f
　proofreading, defects, cancer-prone human syndromes associated with, 200t
　radiation and, 350
sequencing of, 14–15, 15f–17f
　bam file in, 15
　clonal and subclonal patterns revealed by, 310–311, 310f
　fastq file in, 15
　and identification of drug targets, 404
　of irradiated cells, 356
single-strand breaks, repair, 199f
strand breaks, 102
subtelomeric, 213
template, in site-directed mutagenesis, 25, 26f
translesional synthesis of, 197, 198f
unscheduled synthesis of, assay for, 105
DNA alkyltransferase, 197, 452
DNA damage checkpoints, 205–208, 206f, 207f
DNA damage kinases, 178
DNA damage response (DDR), 178, 179, 353, 353f, 363
　disruption, in cancer, 180
　telomeres and, 213, 214f
DNA demethylase, mutations, in cancer, 58

DNA-dependent protein kinase (DNA-PK), 204
DNA-dependent protein-kinase catalytic subunit (DNA-PKcs), 203, 203f, 204, 205
DNA glycosylase
 in base excision repair, 199, 199f
 bifunctional, 199
DNA library, 9
DNA ligase, 9
DNA ligase IV, defect, and radiosensitivity, 362, 362f
DNA methyltransferase(s) (DNMTs), 52–53, 53f
 in de novo methylation, 53, 53f
 in maintenance of methylation, 53, 53f
 mutations, in AML, 58, 58f
DNA methyltransferase inhibitors (DNMTi), 60–61, 60f, 148f
 and immune checkpoint blockade, combined, 61
 toxicity of, 61
 and viral mimicry response, 62
DNA methyltransferases, 149
 microRNAs and, 147
DNA-PK. *See* DNA-dependent protein kinase (DNA-PK)
DNA-PKcs. *See* DNA-dependent protein-kinase catalytic subunit (DNA-PKcs)
DNA polymerase, 6–7, 164, 165f, 171–172
 cytosine arabinoside and, 439
 error-prone, 197
 in polymerase chain reaction, 10–11, 11f
Dnmt1, 53
Dnmt3a, Dnmt3b, 53, 58
DNMT3A gene, 63
DNMTi. *See* DNA methyltransferase inhibitors (DNMTi)
DNMTs. *See* DNA methyltransferase(s) (DNMTs)
Docetaxel, 444–445
 adverse effects, 445
 pharmacokinetics of, 445
 structure of, 444f
Dormancy, cancer-cell, 236
Dose-enhancement ratio (DER), 424
Dose-limiting toxicity, 549
Dose-volume histogram (DVH), for radiotherapy, 372, 372f
DOT1L
 activity, 61
 inhibitors, 61
Double helix, 8f
Double-minute (DM) chromosomes, 195
Double-stranded DNA (dsDNA), 164, 165f
Double-stranded DNA breaks (DSBs), 172, 178–179, 197, 199, 200t, 201–212
Doubling time(s), tumor, 275–276, 277f
Dowling-Degos disease, 128
Doxorubicin, 415, 442–443
 cardiotoxicity of, protection against, 421, 443
 cellular uptake of, pH and, 299
 experimental tumor treated with, growth curves for, 413f
 metabolism of, 443
 pegylated liposomal, 410, 446
  benefits of, 446
  half-life of, 446
  and hand-foot syndrome, 446
 resistance to, 449t
 and second malignancy, 418
 structure of, 443f
 tissue penetration by, 456, 456f
 toxicity of, 443
 uptake, extracellular acidity and, 454–455
DPD. *See* Dihydropyrimidine dehydrogenase (DPD)

Driver mutations. *See* Mutation(s), driver
Drosha, 24, 25f
Drug(s). *See also* Anticancer drug(s); Clinical trials; *specific drug*
 absorption of, 430
 adverse effects of, pharmacogenetic studies of, 89, 89t
 bioavailability of, 430
 cellular uptake of, pH and, 299
 clearance, 430–431, 431t
 concentration-time curve for, 430–431, 430f, 431t
 elimination, 430
 half-life of, 431, 431t
 metabolism of, 430
 renal excretion of, 430
 steady-state plasma concentration of, 431, 431t
Drug activation, decreased, drug resistance caused by, 446t, 447f, 451–452
Drug-antibody conjugates
 indications for, 467t
 mechanism of action of, 463f
Drug catabolism, increased, drug resistance caused by, 446t
Drug distribution, 430
 in relation to blood vessels in solid tumors, 456–457, 456f
Drug efflux, enhanced, drug resistance caused by, 446t, 447f, 449–451
Drug inactivation
 drug resistance caused by, 451–452, 446t, 447f
Drug interactions, 430
Drug resistance, 195, 421–422, 446–458. *See also* Multidrug resistance
 autophagy and, 133
 autophagy upregulation and, 453
 drug distribution and, 455–457, 456f
 hallmarks of, 501
 hypoxia and, 299
 in hypoxic environment, 454–455
 mechanisms of, identification of, 412
 mediated by ABC transporters. *See also* ATP-binding cassette (ABC) transporters; *specific transporter*
  reversal of, 451
 molecular mechanisms of, 446–448, 446t, 447f
 mutations and, 145–146
 and solid tumor environment, 453–457
 tissue penetration by drugs and, 455–457, 456f
Drug therapy. *See also* Anticancer drug(s); *specific drug*
 adjuvant, 403
 advances in (future directions for), 3
 combination, success of, factors affecting, 403
 curative, 403
 palliative, 403
Drug-tolerant persister (DTP) cells, 318, 448
Drug uptake
 impaired, drug resistance caused by, 446t, 447f, 448–449
 mechanisms of, 448
 pH and, 299, 454–455
DS-3032b, 409
DTIC. *See* Dacarbazine (DTIC)
dTMP. *See* Thymidine monophosphate (dTMP)
DTP. *See* Drug-tolerant persister (DTP) cells
DUBs. *See* Deubiquitinating enzymes (DUBs)
DU145 cell line, 23
Ductal carcinoma in situ (DCIS), of breast, 497–498, 497f
Duffy antigen receptor for chemokine (DARC), 232

dUMP. *See* Deoxyuridine monophosphate (dUMP)
Duplication of chromosomes, 144–146, 145f, 146f
Durvalumab, after chemoradiotherapy, in NSCLC, 375
DVH. *See* Dose-volume histogram (DVH)
Dynamic contrast-enhanced computed tomography (DCE-CT), 332
Dynamic contrast-enhanced magnetic resonance (DCE-MR), 335
 of animal models, 339
Dynein, 165
Dyskeratosis congenita, 215
Dyskerin, 213

E

Early genes
 E2, 149
 E5, *E6*, and *E7*, 149
EBV. *See* Epstein-Barr virus (EBV)
E-cadherin, 228–230, 237, 237t, 240, 240f, 241 313
ECD. *See* Electron capture dissociation (ECD)
Echinoderm microtubule-associated protein-like 4 (EML4), 478
ECM. *See* Extracellular matrix (ECM)
Ecologic fallacy, 74
Ecologic studies, 74–75
Ectodomain shedding, 227
Ectosomes, in tumor neovascularization, 262
Edmonton Symptom Assessment Scale, 559–560
EDT, Electron transfer dissociation (EDT)
EF5, 293
E2F1, MYC and, 150, 151f
Effect modification, 85
E2F transcription factors, 171, 171f
 MYC and, 150, 151f
 retinoblastoma protein and, 158
EGF. *See* Epidermal growth factor (EGF)
EGFR. *See* Epidermal growth factor receptor(s) (EGFR)
EGFR gene, 142t, 145
 and angiogenesis, 265
EGFR-SEPT14 fusion gene, 147t
EG-VEGF/PK1. *See* Endocrine gland VEGF/prokineticin 1 (EG-VEGF/PK1)
Electrical waves, 349–350, 350f
Electromagnetic (EM) radiation, 349–350, 350f
Electron capture dissociation (ECD), 32
Electrons, linear energy transfer of, 351, 351t
Electron transfer dissociation (ETD), 32
Electron volts (eV), 350, 350f
Electrophiles/electrophile-generating metabolites, and DNA damage, 99, 99f, 100, 100f, 101f
Electroporation, 23
Electrospray ionization (ESI), 31–32, 31f
ELK1, 119, 119f
Elongin B/C, 295f
Elotuzumab, 532t
EM. *See* Electromagnetic (EM) radiation
Embedded samples, 38
Embryonic stem (ES) cells, 255, 314, 314t, 318, 321
 homologous recombination in, 27, 27f
EML4-ALK gene fusion, 145, 147t, 465f
EMMPRIN, in cancer-related extracellular vesicles, 262
Emprin, 230
EMT. *See* Epithelial-to-mesenchymal transition (EMT)
Enasidenib, 63, 142t, 409, 477–478
 indications for, 468t
 mechanism of action of, 474f

585

Encorafenib, 119–120, 475–476
　indications for, 467t
　mechanism of action of, 474f
Endocrine glands, 258, 278t, 487
Endocrine gland VEGF/prokineticin 1 (EG-VEGF/PK1), 258
Endometrial cancer
　ARID1A mutations in, and sensitivity to PARP inhibitors, 63
　Cowden syndrome and, 156
　K-RAS mutations in, 154, 154f
　oncogenes in, 142t
　PI3-kinase signaling alterations in, 153f
　PTEN loss of function in, 156
　PTEN promoter methylation in, 157, 157f
　smoking and, 87f
　tamoxifen and, 418
　tumor-suppressor genes in, 142t
　WNT signaling in, 126
Endoplasmic reticulum (ER), hypoxia and, 296f
Endoplasmic reticulum–associated protein degradation (ERAD), 133
Endoscopic confocal microscopy, 340
Endoscopy, 332f, 338, 338f
Endostatin, 257t, 260, 265, 268
Endothelial cells, 239f, 249, 250f
　angiogenic, interactions with basement membrane, 258–259, 259f
　functions of, adhesive mechanisms in, 258–259, 259f
　quiescent, 258
　tumor-associated, 249, 267
　in tumor microenvironment, 283–284
Endothelial precursor-like cells (EPCs), 265
Endothelial progenitor cells (EPCs), 249, 251f, 252
Endothelial-to-mesenchymal transition, 265, 282, 297, 297f, 312–314, 318–321, 323
Endothelium, cancer stem cell (CSC)–derived, 261f
Endoxifen, 432, 499, 500f
End replication problem, 213
Energy metabolism, in cancer cells, epigenetics and, 58–60, 59f
Energy transfer
　by ionizing radiation, 350–351
　linear. See Linear energy transfer (LET)
　x-rays and, 350
　γ-rays and, 350
Enhanced permeability and retention effect, and liposomes, 446
Enoticumab, 128
Entactin, 226
Entinostat, 148f
　and exemestane, combined, for breast cancer, 503
Entrectinib, 142t, 469f
Environment, and carcinogenesis, 2
Enzalutamide, 504, 505
　resistance, 508
　structure of, 505f
Enzyme(s). See also specific enzyme
　bioactivation of procarcinogens, 99–100, 99f–101f
　in cancer-related extracellular vesicles, 262
　drug-metabolizing, 99–100, 430
　　and cancer risk, 108
　　chemoprevention strategies and, 109–110
　　genetic polymorphisms, and drug toxicity, 432
　　genetic variation in, 108
　as drug targets, alterations, drug resistance caused by, 446t, 447f

phase I, 99–100, 430
phase II conjugating, 99–100, 430
Enzyme inhibitors, 60f, 408–409
Eosinophilic syndromes, treatment of, 408
EpCAM. See Epithelial cell adhesion molecule (EpCAM)
EPCs. See Endothelial progenitor cells (EPCs)
Ependymoma, CpG island methylator phenotype (CIMP) in, 57
EPHA, targeted therapy and, 469f, 470
EPH receptors, 258
　EPHB4, 257t, 258
　and lymphangiogenesis, 254f, 255
Ephrin(s), 258
　in vasculogenic mimicry, 255–256
Ephrin B2, 257t, 258
EPHRIN-B2, and lymphangiogenesis, 254f, 255
EPICUP, 63
Epidemiologic studies
　of alcohol and head and neck cancer, 87–88
　analytic, designs, 74–81
　　bias in, 80t
　case-control design, 75–76, 75f
　　bias in, 80t
　　hospital-based, 80t
　cohort design, 75–76, 75f, 76–77
　　bias in, 80t
　confounding in, 78–79, 79f
　cross-sectional design, 77–78, 77t
　　bias in, 80t
　ecologic design, 74–75
　familial -sectional design, 78
　of infection and cancer, 85–86
　multiple, analyses across, 92
　nested designs, 75–76
　and random error, 78
　sampling in, 72–73
　of tobacco and cancer, 86–87, 87f
Epidemiology, 1
　analytic, 69–70, 81–85
　definition of, 69
　descriptive, 69–70, 70–74
　emerging areas in, 88–89, 89t
　general approach to, 69–70
　genomic, 88
　in identification of cancer risk, 104, 104f
　interaction analysis in, 84–85, 85f
　molecular, 104f
　　of carcinogenesis, 107–109
　observational studies in, 69–70
　　advantages and disadvantages of, 90, 90t
　　vs. randomized controlled trials, 90, 90t
　pharmacogenomic, 88–89, 89t
　population, of carcinogens, 104
　scope of, 69
　in translational medicine, 70
Epidermal growth factor (EGF), 151–152
　signaling by, steroid receptor activation, 494
Epidermal growth factor receptor(s) (EGFR), 114, 114f, 149, 151–152, 152f, 227
　and angiogenesis, 262f
　dimerization and activation of, 115, 115f
　inhibitors, 70, 471–472
　　adverse effects, 472
　　diarrhea caused by, 472
　　skin toxicity, 472
　monoclonal antibody against, 532t
　mutations of, 70
　small molecule inhibitors, 115, 408, 408f
　targeted therapy and, 467t, 469f

T790M mutation, 464, 467t, 471–472, 551
variant III mutant, 151
Epigenetic enzyme(s)
　erasers, inhibitors, 60f
　readers, inhibitors, 60f
　writers, inhibitors, 60f
Epigenetic inhibitors, 477–478
Epigenetics, 143–144, 145f, 176–177, 224
　and cancer metabolism, 58–60, 59f
　definition of, 20, 51, 146
　and drug resistance, 448
　and heterogeneity of cancer, 225–226, 312–319
　in liquid biopsy, cancer monitoring based on, 63–65, 64f
　metabolic regulation of, 58–60, 59f
　microRNAs and, 147
　and oncogenesis, 51, 54–58, 55f, 146–147
　in profiling of cancers of unknown primary, 63, 64f
　radiation-induced genetic instability and, 356
　research, techniques for, 20–22, 20f–22f, 307
　and treatment targets, 51, 60–62, 146–147, 148f
　and tumor growth and spread, 98, 146–147
Epigenetic therapy(ies), 60–62, 60f
　in combination with other therapies, 62
　emerging, 61–62
　and immunotherapy, combined, 62, 62f
Epigenetic variants
　at anchors of chromatin interactions, 57, 58f
　as biomarkers for precision cancer medicine, 62–65
　in cancer, 54–60
　at gene enhancers, 56–57, 56f
　at gene promoters, 54–56, 55f
Epipodophyllotoxins, 442, 442f
Epiregulin. See EREG
Epirubicin, 442–443
　resistance to, 449t
　and second malignancy, 418
　structure of, 443f
Epithelial cell adhesion molecule (EpCAM), in detection of circulating tumor cells, 233, 317
Epithelial cells, 195, 196f, 226, 240, 240f, 278–279, 281f, 282, 314t, 364, 495, 497–498, 528f
Epithelial-to-endothelial transformation, 255
Epithelial-to-mesenchymal transition (EMT), 229, 240–241, 240f, 265, 282, 313, 313f
　and chemoresistance, 320
　hedgehog signaling in, 129
　hypoxia and, 297, 297f
　and metastasis, 232
　prognostic significance of, 319–320
　signaling pathways in, 313, 314t
Epothilones, 445
Eppendorf probe (oxygen electrode), 293, 298t
Epstein-Barr virus (EBV), 149, 528
　and Burkitt lymphoma, 86
　and cancer, 85–86
　latent membrane proteins, 149
　nuclear antigens, 149
Equipoise, 553
ER. See Endoplasmic reticulum (ER); Estrogen receptor(s)
ERBB1, 151–152, 152f
　humanized antibodies against, 115
ERBB2 (HER2), 114f, 151–152, 152f
　humanized antibodies against, 115
ERBB3, 114f, 115, 151–152, 152f
ERBB4, 114f, 115, 151–152, 152f
ERBB2 (HER2) gene, 142t, 145, 152

ERCC1. *See* Excision repair cross complementation group 1 (ERCC1) enzyme
Erdafitinib, 469f, 471
  indications for, 467t
EREG, and metastasis, 231f, 233
ERG-EWSR1 fusion gene, 147t
Eribulin, 407, 445
ERK. *See* Extracellular signal-regulated kinases (ERK)
Erlotinib, 115, 142t, 152, 268t, 271, 403, 408, 469f
  indications for, 467t, 472
  mechanism of action of, 472
ERM proteins, 230
Erythema, radiation-induced, 386, 386f
Erythropoietin, 279, 382–383, 415, 416f
  and radiotherapy, 299
ESI. *See* Electrospray ionization (ESI)
Esophageal carcinoma
  alcohol and, 87–88
  gastroesophageal reflux and, 102–103
  genetic and epigenetic heterogeneity of, interdependence of, 319
  NOTCH signaling in, 128
  PI3-kinase signaling alterations in, 153
  smoking and, 87f
  tumor-suppressor genes in, 142t
Estradiol
  classical mechanism of action of, 491–494, 492f
  structure of, 499f
Estrogen(s)
  and breast cancer, 488
  cumulative exposure to, and breast cancer risk, 495–496
  nongenomic effects of, 494–495, 494f
  nontranscriptional actions of, 494f, 495
  receptor binding, conformation change induced by, 501f
  synthesis of, 488, 489f, 490f
  transport in blood, 488–489
Estrogen receptor(s), 490f, 491
  activation of, 491–494, 492f
  alternative regulatory pathways for, 494–495, 494f
  classical nuclear, 491
  coactivators of, 501f
  and resistance to hormonal therapy in breast cancer, 502, 504f
  coregulators, and resistance to hormonal therapy in breast cancer, 502, 504f
  corepressors of, 501f
  crosstalk with growth factor networks, 494–495, 502
  DNA binding by, 492, 492f
  estrogen binding, conformation change induced by, 501f
  fulvestrant binding, conformation change induced by, 501f
  immunohistochemistry of, 495, 496f
  modification, and resistance to hormonal therapy in breast cancer, 502, 504f
  nonclassical, 491
  nonclassical mechanism of action of, 494–495, 494f
  phosphorylation, 494
    and hormone resistance, 502
  tamoxifen binding, conformation change induced by, 501f
ETC-159, 126
ETD. *See* Electron transfer dissociation (ETD)
Ethylene vinyl acetate (EVA) polymer, 39

Etoposide
  dosage and administration of, 442
  indications for, 442
  pharmacokinetics of, 442
  resistance to, 446t, 449t
  and second malignancy, 418, 442
  structure of, 442, 442f
  toxicity of, 442
ETS1, 119, 119f
ETV6-NTRK3 fusion gene, 147t
ETV1-TMPRSS2 fusion gene, 147t
Euchromatin, 52, 52f, 54f
European Organization for Research and Treatment of Cancer Core Quality of Life Questionnaire (EORTC QLQ-C30), 560
European Society for Medical Oncology, Magnitude of Clinical Benefit Scale, 558
EVA polymer. *See* Ethylene vinyl acetate (EVA) polymer
Everolimus, 121, 175, 271, 475
  dosage and administration of, 475
  and exemestane, combined, 475
    for breast cancer, 503
  indications for, 475
  and lenvatinib, combined, 475
  mechanism of action of, 463f, 474f, 475
  and sorafenib, combined, 475
  and sunitinib, combined, 475
Evidence, hierarchy of, 552, 552t
Evofosfamide, 299, 455
  cytotoxicity in hypoxic cells, 384
Evolutionary ecology, of cancer, 321, 322f
EVs. *See* Extracellular vesicles (EVs)
Excision repair cross complementation group 1 (ERCC1) enzyme, 200t, 201f, 203f, 205f, 452
Excitation, 350
Exemestane, 498, 499f
  structure of, 499f
Exercise, and cancer prevention, 110
Exons, 7
  single nucleotide polymorphisms in, 14
Exosomes, 235, 242, 248, 261f, 263
  and cancer-associated fibroblasts, 282
  in tumor neovascularization, 262
Experimenter's bias, 80t
Exportin-1 (XPO1), 481
Extracellular matrix (ECM), 284
  cell adhesion to, 124–125
  cell interactions with, 124
  components, and cancer-associated fibroblasts, 282, 282t
  composition of, 226, 282, 282t
  remodeling mediated by CAFs, 282
  in solid tumors, 453, 454f
    and drug resistance, 453–454
  structure of, 226
  and tumor response to radiotherapy, 377
Extracellular signal-regulated kinases (ERK), 117–118, 117f, 119
  activation, 125, 154f
Extracellular vesicles (EVs), 241, 241f, 242, 248, 248f, 265, 363
  categories of, 262
  in tumor neovascularization, 262
Extravasation, in metastasis, 231f, 233
EZH2
  inhibitors, 61
  mutations, 61
  in cancer, 57–58
Ezrin, 229, 229f, 230

EZRIN, MYC and, 151f
EZR-ROS1 fusion gene, 147t

F
FA. *See* Fanconi anemia
Face validity, 560
FACS. *See* Fluorescence-activated cell sorting (FACS)
FACT. *See* Functional Assessment of Cancer Therapy (FACT) Scale
FACT-General, 560
Factor inhibiting HIF (FIH), 294, 295f
FAD. *See* Flavin adenine dinucleotide (FAD)
FADD. *See* FAS-associated death domain (FADD)
FAFs. *See* Fibrosis-associated fibroblasts (FAFs)
FAK. *See* Focal adhesion kinase (FAK)
False-discovery rate (FDR), 43, 548
Familial adenomatous polyposis (FAP), 126, 225f
Familial breast and ovarian cancer, genetics of, 1
Familial cancer syndromes, 178, 195, 210
Familial hypercholesterolemia, 409–410
Familial studies, 78
FANC. *See* Fanconi anemia complementation (FANC) proteins
Fanconi anemia, 200t, 211
Fanconi anemia complementation (FANC) proteins, 204–205, 205f
Fanconi anemia (DNA repair) pathway, 180
FANC proteins. *See* Fanconi anemia complementation (FANC) proteins
FAP. *See* Familial adenomatous polyposis (FAP); Focal adhesion protein (FAP)
Farnesyl transferase inhibitors (FTIs), 118
FAS, 184–185
FAS-associated death domain (FADD), 185
FASL, 183f, 184–185, 453
Fatigue
  antiangiogenic therapy and, 271
  anticancer drug-related, 417
FAZA. *See* [^{18}F]-fluoroazomycin arabinoside (FAZA)
F-box proteins, 132, 133–134, 169, 170
FBXW7, 133, 142t
Fc gamma receptor IIB (FcγIIB), 533
Fc gamma receptor IIIA (FcγRIIIA), 532, 537
Fc receptors (FcRs), 532–533, 534f
FcγIIB. *See* Fc gamma receptor IIB (FcγIIB)
FcγRIIIA. *See* Fc gamma receptor IIIA (FcγRIIIA)
FDG. *See* [^{18}F]-fluorodeoxyglucose (FDG)
FDR. *See* False-discovery rate (FDR)
Ferroptosis, 353f, 354
Fertility preservation, before chemotherapy, 417
Fetal transcriptional programs, in pediatric cerebellar tumors, 19
[^{18}F]-fluoroazomycin arabinoside (FAZA), 294, 298t, 336, 337f
[^{18}F]-fluorodeoxyglucose (FDG), 287, 329, 330f, 336, 337f
  in PET of animal model, 339, 340f
[^{18}F]-fluoromisonidazole (FMISO), 336, 337f
  detection of hypoxia with, 294, 298t
FGF. *See* Fibroblast growth factor (FGF)
FGFR3-TACC3 fusion gene, 147t
FH. *See* Fumarate hydratase (FH)
Fibonacci sequence, modified, for dose escalation in clinical trial, 549
Fibroblast growth factor (FGF), 149
  acidic (FGF-1), 257t
  and angiogenesis, 260, 262f, 265
  basic (FGF-2), 257t
    hypoxia and, 297

Fibroblast growth factor (FGF) (Cont.)
   and cancer-associated fibroblasts, 282, 282t
   FGF-3, 257t
   FGF-4, 257t
   and lymphangiogenesis, 255
   and metastasis, 231f, 232
Fibroblast growth factor receptor (FGFR), 114, 114f
   inhibition of, 471
   small molecule inhibitors, 115
   targeted therapy and, 467t, 469f, 471
Fibroblasts. See also Cancer-associated fibroblasts (CAFs)
   in cancer, 309
   in normal tissue, 281–282
Fibronectin, 226, 228, 229f, 282, 282t
   and cancer-associated fibroblasts, 282–283, 282t
Fibrosis
   radiation-induced, 387
      prevention of, 389
   tumor, 282
Fibrosis-associated fibroblasts (FAFs), 282
FIH. See Factor inhibiting HIF (FIH)
Filter elution, 211, 212t
Finasteride
   as chemopreventive agent, 110, 506
   mechanism of action of, 505f
   structure of, 505f
FISH. See Fluorescence in situ hybridization (FISH)
Flavin adenine dinucleotide (FAD), and epigenetic enzyme activity, 59, 59f
Flavopiridol, 177
FLI1-EWSR1 fusion gene, 147t
FLIP, modifications, and cancer, 185, 188
Flow-assisted cell sorting, 307
Flow cytometry, 40–41, 42f, 277, 277f, 278, 307
   in paraffin blocks, 280
FLT3
   inhibition of, 470–471
   targeted therapy and, 468t, 469, 469f, 470–471
FLT-3 gene, 142t
Fluctuation Test, 446
Fludarabine
   cellular uptake of, 448–449
   dosage and administration of, 440
   indications for, 440
   mechanism of action of, 440
   structure of, 440f
   toxicity of, 440
Fluorescence-activated cell sorting (FACS), 41, 42f, 307
Fluorescence in situ hybridization (FISH), 6, 11–13, 12f, 38, 211, 212t
   of chromosomal abnormalities, 12–13
   of gene translocations and deletions, 12f, 13
   of irradiated cells, 356
   multifluor-, 13
Fluorescence recovery after photobleaching (FRAP), 212
Fluorescent polarization, 406
5-Fluoro-deoxyuridine monophosphate (5-FdUMP), 438, 438f
Fluoropyrimidines, 437–439
   toxicity, DPD deficiency and, 88–89
5-Fluorouracil (5-FU)
   catabolism, 438
   dosage and administration of, 438–439
   folinic acid with, 421
   and hand-foot syndrome, 439
   indications for, 438
   and leucovorin, combined, 438, 438f
   metabolism of, 437–438, 438f
   mucosal damage caused by, 416
   pharmacokinetics of, 438
   resistance to, 446t
   structure of, 437, 438f
   toxicity of, 438–439
      DPD deficiency and, 88–89, 418, 432, 438
5-Fluorouridine triphosphate (5-FUTP), 438, 438f
Flutamide, 503
   resistance to, 449t
   structure of, 505f
FMISO. See [^{18}F]-fluoromisonidazole (FMISO)
FMS-like tyrosine kinase 3. See FLT3
Focal adhesion kinase (FAK), 123f
   integrins and, 125
   upregulation, in cancer, 125
   in vasculogenic mimicry, 255–256
Focal adhesion protein (FAP), 282, 282t
Focal adhesions (FAs), 125
Folic acid, structure of, 436f
Folinic acid
   with 5-fluorouracil, 421
   with methotrexate, 437
Folkman, Judah, 248
Follow-up tests, for treated tumors, 565
Forest plots, 558–559, 559f
Forkhead-associated (FHA) domains, 115
Forkhead Box class O (FOXO), 120
   and oxidative stress, 290, 290f
   and tumor metabolism, 288
Forkhead transcription factor, FOX2c, and lymphangiogenesis, 255
Formalin, tissue fixation using, 38–39
Fosbretabulin, 268t, 271
Founder line, 27
FOXM1, 172
FOXO. See Forkhead Box class O (FOXO)
FOXP3, 523f, 524
FOXY-5, 127
Fractionalism. See Radiotherapy, fractionation
Fragility index, 557
Framingham Heart Study, 76
FRAP. See Fluorescence recovery after photobleaching (FRAP)
Frizzled (FZ) receptors, in WNT signaling, 125, 126f
FSUs. See Functional subunits (FSUs)
FTIs. See Farnesyl transferase inhibitors (FTIs)
FU. See Fused (FU)
5-FU. See 5-Fluorouracil (5-FU)
Fulvestrant
   for breast cancer, 500
   dosage and administration of, 500
   mechanism of action of, 500, 501f
   structure of, 499f
Fumagillin, 268
Fumarate hydratase (FH), 291
Functional Assessment of Cancer Therapy (FACT) Scale, 559
Functional subunits (FSUs), in late-responding irradiated tissues, 387–388
Funnel plot, 558
Fused (FU), 128, 129f
Fusion protein inhibitors, 478–479

G

GADD. See Growth arrest after DNA damage (GADD)
GAGE, 528
Gain of function, 58, 61, 142t, 150–155
Galunisertib, 131
Gamma rays, 349–350, 350f
Ganitumab, 115
GAPs. See GTPase-activating proteins (GAPs)
GARFT. See Glycinamide ribonucleotide formyltransferase (GARFT)
Gastric cancer. See also Stomach cancer
   chromosomal instability (CIN) variant, KRAS in, 404
   EBV and, 149
   endoscopy of, 338f
   ERBB2(HER-2) in, 152
   HER2 in, 568
   monoclonal antibody therapy for, 532t
   oncogenes in, 142t
   tumor-suppressor genes in, 142t
Gastrointestinal cancer, tumor-suppressor genes in, 142t
Gastrointestinal stromal tumors (GISTs)
   oncogenes in, 142t
   targeted therapy for, 468t, 470
   treatment of, 408
Gastrointestinal tract. See also Intestines
   repopulation of irradiated cells in, 390–391
GATA-3, 523f, 524
GCL. See Glutathione cysteine ligase (GCL)
G-CSF. See Granulocyte colony-stimulating factor (G-CSF)
GDC-0449, 129
Gefitinib, 115, 142t, 152, 268t, 271, 408, 450, 466, 469f
   indications for, 467t, 472
   mechanism of action of, 472
   resistance to, 449t
   and tamoxifen sensitivity, 502
GEFs. See Guanine nucleotide exchange factors (GEFs)
Gel blocks, 34
GeLC-MS, 34
Geldanamycin, 300
Gel-enhanced LC-MS, 34
Gemcitabine
   cellular uptake of, 448–449
   indications for, 440
   mechanism of action of, 440
   pharmacokinetics of, 440
   resistance to, 446t
   structure of, 439f, 440
   tissue penetration by, 456
   toxicity of, 440
Geminin (GEM), 172, 172f, 173f
GEMMs. See Genetically engineered mouse models (GEMMs)
Gemtuzumab, 532t
Gemtuzumab-ozogamicin, 534
Gene(s). See also Oncogenes; Tumor-suppressor gene(s); specific gene
   acetylation, and genetic instability, 194, 1894f
   amplification
      and drug resistance, 446, 447f
      and genetic instability, 194–195, 1894f
   cloning of, 8–9, 9f
   conversion, 14, 17
   co-regulation of, 43
   deletions, FISH detection of, 12f, 13
   essentiality in human cell lines, online resource on, 28
   knocked out, 26–27, 27f
   manipulation, in cells, 23–24

manipulation of, with restriction enzymes, 7–9, 9f
methylation, and genetic instability, 194, 1894f
targeted, in pharmacogenetic epidemiology, 89, 89t
translocations, FISH detection of, 12f, 13
Gene editing, 28–30, 29f
Gene enhancer(s), epigenetic variants at, and oncogenesis, 56–57, 56f
Gene expression
  in cancer, 2
  carcinogens and, 109
  epigenetic changes and, 20–22, 20f
  epigenetic mechanisms and, 52–54, 53f, 54f
  growth factor signaling and, 122
  hypoxia and, 294, 298t
  microarrays, 307
  modification, by tumor promoters, 102
  profiles, analysis of, 548
  studies of, RNA sequencing for, 404, 405f
Gene expression profiling, of cancers of unknown primary, 63
Gene fusions
  cancer-associated, 144–145, 147t
  identification of, 404
Gene gun, 23
Gene ontology (GO), 44
Gene promoter(s)
  demethylation at
    and carcinogenesis, 55
    and treatment-resistant cancer, 55
  histone modifications at, and carcinogenesis, 55f, 56
Gene signatures, of -omic data, 43
Gene silencing, 20
Genetically engineered mouse models (GEMMs), for preclinical evaluation of anticancer drugs, 413–414
Genetic instability, 98, 193, 224
  combined treatment and, 421–424, 422t
  in epithelial tissue, 195, 196f
  extrinsic causes of, 196–197
  intrinsic causes of, 194–195, 194f
  and malignant transformation, 194–197
  radiation-related, 196–197, 356
  in stromal tissue, 195, 196f
  UV radiation and, 196
Genetic interaction, 200
Genetics
  of cancer, 1, 2, 176–177, 193, 224
    historical perspective on, 139–140
    therapeutic strategies guided by, 158–159
  of drug resistance, 446–448, 446t
  and tumor angiogenesis, 266
  and tumor growth and spread, 98
Genome, duplication, in S phase of cell cycle, 163–164, 164f, 165f
Genome sequencing analysis, 14
  and molecular signatures of exposure and risk, 108–109
Genome-wide analysis, 15
Genome-wide association studies (GWAS)
  of cancer risk, 88
  in pharmacogenetic epidemiology, 89, 89t
Genome-wide CRISPR screens, online resource on, 30
Genomic analysis, 2, 141, 142t, 547–548, 551
  limitations of, 548
Genomic epidemiology, 88
Genomic instability, 146, 178–181
  hypoxia and, 297f, 298

MYC and, 151f
as therapeutic target, 180–181
Genomics, 547
Genotyping, high-throughput, 548
Geographic variation, in cancer epidemiology, 73, 73f
Gilteritinib, 469f, 471
  indications for, 468t
GISTs. See Gastrointestinal stromal tumors (GISTs)
Gleevec. See Imatinib
GLI
  hedgehog signaling and, 128–129, 129f
  inhibitors, 129
Glioblastoma, 266
  cancer stem cells in, 315–316, 320
  cell cultures, heterogeneity in, 308
  cell line derived from, 23
  cellular radiosensitivity in, 378t
  copy-number variations in, 17
  epigenetic alterations in, 58f
  gene fusion in, 147t
  hedgehog signaling in, 129
  heterogeneity in, 19
  heterogeneity of, and radioresistance, 320
  IDH in, 155
  initiating cells, 314
  NOTCH signaling in, 128
  oncogenes in, 142t
  PI3-kinase signaling alterations in, 153f
  PTEN loss of function in, 156
  radiomics studies of, 344f
  secondary, IDH1/2 mutations in, 477
  somatic mutations and epigenetic factors in, 58f
  transcriptional regulators and, 122
  tumor-initiating cells in, 267
  tumor-suppressor genes in, 142t
  WNT signaling in, 128
Glioma
  CpG island methylator phenotype (CIMP) in, 57, 58f
  ERBB1 mutations in, 151
  gene fusion in, 147t
  IDH in, 155, 291
  IDH1/2 mutations in, 63
  low-grade, NOTCH signaling in, 128
  oncogenes in, 142t
  tumor-suppressor genes in, 142t
GLI transcription factors, 196
Glomeruloid vessels, 261f, 262
Glomus cancer, NOTCH signaling in, 128
GLS2. See Glutaminase 2 (GLS2)
Glucagon-like peptide 1, secretion by tumors, 509
Glucocorticoid receptor(s), DNA-binding motif, 492
Glucose, and epigenetic enzyme activity, 59
Glucose transporter-1 (GLUT-1)
  hypoxia and, 294, 297
  MYC and, 151f
Glucose transporter-2 (GLUT-2), hypoxia and, 297
Glutamate, production, in glutamine metabolism, 289, 289f
Glutaminase 2 (GLS2), and oxidative stress, 290, 290f
Glutamine metabolism, 289, 289f
  and epigenetic enzyme activity, 59, 59f
Glutaminolysis, 284, 287f, 289, 289f
Glutathione (GSH)
  drug binding, drug resistance caused by, 446t, 447f, 451–452
  and MRP1, in drug resistance, 451

production of, 289, 289f
reduced, as antioxidant, 289, 290, 290f
Glutathione cysteine ligase (GCL), 289, 289f
Glutathione S-transferases (GSTs), 100, 447f, 451
Glycinamide ribonucleotide formyltransferase (GARFT), 437, 437f
Glycogen synthase kinase (GSK), 126, 229
Glycolysis
  aerobic, 59, 175–176, 284, 285–287
    molecular regulation of, 285–286, 286f
  hypoxia and, 296–297, 297f
  relation to biosynthetic pathways, 286–287, 287f
GM-CSF. See Granulocyte-macrophage colony-stimulating factor (GM-CSF)
GO. See Gene ontology (GO)
Gonadal-hypothalamic-pituitary axis, 488, 490f
Gorlin (basal cell nevus) syndrome, 480
  hedgehog signaling in, 129
Goserelin, in prostate cancer treatment, 503
GP100, 528, 528f, 534
GPR30, and nongenomic effects of estrogens, 491, 494f
GR. See Glucocorticoid receptor(s)
Grade, of tumor, 3, 329, 330f
Graft-vs-leukemia effect, 539
Granisetron, cellular efflux, 450
Granulocyte colony-stimulating factor (G-CSF), 123, 279, 283, 388, 415, 416, 421, 431
Granulocyte-macrophage colony-stimulating factor (GM-CSF), 283, 297, 315, 388, 535, 535f, 536
Granulocytes, production of, 278–279, 415, 416f
  chemotherapy and, 279, 415, 416f, 421
Granzymes, 283, 523, 525, 531, 538
Gray (Gy), 350
GRB2. See Growth factor receptor bound-2 (GRB2)
Gross tumor volume (GTV), 336, 372, 372f
Growth arrest after DNA damage (GADD), GADD45, MYC and, 151f, 186f
Growth factor(s). See also specific growth factor
  and cancer-associated fibroblasts, 282, 282t
  and cancer progression, 237–238, 237t
  in cancer-related extracellular vesicles, 262
  in cell cycle, 167
  and cell growth, 175–176, 176f
  in cellular signaling, 113–123
  extracellular, and receptor tyrosine kinases, 113–115, 114f, 115f
  and hemopoietic cell maturation and proliferation, 415, 416f
  in irradiated tissue, 385–386
  and metastasis, 231f
  signaling by
    biological outcomes of, 122
    and resistance to hormonal therapy in breast cancer, 502–503, 504f
    steroid receptor activation, 494
    suppression by protein phosphatases, 122–123
  and steroid receptor phosphorylation, 494, 494f
  and tumor response to radiotherapy, 377
Growth factor receptor(s). See also Receptor protein tyrosine kinase(s) (RPTK); specific growth factor
  and metastasis, 233
Growth factor receptor bound-2 (GRB2), 116, 117f, 124, 154f
Growth fraction, 278, 279
GSH. See Glutathione (GSH)
GSK. See Glycogen synthase kinase (GSK)

589

GSTs. *See* Glutathione S-transferases (GSTs)
GS-X pumps, 452
GTPase-activating proteins (GAPs), 118, 118f
GTV. *See* Gross tumor volume (GTV)
Guanine nucleotide exchange factors (GEFs), 117–118, 118f, 154f
GWAS. *See* Genome-wide association studies (GWAS)

H
Hair loss
 alkylating agents and, 432
 antiangiogenic therapy and, 271
 drug-induced, 278, 371t, 417, 442, 469
Hair regrowth, 417
Hairy cell leukemia, 440, 534
 BRAF V600E mutation in, 404
Hajdu-Cheney syndrome, 128
Half-life, of drug, 232, 418, 431, 431t, 446, 469, 479
 stability of radioisotope probes, 336
Halichondrin B, 445
Hallmarks, of cancer, 98, 141–143, 224, 224f
 hypoxia-mediated, 296–298, 297f
 molecular targeted therapies and, 464f
Hand-foot syndrome, 417, 439, 469, 471
 antiangiogenic therapy and, 271
 pegylated liposomal doxorubicin and, 446
HAPs. *See* Hypoxia-activated prodrugs (HAPs)
HATi. *See* Histone acetyltransferase inhibitors (HATi)
HAT/KAT. *See* Histone lysine acetyltransferases (HAT/KAT)
HATs. *See* Histone acetyl transferase(s) (HATs)
H2AX, assays for, 105, 211, 212, 212f
 phosphorylation of (gamma-H2AX), 206, 206f, 207, 207f, 213, 214f
Hayflick limit, 23, 213
Hazard ratio (HR), 556, 566
HB-EGF. *See* Heparin-binding epidermal growth factor (HB-EGF)
HBV. *See* Hepatitis B virus (HBV)
HCC. *See* Hepatocellular carcinoma (HCC)
HCD. *See* Higher-energy collisional dissociation (HCD)
HCV. *See* Hepatitis C virus (HCV)
HDAC. *See* Histone deacetylase (HDAC); Histone lysine deacetylases (HDAC)
HDACi. *See* Histone deacetylase inhibitor (HDACi)
HDM2 gene, 196
Head and neck cancer
 alcohol and, 87–88
  genomic risk study of, 88
 cellular radiosensitivity in, 378
 cetuximab and radiation therapy for, 375
 gene fusion in, 147t
 HPV-negative, hypoxic, prognostic significance of, 381
 human papillomavirus and, 85, 103, 149
 hypoxic
  prognostic significance of, 381, 382f
  radiotherapy for, and prognosis, 381–382, 382f
 NOTCH inhibitors for, 321
 oncogenes in, 142t
 PI3-kinase signaling alterations in, 153
 radiotherapy for, salivary gland radioprotection with, 389
 squamous cell carcinoma
  and cell repopulation during radiotherapy, 391–392, 391f

 hypoxic modification of radiotherapy in, 383–384, 383f
 somatic mutations and epigenetic factors in, 58f
 treatment of, hypoxia and, 298t
 tumor-suppressor genes in, 142t
Health outcomes research, 560–561
 in evaluation of screening test, 565
 population-based, advantages and disadvantages of, 560–561, 560t
Heat shock factor(s), 133
Heat shock protein(s) (Hsp), 491, 492f, 508
 Hsp70, 133
 Hsp90, 133
  inhibitors, 133
Hedgehog acyltransferase (HHAT), 128
Hedgehog interacting protein (HIP), 128
Hedgehog signaling (pathway), 128–129, 129f, 196, 282, 314, 314t, 321, 480
 abnormalities, and cancer, 129
 in development, 125
 inhibitors (HPIs), 129, 480
Helicobacter pylori, and cancer, 85–86
Helix-loop-helix transcription factors, 121f, 122, 128
Helix-turn-helix, of transcription factors, 121, 121f
Helper T cells (T$_H$), 515, 523
 subsets, 523–524, 523f
Hemangioblastoma, tumor-suppressor genes in, 142t
Hemangiocytes, 251, 251f
Hematologic malignancies
 cancer stem cells in, 314–315, 315f
 epigenetic variants in, as biomarkers for precision cancer medicine, 63
 WNT signaling in, 126
Hematopoietic cell(s)
 in cancer, diversity of, 308
 maturation and proliferation of, 278, 415, 416f
Hematopoietic stem/progenitor cells (HSCs), 278, 314, 314t
 and angiogenesis, 251
 growth factors for, 279
Hemolytic uremic syndrome (HUS), mitomycin C and, 445
Hemorrhagic cystitis
 camptothecin and, 440
 cyclophosphamide and, 434
 ifosfamide and, 434
Heparan sulfate proteoglycan (HSPG), 226
Heparin-binding epidermal growth factor (HB-EGF), 152f, 271
 and cancer progression, 237–238, 237t
Hepatitis B virus (HBV)
 and aflatoxin B$_1$, in hepatocellular carcinoma, 102
 and hepatocellular carcinoma, 1, 73, 85–86
 vaccine against, 1, 110
Hepatitis C virus (HCV)
 and hepatocellular carcinoma, 1, 73, 85–86
 vaccine against, 1, 110
Hepatoblastoma, parental smoking and, 86
Hepatocellular carcinoma (HCC)
 aflatoxin B$_1$ and viral infection in, 102
 antiangiogenic therapy for, 270
 cancer stem cells in, 315
 viral hepatitis and, 73, 85–86
 viruses and, 1
 WNT signaling in, 126
Hepatocyte growth factor (HGF)
 and angiogenesis, 260

 and cancer-associated fibroblasts, 282, 282t
 and lymphangiogenesis, 255
 and metastasis, 231f, 232
 receptors for, 114, 114f
HER2. *See* Human epidermal growth factor receptor-2 (HER2)
Hereditary cancer syndromes, 178
 TCA cycle disruption and, 291
Hereditary nonpolyposis colorectal cancer (HNPCC), 200, 210–211, 225f
HER2 gene, 195
 and angiogenesis, 265
HER2/NEU, 2, 89, 502, 527, 528f
 immunity against, 529
 monoclonal antibody against, 532t
Hertig, Artur Tremain, 248
HES, in NOTCH signaling, 127f, 128
Heterochromatin, 20, 52, 52f, 54f
Heterogeneity, of cancer, 3, 225–226, 305–323, 306f
 diagnosis of, liquid biopsy and, 320
 epigenetic, 225–226, 312–319
  models, as aspects of same biology, 318–319
 exploration of, in clinical practice, 320
 genetic, 139, 142–143, 225–226, 306f, 309–312, 312f
 genetic and epigenetic, interdependence of, 319
 in glioblastoma, 19
 imaging of, 329
 interpatient, 306–307, 307f
 intratumoral, 310–311, 310f
 in metastases, 306f
 monitoring, liquid biopsy and, 320
 prognostic significance of, 319–320
 in same organ, 306f
 stromal, 226, 306f, 308–309, 309f
 study of, methods for, 306–308, 308f
 and treatment, 320–323, 322f
HEY, in NOTCH signaling, 127f, 128
2-HG. *See* 2-Hydroxyglutarate (2-HG)
HGF. *See* Hepatocyte growth factor (HGF)
HHAT. *See* Hedgehog acyltransferase (HHAT)
HHV-8. *See* Human herpesvirus 8 (HHV-8)
Hierarchical clustering, 19f, 43, 344f
Hierarchical modeling, 92
HIF. *See* Hypoxia-inducible factor(s) (HIFs)
HIFU. *See* High-intensity focused ultrasound (HIFU)
High-dimensional data, and multiple comparisons, 91–92
Higher-energy collisional dissociation (HCD), 32
Highest non-severely toxic dose (HNSTD), 419
High-intensity focused ultrasound (HIFU), MRI guidance, 342
High mobility group box 1 (HMGB1), 103, 187
High-performance liquid chromatography (HPLC), in DNA analysis, 22
HIP. *See* Hedgehog interacting protein (HIP)
Hippocrates, humoral theory of cancer, 140
Hippo pathway, 176, 176f, 180, 230
Histology, of tumor, 329, 330f
Histone(s), 195
 acetylation, 53, 54f, 144, 146, 195
  and drug sensitivity, 448
  epigenetics and, 59, 59f
  at gene promoters, 55f
  and transcription factors, 122
 core, 52, 52f
 variants, 54, 55f
 H2AX, DNA damage and, 206–208, 206f, 207f
 γ-H2AX intranuclear foci, 211–212, 212t
 hyperacetylated, and drug sensitivity, 448

methylation, 53, 54f, 144, 146
   epigenetics and, 59, 59f
modification, 53, 54f, 146, 307
   and drug resistance, 448
   and epigenetic changes, 20, 20f
   at gene enhancers, and
      carcinogenesis, 56–57, 56f
   at gene promoters, 55f, 56
phosphorylation, 53, 54f, 144, 146
posttranslational modifications, 52, 53, 54f
sumoylation, 53
ubiquitination, 53, 54f
Histone acetyl transferase(s) (HATs), 195
Histone acetyltransferase inhibitors (HATi), 60f
Histone code, 146
Histone deacetylase (HDAC), 195
   in tumorigenesis, 61
Histone deacetylase inhibitors (HDACi), 60f,
      61, 148f, 195, 408, 464, 464f, 477
   mechanism of action of, 61
Histone demethylase, 448
   and phenotypic plasticity, 317–318
Histone lysine acetyltransferases (HAT/KAT), 53
Histone lysine deacetylases (HDAC), 53
Histone lysine demethylases (KDM), 53
Histone methyltransferase, mutations,
      in cancer, 58
Histone variants, 53–54, 55f
   biologic significance of, 54
   core histones and, 54, 55f
   functional roles of, 54
HIV, and cancer, 85–86, 530, 552
HLA. See Human leukocyte antigen(s) (HLA)
HMGB1. See High mobility group box 1 (HMGB1)
HNPCC. See Hereditary nonpolyposis
      colorectal cancer (HNPCC)
HNSTD. See Highest non-severely
      toxic dose (HNSTD)
Hodgkin lymphoma
   ATM gene and, 210
   imaging of, 335
   second malignancy after, 418
   stromal component of, 309, 309f
Holliday junctions, 202
Homeobox, 121, 255, 314t
Homeodomain, of transcription factors, 121, 121f
Homogeneously staining regions (HSRs), 195
Homologous recombination (HR), 26–27, 27f,
      178, 201–203, 202f, 298, 405, 406f
   defects, cancer-prone human syndromes
      associated with, 199, 200f, 452
   and radiosensitivity, 357f, 358f, 361–362
Homologous recombination deficient
      (HRD) cells, 476–477
Honjo, Tasuku, 3, 536
Hormone(s). See also Steroid hormone(s);
      specific hormone
   and breast cancer, 488
   and cancer, 487–488
   classes of, 487
   definition of, 487
   and prostate cancer, 488
Hormone-responsive elements (HREs),
      295, 297, 491–492, 492f, 493f
Hounsfield units (HU), 331
HOXB9, in breast cancer, and
      radioresistance, 320
HOX gene family, 314t
Hoyeraal-Hreidarsson syndrome, 215
HPLC. See High-performance liquid
      chromatography (HPLC)

HPV. See Human papillomavirus (HPV)
HR. See Hazard ratio (HR)
H-RAS, 102, 117, 118
HRAS gene, 142t
   and angiogenesis, 265
   first isolation of, 140
   mutations, in cancer, 154
HRD. See Homologous recombination
      deficient (HRD) cells
HREs. See Hormone-responsive elements (HREs);
      Hypoxia response elements (HREs)
HSCs. See Hematopoietic stem/
      progenitor cells (HSCs)
HS-Damage-Seq, 105
Hsp. See Heat shock protein(s) (Hsp)
HSPG. See Heparan sulfate proteoglycan (HSPG)
HSRs. See Homogeneously staining regions (HSRs)
hTERT gene, 88, 214
hTERT protein, 215
HU. See Hounsfield units (HU)
Human epidermal growth factor receptor-2 (HER2)
   and angiogenesis, 262f
   inhibitors, 472–473
   targeted therapy and, 409, 467t, 469f, 472–473
Human epidermal growth factor receptor
      (HER) family, inhibitors of, 471–473
Human herpesvirus 8 (HHV-8), and
      Kaposi sarcoma, 85
Human leukocyte antigen(s) (HLA), 516, 516f, 526
   HLA-A*0201, 527, 529, 539
Human papillomavirus (HPV), 149, 528
   and cancer, 85–86
   carcinogenicity, 1
      transcriptome and proteome analysis of, 109
   and cervical cancer, 73
   and oropharyngeal cancer, 70
   and replication stress, 149
   vaccine against, 1, 86, 110, 149
Humoral theory, of cancer, 140
Hunter, John, 248
Hutchinson-Gilford progeria, 118
Hyaluronate, 229, 229f
Hybridization, definition of, 7
Hybridomas, 532
Hydrogen peroxide, 101
   radiation and, 351
4-Hydroxycyclophosphamide, 433, 434f
Hydroxyflutamide, resistance to, 449t
2-Hydroxyglutarate (2-HG), 59–60, 155, 291, 463f
   in hypoxic response, 295
   production, by mutant IDH1/2, 59, 63
D-2-Hydroxyglutarate, 477
Hydroxyl radical, radiation and, 351, 352f
4-Hydroxytamoxifen, 499, 500f
Hyperbaric oxygen, and radiotherapy, 299
Hypercalcemia
   from direct osteolytic calcium release, 509
   paraneoplastic, 509
Hypereosinophilic syndrome, targeted
      therapy for, 467t
Hypernephroma, cellular radiosensitivity in, 378t
Hypoglycemia, paraneoplastic, 509
Hypothyroidism, antiangiogenic therapy and, 271
Hypoxanthine phosphoribosyltransferase
      (Hprt) gene, chemical-induced
      mutagenesis in, 106
Hypoxia
   acute (perfusion-limited), 292–293
   and autophagy, 292, 292f
   chronic (diffusion-limited), 292–293
   combined treatment and, 422t, 423–424

   definition of, 263, 292
   and epigenetic changes, 147
   functional imaging in, 294
   gene expression signatures with, 294, 298t
   imaging, PET agents and, 336–337, 337f, 339–340
   intrinsic markers of, 294
   measurement of, 293–294, 298t
   perfusion-related, 292
   and preangiogenic tumor growth, 263
   prodrugs activated by, 299–300, 455, 457
   in solid tumor microenvironment, and
      drug resistance, 454–455
   and treatment outcomes, 297f, 298–299, 298t
   tumor, 284, 292–300, 379–381
      acute, 379–380, 381f
      acute and chronic, coexisting, 380
      and cell survival after radiotherapy,
         380–381, 381f
      chronic, 379–380, 381f
      drugs relieving, and radiotherapy
         response, 299, 383
      exogenous tracers, 293–294, 293f
      heterogeneity of, 293, 293f
      measurement of, 381–382, 382f
      prognostic significance of, 381–382, 382f
      and radioresistance, 298–299, 380–381, 381f
      and radiosensitivity, 380–381, 381f
      and response to fractionated
         radiotherapy, 392–393, 392f
      and targeted therapy for hypoxic cells, 382–384
      therapy targeted to, 299–300
   and tumor angiogenesis, 263–265,
         264f, 295f, 296f, 297, 297f
   in tumor microenvironment, 230
   and tumor response to radiotherapy,
      298–299, 375, 377, 379, 380f
Hypoxia-activated prodrugs (HAPs), 299–300
Hypoxia-inducible factor(s) (HIFs),
      263–264, 294–296
   HIF1, and tumor metabolism, 286f, 288
   HIF1α, 294–296, 295f, 466
   HIF2α, 294
   HIF3α, 294
   HIF1β, 295, 295f
   inhibitors, 300
   isoforms, 294
   structure of, 294
Hypoxia response elements (HREs), 295, 295f, 297
Hypoxic cell radiosensitizers, 299,
      383–384, 383f, 455
Hypoxic cells, in tumors
   and reoxygenation after irradiation,
      392–393, 392f
   targeted therapy for, 382–384
Hypoxic response, 294–298
   hypoxic mechanisms and, 294–296, 295f
   oxygen-dependent mechanisms and, 294, 295f
   therapy targeted against, 300

I

IAPs. See Inhibitors of apoptosis proteins (IAPs)
Iberdomide, 134
Ibritumomab tiuxetan, 532t
Ibritumomab tiuxetan-yttrium-90, 534
Ibrutinib
   adverse effects, 480
   indications for, 480
   mechanism of action of, 463f, 480
   resistance to, 480
   and rituximab, combined, 480
   and venetoclax, combined, 480

ICAMs. *See* Intercellular adhesion molecules (ICAMs)
ICAT (isotope-coded affinity tags), 34, 35f
ICD. *See* Immunogenic cell death (ICD)
ICER. *See* Incremental cost-effectiveness ratio (ICER)
ICIs. *See* Immune checkpoint inhibitors (ICIs)
ICLs. *See* Interstrand crosslinks (ICLs)
Idarubicin, 442–443
Idasanutlin, 409
Idelalisib, 175
   indications for, 475
   mechanism of action of, 475
   side effects of, 475
IDH. *See* Isocitrate dehydrogenase (IDH)
IDH1 gene, 57, 58f, 59, 60, 63, 142t, 155, 291, 295
IDH2 gene, 59, 63, 142t, 155, 291
IDH, inhibitors of, 60f
Idiopathic pulmonary fibrosis, 215
IDO. *See* Indoleamine 2,3-deoxygenase (IDO)
Ifosfamide, 433
   adverse effects, 434
   indications for, 434
   neurotoxicity of, 434
   structure of, 432, 433f, 434
IFP. *See* Interstitial fluid pressure (IFP); Intratumoral fluid proessure (IFP)
IGH-BCL2 fusion gene, 147t
IGH-MYC fusion gene, 147t, 148f, 150
IGRT. *See* Image-guided radiation therapy (IGRT)
IGS. *See* Invasiveness gene signature (IGS)
IHC. *See* Immunohistochemistry (IHC)
ILCs. *See* Innate lymphoid cells (ILCs)
Illumina (Solexa) sequencing, 14, 16f–17f
Image-guided radiation therapy (IGRT), 370, 370f, 372
Imaging, 329–344. *See also* Magnetic resonance imaging (MRI); Positron emission tomography (PET); Single-photon emission computed tomography (SPECT); Ultrasound
   advances in (future directions for), 340–344
   anatomical, 329, 330f
   of animal models in oncology, 338–340, 339f, 340f
   combined with biologic information, 341, 342f
   contrast agents for, 332f
   functional, 329, 330f
   in hypoxia, 294
   general concepts of, 329–331
   guidance, in cancer treatment, 341–342
   hybrid devices for, 331, 336
   Immune-Related Response Criteria (irRC), 341
   limiting spatial resolution in, 331
   microscopic, 329
   molecular, 331, 341, 342, 342f
   molecular probes in, 332f
   multimodal, 331, 341
   nano agents, 340
   nanoparticles in, 342, 343f
   optical, 329
   pixels in, 331
   quality assurance, 340–341
   quantitative methods, 340–341
   recent advances in, 3
   RECIST criteria, 341
   signals in, 329
      endogenous, 329
      exogenous, 329
   signal-to-noise ratio in, 331
   voxels in, 331
   x-ray–based. *See* Computed tomography (CT); Radiography
Imatinib, 2, 142t, 150, 268t, 403–404, 408, 450, 469f, 550
   bound to *c-ABL* kinase domain, x-ray crystallography of, 37
   indications for, 467t, 468t, 470, 478
   mechanism of action of, 37, 463f, 478
   resistance to, 470, 478
      molecular mechanisms of, 37
   side effects of, 470
Imiquimod, 531t, 535
Immediate early genes, 122
Immune-activating agents, for cancer therapy, 531t
Immune cells. *See also specific cell*
   in tumor microenvironment, 283, 309
Immune checkpoint inhibitors (ICIs), 188, 518, 531, 536–539
   and antibodies, combined, 539
   anti-CTLA-4, 536–537, 537f
   anti-PD-1/PD-L1, 536, 537–538, 537f
      acquired resistance to, 538
   for cancer therapy, 531t
   and chemotherapy, combined, 539
   combination, 539
   and DNMT inhibitors, combined, 61
   mechanism of action of, 524
   and radiation therapy, combined, 539
   rationale for, 321, 322f
   resistance to, 321
      acquired, 538
      adaptive, 538
      mechanisms of, 538–539
      primary, 538
   and targeted therapy, combined, 539
   and vaccines, combined, 539
Immune deserts, 538
Immune destruction, avoidance of, 62, 62f. *See also* Immune surveillance
   MYC and, 151f
Immune dysregulation, polyendocrinopathy, enteropathy, X-linked (IPEX), 525
Immune modulation, 531, 538
   for cancer therapy, 531t
Immune-Related Response Criteria (irRC), 341
Immune surveillance, 529–530
   3 Es of, 530, 530f
   and micrometastases, 236
   tumor escape from, 62, 62f, 230
      hypoxia and, 297–298, 297f
      and metastasis, 231f, 232, 233–234
Immune system, 515
   adaptive arm of. *See* Adaptive immunity
   diversity of, 515
   innate. *See* Innate immunity
   memory, 515
   and self vs. non-self recognition, 62, 62f, 515
   specificity of, 515
   and tumor response to radiotherapy, 375
Immunity. *See also* Tumor immunity
   antitumor
      barriers to, 531
      in intercellular response to ionizing radiation, 363–364
      and tumor progression, 529–530, 530f
Immunoediting, 3 Es of, 530, 530f
Immunofluorescence, 41f, 212t, 293, 307
   in hypoxia measurement, 293
Immunogenic cell death (ICD), 181, 186, 187–188
Immunohistochemistry (IHC), 307, 456
   of hormone receptors in tumor tissue, 495, 496f
   in hypoxia measurement, 293–294, 293f
   of tumor, 330f
Immunomodulation, in vivo, 534–536
Immunomodulatory agents, and cytokines, 534–535
Immunoproteasome, 131, 517
Immunoreceptor tyrosine activation motifs (ITAMs), 519, 520f
Immunosuppression
   alkylating agents and, 432
   and cancer, 529–530
   and metastasis, 231f
Immunotherapy, 531–541, 531t, 551. *See also* Immune checkpoint inhibitors (ICIs); *specific agent*
   cancer epigenome and, 60
   combination approaches, 539
   and epigenetic therapy, combined, 62, 62f
   genetic heritage of tumor and, 310
   personalized, 539
   preclinical evaluation, 414
   with radiation therapy, 375
   recent advances in, 2–3
   TGF-β blockade and, 131
Impalefection, 23
Imprinting, 20
IMRT. *See* Intensity-modulated radiation therapy (IMRT)
INCENP, 209
Incidence-density sampling, 76
Incidence rate, 70
   adjusted (standardized), 70–71
   age distribution and, 70
   within age groups, 71
   age-standardized, 70–71, 71f, 72, 72f
   crude, 70
   global trends in, 74
   screening and, 72
Incremental cost-effectiveness ratio (ICER), 561
Indian hedgehog (*IHH*), 128
Indoleamine 2,3-deoxygenase (IDO), 524, 538
   and tumor-related immunosuppression, 538
Infection(s)
   and cancer, 85–86
   chemoprevention strategies targeted to, 110
Infertility
   alkylating agents and, 432
   drug-related, 417
Infiltrated-excluded (I-E) tumors, 283
Infiltrated-inflamed (I-I) tumors, 283
Inflammation
   and cancer risk, 102–103
   chemoprevention strategies and, 110
   in irradiated tissue, 385–386
   and late radiation damage in lung, 387, 388f
   and preangiogenic tumor growth, 263
   TGF-β signaling in, 130
   in tumor microenvironment, 283
   tumor-promoting, MYC and, 151f
Information bias, 79–80, 80t
Informative censoring, 556
Infrared, 39, 40f, 332f, 338, 340, 349–350, 350f
Inhibitors of apoptosis proteins (IAPs), 183f, 184, 453
   modifications, and cancer, 188
INK4, 142t, 164f, 169, 195, 448
INK4a, in familial cutaneous melanoma, 196
INK4B, 175
Innate immunity, 515–519
Innate lymphoid cells (ILCs), 519

Insertion-deletion loops, 197
In situ hybridization (ISH), 307
Instrument(s)
   for assessment of health-related quality of life, 560
   responsiveness of, 560
   validity of, 560
Insulin-like growth factor(s)
   IGF-1
      secretion by tumors, 509
      steroid receptor activation, 494
   IGF-2, secretion by tumors, 509
   and lymphangiogenesis, 255
   and metastasis, 233, 234f
Insulin-like growth factor 1 receptor (IGF1R), 114, 114f
   humanized antibodies against, 115
Integrin(s), 284
   adhesive functions of, 258–259, 259f
   in angiogenesis, 257t
   cell adhesion mediated by, 228–230, 229f
      in solid tumors, and drug resistance, 454
   functions of, 124
   loss of, in tumors, 125
   and lymphangiogenesis, 255
   and metastasis, 235
   mutations of, and angiogenesis, 259
   signaling, 124–125
   subunits, 124–125
   and tumor response to radiotherapy, 377
   upregulation, in tumors, 125
   vascular, 258–259, 259f
Intensity-modulated radiation therapy (IMRT), 370, 370f, 372
Intention to treat, 554
Interaction analyses, 84–85, 85f
Interaction effect, 466
   qualitative, 466
   quantitative, 466
Interaction index, of combined drugs, 419–420
Intercellular adhesion molecules (ICAMs), 259, 282t, 521, 522f
   ICAM-1, MYC and, 151f
Interferon(s) (IFN)
   and angiogenesis, 260
   IFN-α
      adverse effects, 534
      antiangiogenic activity of, 268
      therapy with, 534
   IFN-α(β), 257t
   IFN-γ, 523, 523f
   and immunogenic cell death, 188
Interferon regulatory factor 3 (IRF3), 518
Interleukin(s) (IL)
   IL-2, 523, 523f, 525
      therapy with, 534–535
   IL-3, 416f
   IL-4, 523f, 524
   IL-6, 103, 149
      and angiogenesis, 260, 265
      in angiogenesis, 257t
      and metastasis, 232
   IL-7, and memory T cells, 523
   IL-8, 149
      and angiogenesis, 260, 262f, 265
      in angiogenesis, 257t
      and metastasis, 232
   IL-10, 525
   IL-12, 523
   IL-15, and memory T cells, 523

IL-17, 523f, 524
IL-1β, MYC and, 151f
International Lung Cancer Consortium, 92
Interphase, 12, 12f, 164, 166f, 177, 187, 212t, 353f, 354
Interstitial fluid pressure (IFP), 267, 281, 331, 456
   in tumor microenvironment, 230
Interstrand crosslinks (ICLs), repair, 200, 204–205, 205f, 211
Interviewer bias, 80t
Intestinal bleeding, 279, 416
Intestines
   cell proliferation in, 278t, 279, 279f
   radiation-induced responses in
      early, 386
      late, 387
   repopulation of irradiated cells in, 390–391
Intratumoral fluid proessure (IFP), 283–284
Intravasation, 261f
   and metastasis, 231–232, 231f, 235, 248
Intravital videomicroscopy (IVVM), 232, 233
Introns, 7, 14, 24
Intussusception, in angiogenesis, 252, 261f, 262
Invariant chain, 517
Invasiveness gene signature (IGS), 319
Inversion, 13, 144–146, 145f, 197
Iodine-131, in thyroid cancer treatment, 372–373, 534
Ionizing radiation. See also Whole-body irradiation
   abscopal effects, 363, 375
   biological effects of, 350–351
   bystander effect, 363, 363f
   cellular effects of, 351–353
      direct, 351, 352f
      indirect, 351, 352f
   cellular repair after, 358–362
   definition of, 350
   DNA damage after, assays for, 211–212, 212t
   DNA double-strand breaks, signaling pathways in response to, 206–208, 206f
   dose-sparing effect, 359
   genetic instability caused by, 356
   genetic instability related to, 196–197
   interactions with matter, 349–353
   intercellular responses to, 363–364
      neighboring cells in, 363–364
      signaling molecules/pathways in, 363–364
      timing of, 364
   intracellular signaling after, 363
   and lung cancer, 104
   molecular and cellular responses to, 356–364
   molecular repair after, 358–362
   radiobiological effectiveness of, 355
   sublethal damage from, 358, 359f
Ions (b-ions, y-ions), 32, 32f
Ipafricept, 126
IPEX. See Immune dysregulation, polyendocrinopathy, enteropathy, X-linked (IPEX)
Ipilimumab, 531t, 536–537
   mechanism of action of, 524
IQ. See 2-Amino-3-methylimidazo[4,5-f]quinoline (IQ)
IRF3. See Interferon regulatory factor 3 (IRF3)
Irinotecan, 300, 442
   diarrhea caused by, 417, 432, 442
   with 5-FU and leucovorin, 442
   indications for, 442

   nanoliposomal formulation of, 446
   neutropenia caused by, 432, 442
      pharmacogenetics of, 432
   structure of, 441f
   toxicity, 442
Isobologram analysis, of combined drugs, 419–420, 421f
Isocitrate dehydrogenase (IDH)
   activity, 477
   IDH1
      in hypoxic response, 295
      mutant, in glioma, 57, 58f, 63
      targeted therapy and, 468t, 477–478
   IDH2, targeted therapy and, 468t, 477–478
   IDH1/2 mutations, in cancer, 59–60, 63, 291, 409, 477–478
      and cancer metabolism, 59–60
      selective inhibitors for, 60
   inhibitors, 63, 409, 463f, 468t, 477–478
   mutant, 57, 58f, 409, 477
      and cancer metabolism, 59–60
      and CpG island methylator phenotype (CIMP), 57, 58f
      and glioma phenotype, 57, 58f
      and leukemia risk, 63
Isoeffect, of fractionated radiation treatment, 393
Isoeffect curves, for fractionated radiation treatment, 393, 394f
Isoelectric point (pI), 34
ITAMs. See Immunoreceptor tyrosine activation motifs (ITAMs)
iTRAQ (isobaric tag for relative and absolute quantitation), 35, 35f
Ivosidenib, 63, 477–478
   indications for, 468t
   mechanism of action of, 463f
IVVM. See Intravital videomicroscopy (IVVM)
Ixabepilone, 445
Ixazomib, 133
   adverse effects, 479
   dosage and administration of, 479
   mechanism of action of, 479

J

JAGGED, 127, 127f
Jagged 1 (JAG1), 255, 257t, 258
Jagged 2 (JAG2), 258
JAK. See Janus kinase (JAK)
JAK2 gene, 142t
JAK/STAT
   in EMT activation, 240f
   in development, 125
JAK/STAT inhibitors, 124
Janus kinase (JAK), 123, 123f
   JAK2, 142t, 320, 538
      inhibitors, 124
      mutations of, 124
   JAK3, 149
   structure of, 123f, 124
JARID1B, 317–318
Jensen, Elwood, 488
JNK. See Jun kinase (JNK)
JNK/SAPK, 119
Joules, 350, 350f
Jumonji demethylase(s)
   and cancer metabolism, 59–60, 59f
   inhibitors, 61
Jun kinase (JNK), 149
   activation, 125
   in WNT signaling, 125, 126f

593

K

Kallikreins, 227
Kaplan-Meier method, of survival analysis, 555–556
Kaposi sarcoma (KS)
   in HIV-infected (AIDS) patients, 529
   treatment of, 410
   viral infection and, 85
Karyotyping, 5–6, 6f. See also Spectral karyotyping (SKY)
Kataegis, 14–15
KDM. See Histone lysine demethylases (KDM)
KDMi. See Lysine demethylase inhibitors (KDMi)
KEN-boxes, 168f
Keratoacanthomas, BRAF inhibitor therapy and, 475
α-Ketoglutarate, in hypoxic response, 294, 295, 295f
Ki67, 56, 277–278, 278f, 279, 497
Kidney
   drug elimination by, 430
   repopulation of irradiated cells in, 391, 391f
Kidney cancer. See also Renal cell carcinoma
   hedgehog inhibitors for, 129
   oncogenes in, 142t
   smoking and, 87f
   tumor-suppressor genes in, 142t
KIFC1, 180
Kinase(s). See specific kinase
Kinesin-5 motor (Eg5), 165
Kinetochore(s), 23, 54, 164f, 167, 173f, 174, 178–179, 208–209, 209f
Kininogens, 228
KIP1, 151f, 168f, 169, 170–171, 170f, 171, 177
KIT, targeted therapy and, 468t
KIT gene, 142t
k-mean clustering, 43
KMT. See Lysine methyltransferases (KMT)
KMTi. See Lysine methyltransferase inhibitors (KMTi)
Knudson, Alfred, 17, 140–141, 143f, 155
KRAS, 89, 117, 118, 129, 226, 295, 310, 465f, 467t, 471, 551
   in colon cancer, 551
KRAS gene, 142t
   activating mutations, cancer associated with, 154–155, 154f
   and angiogenesis, 265
   in chromosomal instability (CIN) variant gastric cancer, 404
   first isolation of, 140
Kruskal-Wallis test, 83
KS. See Kaposi sarcoma (KS)
KU70/80, 203, 203f, 204, 206f, 298, 361

L

Label-free peak integration, 36
Lactate, in tumor microenvironment, 284, 286, 286f, 287f
Laminin, 124, 226, 228, 229f, 240, 240f, 282, 284
   in vasculogenic mimicry, 255–256
Lapatinib, 142t, 268t, 469f
   with capecitabine, 473
   indications for, 467t
   mechanism of action of, 473
   prevention of tumor in GEMM, 414
   toxicity of, 473
   with trastuzumab, 473
Larotrectinib, 2, 404, 469f, 479
   indications for, 467t

Laryngeal cancer
   alcohol and, 87–88
   radiotherapy for, with concomitant nicotinamide and carbogen, 383
   smoking and, 87f
Laser capture microdissection, 38, 39, 40f
Late Effects Normal Tissue Task Force Subjective, Objective, Management, and Analytic (LENT/SOMA) system, 384
Latent period, 97, 103, 105t, 418, 442
LC-MS analysis, 32, 33f, 35, 35f, 36
   gel-enhanced, 34
LDHA, MYC and, 151f
Lead-time bias, 80–81, 80t, 564–565, 565f
LECs. See Lymphatic endothelial cells (LECs)
Lectins, c-type, 518
LEF. See Lymphoid enhanced transcription factor (LEF)
Lenalidomide, 134, 407, 479
   antiangiogenic properties of, 268, 268t
   plasma time-concentration curve for, 430f
Length-time bias, 80, 564, 564f
Lentivirus, transfection using, 23–24, 24f, 540f, 541
Lenvatinib, 268t, 469f, 470, 475
LET. See Linear energy transfer (LET)
Letrozole, 121, 476, 498, 499f
   structure of, 499f
Leucine-rich repeat regions (LRR), 518
Leucine zipper transcription factors, 25, 121f, 122
Leucovorin, see also folinic acid, 437
   and 5-fluorouracil, combined, 438, 438f, 439, 442
Leucovorin rescue, methotrexate and, 437
Leukapheresis, 536
Leukemia(s). See also specific leukemia
   acute, as second malignancies, 418
   cancer stem cells in, 314–315, 315f
   cells of origin, 314
   CpG island methylator phenotype (CIMP) in, 57
   cytogenetic analysis of, 6
   cytokine signaling and, 124
   etoposide-induced, 442
   MLL mutations in, 58, 61
   myeloid
      EZH2 mutations in, 61
      hedgehog inhibitors for, 129
      p53 mutations in, 155
   relapse, after bone marrow transplantation, 539
   secondary, 442
   stem cell gene expression in, prognostic significance of, 319
Leukemia stem cells (LSC), 315
Leukocyte function–associated antigen (LFA), 521, 522f
Leukocytes, vascular, 238, 251, 251f, 270, 283, 306f, 309, 309f, 536
Leuprolide, in prostate cancer treatment, 503, 506f
LFA. See Leukocyte function–associated antigen (LFA)
LGK974, 126
LGP2, 518
LGR5, 127
   in colorectal cancer, 317
LH. See Luteinizing hormone (LH)
LHRH. See Luteinizing hormone–releasing hormone (LHRH)
Lifestyle, and cancer risk, 1, 110
Life-table method, for actuarial survival curve, 555, 555f, 555t
Li-Fraumeni syndrome, 1, 155, 200t, 211, 361

Likelihood ratios, 566
Linear energy transfer (LET), 351, 351t, 352f, 380f, 374
   and oxygen enhancement ratio, 379, 380f
Linear quadratic (LQ) equation, and models for isoeffect of fractionated radiotherapy, 394–395
Linear-quadratic model
   of cell survival after radiation, 355f, 356, 368, 368f, 378f
   for isoeffect of fractionated radiotherapy, 394–395
Linear regression, 84, 84t
Linker DNA, 52f
LIN12/NOTCH repeat (LNR), 127, 127f, 128
Lipid(s), synthesis of, 287, 287f
Lipid phosphatase(s), 122–123, 153f, 156
Lipopolysaccharide (LPS), 518
Liposomal drugs, 445–446
Liposomes, 410, 445–446
   enhanced permeability and retention effect and, 446
Liquid biopsy, 63, 65
   and cancer heterogeneity, 320
   in cancer screening, 64–65
   epigenetics in, cancer monitoring based on, 63–65, 64f
Liquid chromatography (LC), 32
Liver cancer. See also Hepatocellular carcinoma (HCC)
   age-standardized incidence rates for, global variation in, 73, 73f
   alcohol and, 87–88
   gene fusion in, 147t
   risk factors for, 73
   smoking and, 87f
   tumor-suppressor genes in, 142t
   viral hepatitis and, 103
   WNT pathway inhibitors for, 127
Liver kinase B1 (LKB1), 153
   and tumor metabolism, 286f, 288
LKB1 gene, 142t
LNCaP cell line, 23, 507
LN229 cell line, 23
lncRNAs. See RNA (ribonucleic acid), long noncoding (lncRNAs)
LNR. See LIN12/NOTCH repeat (LNR)
Local multiply damaged sites (LMDSs), of DNA, 352, 352f
Logistic regression, 84t
Log-rank analysis, 42
Log-rank test, see also Wilcoxon, 556
LOH. See Loss of heterozygosity (LOH)
Lonafarnib, 118
Lorlatinib, 479
   indications for, 467t
Loss-of-function events. See also specific event
   and cancer, 155–158
Loss of heterozygosity (LOH), 15, 196, 476, 477
   copy-neutral, 14
   studies, SNP arrays for, 14
   at tumor-suppressor locus, 140
Low-density lipoprotein receptor-related proteins (LRPs), in WNT signaling, 125, 126f
LPS. See Lipopolysaccharide (LPS)
LQ equation. See Linear quadratic (LQ) equation
LRR. See Leucine-rich repeat regions (LRR)
LSC. See Leukemia stem cells (LSC)
Luciferase, in optical imaging of animal models, 232, 332f, 340, 340f, 413
   in sequencing, 16f, 17f

Lung
  fibrosis
    bleomycin-induced, 445
    radiation-induced, 387, 388f
  functional reserve in, 387
  late radiation damage in, 387, 388f
  volume irradiated, and functional impairment, 387
Lung cancer, 1
  age-standardized incidence and mortality rates for, 72, 72f
  B-RAF mutations in, 154, 154f
  carcinogens and, 104
  chemoprevention of, 110
  computed tomography of, 330f
  copy-number variations in, 17
  EGFR-sensitizing mutations in, and treatment outcomes, 89
  ERBB1 mutations in, 151
  gene fusion in, 147t, 404
  genetic and epigenetic heterogeneity of, interdependence of, 319
  genetic susceptibility for, heterogeneity of, 88
  hedgehog inhibitors for, 129
  incidence of
    sex differences in, 72f, 73–74
    time trends in, 72f, 73–74
  invasiveness gene signature in, 319
  K-RAS mutations in, 154, 154f
  metastasis, principal sites of, 234t
  microRNAs in, 147
  monoclonal antibody therapy for, 532t
  oncogenes in, 142t
  PI3-kinase signaling alterations in, 153, 153f
  prognostic factors in, 70
  PTEN loss of function in, 156
  PTEN promoter methylation in, 157, 157f
  RAS-MAPK mutations in, 119
  risk
    genetic variations in, 108
    nicotine addiction and, genomic epidemiologic study of, 88
  screening, 565
    CT in, 332
    and prevalence, 72
  smoking and, 1, 86–87, 87f
  susceptibility gene for, 88
  treatment of, recent advances in, 3
  tumor-suppressor genes in, 142t
  WNT signaling in, 126
Lung-colony assay, 356
Luteinizing hormone (LH), 488, 490f
Luteinizing hormone–releasing hormone (LHRH), 488, 490f
Luteinizing hormone–releasing hormone (LHRH) agonists
  in breast cancer treatment, 490f, 498
  in prostate cancer treatment, 503
Luteinizing hormone–releasing hormone (LHRH) antagonists, in prostate cancer treatment, 503
LY3039478, 128
Lymphangiogenesis, 241, 254f, 257, 257t, 258, 264f
  definition of, 255
  tumor, 264f, 267
Lymphatic endothelial cells (LECs), 250f, 255
Lymphatics, 249, 250f, 252f, 255, 256, 259, 264f, 267, 283, 308
Lymphatic vessel hyaluronan receptor-1 (LYVE-1), and lymphangiogenesis, 255

Lymphocyte(s). See also B cells (B lymphocytes); T cells (T lymphocytes)
  diversity, generation of, 519, 520f
  in tumor microenvironment, 309
Lymphoid enhanced transcription factor (LEF), in WNT signaling, 125, 126f
Lymphoid malignancy, ATM gene and, 210
Lymphoma(s). See also Hodgkin lymphoma; Non-Hodgkin lymphoma (NHL)
  B-cell
    EZH2 mutations in, 58
    hedgehog signaling in, 129
    MYC upregulation in, 150
    NOTCH signaling in, 128
  cancer stem cells and, 315
  cellular radiosensitivity in, 378t
  cytogenetic analysis of, 6
  diffuse large B-cell, EZH2 mutations in, 61
  endothelial transdifferentiation in, 255
  follicular, EZH2 mutations in, 61
  gene fusion in, 147t
  hedgehog inhibitors for, 129
  large-cell, stromal component of, 308, 309f
  oncogenes in, 142t
  radiosensitivity of, 353
  second malignancy after, 418
  T-cell
    cutaneous, treatment of, 408, 477
    gene fusion in, 147t
    histone deacetylase inhibitors for, 61
    NOTCH signaling in, 128
    peripheral, treatment of, 477
  treatment of, 408, 409, 477
Lynch syndrome, 200t
Lysine demethylase(s), 53
  Jumonji C (JMJC) domain-containing, 59–61, 59f
  KDM1 class
    inhibitors, 60, 61
    metabolic cofactors for, 59, 59f
    overexpression of, 61
Lysine demethylase inhibitors (KDMi), 60f, 61
Lysine methyltransferase(s) (KMT), 53
  activity, 61
  mutations, in cancer, 57–58
Lysine methyltransferase inhibitors (KMTi), 60f, 61

M

mAb. See Monoclonal antibody(ies) (mAb)
MABEL. See Minimal anticipated biologic effect level (MABEL)
MAC. See Membrane attack complex (MAC)
Machine learning,
  in large dataset analysis, 43
  for image reconstruction, prognostics, and predictions, 342–344, 344f
Macrophage(s), 516
  anti-inflammatory M2, and adaptive resistance, 538
  M1, 238
  M2, 230, 238, 265
    tumor-associated, 249
  migration of, 518–519
  tissue-resident, 283
  in tumor microenvironment, 309
Macrophage colony-stimulating factor (M-CSF), 415f
MAD1, 180
MAD2
  and mitotic spindle checkpoint, 208–209, 209f
  MYC and, 151f

MAD2 gene, 180
MAGE, 526, 528
Magnetic resonance imaging (MRI), 3, 329, 330f, 332–335, 332f, 333f, 337f
  advances in (future directions for), 342
  agents for, 332f
  of animal models, 339
  in breast cancer, 334–335
  HIFU guidance, 342
  hyperpolarized ^{13}C in, 339, 339f
  hyperpolarized ^{129}Xe gas in, 339
  quality assurance, 340–341
  radiomics and, 343, 344f
  radiotherapy guidance, 341–342
  spin-lattice relaxation time (T_1), 334
  spin-spin relaxation time (T_2), 334
Magnetic resonance spectroscopy imaging (MRSI), 332f, 334, 336f. See also Chemical shift imaging (CSI)
Magnetofection, 23
Major histocompatibility complex (MHC), 516, 516f
  class II molecules, 516–517, 516f, 517f, 523
  class I molecules, 516–518, 516f, 517f
    in detection of TAA-specific T cells, 529, 529f
  NK cells and, 519
  peptide-binding cleft of, 516–517, 516f, 517f
  and T-cell immunity, 524–525
  and T-cell tolerance, 524–525
Malate production, in glutamine metabolism, 287f, 289, 289f
MALDI. See Matrix-assisted laser desorption/ionization (MALDI)
MALDI-TOF MS. See Matrix-assisted laser desorption/ionization-time of flight mass spectrometry (MALDI-TOF MS)
Malic enzyme 1 (ME1), 289
Malignant melanoma-initiating cells (MMICs), 317
Malignant transformation. See also Carcinogenesis
  in cell culture, assays for, 106
  genetic instability and, 194–197
  growth factor signaling in, 114
Mammalian target of rapamycin (mTOR), 120–121, 123, 124, 125, 133, 175, 271, 363, 416, 473, 502, 503
  functions of, 474f, 475
  in hypoxic response, 295, 296f
  and oxidative stress, 290, 290f
  and tumor metabolism, 286f, 288
Mammalian target of rapamycin (mTOR) inhibitors, 475
  mucosal damage caused by, 417
  toxicity of, 475
Mammaprint, 3, 495
Mammography, screening, evaluation of, 561, 564–565
MaMTH, 30
Mann-Whitney U test, 83
Mantle cell lymphoma (MCL), 188
  ATM gene and, 210
  relapsed, targeted therapy for, 480
  treatment of, 133, 408, 479, 480
MAPK. See Mitogen-activated protein kinase(s) (MAPK)
Marrow-derived suppressor cells (MDSCs), 251
Mass cytometry, 307
Massively parallel signature sequencing (MPSS), 14

Mass spectrometer
    detector of, 30, 31f
    ion source of, 30, 31f
    mass analyzer of, 30, 31f
Mass spectrometry (MS), 30–32, 31f, 307
    in biomarker discovery, 36–37, 36f
    in bottom-up proteomics, 32
    quantitative protein profiling by, isotope labeling used in, 34–36, 35f
Mass-to-charge ratio. See m/z ratio
Mast cells (MCs), and angiogenesis, 251, 265, 283, 386
Matrigel, 267, 269f, 307, 317
Matrix-assisted laser desorption/ionization (MALDI), 31, 31f
Matrix-assisted laser desorption/ionization-time of flight mass spectrometry (MALDI-TOF MS), in DNA analysis, 22
Matrix metalloproteinases (MMPs), 227, 230
    in angiogenesis, 254, 259, 260f
    and cancer progression, 237–242, 237t
    in cancer-related extracellular vesicles, 262
    membrane-type (MT-MMPs), 259, 260f
    and metastasis, 231f, 232, 233
    MMP9, in angiogenesis, 257t
    noncatalytic fragment. See PEX
    in vasculogenic mimicry, 255–256
MAX, 175
Maximum tolerated dose (MTD), 431, 548–549
MCC. See Mitotic checkpoint complex (MCC)
MCCs. See Multilayered cell cultures (MCCs)
MCF-7 cell line, 23, 493, 503
MCL. See Mantle cell lymphoma (MCL)
MCL-1, 182, 184, 185, 188
MCT. See Monocarboxylate transporters (MCT)
MDA-5, 518
MDM2, 155, 156f, 184, 186f, 196, 207, 208f, 296, 409, 453
    targeted degradation of, 134
MDM2-TP53, targeted therapy and, 409
MDS. See Myelodysplastic syndrome (MDS)
MDSCs. See Marrow-derived suppressor cells (MDSCs)
2ME2. See 2-Methoxyestradiol (2ME2)
Mechlorethamine, 432, 434. See also Nitrogen mustard(s) and related compounds
    structure of, 432, 433f
MED1, overexpression, in prostate cancer, 508
MeDIP. See Methyl-specific antibodies (MeDIP)
Medulloblastoma
    cancer stem cells in, 315–316
    cells of origin, 314, 314t
    cellular radiosensitivity in, 378t
    hedgehog inhibitors for, 129
    hedgehog signaling in, 129
    invasiveness gene signature in, 319
    MLL2 and MLL3 mutations in, 58
    WNT signaling in, 126
MEK, 117–118, 117f, 119, 154f, 195, 377, 502
    targeted therapy and, 467t
MEK inhibitors, 322f, 418
    indications for, 475
    for melanoma, 320, 321
    side effects of, 475–476
Melan-A/MART-1, 528, 529
Melanoma, 196
    B16F10 cells from, 235, 235f
    BRAF inhibitor therapy for, 321
        and secondary squamous cell carcinoma, 418

BRAF mutations in, 119–120, 154, 154f, 196, 306–307, 307f, 320, 528, 528f, 568
    and targeted therapy, 158–159, 404
    and treatment, 321
cancer stem cells in, 316f, 317
cell line treated with low-LET radiation, survival curve for, 355, 355f
cellular radiosensitivity in, 377, 378f, 378t
clonal subpopulations in, 310
differentiation antigens in, 528, 528f
driver mutations in, 306–307, 307f
    and treatment, 310
epigenetic therapy and immune checkpoint blockade for, 62
EZH2 mutations in, 58
familial cutaneous, 196
hedgehog signaling in, 129
heterogeneity of, clinical significance of, 320
IDO expression in, prognostic significance of, 538
interpatient heterogeneity of, 306–307, 307f
JARID1B in, 317–318
KIT mutations, 307, 307f
metastatic, adoptive cell therapy with tumor-infiltrating lymphocytes, 539
mutations in, 306–307, 307f, 528, 528f
    and acquired resistance to PD-1 therapy, 538
NF1 mutations, 307, 307f
NRAS mutations in, 154, 154f, 307, 307f
oncogenes in, 142t
RAS mutations, 119
stromal component of, 308, 309f
targeted therapy for, 467t
treatment of
    BRAF and MEK inhibitors in, 321
    recent advances in, 2–3
tumor-suppressor genes in, 142t
uveal, endothelial transdifferentiation in, 255
WNT pathway inhibitors for, 127
Melphalan, 407, 416, 418, 433
    AML caused by, 432
    and second malignancy, 418
    structure of, 432, 433f
    toxicity of, 433
    uptake, extracellular acidity and, 454–455
Membrane attack complex (MAC), 532, 534f
Membrane-bound proteins/receptors, 38, 113, 125, 126, 127, 154, 464, 469, 519
    and cancer-associated fibroblasts, 282, 282t
    and ectoenzymes, 230
    and vesicles, 186
Membrane 2-hybrid system, 30
Mendelian randomization, 91
Meningioma, tumor-suppressor genes in, 142t
Menopause, 495
    chemotherapy-induced, 417
    in men, 488
2-Mercaptoethane sulfonate. See Mesna
Merkel cell carcinoma–associated polyoma virus, 529
Mesenchymal cells, 226, 240, 281
Mesenchymal-to-epithelial transition (MET), 240, 313
Mesna, 434
Mesothelin, 529
Mesothelioma, 1, 437, 468, 529
Messenger RNA (mRNA)
    alternative splicing, 229
    analysis of, 42–43, 108, 307, 404, 405, 405f
    in cancer-related extracellular vesicles, 242, 262
    methods for detection, 38, 39

modulation, and oncogenesis, 144, 145f, 147, 288, 289
stability/degradation, by RNA interference or small non-coding RNAs, 24–25, 25f, 406f
transcription of, 7
reverse transcription of, 7, 11
untranslated regions, 448
MET. See Mesenchymal-epithelial transition (MET)
Meta-analysis, 92, 383, 383f, 558–559, 559f
Metabolic modifiers, mechanism of action of, 463f
Metabolome, and molecular signatures of exposure and risk, 108–109
Metabolomics, 70, 88
Metalloproteinase(s), 226, 226t, 227
Metallothionein, 351
    drug binding, drug resistance caused by, 446t, 447f
Metaphase, 6, 11, 12f, 13, 166f, 167, 170, 172, 173f, 174, 178, 208, 209f
Metaphase plate, 167
Meta-regression, 92
Metastasis, 2, 143, 230–234, 305
    cancer stem cells in, 236
    cancer subclones and, 225–226
    circulating tumor cells in, 232–233. See also Circulating tumor cells (CTCs)
    clonal heterogeneity in, 235, 236f, 242
    colonization in, 231f, 233–234
    definition of, 223
    detachment from primary tumor in, 231–232, 231f
    dormancy in, 236
    dynamics of, 234–236
    extravasation in, 231f, 233
    formation of, 312
    genetic evolution of, 242
    genomic evolution of, 311, 312f
    hedgehog signaling in, 129
    heterogeneity and, 225–226
    hypoxia and, 297, 297f
    inefficiency of, 235, 236f
    intravasation in, 231–232, 231f
    kinetics of, 230
    local invasion in, 231–232, 231f
    molecular mechanisms of, 237–242, 239f
    MYC and, 151f
    organotropism in, 234–235, 234t
    pre-metastatic niche formation and, 233, 241–242, 241f
    prevention of, treatment for, 242–243
    routes of, 230
    steps in, 230–231, 231f, 235
    treatment of, 429
        heterogeneity and, 321
    tumor cell survival in bloodstream and, 231f, 232
    before tumor detection, 276, 277f
    tumor size and, 276
Metastatic dissemination, 224, 238, 241, 262, 284, 465
    linear model, 242
    parallel progression model, 242
Metastatic relapse, 233, 236
Metformin, 288, 289, 299
    anticancer activity of, 407
MET gene, 142t
Methotrexate, 436–437
    adverse effects, 437
    cellular uptake of, 447f, 448
    dosage and administration of, 437
    drug interactions with, 437

596

effects on cellular metabolism, 436, 437f
high-dose, 437
indications for, 437
and leucovorin rescue, 437
mechanism of action of, 437
mucosal damage caused by, 417
nephrotoxicity of, 430
pharmacokinetics of, 437
polyglutamates, 436–437
resistance to, 437, 446, 446t, 447f, 448, 449t, 451
structure of, 436f
tissue penetration by, 456
toxicity of, 437
2-Methoxyestradiol (2ME2), 268
Methylated DNA, in DNA methylation analysis, 20–22, 21t, 22f, 25, 26f
Methylated DNA-binding proteins, in DNA methylation analysis, 21t
3-Methylcholanthrene, potency as carcinogen, 107f
O[6]-Methylguanine-DNA methyltransferase (MGMT), 63, 448, 452, 452f
Methyl methanesulfonate (MMS), potency as carcinogen, 107f
Methylome, 44, 243, 307
Methyl-specific antibodies (MeDIP), 20–22, 22f
  MeDIP-chip, 21t
  MeDIP-seq, 21t
Methyl thiazole tetrazolium (MTT) assay, 356, 411
Metronidazole, potency as carcinogen, 107f
Metronomic therapy, 416
M-FISH. See Multifluor fluorescence in situ hybridization (M-FISH)
MGMT. See O[6]-Methylguanine-DNA methyltransferase (MGMT)
MHC. See Major histocompatibility complex (MHC)
MHC-peptide multimer, 529, 529f
Mice
  bioassays in, 106
  CRISPR used in, 30
  immune-deprived, 1–2
  immunocompromised, 307, 412–413
  immunodeficient, and immune surveillance studies, 529–530
  inbred (syngeneic), 1
  knockout, 25–27
  NOD/SCID, 307, 412–413
  NSG, 307
  SCID, 307
    AML formation in, 315
    DNA-PK studies in, 204
  stem cell biology studies in, 307
  studies of targeted agents in, 462
  telomerase-deficient, 214–215
  telomere dysfunction in, 214–215
  transgenic, 25–27. See also Genetically engineered mouse models (GEMMs)
    in preclinical evaluation of anticancer drugs, 411f, 413–414
  xenografting of human tumors into, in preclinical evaluation of anticancer drugs, 411f, 412–413
  xenografts in, 1–2, 307
Microarrays, 13, 14, 17–19, 19f, 21t, 22, 30, 38, 39, 39f, 307, 548
  analysis, challenges to, 42, 548
  data analysis, web-based resources on, 18
Microcirculation, 252f, 255
  tumor, properties of, 264f, 266–267, 269f

Microenvironment. See Tumor microenvironment (TME)
β_2-Microglobulin, 516, 516f
Microhomology-mediated end joining (MMEJ)/single-strand annealing (SSA), 203f
Micronuclei, 105, 179, 180, 187, 354
  in intracellular response to ionizing radiation, 363
Microparticles, in tumor neovascularization, 262
MicroRNA axes, 149
MicroRNAs (miRNAs), 24, 25f, 145f, 307
  and angiogenesis, 265
  biogenesis of, 24, 25f
  in cancer, 24, 147
  in cancer-related extracellular vesicles, 262
  in EMT, 313
  functions of, 24, 25f
  genomic organization, 24, 25f
  hypoxia and, 295f, 298
  in metastasis, 233
  precursor (pre-miRNA), 24, 25f
  primary transcripts (pri-miRNA), 24, 25f
  PTEN-targeted, 121, 157, 157f
  regulation by circRNA and lncRNA, 149
  as therapeutic focal points, 147
  as tumor suppressors, 24, 147
Microsatellite instability (MSI), 3, 121, 178, 200t, 210–211, 321
  in colorectal cancer, 309–310
Microsatellites, 197, 210–211
Microscope, 1, 6, 40, 41f, 165, 340, 341
Microscopy, 6, 11, 30, 38, 332f, 340–341
Microtubule binding agents (MTBAs), 177, 177f
Microtubules, 164–165, 164f, 166f, 167, 172–174, 175, 178, 179, 205, 208, 209, 209f. See also Antimicrotubular agents
  taxanes and, 444–445
  vinca alkaloids and, 443
Microvesicles, in tumor neovascularization, 262
Microvessels, 255
  in cancer, 309
Midostaurin, 142t, 469f, 471
  indications for, 468t
Minichromosome maintenance complexes (MCMs), 165f, 170
Minimal anticipated biologic effect level (MABEL), 419
miniTurbo, 30
Mipomersen, 409–410
miRNAs. See MicroRNAs (miRNAs)
Misclassification, of exposure, 79–80, 90–91
Mismatch repair (MMR), 197–198, 198f
  defects, cancer-prone human syndromes associated with, 200t, 210
  hypoxia and, 298, 299
  PTEN and, 121
Misonidazole, 294, 299, 336, 337f
Missing self, 519
Mitochondrial cell death pathway, 183f, 184, 480
  targeted therapy and, 474f
Mitochondrial DNA, damage to, 105
Mitochondrial metabolism, 285–286, 286f
Mitogen-activated protein kinase(s) (MAPK), 118–120, 149, 154, 154f, 230
  activation, 118–119, 119f
  core signaling molecule, 118–119, 119f
  dysregulation, and malignancy, 119–120
  in hypoxic response, 295
  inhibitor, 470, 475–476
  mutant EGFRs and, 152
  substrate specificity, 119

Mitogen-activated protein kinase (MAPK) pathway inhibitors, 470, 475–476
Mitomycin C, 197, 202
  adverse effects, 445
  indications for, 445
  metabolism of, 445
  myelosuppression caused by, 445
Mitosis, 163–165, 164f, 166f, 172
  as anticancer therapeutic target, 180–181
  late, daughter cells in, 174–175
  molecular events of, 172–174, 173f
  morphologic events of, 172–174, 173f
  phases of, 165–167, 166f
Mitotic catastrophe, 209–210, 353f, 354, 356, 364, 453
  mechanisms of, 187
  morphologic changes during, 181, 181f
Mitotic checkpoint complex (MCC), 179
  disruption, in cancer, 180
Mitotic errors, 179–180
Mitotic slippage, 187, 208
Mitotic spindle, 6, 132, 164, 165, 167, 174, 179, 180, 187, 443, 445
Mitotic spindle checkpoints, 205, 208–209, 209f
Mitoxantrone,
  indications for, 443
  pharmacokinetics of, 443
  resistance to, 449t
  and second malignancy, 418
  structure of, 443f
  tissue penetration by, 456, 456f
Mixed effects modeling, 92
Mixed-lineage kinase domain-like pseudokinase, 186
MLL-AF9 fusion gene, 147t
MLL-ENL fusion gene, 147t
MLL1 mutations, in childhood leukemias, 58
MLN4924, 133
MMEJ/SSA. See Microhomology-mediated end joining (MMEJ)/single-strand annealing (SSA)
MMICs. See Malignant melanoma-initiating cells (MMICs)
MMPs. See Matrix metalloproteinases (MMPs)
MMTV. See Mouse mammary tumor virus (MMTV)
Moesin, 124, 229, 229f, 230
Molecular cytogenetics, 6
Molecular epidemiology, 88, 92, 104f
  of carcinogenesis, 107–109
Molecular residual disease, detection of, 65
Molecular targeted therapies, 461–481
  advances in (future directions for), 481
  candidates for, identification of, 461
  clinical trials of, 549
  costs of, 461
  development of, 551
  dosage and administration of, 431
  indications for, 467t–468t
  intracellular targets, 474f
  mechanism of action of, 462–464, 463f
  and mitochondrial cell death pathway, 474f
  and oncometabolite pathway, 474f
  resistance to
    acquired (secondary, adaptive), 465
    activation of compensatorty pathways in, 465, 465f
    alteration of targeted protein in, 465, 465f
    bypass activation of signaling pathways in, 465, 465f

Molecular targeted therapies (Cont.)
    intrinsic (primary, de novo), 465
    mechanisms of, 465, 465f
    and SMO/PTCH signaling, 474f
    target identification for, 462
Monocarboxylate transporters (MCTs), and glycolysis, 287
Monoclonal antibody(ies) (mAb), 403
    antiangiogenic, 468–469
    bispecific, 409
    cancer cell targeting by, 462–464, 463f
    for cancer therapy, 2, 531–534, 532t
    and chemotherapy agents, combined, 534
    chimeric, 532, 532t, 533f
    conjugated to cytotoxic agent, 409
    conjugated to radioactive molecules, 534
    and Delta-Like Ligand 4 receptor (DLL-4), 128
    humanized, 532, 532t, 533f
    indications for, 532t
    integrin-blocking, 125
    mechanism of action of, 532–533
    modified, 533–534
    mouse, 532, 532t, 533f
    and NOTCH, 128
    production of, 531–532, 533f
    sequencing of, 33
    target molecules for, 532t
    tissue penetration by, 456
    types of, 532, 532t, 533f
    and WNT-related disease, 127
Monoclonal antibody(ies) (mAb), against angiogenic ligands, 268–270, 268t
Monocytes
    migration of, 518–519
    production of, 415, 416f
    TIE2-expressing, 249, 251f
    tissue-resident, 283
Monopolar spindle 1 (MPS1), see also TTK, 179, 181
Monosomy, FISH detection of, 12–13
Mortality rate, 70, 71, 118, 561, 565
    age-standardized, 72, 72f
    cause-specific, 70
    global trends in, 74
    per person-year, 70
Mother vessels, in angiogenesis, 253, 253f
Mouse mammary tumor virus (MMTV), 414
    mammary carcinoma caused by, NOTCH signaling in, 128
MPS1. See Monopolar spindle 1 (MPS1)
MRE11, 200t, 202–204, 206f, 207f, 213
    and radiosensitivity, 362f
MRI. See Magnetic resonance imaging (MRI)
MRM-MS. See Multiple reaction monitoring-mass spectrometry (MRM-MS)
mRNA. See Messenger RNA (mRNA)
MRN complex, 202, 202f, 203, 203f, 204, 206–208, 206f, 213, 214f
MRP1. See Multidrug resistance protein 1 (MRP1)
MRP2. See Multidrug resistance protein 2 (MRP2)
MRP4. See Multidrug resistance protein 4 (MRP4)
MR-PET, 341
MRSI. See Magnetic resonance spectroscopy imaging (MRSI)
MSI. See Microsatellite instability (MSI)
MTBAs. See Microtubule binding agents (MTBAs)
MTD. See Maximum tolerated dose (MTD)

mTOR. See Mammalian target of rapamycin (mTOR)
mTORC1 kinase, 175
mTOR complex. See TORC1; TORC2
MTT. See Methyl thiazole tetrazolium (MTT) assay
Mucin-1 (MUC-1), glycosylation, in cancer, 528f, 529
Mucositis
    drug-induced, 416–417, 442
    radiation-induced, 386, 386f
Multidimensional protein identification technology (MudPIT), 34
Multidrug resistance, enhanced drug efflux and, 449–451, 449f, 449t, 450f
Multidrug resistance protein 1 (MRP1)
    and multidrug resistance, 447f, 449, 449f, 449t, 450–452, 450f
    physiologic functions of, 451
    structure of, 450, 450f
Multidrug resistance protein 2 (MRP2), 447f, 449f, 450f, 451
Multidrug resistance protein 4 (MRP4), 449f, 450f
Multifluor fluorescence in situ hybridization (M-FISH), 13
Multikinase inhibitors, 269, 271, 408
Multilayered cell cultures (MCCs), 411, 453, 455f
    drug transport studies, 453, 455f, 456
Multiomics analysis, 307
Multiple myeloma (MM)
    cell adhesion–mediated drug resistance in, 454
    drug treatment of, 407
    hedgehog signaling in, 129
    histone deacetylase inhibitors for, 61
    monoclonal antibody therapy for, 532t
    P-glycoprotein increase in, prognostic significance of, 450
    relapsed, treatment of, 408
    thalidomide treatment for, 268
    treatment of, 133, 134
Multiple reaction monitoring-mass spectrometry (MRM-MS), 36–37
Multipolar spindle, 179–180
Multisite variants (MSVs), 17
Multispecific organic anion transporters, 452
Multivariable analysis, 43, 556, 567
Multivariate analysis, 43
Mural cells, of vasculature, 249, 251f
Mutation(s), 194–195, 194f. See also Site-directed mutagenesis
    in cancer genomes, 3
    and carcinogenesis, 2, 97–98, 193, 224–225
    carcinogen-induced, detection of, 105–106, 105f
    caretaker, 143, 144f
    chemical carcinogens and, 102
    classification of, 547–548
    conditionally targeted, 27
    driver, 2, 139, 140f, 141f, 225
        as drug targets, 404
        identification of, 404
        and intratumoral heterogeneity, 310–312, 310f
        in melanoma, 306–307, 307f, 310
        and treatment, 310
    and drug resistance, 446, 448
    frame-shift, 102
    gatekeeper, 143, 144f, 465, 472, 479
    genomic, 144–146, 145f, 146f
    germline, 141, 141f
    identification of, 404

    insertional, 26, 144–146, 145f, 146f
    landscaper, 143, 144f
    missense, 144–146, 146f
    nonsense, 144–146, 146f
    oncogenic, 109, 142–143, 144f, 145f
        cellular context and, 144
        proangiogenic effects of, 265
        properties conferred by, 141–143, 141f, 144
    passenger, 2, 139, 140f, 225
        identification of, 404
    point, 144–146, 145f, 146f
    as predictive markers for targeted therapies, 568
    properties conferred by, 146f
    recurrent, 568
    and response to treatment, 321
    solvent-front, 465, 479
    somatic, 141, 141f
    synonymous, 144–146, 146f
    and tumor growth and spread, 98
    and tumor initiation, 97–98
Mutational signatures, in human cancer, 102, 109
Mutation genotyping, 568
Mutator phenotype, see also hypermutator phenotype, 98, 194, 194f, 211, 310f, 321
MUTYH-associated polyposis, 200t
MYC, 122
    and angiogenesis, 151f
    and apoptosis, 150, 151f
    and avoidance of immune destruction, 151f
    and cell proliferation, 151f
    central regulatory role of, 150, 151f
    and genomic instability, 151f
    and glutaminolysis, 289, 289f
    and metastasis, 151f
    promotion of tumorigenesis, 150–151, 151f
    targets, 150, 151f
    and tumor metabolism, 286f, 288, 289
    upregulation of, in cancer, 150–151, 151f
    UPS and, 132
MYC gene, 142t, 145, 175
    and angiogenesis, 265
MYCL1 gene, 150
MYCN protein, 508
MYCN gene, 12f, 17, 150
Myelodysplastic syndrome (MDS), 61, 63
    after anticancer treatment, 418
    DNMT inhibitors for, 60–61
    targeted therapy for, 134, 467t
    TET2 mutations in, 63
Myeloid bone marrow–derived regulatory cells, 249
Myeloid cells, in tumor microenvironment, 309
Myeloid-derived suppressor cells (MDSCs), 230, 241f, 251, 283
    and adaptive resistance, 538
    hypoxia and, 297, 297f
Myeloid dysplastic syndromes, treatment of, 134
Myeloma. See also Multiple myeloma (MM)
    cancer stem cells and, 315
    cellular radiosensitivity in, 378t
Myelopathy, radiation-induced, 387
Myeloproliferative disease, cytokine signaling and, 124
Myelosuppression, 278, 279,
    alkylating agents and, 432, 433, 436–438
    drug-induced, 414–416, 439–440, 442–446, 475, 476, 478, 480
    mitomycin C and, 445
Myofibroblasts, 282, 309
MZF1 gene, in cancer, 122
m/z ratio (mass-to-charge ratio), 30, 31f, 33f

598

N

Nab-paclitaxel, 445
NADPH. *See* Nicotinamide adenine dinucleotide phosphate (NADPH)
NADPH oxidase (NOX), 103
NAFs. *See* Normal activated fibroblasts (NAFs)
nal-IRI, 446
Nano agents, 340
NANOG, 314, 314t, 318
Nanoparticles
  anticancer drugs entrapped in, 410, 446
  in imaging, 342, 343f
β-Naphthylamine
  as carcinogen, 98, 99f
  metabolic activation of, 100, 101f
Narrowband imaging, 338, 338f
Nasopharyngeal carcinoma (NPC)
  EBV and, 149
  smoking and, 87f
NATs. *See* Arylamine *N*-acetyltransferases (NATs)
Natural killer (NK) cells, 519, 532
  and metastasis, 231f, 233–234
  ubiquitin ligase and, 132
Natural product libraries, 406–407
Nausea and vomiting
  anticancer drug-related, 417, 432
NBS. *See* Nijmegen breakage syndrome (NBS)
NBS1, and radiosensitivity, 362, 362f
N-cadherin, 313
ncRNA. *See* RNA (ribonucleic acid), noncoding (ncRNA)
Necroptosis, 186, 187f
Necrosis, 181, 353f, 354, 453
  hypoxia and, 292
  mechanisms leading to, 186
  morphologic changes during, 181, 181f
  tumor, 284
  in tumors, 279
NEDD8, 132, 133
NEDD8-activating enzymes (NAEs), inhibitors, 133
N-end rule pathway, 132
Neoadjuvant treatment, 429
Neoantigens, 528, 538
  and response to treatment, 321, 322f
Neovascularization, tumor, 230, 259–260, 261f. *See also* Angiogenesis
  constituent processes of, 261f, 262–263
  extracellular vesicles and, 262
  mechanisms triggering, 263
NEPC. *See* Neuroendocrine prostate cancer (NEPC)
Nephropathy, radiation-induced, 387
NER. *See* Nucleotide excision repair (NER)
Neratinib, 142t, 467t, 469f, 473
  adjuvant use of, 473
Nested case-control studies, 75–76
Network analysis, of -omic data, 44
Neuroblastoma
  ABCC1 polymorphism in, 451
  cellular radiosensitivity in, 378t
  heritable germline copy-number variation in, 17
  MRP1 expression in, 451
  MYCN amplification in, 17
  MYC upregulation in, 150
  N-*myc* amplification in, FISH detection of, 12, 12f
  oncogenes in, 142t
  P-glycoprotein increase in, prognostic significance of, 450
  tumor-suppressor genes in, 142t
Neuroendocrine prostate cancer (NEPC), 508
  androgen receptor status, 495, 508

Neuroendocrine tumors, and hypercalcemia, 509
Neurofibroma, tumor-suppressor genes in, 142t
Neuropilin 1 (NRP1), 256, 257t
  in angiogenesis, 254f, 255
Neuropilin 2 (NRP2), 256
  and lymphangiogenesis, 255
Neurotoxicity
  P-glycoprotein deficiency and, 450
  vinca alkaloides and, 443–444
Neurotrophin-3 (NT-3), receptor, 114f
Neurotrophin-4 (NT-4), receptor, 114f
Neutrons
  linear energy transfer of, 351, 351t
  in radiotherapy, 374
Neutrophils
  angiogenic, 251, 251f
  in metastasis, 238
Next-generation sequencing (NGS), 14–17, 16f–17f, 18f, 211, 307
  commercial platforms, performance of, 320
  and targeted therapy, 159
NF1 gene, 142t
NF2 gene, 142t
NGS. *See* Next-generation sequencing (NGS)
NHEJ. *See* Nonhomologous end-joining (NHEJ)
NHL. *See* Non-Hodgkin lymphoma (NHL)
Nicotinamide, and epigenetic enzyme activity, 59, 59f
Nicotinamide adenine dinucleotide phosphate (NADPH), production, in glutamine metabolism, 289, 289f
Nicotinamide adenine dinucleotide phosphate (NAD(P)H) quinone oxidoreductase, 100
Nicotinamide *N*-methyltransferase, in solid tumors, 59
Nicotine addiction, and lung cancer risk, genomic epidemiologic study of, 88
Nidogen, 226
Nijmegen breakage syndrome (NBS), 200t, 204, 210
  radiosensitivity in, 359, 360f, 361
Nilotinib, 142t, 467t, 478
NimbleGen, 18
Nimorazole, 299
  as hypoxic radiosensitizer, in head and neck cancer, 383–384
Nintedanib, 268t
Niraparib, indications for, 467t, 477
Nitroaromatics, 299
Nitrogen mustard(s) and related compounds, 99f, 432–434, 433f, 446t
Nitroimidazoles, 293, 299
Nitrosamines
  as carcinogens, 99f
  metabolic activation of, 100, 101f
N-Nitrosomorpholine, genomic and proteomic response to, in rat liver, 109
Nitrosoureas, AML caused by, 432
NK cells. *See* Natural killer (NK) cells
NLRs. *See* Nucleotide-binding domain and leucine-rich repeat receptors (NLRs)
NMR. *See* Nuclear magnetic resonance (NMR)
N-MYC, 195
NOAEL. *See* No observed adverse effect level (NOAEL)
Noble, Robert, 488
NOD proteins, 518
Non-Hodgkin lymphoma (NHL)
  ATM gene and, 210
  B-cell, radioimmunotherapy for, 374

  in HIV-infected (AIDS) patients, 529
  indolent, treatment of, 475
  monoclonal antibody therapy for, 532t
  WNT pathway inhibitors for, 127
Nonhomologous end joining (NHEJ), 178, 202, 203–204, 203f, 298, 476–477
  and radiosensitivity, 358f, 361–362
Non-nucleoside DNMT inhibitors, 60–61
Nonparametric smoothing analysis, 548
Non-small cell lung cancer
  cellular radiosensitivity in, 378t
  durvalumab after chemoradiotherapy for, 375
  EGFR and *ALK* in, and targeted therapy, 158–159, 466
  EGFR-mutant, 321, 322f, 568
  EML4-ALK gene fusion in, 145
  gefitinib for, 466
  gene expression profile in, prognostic significance of, 43
  heterogeneity of, clinical significance of, 320
  intratumoral heterogeneity of, 311
  neoantigens in, and treatment response, 321
  ROS1 mutations and ALK translocations in, and treatment outcomes, 89
  targeted therapy for, 467t
  xenograft formation, prognostic significance of, 308
Noonan syndrome, 123
Nordling, Carl, 143f
Normal activated fibroblasts (NAFs), 281–282
Normal distribution, 82, 82f
Normal tissue complication probabilities (NTCP), with radiotherapy, 388
Northern blotting, 9–10
  probes for, 9
NOTCH receptor, 127, 127f
NOTCH signaling pathway, 127–128, 127f, 227, 257t, 258, 282, 314, 314t, 321
  in angiogenesis, 254–255, 254f
  antiangiogenic therapy targeted to, 272
  in breast cancer, 128
  and cancer progression, 237–238, 237t
  in development, 125
  germline mutations in, diseases caused by, 128
  inhibitors, 128
  somatic mutations in, and cancer, 128
  in T-ALL, 128
NOXA, 182, 184, 184f
N-oxide banoxantrone (AQ4N), 299
N-oxides, 299
NPC. *See* Nasopharyngeal carcinoma (NPC)
NPM1-ALK fusion gene, 147t
N-RAS, 118
N-RAS gene, 142t
  activating mutations, cancer associated with, 154–155, 154f
  first isolation of, 140
  in melanoma, 154, 154f, 307, 307f
N region diversity, 519
NRF2, and oxidative stress, 290, 290f
NTCP. *See* Normal tissue complication probabilities (NTCP)
NTHL1-associated polyposis, 200t
NTRK gene, 142t
NTRK gene fusion, 404
NTRK receptor gene rearrangements, 479
Nuclear coactivators (NCOA), 502
  overexpression, in prostate cancer, 508, 508f
Nuclear export, selective inhibitors of, 481

Nuclear factor-κB (NF-κB), 103, 149, 184, 479, 518
Nuclear magnetic resonance (NMR)
  spectroscopy, 30, 37–38
  in drug binding assays, 407, 407f
  multidimensional, 38
Nucleic acid(s). See also DNA (deoxyribonucleic
    acid); RNA (ribonucleic acid)
  analysis, principal techniques for, 5–22
  synthesis of, 287, 287f
Nucleoid sedimentation, 212t
Nucleoside analogs, 439
  cellular uptake of, 448
Nucleoside DNMT inhibitors, 60–61
Nucleosomes, 52, 52f, 54f, 55f, 56
Nucleotide-binding domain and leucine-rich
    repeat receptors (NLRs), 518
Nucleotide excision repair (NER),
    200–201, 201f, 452
  defect, cancer-prone human syndromes
    associated with, 200t
  and drug sensitivity and resistance, 452
  global genome repair (GG-NER), 201, 201f
  and radiosensitivity, 362
  transcription-coupled repair
    (TCR), 197, 201, 201f
Nucleotide instability, 178
Null hypothesis, 42, 92, 553
Nurses' Health Study, 76
NUT carcinoma, 61
Nutrient(s)
  and cancer risk, evaluation of, 90–91
  in tumor microenvironment, 284
  uptake, by malignant cells, 284
NY-ESO-1, 527, 528, 528f, 541

O

Obesity
  and cancer risk, 1, 110
  postmenopausal, and breast cancer risk, 495
  and prostate cancer risk, 497
OCT4 gene/protein, 314, 318
ODD. See Oxygen-dependent degradation
    domains (ODD)
Odds ratio, 81–82, 82t, 84
OER. See Oxygen enhancement ratio (OER)
Ofatumumab, 532t
OGG1. See 8-Oxoguanine glycosylase (OGG1)
Olaparib, 142t, 158
  indications for, 467t, 477
  mechanism of action of, 463f
Olaratumab, 469, 469f
Oligodendroglioma, IDH1/2 mutations in, 477
OMI, 184, 528
Omics technologies, and molecular signatures
    of exposure and risk, 108–109
Oncofetal antigens, 528
Oncogenes, 98, 141, 142t, 175
  and angiogenesis, 262f, 265
  cancers associated with, 142t, 144
  cellular, 193
  discovery of, 140
  metabolic, 291
  mutations of, 193
  as potential drug targets, 404
  and targeted treatment, 142t
  UPS and, 132
Oncogenesis
  multistage, 141, 141f, 143–144, 145f
Oncoproteins
  in cancer-related extracellular vesicles, 262
  viral, 145f, 149

Oncotype DX, 243, 495, 566
Ondansetron
  cellular efflux, 450
  for nausea and vomiting, 417
Oophorectomy, in breast cancer
    treatment, 490f, 498
OPG. See Osteoprotegerin (OPG)
OPN. See Osteopontin (OPN)
Opsonization, 445
Optical coherence tomography, 332f
  in animal models, 340
Optical imaging, 338, 338f
  of animal models, 340, 340f
Optical (laser) transfection, 23
Optimal biological dose, 549
Oral mucosa
  radiation-induced responses in, early, 386
  repopulation of irradiated cells in, 391
Orchiectomy, for prostate cancer, 488
Organoid model systems, 23
  in preclinical evaluation of drug response, 412
Origin recognition complex (ORC), 170, 172f
Oropharyngeal cancer, 86–88, 87f
  human papillomavirus and, 70, 86, 149
Osimertinib, 142t, 464, 467t, 469f, 472
Osteogenic sarcoma, P-glycoprotein increase
    in, prognostic significance of, 450
Osteopontin (OPN), 226
  hypoxia and, 294
Osteoprotegerin (OPG), and metastasis, 233, 234f
Osteosarcoma
  cell line derived from, 23
  cell line irradiated with accelerated charged
    particles, survival curves for, 355, 355f
  cellular radiosensitivity in, 378t
  tumor-suppressor genes in, 142t
Outcome(s). See also Health outcomes research;
    Patient-reported outcomes
  assessment of, in clinical trials, 554
  in cohort study, 77
  in evaluation of screening test, 565
  surrogate measures for, 554
Ovarian cancer
  anti-PD-1 therapies for, 62
  ARID1A mutations in, and sensitivity
    to PARP inhibitors, 63
  BRCA1/2 and, 157
  BRCA-deficient, treatment of, 3, 477
  circulating tumor cells in, 320
  DNMT inhibitors and viral mimicry
    response in, 62
  epigenetic therapy combined with
    other therapies for, 62
  ERBB2(HER-2) in, 152
  ERBB1 mutations in, 151
  familial. See Familial breast and ovarian cancer
  gene expression profile in, prognostic
    significance of, 43
  hedgehog inhibitors for, 129
  heterogeneity of, clinical significance of, 320
  K-RAS mutations in, 154f
  MYC upregulation in, 150
  P-glycoprotein increase in, prognostic
    significance of, 450
  PI3-kinase signaling alterations in, 153, 153f
  PTEN loss of function in, 156
  PTEN promoter methylation in, 157, 157f
  serous, p53 mutations in, 155
  smoking and, 87f
  targeted therapy for, 467t
  treatment of, 158

  tumor-suppressor genes in, 142t
  WNT pathway inhibitors for, 127
  WNT signaling in, 126
Overdiagnosis bias, 80, 80t
Oxaliplatin, 417, 435–436, 435f
Oxford NanoPore sequencing platform, 14
Oxidative phosphorylation, 285–286
Oxidative stress, tumor suppressors and, 290, 290f
8-Oxoguanine glycosylase (OGG1), 200
Oxygen
  delivery, to tumors, strategies for
    increasing, 299, 382–383
  diffusion in tissue, 280, 280f, 292, 379, 381f
  gradients, in tumor microenvironment, 284
  high-pressure, as adjuvant to radiotherapy, 383
  as radiosensitizer, 379, 380f
Oxygen-dependent degradation
    domains (ODD), 294
Oxygen electrode, 293
Oxygen enhancement ratio (OER), 379, 380f
Oxygen fixation hypothesis, 299, 379

P

p15, 175, 176f, 196
p16, 55, 142t, 196, 448
p21, 151f, 175, 176f, 178, 183, 195–196, 207,
    208f, 213, 214f
  and cell-cycle checkpoints, 357
  and oxidative stress, 290, 290f
p53, 43, 98, 104f, 122–123, 142t, 143, 176–188,
    183f, 186f, 199, 200t, 206f, 207,
    208f, 209, 211, 213–215, 214f, 226,
    265, 310–311, 409, 479–480, 508
  and angiogenesis, 262f
  and apoptosis, 453
  and cell-cycle checkpoints, 357
  and cell fate determination, 155, 156f
  hypoxia and, 296
  mutations of, 102, 155–156, 196, 361–362
  and oxidative stress, 290, 290f
  phosphorylation of, 149
  and tumor metabolism, 285f, 286f, 288–289
  UPS and, 132
P53, 7, 188
p62, 185
PA. See Photoacoustic (PA) imaging
Paclitaxel, 131, 407, 416, 444–445, 466, 472
  adverse effects of, pharmacogenetic
    studies of, 89, 89t
  nanoparticle albumin-bound, 445
  neutropenia caused by, 445
  pharmacokinetics of, 445
  resistance to, 449, 449t, 451
  structure of, 444f
Paget, S., 305
Paget's soil and seed hypothesis, 234
PAHs. See Polycyclic aromatic
    hydrocarbons (PAHs)
PAK, activation, 125
PALB2 gene, defects, and BRCA-ness, 476
Palbociclib, 177
  and fulvestrant, combined, 476
  with hormonal agents, for breast cancer, 503
  and hormonal therapy, combined,
    for breast cancer, 503
  indications for, 476
  and letrozole, combined, 476
  mechanism of action of, 463f, 476
Palmar-plantar erythrodysesthesia, 417, 439
PAM. See Protospacer adjacent motif (PAM)
Pan-CDK inhibitors, 177

Pancreatic cancer
  BRCA-mutated, 406, 477
  cancer stem cells in, 229–230, 315
  case fatality rate for, 71
  cellular radiosensitivity in, 378t
  clonal subpopulations in, 310
  drug sensitivity, 440, 445–446, 472, 477
  fibroblast component of, 309
  fibrosis in, 226, 282–283
  gene fusion in, 147t
  genomic evolution of, 225, 311
  hedgehog inhibitors for, 129
  hedgehog signaling in, 129
  heterogeneity of, and chemoresistance, 320
  hypoxia in, 293f, 294
  K-RAS mutations in, 154, 154f
  metastasis, principal sites of, 234, 234t, 241–242
  oncogenes in, 142t
  preclinical imaging of, 340, 340f
  RNF43-mutated, Wnt-FZD5 signaling in, 405
  smoking and, 87f
  stromal component of, 308–309, 309f, 320
  tumor-suppressor genes in, 142t
  WNT pathway inhibitors for, 127
  WNT signaling in, 126, 405
Pancreatic Cancer Case-Control Consortium, 92
Panitumumab, 115, 408, 408f, 469f, 471–472, 532t, 550, 551
  indications for, 467t
Panobinostat, 61, 477
Parallel reaction monitoring mass spectrometry (PRM-MS), 37
Paraneoplastic endocrine syndromes, 509
p14^{ARF}, 142t, 156f, 196
Parkinson disease
  DJ1 in, 290–291
  and lower cancer risk, 291
PARP. See Poly-ADP ribose polymerase (PARP)
Particle therapy, 374
Passenger mutations. See Mutation(s), passenger
Patched (PTC), 128–129, 129f, 196, 480
  inhibitors, 480
Patient-derived xenograft (PDX) models, for preclinical evaluation of anticancer drugs, 412–414
Patient-reported outcomes, 559–560
Pattern-recognition receptors (PRRs), 187–188
Paxillin, integrins and, 125
Pazopanib, 268t, 269f, 469–470, 469f
PCAs. See Protein complementation assays (PCAs)
p21CIP1, See p21
PD-1, 2, 62, 62f, 230, 283, 321, 503, 520f, 521f, 524
  immune checkpoint inhibitor targeting, 62, 531, 531t, 536, 537–539, 537f
  ligands. See PD-L1; PD-L2
PD-ECGF/TP. See Platelet-derived endothelial cell growth factor/thymidine phosphorylase (PD-ECGF/TP)
PDFRA, targeted therapy and, 467t
PDK1. See Pyruvate dehydrogenase kinase 1 (PDK1)
PDK gene, cancer-associated mutations in, 153, 153f
PD-L1, 2, 62, 188, 230, 283, 297–298, 375, 524, 531t, 536, 537, 537f, 538
  epigenetic regulation of, 62, 62f
PD-L2, 524, 536, 537, 537f
PDX. See Patient-derived xenograft (PDX) models

PE. See Plating efficiency (PE)
PEDF. See Pigment epithelium derived factor (PEDF)
Pembrolizumab, 3, 121, 270, 503
Pemetrexed, 436f, 437, 437f
Penicillamine, 268
Pentose phosphate pathway, 175, 286–289
Perforin, 519, 521f, 523
Performance status, prognostic significance of, 568
Pericentriolar material (PCM), 164
Pericytes, 238, 239f, 249–255, 250f, 252f, 253f, 255, 261f, 263, 264f, 266, 267, 269f, 282, 283, 308, 309
Period prevalence, 71
Periostin, 228
Perivascular niche, 236, 267
Peroxidase(s), 10, 30, 100, 451, 496f
Peroxisome proliferator-activated receptor gamma co-activator 1α. See PGC-1α
Personalized medicine, 3, 158–159, 320, 481, 539, 547, 550–551
Pertuzumab, 142t, 409, 469f, 532t
  adjuvant, for breast cancer, 558
  adverse effects, 473
  indications for, 467t, 473
  mechanism of action of, 463f, 464, 473, 532–533
PEST sequence, 127, 127f
PET-CT, 333, 336, 337f, 341, 342f
  ^{18}F-FAZA, respiratory gating and, 341
PET-MRI, 336
Pevonedistat, 133
PEX, 257t, 260, 262f
PF-03084014, 128
PFS. See Progression-free survival (PFS)
PGC-1α, and tumor metabolism, 289
p110α gene, 142t, 153, 153f, 473.
  See also PIK3CA
P-glycoprotein
  antagonists, 451
  drug substrates, 442, 449–450
  and multidrug resistance, 447f, 449–450, 449f, 449t, 450f
  structure of, 450, 450f
pH. See also Acidity
  and cellular drug uptake, 299
  in tumor microenvironment, 284
Phagocytosis, 464, 516
Phalanx cells, in angiogenesis, 253–254, 253f, 258, 269f
Pharmacodynamics, 429–431, 462
  and phase II trials, 549
Pharmacoepidemiology, 88–89
Pharmacogenetics, 418, 432, 503
Pharmacogenomic epidemiology, 88–89, 89t
Pharmacogenomics, 431–432
Pharmacokinetics, 429–431, 431t, 451, 462
  and phase II trials, 549
Pharmacology, principles of, 429–432
Pharmacovigilance, 88–89
PHD2. See Prolyl hydroxylase 2 (PHD2)
PH domains. See Pleckstrin homology (PH) domains
Phenobarbital, as tumor promoter, 102, 103f
Phenotypic plasticity, 317–318
Philadelphia chromosome, 2, 6f, 140, 143f, 148f, 150, 410, 478, 551
  FISH detection of, 12f
Phosphatase and tensin homolog (PTEN). See PTEN

Phosphatidylinositol 3-kinase (PI3K), 175
  in hypoxic response, 295
  and tumor metabolism, 286f, 287–288
  in vasculogenic mimicry, 255–256
Phosphatidylinositol 3-kinase (PI3K) inhibitors, 175, 473–475, 474f
PI3Kα, 121
Phosphatidylinositol 3-kinase (PI3K) pathway, 116–118, 117f, 118f, 120, 120f, 122, 124, 149, 152–154, 153f, 473–474, 474f
  alterations, in cancer, 153–154, 153f
  in cancer, 121
  catalytic subunit (p110α), activating mutations/amplification, 153, 153f
  mutant EGFRs and, 152
  mutations and, 153, 153f
  p85 subunit, cancer-associated mutations in, 153, 153f
  regulatory roles of, 153f
Phosphoinositides (PtdIns), in growth factor receptor signaling, 116–117, 116f, 120–121, 120f
Phosphorylation. See also Oxidative phosphorylation
  of PTEN, 157, 157f
  and transcription factors, 122
Phosphotyrosine-binding (PTB) domains, 115–116, 116f
Photoacoustic (PA) imaging, 341, 342f
Photoelectric effect, 350
Photon beam, depth dose curves for, 373f
Photons, 349–350
  linear energy transfer of, 351, 351f, 351t
Photoproducts, 350
Photothermal ablation therapy (PTT), prostate cancer, nanoparticles in, 343f
pI. See Isoelectric point (pI)
Pigment epithelium derived factor (PEDF), 265
  and angiogenesis, 262f
PI3K. See Phosphatidylinositol 3-kinase (PI3K)
PIK3CA, targeted therapy and, 467t
PIK3CA gene, cancer-associated mutations in, 153
PIK3R gene, cancer-associated mutations in, 153
Pimonidazole, 293–294, 293f, 298t
PIN. See Prostatic intraepithelial neoplasia (PIN)
p16^{INK4A}, 142t, see also p16
PKB/AKT, 153
p27KIP1, MYC and, 151f
Placenta growth factor (PlGF), 256–257, 257t, 260
Planning target volume (PTV), for radiotherapy, 372, 372f
Plasmacytoma, murine, MYC upregulation in, 150
Plasma membrane damage, radiation-induced, 363
Plasmid(s), DNA insertion into, 8–9, 9f
Plasmin, 227
Plasminogen activator inhibitor (PAI), 226t, 227, 228
Plasminogen activators, 226t, 227
  tissue type (tPA), 226t, 227
  urokinase type (uPA), 226t, 227, 259, 260f
Platelet(s)
  and angiogenesis, 251f
  and metastasis, 232
  production of, 279, 415, 416f
    chemotherapy and, 415
  and tumor angiogenesis, 260

601

Platelet-derived endothelial cell growth factor/thymidine phosphorylase (PD-ECGF/TP), 257t
Platelet-derived growth factor (PDGF), 256, 258, 313
  hypoxia and, 297, 297f
  PDGF-A, 258
  PDGF-B, 254, 257t, 258
    and lymphangiogenesis, 255
    and vascular maturation, 255
  PDGF-C, 258
  PDGF-D, 258
Platelet-derived growth factor receptor (PDGFR), 57, 114, 114f, 258
  imatinib and, 408
  PDGFRA, in IDH-mutant glioma, 57
  PDGFRβ, 257t
  small molecule inhibitors, 115
  targeted therapy and, 469, 469f
Platelet factor 4 (PF4), 260
Plating efficiency (PE)
  of drug-treated cells, 411
  of irradiated cells, 354–355, 354f
Platinum agents, 435–436
  cellular uptake of, 447f, 449
  pharmacology of, 435
  resistance to, 451
  structure of, 435, 435f
PLDR. See Repair of potentially lethal damage (PLDR)
Pleckstrin homology (PH) domains, 116, 116f, 153
Pleiotrophin, 260
PlGF. See Placenta growth factor (PlGF)
Plinabulin, 268t, 271
PLK1. See Polo-like kinase 1 (PLK1)
PLK4. See Polo-like kinase 4 (PLK4)
PML-RARA fusion gene, 147t
Pneumonitis, radiation-induced, 387
PNKP, 203–204, 203f
Podophyllotoxin, glycoside derivatives of, 442
Podoplanin (PDPN), 255
  and lymphangiogenesis, 255
Point prevalence, 71
Polo-like kinase 1 (PLK1), 166f, 172–174, 173f
  inhibitors, 178
Polo-like kinase 4 (PLK4), 166f
  inhibitor, 181
Polony sequencing, 14
Poly-ADP ribose polymerase (PARP), 199, 199f
  inhibition, 3, 158, 362, 405–406
  targeted therapy and, 467t
  trapping, 463f, 476–477
Poly-ADP ribose polymerase (PARP) inhibitors, 199, 211, 464f, 476–477
  and AML or MDS, 418
  mechanism of action of, 476
  resistance to, 215, 477
  sensitivity to, epigenetic factors and, 63
  side effects of, 477
  in treatment of tumors with DNA repair deficit, 63, 453
Polycyclic aromatic hydrocarbons (PAHs)
  as carcinogens, 98, 99f, 107
  metabolic activation of, 100, 100f
Polyglutamation, 436
Polymerase chain reaction (PCR), 10–11, 11f, 307
  in DNA sequencing, 14, 16f–17f
  inverse, of irradiated cells, 356
  quantitative real-time (qPCR), 11
  in site-directed mutagenesis, 25, 26f

Polymerase proofreading-associated polyposis (PPAP), 200t
Polypeptides, synthesis of, 7
Polyposis-associated colorectal cancer syndromes, 200t
Polysorbate 80, 445
Polytomous ordinal logistic regression, 84t
Pomalidomide, 134
Ponatinib, 142t, 464, 467t, 478
Population epidemiology, of carcinogens, 104
Population stratification, 78
Porcupine (PORCN) inhibitors, 126, 127
Position effect, 20
Positron emission tomography (PET), 3, 329, 331, 332f, 333f, 335–337, 337f
  agents for, 332f, 336
  in animal models, 339–340
  FAZA in. See [^{18}F]-fluoroazomycin arabinoside (FAZA)
  FDG in, 287, 329, 330f, 337f. See also [^{18}F]-fluorodeoxyglucose
    in animal model, 339, 340f
    and quality assurance, 340–341
  FMISO in. See [^{18}F]-fluoromisonidazole (FMISO)
  hypoxia imaging, 294, 298t
  PSMA in, 342
  radiomics and, 343
  standardized uptake value in, 336
Posttest (posterior) probability, 565
Pott, Percival, 1, 98
Power, of clinical trial, 557–558
PPAP. See Polymerase proofreading-associated polyposis (PPAP)
pp90rsk1, and estrogen receptor activation, 502
PRC2, 61
Precision oncology, 320, 321
Predictive factors, 90
Predictive markers, 568, 568f
Predictive test, 566
Predictive validity, 560
Premature chromosome condensation (PCC), 211, 212t
Pre-metastatic niche(s), 233, 241–242, 241f, 282–283
Prenylation, 118
Pre-replicative complex (pre-RC), 164, 165f, 170, 172, 172f
Pretest (prior) probability, 565
Prevalence, 71–72
Prevalence bias, 77
Prevalence studies, 77
Prevention. See also Chemoprevention
  of metastasis, treatment for, 242–243
  of prostate cancer, finasteride and, 506
Primary capillary plexus, 251, 252f
Primary cells, 23
Primer(s)
  in DNA sequencing, 14
  in polymerase chain reaction, 10–11, 11f
PRM-MS. See Parallel reaction mass spectrometry (PRM-MS)
Probability curve, 82, 82f
Procarcinogens, metabolic activation of, 99–100, 99f–101f
PRO-CTCAE. See Common Terminology Criteria for Adverse Events (CTCAE)
Prodrugs, hypoxia-active, 455, 457
Product limit method, of survival analysis, 555–556
Progeria, 118

Progesterone receptor(s), immunohistochemistry of, 495, 496f
Progestin receptor(s), DNA-binding motif, 492
Prognosis, 230, 566–568
  cell proliferation and, 280–281
  patient factors affecting, 568
  tumor characteristics affecting, 567–568
Prognostic factors, 90, 566–568, 568f
Programmed cell death protein 1. See PD-1
Progression-free survival (PFS), 550, 554
Prokineticins, 258
Prolactin (PRL), 16-kDa fragment, 260
Prolyl hydroxylase 2 (PHD2), and vascular maturation, 255
Prolyl-4-hydroxylases (PHDs), in hypoxic response, 295
Prolymphocytic leukemia (PLL), T-cell, ATM gene and, 210
Prometaphase, 166f, 167, 172–174, 173f
Prominin-1 (PROM1), 314
Prophase, 165, 166f, 173f
β-Propiolactone, 99f
Proportional hazards, 556
Propyleneimine, potency as carcinogen, 107f
Prospero homeobox transcription factor (PROX-1), and lymphangiogenesis, 255
Prostate cancer. See also Neuroendocrine prostate cancer (NEPC); Transgenic model of prostate cancer (TRAMP)
  age-standardized incidence and mortality rates for, 72, 72f
  androgen deprivation therapy for, 503–509, 508f
  androgen receptor amplification in, 507, 508f
  androgen receptor status, 495
  androgen receptor variants in, 491
  bone metastases, radionuclide therapy, 373
  brachytherapy for, 371f
    rectal radioprotection with, 389
  BRCA2 and, 157, 496–497
  BRCA-mutated, 477, 496–497
  cancer stem cells in, 315, 498
  castration-resistant, 503
    mechanisms of, 507–509, 507f, 508f
  chemoprevention of, 110, 506
  circulating tumor cells in, 320
  coactivator overexpression in, 508, 508f
  development and progression of, 498
  epigenetic modifications at promoters and, 56
  ERG oncogene in, 145
  gene fusion in, 147t
  hedgehog signaling in, 129
  heritable germline copy-number variation in, 17
  heterogeneity of, clinical significance of, 320
  hormonal therapy for, 503–509, 507f, 508f
  hypoxic, prognostic significance of, 381
  intratumoral androgen production in, 508–509, 508f
  invasive, methylation of uPA promoter and, 55
  invasiveness gene signature in, 319
  metastasis, principal site of, 234t
  metastatic, clonal origin of, 310
  microRNAs in, 24
  molecular evolution of, 44
  natural history of, 497f
  neuroendocrine, 508
    androgen receptor status, 495, 508
  oncogenes in, 142t
  photothermal ablation therapy, nanoparticles in, 343f

602

PI3-kinase signaling alterations in, 153f
prevention of, finasteride and, 506
PTEN loss of function in, 156
radioimmunotherapy for, 374
radiotherapy for, 373f
risk factors for, 496–497
screening, and overdiagnosis, 72
screening for, 565
sex steroids and, 488
SIADH with, 509
sipuleucel-T therapy for, 536
smoking and, 87f
subgroups of, 44
tmprss2-erg abnormalities in, FISH detection of, 12f, 13
tumor-suppressor genes in, 142t
WNT signaling in, 126
Prostate Cancer Outcome Study, 560–561
Prostate-specific antigen (PSA), 528
screening for, 565
serum, and outcomes, 554
Prostate-specific membrane antigen (PSMA)
in PET, 342
radioisotopes conjugated to, 374
Prostatic intraepithelial neoplasia (PIN), 497, 497f, 498
Protease(s). *See also specific enzyme*
angiogenesis-regulating, 259, 260f
Proteasome. *See* 26S proteasome; Ubiquitin proteasome system (UPS)
Proteasome inhibitors, 271, 300, 408, 464, 464f, 479
Protein(s)
adaptor, 116, 117f
basic zipper, 122
degradation, targeted, 133, 134
as drug targets, alterations, drug resistance caused by, 446t
expression, translocations and, 148f
functions of, translocations and, 148f
phosphorylation, in receptor signaling cascade, 114–115, 115f
synthesis of, 7
ubiquitination, 131–132, 131f
Western blotting of, 10, 10f
Proteinase(s). *See also specific enzyme*
catalytic classes of, 226, 226t
cellular, 226–228
inhibitors, 226, 226t, 228
in metastasis
activity at invasive front, 237
activity in microenvironment, 237–238, 237t
Protein complementation assays (PCAs), 30
Protein kinase A (PKA), and estrogen receptor activation, 494, 502
Protein kinase B (PKB), 149
and estrogen receptor activation, 502
and tumor metabolism, 286f, 288
Protein kinase C (PKC)
and estrogen receptor activation, 502
inhibition of, 127
Protein kinase C alpha (PKCα), 120
Protein microarrays, 38, 39f
Protein phosphatase(s). *See also specific enzyme*
suppression of growth factor signaling, 122–123
Protein–protein interactions
databases of, and network analysis, 44
disruption, targeted therapy for, mechanism of action of, 463f, 464
disruptors of, 409, 464
identification of, 30

Protein serine/threonine phosphatase(s), 122–123
PP1 (type I), 123
PP2 (type II), 123
PP2A, 123
Protein tyrosine phosphatase(s), 122–123
Proteoforms, 32, 34
Proteolysis
and cancer progression, 237–238, 237t
mechanisms, in angiogenesis and endothelial cell function, 259, 260f
ubiquitin-mediated, and cell-cycle regulation, 169–170
Proteolysis-targeted chimeras (PROTACS), 134
Proteome
human, 32
proteoforms in, 32, 34
and molecular signatures of exposure and risk, 108–109
Proteomics, 30–38, 30t
biomarker discovery with, challenges for, 36–37, 36f
bottom-up, 32–33
isotope labeling used in, 34–36, 35f
MS-based
spectral matching in, 32
synthetic peptide libraries for, 33
posttranslational modification, 30t
top-down, 33–34
Proteosome, 517–518, 517f
Proteostasis, 133
perturbations in, 133
Proteotoxic stress, 133
Proteus-like syndrome, 156
Proton beam, depth dose curves for, 373f
Protons, 350
Proton therapy, 374
Proto-oncogenes, 140, 193
mutations of, 102
Protospacer adjacent motif (PAM), 28, 29f
PRRs. *See* Pattern-recognition receptors (PRRs)
Pruning, vascular, 251, 261f, 263
PSMA. *See* Prostate-specific membrane antigen (PSMA)
PTB, 123
PTC. *See* Patched (PTC)
PTCH, mutations of, 196
PTCH1, 480
PTEN, 120–121, 120f, 122, 149
and angiogenesis, 262f
in cancer, 120–121
cytoplasmic, 156
deregulation, 156–157, 157f
and glycolysis, 286f, 289
loss
in cancer, 153f, 156–157
nuclear, 156
and oxidative stress, 290–291, 290f
post-translational modulation of, 157, 157f
structure of, 156
transcriptional modulation of, 157, 157f
UPS and, 132
PTEN gene, 142t, 145
and angiogenesis, 265
germline mutations of, 156
promoter methylation, 157, 157f
somatic mutations of, 156
PTHS (PTEN hamartoma tumor syndrome), 156
PTPN11 gene, 123
PTP superfamily, 122–123
PTT. *See* Photothermal ablation therapy (PTT)

PTV. *See* Planning target volume (PTV)
Publication bias, 92, 558
Pulsed-field gel electrophoresis (PFGE), 211, 212t
PUMA, 182, 184, 184f, 188
Punctuated evolution, 311
Purine antimetabolites, 440
P value(s), 42–43, 78, 548, 552, 553, 556, 557, 567
pVHL, targeted degradation of, 134
Pyrosequencing, 14, 16f–17f
Pyruvate dehydrogenase kinase 1 (PDK1), 120, 120f, 153
and glycolysis, 286f, 297
hypoxia and, 297
Pyruvate kinase
isoenzymes, 289
and tumor metabolism, 289

Q

QALY. *See* Quality-adjusted life-year (QALY)
QIN. *See* Quantitative Imaging Network (QIN)
Quality-adjusted life-year (QALY), 561
Quality of life, 554
measures of, 559–560
prognostic significance of, 568
Quantitative Imaging Network (QIN), 341
q values, 43

R

RAC GTPase (i.e. RAC GTPase), 125, 126f
RAD51, 158, 183, 186f, 202, 202f, 203, 203f, 298, 476
RAD52, 202–204, 202f, 203f
Radiation. *See also* Ionizing radiation; Radiotherapy
interactions with matter, 349–353
types of, 349–350
Radiation dose
deposition, 351
measurement of, 350–351
Radiation recall, 424
Radiation sensitizers, 422, 422f
Radiation therapy. *See* Radiotherapy
Radiation Therapy Oncology Group (RTOG)/European Organization for Research and Treatment of Cancer (EORTC) classification of tissue response to radiation, 384
Radiobiological effectiveness (RBE), 355, 374
Radiography, 331–332, 332f
Radioimmunotherapy, 374
Radiomics, 342–344, 344f
Radionucleotides, in cancer treatment, 372–373
Radioprotection, 389
Radioresistance, 203, 359, 361f, 363, 373, 377, 421–422
cancer heterogeneity and, 320
in hypoxic tumor cells, 380–381, 381f
and reoxygenation after irradiation, 392–393, 392f
Radiosensitivity
assays for, 354–356, 354f, 355f, 378, 379f
cell-cycle phase and, 356–357, 357f, 358f
redistribution effects of, 392
DNA double-strand breaks and, 359–360, 360f
epigenetic factors and, 63
genetic factors in, 389
in hypoxic tumor cells, 380–381, 381f
oxygen effect and, 379, 380f
Radiosensitizers, for hypoxic cells, 299, 383–384

603

Radiotherapy, 349, 369–401. *See also* Ionizing radiation
  with anticancer drug treatment, 419, 421–424, 422*t*, 423*f*, 424*f*
  cellular response to, 384–386, 385*f*
  and chemotherapy, 374
    combined, 421–424, 422*f*, 422*t*, 423*f*
  clinical
    heavy particles in, 350
    light particles in, 350
    physical principles of, 350
    principles of, 370–375
  combined with other cancer treatments, 374–375
  combined with targeting of intracellular signaling pathways, 363
  conformal, 370, 370*f*, 372
  curative, 370
  delivery of, 350
  3-dimensional (3D) conformal, 370, 370*f*
  dose, 370–372
    and lethality in mice, 385, 385*f*
  dose-volume, 372, 372*f*
  external beam, 350
    delivery, 369–370, 372
    multifractionated, 369–370
    planning, 372
    target volumes, 372, 372*f*
  fractionation, 390–393
    accelerated, 395–396, 396*t*
    altered schedules for, 395–396, 396*t*
    effects of, modeling of, 393–396
    isoeffect curves for, 393, 394*f*
    linear quadratic (LQ) equation and models for isoeffect, 394–395
    redistribution effects of, 392
    and reoxygenation, 392–393, 392*f*
    and repair, 390, 391*f*
    and repopulation, 390–392, 391*f*, 422–423, 422*t*, 423*f*
    time and dose relationships, 393
  and hormone therapy, 374
  hyperfractionation, 395–396, 396*t*
  image-guided. *See* Image-guided radiation therapy (IGRT)
  and immunotherapy, 375
  inflammatory response in, 385–386
  intensity-modulated. *See* Intensity-modulated radiation therapy (IMRT)
  and molecular-targeted agents, 374–375
  normal tissue complication probabilities, 388
  normal tissue response to, 384–390
    acute (early), 384, 386, 386*f*
    chemotherapy and, 424
    classification/scoring systems for, 384
    dose-response curves for, 389–390, 390*f*
    functional assays, 385, 385*f*
    functional subunits and, 387–388
    in situ assays, 384, 385*f*
    in vivo assays, 384, 385*f*
    late, 384, 386–388
    prediction, 389
  organ response to
    cellular factors and, 385–386
    functional assays, 385, 385*f*
  palliative, 370–372
  planning, 369–370, 393
    imaging in, 330*f*
  plus cetuximab, 375, 376*f*
  plus cisplatin, 375, 376*f*
  recent advances in, 3
  resistance to. *See* Radioresistance
  and retreatment tolerance, 389
  risk–benefit of, 369
  sensitivity to. *See* Radiosensitivity
  side effects, 370, 371*t*, 384
    genetic factors and, 389
  and surgery, 374
  target volumes
    clinical, 372, 372*f*, 373*f*
    planning, 372, 372*f*
  therapeutic ratio of, 369, 389–390, 390*f*, 393
  tolerance dose for specific organs, in rodents, 385, 385*f*
  tumor control after, 375–379
    dose response and, 375–377, 377*f*
    dose-response curves for, 389–390, 390*f*
    prediction of, 377–379, 378*f*, 378*t*, 379*f*
    repopulation of tumor cells and, 390–392, 391*f*, 422–423, 422*t*, 423*f*
Radio waves, 349–350, 350*f*
Radium-223, for metastatic prostate cancer, 373
Radixin, 124, 230
Radon, 104, 194
RAF/MEK inhibitors, 475–476
RAF protein kinase, 117–118, 117*f*, 118*f*, 119, 154–155, 154*f*
  targeted therapy and, 470
RAG recombinase, 519
RALGDS, 117, 118*f*
raloxifene
  for breast cancer, 500
  as chemopreventive agent, 110
  mechanism of action of, 110
Ramucirumab, 115, 268, 268*t*, 468–469, 469*f*, 532*t*
  mechanism of action of, 463*f*
Random error, 78
Randomization, 548
  in evaluation of screening test, 564–565
  importance of, 552–554
Randomized controlled trial(s) (RCT), 77, 89–90, 90*t*, 455, 550, 560–561, 560*t*, 565
  vs. observational studies, 90, 90*t*
RANKL, and metastasis, 233, 234*f*
Rapalogs, 475
RAS genes, activating mutations, cancer associated with, 154–155, 154*f*
ras oncogenes
  activation by carcinogens, site specificity of, 102
  mutations of, 102
RAS protein(s), 154–155, 154*f*
  activation of, 116–118, 117*f*, 118*f*
    by integrins, 124–125
  and angiogenesis, 262*f*, 265
  downstream signaling, 117–118, 118*f*
  mutations of, in cancer, 117–118
  prenylation of, 118
  in TGF-β signaling, 130
  tumor-specific isoforms of, 118
RB. *See* Retinoblastoma
RBE. *See* Radiobiological effectiveness (RBE)
RCT. *See* Randomized controlled trial(s) (RCT)
REA (repressor of estrogen receptor activity), 493
Reactive oxygen species (ROS), 101, 103, 289–291
  and cancer, 290, 290*f*
  cellular damage caused by, 289–290, 451
  chemoprevention strategies and, 110
  and metastasis, 231*f*
  radiation and, 351–352, 352*f*, 353, 385–386
Recall bias, 76, 79, 80*t*
Receiver operating characteristic (ROC) curve, 563, 563*f*
Receptor binding, drug uptake by, 448
Receptor-interacting protein kinase. *See* RIPK1; RIPK3
Receptor protein tyrosine kinase(s) (RPTK)
  dimerization and activation of, 115, 115*f*
  extracellular growth factors and, 113–115, 114*f*, 115*f*
  families, 114, 114*f*
  humanized antibodies against, 115
  inhibitors, 115
  ligand binding by, 114
  and cell growth, 175–176, 176*f*
  and regulation of vascular growth, 256–258
  recruitment of cytoplasmic signaling molecules, 116–117, 117*f*
  signal transmission, formation of multiprotein complexes and, 115–117, 116*f*, 117*f*
  structure of, 114, 114*f*
  types of, 114, 114*f*
  ubiquitination of, 132
Receptor tyrosine kinase(s) (RTKs), *See* Receptor Protein Tyrosine Kinase(s) (RPTK and RTK are the same thing)
Receptor tyrosine kinase inhibitors, 464, 469, 473–476, 474*f*
RECIST. *See* Response Evaluation Criteria in Solid Tumors (RECIST)
Recombinant DNA clone(s)
  generation of, 7–9, 9*f*
  isolation of, 9
Recombination activation gene recombinase. *See* RAG recombinase
Red blood cells, production of, 278–279, 415, 416*f*
  chemotherapy and, 415
Redox status, 289–291
Reed-Sternberg cells, 309, 309*f*
Referral bias, 567
Regorafenib, 268*t*, 270, 469*f*, 470
Regression analysis, 83–84, 84*t*
Regulatory T cells (Tregs), 131, 524, 525*f*
  and adaptive resistance, 538
  hypoxia and, 297–298, 297*f*
  immune checkpoint inhibitor and, 535–537
  induced, 524
  natural, 524
  and T-cell tolerance, 524–525, 525*f*
Relative risk, 81, 81*t*
Relugolix, in prostate cancer treatment, 503
Remission, and residual population of tumor cells, 424
Renal cell carcinoma
  antiangiogenic therapy for, 270
  clear cell
    genetic evolution of, 311
    intertumoral heterogeneity of, 311
    intratumoral heterogeneity of, 311
    stromal component of, 309, 309*f*
  clonal subpopulations in, 310
Reoxygenation, radiotherapy and, 392–393, 392*f*
Repair of potentially lethal damage (PLDR), in irradiated cells, 359–360
Repair of sublethal damage (SLDR), in irradiated cells, 358–359
Repeat variable di-residue (RVD), 28
Replication fork, 164, 165*f*
Replication origin(s), 164, 165*f*
Respiratory burst, 103

Response Evaluation Criteria in Solid
　　　Tumors (RECIST), 341
Response-shift, 560
Responsiveness, of quality-of-life
　　　instruments, 560
Restriction enzymes, 7–9, 9f
　in site-directed mutagenesis, 25, 26f
Restriction point, 122, 164f, 167, 171,
　　　171f, 177f, 180, 476
RET
　inhibition of, 470
　oncogenic activation of, 470
　targeted therapy and, 469f, 470
Retinoblastoma
　progression, tumor-suppressor
　　　genes and, 140–141
　tumor-suppressor gene in, 140–141,
　　　142t, 143f
Retinoblastoma gene (Rb), 141, 142t, 147
Retinoblastoma gene (RB), 1
　mutations, and cancer risk, 108, 176
Retinoblastoma gene (Rb1), See Retinoblastoma
　　　gene (Rb)
Retinoblastoma gene (RB1), See Retinoblastoma
　　　gene (RB)
Retinoblastoma protein (RB or RB1)
　　loss of function, 158, 177, 476
　　and oxidative stress, 290, 290f
　　and synthetic lethal treatment, 3, 476
　RB1 or pRb, functions of, 158
Retinoic acid, 110, 195, 321, 322f
Retinoic acid–inducible gene-like
　　　receptors (RLRs), 518
RET-KIF5B fusion gene, 147t
Retroviruses
　transforming, and discovery of oncogenes, 140
　as vectors, 23
Reverse-phase arrays, 38
Reverse-phase fractionation, 34
RHEB, 118, 153f, 176f
RHO, in WNT signaling, 125, 126f
RHO-A, in TGF-β signaling, 130
RhoC, and metastasis, 231f, 232
Ribociclib, 121, 177, 476, 503
Ribonucleoside reductase, 440
Ribosomal S6 kinase (RSK), 119
Richter transformation, 480
Riddle syndrome, 200t
RIG-I proteins, 518
RIPK1, 186, 187f
RIPK3, 186, 187f
RISC. See RNA-induced silencing
　　　complex (RISC)
Risk factors, 73–74, 76, 90, 495–497,
RIT. See Radioimmunotherapy (RIT)
Rituximab, 409, 475, 480, 532t
RLRs. See Retinoic acid–inducible gene-
　　　like receptors (RLRs)
RNA (ribonucleic acid). See also Nucleic acid(s)
　assays, 548
　closed circular (circRNA), 145f, 149
　crRNA, 28, 29f
　long noncoding (lncRNAs), 145f, 149
　noncoding (ncRNA), 147. See also
　　　MicroRNAs (miRNAs)
　northern blotting of, 9–10
　sequencing, 18–19, 307
　　and identification of potential targets
　　　for anticancer drugs, 404, 405f
　　single-cell, 43
　transcription, DNA lesions and, 197

RNA-induced silencing complex (RISC),
　　　24, 25f
RNA interference (RNAi), 24, 128, 233, 405
　in anticancer therapy, 409–410
　and drug resistance, 448
　functional genomic screens, for identification
　　　of potential drug targets, 405–406
　mechanism of action of, 405, 406f
RNA polymerase, 7, 197, 201, 201f, 443
RNA polymerase II, 121–122, 492–493
RNA-seq, 18–19
RNA silencing, 24
RNF43, in WNT signaling, 125–126, 405
RNF168, 200t, 206, 206f, 362
RO492907, 128
Roberts syndrome, 200t
ROC. See Receiver operating
　　　characteristic (ROC) curve
Romidepsin, 61, 477
RORγt, 523f
ROS. See Reactive oxygen species (ROS)
ROS1, 89, 142t, 147t, 467t, 469f, 478–479, 551f
ROS1-SDC4 fusion gene, 147t
Rous, Peyton, 140, 143f
Rous sarcoma virus, 140
RSK. See Ribosomal S6 kinase (RSK)
RTKs. See Receptor protein tyrosine
　　　kinase(s) (RTKs)
Rucaparib, indications for, 467t, 477
Ruxolitinib, 124
RVD. See Repeat variable di-residue (RVD)

S
S100A4, 313
SAC. See Spindle assembly checkpoint (SAC)
Saccharin, potency as carcinogen, 107, 107f
Saccharomyces cerevisiae, homologous
　　　recombination in, 202
S-adenosylhomocysteine (SAH), and
　　　epigenetics, 59, 59f
S-adenosylmethionine (SAM), and
　　　epigenetics, 53, 59, 59f
SAH. See S-adenosylhomocysteine (SAH)
Salivary gland(s)
　cancer, gene fusion in, 147t
　radioprotection, in head and neck
　　　cancer treatment, 389
Salmonella typhimurium, in Ames
　　　test, 105–106, 105f
SAM. See S-adenosylmethionine (SAM)
Sampling
　for case-control studies, 75
　cumulative incidence, 75
　in epidemiologic analyses, 72–73
　incidence-density, 76
Sampling bias, 79–80, 80t
Sanger sequencing, 14, 307
　automated, 14, 15f
SaOS-2 cell line, 23
Sarcoma, metastasis, principal site of, 234t
Saridegib, 283
SASP. See Senescence-associated secretory
　　　phenotype (SASP)
Savolitinib, 472
Scavenging, by tumor cells, 284, 351
SCF. See Stem cell factor (SCF)
SCF complexes, 168f, 169
SCF-SKP2, 170, 170f
Schwannoma, tumor-suppressor genes in, 142t
SCID. See Severe combined immunodeficiency
　　　(SCID) mice

SCLC. See Small cell lung cancer (SCLC)
SCO2, and glycolysis, 286f, 289
Screening, see also Computed Tomography
　　　(CT) and Magnetic Resonance
　　　Imaging (MRI)
　bias in, 80–81, 80t, 81f
　DNA methylation profiling of
　　　ctDNA and, 64–65
　effects on incidence and prevalence, 72
　lead-time bias in, 564–565, 565f
　length-time bias in, 564, 564f
　liquid biopsy in, 64–65
　and overdiagnosis, 72
　pan-cancer, DNA methylation approach
　　　for, 65
　tests for, 64–65, 564–565
scRNA-seq, 18–19
Scrotal cancer, historical perspective on, 1, 98
SCX. See Strong cationic exchange (SCX)
SDF1. See Stromal-derived factor 1 (SDF1)
SDH. See Succinate dehydrogenase (SDH)
SDS-PAGE. See Sodium dodecyl
　　　sulfate–polyacrylamide gel
　　　electrophoresis (SDS-PAGE)
Seckel syndrome, 200t
Second malignancy(ies), drug
　　　therapy and, 417–418
Second mitochondria-derived activator of
　　　caspases (SMAC), 182, 184
γ-Secretase, in NOTCH signaling, 127, 127f
γ-Secretase inhibitors (GSIs), 128
Securin, 170, 173f, 209, 209f
Selected reaction monitoring-mass
　　　spectrometry (SRM-MS), 36f
Selectins, 259, 259f
Selection bias, 79–80, 80t, 554
Selective estrogen receptor downregulators
　　　(SERDs), 500
Selective estrogen receptor modulators
　　　(SERMs), 499–500, 501f
　as chemopreventive agents, 110
Selective inhibitors of nuclear export
　　　(SINE), 464f, 481
Selenium supplements, 110
Self-seeding, 242
Self-selection bias, 80t
Self-tolerance, 515, 524–525
Seliciclib, 177
Selinexor, 481
　mechanism of action of, 463f
Semaphorin, 256
Senescence, 23, 290f, 453
　cellular, 167, 195, 213–214, 353f, 354
　radiation-induced, 364
Senescence-associated secretory
　　　phenotype (SASP), 143, 364
Senolysis, 195
Sensitizer enhancement ratio (SER), 383
Separase, 166f, 173f, 174, 178, 209f
SEPT9 (Septin9), promoter methylation,
　　　in colorectal cancer, 65
Sequence-specific enzyme digestion, in
　　　DNA methylation analysis, 21t
SER. See Sensitizer enhancement ratio (SER)
SERDs. See Selective estrogen receptor
　　　downregulators (SERDs)
SEREX. See Serological analysis of recombinant
　　　cDNA expression libraries (SEREX)
Serine protease(s), 226t, 227
SERMs. See Selective estrogen receptor
　　　modulators (SERMs)

Serological analysis of recombinant cDNA expression libraries (SEREX), 526f, 527
Serotonin (5HT3) receptors, in nausea and vomiting, 417
Serum- and glucocorticoid-induced kinase (SGK1), 120
Severe combined immunodeficiency (SCID) mice, 307
  AML formation in, 315
  DNA-PK studies in, 204
Severely toxic dose in 10% of animals (STD 10), 419
Sex hormone–binding globulin (SHBG), 488–489
Sex hormone–binding globulin receptor (SHBG-R), 488–489
sFlt-1/sVEGFR1, 257t
SHBG. See Sex hormone–binding globulin (SHBG)
SH2 domains. See SRC homology 2 (SH2) domains
SH3 domains. See SRC homology 3 (SH3) domains
SHE assay. See Syrian hamster embryo (SHE) assay
Shelterin, 214f
  and telomere integrity, 214f, 215
Shieldin, 214f, 215
Short hairpin RNAs (shRNAs), 24
Short-interference RNA (siRNA), 24
SHP. See Src homology domain-containing phosphatase(s) (SHP)
SHP2, 123, 124f
shRNAs. See Short hairpin RNAs (shRNAs)
Signal-to-noise ratio (SNR), 331
Signal transducer and activator of transcription (STAT), STAT1, 3,5: 123–125,149, 203, 239, 240f, 242, 265, 320, 408f, 529, STAT6, 524
SILAC (stable isotope labeling with amino acids in cell culture), 34–35, 35f
Single nucleotide polymorphisms (SNP), 13–14
Single-photon emission computed tomography (SPECT), 332f, 335–337
  agents for, 332f
  in animal models, 339
  SPECT-CT, 336
  SPECT-MRI, 336
Single-strand annealing (SSA), 203f
Single-stranded DNA (ssDNA), 164, 165f
Sipuleucel-T, 536
Sirolimus, 121
Sister chromatids, 6, 164, 164f, 165, 167, 172, 178, 179, 357f
  and chromosome segregation errors, 179
  separation of, 172–174
Site-directed mutagenesis, 25, 26f
  in vivo, 26–27, 27f
Skin
  radiation-induced responses in
    early, 360f, 371t, 386, 394f, 396t
    late, 387, 387f
  repopulation of irradiated cells in, 390–391, 391f
Skin cancer
  metastasis, principal sites of, 234t
  UV damage to DNA in, 196, 200t, 201f, 210
SKP2, 172–174, 173f
SKY. See Spectral karyotyping (SKY)
SLAM7, monoclonal antibody against, 532t
SLC. See Solute carrier superfamily (SLC)

SLDR. See Repair of sublethal damage (SLDR)
Slug, and metastasis, 231f, 240
SMAC. See Second mitochondria-derived activator of caspases (SMAC)
SMAD
  mutations of, in cancer, 131
  in TGF-β signaling, 130, 130f
Small cell lung cancer (SCLC)
  cellular radiosensitivity in, 378t
  Cushing syndrome with, 509
  hedgehog signaling in, 129
  and hypercalcemia, 509
  NOTCH signaling in, 128
  SIADH with, 509
Small intestine, cell proliferation and migration in, 279, 279f
Small molecule inhibitors
  cancer cell targeting by, 462, 463f, 464
  indications for, 467t–468t
  mechanism of action of, 464, 475
  metabolism of, 464
Small ubiquitin-like modifier (SUMO) proteins. See SUMO
SMCs. See Smooth muscle cells (SMCs)
SMO. See Smoothened (SMO)
Smoking
  and adduct levels in white blood cells, and lung cell biomarkers for cancer risk, 108
  and alcohol consumption, and cancer risk, 85f, 88
  and cancer, 86–87, 87f
    by cancer type, 86, 87f
  and carcinogenesis, 1
  carcinogen exposure via, 109–110
  and lung cancer, 86–87, 87f
    carcinogen-adduct formation and, 108, 108f
    genetics and, 108
  and oropharyngeal cancer, 86
  and radiotherapy, 299
  and response to radiotherapy, 383
  secondhand, and cancer risk, 87
Smoothened (SMO), 128–129, 129f, 480
  antagonists, 129
  inhibitors, 480
Smooth muscle actin, 249, 313
  α-SMA, 282, 282t, 309
Smooth muscle cells (SMCs), of vasculature, 249, 250f
SMO/PTCH signaling, targeted therapy and, 474f
SMURF, in TGF-β signaling, 130, 130f
SN-38, 442
  resistance to, 449t
  structure of, 441f
Snai1, 230
  and metastasis, 231f, 232
SNAIL, 313
SNP. See Single nucleotide polymorphisms (SNP)
SNR. See Signal-to-noise ratio (SNR)
Sodium bisulfite conversion, 20–22, 21f, 21t
Sodium dodecyl sulfate–polyacrylamide gel electrophoresis (SDS-PAGE), 34
Soft tissue cancer, gene fusion in, 147t
Solid tumor(s)
  acidity in, 453, 454f
  and drug resistance, 284, 454–455
  blood vessels in, 453, 454f
  drug distribution in relation to, 456–457, 456f

  cancer stem cells in, 315–317, 316f
  cytogenetic analysis of, 6
  drug concentration gradients in, 453, 454f
  and drug sensitivity and resistance, 455–457, 456f
  epigenetic variants in chromatin factors in, 63
  genetic heterogeneity of, 309–313
  heterogeneity of, 143, 144f
  hypoxia in, 263, 292–300, 379
  microenvironment, and drug resistance, 453–457
  oxygen gradients in, 453, 454f
  preclinical evaluation of drug response in, 411–412
  as second malignancies, 418
  targeted therapy for, 467t
  WNT pathway inhibitors for, 127
Solute carrier superfamily (SLC), 448–449
Somatostatin analogs, for neuroendocrine tumors, 373
Sonic hedgehog (SHH), 128, 283
Sonidegib, 129
Son-of-sevenless (SOS), 116, 117, 117f
Sonoporation, 23
Sorafenib, 268t, 270, 408, 469f, 470
  and hand-foot syndrome, 417
Southern blotting, 9–10, 10f
  probes for, 9, 9f
SOX gene family, 314t
Sox2, 318
SP1 (Specificty Protein 1), 119, 119f, 494f
S1P. See Sphingosine 1 phosphate (S1P)
SPECT. See Single-photon emission computed tomography (SPECT)
Spectral counting, 36
Spectral karyotyping (SKY), 13, 13f
  of irradiated cells, 356
SpectraST, 32–33
Spheroid model system, 453, 455f, 456
Sphingosine 1 phosphate (S1P), and vascular maturation, 255
Spindle assembly checkpoint (SAC), 164f, 170, 173f, 174, 177f, 178–179, 180, 208–209
Spin-lattice relaxation time, 334
Spin-spin relaxation time, 334
Spleen-colony assay, 356
Spleen tyrosine kinase (SYK), 479
Spondylocostal dysostosis, 128
26S proteasome, 131–132, 131f, 168f, 169–170, 408
  20S peptidase activity, 131, 133
  inhibitors, 133
Squamous cell carcinoma (SCC), 196
  BRAF inhibitor therapy and, 418, 475
  cellular radiosensitivity in, 378t
  of head and neck
    cancer stem cells in, 315, 319
    and cell repopulation during radiotherapy, 391–392, 391f
    HPV and, 86, 149
    hypoxic modification of radiotherapy in, 383–384, 383f
    somatic mutations and epigenetic factors in, 58f
  and hypercalcemia, 509
  NOTCH signaling in, 128
  of skin, BRAF inhibitor therapy and, 475
SRC, and angiogenesis, 265
SRC, integrins and, 125
Src homology domain-containing phosphatase(s) (SHP), SHP-1, 524

Src Homology 2 (SH2) domains, 115–117, 116f, 117f
　non-catalytic, 116
SRC homology 2 (SH2) domains, 123, 123f
SRC homology 3 (SH3) domains, 116, 116f, 123, 123f
　non-catalytic, 116
SRC kinases, 115–116, 123f
SRM-MS. See Selected reaction monitoring-mass spectrometry (SRM-MS)
SRS. See Stereotactic radiosurgery (SRS)
SSA. See Single-strand annealing (SSA)
ssDNA. See DNA (deoxyribonucleic acid), single-strand
Stage, of tumor, 3, 141f, 230
Stage migration, 553, 553f
Stalk cells, in angiogenesis, 253f, 255
STAMPEDE trial, 550
Standardized uptake value (SUV), in PET, 336
STAR. See Study of Tamoxifen and Raloxifene (STAR)
Starling, Ernest Henry, 487
Statins, 118
Statistical analysis
　of clinical trials, 557–558
　of -omic data, 42–43
　of outcome measures, 556
　of prognostic factor studies, 567–568
　of survival duration, 556
Statistical significance, 556
STATs
　functions of, 124
　STAT3, 230, 240f
　structure of, 124, 124f
STD 10. See Severely toxic dose in 10% of animals (STD 10)
Steady-state plasma drug concentration, 431, 431t
Stefins, 226t, 228
Stem cell(s). See also Cancer stem cells (CSCs); Leukemia stem cells (LSC)
　irradiated, repopulation of, 391–392
　normal tissue, 278–279, 305, 415f
　somatic, signaling pathways in, 314, 314t
　studies in mice, 307
　tumor, 305, 313–318, 414
Stem cell factor (SCF), 263, 415f
Stemness, hypoxia and, 297, 297f
Stereotactic body radiation therapy (SBRT), 370, 396
Stereotactic radiosurgery (SRS), 370
Sterigmatocystin, potency as carcinogen, 107f
Steroid hormone(s)
　metabolism of, 488
　synthesis of, 488, 489f, 490f
　transport in blood, 488–489
Steroid hormone receptor(s), 489–491, 490f. See also Androgen receptor(s); Estrogen receptor(s)
　activation in absence of ligand, 494, 494f
　agonists, coactivators and, 490f, 492–494, 493f
　amino acid sequence homology in, 490f, 491
　antagonists, corepressors and, 492–494, 493f
　binding to DNA, 491–492
　classical mechanism of action of, 491–494, 492f
　and coregulators, interactions of, 492–494, 493f
　DNA-binding domain, 489, 490f
　and gene transcription, in cancer, 495
　hinge region, 490f, 491

　ligand-activated, transcription factor modulation by, 494, 494f
　ligand-binding domain, 490f, 491
　nonclassical mechanism of action of, 494–495, 494f
　phosphorylation of, growth factors and, 494, 494f
　quantification of, 495, 496f
　structure of, 489–491, 490f
　transcriptional activating functions, 489–491, 490f, 493
Steroid receptor coactivator (SRC). See SRC
STING, in intercellular response to radiation, 363–364
Stomach cancer. See also Gastric cancer
　HER2 in, and targeted therapy, 158–159
　incidence of, time trends in, 74
　smoking and, 87f
　WNT signaling in, 126
Stratifying, of groups of patients, 553
Stroma/Stromal cells, 308, 309f
　genetic instability in, 195, 196f
　isolation of, 307
　tumor, angiogenic activation of, 265–266
　and tumor heterogeneity, 226, 306f, 308–309, 309f
　and tumor progression, 239f, 241, 283
Stromal-derived factor 1 (SDF1), 260
Strong cationic exchange (SCX), 34
Study of Tamoxifen and Raloxifene (STAR), 500
Substance P, in nausea and vomiting, 417
Subtelomeric DNA, 213
Succinate, and epigenetic enzyme activity, 59
Succinate dehydrogenase (SDH), 291
Sucrose velocity sedimentation, 211, 212t
SU/FU. See Suppressor of Fused (SU/FU)
Sulfhydryls, drug binding, drug resistance caused by, 446t, 447f
Sulforhodamine B assay, 411
Sulfotransferases (SULTs), 100
SULTs. See Sulfotransferases (SULTs)
SUMO, 133, 156
SUMO isopeptidases, 133
SUMO-targeted ubiquitin ligases (STUBLs), 133
Sumoylation, 30t, 133, 184
　of PTEN, 157, 157f
Sun exposure, 196
Sunitinib, 268t, 269f, 270, 408, 469, 469f, 470
　and hand-foot syndrome, 417
Superoxide, radiation and, 351–352
Superoxide dismutase, 290, 389
Super-SILAC, 34–35
Super state, of cells, 318
Suppressor of Fused (SU/FU), 128–129, 129f, 480
Suramin, 268
Survival
　statistical analysis of, 42
　surrogate measures for, 554
Survival analyses, bias in, 80t
Survival bias, 78, 80t
Survival curves
　actuarial, 555, 555f, 555t
　in clinical trials, 554–557, 555f
　of drug-treated cells, 411, 412f
　radiation and, 422, 422f
　for irradiated cells, 355–356, 355f, 358f, 359, 360f, 361f, 362f
　　with acute dose vs. chronic low-dose rate, 359, 361f
　　dose fractionation and, 390, 391f

　　drug treatment and, 422, 422f
　　linear-quadratic model, 356, 368, 368f
　　multitarget, 367, 367f
　　from normal rodent tissues, 384, 385f
　　single-hit, 367, 367f
　　target-theory model, 356, 367–368, 367f
　Kaplan-Meier, 555–556
Survival duration, 554–555
Survivin, 184, 209
Surviving fraction, of drug-treated cells, 411, 412f
Susceptibility gene(s)
　GWAS for, 88
　for lung cancer, 88
SUV. See Standardized uptake value (SUV)
SWATH-MS, 37
SYBR™ Green, real-time PCR using, 11, 11f
Symptom scales, 559–560
Syndrome of inappropriate antidiuretic hormone secretion (SIADH)
　paraneoplastic, 509
　vinca alkaloids and, 444
Synergy, of combined drugs, 419–420, 420f, 421f
Synthetic lethality, 3, 44, 158, 199–200, 211, 362, 405–406, 406f, 422t, 453, 476
　chemo-genetic, 453
Syrian hamster embryo (SHE) assay, 106
Systemic mastocytosis, aggressive, targeted therapy for, 468t

T

$t_{1/2}$. See Half-life
TAAs. See Tumor-associated antigens (TAAs)
TACE, 227
TAFs. See Tumor-associated fibroblasts (TAFs)
TAK1. See TGF-β activated kinase 1 (TAK1)
Talazoparib, indications for, 467t, 477
TALENs. See Transcription activator-like effector nucleases (TALENs)
Talimogene laherparepvec (T-Vec), 536
Talin, integrins and, 125, 229f, 531t
Tamoxifen, 3
　antiestrogenic effects of, 499
　for breast cancer, 499
　as chemopreventive agent, 110
　and endometrial cancer, 418
　estrogenic effects of, 499
　mechanism of action of, 110, 499, 501f
　metabolism of, 499, 500f
　metabolites, 499, 500f
　pharmacology, altered, and resistance in breast cancer, 502, 504f
　resistance, 494, 500, 501–503, 504f
　　autophagy and, 133
　　response to, CYP activity and, 432
　structure of, 499f
TAMs. See Tumor-associated macrophages (TAMs)
Tandem mass spectrum (MS/MS spectrum), 32, 33f, 34, 35f, 36
Tandem mass tag (TMT), 35
Tankyrase, 126
TAP. See Transporter of antigenic peptides (TAP) complex
Tapasin, 517f, 518
Taq polymerase, 10
Tarextumab, 128

Targeted agents. *See also* Molecular targeted therapies; *specific agent*
and hormonal therapy, combined, for breast cancer, 503
human studies of, 462
mechanism of action of, 462–464, 463f
and personalized medicine, 551
pharmacodynamic/pharmacokinetic relationships of, 462
preclinical development of, 462
target identification for, 462
Targeted genome sequencing, 547
Targeted treatment, 403–404, 407–408, 467t. *See also* Molecular targeted therapies
and *BRCA1/2*, 142t
and chemotherapy, combined, and therapeutic index, 419
development of, high throughput DNA sequencing and, 404
dosage and administration of, 416
genetic variants in chromatin factors and, 63
and oncogenes, 142t
predictive markers for, 568
side effects of, 415, 462
toxicity of, 462
Target-theory model, of cell survival after radiation, 356, 367–368, 367f
TAR RNA-binding protein (TRBP), 25f
TAS-102, 439
Taxanes, 415, 444–445
indications for, 445
resistance to, 446t, 449t, 450
time-concentration curve for, 430
tissue penetration by, 456
toxicity of, 445
Tazemetostat, 61
T-BET, 523, 523f
TCDD. *See* 2,3,7,8-Tetrachlorodibenzo-*p*-dioxin (TCDD)
T-cell lymphoma. *See* Lymphoma(s), T-cell
T-cell receptor (TCR), 519, 520f
complementarity-determining regions, 519
constant (C) domain, 519, 520f
diversity (D) gene segments, 519, 520f
joining (J) gene segments, 519, 520f
structure of, 519, 520f
variable (V) gene segments, 519, 520f
αβ, 519, 520f
γδ, 519
T cells (T lymphocytes). *See also* Adoptive (T-cell) cell therapies; Cytotoxic T lymphocytes (CTL); Helper T cells (T$_H$); Regulatory T cells (Tregs)
activation of, 515–518, 516f, 517f, 518f, 520–523, 521, 521f, 522f
costimulatory molecules in, 518, 518f
modulation of, 524
and adaptive resistance, 538
antigen recognition by, 519
antitumor response, suppressors of, 538
autoreactive, 524
CD4+, 515, 516f, 517, 517f, 520, 522f, 523–524, 523f
hypoxia and, 298
CD8+, 515, 516f, 517, 517f, 518, 520, 521f, 522f, 523
hypoxia and, 298
chimeric antigen receptor, 539–541, 540f, 541f
contraction of, 521, 522f

cytotoxic response, stages of, 520–521, 521f
diversity, production of, 519, 520f
effector, 520–523, 520f, 521f
immune checkpoint inhibitor and, 536–537
expansion of, 521, 522f
gene-engineered, generation of, 539–541, 540f, 541f
interactions with tumor cells, 3
killing, by Tregs, 525
memory, 520, 520f, 521f, 522f, 523
central (T$_{CM}$), 521f, 523
effector (T$_{EM}$), 521f, 523
and metastasis, 231f, 233–234
naive (resting), 520, 521f
negative selection, 524, 525f
N region diversity, 519
positive selection, 524, 525f
selection, 524–525, 525f
TAA-specific, 525, 529, 540f
tumor-infiltrating, adoptive cell therapy with, 539, 540f
tumor infiltration by, prognostic significance of, 530–531
tumor-specific
activation of, 518, 534f
adoptive cell therapy with, 539, 540f
generation of, 539
suppressors of, 538–539
T-cell tolerance, 524–525
TCR. *See* T-cell receptor (TCR)
TDM-1. *See* Trastuzumab-emtansine (TDM-1)
Technetium-99m, 335, 336
Telangiectasia, *see also* ataxia telangiecstasia, 200t, 203–204, 208f, 210, 357
skin, radiation-induced, 387, 387f, 389, 418
TEL-JAK fusion gene, 147t
TEL-JAK fusion tyrosine kinase, 145
Telomerase, 143, 149, 212–216, 214f, 215f
aberrations, and cancer, 215
as therapeutic target, 216
Telomerase reverse transcriptase (TERT), 23, 88, 213–214
MYC and, 151f
Telomerase RNA-TR, 213–215
Telomere(s), 212
aberrant lengthening of, 214–215
dysfunction, 214f
and genome stability, 213
integrity, shelterin and, 214f, 215
maintenance of, 212–213
and cancer, 215–216
and protection of chromosomal ends, 213, 214f
regulation of, in normal cell replication, 213–215, 214f
replication, 213, 214f
shortening of, 214–215
Telomere-dysfunction-induced foci (TIF), 213, 214f
Telomere-repeat containing RNAs (TERRA), 213
Telomere signal-free ends (TSFEs), 213
Telomere trimming, 214
Telophase, 166f, 167, 173f, 174
Temozolomide
indications for, 434
mechanism of action of, 452
pharmacology of, 434
sensitivity to, epigenetic factors and, 63
Temsirolimus, 121, 175, 271, 475
dosage and administration of, 475
mechanism of action of, 474f

Tenascin, 226, 282t
Tenascin C, 228
Teniposide
indications for, 442
pharmacokinetics of, 442
structure of, 442, 442f
Tensin, integrins and, 125
Tension checkpoint, 209
Teratoma(s), 255
TERRA. *See* Telomere-repeat containing RNAs (TERRA)
TERT. *See* Telomerase reverse transcriptase (TERT)
Tertiary lymphoid structures (TLS), in tumors, 283
Testicular cancer
radiosensitivity of, 353
second malignancy after, 417–418
Testosterone
classical mechanism of action of, 491–494, 492f
structure of, 505f
synthesis of, 488, 489f, 490f
Test-review bias, 563t, 564, 567
TET enzymes (TET1/TET2/TET3), 53f
and cancer metabolism, 60
TET2
ascorbate cofactor, and targeted cancer prevention or therapy, 63
mutations, in AML, 58, 63
TETi. *See* TET inhibitors (TETi)
TET inhibitors (TETi), 60f
2,3,7,8-Tetrachlorodibenzo-*p*-dioxin (TCDD), as tumor promoter, 102, 103f
Tetradecanoyl phorbol acetate (TPA), as tumor promoter, 102, 103f
Tetraploidy, 180
TF. *See* Tissue factor (TF)
TF pathway inhibitor 2 (TFPI-2), in vasculogenic mimicry, 255–256
TGF-α. *See* Transforming growth factor α (TGF-α)
TGF-β. *See* Transforming growth factor β (TGF-β)
TGF-β activated kinase 1 (TAK1), in TGF-β signaling, 130
TH-302, 299
cytotoxicity in hypoxic cells, 384
Thalidomide
antiangiogenic properties of, 268, 268t
anticancer activity of, 407
combined with melphalan and prednisone, anticancer activity of, 407
Theranostics, 342
Therapeutic index
of anticancer drugs, 414–415, 414f, 419, 431
directed drug delivery and, 410
modifiers and, 421
with combined radiation and drug therapy, 419, 421–424, 422t, 422f, 423f, 424f
Therapeutic ratio, in radiotherapy, 369, 389–390, 390f, 393–394
Thiols, and cellular effects of radiation, 351–352
Thioredoxin (TRX), 290, 290f
Thrombin, 259, 260
Thromboplastin, 260
Thrombopoietin, 279
Thrombosis
in cancer, 266–267
vascular, 261f, 263

Thrombospondin
　　TSP-1, 226, 257t, 260, 262f, 263, 265
　　　　downregulation of, 143
　　TSP-2, 260
Thymidine monophosphate (dTMP),
　　　436, 437f, 438, 438f, 447f
Thymidine phosphorylase (TP), 439, 439f
Thymidylate synthase (TS), 436–437,
　　　437f, 438, 438f, 439, 447f
Thymine, structure of, 437, 438f
Thymus, T-cell selection in, 524
Thyroid cancer, 372, 470
　　anaplastic
　　　　targeted therapy for, 467t
　　　　V600E mutation-positive, 475
　　B-RAF mutations in, 154, 154f
　　Cowden syndrome and, 156
　　gene fusion in, 147t
　　incidence of
　　　　sex differences in, 74
　　　　time trends in, 74
　　oncogenes in, 142t
　　papillary, incidence of, 74
　　smoking and, 87f
　　tumor-suppressor genes in, 142t
Thyroid receptor(s), DNA-binding motif, 492
TICs. See Tumor-initiating cells (TICs)
TIE, targeted therapy and, 469f, 470
TIE1, 258
TIE2, 251f, 253f, 257t, 258, 270
　　in angiogenesis, 254–255, 254f
　　and angiopoietins, 254f, 258
　　and lymphangiogenesis, 254f, 255
　　and vascular maturation, 255
Tie2 receptor, 115
TIE2 receptor, 249
　　and lymphangiogenesis, 254f, 255
TIF. See Telomere-dysfunction-induced foci (TIF)
TIGAR. See TP53-induced glycolysis and
　　　apoptosis regulator (TIGAR)
TILs. See Tumor-infiltrating lymphocytes (TILs)
TIME. See Tumor immune
　　　microenvironment (TIME)
Time trends, 72f, 73–74
TIMPs. See Tissue inhibitors of
　　　metalloproteinases (TIMPs)
Tip cells, in angiogenesis, 253f, 254–255
Tipiracil, 439
Tirapazamine, 299–300, 455
　　cytotoxicity in hypoxic cells, 384
Tissue factor (TF), 260
　　in vasculogenic mimicry, 255–256
Tissue inhibitors of metalloproteinases
　　　(TIMPs), 226t, 228, 232, 282t
　　and angiogenesis, 259, 260f
　　and cancer progression, 237–238, 237t
Tissue microarray (TMA) technology,
　　　39–40, 41f, 531
Tissue microdissection, 307
Tissues, molecular analysis in, 38–41
TK. See Tyrosine kinase(s) (TK)
TKB, 123
TKIs. See Tyrosine kinase inhibitors (TKIs)
T-loop, 213, 214f, 215
TLR. See Toll-like receptor(s) (TLR)
TLS. See Tertiary lymphoid structures (TLS)
TMA. See Tissue microarray (TMA) technology
TMB. See Tumor metational burden (TMB)
TME. See Tumor microenvironment (TME)

TMPRSS2-ERG fusion gene, 145, 147t
TMT. See Tandem mass tag (TMT)
TNFR-1, 184, 187f, 257t
TNF-related apoptosis inducing ligand
　　　(TRAIL), neutralization, and
　　　metastasis, 184, 188, 234
TNF-related apoptosis inducing ligand receptor
　　　(TRAILR1/TRAILR2), 184
TNF-α. See Tumor necrosis factor alpha (TNF-α)
TNM staging, 230, 567
TNP470, 268
Tobacco. See also Smoking
　　and cancer, 86–87, 87f
　　smoke, as carcinogen, 1, 74, 106, 108, 321
Tobacco control, 87
Toll-like receptor(s) (TLR), 518, 518f
　　agonists, 518, 531, 535, 535f, 536
　　TLR9, 518
　　　in intercellular response to
　　　　ionizing radiation, 363
Topoisomerase I, 7, 440, 441f
Topoisomerase II, 440, 441f
Topoisomerase inhibitors, 201, 300,
　　　432, 440–443, 452
　　leukemia related to, 418
　　mechanism of action of, 440
　　resistance to, 446t
Topotecan, 300, 441–442
　　resistance to, 449t
　　structure of, 441f
TORC1, see also mTORC1, 118, 120–121, 120f,
　　　153f, 175, 176f, 463f, 474f, 475
TORC2, 120
Tositumomab, 532t
Tositumomab-iodine-131, 534
TP. See Thymidine phosphorylase (TP)
TP53, 123, 177, 178
　　and apoptosis, 182, 183f, 184,
　　　185, 186f, 187, 296
　　and cell cycle, 176, 186f
　　and death receptor apoptotic pathway, 185
　　and DNA repair, 186f
　　loss of function, and cancer, 181, 188, 265
　　and metabolism, 186f
　　as multifunctional protein, 186f
　　posttranslational modifications of, 186f
　　targeted therapy and, 409
TPA. See Tetradecanoyl phorbol acetate (TPA)
TP53 gene, 1, 180, 196, 211
　　and angiogenesis, 265
　　mutations of, 7t, 155, 180, 310, 311, 480, 508
TP53-induced glycolysis and apoptosis
　　　regulator (TIGAR), 286f, 288–289
TRAIL. See TNF-related apoptosis
　　　inducing ligand (TRAIL)
Trametinib, 475–476
　　indications for, 467t, 468t
　　mechanism of action of, 474f
TRAMP. See Transgenic model of
　　　prostate cancer (TRAMP)
Transcription activator-like effector
　　　nucleases (TALENs), 28
Transcription factors, 121–122, 121f. See
　　　also MYC; specific factor
　　activation domains, 121–122
　　altered function, and malignant
　　　transformation, 122
　　DNA-binding domain of, 121, 121f
　　homeodomain families, 121, 121f

　　hypoxia and, 295f
　　repression domains, 121–122
　　site-directed mutagenesis, 25
　　WNT signaling and, 125
Transcriptome, 14, 18, 44, 122, 146f,
　　　243, 265, 294, 307, 502
　　and molecular signatures of exposure
　　　and risk, 108–109
Transduced cells, 23, 24f
Transfection, 340, 448
　　of DNA plasmids, 23–24, 24f
　　of shRNA, 24
Transforming growth factor α (TGF-α), 295
　　and cancer progression, 237–238, 237t
Transforming growth factor α receptor
　　　(TGFαR), 114f
Transforming growth factor β (TGF-β), 230,
　　　295, 298, 313, 314, 314t, 319, 525
　　immune suppression and blockade, 538
　　in development, 125
　　functions of, 130
　　and late radiation damage in lung, 387, 388f
　　and metastasis, 231f, 233, 234f, 236, 242
　　mutations of, 130, 131
　　in radiation fibrosis, 377, 385, 387
　　signaling, 129–131, 130f
　　TGFβ1, in angiogenesis, 257t
　　and tumor dormancy and progression,
　　　236–240, 237t, 241
　　and tumor-related immunosuppression,
　　　283, 523f, 538
　　and cancer-associated fibroblasts, 282f
　　and vascular maturation, 255
Transforming growth factor β receptor
　　　(TGFβR), 114, 130
　　mutations of, in cancer, 130–131
　　TGFβRII, 132, 257t
　　type I, 130, 130f
　　type II, 130
Transforming growth factor β superfamily,
　　　signal transduction by, 129–131, 130f
Transgene, 106
　　definition of, 26
　　expression of, 26
Transgenic animals, bioassays in, 106
Transgenic model of prostate cancer (TRAMP),
　　　3D MRSI with hyperpolarized ^{13}C, 339f
Translational medicine, epidemiology in, 70
Translocation(s), see also chromosomes
　　and specific gene(s) involved,
　　　144–146, 145f, 146f
　　effects of, 148f
Transmission disequilibrium test, 78
Transporter associated with antigen processing
　　　(TAP) complex, 517f, 518
Transposable elements, 55, 146, 158
Trastuzumab, 2, 3, 115, 142t, 152, 268t,
　　　269f, 271, 403–404, 409, 462,
　　　466, 469f, 498, 532t, 550
　　adjuvant, for breast cancer, 558
　　cardiotoxicity of, 473
　　indications for, 467t, 473
　　mechanism of action of, 473, 532–533
　　toxicity of, 473
Trastuzumab-emtansine, 409, 464, 469f, 534
　　indications for, 473
　　mechanism of action of, 463f, 473
　　side effects of, 473
TRBP. See TAR RNA-binding protein (TRBP)

Treatment. See Cancer treatment; specific treatment
Treatment-by-biomarker interaction, 466
Treatment effect, 550
Treatment failure
　cancer heterogeneity and, 319–320
　clonal dynamics in, 311–312
Treatment resistance
　cancer heterogeneity and, 320
　clonal dynamics in, 311
Trebananib/AMG386, 270
Tremelimumab, 536–537
Tricarboxylic acid (TCA) cycle, 286f, 287, 287f, 289, 291
Trichloroethylene, potency as carcinogen, 107, 107f
Trichothiodystrophy (TTD), 210
Trifluridine monophosphate (F$_3$dTMP), 439
Trisomy, FISH detection of, 12–13
Tris(2,3-dibromopropyl)phosphate, potency as carcinogen, 107f
TRK, targeted therapy and, 2, 114, 464f, 467t, 469f, 478, 479
Tropomyosin kinase receptors, 2
TS. See Thymidylate synthase (TS)
TSC, and oxidative stress, 290, 290f
TSFEs. See Telomere signal-free ends (TSFEs)
TSP-1. See Thrombospondin-1 (TSP-1)
TTD. See Trichothiodystrophy (TTD)
t tests, 42–43, 83, 548
TTK gene (see also monopolar spindle 1, MPS1), 180
TTK (protein kinase), 177f, 179
　inhibitors, 181
Tucatinib, 469f
Tucidinostat, 477
Tumor-associated antigens (TAAs), 525–529
　cancer-testis, 527–528, 528f
　differentiation, 527–528, 528f
　identification of, 526–527, 526f–527f
　mutation, 527–528, 528f
　overexpressed, 527–528, 528f
　posttranscriptionally modified, 527, 528f, 529
　in therapeutic cancer vaccines, 535–536, 535f
　and tumor-specific T cell generation, 539
　types of, 527–529, 528f
　viral, 527–528, 528f
Tumor-associated fibroblasts (TAFs), 281
Tumor-associated macrophages (TAMs), 238–239, 239f, 283
　hypoxia and, 297–298, 297f
　inhibitor of, 134
　ubiquitination of, 132
Tumor blood vessel(s), 250f, 264f, 266–267
　viable cells surrounding, 280, 280f
Tumor cells. See also Circulating tumor cells (CTCs)
　arrest in first-pass capillary beds, 232
Tumor cords, 279–280
Tumor cure, and therapeutic ratio, 424
Tumor desmoplasia, 282, 283
Tumor doubling time(s), 275–276, 277f, 413f
Tumor evolution
　clonal, models of, 223, 224f, 310–311, 310f
　genomic, 311
Tumor growth, 275–276, 276f, 277f
　exponential, 275–276
　heterogeneity of, 275
　measurement of, limitations of, 275

Tumorigenesis, basis of, 140f, 143–149
Tumor immune microenvironment (TIME), 283
Tumor immunity
　cancer-associated fibroblasts and, 283
　hypoxia and, 297–298, 297f
Tumor immunology, 519, 525–531
Tumor-infiltrating lymphocytes (TILs), adoptive cell therapy with, 539, 540f
Tumor-initiating cells (TICs), 236, 267, 314
　hedgehog signaling and, 129
Tumor initiation, 97, 109 142t, 313, 404, 414, 497
Tumor invasion
　hedgehog signaling in, 129
　hypoxia and, 297, 297f
　and metastasis, 231–232, 231f
Tumor markers. See also Biomarker(s)
　and treatment outcomes, 89, 554
Tumor metabolic phenotype, determinants of, 284–285, 285f
Tumor metabolism, 284–292
　hypoxia and, 295f
　regulation of, 287–289
　reprogramming, hypoxia and, 296–297, 297f
Tumor mutational burden (TMB), 310, 538
Tumor microenvironment (TME), 226–230, 281–284. See also Extracellular matrix (ECM)
　and carcinogenesis, 2
　cellular components of, 281–284, 281f
　and drug resistance, 453–457
　and drug response, 411–412
　endothelial cells in, 283–284
　and epigenetic changes, 147
　immune cells in, 283
　metabolites in, 284, 285
　nutrient concentration in, 284
　pathophysiological, 230
　pH in, 284
　and preangiogenic tumor growth, 263
　protease activity in, and metastases, 237–238, 237t
　spatial heterogeneity in, 230, 281
　temporal heterogeneity in, 281
　and tumor growth and spread, 98
　and tumorigenesis, 143, 144f
　and tumor response to radiotherapy, 375, 377
　variability of, 308–309, 309f
　vascular network in, 283–284
Tumor necrosis factor alpha (TNF-α), 103, 385, 523, 523f
　in angiogenesis, 257t
Tumor necrosis factor alpha (TNF-α) converting enzyme. See TACE
Tumor necrosis factor (TNF) superfamily, 183f, 184–185
Tumor progression, 97–98, 223–226
　angiogenesis in, 260, 262f
　antitumor immunity and, 529–530, 530f
　cancer-associated fibroblasts and, 283
　cellular aspects of, 223–224
　clonal evolution in, 223, 224f, 310–311, 310f
　definition of, 223
　immunoediting during, 3 Es of, 530, 530f
　molecular genetics of, 224–226
　preangiogenic, 263
　vascular interface in, 247–248, 248f
Tumor promoter(s), 102, 103f
Tumor promotion, 97–98, 109
Tumor response rate, 549–550, 554

Tumor scar, 282
Tumorspheres, 308, 317
Tumor stem cells, 305, 377f, 392, 414
Tumor-suppressor gene(s), 98, 141, 142t, 176, 193
　and angiogenesis, 262f, 265
　cancers associated with, 142t, 144
　deletion of, 17
　first isolation of, 140–141
　hypermethylated, 55
　mutations, 102
　　and cancer risk, 1, 108
　promoter hypermethylation, as therapeutic target, 60–61
　rare, 17
　reactivation, as therapy target, 148f
　UPS and, 132
Tumor suppressors
　metabolic, 291
　and oxidative stress, 290, 290f
Tumor-vascular interface, 247–248, 248f
Tumor volume, and limit of detection, 424
Tumstatin, 257t, 260, 265, 269f
TurboID, 30
Turcot syndrome, and risk from carcinogen exposure, 108
T-Vec. See Talimogene laherparepvec (T-Vec)
TWIST, 295f, 313, 320
　and metastasis, 231f, 232
Two-dimensional gel electrophoresis (2-DE), 34
Two-hit hypothesis, see also Knudson, Alfred, 17, 140, 143f
Tyrosinase, melanoma-associated, 528, 529
Tyrosine kinase(s) (TK), see also specific tyrosine kinase
　cytoplasmic, 123, 123f
　　in cytokine signaling, 123–124, 124f
　integrins and, 125
　in integrin signaling, 124–125
　receptor. See Receptor protein tyrosine kinase(s) (RPTK)
Tyrosine kinase inhibitors (TKIs), 152, 464
　antiangiogenic receptor, 268t, 269–270, 271, 466–471
　antiangiogenic small molecule, 469–470, 469f
　dosage and administration of, 416
　mechanism of action of, 463f
　mucosal damage caused by, 417
　resistance to, 446t, 465
　small molecule, 408

U

UBDs. See Ubiquitin binding domains (UBDs)
Ubiquitin, 168f
Ubiquitin-activating enzyme (E1), 131–133, 131f, 168f, 169–170
Ubiquitination, 145f
　in cell-cycle regulation, 169–170
　of PTEN, 157, 157f
Ubiquitin binding domains (UBDs), 131f, 132–133
Ubiquitin code, 131f, 132–133
Ubiquitin-conjugating enzyme (E2), 131–133, 131f, 168f, 169–170, 295f
Ubiquitin ligase (E3), 131–133, 131f, 155, 158, 167, 168f, 169, 169f, 170, 172f, 185, 205, 206, 206f
　and cell-cycle regulation, 169–170, 174, 179, 208
　cullin-RING, 132

HECT domain, 132
RING between RING, 132
RING domain, 132
SMADs, 130, 130f
SUMO-targeted (STUBLs), 133, 156
targeted therapy and, 170, 294, 294f, 295
Ubiquitin proteasome system (UPS), 125, 126f, 131–132, 131f
  clinical significance of, 133–134
  proteasome inhibitors, 479
U-box, 132
UDH. See Usual ductal hyperplasia (UDH)
UGTs. See Uridine diphosphate (UDP)-glucuronosyltransferases (UGTs)
UHPLC. See Ultra-high performance nano-flow liquid chromatography (UHPLC)
Ulcerative colitis (UC), TGF-β signaling in, 130
Ultra-high performance nano-flow liquid chromatography (UHPLC), 34
Ultrasonography. See Ultrasound
Ultrasound, 333f, 337
  agents for, 332f
  of animal models, 340
  high-intensity focused, MRI guidance, 342
Ultraviolet photodissociation fragmentation (UVPD), 32
Ultraviolet radiation, 74, 97, 321, 350, 350f
  damage caused by, 362, 362f
  genetic instability related to, 196
Umbrella trials, 481, 551, 551f
Unfolded protein response (UPR), 133, 187
  in hypoxic response, 295, 296f
Uniparental disomy, 14
Unsupervised clustering, 19
  of -omic data, 42, 43
uPA. See Plasminogen activators, urokinase type (uPA)
UPR. See Unfolded protein response (UPR)
UPS. See Ubiquitin proteasome system (UPS)
Uracil, see also 5-fluorouracil, structure of, 437, 438f
Urethane, potency as carcinogen, 107f
Uridine diphosphate (UDP)-glucuronosyltransferases (UGTs), 100, 432, 442
Urothelial cancer, 435, 471
  NOTCH signaling in, 128
  transitional cell, cyclophosphamide-related, 418
US. See Ultrasound
Usual ductal hyperplasia (UDH), of breast, 497–498
Uterine cancer, 499, PI3-kinase signaling alterations in, 153, 153f
Uveal cancer, 255
  metastasis, principal site of, 234t
UVPD. See Ultraviolet photodissociation fragmentation (UVPD)

V
Vaccine(s)
  anticancer, 531, 531t, 535–536, 535f
  antiviral, 1
Vadimezan, 268t, 271
Validity, 560
Vandetanib, 268t, 271, 469f, 470
Vantictumab, 126
Variant enhancer loci (VELs), 56–57, 56f
Vascular aging, and tumor angiogenesis, 266
Vascular co-option, 256, 261f
  antiangiogenic therapy targeted to, 272

Vascular disrupting agents (VDAs), 268t, 269f, 270–271
  adverse effects, 271
Vascular endothelial growth factor (VEGF), 149, 261f, 468
  in angiogenesis, 253–255, 253f, 254f, 260, 262f, 265
  and cancer-associated fibroblasts, 282, 282t
  and cancer progression, 237–238, 237t
  hypoxia and, 297, 297f
  and metastasis, 231f, 232
  monoclonal antibody against, 532t
  MYC and, 151f
  in tumor neovascularization, 263
  upregulation of, 143
  and vascular growth, 256–257, 257t
  vascular maturation and, 255
  VEGF-A, 256–257, 257t, 265
    and lymphangiogenesis, 254f
  VEGF165b, 257t
  VEGF-B, 256–257, 257t
  VEGF-C, 256–257, 257t
    and lymphangiogenesis, 254f, 255
  VEGF-D, 256–257, 257t
    and lymphangiogenesis, 254f, 255
Vascular endothelial growth factor receptor (VEGFR), 114, 114f, 468
  in angiogenesis, 254–255, 254f
  humanized antibodies against, 115, 268t, 269–270
  targeted therapy and, 469, 469f
  tyrosine kinase inhibitors targeted to, 268t, 269–270
  VEGFR-3/FLT-4, and lymphangiogenesis, 254f, 255
  VEGFR2, monoclonal antibody against, 532t
Vascular endothelial receptor tyrosine phosphatase (VE-PTP), 258
Vascular growth, molecular regulators of, 253f, 256–262, 256f, 257t, 259f–262f
Vascular maturation, 251, 252f, 253f, 255
Vascular network, in tumor microenvironment, 283–284
Vascular normalization, as therapeutic strategy, 272
Vascular permeability factor (VPF), 256–257, 257t, 260
Vascular regression, 251, 261f, 263
Vascular remodeling, 251, 252f
  treatment-induced, 270
Vascular repair, 251–252
Vascular system
  constituents of, 249–251, 250f
  development of, 251, 252f
Vasculature, and tumor response to radiotherapy, 377
Vasculogenesis, 261f
  developmental, 251, 252f
  tumor, 265
Vasculogenic mimicry, 255–256, 261f, 262, 270
V_d. See Volume of distribution
VDAs. See Vascular disrupting agents (VDAs)
VE-cadherin. See Cadherins, vascular endothelial
Vector(s)
  for gene cloning, 8–9, 9f
  transfection using, 23–24, 24f

VEGF. See Vascular endothelial growth factor (VEGF)
VEGFR. See Vascular endothelial growth factor receptor (VEGFR)
VEGF-trap. See Aflibercept
VELs. See Variant enhancer loci (VELs)
Vemurafenib, 2, 119–120, 142t, 155, 404, 462, 467t, 474f, 475–476
Venetoclax, 188, 403–404, 407, 409, 463f, 467t, 474f, 480
  adverse effects, 480
Venogenesis, 261f
VE-PTP. See Vascular endothelial receptor tyrosine phosphatase (VE-PTP)
Verapamil, 451
v-ErbB, 140, 152
Vessel abnormalization, 250f, 263–264, 264f
VHL. See von Hippel-Lindau (VHL) protein
VHL gene, 142t
  and angiogenesis, 265
v-h-ras gene, 140
Vimentin, 313
Vinblastine, 409, 415, 443–444, 444f
  resistance to, 449t, 451
Vinca alkaloids, 443–444, 444f
  resistance to, 446t, 449t, 450
Vincristine, 409–410, 415, 443–444, 444f
  resistance to, 449t
Vindesine, 443–444
Vinorelbine, 443–444, 444f
Viral mimicry, DNMT inhibitors and, 60, 62, 62f
Viral transduction, 23, 24f
Virchow, 1
Viruses. See also specific virus
  bacterial, DNA insertion into, 8–9, 9f
  and carcinogenesis, 1, 149
    proviral integration and gene upregulation in, 150
  immune detection of, 518
  oncolytic, immunotherapy using, 536
  transfection using, 23–24, 24f
Vismodegib, 129, 321, 474f, 480
Vitamin E, 110
Vitronectin, 226, 228, 229f
v-k-ras gene, 140
VM-26. See Teniposide
v-myc gene, 140
Volume of distribution, 431, 431t
von Hippel-Lindau (VHL) protein, 262f
  in hypoxic response, 295, 295f
Vorinostat, 61, 463f, 477
Voxels, 331
VP-16. See Etoposide
VPF. See Vascular permeability factor (VPF)
v-src gene, 140

W
Warburg effect, 59, 175, 285–287
Warsaw breakage syndrome, 200t
WEE1 gene/protein, 178, 181, 357
WEE1/MYT1, 168f, 169, 172
Werner syndrome, 108, 200t
Western blotting, 10, 10f, 307
WGS. See Whole-genome sequencing
White blood cells, of smokers, carcinogen-adduct levels in, as biomarker for cancer risk, 108
White light imaging, 338, 338f

Whole-body irradiation, 388–389
Whole-genome sequencing, 547
  of circulating tumor cells, 320
Whole transcriptome sequencing, 18–19
Wilcoxon rank-sum test, 83, 556
Wilms tumor-1 (WT-1), 528
WNT signaling pathway, 123, 125–127, 126f, 282, 313, 314, 314t
  antagonists of, 126
  in development, 125
Workup bias, 564, 567
WT1-EWSR1 fusion gene, 147t

X

X chromosome, inactivation, 20
Xenograft-initiating cells, 314
Xenografts, 1–2, 307–308, 339
  experiments with, criticisms of, 317, 318f
  formation of, cancer stem cells and, 313–314
  in preclinical evaluation of anticancer drugs, 411f, 412–413
Xeroderma pigmentosum (XP), 200–201, 200t, 201f, 210, 362, 362f
  and anticancer drug toxicity, 418
  and risk from carcinogen exposure, 108
  and skin cancer risk, 196
X-linked inhibitor of apoptosis protein (XIAP), 184
XP. *See* Xeroderma pigmentosum (XP)
XPO1. *See* Exportin-1 (XPO1)
X-ray crystallography, 30, 37
X-rays, 349–350, 350f. *See also* Ionizing radiation; Radiotherapy
XRCC4, 203f, 204

Y

YAP/TAZ, 176, 176f
Yeast, homologous recombination in, 202
Yeast 2-hybrid system, 30

Z

Zinc finger nucleases (ZFNs), 28
Zinc-finger (ZFN) transcription factors, 121–122, 121f
ZNF143, and chromatin interactions, 57, 57f
ZNRF3, in WNT signaling, 125
ZSCAN proteins, 122